C000089693

1 MONTH OF
FREE
READING

at
www.ForgottenBooks.com

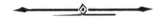

ISBN 978-0-260-89892-0
PIBN 10983700

This book is a reproduction of an important historical work. Forgotten Books uses
state-of-the-art technology to digitally reconstruct the work, preserving the original format
whilst repairing imperfections present in the aged copy. In rare cases, an imperfection in
the original, such as a blemish or missing page, may be replicated in our edition. We do,
however, repair the vast majority of imperfections successfully; any imperfections that
remain are intentionally left to preserve the state of such historical works.

THE

AMERICAN YEAR-BOOK

OF

MEDICINE AND SURGERY

BEING

A Yearly Digest of Scientific Progress and Authoritative Opinion
in all Branches of Medicine and Surgery, drawn from Journals, Monographs, and Text-Books, of the Leading
American and Foreign Authors and Investigators

COLLECTED AND ARRANGED

WITH CRITICAL EDITORIAL COMMENTS

BY

SAMUEL W. ABBOTT, M.D.,
JOHN J. ABEL, M.D.,
J. M. BALDY, M.D.,
CHARLES H. BURNETT, M.D.,
ARCHIBALD CHURCH, M.D.,
J. CHALMERS DaCOSTA, M.D.,
W. A. NEWMAN DORLAND, M.D.,
LOUIS A. DUHRING, M.D.,
VIRGIL P. GIBNEY, M.D.,
HOMER W. GIBNEY, M.D.,
HENRY A. GRIFFIN, M.D.,
JOHN GUITÉRAS, M.D.,
C. A. HAMANN, M.D.,

HOWARD F. HANSELL, M.D.,
BARTON COOKE HIRST, M.D.,
E. FLETCHER INGALS, M.D.,
WYATT JOHNSTON, M.D.,
W. W. KEEN, M.D.,
HENRY G. OHLS, M.D.,
WILLIAM PEPPER, M.D.,
WENDELL REBER, M.D.,
DAVID RIESMAN, M.D.,
LOUIS STARR, M.D.,
ALFRED STENGEL, M.D.,
G. N. STEWART, M.D.,
J. R. TILLINGHAST, JR., M.D.,

THOMPSON S. WESTCOTT, M.D.

UNDER THE GENERAL EDITORIAL CHARGE OF

GEORGE M. GOULD, M.D.

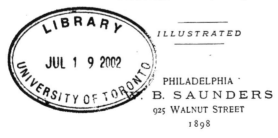

ILLUSTRATED

PHILADELPHIA
W. B. SAUNDERS
925 WALNUT STREET
1898

PRESS OF
W. B SAUNDERS, PHILADA.

LIST OF CONTRIBUTORS.

SAMUEL W. ABBOTT, M. D.,   BOSTON, MASS.
    Secretary of the Massachusetts State Board of Health.

JOHN J. ABEL, M. D.,   BALTIMORE, MD.
    Professor of Pharmacology, Johns Hopkins Medical School, Baltimore, Md.

J. MONTGOMERY BALDY, M. D.,   PHILADELPHIA, PA.
    Professor of Gynecology, Philadelphia Polyclinic; Surgeon to the Gynecean Hospital, Philadelphia.

CHARLES H. BURNETT, M. D.,   PHILADELPHIA, PA.
    Clinical Professor of Otology, Woman's Medical College; Emeritus Professor of Diseases of the Ear, Philadelphia Polyclinic.

ARCHIBALD CHURCH, M. D.,   CHICAGO, ILL.
    Professor of Mental Diseases and Medical Jurisprudence, Northwestern University Medical School, Chicago, Ill.

J. CHALMERS DACOSTA, M. D.,   PHILADELPHIA, PA.
    Clinical Professor of Surgery, Jefferson Medical College, Philadelphia; Surgeon to the Philadelphia Hospital.

W. A. NEWMAN DORLAND, M. D.,   PHILADELPHIA, PA.
    Assistant Demonstrator of Obstetrics, University of Pennsylvania; Consulting Obstetrician to the Southeastern Dispensary, Philadelphia.

LOUIS A. DUHRING, M. D.,   PHILADELPHIA, PA.
    Professor of Diseases of the Skin, University of Pennsylvania, Philadelphia.

VIRGIL P. GIBNEY, M. D.,   NEW YORK CITY.
    Clinical Professor of Orthopedic Surgery, College of Physicians and Surgeons, New York City.

HOMER W. GIBNEY, M. D.,   NEW YORK CITY.
    Clinical Assistant in Orthopedic Surgery, Vanderbilt Clinic, College of Physicians and Surgeons, New York City.

HENRY A. GRIFFIN, M. D.,   NEW YORK CITY.
    Assistant Physician to the Roosevelt Hospital, Out-Patient Department, New York City.

JOHN GUITÉRAS, M. D.,   PHILADELPHIA, PA.
    Professor of General Pathology and Morbid Anatomy, University of Pennsylvania, Philadelphia.

C. A. HAMANN, M. D.,   CLEVELAND, OHIO.
    Professor of Anatomy, Western Reserve University, Cleveland, Ohio.

HOWARD F. HANSELL, M. D.,   PHILADELPHIA, PA.

    Professor of Diseases of the Eye, Philadelphia Polyclinic; Clinical Professor of Ophthalmology, Jefferson Medical College, Philadelphia.

BARTON COOKE HIRST, M. D.,   PHILADELPHIA, PA.

    Professor of Obstetrics, University of Pennsylvania, Philadelphia.

E. FLETCHER INGALS, M. D.,   CHICAGO, ILL.

    Professor of Laryngology and Diseases of the Chest, Rush Medical College, Chicago, Ill.

WYATT JOHNSTON, M. D.,   MONTREAL, CAN.

    Assistant Professor of Public Health and Lecturer on Medico-Legal Pathology, McGill University, Montreal, Canada.

W. W. KEEN, M. D.,   PHILADELPHIA, PA.

    Professor of the Principles of Surgery and of Clinical Surgery, Jefferson Medical College, Philadelphia.

HENRY G. OHLS, M. D.,   CHICAGO, ILL.

WILLIAM PEPPER, M. D.,   PHILADELPHIA, PA.

    Professor of the Theory and Practice of Medicine and of Clinical Medicine, University of Pennsylvania, Philadelphia.

WENDELL REBER, M. D.,   PHILADELPHIA, PA.

    Ophthalmic Surgeon to the Franklin Dispensary and to the Methodist Episcopal Orphanage, Philadelphia.

DAVID RIESMAN, M. D.,   PHILADELPHIA, PA.

    Adjunct Professor of Clinical Medicine and Therapeutics, Philadelphia Polyclinic; Demonstrator of Pathologic Histology, University of Pennsylvania, Philadelphia.

LOUIS STARR, M. D.,   PHILADELPHIA, PA.

    Late Clinical Professor of Diseases of Children in the Hospital of the University of Pennsylvania; Late Physician to the Children's Hospital, Philadelphia.

ALFRED STENGEL, M. D.,   PHILADELPHIA, PA.

    Physician to the Philadelphia Hospital; Professor of Clinical Medicine, Woman's Medical College; Physician to the Children's Hospital; late Pathologist to the German Hospital, Philadelphia.

G. N. STEWART, M. D.,   CLEVELAND, OHIO.

    Professor of Physiology and Histology, Western Reserve University, Cleveland, Ohio.

J. R. TILLINGHAST, JR., M. D.,

    Assistant Physician to the Roosevelt Hospital, Out-Patient Department, New York City.

THOMPSON S. WESTCOTT, M. D.,   PHILADELPHIA, PA.

    Instructor in Diseases of Children, University of Pennsylvania; Visiting Physician to the Methodist Episcopal Hospital, Philadelphia.

PREFACE.

THE largely increased demand for the 1897 *Year-Book* leaves no doubt as to the usefulness of our work and of appreciation on the part of the profession; these facts have increased the endeavor of all concerned in the preparation of the volume for 1898 to bring it more nearly to our ideal of perfection. With the growing clearness of conception, on the part of the editors, of the exact nature of the professional need there has been a corresponding recognition of the necessity of keeping the epitomization within the limits allotted to previous issues. The vast and increasing literature has this year rendered the task of the editors of especial difficulty; but we believe it has been more thoroughly carried out than ever before, despite the protests of most of the editors that any possible sins of omission must be charged to "insufficient space," and not to neglect.

Several changes in the editorial staff have been caused by reasons that seem almost inevitable in a profession as active as ours. Among these I regret to chronicle the resignation of Professor Leffmann. The growing importance of the subjects heretofore so ably edited by him has warranted the creation of three departments, of which three distinguished specialists have kindly consented to take charge. These are: 1. That of Physiologic Chemistry, by Prof. John J. Abel, of Johns Hopkins Hospital; 2. That of Public Hygiene and Preventive Medicine, by Dr. Samuel W. Abbott, Secretary of the Massachusetts State Board of Health; 3. That of Legal Medicine, by Dr. Wyatt Johnston, of Montreal, Canada.

To these gentlemen especially, and to all the other editors, who, without exception, have labored so loyally, I wish to acknowledge my heartiest appreciation of many courtesies and sacrifices.

GEORGE M. GOULD.

CONTENTS.

GENERAL MEDICINE.

By WILLIAM PEPPER, M. D., and ALFRED STENGEL, M. D.,

OF PHILADELPHIA.

General Summary of the Year's Work.—The most important contribution to the progress of internal medicine is the serum-test for typhoid fever, the Widal test as it is now commonly designated. The reaction which is the fundamental basis of this test was first recognized by Pfeiffer, but was applied to the uses of the practical physician by Widal. Grünbaum almost at the same time, and apparently independently, described the same method, though his contribution lacked the definiteness and finish of that of Widal. Details regarding this method will be given in the appropriate place, but it is fitting to refer here to some of the general bearings of the subject. In previous volumes of the *Year-Book* we have had occasion to deplore the lack of a distinctive test by which typhoid fever might be recognized and differentiated from other febrile affections. This need was particularly emphasized in the discussion of Elsner's method last year. At that time Widal's communication had just appeared, and its value remained to be determined. In the year which has elapsed investigators in every part of the world have tested its value, and, with remarkable consonance, declare it a diagnostic method of the very greatest importance. It is true that dissenting voices have been heard, but these, for the most part, represent no considerable authority or following. A careful and scientific analysis shows that in thousands of cases of typhoid fever, in which the diagnosis was established beyond peradventure, the test, when applied in an approved manner, has seldom failed. In almost equally numerous cases of other diseases the test has rarely resulted positively. Many reported cases must be excluded from such an analysis. In the case of certain typhoid with negative results it has often happened that the proportion of blood-serum to culture has been incorrect, that the cultures were unreliable, or that the test was not repeated at suitable times. In the case of positive results in other diseases it has happened that previous attacks of typhoid fever have not been excluded, that the nonexistence of typhoid infection at the time has not been satisfactorily determined, or that the proportion of serum to culture was so great that even a normal serum might have given a more or less definite reaction. With regard to the positive exclusion of typhoid infection, it is of interest and great importance to note that several cases have been studied in which typhoid fever did not exist (that is, the local intestinal lesions and the typical symptoms), and yet the bacillus was present in the spleen and other organs. This is of interest in connection with the rare cases of general typhoid septicemia, and especially important in its bearing upon reported instances of positive Widal reactions in the absence of typhoid fever (as determined by course, symptoms, and lesions). For our own part, we have become so thoroughly convinced of the value of the test that we should hesitate to diagnose typhoid fever in any case in which repeated examinations, made in approved fashion, failed to reveal agglutination. If further experience shows these views to be well founded, the possibility will be afforded of distinguishing typhoid fever from a number of doubtful diseases having some resemblance to it. The certain determination of the nature of these has hitherto proved difficult, because fatal cases have not been admitted as instances (typhoid lesions having been discovered in some of these), and the nonfatal cases could not be surely distinguished from typhoid fever. The same method of diagnosis has been extended to cholera, diphtheria, plague, glanders, pyocyaneous infection, and other conditions, and there are no doubt still greater possibilities to be discovered.

In the domain of treatment we note the further advances of serum-therapeutics. The brilliant discovery of the plague bacillus by Kitasato has been followed by the extensive investigations of Yersin and others of the serum-treatment, and the results justify great hopefulness. The same may be said of cholera-vaccination. In the case of tuberculosis there is little certainty, notwithstanding the favorable reports of the followers of Maragliano, of Paquin, and of Koch. The untimely publication of Koch's original method, and the unfortunate element of commercialism manifest in the whole matter of preparation of serum, have begotten a proper feeling of conservatism and doubt.

The physiologic chemist continues as an active factor in medical progress. Despite much careful investigation, however, the pathology and therapeutics of gout have not been materially advanced during the year. In the case of other diseases in which abnormal metabolic processes are concerned many details have been studied, and some cleared up, but no striking progress can be recorded.

INFECTIOUS DISEASES.

TYPHOID FEVER.

Although the larger part of the literature upon this disease during the past year has been devoted to the investigation of the Widal reaction, numerous other papers of considerable importance have been published.

Remlinger and Schneider,[1] having become convinced that it was possible by using in conjunction the method of Eisner, the reaction of Widal, and inoculation-tests upon immune animals, to diagnose positively the presence of the typhoid bacillus, undertook a series of experiments to determine whether it existed in nature **outside the human body.** Their results were quite unexpected. In 37 specimens of water drawn from various sources (sewers, springs, and rivers) they were able to recognize its existence 9 times. Of these specimens only 2 came from regions where an epidemic of typhoid fever existed. In 13 specimens of dust and earth they found it 7 times—once from the dust of a room where typhoid fever had not existed for a long time. The bacteria obtained from 3 of these specimens were pathogenic for animals; 10 patients not suffering from typhoid fever were also examined, and in 5 cases organisms were found in the feces, 1 being a case of leukemia of febrile type with intermittent diarrhea. Of these 5 specimens, 4 were pathogenic for guinea-pigs, and their pathogenic action was prevented by previous injection of antityphic serum. In view of the ubiquity of the typhoid bacillus the authors ask if it be not possible for infection to be greatly favored by the presence of other microorganisms.

Etiology.—Boyer[2] finds that in Beyrouth the local epidemics of typhoid fever are closely related to the **rainfall;** this is explained by the fact that the

---

[1] Ann. de l' Inst. Pasteur, Jan. 25, 1897.   [2] Lyon méd., No. 46, 1896.

water washes the typhoid bacillus from the ground into the canals, causing infection in all regions through which they pass. From the ground he believes the bacillus is occasionally **transmitted** to the inhabitants **through the air,** but most commonly by the water. [Although favorably considered also by the following writer, the possibility of transmission through the air is more than doubtful.] Wolff[1] reports an epidemic of typhoid fever occurring upon Neuhof Island. As the possibility of infection by water and milk was excluded, it was decided that the cause must reside in an open sewer, and was probably distributed by the atmosphere. Henrot[2] reports an epidemic of typhoid fever that attacked only members of a dragoon regiment, numbering 1200 men, that lived in garrison with 4000 other soldiers in a town of · 30,000 inhabitants. The only cause of infection that could be found was the **dust** of a field upon which human manure had been used, and which had recently been ploughed. [In this and the following article infection from water contaminated by the soil is at least as likely as transmission by the dry dust.] Gibert,[3] having been called to investigate the causation of endemic typhoid fever in Havre, found that the water-supply was quite pure, and was therefore inclined to find the source of infection in the **soil** upon which the city was built. He was more inclined to believe this on discovering that in the part of the city built upon pebbly soil there were few cases of typhoid, while in the section, inhabited chiefly by the rich, that was built upon a less hygienic foundation many cases occurred.

Achille Hauser[4] believes that typhoid fever by **direct contagion** is not so uncommon as is generally supposed; he also believes that it may be transmitted by a third person who does not acquire the infection. He therefore lays down the following rules for the management of typhoid-fever patients: a special nursing-personnel which should itself be immune to the disease and isolated from other patients; the isolation of the typhoid patients; and the frequent and careful disinfection of all the objects that are used by or for them. [The author does not sufficiently establish his contention regarding contagion. Of course, this term is a relative one, and he may apply it to the transmission of the disease by close personal contact in which the germs may somehow reach the alimentary tract of the second person.]

Chantemesse[5] alludes to the danger of infection with typhoid fever through **oysters.** He cites particularly an instance in which 14 persons in 6 families became affected. The other members of these families who did not eat the oysters remained healthy; 8 of the patients had mild symptoms (pain in the stomach, vomiting, diarrhea, loss of appetite, and tympany) for 2 or 3 days; 4 younger members, who had eaten only a little, had severe symptoms of the same general character, with dejections of dysenteric appearance; 2 others of 20 and 21 years had severe typhoid fever, and 1 died. The illness was not one of simple poisoning, such as occurs after consumption of ordinary shellfish. Finally, the author was able to show by direct experiment that typhoid germs become incorporated in the body of oysters when the latter are placed in infected water. [This subject has been discussed in previous numbers of the *Year-Book*, and the truth seems quite well established.]

Symptomatology.—M. A. Bunce[6] reports 2 cases of typhoid fever in which the **onset** was marked by symptoms **resembling influenza.** Among these were the usual languor, drowsiness, muscular soreness, pain in the eyeballs, coryza, and cough. The patients were at first treated as cases of

[1] Berlin. klin. Woch., No. 39, 1896. [2] Bull. de l'Acad. de Méd., No. 26, 1896.
[3] Ann. Micrograph., No. 6, 1896. [4] Gaz. hebdom. de Méd. et Chir., No. 11, 1897.
[5] Gaz. des Hôpitaux, No. 64, 1896. [6] Phila. Polyclinic, Aug. 15, 1896.

influenza, but the persistence of the symptoms later made the diagnosis clear. [We have seen a number of instances during the past year in which the difficulty of diagnosis between these diseases at the onset was quite considerable. In two cases very marked coryza and conjunctivitis, with injection of the conjunctival blood-vessels and fine contraction of the pupils, gave a striking resemblance to influenza. Both of these patients had epistaxis, but, as a rule, we have found this more copious when it occurs in influenza than when it occurs in typhoid fever.]

Wallace Beatty [1] reports a case of typhoid fever commencing suddenly with nausea and pain in the back, followed by rapid development of profound **jaundice.** Death occurred on the 6th day. At the autopsy a large spleen and enlarged mesenteric glands were found. The intestines were free from lesions. Typhoid bacilli were found in the spleen. [The typhoid bacillus does not always give rise to a characteristic clinical or pathologic picture.]

A. G. Nicholls [2] discusses the question of **hemorrhagic typhoid fever,** and particularly the hemorrhagic eruptions. These are especially frequent about the joints. The spots are usually small, but large suffusions may occur. Referring to the more serious hemorrhagic manifestations, he mentions hemoptysis, hematemesis, and severe hemorrhages from the bowels. The tendency to hemorrhage is probably due to the action of the typhoid bacillus in conjunction with pyogenic microorganisms, and to the coincidence of general cachexia. He has observed 2 cases, 1 of which showed a staphylococcus in the abscesses; the other, the microorganism of hemorrhagic septicemia in the organs. Altogether, the author refers to 4 cases of his own, in which the hemorrhagic diathesis developed on the 13th, 28th, 36th, and 40th day of the typhoid fever, respectively. Three of the patients recovered.

J. Comby [3] calls attention to the fact that more or less extensive **desquamation of the skin,** occurring in small branny particles or in large flakes, is frequently met with at the time of defervescence in typhoid fever of childhood. It begins at the neck and spreads over the body, but the hands and feet are unaffected. The sudamina usually occur previous to this, and both the latter and desquamation may be met with in defervescence of other febrile diseases. They are favorable in prognostic significance. [We have repeatedly observed desquamation of marked character in patients who had been treated by cold bathing or frequently sponged.]

E. McD. Cosgrave [4] reports 5 cases in which **scarlet fever and typhoid fever** were coincident. All had the symptoms of enteric fever and of scarlatina, with general desquamation. In all, the incubation-stages were concurrent, the scarlatinal infection being secondary to the typhoidal infection, so that the two diseases started almost at the same time. It was interesting that neither disease apparently aggravated the other; indeed, the typhoid fever appeared to have a mitigating effect on the scarlatina. In the discussion, Dr. Moore referred to the fact that desquamation may occur in typhoid fever, and stated also that he has seen certain papules on the skin in scarlatina very closely resembling the spots of typhoid fever. [In examining this paper we cannot feel certain that the cases are free from all reasonable doubt as to diagnosis.]

Kühnau [5] records a case of typhoid infection in which the clinical history was that of a **septicopyemia.** The diagnosis of typhoid was supported by a gradual onset and the discovery of roseolæ and hypoleukocytosis. Bacilli were obtained from the lymphatic glands and from the spleen that had the

[1] Dublin Jour. Med. Sci., Feb. 1, 1897.   [2] Montreal Med. Jour., June, 1896.
[3] Gaz. des Hôpitaux, No. 39. 1896.   [4] Brit. Med. Jour., Jan. 16, 1897.
[5] Berlin. klin. Woch., No. 30, 1896.

characteristics of Eberth's bacillus. The author states that there are two possibilities: first, that the infection occurred from the endometrium, from which the virus entered the circulation, or, second, that the infection occurred from the intestinal tract, with absence of local lesions. [It seems to us that the typhoid nature of this case admits of considerable question. The occurrence of ascending infection of the urinary tract was highly suggestive of the bacillus coli communis, and the difficulties of distinguishing this organism from the typhoid bacillus are well known. The clinical facts upon which the author bases his diagnosis are most uncertain; roseolæ occur in other conditions or accidentally at times, while gradual onset and reduction of the leukocytes are by no means distinctive.]

Complications.—Dieulafoy[1] discusses **perforative peritonitis** in typhoid fever. This occurs during the height of the disease or during a relapse. It may occur in mild as well as severe cases, and the most constant and significant sign is sudden fall of temperature, although this does not always indicate this accident, as some cases terminate by crisis and hemorrhage is similarly accompanied by rapid decline. In the latter, however, the fever rises quickly again. Peritonitis from perforation usually lasts from 3 days to a week, and deceptive remissions may occur. In rare cases protective adhesions form and recovery ensues. When peritonitis is due to propagation of the infectious process through the ulcerated but not perforated intestines, there may be a lesion in the vermiform appendix. The symptoms are the same as those of other typhoid perforation. The term paratyphoid peritonitis may be applied to cases in which there is a sudden rise of the temperature due to late perforation resulting from a remnant of the typhoid lesion in the appendix. When the occurrence of perforation has been established operation holds out some hope of success. Lerboullet[2] reports several cases of typhoid fever in which perforation was accompanied by increase in the temperature. A case of unusual interest, though not entirely unique, is the following: Heagler[3] reports a case of typhoid fever that occurred in a woman suffering from **ventral hernia.** Perforation of the ileum contained in the hernial sac occurred, and also pierced the epidermis, giving rise to a fecal fistula. This gradually increased in size until it formed an opening 6 by 2 cm. The nutrition of the patient was profoundly depressed; she became greatly emaciated, but subsequently there was some improvement and she ultimately recovered. E. B. Steel[4] reports a case of supposed enteric fever complicated by perforation, peritonitis, and perityphlitic abscess. The onset was sudden, with severe abdominal pain and the signs of peritonitis. Later collapse occurred, and subsequently well-defined typhoid spots appeared. Finally, a local mass developed in the right iliac fossa. It was regarded as a perityphlitic abscess, and was drained. [The author reports this as a case of typhoid fever with perforation, but we must confess that the history is far from satisfactory. It seems to us rather an instance of appendicitis. The presence of spots and the history, upon which the author lays great stress, are insufficient for the purpose of making a positive diagnosis.]

J. B. Herrick[5] reports a case of typhoid fever occurring after an attempt to produce abortion that was supposed, at first, to be septic in nature. Death occurred as a result of hemorrhage, and at the autopsy, besides the lesions of typhoid fever which were confirmed by bacteriologic examination, an **extrauterine pregnancy** was discovered.

[1] Sem. méd., Oct. 30, 1896.   [2] Bull. de l'Acad. de Méd., Nov. 3, 1896.
[3] Korrespondencebl. f. Schw. Aerzte, No. 17, 1896.   [4] Brit. Med. Jour., Jan. 2, 1897.
[5] Med. News, Oct. 17, 1896.

[The more general application of bacteriologic methods is bearing fruit in the way of showing the frequency of secondary and mixed infections in typhoid fever. No useful rules for treatment or prevention can as yet be formulated.] Nicholls[1] reports a case of typhoid fever with **septic infection.** The rarity of the condition is manifest from the absence of reported cases even in extensive statistics, although a number of cases of general septicemia have been reported in which the typhoid germ and some other germ or germs were found in the various organs, or in which a simple secondary infection had occurred in the course of typhoid. The latter is more often the case. These cases run an atypical course, and are usually marked by great prostration, stupor, at times low delirium, subsultus, lividity, high fever, chills, and local septic processes. These symptoms, while they are at times met with in uncomplicated cases, are exceptional when the bath-treatment is used. His own case, a man of 30, had been ill 6 weeks before admission with vague prodromes of typhoid. When admitted his temperature was 104.8°, the skin was slightly livid, his tongue was swollen, and the pulse was dicrotic. The cyanosis increased and a membranous patch developed on the soft palate; the cultures from this showed micrococcus tetragonus and a few short bacilli not resembling the diphtheria bacillus. Bronchopneumonia developed and the patient died. Cultures from the blood during life showed a mixture of the streptococci, staphylococci, and 2 bacilli, 1 conforming to the tests for the typhoid bacillus. At the autopsy cultures were made from all the viscera, and these confirmed the examinations of the blood.

A. Schmidt[2] reports a case of typhoid fever which was followed by the development of **suppuration** beneath the diaphragm. When the abscess was opened by an operation 3 liters of clear brown liquid pus were evacuated, containing a pure culture of typhoid bacillus. The origin of the lesion was either an abscess of the spleen or a suppurated mesenteric gland. He also reports another case in which, after a severe colitis, particularly affecting the transverse and descending colon, a left-sided pleural empyema developed, which contained only the bacterium coli communis. He adopts the explanation of Cürschmann, that the organisms find their way into the pleura along the retroperitoneal space. H. B. Anderson[3] reports a case of suppurative **cholecystitis following typhoid fever.** A man of 67 was attacked suddenly with chill, fever, diarrhea, and pains in the abdomen. He recovered somewhat, but recurrence of similar symptoms followed. Malarial plasmodia could not be detected and the spleen was little enlarged. The right side of the abdomen was tense and very tender, so that the edge of the liver could not be felt. The history gave no indication of previous occurrence of gall-stone or jaundice. A probable diagnosis of abscess of the liver following some form of intestinal lesion was made. The patient died in coma. The autopsy showed an acute peritonitis due to rupture of the gall-bladder. The solitary follicles of the intestine were swollen, and there was ulceration of several of Peyer's patches in the lower part of the ileum. The cystic duct was obstructed by a gall-stone and there were a perforating ulcer and dilatation of the gall-bladder. Typhoid bacilli were obtained from the peritoneal liquid. The author concludes, therefore, that the original disease was typhoid fever. [The diagnosis in this case is not entirely free from doubt. The following case is, however, more satisfactory:] A. L. Mason[4] reports a case of typhoid fever in which, toward the end of the third week, there was pain in the right hypochondrium, followed by development of a tumor in this region. There was partial collapse, and a diagnosis of suppurative distention of the gall-bladder was made. This was tapped, and several ounces of sero-

[1] Montreal Med. Jour., Aug., 1896.   [2] Deutsch. med. Woch., No. 32, 1896.
[3] Med. News, Aug. 8, 1896.   [4] Boston M. and S. Jour., May 13, 1897.

purulent fluid withdrawn that was found to contain the typhoid bacillus. The patient recovered. Fernet[1] reports a case of typhoid fever in a patient suffering from intermittent hydronephrosis. Toward the end of the disease a fluctuating tumor developed in the abdomen, and this was punctured and found to be a **pyonephrosis,** the pus containing a pure culture of typhoid bacilli. As a result of the operation peritonitis developed, and this was apparently due to infection with bacterium coli. During the course of the pyonephrosis there was no pyrexia.

Widal[2] describes a case in which an **exostosis** appeared on the posterior part of the 9th rib, and grew to the size of an egg, beginning on the 27th day of a case of severe typhoid fever. The mass was bony-hard and appeared quickly, but disappeared just as quickly with the improvement in the general condition, and by ·the 41st day there was no visible swelling. The skin over the seat of the tumor remained slightly discolored for a long time. [The appearance and disappearance of swellings of this character are sometimes remarkable. In a recent case under our care a mass appeared on the outer side of the left humerus, and suppuration seemed inevitable. Unexpectedly resolution occurred, complete disappearance of the mass, which had reached the size of a small lemon, speedily following.] Tuffier and Widal[3] report a case of periostitis following 16 months after a mild attack of typhoid. Both tibiæ were affected, and an abscess occurred in the left. This was incised, but no typhoid bacilli could be detected in the pus. The authors ascribe this to the death of the organisms having occurred, such as is known to take place at times in postpneumonic abscesses. Bruni[4] reports a case of **osteomyelitis** in which typhoid bacilli were found, occurring six years after the patient had had typhoid. The patient, aged 36, had chronic afebrile osteomyelitis involving the left tibia and resembling that met with in tuberculosis. The bacteriologic study showed typhoid bacilli.

Salles and Borjon[5] describe a case of **orchitis** in the course of typhoid fever. The case is of special interest from the fact that the epididymis and the body of the testicle, as well, were involved. The tunica vaginalis at the same time was the seat of exudation, this being rather common in cases occurring in typhoid orchitis. The typhoid bacilli were found on the 6th and on the 17th days in some of the serum that had been removed.

Bresler[6] reports a case of **thrombosis** of the vena cava inferior which occurred in a patient who had had typhoid fever 17 months previously. The swelling of the abdominal veins became quite marked, and the upward current of blood was easily demonstrated. As this dilatation was only moderate, and there had been very slight edema of the feet, the author was inclined to the belief that the occlusion was only partial. [This complication is infrequent. Its termination in abscess of the liver was referred to in the last *Year-Book.*] Etienne[7] reports the case of a young man of 18 who on the 51st day of an attack of typhoid fever went into a state of collapse and died 3 days later. At the autopsy a thrombus was found in the coronal vein.

C. S. Bull[8] describes the following **ocular complications** of typhoid fever : conjunctivitis, which may be catarrhal or phlyctenular and combined with keratitis, loss of accommodation, and dilatation of the pupil from paresis of the ciliary muscle, retinal hemorrhage, paralysis of the external muscles, neuroretinitis, and inflammations of the uveal tract.

[1] Gaz. des Hôpitaux, No. 10, 1897.
[3] Ibid., No. 50, 1896.
[5] Gaz. des Hôpitaux, No. 45, 1896.
[7] Sem. méd., p. 321, 1896.

[2] Ibid., No. 48, 1896.
[4] Ann. de l'Inst. Pasteur, No. 10, 1896.
[6] Deutsch. med. Woch., Mar. 18, 1897.
[8] Med. Rec., Apr. 24, 1897.

M. L. Griffin[1] reports a case of enormous **enlargement of the spleen,** following typhoid fever and progressing for 15 years. Upon the administration of arsenic the organ returned to its normal size in the course of 2 months. [It is, of course, very doubtful whether the typhoid bacillus was responsible for this condition.]

Diagnosis.—[Our knowledge of the reaction that takes place between the blood-serum of an infection and the infecting microorganism is based upon the work that has been done by many investigators during the past years. Pfeiffer pointed out the peculiar reaction, which bears his name, that occurs when the microbe is injected into the body of an immune animal. Further investigation proved that a similar reaction took place outside of the body, in the test-tube, with serum from the immune animal. Others found that the reaction occurred also with the blood of convalescents, and even of cases in the acute stages of the infection. Its great practical value in the diagnosis of typhoid fever was discovered by Widal; and, although Grünbaum in Vienna at the same time and independently published similar results, the investigations of the former have been much more useful.

The **Widal reaction** is manifested on adding to a fresh bouillon-culture of typhoid bacillus a small amount of the serum; after a certain time (8–16 hours) the turbidity of the medium disappears. The liquid becomes clear, and the microbes settle to the bottom of the tube as a flocculent deposit. The cause of this, as witnessed under the microscope, is due to a complete loss of the natural motility and an agglutination of the bacilli—a clumping into more or less large masses.

This method of Widal gives such brilliant promise that the more cumbersome bacteriologic methods have received little attention during the year. Clinicians in many quarters incline to make the diagnosis too readily. This tendency is especially marked among some of those who report remarkable results for new " cures." It is hoped that the serum-test will prove a reliable indication, if for no other reason than to serve as a check to reckless laudation of methods of treatment based upon speedy cure of doubtful cases.]

Widal[2] reports the examination of the serum of 6 cases of typhoid on the 7th, 12th, 15th, 16th, 19th, and 21st days of the disease. All gave **characteristic immobilization and agglutination.** With a sterilized syringe a small quantity of blood was withdrawn from the median cephalic vein, and a few drops of the serum thus obtained added to a fresh bouillon-culture of the typhoid bacillus in the proportion of 1 : 10 or 1 : 15. After 24 hours in the incubator the cloudiness had mostly disappeared and the microbes had sunk to the bottom of the tube in flocculent masses. The serum of cases other than typhoid did not have this action. The coli bacilli behaved in the same way toward 2 cases that had had typhoid; but in cases of other diseases they retained their motility and remained free. Achard[3] reports 6 cases, 3 positive and 3 negative. Of these latter, 2 were of doubtful diagnosis, and the course of the disease disproved typhoid; the third was some febrile gastric trouble. Of the 3 positive cases, the first was examined on the 8th day after a relapse; the second was a typical case of typhoid; and the third was a patient with fever and diarrhea, but no stupor nor adynamia. Splenic puncture gave a culture of the bacillus typhosus. Lemoine[4] studied an epidemic of " *typhoidette* " and gastric disturbance: 3 cases of the former gave positive serum-reactions; 7 cases of the latter gave 6 negative results. The one positive reaction was in a case simulating, in some respects, typhoid, which was ren-

---

[1] Dublin Jour. Med. Sci., Apr., 1897.   [2] Sem. méd., p. 259, 1896.
[3] Ibid., p. 295, 1896.   [4] Bull. de la Soc. méd. des Hôp., July 24, 1896.

dered probable by the course of the disease. Siredey[1] gives a ease of typhoid of 31st day, with positive reaction. The patient had fetid diarrhea and a scarlatiniform erythema, and the disease ran a rather abnormal course. Lemoine[2] reports a case of acute tuberculosis in whose stools a bacillus identical with Eberth's bacillus that gave a reaction with typhoid serum was found by Elsner's method. The serum of this patient gave no reaction with the typhoid bacillus. It is interesting to note that this patient had had typhoid fever 17 years before. Widal[3] reports 14 positive cases. In 4 it existed on the 8th day; in 1 it appeared on the 5th; in 1, absent on the 6th day, it appeared on the 7th; 11 cases of gastric disturbances were without result, and the clinical history confirmed this. 1 case for a while was suspicious, but a bacteriologic examination of the spleen gave a culture of staphylococcus. In another very light case the reaction was positive. In association with Sicard he found that the reaction sometimes occurred in the urine, but that this was a very inconstant phenomenon. Chantemesse[4] examined many febrile cases with negative results. In every one of 11 cases of typhoid there was a positive reaction (9th day to convalescence). The serum of these had no effect on the bacillus eoli communis.

Achard and Bensaud[5] observed **agglutination in the milk** of typhoids. A ease of 15 days with a 2 months' child had all the typical signs of typhoid, with positive reaction. The milk gave a good reaction with 1 : 10 dilution. The milk of 6 nursing-women with other diseases gave no reaction; 2 of these had had typhoid 16 and 15 years before. A slight alkalinization or acidification produced no alteration in the reaction. A temperature of 60° C. did not alter it; one of 100° diminished it; and one of 120° for 15 minutes destroyed it. Filtration through a Chamberlain bougie caused its disappearance. The ease with which milk is decomposed makes its use undesirable for the clinical application of the test. Widal and Sicard[6] found that the serum dried on different substances retained a certain amount of its agglutinative action. The best reaction was obtained from that dried on small pieces of **sponge;** 3 cases of typhoid gave a positive result with such serum—1 case at the height of the disease and 2 during the decline. A person who had had typhoid 7 years previously still gave a positive result. Other eases remained negative. The serum obtained from vesicles also gave a distinct reaction.

Widal[7] says the serum of **coli-infection** differs in no way from that of other diseases. Hypothetically, the serum of typhoids whose intestinal lesions have permitted a secondary infection from the intestinal tract may show some reaction with the bacillus eoli communis. But this does not affect the specificity of the typhoid-serum reaction. Vedel[8] reports a case of typhoid of 28 days' duration, whose serum gave the reaction. It had also a slight action on a fresh culture of eoli communis. Another ease, apparently typhoid, gave a negative result. These tests were confirmed by the clinical course. In the second case defervescence took place on the 10th day. Haushalter,[9] among many positive results, reports that the serum of a newborn child of a typhoid mother with positive reaction was negative.

Dieulafoy[10] reports that Widal and Sicard have shown that the **fibrinogen and seroglobulin** of the blood when separated retain the whole of the agglutinative substances. The same is true of other fluids of the body, pericardial and peritoneal, edematous and vesicular. In milk the casein is the active principle.

[1] Bull. de la Soc. méd. des Hôp., July 24, 1896. [2] Ibid., July 31, 1896. [3] Ibid.
[4] Ibid. [5] Ibid. [6] Ibid. [7] Sem. méd., 1896, p. 312. [8] Ibid. [9] Ibid.
[10] Bull. de l'Acad. de Méd., 346, 1896.

A. S. Grünbaum[1] says that, " although anticipating matters, it may be stated that hitherto it is only in cases of enteric fever that the serum shows a distinct agglutinative action within 30 minutes **when diluted** 16 times." Owing to the rarity of typhoid fever in Vienna, he is able to report only 8 cases, in all of which a positive reaction was obtained—2 with a dilution of 1 : 25 ; 4 with 1 : 64 ; 1 with 1 : 100 ; and 1 with 1 : 128. The blood taken from the ear or finger into a V-shaped capillary tube and centrifugated, is broken at the junction of the serum and corpuscles, and the drop or so of serum blown out. A number of tests were made with dilutions of 1 : 4 and 1 : 8, and positive results were obtained in many cases of diseases other than typhoid fever, and in healthy persons.

Achard and Bensaud[2] claim that the agglutinative power does not reside in the leukocytes. Plasma obtained from blood by addition of extract of leeches and centrifugating gave a reaction in no way less complete than plasma containing many leukocytes. Leukocytes separated by filtration through cotton, though living and capable of phagocytosis, had no effect on a culture of typhoid bacillus. This power, then, exists in the **plasma.** It can be dialyzed. It also exists in milk, tears, hydatid-cyst liquid, saliva, gastric juice, and bile.

Pugliesi[3] reports 44 observations of Widal's reaction. In the author's cases the serum was obtained from **blisters,** although in a small number the reaction was confirmed by serum drawn directly from the blood. In the most typical cases the reaction was noticed in from 5 to 6 hours ; sometimes, however, not until 48 hours had elapsed. In 16 cases of typhoid the result was positive in 13, while in 11 cases of other diseases the reaction was negative in 8 and uncertain in 3. He details 6 cases in which the diagnosis was doubtful ; in 4 of these the reaction was positive and in 2 negative : 1 of these was believed to be puerperal fever, but at the autopsy typhoid lesions were found. Widal's reaction was positive. On the other hand, a case diagnosed as typhoid fever gave no reaction, and post mortem there was no evidence of typhoid.

Widal and Sicard[4] think that in general the reaction is less intense in **mild cases** and in convalescence, but that this is not absolute.

Achard[5] found that serum that had lost its agglutinative action on the 16th day of **defervescence** differed in nothing, as regards its immunizing power, from the same serum during the febrile stage. He also noticed an increase of the reaction after relapses. Widal[6] found that the agglutinative action generally decreased after defervescence, but completely disappeared in only 2 cases of 16 on the 18th and 24th days of fever. It existed in 3 cases who had had typhoid 6 months, 3 years, and 7 years previously. During the febrile period the reaction may vary from 1 : 60 to 1 : 80, while in the convalescent stage it drops to 1 : 20, 1 : 10, or even lower. It thus appears to be greatest during infection, and to diminish at the beginning of immunity : it is therefore a phenomenon of infection, not of immunity.

Catrin[7] reports 2 cases of typhoid fever : 1 was followed after convalescence by rise of temperature and subsequent development of a phlegmon on the right arm, containing staphylococcus pyogenes aureus. The **pus** itself gave the typical reaction of Widal. The second case developed a phlegmon on the anterior surface of the thigh, giving the same cultures and having the same effect upon the typhoid bacillus.

[1] Lancet, Sept. 19, 1896.   [2] Sem. méd., 1896, p. 393.
[3] Riforma med., Oct. 2, 1896.   [4] Bull. de la Soc. méd des Hôp., Oct. 16, 1896.
[5] Ibid., Oct. 9, 1896.   [6] Ibid.   [7] Gaz. de Méd. de Paris, Oct. 15, 1896.

Haushalter[1] reports 15 cases of typhoid fever with positive reaction; in 2 cases, however, it was incomplete. Of 8 cases of gastric disturbance, 5 gave a positive reaction; 4 cases of bronchopneumonia were negative.

Thiroloix[2] found that with 1 : 10 dilution the reaction began in 10–20 minutes on the 4–13th day of disease. Once it was negative on the 3d day, and appeared on the 5th. 28 cases of other diseases were negative. In 3 cases of typhoid it persisted for 3, 6, and 8 months. The prognosis does not depend upon the intensity of the reaction.

Villiez and Battle[3] say that in 6 undoubted cases of typhoid the reaction was positive. In 3 of malaria from Madagascar a constant positive reaction occurred in 1 [possibly typhomalaria (?)]. Some cases of simple gastric catarrh gave positive results, and these convalesced slowly; others were negative, and these convalesced rapidly. [The careless manner in which the term **simple gastric catarrh** is employed by some French writers is exceedingly confusing.]

R. Breuer[4] gives a very interesting review of the subject. In his cases he makes use of the second method of Widal. In 43 cases, the diagnosis of which was verified by the course of the disease, and in 3 cases by section, there were marked and undoubted positive reactions: 27 nontyphoids were examined, and 22 gave completely negative results. In some there was a slight agglutination, shown macroscopically by a dust-like cloudiness of the bouillon, without flocculent deposit. The same occurred in 3 cases of short febrile attacks which somewhat simulated typhoid, but which were finally diagnosed as cases of autointoxication. 9 convalescents were tested at periods of from 5 days to 3 months after recovery. In 2 only was the result negative. No relation was observed between the severity of the attack and the intensity of the reaction.

Achard and Bensaud[5] report 2 cases—1 of suppurative arthritis, and the other of paratyphoid, a case with characteristic typhoid symptoms excepting roseolæ and splenic enlargement. The urine gave cultures of the bacillus paratyphosus. No typhoid bacilli were found in spleen or stools. These **paratyphoid** bacilli were akin to the typhoid microbe, but were a different species: they fermented glucose and maltose, but not lactose and saccharose. Inoculations on cultures of Eberth's bacillus acted like the bacillus coli communis. Typhoid serum agglutinated 12 of 14 specimens of bacillus paratyphosus. Paratyphoid serum may agglutinate under some conditions the bacillus typhosus. The serum on the 21st day agglutinated both the bacillus typhosus and paratyphosus. The reaction persisted until the 53d day with the paratyphoid bacillus, but with only 3 out of 13 specimens of the typhoid.

Widal and Sicard[6] claim that the reaction can definitely differentiate the bacilli of typhoid and of **psittacosis.** In dilutions of 1 : 10 the reaction occurs in both, but the masses of bacilli of psittacosis are smaller and more crowded. In dilutions of 1 : 20, 1 : 30, 1 : 40, there arrives a moment when the bacillus psittacosis no longer reacts. With fresh cultures the difference is most marked with 1 : 40–1 : 60, both in test-tube and microscopically. Grüber obtained agglutination with bacillus entericus, but only in concentrated solutions; with dilute solutions there was a distinct difference. They noticed a variation in some of the specimens according to their virulence, transplantation, medium, age, etc.

E. B. Block[7] gives the results in 20 cases of typhoid tested in Dr. Osler's

[1] Presse méd., No. 80, 1896. [2] Ibid., Nov. 4, 1896.
[3] Ibid., No. 84, 1896. [4] Berlin. klin. Woch., Nov. 23 and 30, 1896
[5] Bull. de la Soc. méd. des Hôp., Nov. 27, 1896.
[6] Compt. rend. de la Soc. de Biol., No. 21, 1896.
[7] Bull. Johns Hopkins Hosp., Nov. and Dec., 1896.

wards. The dilution was 1 : 16, and the reaction was complete in only 11 cases. In 6 it was partial. In 3 it was but slight, and these were very mild cases. Grünbaum's method for collecting the serum was used. The dry method was employed in 17 cases, with marked reaction in 9.

Menetrier[1] observed a case of typhoid complicated with pleurisy in which the **pleural effusion** did not give the reaction on the 35th day. At the same date the serum was not examined, but on the 8th day it had given a decided reaction. Achard[2] has found many times a positive reaction with pleural effusions, but has found it wanting in the **pericardial fluid.**

Wyatt Johnston and D. D. McTaggart[3] have contributed papers upon the diagnostic value of the **serum-reaction in typhoid fever,** using the drop-method described by Johnston. The blood is received in drops upon sterilized paper; these drops are afterward treated with distilled water, and the reaction tested with the solution so obtained. The blood used had usually been sent to them from a distance. The reaction occurred usually in a few minutes, but sometimes 3 or 4 or even 24 hours were required. It was best obtained with fresh, active cultures. The following are the results in 143 cases: positive results on first examination, 118, of which the reaction was complete in 112 and partial in 6, 3 of these being about the 3d day. The reaction was doubtful on the first examination in 5 cases, 4 of which were examined about the 6th day. Negative results were as follows: decisively negative, 14 cases; all were proved afterward to be other diseases; doubtfully negative, 3 cases; these were mild cases of typhoid first examined during convalescence; 2 cases with clinical history of typhoid in which no reexamination was made, and the primary examination was negative; 1 case of severe fever of typhoid type in which Widal's method and the dry method (3 times) gave negative results. This makes the total negative results in cases of possible typhoid 6 in 143 cases. The authors have also studied the serum of dry blood in experimental cholera and found that it gave positive results. They were able to demonstrate that the blood of guinea-pigs after a single intraperitoneal injection becomes positive in action. They substantiate the statement of Bordet that the blood of horses produces clumping.

Stern[4] has examined the blood in typhoid-fever patients with regard to leukocytosis and the presence of the typhoid bacilli. Considerable quantities of blood should be used, as the number of bacilli present is always small. The author has also investigated Widal's serum-test in 16 cases. He has taken blood from the finger-tip and added it to a bouillon-suspension of the typhoid bacillus, and then separated the red corpuscles by the centrifugal machine. The exact quantitative estimation of the effective substance in the blood cannot be made by this method. The earliest time that he obtained successful results was the 9th day of the disease, and he invariably obtained negative results in other diseases, excepting in 1 case of otitis, where there was a slight but distinct reaction obtained after 1 hour. The patient had never had typhoid fever. It is necessary, the author states, to determine the proportion of serum to culture that is powerless to give a reaction with blood-serum of other cases than those of typhoid fever. This proportion he found in his cases was 1 to 100, and even 1 to 200; Widal gives it as 1 to 60. The negative result in the early stages of typhoid fever must not be forgotten, and repeated testing of suspicious cases should be practised.

[1] Bull. de la Soc. méd. des Hôp., Dec. 4, 1896.   [2] Ibid.
[3] Brit. Med. Jour., Dec. 5, 1896 ; N. Y. Med. Jour., Oct. 31, 1896.
[4] Centralbl. f. innere Med., Dec. 5, 1896.

C. L. Greene[1] gives a further report of cases tested : 16 cases of typhoid reacted positively, and 19 cases of diseases other than typhoid were negative. He uses both the dried blood and the serum methods. He also observes that the diagnosis may be made by the naked eye, a fact which might sometimes be of service. Thiercelin and Lenoble[2] report a case of fever lasting 4 weeks that reacted during this period ; on the 4th day of normal temperature there was a reaction in 3 minutes in 1 : 10. A relapse occurred 5 days after this and lasted 10 days ; 20 days afterward no reaction occurred even in 2 hours.

Widal and Sicard[3] found the reaction in the **pleural fluid** of 3 cases, although it may be wanting in large effusions. This is not due to the presence of the bacillus, for pus containing bacilli may give a very active reaction. The fact may be due to the rapidity of the formation of the effusion in some way. **Tears** give the test in 1 : 10 and 1 : 5 ; but with artificial lacrimation due to ammonia the reaction does not occur.

Thoinot and Cavasse[4] report a case of mild typhoid or typhus levissimus. The reaction until the period of defervescence was always negative. After 7 days of apyrexia, during which the spleen remained enlarged, a **relapse** occurred of 15 days' duration, with classical symptoms. 2 days after defervescence the reaction by culture-method gave positive result ; none, however, by the extemporaneous method. A second relapse took place 1 month later. On the 8th day the reaction was slow, but positive ; by culture in only 48 hours. 1 day after defervescence the reaction occurred in 10 minutes. The serum from vesicles also gave positive results.

Thiercelin and Lenoble[5] record a case of typhoid in which blood and milk reacted, but the spontaneous **sweat** did not.

Widal and Sicard[6] discuss the **limits of the agglutinative action** of the serum of typhoid-fever patients, and state that it usually occurs on the first day of the infection. Its disappearance may occur as early as the 18th day after convalescence. In the cases that they observed, the disappearance usually took place at the end of a year; although immunity still exists at this time. However, in 22 cases that had had typhoid fever at varying times up to 26 years before the examination the agglutinating reaction was observed 6 times; three of these showing it very markedly in dilutions of 1 to 10 ; one had been well for 3 years, another for 7 years, and the third for 9 years. In other cases it required a larger proportion to obtain this result. They insist again that serum presenting this agglutinating action is not necessarily bactericidal, as they have been able to maintain cultures in it for 2 months without destroying their vitality. They believe, however, that this reaction is one of defence on the part of the organism, especially during the period of infection.

Charrin[7] holds that the Widal reaction is **a defensive action;**—in other words, that it is the beginning of an immunity.

Charrier and Apert[8] report 5 cases of typhoid with positive results. They also report the examination of the tissue of an embryo—from a mother in the third week of typhoid fever. They found that there was total absence of agglutinating action in the tissues of the fetal organism, and that in the placenta this property was present with a dilution of 1 to 15. They conclude that **the placenta** acts as a sort of filter and retains in the maternal organism not only the agglutinating substance, but probably also the toxins, whose dis-

[1] Med. Rec., Dec. 5, 1896. [2] Compt. rend. de la Soc. de Biol., No. 32, Dec. 11, 1896.
[3] Bull. de la Soc. méd. des Hôp., Dec. 11, 1896. [4] Ibid.
[5] Compt. rend. de la Soc. de Biol., No. 33, Dec. 19, 1896.
[6] Ibid. [7] Ibid. [8] Ibid., Jan. 1, 1897.

charge into the fetal circulation would doubtless cause the development of the agglutinating property. [We have knowledge of a case, not yet published, that occurred in the service of one of our colleges, in which the Widal test was positive for the infant blood. Moreover, positive demonstrations have been made of the transmission of typhoid bacilli through the placenta to the fetal circulation.]

Jez[1] reports a case in which reaction by the cultural method took place in 24 hours; by the microscopic in 15 minutes. A control-test was negative. The patient, a woman of 23 years, gave no history of typhoid. The test was made on the 13th day of the disease. The postmortem showed a basilar **tuberculous leptomeningitis.** [It is worth noting that no cultures from the organs were made for typhoid bacilli.]

Fränkel[2] hastened to confirm **Widal's method** as soon as published, and by great good fortune was enabled to study two epidemics, using in every case the three methods—the culture, the hanging-drop, and the test-tube. He believes that the microscopic investigations of the hanging drop give the most delicate, the most accurate, and the most rapid diagnosis of typhoid fever that could be desired. In a large number of investigations he obtained no reaction in only a few cases; they were either doubtful or in persons that had been convalescent for 5 weeks or more. In the latter class of cases he also found some whose blood gave a positive reaction. He also investigated a number of cases that were probably suffering from infection with the bacterium coli communis, and in all cases the result was negative, nor did cultures of the bacterium coli communis ever show the reaction in serum from typhoid fever. He naturally speaks highly of the trustworthiness of Widal's method, and simply raises the question whether the rapidity with which the reaction takes place and its completeness bear any relation to the severity of the infection. In conclusion, he triumphs over those " independent " and " cautious " investigators who have hitherto doubted the specific nature of the bacillus of Eberth.

Pfuhl[3] has employed Widal's method of serum-diagnosis for typhoid fever in a number of cases, and found that it occurred in all cases of typhoid fever, and in no others, excepting in one of so-called gastric fever, which he looks upon as a case of mild typhoid. He suggests as a **simplification of the method** the mixture of 1 drop of blood with 10 drops of water ; 1 drop of this then being mixed with 1 drop of bouillon-culture and examined in the hanging drop.

Jemma[4] agrees that promptness and character of the reaction depend upon the **intensity of the infection.** Jemma's experiments show that the reaction is greatest during the period when the bactericidal power of the blood-serum is greatest—at the febrile acme. Also, the quantity of serum used is less in this stage. Widal and Sicard show that the agglutinative effect and bactericidal power are in part related. Dieulafoy, Widal, and Sicard claim that it is not the serumalbumin, but the serumglobulin and fibrinogen to which the action is due. Devoto isolated the globulin with a saturated solution of ammonium sulfate, and dried the filtrate at low temperatures. When dried at 55° C. it lost its bactericidal property, but the ordinary room-temperature did not destroy this. Under this condition the test occurred with especial rapidity on the addition of the globulin. The same property exists in the urine, milk, tears, and all exudates. Widal and Sicard hold that the reaction is a phenomenon of infection, while others (Maragliano) ascribe it to immuniza-

---

[1] Wien. med. Woch., Mar., 1897.   [2] Deutsch. med. Woch., Jan. 14, 1897.
[3] Centralbl. f. Bakt. parasit. u. Inf'kr., Jan. 20. 1897.
[4] Centralbl. f. innere Med., Jan. 23, 1897.

tion. Jemma says that a temperature of 37° for 24–96 hours has no detrimental effect; also that 40° for 18–50 hours, 55° for 40 minutes, and 60° for 20 minutes diminishes, and 70° for 10 minutes destroys, the agglutinative action completely. It withstands the ordinary temperatures of 12°–15° for 40 days.

Pick[1] gives a **brief resume of the literature** to date. A series of cases were tested to find the most practical method. Venesection proved not to be a good routine practice. He then used blood from the sterilized finger, drawn into a small glass tube. The coagulum was removed and $\frac{1}{2}$–$\frac{3}{4}$ c.c. of pure serum obtained. Mixing 1 part of this with 10 parts of 24–48 hours' bouillon-culture, examination was made under the microscope in hanging drop. He also used the dried blood. Among 20 healthy persons and those with febrile diseases he never found a positive reaction. Sometimes there was a slight agglutination, but the masses never increased in size and the bacilli retained their motility. 20 cases of typically typhoid course and symptoms gave positive reactions. In 16 on the 3d to 21st day of the disease the reaction was immediate; in 4 it occurred in 10–30 minutes; in 12 cases the culture-test was complete in 8–16 hours; in 3, with less than 1 : 20 of serum, it was incomplete. The earliest period at which the reaction appears was on the 3d day. In 4 cases on the 5th day a dilution of 1 : 80 was sufficient; in 2 it took place, but only after 10 minutes; and in 1 a dilution of 1 : 5 was necessary; 1 case gave slow (30 minutes) reaction with 1 : 5 on the 6th day, and a slight one on the following day with 1 : 10. Another gave on the 7th day none; on the 9th day a slight one; and on the 11th an immediate and typical reaction; 12 suspicious and doubtful cases were examined; 3 gave immediate positive reactions, and the course of the disease confirmed the results; 9 were negative. Of these, 3 proved to be pneumonia; 2 tuberculosis and sepsis; 1 meningitis. In 1 the reaction was negative with 1 : 10 and 1 : 4 from the 6th day on by repeated tests, and only on the 34th day with 1 : 2 was there a reaction; 2 cases are worth details. A girl, aged 19, had been sick for a week; there were pain in the head and neck and a temperature of 39.5°. The condition resembled typhoid, but the serum-test was negative. Later symptoms of meningitis developed. A woman, aged 23, had been ill for 16 days with a temperature of 39.3° C., bronchitis and constipation: she had no tumor of the spleen and no roseolæ. The test was markedly positive on the 21st day of the disease. A general low typhoid developed and she died on the 24th day. The section showed no typhoid intestinal lesions, no splenic enlargement. Cultures gave the bacillus typhosus. Blood from the veins and extract of the lymph-glands gave positive reactions. Extract from the lungs and muscles gave only a slight reaction, that from the spleen none at all. Blood after the action of alcohol was negative. He also examined the blood of persons who had had the disease previously. 3 cases after 1½ years and one after 9 days gave an incomplete reaction; 2 after 12–16 years gave none; 1 after 14 days gave a complete reaction. Tests with the cultural method in the 12 negative cases gave the same results as with the microscopic examination. The dry method gave identical results, but he notes two objections—the masking of the reaction due to the coloring, and the difficulty of determining the exact quantity of serum used.

A. E. Wright and D. Semple,[2] in the course of their experiments on the effect of **typhoid vaccine,** tested the blood of their patients for the Widal reaction. The vaccine used was sterilized cultures. In 17 healthy persons that had been injected the reaction appeared almost immediately with 1 : 10 dilution

[1] Wien. klin. Woch., No. 4, 1897.   [2] Brit. Med. Jour., Jan. 30, 1897.

of the serum. The maximum reaction, however, did not develop until a much longer period—2 to 5 weeks—and sometimes even only after repeated injections of the vaccine.

Mesnil de Rochemont [1] reports 2 cases in which an **early diagnosis** of typhoid fever was made. One on the 2d day from the initial chill gave a reaction, microscopically, with a 1 : 10 and, macroscopically, with 1 : 100 dilution. The other on the second day was positive with 1 : 10 and 1 : 40 dilutions. The diagnosis was in both cases confirmed by the subsequent course of the disease. 3 cases of typhoid complicating other diseases gave positive results by the microscopic method with 1 : 10, 1 : 40, and 1 : 40 dilutions; by the macroscopic, 1 : 30, 1 : 40, and 1 : 60 dilutions. Another case, which always was negative by the macroscopic culture-method, gave a positive reaction with 1 : 10 dilution under the microscope, and proved at the autopsy to be purulent meningitis and follicular enteritis. The author concludes that with high dilutions a positive reaction renders the diagnosis absolutely certain.

A. H. Appel and F. J. Thornbury [2] never observed any effect on the **bacillus coli communis,** even with serum that reacted strongly with the typhoid bacillus. With the **bacillus pyocyaneus** they obtained a slight reaction with typhoid serum, but were unable to find any other organisms, pathogenic or saprophytic, that were at all affected by it. Fifty cases of typhoid fever were tested upon attenuated cultures, and more or less typical reactions obtained. With virulent cultures cases which were convalescent for a number of years under the same conditions gave constant negative results; 25 persons in health or suffering from diseases other than typhoid were examined with varying results.

Courmont [3] reports the results of examination of **7 cases of typhoid.** In 4 a mixture made of 1 : 10 of body-juices and culture, the heart's blood and pericardial, pleural, and peritoneal serous fluids gave distinct positive reactions. The liver and spleen gave very feeble ones; in 1 case the latter was negative. The other 3 cases were examined by exact dosage, and it was found that the blood gave the strongest reaction, whilst that of the splenic pulp was always very weak; in other words, those organs in which the bacillus was localized contained little or no agglutinin, whilst the abnormal presence of the bacillus in any situation caused its disappearance. Menetrier [4] found a pleural fluid containing bacilli that did not agglutinate. Other germs have no such effect. Pleural effusions due to pneumococcus and to tubercle-bacillus gave the reaction in cases of typhoid fever.

Stern [5] points out certain **sources of error** in the manipulation of the test. There are sera of nontyphoids which, when used in the dilution originally recommended by Widal, give a distinct reaction. He agrees with Grüber that even normal serum will agglutinate when used with equal parts of culture. In practice he obtains the limit of reaction for the particular culture that he uses. A young culture is necessary, from 8–12 hours old. He also recommends the microscopic method. The cultural reaction, he claims, does not depend wholly upon the agglutination, but "upon the energy of the growth of the culture, the quality of the medium, and, with low dilutions, the bactericidal power of the blood-serum." He fixes the time-limit of observation at 2 hours. In 20 of 70 nontyphoid cases there was a reaction after 2 hours with a 1 : 10 dilution; in 5 with 1 : 20; in 2 with 1 : 30; and in none with 1 : 40. Of 50 cases in which there was no reaction with 1 : 10 dilution, some reacted with 1 : 5; others did not even with equal parts of serum and culture. He reports a

[1] Münch. med. Woch., No. 5, 1897.   [2] Jour. Am. Med. Assoc., Feb. 6, 1897.
[3] Compt. rend. de la Soc. de Biol., No. 7, 1897.
[4] Bull. de la Soc. méd. des Hôp., xii., June, 1897.   [5] Berlin. klin. Woch., No. 11, 1897.

case which, at the beginning of the 9th week, reacted with 1 : 1000. A relapse occurred a few days after and a reaction could be obtained with 1 : 5000. This, he thinks, speaks against the theory that agglutination bears a relation to immunity. Stern can find no relation between the strength of the agglutination and the severity of the attack : the test is of no value in prognosis. He also calls attention to the fact that the reaction may not appear until the disease is advanced to the 2d, 3d, or even 4th week. Also, that it lasts for months, even years, after convalescence. The following case is of interest : of a family of 8, the parents and 3 children were attacked with typhoid and taken to the hospital. The seroreaction was present in all. 2 of the children remaining at home also had symptoms of light typhoid, with positive reactions. The sixth child was never in the least unwell, but his blood showed a reaction with 1 : 50. Stern considers the possibility of an individual immune to typhoid becoming infected and revealing the specific reaction without showing any symptoms.

Scheffer[1] reports 21 cases of typhoid with positive reactions. The reappearance of the agglutination so markedly during the relapses seems to him to confirm Widal's idea that it is a phenomenon of infection rather than one of immunity. Two positive cases are given in some detail. In both the clinical signs of typhoid were slightly marked. In the first the eruption, which quickly disappeared, was the only diagnostic sign. There was no tumor of the spleen, no typical fever, and no intestinal symptoms. In the second case the spots were also wanting, and the case reminded one of tuberculosis of the peritoneum. H. M. Biggs and Wm. H. Park[2] report their experience in the laboratories of the New York Board of Health. As the most practical method the dried blood is used. A test is made with virulent culture of typhoid bacillus. If a reaction takes place with a dilution of 1 : 10, then a higher dilution is employed. In all, 200 cases were examined. In 140 in which the final diagnosis was typhoid, there was a reaction in 100. In 57 in which the final diagnosis was other than typhoid there were 57 negative results ; 3 doubtful cases, which were not regarded as typhoid by the clinical observers, gave positive reactions. They observed clumping and immobilization in other than typhoid bacilli, even when high dilutions were used. They claim that a positive diagnosis may be made in 50 % of cases, and a probable one in half the remaining.

Mossé and Daunic[3] report the case of a woman that had typhoid fever in the 8th month of pregnancy. At delivery the blood and colostrum of the mother and blood taken from the placenta and the child gave immediate positive reactions, and the reaction was still found in the **child's blood** 33 days later. The placenta was normal, and a bacteriologic examination was negative.

Siegert[4] regards the Widal reaction as of great value in the diagnosis of the often **abnormal typhoid fever of children.** He gives as examples the cases of 2 brothers, $9\frac{1}{2}$ and $10\frac{1}{2}$ years old. The first came to the hospital with the diagnosis of perityphlitis. He had high remittent fever, small, frequent pulse, constipation, enlarged inguinal glands, and none of the usual typhoid symptoms. Tuberculosis of the mesenteric glands was thought of. The history of the case inclined to typhoid fever. The other brother was more like typhoid ; he had roseola and meningeal symptoms. Widal's reaction with 1 : 25 and 1 : 100 dilution cleared up the diagnosis. The similarity of the cases, and the fact that the first case gave the Widal reaction 6 weeks after recovery, made it probable that it also was one of typhoid fever.

[1] Berlin. klin. Woch., No. 11, 1897.　　　　[2] Am. Jour. Med. Sci., Mar., 1897.
[3] Compt. rend. de la Soc. de Biol., No. 8, Mar., 1897.
[4] Münch. med. Woch., No. 10, p. 250, 1897.

Guinon and Meunier,[1] *apropos* of certain positive results obtained with the Widal reaction in **tuberculosis,** report a case of acute tuberculosis associated with typhoid fever in a boy aged 8. He had fever (39°–39.2° C.) and characteristic physical signs. Six days after admission the temperature began to rise by oscillations to 40°, where it remained for 10 days. The symptoms corresponded to a pulmonic exacerbation. There were no intestinal signs of typhoid, nor diarrhea. The temperature fell somewhat, and this was followed by frequent, slightly yellow half-formed stools. After 12 days of fever a few roseolæ appeared. There was some splenic enlargement. The diagnosis of typhoid fever was made, and Widal's test gave positive results on the 11th and 17th days of the infection. Defervescence was followed 16 days later by a relapse terminating in death. The postmortem showed tuberculosis of the liver, intestines, mesenteric glands, kidneys, pleura, lungs, spleen. The tubercle-bacillus was present. Cultures from the spleen, pleura, and lungs demonstrated the presence also of the bacillus typhosus. In answer to M. Rendu, who expressed doubt as to the absolute diagnostic signification of the presence of typhoid bacillus after death, the author gives his reasons for believing the case to be one of typhoid fever. The roseolæ, the splenic tumor, the temperature-curve point to such a diagnosis. The age of the patient explains the absence of any typhoid intestinal lesions. [The Widal test and the presence of typhoid bacilli in the spleen are certainly significant. M. Widal also supports this view, and records a similar case of his own.]

J. B. Thomas, Jr.[2] examined 28 cases of typhoid, with 4 negative results. These last were tested on the 6th, 7th, and 9th days respectively. It is probable that in these the reaction had not yet developed. In 8 cases the clinical diagnosis at the time of the test was doubtful, but the course of the disease confirmed the reaction. Of 29 diseases other than typhoid, 5 gave the reaction (phthisis, rheumatism, malaria, and 2 old typhoids of 3 and 6 years). He uses the dried blood. A drop of water is added to this, the mixture transferred to a cover-glass, and a drop of typhoid emulsion added to it. It is examined during 2 hours and at the end of 24. [It is seen that the dilution used must have been too low. This criticism is further warranted by his results with the colon-bacillus.] Eleven typhoids and 11 nontyphoids were tested with this microbe with positive results—in all 22 cases. [This certainly throws some doubt on the positive results of the reaction obtained in the nontyphoid cases with the bacillus typhi.] Gruber[3] reports 36 cases, 34 typhoids and 2 of other diseases. With a dilution of 1 : 1 of serum 25 examinations gave 3 negative results. Two were not typhoid fever, and the other a very light case, the temperature of which rose only to 38.9° C., and which was examined on the 11th day. With 1 : 32 dilution he found 12 negative results, 2 being nontyphoids. The period of examination was from the 5th day to the 5th week. The serum was diluted with distilled water and the time of observation was ½ to 1 hour. He concludes that the reaction is a most useful aid to our diagnosis, but that it is not in any way absolute. [It is worth noting that the 1 : 1 dilution he uses is too low, and that the negative cases might have reacted to one less than 1 : 32.]

C. A. Elsberg[4] used the dried blood, employing an approximately definite dilution of 1 : 8 by means of measured wire loop. Clumping and cessation of all motility should take place in 15 minutes for a complete and positive test. With this dilution he never found any agglutination with normal serum ; 3

[1] Bull. de la Soc. méd. des Hôp. de Paris, No. 13, Apr. 2, 1897.
[2] Med. News, Apr. 3, 1897.   [3] Münch. med. Woch., Nos. 17 and 18, 1897.
[4] Med. Rec., Apr. 10, 1897.

specimens of the typhoid bacillus were used, 2 of low virulence, and these he found to give the best results; 262 examinations of 36 cases of typhoid were made. The reaction appeared on the 4th day in 1; on the 5th in 2; on the 7–12th days in 20; on the 12–14th in 8; on the 14–17th in 2; and on the 24th, 27th, and 32d in 3. Out of 148 cases of other diseases but 1 gave the reaction. This case was considered one of biliary calculus. Splenic cultures were negative. At one time it was thought that there might have been a mild typhoid before admission to the hospital, but this was eliminated. The author concludes that the reaction is in no sense absolute, but that it is of value in doubtful and irregular cases.

Wyatt Johnston [1] states that he was the first to suggest the use of **water as a diluting-fluid** for the dried blood of typhoid cases that was to be submitted to the Widal method. He also declares that attenuated cultures react less delicately than those that are virulent.

H. M. Bracken [2] reports his results in 47 cases examined for the Minnesota State Board. In 28 the clinical diagnosis was that of typhoid: of the 19 not typhoid, none gave the reaction. Of the typhoids, 3 did not react: 2 of these results the author blames on poor technic in collecting the serum. The 3d case had been classed as an aborted or cured typhoid by the attending physician. The diagnosis, judged from the history of the case, was undoubtedly wrong. The earliest date at which the reaction was obtained was the 4th day. The dry serum was used.

Kuhnau [3] points out the importance of using as nearly as possible the same **concentration of bacilli.** He calculates that there are 120 millions of microbes in 1 c.c. of an emulsion made from a fresh agar-culture; 50 specimens of normal serum gave the reaction with low dilutions (41 with 1:3; 8 with 1:10–1:20; 4 with 1:30; 3 with 1:35; and 1 with 1:50). With 4 cases of typhoid fever the reaction occurred respectively with 1:30, 1:30, 1:40, and 1:100. With 11 more cases the same result obtained. Coli bacilli were affected by both normal and typhoid sera only in strong solution —1:5–1:10. His experiments also seem to show that the reaction with non-virulent cultures is nearly double that with virulent ones.

J. L. Miller [4] reports 43 cases examined by the culture-method. Of these, 15 typhoids gave the complete reaction within 20 minutes; 20 sera from healthy persons and 8 from cases of acute disease failed to give any reaction. Thirty more cases were examined by the dry method. The dried blood was dissolved in water, and to it was added a drop of the bouillon-culture. No attempt was made at accurate dilution: 3 typhoids gave the reaction; 22 nontyphoids were negative; and 5 gave a more or less complete reaction. Further, 63 cases were examined with a dilution of 1:10 by removing the blood in a hematocrit-tube and adding a definite quantity to the bouillon-culture. Of 13 typhoids, 10 gave a complete reaction, 2 a partial, and 1 was negative. This last was a mild case; 42 nontyphoids were negative, 3 doubtful, 3 slight, and 2 typical.

Courmont [5] reports the results of the Widal test in 240 cases. He used the rapid method, with blood taken from the finger-tip, the same specimen of typhoid bacillus from a sugar-containing medium, and a 1:10 dilution; 169 cases were examined during the febrile period. The reaction was present before the 6th day in 13; from the 7th to 8th days in 40; 9th to 15th in 73; 16th to the defervescence in 41. In 7 cases only did the reaction, which was absent at first, appear at a subsequent examination. The reaction was positive,

[1] Centralbl. f. Bakt. u. Parasit. Inf'kr., Apr. 24, 1897.
[2] N. Y. Med. Jour, Apr. 24, 1897. [3] Berlin. klin. Woch., No. 19, May 10, 1897.
[4] Chicago Med. Recorder, May, 1897.
[5] Compt. rend. de la Soc. de Biol., No. 19, June 4, 1897, p. 528.

then, in 167 cases. In 2 only was it negative. In 1 of these splenic puncture gave negative cultures; in the other the symptoms were by no means those of typical typhoid. Of 72 convalescents, 58 were examined during the first 6 months. Twenty-three gave positive results during the 1st month; 11 during the 2d; and 2 during the 3d, 4th, and 6th months. The rest were negative. Fourteen other cases were examined at periods of at least 1 year after convalescence: 2 were positive (1 and 2 years); 7 were negative (1–25 years); 5 gave a slight reaction (1–10 years). In 71 cases of disease other than typhoid (mumps, scarlatina, grippe, erysipelas, diphtheria, pneumonia, dysentery, pleurisy, meningitis, etc.) the reaction was absent in all but 1. In 7 there was formation of very small clumps with incomplete immobilization. In 1 case (scarlatina) there were typical clumping and nearly complete immobilization, which disappeared upon convalescence.

Wyatt Johnston[1] calls attention to the necessity of **accurate technic.** Among other things, he points to the importance of the alkalinity of the culture employed. A slightly acid medium may give no clumping, but slight alkalinization may cause this phenomenon. He recently found spontaneous clumping in his cultures, which upon investigation, proved to be due to excessive alkalinity of the bouillon. He also calls attention to the personal equation. What one would call a reaction another would regard as incomplete. He looks upon the coincident occurrence of the gradual cessation of motion and clumping as characteristic. One without the other is a pseudo or partial reaction. He has never seen a typical reaction in a case in which there was not strong ground for believing it was typhoid.

Finally, we cannot do better than to quote in abstract **the last article**[2] **by Widal,** in which he very thoroughly reviews the whole subject. The method originally employed by Widal was to add either to a fresh bouillon-culture or to one 24–48 hours old a certain proportion of serum (1 : 10). A more simple procedure, and one that does not require any venous puncture, is to collect the blood in a glass tube of small caliber, which can be sent to a bacteriologist for examination. In a watch-glass 1 drop of the serum is added to 10 or more drops of fresh bouillon-culture, and the mixture examined under the microscope; or the blood may be added directly without waiting for the separation of the serum. In this way, too, a measurement of the agglutinative action may be made; and this should never be omitted, especially in doubtful cases. As was shown in a previous article by Widal, a good reaction can be obtained by the use of dried blood. This was put to practical use by Johnston and McTaggert (q. v.), and has since been employed almost universally. Bordet found that the reaction took place with cholera-serum and vibriones that had been killed by chloroform. Widal has also showed that typhoid bacilli destroyed by heat or by antiseptics remain capable of producing agglutination. From a practical point of view formol seems to be the most useful agent for this purpose. The **phenomenon of agglutination** is, then, not a vital reaction, but rather a passive one on the part of the protoplasm of the microbe. Although the blood contains the largest amount of the agglutinating material, it is not confined to this fluid. It has been found in the urine, the serous fluid of blisters, of the pericardial, pleural, and peritoneal cavities, milk, the bile, liquid of the seminal vesicles, the aqueous humor, tears, pleural exudates, and to a less extent in the spleen, liver, mesenteric glands. In other words, it is found in almost all of the fluids of the body, even in those which do not contain leukocytes. Outside of the body at least, experiments show that the

[1] Jour. Am. Med. Assoc., July 17, 1897.
[2] Ann. de l'Inst. Pasteur, No. 5, May, 1897.

leukocytes do not secrete agglutinin. Filtration through a porcelain filter diminishes the amount of the agglutinative substance in urine and in milk; and Widal and Sicard have shown the same to be true of the serum and other body-fluids. Filtration retains most of the albuminoid bodies. Fluids that are poor in these, such as the saliva and the cerebro-spinal fluids, are poor in agglutinating properties. Addition of 15 per cent. of sodium chlorid precipitates the fibrinogen, which has strong agglutinative action. Further precipitation by saturation with magnesium sulfate gives the globulins, which also contain much of the agglutinin. The authors never obtained the reaction with a liquid rendered nonalbuminoid by dialysis, nor were they able to separate albuminoid substances that did not give a reaction. **The agglutinating substance** has a great resistance. Serums have been kept for months. Impurities do not destroy the reaction. Relative high temperatures (50° C.) have no effect; only at 60° is there some diminution, and 80° destroys the action. Even direct sunlight does not affect it (Achard). These agglutinative are not identical with the bactericidal substances: often the pure serum from a typhoid patient, which possesses high agglutinative power, has no effect on the vitality of the bacillus. Neither has it any attenuating action. The bactericidal, attenuating, immunizing, and agglutinative properties of sera, although generally present at the same time, because they are derived from the same cause, are, however, mutually independent.

Examination of 26 different varieties of bacilli showed but faint and unimportant differences in agglutinative power. This result is somewhat different from that of some other investigators.

As to the **time of appearance of the reaction,** it is generally on the 7th day; it may, however, appear much earlier or much later. They have seen it on the 5th day. Its precocity bears no relation to the intensity of the infection. Injection of agglutinative serum into another animal produces agglutinative serum in it. As in immunity, this passively acquired agglutination is very transient. By repeated inoculations they obtained a serum which possessed the reaction to a high degree—an ass's blood that reacted in 1 : 43,000 dilution. The agglutinative property is generally lost during the first weeks of convalescence. The possibility of this gives us further proof that it is a reaction of infection (?). It may, however, last for years. It may occur in cases of typhoid without fever or other typhoid symptoms.

We quote at some length, in regard to the **specificity of the reaction,** the opinion of the author: "When, under the influence of an infection, the serum of an animal agglutinates the infecting microbe, this agglutinating action thus acquired, or exaggerated if absent a few days before, is specific for that microbe, in the rigorous acceptation of the term." If such serum is added to microbes which belong to the same family group, there is also a reaction, but to a less degree and proportionate one might say to the degree of relationship. "Again, passing from theory to practice, the bacteriologist in employing the reaction for purposes of diagnosis must recognize that this action is not limited to the infecting microbe—that it can occur, but in different degree with related species."

The following **technic** is proposed. Small glass pipets are prepared which give drops of equal size. With these the serum- and bouillon-cultures of the bacillus are mixed in the required proportions. A preliminary examination is made with a dilution of 1 : 10. If a reaction occurs, further dilutions of 1 : 50 and 1 : 100 are taken. If 1 : 50 does not give the reaction, then the serum is diluted 1 : 40, 1 : 30, etc.; or if it is negative only with 1 : 100, then 1 : 60, 1 : 70, 1 : 80, etc. In this way even higher dilutions may be made until the limit of reaction is obtained. The time that a specimen should be observed is given at two hours.

Widal, in following out these methods, examined some 500 cases. Among these were 162 cases of typhoid, in which he obtained universally positive reactions. In no case of the whole 500 did he make an error in the diagnosis.

The **conclusions** the author draws are as follows :

1. The agglutinative action is a phenomenon of infection. It makes its appearance during the first days of the disease, but may be retarded or even (rarely, however) absent.

2. It is not a vital reaction of the microbes.

3. A negative reaction furnishes a probability against the diagnosis of typhoid fever, but it is only a probability. This is especially the case when the test is made during the early days of the disease : the examination should always be repeated during the following days.

4. A positive reaction, obtained by following the rules laid down, should be considered as a sign of certitude of typhoid fever.

[From the foregoing it may be seen that the test of agglutination and loss of motility of the microbe of typhoid fever occasioned by the addition of a certain quantity of the serum of a typhoid patient is a most important addition to our means of diagnosis. The most important articles have been given in abstract. It is impossible to quote all of the cases that have been reported. About 4000 typhoids and nontyphoids have been examined, with successful results in 96%. To eliminate as far as possible the negative results a most careful technic must be acquired. Lack of this is a most frequent source of error. A reaction with a 1 : 10 dilution does not indicate typhoid fever, and the absolute limit of the reaction must be obtained by repeated dilutions. The value of pseudoagglutinations and of partial reactions must be appreciated, and must not be mistaken for the complete positive reaction. The lack of a careful clinical diagnosis is possibly the cause of the low percentage of positive reactions obtained by workers in the various boards of health. Typhoid infection must be absolutely eliminated by a bacteriologic examination, even when at the autopsy there are no gross lesions of typhoid present. The importance of this is manifested in the cases described by Pick, by Guinon and Meunier, and by Du Mesnil de Rochemont. Those of the last named lose their value as evidence when we consider that no bacteriologic examination is reported as having been made. The presence of typhoid fever may be masked by other pathologic conditions, especially by tuberculosis. The absence or retarded appearance of the reaction during the first days, or even weeks, of the disease should be remembered, and that a previous attack of typhoid may cause a reaction that can lead one into error. If the rules as laid down by Widal be carefully followed, those contradictory results which even now are exceptional will be reduced to a minimum.]

[The following experiments, although made with the **cholera microbe,** bear such a close relation to the Widal reaction that it has been thought best to mention them at this place :]

Taurelli Salimbeni[1] criticises Gruber's assertion that the destruction of microbes *in vitro* or in the body of actively or passively immune animals is produced by the combined action of the alexins and agglutinin—that the agglutinin modifies the cell-membrane and permits the penetration of the alexins. Pfeiffer, and also Bordet, hold that this is entirely hypothetical, and that there is no alteration of the agglutinated microbes toward stains or in the fresh state. They used the serum of an immune horse, of which $\frac{1}{25}$ mg. will

[1] Ann. de l'Inst. Pasteur, Mar. 3, 1897.

protect a guinea-pig against a surely fatal dose of virulent cholera vibrio : $\frac{1}{20}$ mg. of this will give a reaction *in vitro* in 1 hour with $\frac{1}{10}$ of a 24-hour culture of the vibrio diluted in 1 c.c. physiologic salt solution. With the same emulsion $\frac{1}{30}$ mg. reacts in 24 hours. If 5 minutes after the subcutaneous injection of the culture into a guinea-pig a drop is removed and examined, there is seen a certain amount of immobilization, but no agglutination ; but in the course of 2–6 minutes the reaction takes place *in vitro*. Examination of the exudate withdrawn 15–20 minutes after inoculation shows no preexistent agglutination. They therefore hold that the phenomenon of agglutination does not occur in the subcutaneous tissue of horses and goats immunized against the cholera vibrio. Guinea-pigs were injected with immunizing serum, and 12 hours after with more than a fatal dose of cholera culture. Peritoneal lymph and blood of this animal gave the characteristic reaction *in vitro*. Immediate examination of the peritoneal fluid 2 minutes after injection showed most of the microbes immobile, but free and isolated, agglutination occurring under the microscope in 2–3 minutes at most. After 10–15 minutes in the peritoneum the vibriones are seen to be granulated (Pfeiffer's phenomenon), but retain their form and are perfectly free. The agglutination becomes slower in proportion as the Pfeiffer's granulations increase. After a time the exudate contains but a few masses of granules and some rare leukocytes. On sacrificing the animal it is easy to determine a coagulation of the exudate, which contains the microbes and is deposited upon the peritoneum. The phenomenon of agglutination does not occur when the microbes are injected subcutaneously or intraperitoneally into actively or passively immune animals. Agglutination, at least of the cholera vibrio, is a phenomenon that is produced exclusively outside of the organism.

[A definite reply to the above hypothesis put forth by Grüber is at present impossible. For Bordet's idea that the reaction is purely physical, there is not sufficient proof. Grüber's assertion, on the other hand, is at variance with certain morphologic and biologic considerations.]

The following table has been collated from the preceding abstracts and a number of other tables. No attempt has been made to eliminate doubtful results, nor does it contain all of the great number of cases that have found their way into the literature of the past year. It includes, however, many results that we look upon as erroneous, due either to ignorance of the diagnosis or to imperfect technic. Yet, in spite of these defects, it demonstrates very conclusively the great diagnostic value of the reaction :

Table of Results of the Widal Test.[1]

		Typhoid		Nontyphoid.	
		Positive.	Negative.	Positive.	Negative.
Dieulafoy	Sem. méd., p. 266, 1896	2			
Rendu	Bull. de la Soc. méd des Hôp., July 9, 1896	. .	.	.	1
Achard		3	. .	.	3
Lemoine	Bull. de la Soc. méd. des Hôp, July 24, 1896	4	. .		7
Menetrier	Ibid.	2	. .	.	1
Siredey		1			
Courmont	Sem. méd., Aug. 29, 1896	167	. .	1	72
Chantemesse		11			
Catrin	Bull. de la Soc. méd. des Hôp., Oct. 16, 1896	36	. .	12	19
Greene	Med. Rec., Nov. 14, 1896	27	. .	.	33
Jemma		12	. .	.	15
Vedel		6			

[1] The review of the literature of the Widal test and the accompanying table were prepared by Dr. Samuel S. Kneass, to whom we desire to express our thanks in this place.

Table of Results of the Widal Test.—Continued.

		Typhoid		Nontyphoid	
		Positive	Negative	Positive	Negative
Thiroloix		21	. .	. .	28
Charrin and Apert		1			
Stern		16	. .	. .	70
Haushalter		45	. .	. .	12
Achard and Bensaud		1	. .	. .	6
Pugliesi		33	. .	. .	6
Villiez and Battle		6	. .	1[1]	2
Thoinot and Cavasse		1			
Johnston and McTaggert		123	6	.	14
Durham	Lancet, Dec. 12, 1896	6	4	.	1
Pfuhl		8	.	.	2
Haedke		20	.	.	20
Pick		23	.	.	9
Mossé and Daunic		1			
Du Mesnil de Rochemont		6			
Beco	Bull. de l'Acad. Roy. de Méd. de Belge, 1896	11	5		
Jez					
Thiercelin and Lenoble		1			
Delepine		25	.	.	10
Uhlman and Woehnert	N. Y. Med. Jour., Feb. 20, 1897	18	.	.	5
Dupaquier and Pothier	New Orl. M. and S. Jour., Feb. 9, 1897	14	.	.	3
Gehrmann	Chicago Med. Rec., May, 1897	129	5	.	50
Breuer		43	.	.	27
Kühnau		11			
Appel and Thornbury		50			
Mackenzie	Canadian Pract., Dec.,1896	57	4	.	21
Cabot	Boston M. and S. Jour., Feb. 4, 1897	70	1	.	89
C. Fränkel	Deutsch. med. Woch., Nos. 3 and 16, 1896	65	2	.	28
Scheffer		2			
Craig	N. Y. Med. Jour., Feb. 6, 1897	7	1	.	18
Siegert		2			
Ziemke	Deutsch. med. Woch., No. 15, Apr. 8, 1897	6	. .	6	22
Guinon and Meunier		1			
Theolin and Mills	La Clinique, Aug. 9 and Sept. 8, 1896	12			
Sabrazes and Hugon	Sem. méd., Jan.16, 1897	13	3	.	6
Coleman	Lancet, Jan. 16, 1897	11			
Dempsey	Ibid.	12	2		
Wright	Ibid.	15			
Ellsberg	Med. Rec., Feb. 6 and Mar. 27, 1897	261	1		
Lefevre	Ibid., Feb. 6,1897	15			
Wynkoop	Med. News, Mar. 6, 1897	99	5	.	54
Aaser	Jour. Am. Med. Assoc., Apr. 24, 1897	96	.	.	54
Shattuck	Med. Rec., May 8, 1897	124	1		
Abbot	Ibid.	66	2	.	47
Kolle	Deutsch. med. Woch., No. 9, 1897	2			
Cordt	Münch. med. Woch., No. 13, 1897	10	1		
E. Fränkel	Ibid., No. 5, 1897	7	1	.	1
Widal		162	1	.	340
Block	Jour. Am. Med. Assoc., July 3,1897	46	3		
Guerard	Ibid.	129	44	.	98
Kneass	Ibid.	59	3[2]	.	41
Braunau	N. Y. Med. Jour., Mar. 27, 1897	18	2	1	130
Grünbaum		8			
Thomas	Med. News, Apr. 3, 1897	24	4		
		2283	109	22	1365

Reactions in typhoid cases in   95.5%.
No reactions in nontyphoid cases in 98.4 "
Correct results in   96.5 "

Jez[3] divides the diseases in which **Ehrlich's diazo-reaction** occurs into
3 groups—those in which it occurs constantly, those in which it occurs occa-

[1] "Typhomalaria."   [2] Two were convalescents.   [3] Wien. klin. Woch., Dec. 19, 1896.

sionally, and those in which it has never been obtained. According to his experience, the 1st group contains only typhoid fever and miliary tuberculosis; the 2d, especially pneumonia and pulmonary tuberculosis; and the last, acute articular rheumatism, malaria, epidemic cerebro-spinal meningitis, erysipelas, and perityphlitis. The test, therefore, has a negative diagnostic value. The author claims that it is also an aid to the prognosis. If found on the 1st, 2d, or 3d days, or if it disappears by the end of the 2d or 3d week, the prognosis is favorable. If constant to the end of the 4th week, it is more uncertain and relapse likely. The sudden disappearance of the reaction should lead to the suspicion of some complication, as pneumonia. He holds that it depends upon the presence of a toxin. Courmont[1] performed a number of experiments by the **method of Elsner** in order to determine its value for detecting the presence of the typhoid bacillus in the feces, and found that, although the differences in growth were very distinct in this culture-media, nevertheless they were not absolute, and often disappeared, particularly in cultures from typhoid patients, where the bacillus coli frequently assumes a typhoid aspect. In 9 cases of typhoid fever the bacillus of typhoid was only isolated twice. In 11 cases suffering from other diseases it was not found at all.

P. H. Smith[2] has investigated the occurrence of **typhoid bacilli in the urine** in cases of typhoid fever. He examined 7 cases, making 61 observations in all. His method was to implant small and large quantities of urine, obtained aseptically, upon the surface of gelatin plates. The suspicious colonies were examined by all of the ordinary methods and also by certain special tests: (1) The cilia-test; (2) The serum-test; (3) The power of forming slight acidity in milk after 24 hours. These examinations showed typhoid bacilli at some period of the disease in 3 out of 7 cases, sometimes in enormous quantities. The bacilli were never found in the 1st or 2d week (17 observations), appearing first in the 3d week or later. In 1 case they persisted until 22 days after the temperature had become normal.

Treatment.—The search for a specific **antitoxic treatment** is still pursued with vigor, though, it must be confessed, the results are unsatisfactory. Brilliant successes have been reported only to be followed by failures with the same plan. T. M. Pope[3] reports 4 cases in which antitoxic serum was used in the treatment of typhoid fever. In 2 cases the fever steadily declined after the injection, but the decline was gradual, and possibly the disease was scarcely shortened. The symptoms, however, during the 3d week were much less serious than is customary. In 2 of the cases there was an urticarial rash. E. B. Steel[4] reports a case of typhoid fever which, on the 5th day after the development of the disease, was injected with 10 c.c. of antityphoid serum. In the next 2 days there was considerable improvement; nevertheless 10 c.c. of serum were again injected, and this was repeated twice. On the 15th day of the disease the temperature was normal in the morning and evening, after which improvement steadily progressed toward an uninterrupted recovery. The diagnosis was confirmed by the Widal test. P. R. Cooper[5] reports a case of typhoid fever of exceedingly severe type, which on the 32d day was considered hopeless, and therefore injected with antityphoid serum procured from Burroughs Welcome & Co. The following morning the temperature was only 98.8°. The patient, however, began to hiccough, and was apparently in a desperate condition, when renewed injections of serum were given, with immediate and permanent improvement.

[1] Compt. rend. de la Soc. de Biol., July 3, 1896.   [2] Brit. Med. Jour., Feb. 13, 1897.
[3] Ibid., p. 259, 1897.   [4] Ibid., Apr. 17, 1897.
                        [5] Ibid., Feb. 27, 1897.

Pollak[1] reports the results of experiments upon 18 cases of typhoid fever into which the **blood-serum** of patients convalescent from the disease was injected in quantities of from 2 to 45 c.c.   In 3 very mild cases favorable action was noticed, and the fever disappeared permanently after numerous injections; but, as a rule, there was sudden rise of temperature immediately after the injection and no subsequent improvement.   In 1 case, indeed, collapse occurred after this post-injection hyperpyrexia.   In nearly all cases leukocytosis developed in the course of the treatment.

Weispecker[2] reports the result of the treatment of typhoid fever, scarlet fever, and pneumonia, with the serum of patients convalescent from these diseases; 2 cases of typhoid fever showed rapid reduction of temperature and disappearance of all the characteristic symptoms.   Cure seemed to be complete within 48 hours, although in the first case the injection was made upon the 9th day, and in the second on the 8th day.

Pfeiffer and Kolle[3] injected 3 persons with an attenuated culture of typhoid bacillus.   Within 2 or 3 hours after the injections the subjects had chills, dizziness, malaise, and pain in the site of the punctures.   In the evening the temperature reached $38\frac{1}{2}°$ C.   All the disagreeable symptoms rapidly subsided, and 11 days later the blood contained specific bactericidal substances that had not been found in it previously.   The authors believe that this method is practically applicable for the **immunization** of large numbers of persons, such as troops, or the inhabitants of neighborhoods where the disease has become epidemic.

C. H. Richmond[4] reports 9 cases of typhoid fever treated with **salol,** the average duration being $12\frac{1}{2}$ days.

[The **purgative** treatment appears to be diminishing in popularity, but a few advocates are still found.]   W. B. Thistle[5] advocates the treatment of typhoid fever with **calomel** and **salines,** believing that it sweeps the intestines clear of bacilli and counteracts the augmentation of toxins in the body.   T. B. Heimstreet[6] recommends the protiodid of **mercury** in $\frac{1}{5}$ gr. pills for typhoid fever, and reports a case that he was able to abort by this treatment.   J. E. Woodbridge[7] reports 4 cases of typhoid fever treated according to **the Woodbridge method** in the Bellevue Hospital, all of which were apparently aborted.

The Cold-water Treatment.—Robin[8] has investigated the respiratory exchange taking place in health and in typhoid fever.   These studies show that the processes of oxidation are decidedly reduced during the course of this disease, the reduction depending upon the severity of the case.   He then investigated the effect of cold baths upon the oxidation, and found that there was a distinct increase in the exchange of gases and in the whole process.   This was commensurate with the reduction brought about in the temperature, and he found that when the latter was not reduced the beneficial effect of the bath upon the chemical processes was also wanting.   He holds, therefore, that the occurrence or nonoccurrence of decline of temperature may be taken as a standard by which the usefulness or uselessness of bathing may be measured.   The beneficial effects of bathing, he believes, are due to this increase of oxidation, whereby the toxic products of the tissue-destruction are reduced to harmless excrementory bodies.   This effect is accomplished by the intermediation of the nervous system.   [Clinicians have long been aware that the bath-treatment

[1] Zeit. f. Heilk., Bd. 17, Heft 5, No. 6.
[2] Zeit. f. klin. Med, Bd. 32, II. 1 and 2.
[3] Deutsch. med. Woch., 1896, No. 46.
[4] Buffalo Med. Jour., Mar., 1897.
[5] Med. Rec., Oct., 1896.
[6] Jour. Am. Med. Assoc., Apr. 17, 1897.
[7] Med. Rec., Jan. 16, 1897.
[8] Bull. de l'Acad. de Méd., Oct. 27, 1897.

exercises a powerful effect upon the process of respiration.] Thornley[1] gives the statistics of the cases of typhoid fever admitted to the Presbyterian Hospital of New York during the 1st and 2d weeks of the disease: 47 were treated with tub-baths, 25 by sponge-baths, 58 by sponge-baths and tub-baths, and 14 without baths: the latter were very mild cases. Of the 1st group, 4.1% died and 37.5% suffered from complications or relapses; for the 2d group the figures were 11.5% and 34.6%; and for the 3d group, all prolonged and severe cases, 13.7% and 55.1%. T. E. Hare[2] reports the results of Brand's treatment in the Brisbane Hospital. From 1882–86, 1828 cases were treated expectantly, with 14.8% mortality; from 1887–96, 1902 cases were treated by baths, with 7.5% mortality. Careful examination of the causes of death shows that the percentage due to perforation and hemorrhage was little, if at all, affected by the new treatment; but the deaths from other causes were reduced from 9.07% to 3.4%. The most beneficial effects were exhibited in the female wards, where the mortality diminished from 16.02% to 5.6%.

G. E. Armstrong[3] contributes a paper upon **operative interference** in **typhoid perforation.** The author estimates that about 1 or 2% of typhoid cases are complicated by perforation, and about 6% of the mortality of the disease is due to this cause. The majority of the cases occur between the ages of 10 and 40, and more in the male than in the female sex. Regarding the recognition of the condition, the author points out that the symptoms are often obscure, though it is generally held that they are characteristic. Too much reliance should not be placed upon the disappearance of the liver-dulness, though the lessening in the dulness previously determined is significant. The symptoms somewhat resemble those of acute appendicitis, but are, as a rule, less marked. The temperature is usually lowered, but soon rises. In some cases symptoms are almost wholly absent. The author has collected 30 cases treated by operation, including some doubtful ones; there were 6 recoveries. Excluding the doubtful cases, there were 23 operations and 4 recoveries. He feels that the operations are less successful than these figures would indicate, as it is probable that many unsuccessful cases have not been published, while most of the successful ones are recorded. Five cases have recovered after incision and evacuation of local collections of pus, and 1 after aspiration of a collection of pus and gas in the cecal region. The author includes in these statistics 6 from the Montreal General Hospital, 3 of which were operated upon by himself. None of these recovered. He further refers to a case, not included in his series, the result of which was still undetermined. The perforation occurred on the 13th day in a severe case of typhoid. Pain and collapse were not marked, but there was some vomiting. Operation was performed 18 hours after the first symptoms; the perforation was found 6 inches above the ileocecal valve, and was readily closed. The patient 20 days after the operation was in good condition, passing firm stools, sleeping well, and taking nourishment freely. The abdomen was soft and painless, and the outlook favorable. Lerboulet[4] believes that in cases of perforation, occurring in the course of typhoid fever, laparotomy still offers some hopes, providing the pulse is strong and not too frequent.

A. G. Barrs[5] describes 2 cases of typhoid fever in which the use of a **freer diet** than is ordinarily permitted was followed by prompt improvement. In the 1st case the patient had been ill 8 weeks, and the temperature remained a little

[1] Med. News, Mar. 13, 1897.   [2] Intercol. Med. Jour. of Australia, Mar. 20, 1897.
[3] Brit. Med. Jour., Dec. 5, 1896.   [4] Bull. de l'Acad. de Méd., 1896, No. 43.
[5] Brit. Med. Jour., Jan. 16, 1897.

above the normal in the evenings, falling to normal in the morning. Any attempt to get the patient out of bed was followed by temperature disturbance. In the 2d case there were great weakness and diarrhea, and the patient was at about the 22d day of the disease when a freer diet was administered. There was some tendency to decline of temperature at the time, and this continued without intermission. Reasoning from these cases, the author argues for a freer diet throughout the disease, and states that of 28 cases under his own care fed in this way only 1 died, but relapse occurred in 2. [We have seen a number of instances in which persistence of the temperature during convalescence has occurred, and in which a more liberal diet has been advantageous. This is particularly true of cases in which the general vitality has been reduced, and in which the gastrointestinal tract has not suffered greatly. In these cases the temperature apparently remains elevated from weakness, impoverished blood, and other causes, more than from the persistence of local lesions. The term "bed fever" has sometimes been given to these cases. It is scarcely justifiable, however, to conclude from instances of this kind that a more liberal diet is proper throughout the course of typhoid fever.]

H. L. Williams[1] has constructed a frame with a pulley arrangement and a swinging **hammock,** to be used **for lifting typhoid patients** from the bed and lowering them into the tub-bath. The frame is so constructed that it readily rolls over the bed, and then, carrying the patient, it may be rolled over the tub. [We have seen this frame in actual service, and have found, as the author claims, that two nurses are enabled by this means to administer the bath with practically no exertion.]

Infections Resembling Typhoid Fever.—R. S. Woodson[2] reports 2 cases of febrile disease of doubtful nature occurring during the heated period in soldiers stationed in Texas. The 1st case, a man of muscular development and gouty diathesis, exercised violently at baseball during intensely hot weather, and was much exhausted; on the following day he had general muscular soreness and fever. His temperature was 103°; his skin was dry, bowels constipated, and the urine loaded with uric acid. The disease dragged on with irregular febrile movement for 2 months, during which period the subjective sensations were excellent. There was very little emaciation. The 2d case, a man of similar physique and gouty diathesis, after playing baseball on a very hot day was very much exhausted and suffered with symptoms similar to those of the above. The temperature steadily declined, and reached the normal in about 8 days. The author regards these cases as being instances of a thermic fever in which the gouty diathesis of the patients also plays a part. He suggests the term "febris autointoxica." [It seems difficult to determine positively from the report what the nature of these cases was. It may have been typhoid in the 1st, and even in the 2d, despite the atypical symptoms. The author inveighs against the usual readiness with which "continued fevers are classed as typhoid or malarial when the nature of the cases is obscure; but in his own cases the former of these diseases is not positively excluded.]

Guirand[3] reports an epidemic that occurred in Lauraguais that resembled typhoid fever, but was peculiar in the fact that only 2 persons died out of 68 attacked, and that very frequently the symptoms of cerebrospinal meningitis were also present. As all the inhabitants obtained their water from a common reservoir situated in a depression in the village, the author made careful bacteriologic examination, but was unable to find the bacillus of Eberth. On the other hand, he discovered the coli bacillus in abundance, and also a strepto-

---

[1] Univ. Med. Mag., Sept., 1896.   [2] Jour. Am. Med. Assoc., Mar. 20, 1897.
[3] Compt. rend. de la Soc. de Biol., Feb. 19, 1897.

coccus. This was moderately virulent, killing mice but not rabbits. In addition he also obtained a diplococcus somewhat resembling the pneumococcus of Talamon-Fränkel, but differing from it in its cultural peculiarities. He believes that the peculiar character of the epidemic was due to the presence of the streptococcus.

INFLUENZA.

Lindenthal[1] reports 8 cases of **sporadic influenza** with autopsies, in all of which the diagnosis was confirmed by bacteriologic examination. From these he concludes that influenza may occur in periods when no epidemic exists, and then in no way differs from the ordinary epidemic form; also that the influenza bacillus is capable of giving rise to fibrous or serous, or even hemorrhagic, exudate in the lungs, which may become purulent—that when the sinuses communicating with the nose are inflamed it is nearly always a result of infection with the influenza bacillus.

Fränkel[2] reports some **complications and sequelæ** following influenza that he observed in an epidemic. These consisted of arhythmia, which occurred especially during convalescence, and was either associated with tachycardia or bradycardia; arterial thrombosis, of which he observed 3 cases, 1 involving the right axillary artery, 1 the right iliac, and 1 the right central artery of the retina; and angina pectoris, which occurred in a few cases.

Batz[3] also discusses the **cardiac complications** of influenza, as well as cardiac influenza, the distinction between these being that the former includes peri-, endo-, and myocarditis as distinct complications, and the latter a series of changes in the heart-action due to nervous disturbances. The cardiac rhythm is altered and the pauses become equal. The beats become accelerated, and the sounds resemble each other, so that the condition known as embryocardia is developed. Intermittence and bradycardia may occur, or, on the other hand, a high grade of tachycardia. Cardiac weakness and syncope may be noted, but angina due to influenza is of special importance. The latter resembles closely angina pectoris, and indeed is probably induced by the same conditions. The paroxysms are variable in duration, but usually last for some time. The author ascribes the variability of the cardiac conditions to the affection, in different cases, of different nervous structures (sympathetic, intracardiac ganglia, or the vagi). They may even have a bulbar origin.

Kamen[4] reports 3 cases of influenza. The first had a temperature very like that of relapsing fever, a peculiar symptom being a stiffness of the neck during each febrile period. The second suffered from severe pains in the head, but also recovered. The third presented similar symptoms, and at death a purulent leptomeningitis was found. In all 3 the diagnosis was confirmed bacteriologically.

Reverdin[5] reports a case of **multiple abscesses** after grippe. The patient, a young man of 18, had a large abscess beneath the left breast some weeks after the attack. Subsequently others appeared on the left arm and in the left gluteal region. For weeks he had suffered with pain in the right lumbar region and obstinate constipation, but no abscess was formed. Cultures developed only the streptococcus pyogenes.

G. V. I. Brown,[6] a practitioner of dentistry, urges **care of the mouth** in grippe. He refers to cases in which examination showed unhealthy conditions of the oral mucous membrane and the necks of the teeth, and ascribed the continuation of sore throat, bronchitis, etc., to this cause.

[1] Wien. klin. Woch., April 15, 1897.
[3] Thèse de Bordeaux, 1896.
[5] Revue méd. de la Suisse romaine, No. 8, 1896.
[2] Deutsch. med. Woch., Apr. 1, 1897.
[4] Wien. klin. Woch., May 22, 1897.
[6] Jour. Am. Med. Assoc., Jan. 9, 1897.

Delius and Kolle[1] have carried on a number of experiments with the influenza bacillus in order to decide whether it is possible to produce **immunity** either active or passive, or to obtain an efficient antitoxin. They conclude that a specific substance is to be found only in bodies of the microorganisms, and that neither active nor passive immunity can be produced, all their experiments having been absolutely negative. They admit, however, that it is not impossible that a brief period of immunity exists after convalescence from an attack.

CHOLERA.

E. H. Hankin[2] reports a **curious epidemic** of cholera that broke out in an officers' mess in Central India. Rigid antisepsis was employed in the kitchen, and it was difficult to ascertain the source of the infection, but it was finally traced to a chocolate pudding that had been infected either by a muslin-strainer or a dish-cloth used to carry the vessels containing boiled water, both of which had been washed in a stream in which cholera bacilli were found. F. Smith[3] reports an epidemic of cholera that broke out in Penang, and was apparently due to the **aerial transmission** of the germs from the patients in the quarantine station to others that were detained with them. [The effort to exclude transmission in other ways was not sufficiently rigorous.]

Sonsino[4] has noticed the frequency with which **intestinal lesions**, either dysenteric or parasitic, are found in persons that have died of cholera in Egypt.

Engel[5] has criticised the statement of Bachstein's in regard to the diagnostic value of **chrysoidin** in the recognition of cholera. He finds that although it produces agglomeration in vibrio cultures, the vibrio of Asiatic cholera is by no means the most sensitive, and that it is most efficient in those cultures that, through prolonged growth upon artificial media, have lost their virulence.

Treatment.—Kolle[6] carried out 3 series of experiments upon **immunization** against cholera. In the first Haffkine's method was employed; that is, a definite quantity of sterilized culture was injected; 5 days later a small dose and in 5 days more a larger dose of the living virulent culture. The second series was made with 1 injection of a freshly prepared sterilized culture, and the third with a sterile culture that had been kept 4 weeks. The results were essentially the same by all methods. The effects of the injection were swelling and pain at the site, sensitiveness of the neighboring lymph-glands, chills, fever, malaise, and anorexia. The reaction was complete in 3 days; the immunity appeared at the end of the 5th day, and reached its maximum at the end of the 20th day. It then decreased gradually, but was still quite marked at the end of the year. Kolle concludes that it is possible to prepare effective sterile cultures in large quantities at laboratories, and the protective results of the inoculation can be counted upon as lasting for a year after inoculation. He believes that he has furnished convincing proof of the effectiveness of Haffkine's method, and warmly recommends it wherever cholera is endemic or in communities that must necessarily remain isolated and exposed; as, for example, on shipboard.

A. Powell[7] summarizes the results of all of Haffkine's observations in **cholera-inoculations.** He concludes that the largest dose hitherto used

[1] Zeit. f. Hyg. u. Inf'kr., Apr. 13, 1897.   [2] Brit. Med. Jour., Dec. 26, 1896.
[3] Lancet, Jan. 30, 1897.   [4] Ibid., July 18, 1896.
[5] Centralbl. f. Bakt. u. Parasit. u. Infek., Jan. 30, 1897.
[6] Deutsch. med. Woch., Jan. 1, 1897.   [7] Lancet, July, 1896.

does not confer complete immunity, but it is quite marked if there is considerable febrile reaction, and insignificant if not.

Nakagawa[1] reports the results of the treatment of cholera with the anticholera **serum of Kitasato.** In 270 cases the total mortality was 51.1 %. Of these, 163 were treated with the serum, with a mortality of only 33 %. The cases were nearly all mild.

Chauvin[2] believes that it is impossible to secure **antisepsis in the intestinal canal.** The object of the treatment, therefore, in choleraic diseases should be to render the intestinal contents as unfavorable a culture-media for the growth of the organism as possible. This he obtains by the administration of small doses of bichlorid of mercury and a special mixture of his own, of which the essential ingredients are HCl, pepsin, and tincture of opium. He reports 23 cases treated in this manner, in some of which the vibrio of Koch had been found, without a single unfavorable result.

THE BUBONIC PLAGUE.

[The bubonic plague has been the subject, during the past year, of considerable careful scientific investigation. Viegas, Cantlie, Lowson, and the German Plague Commission have studied the epidemic at Bombay and discriminated various clinical forms; Ogata, that at Formosa, particularly from a bacteriologic standpoint. The most important advance, however, is the introduction of successful serum-therapy, for which the whole credit should undoubtedly be given to Yersin. Haffkine has experimented with preventive inoculations according to the methods he has employed for cholera, but it is as yet too early to criticise his results. Finally, it appears that Widal's method of serum-diagnosis may be applied to this disease with as much accuracy as in typhoid fever.]

Epidemics and General Considerations.—A. G. Viegas[3] discusses the outbreak of bubonic plague **in Bombay,** which he was the first to report. He does not believe that it was imported from Hong-Kong, either along with sugar and dates, by infected clothes, or by live or dead plague-stricken rats. Neither can the grain be accused, as nothing whatever suspicious was found in the granaries, and dead rats were found at least as frequently in other places. As all classes of inhabitants have been affected, it cannot be said to be due to a vegetable diet or any particular racial characteristic. Viegas' opinion is that the disease is due to, or at least favored by, the accumulation of sewerage filth. He believes that the plague-bacillus, like that of tetanus, is widely spread, and that its virulence is subject to great alterations, under favorable conditions reaching a point that renders an epidemic possible. The chief predisposing causes are a warm climate, poverty, and youth. Sex does not seem to exert any particular influence. He does not believe that the contagium frequently enters through the skin, only 5 out of the 79 cases he examined showing lacerations of any form. Personally, he thinks that it is most frequently introduced through the respiratory tract, and occasionally he has been able to trace transmission by direct contact. In the 2 cases in which the period of incubation could be determined it was exactly 5 days. He recognizes 3 varieties of the disease, the pestis minor, the pestis major, and the pestis siderans. Generally, the patient has only 1 bubo, but occasionally there are 2. The commonest seat is in the groin, although quite a number occur in the axillary region. He lays great stress upon the physiognomy of the disease, which he

---

[1] Brit. Med. Jour., July, 1896.   [2] Revue de Méd., July 10, 1896.
[3] Indian Med. Rec., Mar. 1, 1897.

describes as that of a person who has been taking hypnotics for persistent insomnia without obtaining any sleep. The eyes are red and injected, and slightly retracted. The face generally is of a bluish-yellow hue. The pulse and respiration are both rapid. In 4 cases there were petechiæ. The nervous system was usually affected between the 4th and 6th days, but there were no paralyses. Insomnia occurred occasionally, often associated with drowsiness, and coma usually developed in the later stages. Some cases had quiet delirium. The prognosis is most unfavorable, the mortality among the native patients being from 95 to 99% in the early part of the epidemic, and falling to 85% toward the end. Treatment is symptomatic, the important thing being to place the patient in favorable hygienic conditions and to commence stimulation as soon as possible. Hypnotics are of no use in combating the insomnia.

B. F. Willoughby[1] describes the epidemic of plague that commenced in Bombay on the 23d of September, 1896. He holds that it was much more severe than reported, as the European as well as the native physicians frequently, at the request of relatives, ascribed death to some other cause, usually remittent fever. Thus in December the death-rate from malaria is officially stated to have been 50 per day—an utterly incredible number. He criticises rather severely the utter lack of method employed by the authorities. He believes that the disease is endemic, the interepidemic periods being always characterized by the existence of an attenuated form called pestis minor. [The term "pestis minor" is indefinite, although well established, and apparently includes a number of totally dissimilar conditions.]

Ogata[2] reports the results of his investigation of the plague that occurred **in Formosa** in Oct., 1896. He first calls attention to the difference between the bacillus of Kitasato and the bacillus of Yersin: the 1st is found in the blood, colors by Gram's method, is motile, encapsulated, appears as irregular grayish-white colonies, and forms chains. The 2d occurs rarely in the blood, but always in the swollen lymph-glands, decolorizes by Gram's method, is not motile, forms white colonies with iridescent edges, and forms chains in bouillon-cultures. Altogether, Ogata examined 27 cases. Blood from the finger-tip, 19 to 65 days after the disease, failed to give any cultures of the bacilli, but killed mice, from whose tissues the bacilli were obtained in pure culture. In acute cases bacilli could be found in the blood both microscopically and in culture. Curiously enough, he also found in the blood of these acute cases a second microorganism resembling morphologically the pneumococcus of Fränkel, but not pathogenic for mice. In the blood of 2 cases examined post mortem the bacillus subtilis and the staphylococcus aureus were also found. In the urine and bile of 2 bodies examined after death plague-bacilli were found in great numbers. In all the cases these bacilli resembled in all respects those described by Yersin; he also examined several rats that had died of the disease, and found in their tissues pure cultures of the same organism. A very interesting observation was the fact that bouillon, in which fleas obtained from these rats had been crushed, was capable of killing mice, and from their tissues the plague-bacillus was obtained. In conclusion, he reports his results with antiseptics, to which, even in dilute solutions, the bacillus of the plague is extremely susceptible. He advises destruction of all rats and hogs that seem to be suffering from the disease, and the disinfection of all objects that come in contact with the invalids. [Two facts deserve particular attention in this valuable paper: first, the existence in the blood of convalescent and immune patients of virulent bacilli; and second, the role that suctorial insects play in

[1] Am. Jour. Med. Sci.. Mar. 27, 1897.
[2] Centralbl. f. Bakt. Parasit. u. Infek., June 24, 1897.

the distribution of the disease—a role apparently not confined to plague and filariasis.]

J. Cantlie[1] suggests that the term *malignant polyadenitis* would be more appropriate for plague. He then discusses **the varieties and spread of the plague.** Of the former he recognizes 3—fulminant, typical, and pestis minor. The latter is the form of disease that sometimes precedes or follows severe epidemics. This disease, as he has observed it, consists of a slowly developing, nonvenereal bubo, attended by general weakness, anemia, and fever. There are, however, 2 other varieties—the idiopathic enlargement of one or more glands in the necks of children, associated with fever and without sore throat or swelling of the parotid, but undoubtedly infectious; and the form that prevailed in Hong-Kong in 1893–94, in which cases of fever of typhomalarial type frequently presented a general enlargement of the lymphatic glands in the 3d or 4th week, lasting for 10 days and then subsiding. He calls this condition benign polyadenitis, and holds that it may coexist or not with malignant polyadenitis. That it is sometimes of the same nature seems to be proved by the occasional discovery of the plague-bacillus. The animals most likely to be affected are rats, and they always suffer from the disease when it is epidemic among the human race, but do not die when only pestis minor exists. The fulminant and ordinary types may undergo sudden transformation from one into the other. In regard to the contagiousness of the disease, he finds that Europeans exposed to the most concentrated forms of poison are usually unaffected. The disease is not extremely contagious, as persons attending plague-patients under favorable sanitary conditions usually escape. Ordinarily, the disease is communicated by dust from the dwellings which plague-patients have inhabited. The plague spreads slowly. It is endemic in a definite area of Asia, with its chief source in Mesopotamia and adjacent countries. The length of the incubation-period is very doubtful. It seems probable that the patients may be affected with pestis minor, and that the bacilli subsequently become more virulent and give rise to the true form of plague.

J. A. Lowson[2] recognizes **3 varieties of plague**—pestis minor, pestis major, and pestis ambulans. The first includes those cases of bubonic disease which precede an outbreak of plague proper; they are of very mild character and usually disappear in a short time. He believes that these cases are exceedingly rare, the majority being venereal in character, although some cases have been described in which the bacillus was found. Pestis ambulans is again a mild form, which occurs after the main epidemic has subsided. As in the others, a great variety of diseases may be included under this definition, 1 case of filariasis being recorded. In regard to the way in which the infection leaves the body, he recognizes 4 channels: from the pus of a suppurating bubo; by the feces; by the saliva; and occasionally, if there are renal lesions, by the urine. He is quite convinced that the bacilli are not exhaled by the breath and are not carried by the atmosphere. Infection may take place by inoculation, inspiration, or introduction into the alimentary tract. He records 3 interesting cases of the first method—1, Professor Aoyama, who scratched himself twice while performing a postmortem; another, Dr. Ishigami, Kitasato's assistant, who had inoculated himself in the same way; and the third, a woman with an open sore upon the foot, who suffered from mixed infection with plague and streptococcus.

The Plague Commission of the Imperial Academy for Sciences of Vienna,[3]

[1] Lancet, Jan. 2, 1897.   [2] Ibid., Feb. 15, 1897.
[3] Wien. klin. Woch., May 20, 1897.

in a preliminary report, gave the following results of their investigations of
the bubonic plague at Bombay : They recognize three varieties: first, the sep-
ticemic-hemorrhagic form, characterized by the development of hemorrhagic
buboes, in the neighborhood of which there is often extensive edema, and the
presence of hemorrhages in the various organs; second, the septicemic-pyemic
form, characterized by numerous metastases into the internal organs, particularly the lungs, liver, and kidneys; and third, a primary plague-pneumonia
which appears as a confluent lobular pneumonia of characteristic appearance
and usually without swelling of the lymphatic apparatus.   The contagion
usually enters through the skin, although the exact point of introduction can
only occasionally be discovered.   It may, however, get into the system either
through the tonsils or the lungs.   They have never been able to recognize a
case where it entered from the gastrointestinal tract.   The clinical course is
that of an exceedingly severe infectious disease, and often the enormous buboes
add a peculiar and characteristic appearance.   Death may occur during the
first 24 hours.   The pulse and respiration are both greatly increased, and the
former usually becomes soft and feeble.   Consciousness is sometimes preserved
until death ; in other cases there is wild delirium.   The fever is usually intermittent.   Of points that aid in diagnosis, they call attention to the invariable
absence of herpes and the rarity of cutaneous petechiæ.   The spleen is swollen
and soft, and the urine contains small quantities of nucleoalbumin.   In 2 cases
neuritis was observed as a sequel of the disease.   They regard the bacillus of
Yersin and Kitasato as the specific cause of the disease, and were able to obtain
cultures of it in many cases from the blood.   When it could be recognized
microscopically in the latter element the prognosis was exceedingly grave.
Mixed infection is frequent, among the organisms found being the streptococcus, diplococcus pneumoniæ, and the staphylococcus.   The disease is communicated either by direct contact with other patients or by contact with
infected lower animals, or by contact with objects that have conveyed the
poison from other persons.   They reserve their opinion upon the value of
serum-therapy.   Drugs have been useless.   Prophylactic measures, however,
particularly the isolation of all cases, should be rigidly enforced.

The German Plague Commission (communication from Bombay, Mar. 19,
1897)[1] has been able, as a result of a careful examination of about 100 cases,
to determine the various **routes by which the plague enters the body.**
In the great majority of cases this is unquestionably through small wounds in
the skin; the organisms often entering by several of these at the same time,
giving rise to those curious symptom-complexes in which primary glandular
swellings occur simultaneously in various parts of the body.   So long as the
glands are not penetrated by the bacillus general septicemic symptoms do not
arise.   When suppuration takes place in the glands it ordinarily produces
rapid destruction of the microorganisms, but in very light cases resolution
may occur.   When, however, the glandular filter has been passed an almost
invariably fatal septicemia develops and plague-bacilli are found in the blood
and internal organs.   It seems not likely that the contagion is transmitted by
suctorial parasites; at any rate, the mosquito does not seem to be guilty.   The
second mode of entrance is through the respiratory tract, giving rise to pneumonic areas in the lungs, where the organism is found either as a pure culture
or mixed with diplococci or streptococci.   This form is not only of itself
usually fatal, but it is also extremely dangerous for all in the neighborhood
of the patient, as the sputa contain numbers of virulent bacilli.   It does not
appear that infection ever takes place by the digestive tract.   In 2 cases, how-

---

[1] Deutsch. med. Woch., Apr. 22, 1897.

ever, it appeared that a primary infection took place through the tonsils, leading to a rapid general infection. The diagnosis of the disease cannot be made invariably by microscopical examination of the blood. Cultures develop with sufficient rapidity to be characteristic in 48 hours. It is probably dangerous to puncture a bubo in order to get material for these cultures, as by this procedure bacilli may be introduced into the general blood-current. A method that promises greater accuracy is that which corresponds exactly to Widal's reaction for typhoid fever. It can be employed in exactly the same way and gives identical results. The commission refrain, on account of insufficient clinical observation, from expressing opinion upon either Haffkine's prophylactic inoculations or Yersin's curative injections of antitoxic serum.

The German Plague Commission [1] as a result of their further observations and studies recognize the following **varieties of plague** : the bubonic form ; the pustular form, in which the primary lesion appears to be a carbuncle situated in the skin (in both of these varieties the swollen glands may undergo resolution or suppuration, with or without development of general septicemia) ; the true septicemic form, commencing with high fever, delirium, and collapse ; and the pneumonic form, commencing with chill, rapidly increasing dulness in one or more lobes of the lung, and serous, white, or rusty sputum, to be distinguished from croupous pneumonia by the extreme prostration and a considerably enlarged spleen. Besides these, there is a milder form with fever lasting a day and swelling of one or more glands. Among the peculiar complications they mention an inflammation of the cornea, which usually leads to iridocyclitis or even complete suppuration of the eye, and the appearance of a pustular eruption, with sometimes the formation of multiple abscesses. The prognosis they regard as unfavorable. The septicemic form is invariably fatal ; the pneumonic form in the great majority of cases, for even after apparent crisis death may occur from vasomotor paralysis, cachexia, or septicemia ; but, on the other hand, patients apparently moribund or even dead may recover. The treatment is purely symptomatic. Among the pathologic lesions they mention the number of bacilli found in the lungs in the pneumonic form, and the presence of necrotic foci in the liver, and packing of the lymphatic tissues with bacilli in the septicemic form. The organism is very easily destroyed.

Patrick Manson [2] states that the bubonic plague occurs in the lower animals ; assumes two forms, benign and malignant ; is caused by microorganisms, the virulence of which is susceptible to great modification ; and can be both prevented and cured by practical serum-therapy.

Drasche [3] calls attention to the fact that the present type of bubonic plague differs from those types that are recorded in history by the fact that it shows no tendency to become endemic.

Waters,[4] in discussing the **etiology** of the plague, rejects the theory that it is distributed by insects or rodents. He believes that its development is favored by a certain emanation from fermenting grain, particularly the different varieties of millet, because the disease was only found among persons using this substance. Europeans using wheat and Asiatics using rice escaped completely ; and, furthermore, whitewashing the granaries produced an immediate and notable diminution in the number of cases. In regard to the prophylaxis he suggests whitewashing of the native houses and the interdiction of the importation and the consumption of old or long-buried millet-grain. [These conclusions are very sweeping in character, and it seems doubtful whether they will be sustained by further observations.]

[1] Deutsch. med. Woch., May 6, 1897.
[2] Practitioner, Jan., 1897.
[3] Wien. klin. Woch., Mar. 13, 1897.
[4] Indian Med. Rec., Feb. 15, 1897.

S. Flexner[1] gives a *résumé* of the plague literature, and calls attention to the fact that streptococci and staphylococci, as well as the specific bacillus, are frequently found in the glands.

W. Wyman[2] reports some experiments with **disinfectants** upon the plague-bacillus. Formaldehyd in solutions of less than 1 : 1000 is not effective. The most effective antiseptics appear to be corrosive sublimate and trikresol (1 % solution).

L. F. Child[3] reports a case of plague in which the only lesions found were patches of **bronchopneumonia** in the lungs. The lymphatic glands were not enlarged. The peculiar symptoms of this condition are the great prostration, out of all proportion to the amount of pulmonary tissue involved, and the yellow serous expectoration.

Zaboltony[4] has investigated the **agglutinating action** of the serum of patients suffering from the plague, and finds that it only commences to be manifest toward the end of the 2d week ; becomes more distinct and is at its maximum during the 4th week. It is most marked in the grave cases and disappears after death.

Treatment.—Yersin[5] reports the result of his experiments with the **serum-therapy** of bubonic plague. The immunizing serum was obtained by injecting a horse subcutaneously with minute portions of a virulent culture. Each injection was followed by a very powerful reaction, and the fever reached 41.5° C. ; the horse became feeble, trembled, refused to eat, and emaciated rapidly, but ultimately, when completely immunized, recovered its normal health. With the serum obtained from this horse it was possible to prevent infection in mice inoculated with virulent culture : 0.1 c.c. sufficed to produce immunity if injected 12 hours before the inoculation ; if, however, the mouse had been already inoculated, from 1 to 1.5 c.c. of serum were required to obtain a certain cure. Yersin returned to Indo-China in 1895, organized a Pasteur institute, and set about immunizing a number of horses. This required some time, but finally he obtained a supply of serum properly prepared, which was further increased by an invoice from Paris. He immediately departed for Canton, where, after some difficulty, he obtained permission to treat a young Chinaman, 18 years old, whose case was considered hopeless : 3 injections of 10 c.c. each were made at 5, 6, and 9 in the afternoon, and the next morning the patient seemed to be almost well. The temperature had fallen, lassitude and other serious symptoms had disappeared, and the swollen glands in the groin were no longer painful. Two other patients were treated with the serum at Canton after Yersin's departure, with equally good results. At Amoy he was able to make an extensive trial of the serum in the charity hospital, and so great was his success that the Chinese themselves called upon him to treat them. Altogether, 23 cases were treated. Of these, 6 were injected on the 1st day of the disease with from 20 to 30 c.c. of serum : cure occurred within 12 to 24 hours without suppuration of the buboes ; 6 were injected on the 2d day with from 30 to 50 c.c. of serum : cure occurred in 3 or 4 days without suppuration ; 4 were injected on the 3d day with from 40 to 60 c.c. of serum ; all recovered, but fever usually persisted for a day or two ; and in 2 cases there was suppuration of the buboes ; 3 were injected on the 4th day with from 20 to 50 c.c. of serum ; all recovered within 6 days ; suppuration occurred in 1 case ; 4 were injected on the 5th day with from 60 to 90 c.c. ; 2 died, and they were apparently moribund when the injection was made ; the

[1] Johns Hopkins Hosp. Rep., Sept., Oct., 1896.   [2] Am. Jour. Med. Sci , Mar , 1897.
[3] Brit. Med. Jour., May 15, 1897.   [4] Compt. rend. de la Soc. de Biol., June 4, 1897.
[5] Ann. de. l'Inst. Pasteur, Jan. 25, 1897.

other 2 recovered. Altogether, 26 cases were treated and 2 died—a mortality of 7.6 %. The average mortality is rarely less than 80 %. Yersin, although he admits that the number of cases is too small to enable him to make positive conclusions, feels sure that the rapid convalescence of the patients, so unlike the convalescence from plague, indicates that, in some way, the serum exercises a specific action. Not only had the serum that he used been kept a long time, but it is probable that none of the horses had reached the maximum degree of immunity. The only disagreeable result was a certain amount of pain at the site of injection. In view of its high protective action in the lower animals he believes that the serum should be used in the course of epidemics to protect those not yet affected. In the discussion of the nature of plague he recalls the fact that in an epidemic rats seem to be the first affected, then the larger domestic animals, and finally human beings. He therefore suspected that the microorganisms existed in the soil, and, indeed, was able to find in the earth of affected localities a bacillus similar to that of the plague, though not as virulent as that taken from the buboes.

Money Shewan [1] reports some experiments that he helped to perform at the Pasteur Institute for the purpose of producing **an antiplague serum.** The cultures were sterilized by exposure for 1 hour to 58° C., and then injected into rabbits and guinea-pigs. If only enough were employed to make the animals temporarily sick, it was found that they had acquired immunity, although this did not appear until the reaction had ceased ; the serum of these animals would protect other animals against the subcutaneous inoculation of virulent cultures.

C. B. Fitzpatrick [2] first inoculated a horse with virulent cultures of the plague-bacillus, and then, after apparent immunity had been attained, used its serum to prevent or cure **experimental inoculation** in guinea-pigs. The results were entirely successful.

Lustig and Galliotti [3] have prepared a **toxin** from agar-cultures of the bacillus of bubonic plague by dissolving the bacilli in 0.75 % solution of caustic potash, and then precipitating with ammonium sulfate or acetic acid. This precipitate gave the reactions of a nuclear proteid, was highly virulent, and when injected in less than lethal doses protected susceptible animals against the general and local manifestations of the disease.

W. M. Haffkine [4] reports the results of the **inoculation** of healthy persons with sterilized bouillon-cultures of plague-bacillus : 154 prisoners out of a total of 345 were thus inoculated. On the day of inoculation 6 cases occurred in the noninoculated and 3 in the inoculated. Subsequently, 12 cases occurred among the noninoculated, of which 6 died, and 2 among the inoculated, both of which recovered. Besides these cases, 11,362 persons from the infected areas were inoculated, of whom only 45 were attacked by the plague, 12 dying.

J. Cantlie [5] discusses the treatment of the bubonic plague, which, according to him, consists of **purgation and stimulation** from the onset ; control of the delirium and pain by hyoscin or morphin ; control of the temperature by tepid sponges and, if necessary, antipyrin. He does not believe in local treatment of the buboes before suppuration occurs, although he has observed good results to follow injections of bichlorid and potassium iodid. Camphor is recommended as a stimulant.

Prophylaxis.—Harvey [6] gives a very thorough history of the various epidemics of bubonic plague. He concludes from these and the study of the

[1] Indian Med. Rec., Nov. 1, 1896.   [2] N. Y. Med. Jour., Apr. 10, 1897.
[3] Deut. med. Woch., Apr. 8, 1897.   [4] Brit. Med. Jour., June 12, 1897.
[5] Indian Med. Rec., May 16, 1897.   [6] Ibid., Jan. 1, 1897.

Indian epidemic that it is chiefly occasioned by unsanitary habits, and that the danger may be greatly reduced by the careful isolation of the sick and effective quarantine. A. H. Doty[1] considers that the short period of incubation of plague is the greatest safeguard against its introduction into any country where the disease does not exist. The virus may, however, be transmitted by clothing, articles of merchandise, etc., and it is therefore necessary to disinfect most carefully all articles coming from a suspected point.

VACCINIA.

Kaempffer[2] records an **epidemic of cowpox** among milkmaids. The disease first appeared in a cow that had been on the farm for 2 years. It became ill without any discoverable source of infection. In a short time 60 cows out of 90 were affected, the pocks being only on the udders and forming sluggish ulcers when broken. Of 16 milkmaids, 10 acquired cowpox without regard to the length of time after revaccination. The incubation was usually from 3 to 4 days, but 9 to 10 in 2 cases. General symptoms occurred only in cases in which complications like phlegmon occurred. In 6 cases there was only 1 pock, in the others from 2 to 6. They appeared especially on the flexor side of the fingers and on the back of the hand, and ran the same course as those in vaccination, except that the time was shortened to 12 days and the cicatrices were not so deep.

W. M. Jones[3] reports a case of vaccinia that was contracted by a farmer from a cow that he was milking. The pustules developed upon the arm in localities where it had rubbed against an abdominal crust. Subsequently his father, who had had smallpox, developed a similar vaccine pustule.

C. F. Sutton[4] reports a case of **vaccination of curious type.** The child was vaccinated in March with calf's lymph. After the usual course four perfectly healed marks were left. About a month later the same spots rose again, and resembled in every way a newly vaccinated arm, and ran the usual course; after complete healing the same thing occurred a third and fourth time in June and late in July; another attack occurred in October. The child suffered no inconvenience, and was subsequently perfectly healthy.

Weber[5] has observed in several cases of **revaccination** in the Reserve Hospital at Warsaw that, instead of the typical vaccine pustules, one or more dark-red, smooth, shining nodules about the size of a pea appeared about the site of the inoculation, and finally disappeared after slow desquamation, leaving a pigmented area in the skin. In drops of blood taken from such nodules he observed amebæ varying from 10 to 16μ in diameter. These contained granules which moved slowly about in a cloudy protoplasm. Sometimes the pustules undergo suppuration, and then he has observed the siren forms that he himself had previously described. Amebæ, however, are found in the blood taken from the surrounding areas of congestion.

F. H. Payne[6] discusses the **history of vaccination,** and notes particularly the record of Chicago, where only 17 cases of smallpox have occurred in the last 15 years among the school-children, whose average number exceeds 200,000, and among whom vaccination is compulsory. C. S. Patterson[7] calls attention to the report of Surgeon Hinde of the epidemic of smallpox that broke out among the soldiers of the Congo Free State. Altogether, there were 366 sol-

[1] Am. Jour. Med. Sci., Mar., 1897.   [2] Med. Woch., No. 50, 1896.
[3] Quart. Med. Jour., Jan., 1897.   [4] Lancet, Oct. 24, 1896.
[5] Medycyna, No. 20, 1896.   [6] Pacific Med. Jour., Nov., 1896.
[7] Lancet, Oct. 24, 1896.

diers; of these, 158 had been vaccinated, and only 2 took the disease, neither of whom died. Of the 208 that had not been vaccinated, 105 took the disease, and among them the death-rate was over 76%. [Statistics such as these seem very conclusive.] Queirel[1] states that smallpox is endemic in Marseilles, because a considerable number of strangers, particularly Italians, inhabit the city and refuse all forms of vaccination. He advocates, therefore, **compulsory vaccination** of all persons.

VARIOLA.

Coste[2] reports an epidemic of smallpox that occurred at Marseilles in 1896, and was characterized by the appearance of a **secondary eruption** from 6 to 37 days after the commencement of the disease, after the pustules of the previous eruption had completely disappeared. All of the 33 cases that he observed recovered. The second eruption was usually milder than the first, and Coste holds that it is probably no reinfection, but simply a continuation of the original disease.

A. Newsholme[3] reports a case of **recurrent smallpox** that was taken to the High Gate Smallpox Hospital and there treated. The patient apparently recovered and returned to his rooms. Shortly afterward 2 charwomen employed in cleaning the rooms and living in entirely different localities contracted the disease; 3 days after his return he developed a papillary rash that subsequently became pustular.

Prophylaxis.—E. H. Sargent[4] reports an epidemic of smallpox that occurred in the Detroit House of Correction; 4 of the cases were very severe, 3 of them being confluent and hemorrhagic and terminating in death. One was partially confluent, and convalescence was retarded by an attack of furuncles. Only 1 patient had been vaccinated, and he when a child. Two other patients, both of whom had been frequently vaccinated, had the disease in a very mild form, 1 of these passing through her second attack. Two other cases, occurring in sisters, were remarkable for their virulence and the apparent susceptibility of the patients; 1 of these apparently contracted the disease at the hospital, and developed the symptoms after her return home. Her sister was then vaccinated very successfully, and whilst the vaccine pustule was still on the arm she was attacked with headache and fever, and a rash appeared over her face and body. She recovered perfectly from this affection, which was diagnosed variously as varicella and varioloid. Shortly afterward she was attacked by malignant, confluent variola, that became hemorrhagic, and from which she died. The mother of these children had been vaccinated a number of times unsuccessfully. A very severe case occurred in a man who had been successfully vaccinated $1\frac{1}{2}$ years previously. Another case occurred in a girl of 7 who had never been vaccinated successfully, and subsequently appeared in a mild form in her parents, although both had been successfully vaccinated when she was first taken ill. [Some of these cases would seem to argue against the efficiency of vaccination. It must be recalled, however, that the histories as to successful vaccinations should not be too readily accepted in persons of this class.]

Weber[5] has found in the **blood of patients** suffering from variola various round bodies, usually of high refractive index and measuring from 1.8 to 7.2 μ in diameter. There were also certain siren forms enclosed in the blood-

[1] Bull. de la l'Acad. de Méd.. Oct. 20, 1896.   [2] Rev. de Méd., Dec. 10, 1896.
[3] Brit. Med. Jour., Oct. 10, 1896.   [4] The Physician and Surgeon, Sept., 1896.
[5] Medycyna, 1896, No. 14.

cells. All these forms could be stained by methylen-blue, the round bodies, however, taking that stain more deeply than the siren forms. The latter he was able to cultivate upon partially solidified alkaline agar. They have been found, however, in other diseases, such as measles and scarlet fever ; in variola they appeared to increase toward the period of suppuration, and at the same time to grow larger, sometimes attaining the diameter of 15 μ. They resemble esinophile-cells very closely, and can only be distinguished from them by the rapid movements of the granulations. [It appears to be so easy to find peculiar bodies in the blood and tissues of various diseased conditions that all such descriptions must be regarded with a certain degree of conservatism ; the author, however, makes no claims for the pathogenicity of those he found.]

V. During[1] gives the statistics of the **mortality** from smallpox in Constantinople for the last 10 years. The deaths range from 659 in 1887 to 30 in 1889. Vaccination is not obligatory, and he explains the great variations by supposing that in times of epidemic all the children have the disease, and it requires a certain length of time for the births to increase the number of the susceptible population until the epidemic can again break out.

Treatment.—Bryan[2] reports a case of discrete smallpox to which he applied his method of **sterilization of the epidermis.** This consists of careful scrubbing with a strong alkaline soap, washing in alcohol, and the subsequent application of some mild antiseptic. The parts treated were only the forearms. No pustules developed here, whereas on the other parts of the body the vesicles became pustules and left pits.

F. S. Furman[3] has treated 2 cases of discrete smallpox according to **Bryan's method** for arrest in the vesicular stage. He carefully sterilized the surface, and then, having opened each vesicle, touched its interior with carbolic acid. Only a few pustules appeared, the vesicles drying up without the formation of a pit. Casrellvi,[4] in order **to prevent pitting** after smallpox, recommends the spraying of the face with a solution of corrosive sublimate in alcohol and ether, and subsequently painting the face with sublimate of glycerin.

J. F. O'Leary[5] reports 53 cases of smallpox treated with **muriate of cocain.** There were 11 deaths, 6 of the patients suffering severe complications. All the others recovered, and had very satisfactory convalescences. The dose was usually $\frac{1}{4}$ of a grain every 4 hours.

SUNDRY INFREQUENT INFECTIONS.

Relapsing Fever.—Tictin,[6] having had occasion to observe an epidemic of relapsing fever in Odessa in which 10,000 cases occurred, was struck by the fact that it seemed to originate in the small inns near the wharves. It occurred to him, therefore, that the **medium of transmission** might possibly be **through suctorial insects.** In order to test his theory he allowed hungry bedbugs to bite a monkey that had the spirilli in his blood, and then examined the blood that was obtained by crushing them. In this he found organisms that were active for some time ; he then collected the blood from the bedbugs, and with it injected another monkey, which rapidly developed the disease. He suggests that infection might take place directly from the bedbugs in 2 ways : either from the proboscis of a parasite that had fed upon the patients in whose blood the spirilli were present, or as a result of scratching the skin where one of these animals had been killed.

[1] Deutsch. med. Woch., 1897, No. 15.   [2] Med. Rec., July 8, 1896.
[3] Ibid , Sept. 5, 1897.   [4] Gac. Med. Cat., Dec. 15, 1896.
[5] New Orleans M. & S. Jour., June 1, 1897.
[6] Centralbl f. Bakt. Parasit. u. Infek., Feb. 15, 1897.

Gabritchewsky [1] has carefully examined the blood of monkeys and human beings affected with recurrent fever, and finds that as the crisis approaches it becomes possessed of marked bactericidal power. He finds that the spirilli will live in normal blood for 160 hours at a temperature of 37°. In the blood of a person who has just passed through a crisis they die often within an hour at this temperature. These facts led him to experiment whether it would be possible or not to treat the disease with the **serum of monkeys** that had been cured of it, and in which a considerable degree of bactericidal power had been found. In a single experiment he found it was possible by injecting such serum to limit the pyrexial period to 2 days and to avoid absolutely the relapse. Metchnikoff in the same journal criticises the theoretic consideration upon which this treatment is based, but admits the partial bactericidal action of such serum.

Mamurowski [2] reports a case of **relapsing fever in a pregnant woman** who aborted in the 4th month. In the blood of the fetus numerous spirilli were found.

Typhus Fever.—Lewaschew [3] has found in the venous blood of patients suffering from typhus fever small bodies from 2 to 5μ in diameter, occasionally with a long cilium. These grow on human ascitic fluid and form small grayish-white colonies. No details are given concerning the differential staining, nor records of any attempt to test the virulence of the organism in lower animals.

Spillman [4] reports **an epidemic of typhus fever** that occurred in Nancy in 1893. The disease was remarkable for its fatality (5 of 9 cases dying) and for the nervous and secondary complications. The former consisted of abolition of the reflexes, paresis or ataxia of the lower limbs, anesthesia, and trophic disturbances. The latter were divided into 2 groups, local and general. The former consisted of otitis media, bronchopneumonia, and suppurative parotiditis. The general infection was septicemia, resulting from a local lesion. The toxicity of the urine was diminished. Bacteriologic investigations were largely negative, although in many of the secondary lesions the staphylococcus anreus was found. At the autopsies the spleen and liver were found to be enlarged ; there were acute parenchymatous nephritis and changes in the central nervous system.

Yellow Fever.—Havelburg [5] has carefully studied the **pathology and bacteriology of yellow fever.** He found that in the liver there were considerable fatty degeneration and some areas of necrosis. In the kidneys he found marked parenchymatous degeneration of the epithelium of the renal tubules. The spleen showed no alteration ; the mucous membrane of the gastrointestinal tract was pale, rather thin, congested, and blood was found in the lumen. Occasionally the lymphatic follicles were swollen. Cultures were made from nearly all the organs, and all the known staining-methods employed in order to determine the presence of microorganisms. In the contents of the intestinal tract he finally found very constantly a certain bacillus pathologie for guinea-pigs, and very similar to the bacillus coli communis ; but it could be distinguished from it by its peculiar action upon guinea-pigs, causing death in from 8 to 24 hours. Its characteristics are as follows : its size is $1 \times 0.3\mu$; it is straight, usually isolated, and more distinct at the poles. It is apparently motile. On a gelatin plate the growth appears as a fine white point at the end of 24 hours ; 2 days later it is somewhat larger and shows a

[1] Ann. de l'Inst. Pasteur, Nov. 25, 1896.   [2] Medicin. Obosrebje, 1896, No. 20.
[3] Arch. des Sci. Biol., 1896, No. 4.   [4] Rev. de Méd., Aug. 10, 1896.
[5] Berlin. klin. Woch., June 7, 1897.

yellowish discoloration. It renders bouillon turbid, ferments sugar solutions, and coagulates milk. Injected into guinea-pigs, it causes lesions not unlike those found in yellow fever. Although he did not obtain a reaction with it similar to the Widal reaction of typhoid fever, he concluded that this was the specific germ of the disease, and, furthermore, that the prospects for effective serum-therapy are very promising, because injections of the blood of yellow-fever patients into guinea-pigs protected them against its pathogenic action.

J. Sanarelli [1] has studied the pathology of yellow fever with especial reference to the **bacteriology.** He summarizes the morbid anatomy as follows : hyperemia, infiltration and even hemorrhage of the serous membranes, fatty degeneration of the organs, catarrhal inflammation of the mucous membranes, enlargement of the lymphatic structures, moderate disintegration of the red blood-cells, and the presence of urea in the blood. He made cultures in a number of cases from the blood antemortem, from the organs postmortem. In the second case he was able to isolate a peculiar bacillus that he designates as the **bacillus icteroidis,** and obtained the same organism repeatedly in subsequent cases. It has the following characteristics: it is from 2 to 4μ long, motile and ciliated; it decolorizes by Gram's method, and grows readily at room-temperature upon the ordinary media. Under certain circumstances the growth is sufficiently peculiar to render it possible to make a diagnosis within 24 hours. This occurs when an agar-culture is kept at 37° for several hours and then at room-temperature, when the colonies will be found to have raised edges and a depressed center, or, if the process be reversed, depressed edges and a raised center. Occasionally some difficulty may be caused by the tendency of the bacillus to pleomorphism. This microorganism is pathogenic for most of the lower animals, giving rise to a disease with characteristic stages, and causing fatty degeneration in the organs, especially in the liver and kidneys. In human beings it is often associated with other microorganisms, giving rise to abnormal clinical types of the disease. When inoculated it may cause an intoxication due to the development of a toxin, and this is especially apt to be the ease in the lower animals when the infection takes place through the respiratory tract; in these cases it is usually found in relatively pure cultures throughout the body; or there may be a condition of septicemia due to mixed infection, in which case only other microorganisms are found; or death may be due to uremia, the tissues giving no cultures and the proportion of urea in the blood being greatly increased. This bacillus appears to have 3 specific properties—emetic, hemorrhagic, and steatogenic, the two former giving rise to the black vomit, and the latter to the icterus. [It is to be regretted that Sanarelli has not described experiments for the production of immunity in this paper; although it is stated that the serum of the one animal that survived inoculation (a dog) possessed some slight protective powers. Reasoning from analogy, there would seem to be few diseases more adapted both to inoculation and to serum-therapy than yellow fever. It is unfortunate also that he has not tried the Widal reaction, for it would add much to the presumptive evidence in favor of the specific pathogenicity of the bacillus icteroïdis.]

Malta Fever.—M. L. Hughes [2] suggests the term **febris undulans** for the disease variously known as Malta fever, pseudotyphus, etc. It is a specific endemic and sometimes epidemic malady of long duration, and is marked by characteristic undulations in the fever. Constipation, neuralgic pains, swelling of the joints, and profuse sweating are frequent symptoms. The lesions of

[1] Ann. de l'Inst. Pasteur, June, 1897.   [2] Lancet, July 25, 1896.

typhoid fever are absent. Wright and Smith[1] treat of the **diagnosis** between cases **of typhoid, Malta fever, malarial fever,** and other varieties of continued fevers. The means at our disposal are the examination of the blood in malaria; of the stools in typhoid and possibly Malta fever; and, lastly, the sero-diagnosis in typhoid and Malta fever, using a modification of the first method of Widal. Eight cases of Malta fever gave positive reactions with dilutions of 1 : 10 and 1 : 25; 1 with as high as 1 : 1000; 15 eases, diagnosed as typhoid, gave a positive reaction with a 1 : 25 dilution; 3 cases, diagnosed as typhoid, were negative with the typhoid culture, but gave a reaction with the microbe of Malta fever; 1 case, supposed to be Malta fever, was negative with the organism of that disease, but reacted with that of typhoid fever; 3 cases, supposed to be malaria, reacted with the Malta-fever organism. Finally, 14 cases, diagnosed as typhoid fever, were without result on either the typhoid or Malta-fever microbe. [These results show the importance of this test in distinguishing between certain tropical and subtropical febrile conditions. They also strengthen the assertion of Bruce that his micrococcus Melitensis is the true cause of Malta fever.]

A. E. Wright[2] has tested the blood of 10 soldiers invalided home from India for the **reaction with the micrococcus Melitensis.** In 7 cases agglutination occurred in a proportion of 1 to 150 or 300; in 2 cases in a proportion of 1 to 1000; and in 1 case in a proportion of 1 to 10, although in this case higher dilutions were not tried. Only 6 of these patients had previously served in the Mediterranean, and only 1 had fever whilst on this service. Wright therefore believes that Malta fever is endemic in India. [It is not unlikely that the disease is even more widely distributed.]

G. E. MacLeod[3] reports a case of rapidly fatal **purpura hæmorrhagica** that followed an attack of Malta fever. [It does not appear, however, that the diagnosis was confirmed by bacteriologic examination.]

Foot-and-mouth Disease.—Bussinius and Siegel[4] in the blood and tissues of a patient who died, apparently, of foot-and-mouth disease found, among various other microorganisms, a small oval bacillus that was pathologic for animals. The results, however, were not entirely satisfactory until they were able to obtain the same microorganism in the saliva and fluid from pustules in the mouths of 3 children suffering from the same disease. With this saliva they inoculated a calf, some chickens, a cat, sheep, and dog. Of these, the calf became affected apparently with typical foot-and-mouth disease, and from its blood the same oval bacillus was obtained in pure culture. Later they were able to study 2 epidemics of foot-and-mouth disease in cattle, and again found the same bacillus. Subsequently, with the material thus obtained, they inoculated 3 calves and a young pig, all of which became diseased and were certified as suffering from foot-and-mouth disease by a qualified veterinarian. The authors therefore believe that they have discovered the common cause of foot-and-mouth disease in man and the lower animals, but reserve their description of its morphologic and biologic characteristics for a later paper.

Cerebrospinal Fever.—Diagnosis.—Heubner[5] has recently demonstrated the meningococcus intracellularis of Weichselbaum during life in several cases of meningitis. The organism was found in the liquid obtained by puncture of the spinal membranes. The specific properties were demonstrated by the action of the cultures upon goats, rabbits and guinea-pigs being immune.

---

[1] Lancet, Mar. 6, 1897. [2] Brit. Med. Jour., Apr 10, 1897.
[3] Lancet, May 22, 1897. [4] Deutsch. med. Woch., Feb. 4, 1897.
[5] Ibid., No. 27, 1896.

The inoculations were made into the spinal canal, and showed that the organism is of lesser virulence than the pneumococcus. Jemma[1] describes a case of meningitis in which the microscopic examination and cultures showed the presence of diplococci (regarded as pneumococci by the author) in the liquid obtained by spinal puncture. Fürbringer[2] describes an instance of meningitis in which a diplococcus was demonstrated in the liquid obtained by spinal puncture. It was probably the meningococcus. [These cases are of great interest in the differential diagnosis of cerebrospinal fever and tuberculous meningitis, and illustrate the value of puncture of the spinal membranes in diagnosis.]

Weil's Disease.—Bignone[3] reports a case in which a man, after dietetic error, had chill, acute pharyngitis, then icterus at first, with typhoid, and finally hemorrhagic symptoms. At the end of 7 days there was critical discharge, and 5 days later a typical relapse. The author concludes that the case is one of Weil's disease, and believes that the best theory of its pathogenesis is the formation of a toxalbumin by some infectious agent that irritates the epithelium of the biliary passages and the cells of the liver.

Streptococcus Infection.—Jemma[4] reports a case of **meningitis** due to streptococci and **secondary to facial erysipelas.** He first points out that meningitis is less frequently present than is diagnosed in erysipelas; and in the cases in which meningitis is actually present other microorganisms are usually associated with the streptococcus. In his own case the patient, who had erysipelas in January, developed bronchopneumonia in February, and finally, on March 4th, symptoms of meningitis. Fluid removed by lumbar puncture 24 hours before death gave pure cultures of streptococci. The same result was obtained from the exudate on the brain and from the liquid obtained by puncture of the spleen. The examination of the blood was negative; nevertheless, Jemma believes that the meningitis resulted from infection through the circulation, and not through the lymphatics. [It is to be observed that the erysipelas had subsided more than a month previous to the development of the meningitis. This does not, however, exclude the direct etiologic relation between the two diseases.]

Two cases are reported from the Royal Infirmary of Edinburgh[5] of chronic recurrent erysipelas, 1 having lasted 12 and the other 2 years. Both were greatly improved by the use of antistreptococcic serum.

Infection with the Bacillus of Friedländer.—Brunner[6] records a case of general infection due to the bacillus of Friedländer. The patient, previously a healthy person, suffered with suppurative middle-ear disease, from which abscesses of the mastoid sinuses developed. Operation was undertaken, but suppurative meningitis with general pyemia occurred. The patient died after 14 days. Pure cultures of the bacillus of Friedländer were obtained from the pus obtained at the operation and from the various organs postmortem. Reichel[7] reports a case that commenced suddenly with fever, profound stupor, and slight meteorism. On the 3d day of his admission to the hospital and on the 17th day of the disease extreme indicanuria developed, and a thick, confluent papillary eruption appeared upon the breast and soon spread to the whole body. There was slight leukocytosis. Acetone and diacetic acids were not found in the urine, but there were slight albuminuria and considerable in-

[1] Gaz. degli Osped. e delle Clin., No. 39, 1896.
[2] Deutsch. med. Woch., No. 27, 1896.
[3] Resoconto clinico statistico degli Ospedali di Geneva, 1895.
[4] Gaz. degli Osped. e delle Clin., 1896, No. 66.
[5] Brit. Med. Jour., Feb. 27, 1897.   [6] Münch. med. Woch., Nos. 13 and 14, 1896.
[7] Wien. med. Woch., Jan. 9, 1897.

crease in the ethereal sulphates. A diagnosis was made of autointoxication from the intestinal tract, and was apparently confirmed by the autopsy, which showed parenchymatous degeneration of the kidneys, hemorrhagic cystitis, and a chronic gastrointestinal catarrh, with several transverse ulcers in the colon. Bacteriologic investigations of the intestinal contents showed that they contained a pure culture of a long, thick bacillus resembling the bacillus of Friedländer, and markedly pathogenic for guinea-pigs.

Pyocyaneus Infection.—Charrin [1] reports a curious case observed by Dr. Bardom, in which the patient, a woman of 45, could voluntarily cause a greenish liquid to issue from the breast. This, when examined bacteriologically, was found to contain the bacillus pyocyaneus.

Hydrophobia.—Kraïouchkine [2] states that in the year 1895 269 persons were treated in St. Petersburg for hydrophobia by Pasteur's method. In 2 cases the disease developed before the treatment was completed; 1 other patient died after the treatment, giving a mortality of 0.4%.

Febrile Diseases of Unknown Nature.—Ruge [3] describes a peculiar fever that occurs on the east coast of Africa and is characterized by a painful **swelling of the inguinal glands.** The course was variable. In the acute forms the fever was very high; in the more chronic forms, which lasted sometimes for months, the fever was lower or entirely absent. The temperature is not typical, but approximates the remittent type. Swelling is sometimes extreme and the local pain intense, and there is often infiltration of the periglandular tissues. In 38 cases resolution without suppuration occurred 23 times, suppuration occurred 3 times during the stage of decline, and in 12 cases early incision was necessary. The conditions must be distinguished from venereal, tubercular, leukemic, and pseudoleukemic buboes, and the bubonic plague, although the latter condition can usually be easily excluded. In regard to the etiology, it appears that it cannot be a malarial condition, as the fever disappears as soon as the glands are removed and it is not influenced by quinin. [This is probably one of the conditions that have been included among the group known collectively as pestis minor.]

D. J. Caddy [4] reports the case of a ship's captain on the west coast of Africa. The disease commenced with chills and moderate rise of temperature, apparently producing no great exhaustion and not influenced in the least by large doses of quinin. Subsequently some blood was vomited, the temperature rose to 107°, the patient became delirious, then rapidly passed into a state of collapse, and died. [It is unfortunate that a microscopic examination of the blood was not made.]

E. Way [5] describes the so-called **fish-slime disease** endemic at Cape May, which is apparently a peculiar form of septicemia resulting from punctured wounds by fish-spines.

Beri-beri.—A. Beale [6] reports an epidemic of beri-beri that broke out amongst Mohammedans of a crew of native sailors in an English ship. Altogether, 19 were attacked. The Hindoos and Christians escaped entirely. No cause was discovered for this peculiar selection, as the men lived under the same conditions and had the same diet. He divides the cases into 4 types: the incompletely developed or rudimentary form (5); the atrophic form (2); the dropsical form (6); the pernicious form (6). The first was characterized by edema of the legs and fever, some numbness of the lower extremities, and

---

[1] Compt. rend. de la Soc. de Biol., July 11, 1896.
[2] Arch. Sci. Biol. de St. Petersburg, vol. 4, No. 5.
[3] Arch. f. Dermat. u. Syph., H. 3, 1896.   [4] Lancet, May 22, 1897.
[5] Jour. Am. Med. Assoc., May 29, 1897.   [6] Indian Med. Rec., Mar., 1897.

profound anemia ; the second by anemia, edema, and fever that persisted in 1 case for 30 days ; the third type by symptoms of scurvy in addition to those before described and a subnormal temperature ; the pernicious form by an exceedingly severe anemia, violent palpitation of the heart, great anxiety, and collapse. All 6 of this pernicious form died. Ankylostoma duodenalis was suspected, but no eggs nor ova were found, and treatment by thymol had no effect.

Gibbs [1] describes a disease, endemic in the Singapore Lunatic Asylum, that he names **"pseudo-beri-beri."** It is noncontagious, prevails during the wet season, and, for the most part, in the damp, low-lying levels. Clinically, it is characterized by slight anemia and considerable soft anasarca, and a tendeney to sudden death from shock. The hygienic conditions surrounding the asylum are most unfavorable, and, on account of the fact that those most frequently affected drank well-water which contained numerous living organisms, it was supposed that this might be the cause. However, it attacks exclusively Asiatics, and continues to attack them when the water-supply is changed. The urine is normal, which serves to distinguish the disease from nephritis. Ankylostoma are not found. It can be distinguished from beri-beri by the softness of the edema and absence of spastic and paralytic conditions of the muscles and by the rapidity of recovery. The period of incubation apparently lasts from 1 to 2 days, and is characterized by malaise. There is some fever, and edema develops, commencing in the feet and spreading very rapidly. The blood contains irregular masses of pigment free and in the leukocytes ; no malarial organisms have been found. Cultures of the blood showed the presence of a bacillus forming yellowish-brown colonies, and a micrococcus forming yellow colonies. These were possibly contaminations. The treatment consists in removal to a more favorable locality and free purgation. Subsequently iron and stimulants may be of use.

Intoxications Resembling Infections.—F. W. Burton Fanning [2] describes a number (11) of cases of what he regards as **sewer-air poisoning.** He admits the difficulty of proving that these are really instances of sewer-air poisoning, but was led to believe them such from the facts that they did not correspond to any definite disease ; that they presented many features in common ; that some grave sanitary defect was found in all cases, and most of them recovered after this was removed. As to the clinical features, most of them presented fever, this, as a rule, being of the hectic type, and in 3 cases distinguished by remarkable abatement of the symptoms during the febrile remissions. Rigors were met with in 3 cases ; headache quite generally ; but pains in the limbs were more significant. Epigastric pain was found in 2 children, petechiæ on the legs occurred in 3 severe cases, and erythema annulare in 1. Of the 8 adult cases, 5 had lymphangitis on the legs or arms and glandular enlargement without wounds or local injury. In 1 case there was phlebitis ; in 2 a suspicion of endo- and pericarditis. In 3 cases the spleen was enlarged, and in 6 of 10 in which the urine was examined at the height of the disease albumin was discovered. Regarding diagnosis, he states that ulcerative endocarditis, typhoid fever, and rheumatism are most difficult to exclude. In 1 of his cases bacteriologic examination showed the presence of staphylococci and an undefined bacillus in the blood. [While there are interesting points in this paper, it furnishes no data for the solution of the question, whether or not sewer-air poisoning occurs. Other possibilities in the way of etiologic factors were not excluded.]

[1] Indian Med. Rec., Feb. 15, 1897.   [2] Lancet, Oct. 24, 1896.

A. Crawford[1] reports an epidemic of **food-poisoning** that occurred in Iowa in 1895. More than $\frac{1}{3}$ of 300 guests assembled at a wedding were affected, and there were 7 deaths. The first cases occurred 3 days after partaking of the food, and the last cases about 28 days. The symptoms were those of intense gastroenteritis or gastritis. In many there was severe pain in the limbs with tenderness in the muscles. All the patients appear to have suffered from fetid sweating. There were 2 autopsies, in both of which the liver and spleen were enlarged and soft. In 1 there was hyperemia of the cecum ; in the other, ulceration. Both of these cases were examined microscopically, and the pathologist made a diagnosis of typhoid fever. It is also stated that another pathologist made a diagnosis of trichina-poisoning from the examination of the muscles. [The symptoms certainly resembled those of trichina-poisoning more closely than those of typhoid fever, but the description of the cases is so unsatisfactory that it is difficult to draw any conclusions.]

J. Dixon Mann[2] considers the subject of **meat-poisoning,** and notes that, aside from parasitic diseases and accidental poisoning, meat may be injurious from —(a) preexistence of disease in the animal prior to its slaughter, or (b) from the invasion of microorganisms in the meat subsequent to slaughter, and (c) from the presence of toxalbumoses or ptomaïns. The symptoms may be either infectious or toxic. In the first group the characters of the disease are those of any infection, as in an instance in which the symptoms suggested typhoid fever in 600 people who had eaten from an animal killed while moribund. In the second group of cases the symptoms resemble those due to acute gastro-enteritis, among these being violent vomiting and purging, rapid loss of strength, and cramps in the legs, subnormal temperature with general cold-ness, although occasionally there is fever. The symptoms are variable accord-ing to the form of poison, and sometimes also in different persons poisoned with the same meat. The latter fact may be explained by the unequal distribution of the poison in the meat or by the fugitive nature of the poison. Prolonged cooking does not necessarily render the poisons harmless, as many of these resist heat. Sometimes the flesh of animals having some form of infection is not toxic immediately after slaughter, but becomes so when kept, and the flesh of healthy animals may readily become contaminated by various microorgan-isms when it is kept.

Van Ernengen[3] reports investigation of some **sausage and smoked beef** that had produced severe symptoms similar to those of cholera nostras in a number of persons. Portions of these submitted to a skilled investigator appeared so tempting that, in common with several of his assistants, he par-took of them, and soon developed symptoms of violent enteritis and nephritis, leading to death in 6 days. At the autopsy there were found gastroenteritis, acute nephritis, and fatty degeneration of the liver. In the feces and tissues a peculiar bacillus was found, morphologically and culturally similar to the bacillus enteritidis of Gärtner, and the same organism was found in the meat. It remains to be shown whether the flesh of the animal from which the sausage had been made was diseased or not, or whether the sausage had been subse-quently infected.

Hick[4] holds that the disposition to **autointoxication** consists of a pecu-liar reaction of a special organism to a definite irritant. As soon, however, as the products of the decomposition of albumin have entered the organism and produced toxic effects microorganisms unquestionably begin to act in con-junction with them.

[1] Jour. Am. Med. Assoc., June 19, 1897.   [2] Med. Chron., July, 1896.
[3] Rev. de Hyg., 1896, p. 761.   [4] Wien. med. Woch., No. 1, 1897.

E. D. Fergussou [1] reports 8 cases which he believes to be due to **autointoxication** with ptomaïns from the intestinal tract. The symptoms consisted of sudden onset with regurgitation of food. The regurgitated material subsequently became more serous in character, contained brown specks, and finally became coffee-ground in character. There were great prostration and rapid, feeble pulse and some fever. In those cases in which autopsy was obtained the intestinal tract was found to be hyperemic and the liver softened and fatty. He finally reports a 9th case in which vomiting became stercoraceous; he succeeded in washing out the intestinal tract by continuous rectal injection until the vomited material was clear. This patient recovered.

C. J. Whitby [2] discusses **self-poisoning,** of which he reports 4 cases. He assumes that the toxins are ordinarily produced in the intestinal tract, and in normal conditions chiefly eliminated by the kidneys. He therefore advocates treatment by intestinal antisepsis, diuretics, and especially by Turkish baths.

W. G. Thompson [3] believes that **hysterical fever** is due to pure malingering, the patients causing the mercury to rise by some manipulation akin to prestidigitation. He mentions several cases in which, upon taking the temperature himself, the rise failed to occur.

TUBERCULOSIS.

Etiology.—Kelsch [4] gives a *résumé* of 7 theses upon "**Heredity and Contagion in Tuberculosis.**" The authors attempted to solve the question in various ways, and agree that contagion is by far the most important element in the spread of tuberculosis. They, however, differ very much as to the part played by heredity, most of them believing that it is of little or no significance, although one, who based his conclusions chiefly upon laboratory experiments, concluded that it was more important than was generally believed. [Reliance on experimental work must not be too implicit, as the dosage and general conditions differ from those in spontaneous infection; but with clinical and pathologic evidence pointing in the same direction it may be confidently asserted that occasional intrauterine transmission does occur.]

I. H. Hance [5] has performed a number of experiments upon the **infectiousness of dust in dwellings and public conveyances,** with the following results: of 16 guinea-pigs inoculated with dust taken from 4 tenement-houses, where the families had paid attention to the instructions and regulations given them, 5 died of acute infection, and none were affected with tuberculosis. Of 12 pigs inoculated with dust from suspected rooms, 2 died from acute infection, 1 was indicative of tuberculosis, and 5 were tuberculous; 2 tenements out of 3 were found not infected. In the Bellevue and Charity Hospitals 11 wards were examined with negative results. Of 4 animals inoculated with dust from the waiting-rooms of the out-door poor department, 2 died of acute infection and 1 was tuberculous. Tubercle-bacilli were found in none of the elevated railroad cars, but the dust contained other highly infectious germs, which rapidly proved fatal. Of the street-cars, 1 of the 2 examined was infected with tubercle-bacilli. Two experiments with dust kept sealed in a dark drawer for 2 months showed that the acute infectious nature of the material had died out. The small amount of dust obtainable for the experiments (averaging but little over 3 sq. in. per room) makes these results all the more striking. A large number of the animals that died of acute infection might,

---

[1] Med. Rec., Oct. 31, 1896.								[2] Bristol Med.-Chir. Jour., Dec., 1896.
[3] Med. News, Jan. 2, 1897.								[4] Bull. Acad. de Méd., Oct. 13, 1896.
								[5] Med. Rec., Feb. 15, 1897.

had they lived, have increased the number of positive results. The great contrast between the clean tenements and those where more carelessness was exhibited shows emphatically the value of the work being done by the N. Y. Board of Health. He advocates the establishment of State sanitoria for the segregation and treatment of all cases of consumption.

Bay[1] examined 351 separate specimens of **cow's milk** by centrifugation, and in 51 found tubercle-bacilli. In 204 mixed specimens he found tubercle-bacilli 4 times.

Wolff[2] suggests the following rules in order to determine the source of **hereditary tuberculosis :** If several children of the same family become diseased, the mother remaining healthy, she is not the original source; if, however, only the younger children become diseased, whilst the parents remain healthy, she possibly has a latent form of the disease. If the elder children alone are affected, the father has been the cause of transmission. He analyzed 250 cases, and found that one or both of the parents died of tuberculosis in 80, and in 2 cases had tuberculosis without fatal result. There were 38 cases in which brothers and sisters were tuberculous, and 64 in which there was a tendency on the part of other children of the family to die young. Malignant tumors occurred in the parents of 25, and mental or nervous diseases in those of 8 of the patients; 33 patients were without hereditary history. Of these, however, 22 were either sickly or had tubercular habitus.

[The following paper, which is only a confirmation of previous work, demonstrates very clearly the fact of direct transmission.]

Bugge[3] has had an opportunity to examine the **fetus and placentas** of 5 tuberculous mothers. In 2 of the cases the examinations of the infants alone were negative; in 2 other cases both infants and placenta were negative; in the fifth case the child was born at the eighth month and died in thirty hours; the placenta could not be examined; but at the site of its insertion numerous bacilli were found in the wall of the uterus. Tubercle bacilli were also found in the blood of the umbilical vein and in the vessels of the infant's liver, but there were no gross tubercular lesions.

Charrin and Riche[4] have carefully examined **3 children born of tuberculous mothers,** and found that they presented anomalies in weight, growth, nutrition, and the toxic qualities of the urine. The latter were increased, which they take to indicate a sort of humoral toxicity—that is, a condition favoring infection.

Otto[5] discusses the relation of **phthisis and heart-disease.** He holds that there is truly an antagonism between left-sided disease and phthisis, phthisis rarely developing in a person suffering with left-sided valvular disease, especially if it is advanced to the stage in which passive congestion of the base of the lung is occasioned. Previous publications are contradictory. He himself has studied a number of cases, and in particular has searched carefully their histories to determine, if possible, whether, in the case of coincidence, the valvular lesion was first in development. He reports a case where the phthisis was primary, and where the appearance of the anatomical lesion was such that one might suppose the reverse. In other cases the cardiac lesions seemed to have impeded the extension of phthisis, for he found ancient tuberculous foci. In women he found, on the contrary, some cases in which phthisis developed in persons suffering with valvular disease ; but he also found some cases of arrest of tuberculosis under the influence of cardiac lesions. In 2 other cases the mod-

---

[1] Annual Report of Iowa State Mission, 1896.   [2] Münch. med. Woch., No. 40, 1896.
[3] Ziegler's Beiträge, vol. 19, p. 432.   [4] Compt. rend. de la Soc. de Biol., Apr. 16, 1897.
[5] Virchow's Archiv, Bd. 144, H. 1.

erate degree of cardiac trouble had not even occasioned hypertrophy. From his observations he concludes that there are rare exceptions to the rule that phthisis is not apt to develop in the course of cardiac disease. The exceptions are explained for the most part by the poor development of the cardiac lesions or by cases of general debility which have rendered the cardiac muscle insufficient. It is also well to note that the antagonism manifests itself less strikingly in the female. [This subject has been studied and restudied. It may be true that valvular disease with failing compensation impedes or prevents the occurrence of tuberculosis ; but the statistical evidence should take into account the limitation of individuals. It might, for example, be found that the number of cases of phthisis in any other condition (in a small number of cases) would be small as compared with the bulk of humanity; and yet no real antagonism could be asserted. It must be admitted, however, that there is considerable evidence to prove that congestion is antagonistic to the growth of tubercle.]

Rendu [1] reports the case of a man of 25 suffering from chronic cyanosis due to congenital narrowing of the pulmonary artery. In spite of the fact that he had spent all his life in hospitals exposed to tubercular infection, his lungs were free from the disease. [A single case of this kind proves little. There is undoubtedly evidence to prove greater susceptibility on the part of persons suffering with pulmonary stenosis.]

Jaccoud [2] contributes an interesting paper upon the **contagiousness of pulmonary tuberculosis.** Though the infectiousness of the disease is practically admitted by all, certain practical questions enter into the discussion of its contagiousness, and the experience of hospital managements must be taken into account. Regarding cases in which it has been alleged that infection has taken place within the hospital, he urges great care, and cites three instances in which the first consideration of the cases seemed to warrant this deduction, but in which subsequent study disproved the view. He particularly directs attention to autoinfection, as it might be called—that is, infection of the body by bacilli that previously existed somewhere in the body, though in a quiescent state. The tuberculosis itself may not appear until the patient has been reduced by some other affection or brought to the hospital with some form of injury. The author opposes the isolation in the hospitals of tuberculous cases, and states that there is greater danger to the tuberculous near to the phthisical than to the healthy near to either. He bases this upon the ground that infection with pyogenic micrococci occurs more readily than with the bacillus of tuberculosis, and that symbiosis of the former organisms with the latter renders the tuberculous process in the lungs or elsewhere particularly rapid and severe, while the pure tubercular bacillosis is less serious. In discussing this paper Pean rather favored the idea that infection frequently occurs in the hospital, and Terrier held that tuberculosis is exquisitely contagious, though this is not usually striking, from the fact that the symptoms of the disease are not marked at first. Debove took the same ground. Dumontpallier, on the other hand, stated that in his 40 years of experience in hospitals he had not been able to observe any marked contagion in this disease. In closing the discussion Jaccoud alluded to the investigations of Bollinger and Loomis, both of whom demonstrated the frequency of latent tubercular disease of the bronchial lymphatic glands.

W. Murrell [3] reports a case of **phthisis acquired** by a woman, previously healthy and without tubercular family history, from her husband, who had died

---

[1] Bull. méd., Feb. 24, 1897.   [2] Bull. de l'Acad. de Méd., No. 4, 1896.
[3] Lancet, Apr. 10, 1897.

from the disease, and in nursing whom she had taken no precautions. [It is only from a collection of a number of such cases that any definite results can be drawn, although it must be admitted that the present instance is very suggestive.]

R. Menger[1] has studied the **statistics** of tuberculosis at San Antonio, Texas, and concludes that the influx of consumptives has had no injurious effect upon the health of the inhabitants, as the mortality shows a relative decrease. Elaborate precautions to prevent infection, however, are exacted in the hospitals.

S. W. Abbott[2] states that the **death-rate** of consumption has been reduced ½ in the State of Massachusetts in the last 50 years. [These conclusions are unsatisfactory, because it is impossible to place great faith in the diagnoses made at a period when autopsies were even less common than at present, and the tubercle-bacillus had not been discovered.]

Surmont and Predhomme[3] find that the **mortality** from pulmonary tuberculosis has diminished from 1893, when it was 47.5%, to 25.7% in 1895. The general mortality-rate has not been affected. [These figures cover too short a period of time to be of value.]

Pathology.—The determination of the frequency and forms of secondary infection in tuberculosis is a matter of growing interest and importance.

Lannelongue and Achard[4] have studied the question of **microbic association** in cases of **tubercular suppurations** and other tubercular affections. Sixty-two cases presented the clinical appearance of tuberculosis; in 16 of these positive proof was furnished by injections of pigeons and in 2 by injection with tuberculin. In 57 of these cases there were suppurative collections wholly closed to the external air, while in the other 5 similar collections communicating with the outer air were found. Of the first 57 cases, 51 were negative on culture; in 4 the staphylococcus aureus was found, and in 2 streptococci. In the 5 open cases the staphylococcus aureus was found in 2, the streptococcus in 2, and both forms with saprophytes in 1. Referring to the question of the bearing of these micrococci on the febrile movement, the authors point out that opinions have differed greatly. In their own investigations febrile movement was found in 14 cases, including 6 in which micrococci were found, but also 8 in which the culture was negative. They therefore hold that the fever is not connected with micrococcic infection. [This opinion is not by any means definite, as the absence of microorganisms from cultures does not exclude the existence of such. It is unnecessary to instance lesions in which microorganisms are difficult to demonstrate in culture, but in which they are known to exist.]

Luzetto[5] has examined 15 cases of senile tuberculosis in order to determine the nature of the mixed infection. In 8 cases streptococci were present. These always presented the same characteristics, but were apparently either not pathogenic or only slightly so. Staphylococci were also present, and in all cases the following saprophytic types : the micrococcus candicans, the bacillus fungoides, and a motile bacillus. There appeared to be no definite relation between the streptococci and the fever, nor were these organisms found in patients over 60 years of age. The virulence of the tubercle-bacillus was normal, and the author concludes that senile tuberculosis resembles that of early life, excepting that mixed infection is rarer and the microorganisms usually show slight vitality and virulence.

---

[1] Texas Med. Jour., Mar., 1897.   [2] Jour. Am. Med. Assoc., Apr. 10, 1897.
[3] Rev. de Hyg., p. 591, 1896.   [4] Compt. rend. de la Soc. de Biol., No. 6, 1896.
[5] Centralbl. f. Bakt. Parasit. u. Inf'kr., Jan. 20, 1897.

Schabad [1] discusses mixed infection of phthisis, and includes only those microorganisms, other than tubercle-bacilli, that he has found in the blood, bronchi, and alveoli. These adventitious organisms frequently complicate the last stages of the disease and hasten death, though the hectic fever may exist when they are absent.

Complications.—Haushalter and Etienne [2] report 3 cases of pulmonary tuberculosis complicated by thrombosis of the ascending vena cava. In 1 of these cases staphylococci were found in the clot. [Thrombosis in the late stages of tuberculosis is probably less uncommon than is generally supposed ; we recall 2 striking cases, 1 of which was discovered accidentally at the autopsy.]

H. J. Godlee [3] contributes an interesting study of the changes in the **bones and joints** that occur in connection with thoracic disease. He first refers to caries of the spine and chronic tuberculous joints ; then to caries of the ribs in connection with phthisis, and to carious conditions of the lower jaw following disease of the teeth. A rare affection which has once come under his observation was " perforating necrosis of the skull." A number of fluctuating areas appeared on the head, and when these were opened small sequestra involving the whole thickness of the skull were discovered, whose rapid separation was in marked contrast with the tedious course met with in syphilitic cases. Finally, he discusses at much greater length the subject of pulmonary osteoarthropathy (*q. v.*).

Diagnosis.—A. M. Holmes [4] contributes a paper on the diagnosis of tuberculosis from the **morphology of the blood.** He begins with the assumption that the processes affecting the body as a whole are accompanied by analogous processes involving the leukocytes; or, in other words, that individual cells present changes comparable with those involving the whole organism. He then details the blood-examinations with differential counts of the leukocytes in 35 cases, calling attention to the fact that there is not a single characteristic which permits of the diagnosis of tuberculosis, but that a number of conditions must be brought into relation. The relative proportion of the leukocytes and the occurrence of beginning or advanced degeneration of the same cells are the factors of importance. He finds that there is reduction of the relative number of small lymphocytes and increase of polymorphous elements ; that the large mononuclear cells usually increase in number, and that giant lymphocytes with irregular outline and globules of hyaloplasm in the state of extrusion are frequent. The eosinophile cells are wanting, or reduced in number only in severe cases. Occasionally myelocytes may be found. Various degenerated forms of leukocytes may be observed. He then goes on to state the character of the blood in different stages. Beginning with the earlier and proceeding to the advanced stages of the disease, the number of lymphocytes decreases, while the polymorphous elements increase. [The paper is filled with crude speculations, and is marked by a disregard of known causes of alteration in the proportions of leukocytes. An increase in the polymorphous elements in such a condition as advanced phthisis is scarcely distinctive. The degenerations of leukocytes to which he calls attention are often due to the method of staining.]

Terrile [5] injected the sputum of 33 patients suffering from acute disease of the respiratory tract, but none of whom were suspected of tuberculosis, into guinea-pigs, 11 of which developed **experimental tuberculosis.** Of these 11 patients, 10 were cured and 1 showed an old sclerotic focus at the autopsy.

[1] Rev. de la Tuberculose, Dec., 1896.   [2] Gaz. hebdom. de Méd. et Chir., Aug. 27, 1896.
[3] Brit. Med. Jour., July 11, 1896.   [4] Med. Rec., Sept. 5, 1896.
[5] Arch. Ital. klin. Med., 1896, anno 35, punt. 3.

Combelale and Raviart[1] employed **tuberculin** in doses of 0.2 to 0.3 mg., and found that the reaction was sufficient for the purpose of diagnosing tuberculosis, and without any bad effects upon the patient. In 2 cases, however, where 0.5 mg. was employed there resulted a maculopapular eruption, commencing on the third day after the injection and lasting from 3 to 5 days. In these cases the tubercular lesions were very extensive. They conclude that injections of 0.25 mg. may be of much use in obscure cases and cannot prove dangerous to the patient.

E. L. Trudeau[2] has used tuberculin for the purpose of diagnosing incipient tuberculosis in 14 cases. The highest dose given was 3 mg., but in 6 cases the reaction was obtained with 2 mg. or less. The symptoms usually occurred within 12 hours, although in 1 case they did not appear until 22 hours after the injection. Of the 7 negative cases, 5 have since been under observation, and remain perfectly well. [As this method appears to be perfectly safe when carefully employed, and as the results of various investigators agree that it is fairly accurate, it seems justifiable to employ it in doubtful cases where tubercle-bacilli cannot be found.]

Pulmonary Tuberculosis.—Symptoms.—Samuel West[3] records a case of **acute phthisis** in a man of 20, remarkable for the **absence of fever.** The patient, a polisher by occupation, was in perfect health until 6 weeks before, when he got a slight cough. A month later pain in the left axilla developed, and he began to expectorate thin mucus and to emaciate. When he was admitted signs of pleurisy were discovered, and a few days later slight dulness. The sputa were thin, greenish, and frothy, slightly blood-stained, and contained tubercle-bacilli. On the first day his temperature was from 99.8° to 100.8°, on the 10th day between 99° and 100°, and from this time until the end of his illness rarely above normal, reaching 99° only once or twice. The physical signs made rapid progress, and the general condition rapidly deteriorated. Two months after his admission there was marked dulness down to the middle of the axilla, with defective entry of air and sharp crepitations. In spite of increase of physical signs, however, he began to improve, did not sweat so much at night, and gained 2 pounds in 5 weeks. He finally left the hospital 11 weeks after admission in an apparently subacute or chronic state.

J. P. Arnold[4] reports 2 cases in which he detected **cog-wheel inspiration** in the apices. In the course of a few months both developed tuberculosis. He regards the sign as almost pathognomonic of a pretubercular state. [We can hardly agree with this sweeping conclusion, having observed this sign in a number of cases that certainly did not develop tuberculosis within the period he mentions.]

D. Riesman[5] reports a case of miliary tuberculosis that during life had presented a **pleural friction-sound,** from the presence of which the diagnosis was made.

Potain[6] states that in the first stage of tuberculosis, before the disease has been fully developed, **gastric disturbances,** such as pain, vomiting without nausea, but with cough, and occasionally dilatation of the stomach, are not infrequent. These disappear with the development of the second stage. They appear to be due to depressed gastric action.

Rumpf[7] has studied the **diaphragm-phenomena** in 70 cases of tuber-

[1] Bull. méd. du Nord, Sept. 11, 1896.   [2] Med. News, May 29, 1897.
[3] Brit. Med. Jour., Aug. 29, 1896.   [4] Med. News, Mar. 20, 1897.
[5] N. Y. Med. Jour., Apr. 17, 1897.   [6] Tribune méd., Feb. 3, 1897.
[7] Berlin. klin. Woch., Feb. 8, 1897.

culosis of the lungs. In 5 of these cases it was totally normal, and in a 6th it was practically so. It was practically equal on the two sides, though reduced, in 29 of the 70 cases, and was completely absent on the two sides in 1 person, a young man, emaciated, with double pleurisy and beginning inflammation of the right apex. It was reduced upon one side only in 34 cases of the 70, and was practically absent on the one side, while the other side was nearly normal in 6 cases. In these there was combination of pleurisy with involvement of the apices. The material furnished in the institution in which the author worked does not include cases of advanced phthisis. The phenomenon has no special diagnostic value, according to his observations. [Our own experience accords with this conclusion, not only in pulmonary tuberculosis, but in other diseases as well.]

David Newman [1] reports 6 cases of **hemoptysis,** in all of which tuberculosis was suspected, but which proved upon careful examination to be cases of laryngeal disease, and yielded to appropriate treatment. [It cannot be too strongly urged that all other conditions should be excluded before hemoptysis is ascribed to tuberculosis.]

Hanot [2] discusses the **termination of pulmonary phthisis.** He holds that it is curable, even spontaneously, and has himself observed a case in which complete recovery apparently took place. One of the signs of improvement, after cavity-formation has taken place, is dislocation of the heart, due to cicatricial retraction of the tubercular areas. He holds that the only satisfactory treatment, so far discovered, is climatological, and believes that if means were provided for the treatment of cases from their incipiency, 60 per cent. of those who annually die of the disease could be saved. Among the peculiar features of tubercular cachexia is the fact that, even though it be extreme, the assimilation may be undisturbed and decubitus rarely occurs. A symptom that almost invariably announces imminent death is a melalgia described by Beau. It consists of an exquisitely sensitive point just above the knee, due, Hanot believes, to a form of neuropathy.

Treatment.—[Greater attention is constantly given to **prophylaxis,** and we select the following as representative opinions upon this point:]

Granjux [3] makes an exhaustive study of **tuberculosis in the French army,** and finds that it affects 7 men in every 1000, a greater proportion than occurs among the civilians. The statistics show that it is gradually increasing from year to year, this increase corresponding to the proportion of young soldiers and the obligations imposed upon them to learn their duties in the least time possible. In order to diminish this comparatively large proportion he recommends that the medical examination should be stricter and more thorough, in order to exclude those who become tubercular on account of predisposition or the development of a latent form of the disease—that this medical examination should take special account of tubercular heredity. Further, the circumference of the thorax should be carefully noted and its proportion to the height and weight of the individual; and in those cases where instead of increasing, as is usual in military life, it decreases, the individual should be discharged from the army. Finally, in order to prevent those cases that are due to contagion, he recommends the periodical disinfection of the barracks, a supply of spittoons, and the enforcement of the ordinary measures of hygiene, such as the restriction of crowding and the careful examination of food.

Grancher and Thoinot [4] have reported to the Commission de l'Assistance publique of Paris their conclusions regarding the **prophylaxis of tuber-**

---

[1] Brit. Med. Jour., May 29, 1897.   [2] Sem. méd., 1896, p. 289.
[3] Rev. de la Tuberculose, July, 1896.   [4] Ibid., Dec., 1896.

culosis. These are as follows: the best way of combating and treating tuberculosis is to isolate the patient, for the reason that by this means only is the risk of contagion diminished and better therapeutic conditions obtained. In the special hospitals every effort should be made to secure thorough antisepsis: the floors should be washed with an antiseptic solution; the sputum should be collected and carefully destroyed, and it should never be permitted to fall upon the floor; all the objects that the patients touch or use should be subjected to the same precautions, which should also extend to the furniture; and in order to make this as effectual as possible it is suggested that the mattresses be made of fireproof material. The patients should only wear clothing provided by the hospital, which should be washed at stated intervals. In regard to the personnel of the hospital, they regard it desirable to obtain better service than has hitherto been employed, and admit that for this purpose salaries must be considerably increased. As the risk of infection on the part of the nurses is very great (at least one-third die of this disease in France), they advise that only unmarried persons should be selected, or, at least, that they should be given the preference. In those unfortunate cases where it is still necessary to treat the patient at his house the rules should be all the more rigorously insisted upon.

In the congress of Russian physicians held at Kieff in the spring of 1896[1] Kostkevitch urged the **isolation of tuberculous patients** in special sanitaria, particularly cases in the advanced stages of the disease, when mixed infection exists, and not only the tubercle-bacilli, but also other pyogenic microorganisms are liable to be disseminated. He holds that the climate is of little consequence, as the sanitaria of the north give as good results as those of the south, the essential conditions being life in the open air, superalimentation, and complete change of habits. Helmann, in the same meeting, distinguished 2 categories of patients: those with slight expectoration and those with abundant expectoration; the latter, being the more dangerous, should be especially isolated. He believes that it is important to keep the two classes separated.

In a discussion on tuberculosis held in the Dublin Medical Society Moore[2] laid emphasis upon the necessity of closer government supervision of the disease, and urged particularly that in case of death the local health board should be notified and the dwelling be disinfected.

H. T. Tillotson[3] objects to the **segregation of consumptives,** and also to the deteriorating effects of too much **isolation.** He suggests, as a compromise, the establishment of small camping-parties in some favorable climate.

E. A. Edlen[4] believes that the popular opinion can be educated to object to the unrestricted **association with tuberculous patients,** and suggests the following rules: the destruction of all tuberculous cattle; the registration of all cases of tuberculosis, which shall then be instructed how to prevent infection; forbidding all tuberculous patients to marry until all signs of the disease have disappeared; and, finally, the disinfection of all houses in which tuberculous patients have died.

T. C. Craig[5] calls attention to the close **analogy between tuberculosis and leprosy,** and to the great inconsistency in the municipal control exercised over the two diseases. He thinks that it is very important that more precautions should be taken to prevent the spread of tuberculosis; particularly all food capable of conveying germs should be carefully investigated, and meas-

[1] Rev. de la Tuberculose, Dec., 1896. [2] Brit. Med. Jour., Oct. 10, 1896.
[3] Jour. Am. Med. Assoc., Apr. 3, 1897. [4] N. Y. Med. Jour., Apr. 17, 1897.
[5] Med. Rec., Jan. 23, 1897.

ures taken to prevent reckless expectoration either in dwellings or in public conveyances.

[The efforts to obtain an efficient antitubercular serum are being continued with great enthusiasm. Confidence is, however, somewhat shaken by the fact that the best results are usually obtained by the persons that have produced the serum, although Maragliano's report appears to be both sincere and frank.]

Maragliano[1] gives a summary of all the cases of tuberculosis that have hitherto been treated in Italy by his antitubercular serum. A cure is to be understood when all the symptoms of the disease have disappeared and remained absent permanently as determined, where possible, by frequent control-observations of the discharged patients. Altogether, 712 cases are reported. These are divided into 6 groups, according to the nature of the lesions : 168 cases suffered from bronchopneumonia with cavity-formation, of which 129 are reported to have had fever ; this latter symptom disappeared after treatment in 55 cases, was diminished in 22, and remained stationary in 52. The expectoration disappeared in 27, was considerably improved in 75, and was unaffected in 66. In only 59 cases are there records of the discovery of tubercle-bacilli. These disappeared in 10 cases, were diminished in 27, remained as before in 19, and were increased in 3. In 129 of these cases the body-weight was increased ; in 38 it was unaffected, and in 16 it was diminished. Altogether, 14 cases are recorded as cured, 75 as improved, 50 as stationary, and in 29 the symptoms grew worse. 127 cases are classified as destructive bronchopneumonias without cavity-formation or with mixed infection. In 94 of these cases temperature-records are given ; in 54 cases the fever disappeared, in 15 was diminished, and in 25 was uninfluenced. In 22 cases all expectoration disappeared, in 66 cases it was diminished, and in 39 was unaffected. In 52 cases there are records of the bacilli, in 13 they disappeared after the treatment, in 27 they were diminished, and in 12 unaffected. In 13 cases there are records of the body-weight. This was increased in 74, unaffected in 35, and diminished in 4. Altogether, 12 of these cases were cured, 71 improved, 35 remained stationary, and 9 became worse. The third group included diffuse febrile bronchopneumonias with or without destructive symptoms. Altogether, there were 220 cases collected. Fever disappeared in 107, remained stationary in 60, was diminished in 37, and became worse in 16. Expectoration disappeared in 36, was diminished in 93, was unaffected in 72, and grew worse in 19. Of 81 cases in which examination for bacilli was undertaken, these disappeared in 31, diminished in 53, remained stationary in 12, and increased in 3. The body-weight is reported for 151 cases : it was increased in 90, remained constant in 49, and diminished in 12. Of the whole number, 10 were completely cured, 120 improved, 67 unaffected, and 22 grew worse. The fourth group included diffuse apyretic bronchopneumonias with or without symptoms of destruction of pulmonary tissue. Of 68 cases, the catarrhal symptoms disappeared in 13, improvement took place in 41, and 14 remained stationary. In only 17 cases were bacillary examinations made. Of these they disappeared in 7, were diminished in 9, and remained as before in 1. Of 58 for whom there are records of the body-weight, 43 increased and 15 remained stationary. The total result was 2 cures, 54 improvements, and 12 unimproved. Group five were cases of circumscribed bronchopneumonia with fever. Of 81 cases, fever disappeared in 69, was diminished in 7, was stationary in 4, and increased in 1. The catarrhal symptoms disappeared in 46, were improved in 31, were unaffected in 3, and grew worse in 1. Of 44 cases where records are given, the tubercle-bacilli disappeared in 27, were dimin-

---

[1] Gaz. degli Osp., Nos. 125, 126, 1896.

ished in 16, and unaffected in 1. Thirty-three cases are reported as cured, 45 as improved, and 30 as stationary. The sixth group included 48 patients affected with circumscribed apyretic bronchopneumonia. All signs of catarrh appearances disappeared in 35, in 11 they were improved, in 2 remained stationary. Of 36 cases, the bacilli disappeared in 33 and were diminished in 3 ; of 45 cases, there was increase in the body-weight in 44 ; in 1 it remained stationary. Altogether, there were 33 complete cures, 13 cases of improvement, and 2 unaffected. That is to say, of the 712 cases, 104 appear to have been completely cured, 379 improved, 169 remained stationary, and 60 grew worse. Maragliano contends that in many of these cases the fact that no deterioration appeared must be taken as in some sense a positive result. The best results appear to have followed the regular injection of from 1 to 2 c.c. The most unfavorable for the treatment appeared to be cases of mixed infection.

Among the other papers dealing with the **antituberculous serum** of Maragliano, the following may be briefly alluded to : Derenzi[1] injected 22 cases, and has found no disadvantages or dangers. The patients improved in appetite and general feeling. In some cases the disease appears to be arrested. The improvement is slow, and increasing the dose does not render it more rapid. The best results are obtained in circumscribed and uncomplicated cases without high fever. Regnier[2] describes 3 cases in which he obtained good results. De Bernardi[3] claims to have cured an advanced case in a relative. After 40 injections in 1 month the cough ceased and the weight increased 1800 gm. F. Carlucci[4] has used the serum in 5 cases, and has found it of use in bronchopneumonia. It is harmless, and to be preferred in cases of phthisis to any medicinal treatment. The action is gradual. Cattaneo[5] reports 2 cases in children, aged 3 and 5, in which he obtained useful results. Crescinano[6] reports a case of laryngeal and pulmonary tuberculosis that was cured. Tubercle-bacilli had been found in the sputum.

[Unfortunately, in some of these instances showing remarkable success the exact details of the cases are not furnished, and doubt may exist as to the definiteness of the diagnosis. In many of them tubercle-bacilli had not been demonstrated.]

De la Jarrige[7] reports an interesting case of pulmonary tuberculosis. The patient, a young girl, had had a dry cough at the age of 17 years, and at the age of 20 presented the symptoms of cavity at the left apex, a tuberculous infiltration of the larynx, and multiple cavities in the lower third of the left lung. The treatment at first instituted having been interrupted, the disease progressed rapidly. It was then determined to employ subcutaneous injections of the **antitubercular serum of Richet and Hericourt.** Neither the first nor the second injections were followed by any reaction. The third, however, produced intense general urticaria with violent headache, high temperature, and intense congestion of the right lung. Death appeared imminent, but gradually the temperature fell, and in 8 days the patient had resumed her previous condition. New injections were practised, in spite of the serious symptoms that had been previously produced, usually without result, but occasionally giving rise to inflammatory action less marked than before. In 2 months improvement was manifest, particularly in the larynx. Finally, the girl seemed to be cured. The cavity in the left apex persisted, but was appar-

[1] Riforma Med., No. 8, 1896. [2] Progrès Méd., No. 6, 1896.
[3] Gaz. degli Osped. e delle Clin., No. 6, 1896. [4] Med. Rec., No. 15, 1896.
[5] Gaz. degli Osped. e delle Clin . No. 32. 1896. [6] Riforma Med., No. 67, 1896.
[7] Compt. rend. de la Soc. de Biol., July 3, 1896.

ently dry. She became stout, vigorous, and capable of enduring considerable exposure.

P. Paquin,[1] referring to his results in the treatment of tuberculosis with the **antitubercle-serum of horses,** summarizes his cases up to September 1, 1896. There are 226 cases tabulated; among these 37 were bronchopneumonias with cavities; 66 destructive bronchopneumonias without cavities; 19 diffuse febrile pneumonias with or without destructive processes; 19 diffuse nonfebrile pneumonias with or without cavities; 35 circumscribed febrile bronchopneumonias; 13 circumscribed apyretic pneumonias; 32 indefinite; 2 hip-joint disease; 2 laryngeal tuberculosis; 1 ovarian. The fever subsided in 60 and was reduced in 56; the night-sweats subsided in 69; the weight increased in 125; strength increased in 54; the appetite was improved in 114; the local signs disappeared in 46, improved in 58; the tubercle-bacilli disappeared in 40, diminished in 103. As to the results, the following summary may be made: recoveries, seemingly complete and permanent, 40; apparent recoveries with existing lesions, 3; improved cases capable of returning to work, 41; improved to less degree, 69; deaths, 32; disappeared or ceased treatment, 41. The author points out that most of the cases coming under this treatment are in the late stages, and that in the vast majority of such cases nothing can cure the disease.

W. H. Prioleau[2] reports 13 cases of tuberculosis treated with Paquin's antituberele-serum. Of these, 2 cases are reported as practically cured. In the sputum of 1 no tubercle-bacilli were ever found, and it is doubtful if the case was really tubercular in character. The other suffered from hemorrhages, and, although he improved considerably, still had cough and continued the treatment. Of the remaining 11 cases, it is stated that all but 1 were benefited; 6 died, and in 5 the ultimate result was not known. [It is difficult to discover what grounds the author has for his very favorable conclusions as to the value of this treatment.]

Allen[3] also reports 4 cases treated with Paquin's antitubercular serum: 1 case was apparently cured; 2 improved, but 1 of these died of femoral thrombosis; and 1 patient was not improved and died.

A. Woreester[4] reports the results of a year's treatment of various cases of tuberculosis with **antiphthisin** and **tuberculin.** Of 7 cases treated with tuberculin, 3 improved; 3 were obliged to change to antiphthisin; 2 are still under treatment: of these 7, 4 were in an advanced stage. Of 22 cases treated with antiphthisin, 10 were in advanced stages, and yet 4 of these improved markedly; 9 in less advanced stages showed no special improvement. Altogether, he believes that the patients that improve under tuberculin do better afterward and show less tendency to relapse than those which improve under antiphthisin.

[The results of experimental work in serum-therapy are more definite and satisfactory than the reports of its clinical use. The following papers are not favorable to its employment:] Tourkine[5] has carried out a number of experiments with the design of testing the **value of serum-treatment** in tuberculosis. He finds that the horse withstands very well the injection of the living bacilli, and that its serum becomes in time, to a certain extent, resistant to the action of the organism. When this serum was injected into animals that had previously been inoculated with tuberculosis he noticed some favorable results, indicated by the diminution of the temperature and a longer duration of life.

[1] N. Y. Med. Jour., Oct. 24, 1896. [2] Ibid., June 26, 1897.
[3] Jour. Am. Med. Assoc., May 29, 1897. [4] Boston M. and S. Jour., Aug. 2, 1896.
[5] Wratch, Oct 2, 1896.

However, all these animals finally died as a result of fatty degeneration of the viscera, and he concludes that the serum, as far as cats and guinea-pigs are concerned, has only a retarding action upon the invariably fatal result, and that therefore Maragliano's proposition to treat human tuberculosis with antitubercular serum is, at the least, premature.

Peron[1] immunized 10 guinea-pigs by inoculating them in the peritoneal cavity with small quantities of tubercular pus that had been heated for ¼ hour to 150° C. These and 6 control-animals were then injected with caseous material that had been heated to 150°. All of the 6 control-animals showed tumefaction. Of the 10 that had been immunized, 2 only showed a manifest induration after 17 and 24 hours respectively. Somewhat later all were injected with living cultures of tubercle-bacilli, and it was found that the protected animals became infected more rapidly and more severely than the control-animals. He concludes, therefore, that it is possible to vaccinate the guinea-pig in a certain measure against the toxins contained in the tubercle-bacillus, but that this **vaccination** does not give **immunity** against living virulent organisms.

Koch[2] obtained a **new form of tuberculin** by rubbing dried cultures in a mortar until only few tubercle-bacilli were left, adding serum and removing those remaining by centrifugation ; the resulting product is completely absorbed by the tissues and never gives rise to abscesses. This liquid could be separated into two portions—*i. e.* that obtained after the first centrifugation, which Koch speaks of as T. R., and that in the following centrifugations, which he speaks of as T. O. The former contains those constituents of the tubercle-bacilli which are insoluble in glycerin ; it has a distinct immunizing action, although it produces a slight reaction when injected into tuberculous patients. A curious effect, showing that it contains all the immunizing principles of tuberculin, is that the patient immunized by it fails to give the reaction when treated with ordinary tuberculin. The technic for the production of immunization in animals is as follows : in healthy guinea-pigs the dose may be as high as 2 or 3 mg. ; in those suffering with tuberculosis it must be very much less, in order to avoid, as far as possible, any reaction. The object to be attained is the giving of doses as large as possible in the shortest possible time. In tuberculous pigs more or less pronounced retrogressive changes could always be found in the tubercular lesions. Upon human beings it has already been used quite extensively in cases of pulmonary tuberculosis and lupus. In the latter, although there was but slight local reaction, progressive improvement always occurred.

Buchner[3] discusses the **new preparation of tuberculin** that has been described by Koch, and concludes that we are justified in expecting much greater success with it than with the older form, because it ought to be possible to produce specific immunization. He, however, claims the priority of the suggestion for his brother, and believes that his brother's method is infinitely better, as it does not subject the preparer to the same amount of danger.

V. C. Vaughan[4] reports the further history of 12 of the 24 cases of **tuberculosis treated with nucleinic acid** that he had reported 2 years previously. In 1894, 12 cases had died ; of the 12 then living, 2 have since died ; 3 are still affected ; 5 now show no evidences of the disease ; and in 2 the result is unknown. He reports 52 additional cases, making in all 76. Of these, 70 were suffering from pulmonary tuberculosis, and 3 have died ; 17 have been continuously free from the bacilli, and are apparently cured ; 2 more are appar-

[1] Compt. rend. de la Soc. de Biol., May 7, 1897.
[2] Deutsch. med. Woch., Apr. 1, 1897.
[3] Berlin. klin. Woch., No. 15, 1897.   [4] Med. News, Feb. 27, 1897.

ently well, but have not been examined; 20 were still affected at the last examination. Of these, 16 had been apparently improved: 5 were cases of urinary tuberculosis; 4 have been apparently cured; 1 developed acute miliary tuberculosis; and the 1 case of joint-tuberculosis was benefited. Vaughan, as a result of his studies in these and in some 40 more recent cases, concludes that in the advanced stages of disease, in which the area of inflammation is great, only temporary improvement, if any, occurs. In initial cases it not only arrests the progress of the disease, but may act as a curative agent.

H. M. King [1] has treated 37 cases of pulmonary tuberculosis with hypodermic injections of **nuclein**; of these, 7 were in the incipient stage, 15 in the advanced stage, and 15 in a far-advanced stage; 8 were apparently cured, 7 arrested, 6 improved, and 16 were unimproved, of whom 3 died. He observed that during the treatment the number of red blood-corpuscles was almost invariably increased.

[**Röntgen Rays.**—It has been claimed that these rays have decided bactericidal power, though experiments have not borne out the assertion uniformly. The experiments in tuberculosis have been fragmentary and inconclusive.] Lortet and Genoud [2] exposed some guinea-pigs that had been inoculated with tuberculosis to the Röntgen rays, and found that at a time when some control-animals were seriously affected these remained comparatively well.

Fiorentini and Luraschi [3] also believe that the resistant power of the animals was increased, although their results were not conclusive.

Ravillet [4] reports a case of pulmonary tuberculosis occurring in a young man of 18 with tubercular family history, treated by the Röntgen rays. During a *séance* the patient always slept quietly and the fever was diminished. Tubercular laryngitis was noticeably improved. All these symptoms reappeared when, on account of the breaking of the apparatus, the treatment was suspended for a short time. The local results were the appearance of an erythema upon the anterior and posterior surfaces of the body, which subsequently became vesicular. In spite of transient benefit the patient subsequently died.

Rendu [5] reports the case of a man of 20 who became ill with the symptoms of beginning typhoid fever, changing to those of an infective pneumonia. The sputum contained pure cultures of staphylococcus. The fever declined partially, but returned, and the evidences of suppuration of the pleura or lung were discovered. Another examination of the sputum showed a few tubercle-bacilli. At the end of 6 weeks the patient seemed nearing the end. He was exposed to the **Röntgen rays** at this time for 55 minutes every day. After the fourth exposure the temperature fell and did not arise again. There were diuresis and diaphoresis, and the patient became quite well. The author does not believe the result to have been purely coincidence. After 10 of the applications erythema and ulceration of the skin were found, and he holds that equally marked trophic changes may have taken place in the deeper tissues. [The typical decline of the symptoms so strongly suggests a pneumonic process that we should hesitate to accept the reporter's statement without further confirmation.]

Jakoby [6] has endeavored to produce hyperemia of the pulmonary apices by means of his thermo-therapeutic apparatus, which consists essentially of the local application of heat. He hopes by this method to increase the collection of the alexins in this region and thereby hinder the development of tuberculosis.

[1] Med. News, May 29, 1897.   [2] Sem. méd., p. 266, 1896.
[3] Atti della Assoc. médica Lombarda, No. 1, 1897.   [4] Rev. de la Tuberculose, Apr., 1897.
[5] Sem. méd., Jan. 20, 1897.   [6] Munch. med. Woch., No. 89, 1897.

J. K. Crook [1] reports 45 cases of pulmonary tuberculosis treated with large doses of **creasote.** Of these, 5 were apparently cured—that is, there was complete disappearance of the symptoms and physical signs of phthisis; 5 showed marked signs of improvement, and 8 received some degree of benefit; 13 showed no influence at all from the treatment, and 8 died. The remainder were not treated long enough to enable the author to draw any positive results. Of the 5 cases that were cured, 2 were in the 2d stage and 3 in the 1st stage; of the 5 that were benefited, 2 were in the 1st stage and 3 in the 2d. Crook believes that creasote is a remedy capable of arresting certain cases of tuberculosis.

A. Chaplin and F. W. Tunnicliffe [2] have employed **guaiacolate of piperidin** in 14 cases of pulmonary consumption. There was some improvement in the cough, and often the lungs seemed dryer. The temperature was usually unaffected. While under its influence the patients improved in appetite and general strength. As much as 30 gr. was given 3 times daily without bad effects.

Leannau [3] has employed **ichthyol** in the treatment of pulmonary phthisis. He gives it in capsules that contain .025 of a cgm., and administers from 4 to 24 of these per day. All the symptoms improve; the cough becomes less severe, the dyspnea less, excepting in those cases complicated with valvular heart-disease; the intercostal pains disappear, and physical signs are altered for the better. All the general symptoms improve; weight is increased, and the sweating greatly diminished. In conclusion, he reports 10 cases, in all of which great improvement occurred.

J. H. Thompson [4] reports 5 cases in which he has used inhalations of **cinnamon oil** in the treatment of consumption. Expectoration and cough were the first symptoms to improve; then the temperature tended to become normal, and finally the weight began to increase. These changes were accompanied by a gradual diminution in the number of tubercle-bacilli in the sputum.

Schröder [5] suggests **peronin** for the treatment of the **irritating cough** of pulmonary tuberculosis. It appears to be almost equally effective as codein, and very rarely causes disagreeable symptoms. It is particularly valuable when the patients have become accustomed to the use of the latter drug or to morphin.

Joquet [6] has used **sodium tellurate** in the treatment of the **night-sweats** of phthisis. The drug is given in the form of a pill or solution, the sodium salt being readily soluble in water or alcohol. The dose is $\frac{3}{10}$ gr., but in bad cases $\frac{3}{4}$ gr. may be taken daily. For a lasting effect the drug should be administered 3 days. Large doses tend to disturb the stomach.

Hemoptysis.—R. H. Babcock,[7] in a paper on the treatment of hemoptysis, records the opinions of 27 physicians of experience in Chicago. Of these, 18 insisted upon absolute rest; 13 apply cold to the chest; 17 use opium and morphin to allay cough or promote calm; 15 use ergot, though some state that they have doubts of its utility—11 others are positive that ergot is not efficient; 6 use acetate of lead, either with or without opium; 2, tannic acid; 2, gallic acid; 1, dilute sulphuric and 1 aromatic sulphuric acid; 6 use ipecac; 4, aconite; 2, veratrum viride. Finally, the author states his own views. He quiets cough with phosphate of codein, $\frac{1}{4}$ to $\frac{1}{2}$ gr. hypodermically, or $\frac{1}{2}$ to 1 gr. by the mouth. He gives ipecac in frequent doses until nausea is produced, and a saline aperient like Hunyadi water. When the

[1] Med. Rec., Mar. 27, 1897.
[2] Brit. Med. Jour., Jan. 16, 1897.
[3] Jour. de Méd. de Paris. Aug., 1896.
[4] Brit. Med. Jour., Nov. 7. 1896.
[5] Thérap. Monatsh., 1897, p. 4.
[6] Jour. de Méd., Aug. 10, 1896.
[7] Medicina, Sept., 1896.

hemorrhage occurs from a cavity, he gives an immediate injection of gr. $\frac{1}{50}$ to even gr. $\frac{1}{25}$ of sulfate of atropin. Absolute rest is always insisted upon.

C. E. Quimby[1] advocates the employment of his **pneumatic cabinet** for the arrest of **pulmonary hemorrhage.** The patients are obliged to expire into a negative pressure of from $\frac{1}{2}$ to $\frac{3}{4}$ inch of mercury. This produces a general capillary dilatation and lowering of the systemic vascular tension, so that the venous system is distended, while the pulmonary vessels suffer corresponding depletion and slowing of their circulation—a condition that favors clotting. The statistics of 50 cases suffering from hemoptysis are reported, and in only 2 this treatment failed to prevent recurrence, 1 of these being acute phthisis involving the larger part of the right lung, and the other acute diffuse infiltration of both lungs; 2 cases in particular had hemorrhage while under observation, which was immediately arrested by treatment in the cabinet, and after systematic treatment failed to return.

J. W. Brannan[2] recommends morphin, gallic acid, ergot, etc., and lays particular emphasis upon careful respiratory gymnastics in the interval between the attacks.

V. Y. Bowditch[3] discusses the treatment of phthisis in **sanitaria near our homes.** He refers to his previous papers upon the results obtained in 40 cases of consumption treated at Sharon : 10 of these cases were reported as arrested, Since that time (that is, during the last 2 years) 26 cases have been admitted, but 2 remained only a short time. Of the 24 remaining cases, 7 left the sanitarium as "arrested" cases; of the remaining 17, 1 was an uncertain case, which was apparently cured ; 12 others were more or less advanced and little was expected of the treatment ; 8 of these improved somewhat ; 4 were not benefited.; 4 other cases were really incipient cases, and 2 of them left for Colorado, and after $3\frac{1}{2}$ and 6 months decidedly improved. One other left in 2 months much improved, and the 4th is still at the sanitarium the picture of health, with little cough and no bacilli in the sputa. In addition to the 10 arrested cases previously reported, 5 who were then under treatment, classed as "much improved," have been since discharged as arrested. Altogether, of 64 cases treated at the sanitarium in the last 5 years, 22 are classed as arrested ; of these, 4 have since died, and in 2 others the symptoms of the disease soon returned after leaving Sharon, though they are still living : 1 of the 4 that died succumbed to an operation. Good accounts are obtained of all the others.

Lymphatic Tuberculosis.—Duclion[4] believes that the greater number of **enlargements of the lymph-glands** are due to either lymphosarcoma or tuberculosis. The differential diagnosis is important, as in the latter case operative procedure is indicated, but is almost impossible clinically, and even histologically very difficult. He therefore recommends excision of a suspected gland and inoculation into some lower animal, a method he regards as the only positive one.

Frouz[5] discusses the dangers which may arise from the **rupture of tubercular glands** into the air-passages. These he holds to be nothing more serious than the development of a putrid bronchitis, unless incomplete liquefaction of the glands has taken place, when the caseous masses may form serious obstructions, and occasionally require tracheotomy for their removal, as in 2 cases that he cites. He also suggests that hemoptysis without pulmonary lesions is probably due to the rupture of a small artery in one of these glands.

[1] N. Y. Med. Jour., Aug. 1, 1896.   [2] Ibid., Aug. 15, 1896.
[3] Boston M. and S. Jour., Aug. 6, 1896.   [4] Thèse de Bordeaux, No. 32.
[5] Jahrb. f. Kinderh., Feb. 5, 1897.

In conclusion, he urges the importance of the earlier diagnosis of these conditions, and suggests the use of mercurial inunctions in treatment.

Pluder and Fischer[1] have examined 32 cases of **hyperplasia of the faucial tonsils,** in 5 of which they found tuberculosis limited to the mucous layer. They consider that this condition represents a latent primary form of the disease.

Cardiac Tuberculosis.—Labbe[2] reports 2 cases of tuberculosis of the **heart-muscle,** and alludes to 36 previously published cases. Tuberculosis of the myocardium occurs in 4 forms: (1) small miliary tubercles, (2) large solitary tubercles, (3) the diffuse form, (4) tubercular myocarditis with diffuse sclerosis and miliary tubercles, but without caseation. The pericardium may or may not be involved; the endocardium is generally unaltered except in the diffuse form. The disease is most frequent in young subjects, 17 of 29 cases being under 15 years; and is usually secondary. The infection may occur by dissemination through the blood coming in the pulmonary veins or by direct extension from the tuberculous pericardium; the most frequent method, however, seems to be by way of the lymphatics—a fact which explains the deeply seated affection of the cardiac muscle and the secondary involvement of the mediastinal glands. The author's 2 cases are as follows: (1) A boy of 6 developed a persistent cough after bronchopneumonia. The heart-area was increased; the heart-action irregular, and later enlarged, and ascites prominent. Cardiac symptoms (pain, irregular pulse, and general edema) increased and sudden death resulted. Postmortem tuberculosis of the third form was discovered, the pleura and pericardium being adherent, and the latter much thickened and containing cheesy nodules. The heart-musele was hard and lardaceous in appearance. (2) The second case, a girl of 1 year, had suspicious bronchitis and enlarged glands; had whooping-cough and chicken-pox, and died with the symptoms of pulmonary tuberculosis. At the autopsy a large cavity was found in the middle lobe of the right lung, with tubercles in both lungs. A cheesy tubercle penetrated the myocardium, being visible beneath the pericardium. Tubercle-bacilli were demonstrated in both cases. The latter case belongs to the second form of tuberculosis.

Renal Tuberculosis.—Plicque[3] discusses **uremia** in tuberculous patients. He classifies the various forms into acute and massive tuberculosis of the kidneys. In addition to these, epithelial and renal lesions and albuminuria are exceedingly common. All these lesions favor the occurrence of uremia, and in addition fatty and amyloid degeneration occurs frequently. Uremia is, nevertheless, not frequent, chiefly because there are so many other methods of elimination that are active in these conditions, as, for example, the sweats, the sputum, etc.; and in addition there is a gradual development of tolerance of the alteration of the kidneys.

Louis-Dubois[4] believes that the **pretubercular albuminuria** is not due to the elimination of the poison, but rather to a direct infection of the kidneys by the tubercle-bacilli, liberated for some reason or other from a latent focus and circulating in the blood. He supports this hypothesis by 2 series of experiments: in 1 he injected considerable quantities of toxin into rabbits without producing albuminuria; in the other he injected virulent cultures, and was frequently able to recover the bacilli from the kidney.

Intestinal Tuberculosis.—R. B. Shaw[5] reports a case of pulmonary

[1] Arch. f. Laryng. u. Rhin., p. 372, 1896.
[2] Rev. mens. des Mal. de l'Enfance, June, 1896.
[3] Rev. de la Tuberculose, Apr., 1897.
[4] Compt. rend. de la Soc. de Biol., Jan. 1, 1897.
[5] Montreal Med. Jour., Jan., 1897.

72   *GENERAL MEDICINE.*

tuberculosis suffering from persistent diarrhea in which **tubercle-bacilli** were discovered **in the feces.** At the autopsy no anatomical changes were discovered in the intestinal tract. [The diagnosis of intestinal tuberculosis would doubtless be made in such a case, and would be justified. A warning, however, should be sounded that smegma-bacilli be as carefully distinguished as possible.]

Nové-Josserand [1] reports a case of **tumor in the right ileocecal** region about the size of a fist, easily movable and with irregular nodular surface. Exploratory incision showed that this consisted of a tubercular cecum. Although no treatment was undertaken, there was great improvement after the operation, and in less than 3 weeks the tumor had almost entirely disappeared.

Claud [2] describes a case in which severe **tuberculous ulcers** were found **in the duodenum.** This occurred in a patient who had not suffered with vomiting or diarrhea: 1 ulcer was found within a centimeter of the pylorus, and 7 others below this. The appearance of these was not like that of the ordinary tuberculous ulcers found in the small intestine in the same case. The histological examination, however, showed their nature, and tubercle-bacilli were demonstrated.

Peritoneal Tuberculosis.—Marchthurn [3] reports 19 cases of tuberculosis of the peritoneum treated by laparotomy, and adds to these 17 cases that had been previously treated by this method : 21 were permanently cured ; in the others, in which tuberculosis of other organs existed, the results were only temporarily favorable. Fever did not occur after the operations in those cases in which asepsis had been most rigid. Diagnosis was confirmed in all cases by microscopical examination.

Ovarian Tuberculosis.—Prochownik [4] reports the case of a woman who, in the lower third of the abdomen, developed a tumor that was about two-thirds of the diameter of the colon. It was nodular and pedunculated. At the autopsy it was found to be tubercular in nature, probably springing from the left ovary.

LEPRA.

Etiology.—Ehlers [5] in discussing the etiology of leprosy, particularly as it occurs in Iceland, shows that the disease has increased somewhat in recent years, and in particular has collected statistics bearing upon the transmission of the disease. He found 158 cases on the island in 1894–95, and of these he was able to examine personally 119. In 56 cases there was a history of the disease in the family. Of these, the father and mother were affected in 3 ; father alone in 15 ; mother alone in 4 ; sisters or brothers in 4 ; distant relatives in 14.

K. Grossman [6] has also studied the etiology of leprosy in Iceland, which country he considers the most favorable field for such an investigation. The inhabitants themselves, according to him, appear to pay no regard to the possibility of contagion, associating freely and intimately with advanced cases. The natives take great pride in their ancestry and keep family records. He concludes, from a study of these, that leprosy is certainly not hereditary, and can only be spoken of as possibly contagious, an absolute demonstration of infection from direct contact being still lacking. He suggests the possibility that human beings are but temporary hosts of the parasite, it having possibly some extra-human habitat, in the same manner as the bacillus of tetanus.

[1] Lyon méd., 1896, No. 20.　　[2] Bull. de la Soc. anat. de Paris, No. 8, 1896.
[3] Wien. klin. Woch., Mar. 4, 1897.　[4] Münch. med. Woch., No. 49, 1896.
[5] Derm. Zeit, No. 3, 1896.　　[6] Brit. Med. Jour., Dec. 5, 1896.

Havelburg[1] as a result of extensive observations in Rio Janeiro, where there are about 3000 cases of leprosy, has reached the conclusion that the disease is **contagious**; even in the hospitals some of the attendants have been attacked in spite of thorough precautionary measures. The period of incubation appears to be, in some cases at least, as much as 2 years, and may possibly be longer. The disease is frequently associated with tuberculosis; indeed, nearly all his patients ultimately die of phthisis. He holds that it is important to prevent the subjects of leprosy from travelling, and particularly to prevent them from entering countries where the disease is rare or practically unknown.

Diagnosis.—Gravagna[2] has been able to demonstrate the lepra-bacilli upon the skin in cases of leprosy with cutaneous manifestations. The bacilli are absent from the skin when cutaneous manifestations are wanting. He was able to demonstrate the bacilli in the fluid of blisters raised upon healthy portions of the skin of leprous patients, but was unable to find them in sweat induced by pilocarpin or in fresh sperma.

Faber[3] has examined the secretions and tissues of a case of leprosy, and found bacilli in the blood of diseased tissue, sweat, epidermis, and sperma, and failed to find bacilli in the blood of healthy tissues, in the urine and sputum.

Visceral Lepra.—Scageliosi[4] examined the so-called lepra-nodules of the lungs occurring in a case of leprosy, but found only staphylococci and streptococci.

Doutrelepont and Wolters[5] describe a case of leprosy with widespread visceral lesions. The lepra-bacilli were found in the lungs, mesenteric glands, intestines, bone-marrow, and the kidneys. The diagnosis of lepra may be made by the intracellular position and peculiar arrangement of the bacilli, by the abundance of vacuolated cells in the different tissues, and by the absence of structures resembling tubercles and of evidence of necrosis. They found the bacilli in the cavities of the heart, and therefore conclude that the disease is transmitted through the circulation.

Von Reisner[6] describes 3 cases of lepra with **ulcers in the intestines.** In 2 of these there was at the same time tuberculous disease of the lung, as in the 13 cases described by Hansen and Looft. The ulcers, however, were distinguished by great thickening and bluish coloration of the edges. In the 3d case the ulcer was flat, rounded, and with a sharp edge. No tuberculosis of other organs could be discovered. Microscopically lepra-bacilli were found in the third case, while in the ulcers of the first and second bacilli could only be found after staining the length of time that would also stain tubercle-bacilli. The author believes that the third case was a true instance of leprous ulcer of the intestine.

Treatment.—Prophylaxis.—P. A. Morrow[7] urges that leprosy is not only exceedingly rare, but also very slightly contagious, and that the precautions taken to isolate patients are absurd when contrasted with the freedom accorded to consumptives and syphilitics.

Serum-therapy.—Juan de Carrasquilla[8] injected animals with serum obtained from leprous patients, then bled these animals and used their serum in the treatment of leprosy. He found that it caused discoloration of the spots, restoration of sensation in the anesthetic patches, and notable improvement in

[1] Berlin, klin. Woch., Nov. 16, 1896.
[2] Riforma med., No. 138, 1896.
[3] Deutsch. med. Woch., June 1, 1897.
[4] Riforma med., No. 189, 1896.
[5] Arch. f. Dermat. u. Syph., Bd. xxxiv. H. 1.
[6] Monatsch. f. Prakt. Dermatol., No. 5, 1896.
[7] N. Y. Med. Jour., Nov. 7, 1896.
[8] New Orl. M. and S. Jour., Nov., 1896.

the general condition of the patients. Occasionally there was reaction. In the nodular form there were desquamation and subsequent return of the skin to a normal condition. [There is not the slightest proof offered that the animals employed became more than normally immune, or that their serum acquired any curative properties. This method of preparing serum has not given satisfactory results in any other infectious disease.]

C. B. Maitland [1] reports 2 cases of leprosy treated by the **thyroid-gland** substance, in both of which there was considerable improvement in the local lesions and general condition.

H. R. Croeker [2] has treated 2 cases of leprosy with **corrosive sublimate** injected hypodermically. In both there was improvement in the general condition and no bad effects from the treatment.

Tuberculosis and Leprosy.—A. Ransome [3] has made a careful comparative study of tuberculosis and leprosy, and concludes that the latter disease is limited mainly by general sanitary measures, and that it is scarcely affected by direct efforts to prevent contagion.

Ainhum and Leprosy.—Zambaco-Pacha [4] considers the relations of ainhum and lepra, and concludes that the former is really a form of the latter. He reaches this conclusion from the consideration of cases described in Europe, as well as from the similarity in the clinical history and the localization of the disease to restricted districts for a long period.

De Brun [5] denies the identity of these diseases, as a result of his experience in Syria. He admits that the mutilations of leprosy may resemble those of ainhum, even to the formation of a distinct line of demarcation; but points out that such resemblance is rare, that ainhum fails to affect the fifth toe of the foot in only exceptional cases, and that it never causes other manifestations suggesting leprosy.

A. S. Ashmead [6] also points out the dissimilarity of leprosy and ainhum, and alludes to **quigila,** another infectious and contagious disease of the skin occurring in Brazil. The author states that leprosy was carried to Brazil from Europe and Africa. The black race is particularly liable.

Berger-Lardy [7] believes that ainhum and leprosy are the same disease, and describes a skiagraph of a diseased foot which showed that the soft parts were present, but that the bones had been absorbed.

Psittacosis.—Gilbert and Fournier [8] have studied an epidemic of psittacosis. This is a disease transmitted from birds, particularly parrots, to man. In birds it is characterized by marked diarrhea, loss of appetite, depression, and loss of feathers. In man it runs the course of an intense typhoid fever, without abdominal symptoms but with marked pulmonary disturbances, resembling a severe infectious pneumonia. A marked epidemic occurred in Paris in 1892, affecting 50 persons or more. The cases studied by the authors occurred in February, 1896, and affected 5 persons, of whom 2 died. They were able to confirm the observation of Nocard regarding the occurrence of a definite bacillus, having found it in the cases under their observation as well as in the bone-marrow of the birds. They could not find the organism in the blood of the patients during life, but they did find it in one case in the blood of the heart postmortem. The organism resembles the bacillus of Eberth in a number of particulars. It is extremely virulent, causing death in rabbits, mice, and pigeons within 14 to 48 hours.

[1] Lancet, Oct. 31, 1896.
[2] Ibid., Aug. 8, 1896.
[3] Ibid., July 11, 1896.
[4] Bull. de l'Acad. de Méd., July 28, 1896.
[5] Ibid., Aug. 25, 1896.
[6] Med. News, Oct. 18, 1896.
[7] Bull. de l'Acad. de Méd., No. 32, 1896.
[8] Ibid., Oct. 21, 1896.

An editorial in the *Gaz. heb. de Méd. et Chir.*, Apr., 1897, discusses psittacosis. It was introduced into Paris in 1891 by some parrots from South America. It may be transmitted either from the parrots to man directly, or through intermediate objects, or from other men. The period of incubation is from 7 to 12 days; the disease commencing with malaise, epistaxis, and disturbances of the digestion. This is followed by bronchitis or bronchopneumonia, with slight albuminuria; and finally there is high fever, which appears very early, and lasts 3 to 4 days, and terminates by crisis. These phenomena may recur several times; defervescence finally taking place by lysis. During the course of the disease the spleen is enlarged, and the signs of pneumonia may be more or less pronounced. In some cases an eruption has been present; at first roseolar, and subsequently petechial. Three forms are recognized : the slight, nervous, and ordinary. The duration of the whole disease is about 30 days. If no complications occur, recovery is the rule; but the mortality is about 37 %. The cause appears to be the bacillus discovered by Nocard, which closely resembles the bacillus of typhoid fever. Curiously enough, a reaction analogous to that of Widal does not seem to occur in this disease. The treatment is purely symptomatic, prophylaxis being by far the most important part.

Actinomycosis.—Ruge[1] reports the results of the investigation of 25 tonsils, in 4 of which he found peculiar bodies that resembled the ray-fungus. These were not found in the tissue, but only in the crypts, which were sometimes surrounded by inflammatory changes. [These bodies are doubtless similar to those observed about carious teeth. Their exact nature is not as yet determined.]

Abée[2] reports 3 cases of fatal actinomycosis. The first patient was probably infected from the month. In 1887 he had pneumonia; in 1888 he developed a dry pleurisy on the right side, from which time he had suffered continually from cough, pain in the side, and pressure upon the chest. In December of the same year he developed an abscess over the sternum that did not heal after evacuation; at the same time infiltration of the right lung developed; the sputum became bloody, and death followed about 6½ months after the first symptoms. At the autopsy multiple abscesses were found in the lung and a large phlegmon in front of the cervical vertebræ, which had destroyed their substance and produced a pachymeningitis cervicalis. All the lesions were actinomycotic in nature. The second patient had pneumonia in 1882 ; in 1884 he injured his right side; several months later he had a chill and pain in the right side and expectorated yellowish masses. The condition rapidly grew worse, the expectoration became bloody, and there were signs of infiltration in the right lung. Later, abscesses developed on the shoulders. The patient from time to time had paroxysms of severe dyspnea, and finally died during an attack of hemoptysis. At the autopsy there was found a posterior mediastinitis with lesions of the spinal column and the meninges, and rupture into the esophagus ; also a large actinomycotic abscess in the lung and thrombosis of the inferior vena cava. The third patient had influenza in 1895, since which time he had suffered from cough with occasional hemoptysis. When examined he was found to have infiltration in the lower part of the right lung, and shortly after that a large abscess developed in the thoracic wall. This was opened, but the patient rapidly became worse with severe intermittent fever. At the autopsy actinomycotic phlegmons were found in the retroperitoneal and mediastinal cavities. The vertebral column was involved and there was, as in the other cases, a peripachymeningitis. In all the cases very

[1] Zeit. f. klin. Med., vol. xxx., 1896.   [2] Ziegler's Beiträge, vol. xxii., H. 1, 1897.

accurate pathological studies were made. [In all of these cases there was history of previous disease or injury of the lung; but it is difficult to trace the connection between this and the subsequent infection.]

Habel[1] reports 5 cases of actinomycosis, with autopsy. In 3 there was simulation of tuberculosis of the lungs with complications in other organs; 2 gave the appearance of perityphlitis or peritonitis. In 2 of these cases there was a history of tuberculosis in the family, and in 1 tuberculosis coexisted with the other disease. [Sufficient attention has not been paid in the past to the cases simulating pulmonary tuberculosis; and the frequency of this form cannot as yet be properly estimated.]

Ducor[2] reports a case of actinomycosis that commenced in 1888 with moderate pains just back of the inferior angle of the right jaw; subsequently a tumor developed. This continued, varying in size for some time, and finally gave rise to a huge abscess, with all the symptoms of severe septic infection. This was relieved by the discharge of an enormous quantity of pus. Diagnosis, however, had not been made, but examination of the pus showed the typical ray-fungus and the presence of numerous streptococci. Treatment with potassium iodide and Marmorek's antistreptococcic serum resulted in rapid improvement in all the symptoms. The causation of the condition proved to have been a habit that the patient acquired when a pupil in a convent of cleaning her teeth with various forms of grain.

Galli-Valerio[3] reports a case of pseudoactinomycosis of the lower jaw characterized by the presence of a fungus that resembled somewhat the streptothrix maduræ, but which occurred in small masses.

Glanders.—Errich[4] reports a case of glanders which was remarkable for the fact that the large joints—i. e. the elbow, the knees, and the ankles—showed suppurative inflammation, whilst the multiple abscesses in the muscles were absent.

A. G. R. Foulerton[5] has applied the **serum-test** to the diagnosis of glanders, using it as Widal does in typhoid fever, and with the same results. The bacilli were obtained from the patient himself, and cultivated upon agar. They agglutinated very promptly at a dilution of 1 to 20. The reaction, however, was found to be not specific for glanders, diphtheritic serum and serum from 4 cases of typhoid fever producing agglutination in an emulsion of the bacilli. Normal human or equine serum had no effect. [It is possible that the reaction would have proved to be specific if higher dilutions had been used.]

Forestier[6] reports a case of **acute glanders** which was characterized by the development in all the extremities of fluctuating tumors that contained hemorrhagic pus. There were numerous bronchopneumonic foci in the lungs. Toward the end of the disease a general pustular eruption appeared and periostitis developed over the frontal bones. The diagnosis was confirmed by bacteriologic investigation.

Brault and Rouget[7] report a case of glanders which was characterized by 17 subcutaneous muscular abscesses and suppuration in 4 joints. Miliary nodules were not found in the lungs. A microorganism was found which in many respects resembled the bacillus of glanders, but was not absolutely typical.

[1] Virchow's Archiv, vol. cxlv., 1896.   [2] Bull. de l'Acad. de Méd., Aug. 4, 1896.
[3] Gaz. degli Osped. e delle Clin., No. 149, 1896.   [4] Beitr. z. klin. Chir., vol. xvii., sec. 1.
[5] Lancet, May 1, 1897.   [6] Lyon méd., No. 6, 1897.
[7] Gaz. hebdom. de Méd. et Chir., No. 102, 1896.

MALARIAL FEVER.

Etiology.—J. M. Anders[1] contributes a statistical paper on the occurrence of malaria. He has collected 5044 cases from the records of 5 hospitals in Philadelphia. In tabulating these he finds that there has been a decline in the number of cases during the last half century and more especially during the last 25 years. Alluding to the statement sometimes made that malaria is increasing in certain localities, he states that investigation in all of the large cities, here and abroad, would probably show that increase is found in comparatively few places. He shows that there is no increase of the disease in the spring as there is in the fall. It grows progressively throughout the summer, reaching the maximum in September and then declines rapidly during October and November, and reaches the minimum in January and February. The figures are as follows: January, 134; February, 103; March, 155; April, 216; May, 304; June, 340; July, 408; August, 683; September, 969; October, 868; November, 409; December, 254. This table agrees almost entirely with that of Thayer and Hewetson.

[The evidence in favor of the role of the mosquito in conveying the plasmodia is increasing. Whether the insect acts as an intermediate host is more doubtful.]

Laveran,[2] after a critical study of the theories that attempt to explain the **transmission of the malarial poison,** concludes that the most rational is that it is conveyed by the mosquito; since all those precautions that are taken against malarial infection are likewise precautions against the mosquito. He still insists upon the unity of the various forms of the plasmodium. Patrick Manson,[3] in a letter to the *Lancet,* makes a vigorous answer to Dr. Bignami, who had criticised his theory of the mosquito as an intermediate host for the malaria parasite. He declares that the movements of the flagellated form of parasite have nothing in common with the movements of dying protozoa; he also thinks that Mauritius and Reunion furnish good examples of the dissemination of malaria. The disease spread rapidly after its introduction from outside. Suctorial insects had always been present. He then takes occasion to express skepticism in regard to Bignami's hypothesis that the disease is spread directly by the mosquito from one patient to another, the organisms remaining adherent to the proboscis.

D. P. Ross[4] also retorts against Bignami's criticism in regard to Manson's theory of the vital nature of the flagellate bodies. He maintains that the only valuable argument is the absence of chromatin, but contends that this absence is by no means universally acknowledged. Against the degenerative theory he urges the other forms of degeneration that may be noted in the crescents and spheres when they are kept in sealed tubes; furthermore, he has observed flagelli in the interior of living spheres. Moreover exflagellation never occurs in dying fever-forms or crescents, and invariably occurs in forms that we might suppose to be favorable to the continued existence of the organisms. Ross has devised a number of interesting experiments, all of which tend to prove his assertion, the most important being the behavior of crescents collected under vaselin and not exposed to the air. Under these circumstances neither spheres nor flagellate bodies develop. As a final result, he concludes that spherulation is produced as the result of abstraction of water from the blood, and thinks he proves this by permitting some evaporation of the blood collected under vaselin, when the spheres develop rapidly. He therefore builds the

[1] Univ. Med. Mag., May, 1897.   [2] Rev. de Hyg., Bd. 18, No. 12.
[3] Lancet, Dec. 12, 1896.   [4] Brit. Med. Jour., Jan. 3, 1897.

theory that the flagella represent the reaction of the parasite to the increased viscidity of the media in which it finds itself, and supposes that the organism changes into this form as a result of its possibility to further development. In regard to Bignami's arguments against the mosquito water theory, Ross states that in 2 cases, after 21 experiments, he was able to produce a slight malarial reaction by administering to patients the mosquito water; and in 3 persons who had allowed themselves to be bitten by mosquitoes which had previously bitten patients in febrile condition no reaction resulted. In conclusion, he speaks of the observations of Dr. Marshall, who reported that malarial crescents become spheres after the blood is diluted with water. This Ross claims to be due to degenerative changes, and not similar to that produced by increased density of the blood.

Ross[1] has performed a number of experiments as to malarial infection. In some he allowed **mosquitoes** that had bitten malarial subjects to die in water and then gave this water to other subjects to drink; in others he allowed mosquitoes to bite first malarial and then healthy patients. The results in the 2d series were negative (3 experiments). In the others there were, on 3 occasions, slight febrile reaction and twice very doubtful parasites were found in the blood. In no case was the febrile reaction persistent.

G. M. Sternberg[2] criticises Manson's **mosquito theory** of the intermediate existence of the malarial organism, and suggests that possibly the plasmodia finds its normal habitat upon the stems of water plants, urging in favor of this view the fact that contagion does not take place when these plants are submerged and that the mosquito, whose normal food is plant juice, could easily obtain them from this situation. Intermediate hosts, if we assume the necessity for their existence, can easily be found in other animals besides man; but if the analogy of tse-tse disease of South America be accepted as valid for the malarial organism, it is probable that the mosquito merely serves as a carrier of the contagion.

Rupert Norton[3] discusses the evidence for and against the possibility of malarial infection being conveyed by **drinking-water,** and decides that all cases alleged in favor of it are at least doubtful and susceptible of other explanation.

Corinado[4] found, beside the ordinary infusoria, numerous Laveran organisms in the water of a ditch that runs through the city of Havana. He was also able to cultivate organisms taken from the blood of malarial patients in the same water. No inoculation-experiments were made.

S. F. Mayfield[5] believes that **drinking-water** invariably contains the sources of malarial infection, especially as, in those localities where the inhabitants have commenced to use artesian water exclusively, malaria has practically disappeared.

K. Winslow[6] reports the case of a woman who, for two weeks before delivery, suffered from quotidian malaria. After the child was born it seemed weak and took its nourishment badly. Examination of its blood showed the presence of plasmodia.

The Plasmodium.—J. G. McNaught[7] has studied the blood in malarial fever in Northern Deccan. He found the parasite in 50 cases, 130 examinations being made. When he found large intracorpuscular pigmented forms, the

[1] Indian Med. Rec. May 1, 1897.   [2] Am. Med. and Surg. Bull., Apr. 10, 1897.
[3] Bull. Johns Hopkins Hosp.. Mar., 1897.
[4] Cron. Med. Quir. de la Habana, 1896, No. 9.
[5] New Orl. M. and S. Jour., Aug., 1896.   [6] Boston M. and S. Jour., May 27, 1897.
[7] Brit. Med. Jour., Sept. 26, 1896.

corpuscles being swollen, he diagnosed tertian fever; but there were only 3 cases of this description. When he found hyaline intracorpuscular forms, the corpuscles not markedly enlarged and the pigmented intracorpuscular forms small and few in number, he diagnosed Summer-Autumn fever; 46 cases were of this type, and in 16 of these crescents were found. It is perhaps of some interest to note the relative frequency of the different pigmented forms. The numbers refer to separate examinations. Crescents alone occurred in 14; crescents and spheres in 17; crescents, spheres, and flagellated bodies in 12; spheres alone in 29; spheres and flagellated bodies in 4; crescents and flagellated bodies in 2; flagellated bodies only in 1.

W. B. French[1] has studied the cases of malarial fever occurring at the Washington Asylum and the Government Hospital for the Insane in the District of Columbia. Among these were 41 tertians, 50 of the estivo-autumnal, and 3 of the combined type. In 2 of the latter the tertian organism predominated. No cases of quartan infection were discovered.

W. Fisher,[2] who was stationed in upper Zambesi, found plasmodia in 40 cases of malaria, which were peculiar for the reason that none of the parasites contained any pigment. In general, the course of the disease was irregular, the attacks of fever occurring at intervals of from a few hours to several days. In some cases icterus was present without hemoglobinuria.

Hehir[3] has looked for the malarial organisms in marsh-water and has been able to stain them by fixing first with osmic-acid vapor and then using a diluted solution of Löffler's alkaline staining-fluid. An interesting observation that he has also made is the fact that the malarial organism can retain its vitality a long time after the specimen has been dried. [Unfortunately no details are given of the appearance of the organism as found outside the body.]

Symptomatology.—A. Plehn[4] describes the various forms of **acute malaria** that occur in **Cameroon.** These are the continuous, the remittent, and the intermittent types, and the blackwater fever. An effort was made in the first 3 groups to give the quinin in accordance with the results of microscopical examinations of the blood—that is, only when the small endoglobular forms were found. From 1 to 1½ gm. was given during the decline of the fever, and this sufficed to destroy the younger of the two generations that coexisted in the blood. Crescents were very rare, and only once were the flagellate forms discovered. Plehn regards these as retrogressive forms of the plasmodia, stating that they were found either in those entirely free from symptoms, or in those in whom the relapses occurred infrequently. Blackwater fever is the most frequent form in which malaria appears, and, according to the author, is due to an excessive destruction of the red blood-cells, although he admits that it is difficult to demonstrate this destruction under the microscope, the color-index being normal and poikilocytosis rare. Aside from the presence of hemoglobin, the urine is variable; albumin and tube-casts are present in some cases, but fail in others. A most important statement is that in all cases of this disease the active parasites die during the disintegration of the blood-cells. He therefore agrees with F. Plehn that quinin is superfluons, and, indeed, not without danger, because it predisposes to fresh paroxysms of corpuscular destruction.

C. E. Skinner[5] describes a fever that is endemic in the malarial regions of **Corsica.** The chief etiologic factor is exposure to cold and wet toward sundown in a region where it is common. It attacks all ages and both sexes.

[1] N. Y. Med. Jour., Apr. 24, 1897.　　　　[2] Lancet, Jan. 16, 1897.
[3] Indian Med. Rec., Feb., 1897.　　　　[4] Dissert. Berlin, 1896.
[5] N. Y. Med. Jour., Dec. 12, 1896.

The commonest forms are the remittent, continued, and frankly intermittent, the latter being usually quotidian. The prodromal symptoms consist of marked malaise lasting for a day or two, then a chill or sensation of chilliness, and, finally, a rise in temperature. Anorexia and thirst are common, and, if the disease is not promptly treated, considerable emaciation takes place. The spleen is not necessarily enlarged. The complications that have been observed are cystitis, pleurodynia, and megalosplenia, without fever. The disease usually yields readily to quinin; although this remedy, in cases of long standing, must sometimes be administered hypodermically in order to obtain any result. The prophylactic measures to be observed are to avoid Corsica between the months of April and November, to keep indoors at sunset, and to keep the windows shut at night. The author very naturally concludes that the disease is simply a peculiar form of malaria, although, most unsatisfactorily, he fails to mention the result of hematological investigations.

Doorga Das Sen [1] discusses malarial fevers of India, describing among others a **remittent fever** whose only peculiarity is that the temperature does not fall to normal. Boisson [2] reports 3 cases of malaria in the course of which **icterus** developed. He found no bile-pigment in the urine, but did find oxyhemoglobin, methemoglobin, and urobilin; he concludes that it was hemoglobinuria. Two cases were cured, in both of which there was great diminution of the red cells. Microscopically, the blood showed a small amount of black pigment partially free and partially in the leukocytes. In the third case an autopsy was made and the biliary passages found to be normal, but there were parenchymatous hepatitis and nephritis.

D. W. Torrance [3] reports a case of malaria in which the temperature reached 109.2° during the second paroxysm. Recovery occurred promptly after administration of quinin.

Lodigiani [4] holds that the ordinary form of **cirrhosis of the liver** may occur in cases of malaria. He is at variance in this view with Frerichs, Colin, and Liebermeister. This view is based upon a case of chronic malaria in which operation for enlargement of the spleen was undertaken, and the patient succumbed. At the autopsy cirrhosis of the liver was found, and this resembled that occurring in alcoholic subjects or from other causes. The author notices that some authorities have stated that the cirrhosis following malaria differs from that due to other causes. His own case does not justify this view. Regarding the cause, he holds that the products of the metabolism produced by the malarial plasmodium are the active agents. [In a case of our own in which malaria was the only likely causal factor, cirrhosis of the liver presented the ordinary appearances of the alcoholic variety.]

De Brun [5] describes the clinical forms of malarial ascites. These he separates into three distinct varieties: 1st, those resulting from malarial atrophy of the liver—in this form the liver presents, microscopically and macroscopically, all the features of the alcoholic cirrhosis of Laennock. He reports 2 cases occurring in women coming from a region where malaria is frequent in its most obstinate forms; both had suffered all their lives from various manifestations and neither had ever indulged in wine. The 2d variety results from the perisplenitis that occurs in the course of malarial splenomegaly. It is characterized by violent pains in the splenic region and by the gradual accumulation of peritoneal fluid. The 3d variety results from peritoneal congestion. It is indolent, develops insidiously, and gives rise to no subjective manifes-

---

[1] Indian Med. Rec., Nov., 1896.   [2] Gaz. hebdom. de Méd. et de Chir., No. 28, 1896.
[3] Brit. Med. Jour., May 1, 1897.   [4] Morgagni, Jan., 1896.
[5] Sem. méd., p. 344, 1896.

tations. It can be distinguished from tubercular peritonitis by the absence of abdominal pain or peritoneal friction. It yields readily to the action of quinin.

Brault[1] reports 2 cases of malarial cachexia, with hypertrophy of the liver, spleen, and heart; chronic bronchitis, and **enormous ascites.** Both suffered extremely from dyspepsia. The ordinary malarial treatment having failed, they were both treated by laparotomy and the evacuation of ascitic fluid. Improvement was immediate, and within 3 weeks both patients were out of bed. Subsequent treatment consisted, in addition to the ordinary tonics, of the extract of bone-marrow, which apparently gave very good results.

Vidal[2] has made a clinical study of **malarial cachexia** and notes particularly **hypertrophy of the heart.** The heart-sounds are feeble; often instead of a systolic bruit at the apex there is a murmur heard after the muffled second sound. These signs he attributes to myocarditis, and this he holds is largely the cause of the symptoms. He therefore advocates a form of treatment directed to the heart: diuretic medication and the employment of absolute milk-diet in those who can tolerate it. If the heart is feeble, digitalin in doses of 15 drops of a 0.1 % solution of the crystallized substance. [The use of the milk-diet in a case in which the heart is weakened by myocarditis is scarcely rational.]

Topi[3] emphasizes the importance of **lesions of the gastric mucous membrane** in malaria. Recalling the fact that gastric lesions have been met with in cases of severe pernicious anemia, he concluded that the same may occur in individuals presenting the malarial cachexia, and states that in these cases lesions of the gastric walls are not rarely found. The glands are found to be contracted and degenerated in the capillaries surrounding them—he has found, in a number of cases, large numbers of malarial parasites in various stages of development. He regards it as probable that the organism enters by way of the gastro-intestinal mucous membrane in such instances.

Diagnosis.—Wm. Osler[4] calls attention to the frequency with which malaria is diagnosed as other diseases north of Mason and Dixon's line, and other diseases are diagnosed as malaria south of this boundary. Considering the facility with which a positive diagnosis can be made by blood-examination, or by a therapeutic test, he considers it very unfortunate that this disease should be the cause of so much inaccuracy in the vital statistics. Regarding the frequency with which infection with the bacillus of Eberth and the plasmodium malariæ occurs simultaneously, he has himself observed but 1 doubtful case in 1500 patients suffering from one or the other disease.

Treatment.—Jancso and Rosenberger,[5] in a paper upon the study of blood in malarial fever, based upon 100 cases, state that the use of quinin 4 or 6 hours before the attack reduces the number of parasites quite notably 1 hour or 3 hours later. The new generation is weak and represented by a few young spherules. These are roughly granular and without ameboid movements. When quinin is given 12 to 10 hours before the attack the number of parasites diminishes, but not so notably. The remedy has least effect upon the crescents. Quinin would seem to have least effect upon the organisms that are somewhat advanced in their growth, though 23 to 40 gr. serve to destroy these. In those in which sporulation had begun the spores of only a few proved to be devitalized.

Hemorrhagic Forms.—Luke Fleming[6] records a case of malaria in a ser-

---

[1] Compt. rend. da la Soc. de Biol., Jan. 15, 1897.   [2] L'Union méd., No. 24, 1896.
[3] Gaz. degli Ospidali, No. 83, 1896.   [4] Med. News, Mar. 16, 1897.
[5] Pest. med.-chir. Presse, No. 8, 1896.   [6] Med. Rec., Sept. 19, 1896.

vant 42 years old, in which purpura hemorrhagica covering a large part of the body was the principal manifestation. There were also hemorrhages from the mucous membrane of the month and of the vagina. For 3 or 4 days before she came under observation she had suffered with symptoms of malaria and had taken 15 gr. of quinin 24 hours previous to her first visit. Hemorrhagic symptoms soon appeared. The quinin in large doses was discontinued, and arsenic with Warburg's tincture was given instead. After a convalescence of 2 weeks she recovered. Five months later she suffered with malaria, and the same symptoms occurred on attempting to check the disease with quinin. The hemorrhages did not appear until the drug had been administered. The following summer she came under observation for the third time suffering with malaria. The author himself administered quinin to determine whether it was the cause of hemorrhage, and found that bleeding soon followed its administration. [Similar observations have frequently been made, especially in tropical climates, and some writers condemn quinin entirely. Cases in point are the following:]

C. D. Simmons[1] reports 3 cases of **hemorrhagic malaria** occurring in **pregnancy.** In the 1st case he administered quinin in spite of the fact that the patient stated that this drug had increased the hemorrhage in a previous attack. The next day the disease was more pronounced and the quinin was abandoned. Calomel followed by arsenic and digitalis was ordered and the patient gradually improved. In the 2d case, a woman who had chronic splenic enlargement was seized very suddenly with the symptoms of hemorrhagic malaria. Quinin was given freely during 2 days without good effects; arsenic and digitalis were also administered. There were no alarming symptoms until without warning the uterus expelled its contents. The patient died. In the 3d case the uterus was irritable and the author therefore administered morphin. The attack was cut short and the patient finally recovered, the pregnancy continning. The author believes that when abortion or premature labor comes on death is almost sure to follow. Quinin he believes to be useless and often harmful in this form of malaria. In the acute forms with chills and fever pronounced and regularly recurring, and when the kidneys are active, quinin often does good.

Baccelli[2] discusses **hemoglobinuria** in its relations to malaria. In 1 group the hemoglobinuria is due to malarial infection and is cured by the administration of quinin; in another group the hemoglobinuria is independent of malarial infection and may be due to the quinin administered. In the latter cases individual idiosyncrasy is important. He offers no explanation of the mode in which this is brought about. The treatment of hemoglobinuria must be active. The author has found the persulphate of iron combined with inhalations of oxygen and careful hygienic regulations most useful.

W. D. Bush[3] and H. Meek[4] object to the administration of quinin in malarial hematuria.

Naame[5] has treated 5 cases of malarial cachexia with hypodermic injections of **citrate of iron.** Four cases recovered completely. The 5th was greatly improved; but, probably on account of extreme sclerosis and hypertrophy of the spleen, it was impossible to restore the blood to the normal condition; 2 of the cases were examined 2 months after discharge and found to be well.

Celli and Santoni[6] have employed the **serum** of animals that had been exposed to malarial infection in the neighborhood of Rome, for the pro-

[1] New Orl. M. and S. Jour., Oct., 1896.
[2] Gaz. degli Osped. e delle Clin., Feb. 15, 1897.   [3] Med. Rec., Aug. 8, 1896.
[4] Therap. Gaz., May 15, 1897.   [5] Rev. de Méd. de Paris, Mar. 10, 1897.
[6] Centralbl. f. Bakt. Parasit. u. Infek., Jan. 20, 1897.

duction of immunity. In the first series of experiments they injected 6 individuals that had never had malaria with 10 c.c. of serum at intervals of several days for some weeks, the serum being obtained from buffaloes, oxen, and a horse. At the end of this time 3 were inoculated with blood from a quartan case, and a control-person was inoculated at the same time. In the inoculated subjects fever occurred after 6 and 17 days. In the control-patient it occurred on the second day. Three were also inoculated with the parasite of the estivo-autumnal type. Fever did not occur until 25 days later, and at first was very light. As the longest hitherto recorded incubation-period for this type was 15 days, they ascribe the delay to the treatment. Finally, a family that was compelled to live in an excessively malarial district was treated with this serum, and but one member was attacked by malaria; in a neighboring family, not treated with the serum, all the members were attacked. [It seems doubtful, in spite of the success of these investigators, whether much can be expected from serum-therapy in malaria.]

Treille[1] has employed **Roux's serum** in 2 cases of quartan fever. In the first case there were 2 subsequent rises of temperature and then complete cure. The second case, even after a second injection, showed no beneficial result.

General Considerations upon Infectious Diseases and Fever.—G. M. Sternberg[2] classifies **infectious diseases**, according to the mode of infection, into (*a*) traumatic; (*b*) infection by contact; (*c*) infection through ingesta; (*d*) infection through the respiratory tract; according to the nature of the infections agent, into diseases due to infection by vegetable parasites and those due to infection by the animal parasites; and finally, according to the special tissues of the organs involved, into general blood-infections and localized infections.

Lode[3] has performed a number of experiments upon animals in order to test whether **diminution of the bodily temperature** produces susceptibility to infection. Diminution of the temperature was obtained in 3 ways. First, the animals were shaved, heated, and then exposed to a current of air, or they were simply shaved, or they were simply exposed to influences diminishing bodily temperature. Guinea-pigs, rats, and chickens were employed, the two latter being used for experiments with the anthrax-bacillus; the other organisms tested were the pneumobacillus of Friedländer, the vibrio of cholera, the staphylococcus pyogenes aureus, and sputum containing numerous tubercle-bacilli. The results in general were that, of 99 animals, 54 artificially cooled and 45 used for control, 46 of the former and 9 of the latter died from the infectious process, and 8 of the former and 36 of the latter survived. Of 9 animals exposed to air laden with tubercle-bacilli, the 5 cooled animals died, and of the control-animals, 2 died and 2 survived. As a result, Lode concludes that animals so treated are more susceptible to artificial infection than normal animals handled in the same manner.

[The author proceeds next to the consideration of various theories that may be advanced in explanation of the facts he demonstrated. We are less interested for the present in this side of the question. It is of greatest moment to have actual demonstration of an old belief that reduction of temperature causes increased susceptibility to infection. There has been an expansion of this thought of late, to the effect that authors assign a distinct conservative property to fever. This is seen in the following :]

Löwy and Richter[4] contribute an experimental paper on the **curative influence of fever** from which certain deductions regarding treatment seem proper. They injected certain microorganisms into animals in which artificial

[1] Sem. méd., 1896, p. 312.
[3] Arch. f. Hyg., vol. xxviii., H. 4, 1897.
[2] Am. Jour. Med. Sci., Dec., 1896.
[4] Berlin. klin. Woch., Mar. 1, 1897.

fever had been induced, and noted the results as compared with control-animals not previously rendered febrile. The artificial fever was produced by puncture of the corpus striatum, rabbits being used. The fever following this is marked by elevation of temperature, increased destruction of tissue, and increased respiratory exchange; but differs from ordinary fever in that the animals seem well and preserve their appetite. It is, therefore, analogous with the so-called aseptic fever. They used cultures of the pneumococci, of the microorganisms of fowl cholera, and of hog cholera. They also injected the toxin of diphtheria. In the case of pneumococci they found that life was preserved from 1 to 3 days longer in the febrile than in the healthy animals; in 2 cases the trephined animals survived the infection, which in 1 case was caused by 4 times the fatal dose. In the experiments with hog cholera the increased length of life was from 3 to 4 days, and 1 animal survived. The experiments with chicken cholera were unsatisfactory, probably because the virulence of the organism was so great that very small doses sufficed to kill the animal, and the minimal dose could not be ascertained. When diphtheric toxin was used life was preserved 1 to 3 days longer in the febrile animals, and 1 of them recovered.

The authors do not deny that an objection might be offered to their work on the ground that this artificial fever is not, after all, natural fever; but they point out that it resembles natural fever in several particulars, and the definition of the term fever is still uncertain. They conclude, therefore, that, with this reservation, it may be said that fever does exercise a curative influence, and that the administration of remedies merely to reduce the fever, without regard to their other actions, is not justified. The favorable action of quinin in malaria and of salicylate of sodium in rheumatism is connected with the specific action of these remedies rather than with their antipyretic action, and the same may be said of the beneficial influence of cold bathing, the more important influence being that exercised upon the nervous system, circulation, and the respiration. They particularly hold that the artificial hyperleukocytosis induced by cold may play an important part in combating infection. [Clinicians have frequently maintained that fever is often a conservative process, and that its reduction may be harmful in some cases. This contention, however, has always been answered by the objection that antipyretic drugs used in the reduction of the temperature may have been the real cause of untoward symptoms. The facts brought out in the present paper are not entirely new and do not as yet definitely settle the question.]

Blumreich and Jacoby [1] found that animals from which the **spleen** had been removed exhibited greatly increased resistance to injections of virulent living bacilli, but the reaction to injections of toxins was unaltered.

Piccinino [2] has performed some experiments upon animals in order to test the influence of the **nervous system** upon the susceptibility to infection, using dogs refractory to tuberculosis, cutting the vagi nerves, and then subjecting them to tubercular infection. The results were negative.

H. A. Hare [3] advocates the **intravenous injection of saline solutions** for the purpose of washing the blood in toxemic conditions, and reports 2 cases, 1 of acute toxemia and 1 of uremia, in which it produced excellent results. The first case, however, died of gangrene.

[1] Berlin. klin. Woch., May 24, 1897.   [2] Riforma Med., Nos. 11, 12, 1896.
[3] Therap. Gaz., Apr. 15, 1897.

CONSTITUTIONAL DISEASES.

Rheumatism.—Etiology.—Chauffard and Ramon [1] report certain examinations to determine the infectiousness of articular rheumatism. They examined the glands in the neighborhood of the affected joints, and found that sometimes those in the immediate neighborhood became swollen at the time of the attack. In most of the cases there was some pain in the glands, and at times the enlargement was so considerable that the patients themselves noticed it, and also that it increased with exacerbations of the disease. Cultures made on various media from 1 of the cases were negative, but cover-slips from the fluid in the joint and from the neighboring enlarged glands both showed a bacillus. The authors regard the glandular condition as evidence of the infectiousness of rheumatism. [A majority of modern writers agree with this view, but we must refer to the great variance in the bacteriologic studies. The authors quoted above and others presently to be referred to find bacilli, whereas many previous investigators report the discovery of micrococci of various kinds. No reliance can, therefore, be placed on any of the claims to the discovery of the specific cause.]

Jaccoud [2] discusses the infectious nature of rheumatism, pointing out that local lesions of some kind or other have frequently been found preceding rheumatism, and that these may constitute the nidus from which the infection has occurred. Tonsillitis is by far the most common, and he calls particular attention to the fact that the microorganisms found in the pharynx are the same as those seen in the diseased tissues. He refers to a case in which a wound of the foot seemed to be the exciting cause. He believes the infectious nature of the disease to be beyond doubt, taking into consideration its mode of development, its character, and the occurrence of intrauterine transmission. In this connection he refers to a case in which a mother suffering from a severe attack of rheumatism gave birth to a child, which, in 12 hours developed fever, swelling, and pain in the joints; under treatment with salicylate of sodium the symptoms subsided. [As an illustration of the connection or coincidence of local lesions and the development of rheumatism we may cite a recent case in which violent polyarticular arthritis involving many of the large and some of the small joints occurred in a boy of 18 who had received a wound of the hand which was badly treated. When he was admitted to the hospital a wound was found which had been sutured, but was almost hidden from view by a filthy crust. On removal of the stitches about a dram of pus escaped. The patient had decidedly irregular fever and marked symptoms of general infection with glandular enlargement. After relief of the local lesion antirheumatic treatment caused speedy recovery.]

Achalme [3] has examined the body of a woman dying of acute articular rheumatism, making anaërobic cultures of the blood, the cerebrospinal and the articular fluid, and found a bacillus similar to that described by him in 1891.

Thiroloix [4] has examined the blood of two persons suffering from acute articular rheumatism. Anaërobic cultures were made, and in both cases there was a voluminous growth, which was found to consist of pure cultures of an anaërobic bacillus, slightly motile, which stained by Gram's method and was pathogenic for guinea-pigs, but not for dogs, rabbits, or mice. He holds that it is identical with the bacillus already described by Achalme.

---

[1] Rev. de Méd., Sept., 1896.   [2] Jour. de Méd., Feb. 10, 1897.
[3] Compt. rend. de la Soc. de Biol., Mar. 17, 1897.   [4] Ibid., Mar. 19, 1897.

In a discussion in the Congress for Internal Medicine in Berlin [1] Chvostek held that not only was acute articular rheumatism not a microorganismal disease, but that in fact there was no such disease, a number of conditions being included under this name. Singer, on the contrary, investigated 92 cases and frequently found streptococci and staphylococci in the urine. In 3 cases upon which autopsies were obtained he was able to find the same bacteria in 2. He holds that the pyogenic cocci are causes of the disease. Schuller has also found bacteria, particularly a form that caused villous swelling in the joints of rabbits. Michaelis reported that in 3 cases of endocarditis following rheumatism a diplococcus was found in the blood that could be cultivated upon blood-serum. In no case in Leyden's clinic was it possible to find bacteria either in the blood or joints.

McClymont [2] believes that the opinion that men are more frequently affected than women with acute articular rheumatism is probably incorrect. When the disease is hereditary it is usually derived from the mother.

Complications.—Widal and Sicard [3] report a case suffering from recurrence of generalized polyarticular rheumatism. On the 31st day a sudden rise of temperature occurred; edema developed in the right arm, which gradually extended upward until it involved the shoulder. Palpation showed thickening of the humoral vein. At the autopsy this proved, as was expected, to be a **thrombosis of the vein** extending into the finest radicles of the hand.

Steiner [4] calls attention to a complication of acute articular rheumatism that he claims has been hitherto seriously neglected. This consists of a **multiple peripheral perineuritis,** which may be subordinate to severe inflammation of the joints or else itself form the most prominent clinical manifestation, joint-affection being simply indicated by pain without swelling or other signs of inflammation. Of the first group he has observed 28 cases in which one or more joints were acutely involved, and many of the peripheral nerves were exquisitely sensitive to pressure. Of the second group he found 7 cases in which the nerve-involvement was exceedingly general. As none of these cases died, it was impossible to make any investigations in regard to the pathology of the disease; but he is inclined to believe that it is a perineuritis.

W. H. Washburn [5] reports 5 cases, with 3 autopsies, of **pulmonary complications** in acute rheumatism. The postmortem findings were: in 1 case bericarditis with edema of the lungs; in another acute catarrh of the lungs; and in the 3d congestion and edema. In the 4th case the patient died with symptoms of edema of the lungs, but no autopsy was obtained.

F. Krauss [6] reports a case of acute articular rheumatism, limited to the right side, occurring in a girl of 16, who subsequently developed **chorea,** also limited to the right side and associated with a rise of temperature.

M. L. B. Rodd [7] reports a case of acute articular rheumatism in which, after the temperature had become normal under salicylates, there was a sudden rise to 110° F. In spite of the ice-pack the **hyperpyrexia** persisted until death.

V. Hanot [8] includes among some of the varieties of acute articular rheumatism those which commence with syncope without localized symptoms, and those whose initial symptoms are purely visceral.

Salman [9] reports a case of scarlet fever that after a normal course was fol-

[1] Centralbl. f. innere Med., June 26, 1897.		[2] Lancet, Nov. 21, 1896.
[3] Sem. méd., p. 321, 1896.		[4] Deutsch. Arch. f klin. Med., Mar. 15, 1897.
[5] Chicago Clin. Rev., July, 1896.		[6] Med. News, July 25, 1896.
[7] Brit. Med. Jour., May 8, 1897.		[8] Presse méd., Dec. 2, 1896.
[9] Deutsch. med. Woch., Dec. 24, 1896.

lowed first by acute nephritis. After this was cured the fever continued, and the joints of the right upper extremity showed an apparently serous exudate and excessive pain upon movement. Later the hip and knee became also involved—the former undergoing spontaneous luxation, the latter presenting the appearance of tumor albus. Salman believes that the disease was infectious, but excludes tuberculosis on account of the rapidity and completeness of the cure that took place in the hip through ankylosis as soon as the process ceased to advance. Salicylates were not used until late in the disease, when they gave immediate relief to the pain and produced marked improvement in the general condition.

Diagnosis.—G. Parker [1] discusses the various diseases which have recently been differentiated from rheumatism, and enumerates (1) Henoch's purpura, of which he reports an interesting case that commenced with sharp pain in the gastric region, followed by swelling of the wrists and then vomiting and diarrhea. Later there was edematous swelling over the right side of the scalp and later a purpuric eruption upon the legs. Salicylates had no effect, and no satisfactory cause could be discovered. (2) Angioneurotic edema, of which he also reports a case; (3) rheumatoid arthritis; (4) the various septic arthritides and the joint-affections that occur in infectious endocarditis. Finally, he speaks of the hemorrhagic diseases—hemophilia, erythema multiforme, and purpura hemorrhagica.

Treatment.—Boucheron [2] believes that, in addition to the bacillus of Achalme, staphylococci and streptococci invade the organism in acute rheumatism. In accordance with this theory he has used Marmorek's antistreptococcic serum in 6 cases with excellent results. [The number of cases is too small to furnish reliable data. All efforts in the direction of serum-therapy, using serum of convalescent patients, have thus far failed.]

E. Lee [3] recommends hydrotherapy for rheumatism, using the following methods: (1) the administration of pure, soft water at frequent intervals, about 4 liters being given to an average man per day; (2) irrigation of the intestinal tract with water to which a little liquid soap has been added; (3) thorough moistening of the body, either by bathing, the wet pack, or by sprinkling. [It seems to us that the second element of this treatment at least might well be omitted.]

Jaccoud,[4] in discussing the **contraindications** of the treatment of acute articular rheumatism with **salicylic acid,** states that he never gives the drug in the presence of endocarditis, believing, as he does, that it only exercises an influence upon the articular manifestations of the poison. This limitation of its use applies also to the other internal viscera.

Soulages [5] reports a case of acute articular rheumatism treated with **electric currents** of high frequency. After the first 2 or 3 applications the pain was greatly diminished, and subsequently complete cure obtained.

J. R. Philpots [6] recommends **methylen-blue** in acute articular rheumatism, claiming that it has a favorable effect upon the local inflammatory process in the joints and upon the general condition of the patients.

Myositis.—Risse [7] reports a case of "acute polymyositis" that followed several attacks of acute articular rheumatism. The disease involved first the right, then the left leg, and spread slowly upward by a strictly continuous process until it involved also the muscles of the abdomen. The affected

---

[1] Lancet, June 26, 1897. [2] Compt. rend. de la Soc. de Biol., April 9, 1897.
[3] Jour. Am. Med. Assoc., July 25, 1896. [4] Sem. méd., p. 431, 1896.
[5] Compt. rend. de la Soc. de Biol., July 11, 1896.
[6] Brit. Med. Jour., March 27, 1897. [7] Deutsch. med. Woch., April 8, 1897.

muscles were swollen, painful, hard, and the skin over them edematous. After recovery had taken place a moderate degree of muscular wasting was observable, but the muscular power was apparently unimpaired.

Laquer[1] reports a case that at various times within the course of 15 years presented a marked **swelling of the right upper arm.** This was accompanied by the symptoms of inflammation—that is, pain, reddening, and edema, and the general symptoms of fever and malaise. The only treatment that seemed to be of use in any of the cases was a deep incision through the periosteum. On one occasion a portion of the muscle was excised and examined, but appeared to be normal. The author regards the disease as an acute intermittent interstitial monomyositis. As all forms of intoxication could be excluded, he believes that it is probably due to an infectious poison which may be similar to that of rheumatism.

RHEUMATOID ARTHRITIS.

Chauffard and Ramond[2] found disease of the **lymphatic glands** in the neighborhood of the affected joints in 7 cases of chronic deforming polyarthritis. These were sensitive, particularly when the joints were painful, and showed alterations in size. In 1 case bacteriologic investigation was made of the contents of one of the joints, and a diplococcus was found that did not decolorize by Gram's method. It was impossible to cultivate it.

Potain[3] points out that **the deformities** that occur in rheumatoid arthritis may be due to alterations in the extremities of the bones and to abnormal muscular action. The thickening of the head of the bone may impede the movement, but does not cause ankylosis. The ligaments are rarely involved, though they are sometimes relaxed. The irregular swelling of the bones is only an accessory cause of the deformity, the contraction of the muscles with paresis or atony of certain groups being the principal cause. Then loss of muscular power is not dependent upon nerve-changes, but probably is reflex, as is suggested by the fact that sometimes similar paresis occurs in cases of traumatic injuries of the joints.

G. A. Bannatyne[4] remarks that marked anemia is seldom found in **rheumatoid arthritis** except in the advanced and acute cases, but he has found a slight amount of blood deficiency in about 95 per cent. of the cases. Hemorrhages due to anemia are rare, but he refers to a case under his care, in a woman of 22, with advanced rheumatoid arthritis, in whom hematemesis developed without obvious gastric disease. The blood showed the following characteristics : red corpuscles 4,000,000 to 3,000,000 ; hemoglobin 80 to 40 % ; slight leukocytosis ; the red corpuscles varied in size and shape, but there were no microcytes or erythroblasts. The hemoglobin seemed to be less firmly attached to the stroma ; it crystallized out very readily and was more easily acted upon by such substances as common salt, acetic acid, and sulphate of sodium in solution.

Treatment.—W. K. Sibley[5] reports a case of arthritis deformans treated by the Tallerman-Sheffield localized hot-air apparatus. After 9 baths the patient was able to resume her former occupation of dressmaker, and after 20 baths considered herself cured. [Others have reported favorable results in the same condition. In our own experience with some half dozen cases the effect of the baths was only temporary, and even then often slight. There was not the least general or lasting improvement.]

[1] Deutsch. med. Woch., No. 28, 1896.   [2] Rev. de Méd., Bd. 16, p. 345, 1896.
[3] Sem. méd., Dec. 18, 1896.   [4] Lancet, Nov. 28, 1896.
                        [5] Ibid., Aug., 1896.

W. E. Burtless [1] suggests the treatment of chronic articular rheumatism with **plaster-of-Paris casts,** using the following *modus operandi:* the joints are packed in hot mineral water, and kept so during an entire night; the cast is then permitted to remain from 6 to 24 hours, according to the endurance of the patient, removed, and the joints of the leg thoroughly kneaded. He reports a case that had been suffering for 3 years, in which perfect cure was obtained.

W. Armstrong [2] has used **methylen-blue** in rheumatoid arthritis and found that it was particularly valuable in those forms due to autointoxication from the intestinal tract.

PULMONARY OSTEO-ARTHROPATHY.

[We consider this condition in this place from the conviction that it is caused by toxemia, and that it is akin to rheumatoid arthritis in this respect. Furthermore, the clinical features require differential diagnosis from rheumatoid diseases, and are therefore advantageously considered here.]

H. G. Godlee [3] holds that the cases described under the name pulmonary osteo-arthropathy, or under the formidable title bestowed on these conditions by Marie in 1890, form a heterogeneous group of diverse conditions. He analyzes the symptoms as they have been described by Marie and others, and refers in particular to the conditions found about the ends of the bones. The hand proper is said not to depart perceptibly as regards size from the normal hand, except that there may be a little hypertrophy of the ends of the metacarpal bones possibly due to some thickening of the soft parts in the neighborhood. Where this occurs, as it certainly did in some cases that have

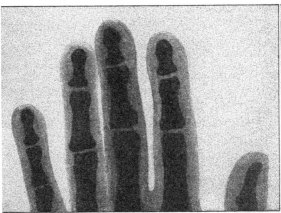

FIG. 1.—From a skiagram of the fingers of a marked case of pulmonary osteo-arthropathy (Brit. Med. Jour., Apr 24, 1897).

come under his observation, though most observers deny its existence, it is most difficult to estimate the size of the subjacent bones. The Röntgen rays alone will prove satisfactory in the absence of postmortem examinations. He

[1] Am. Med. and Surg. Bull., Nov. 28, 1896.   [2] Brit. Med. Jour, April 24, 1897.
[3] Ibid., July, 1896.

alludes to a few postmortem examinations recorded in the literature, quoted from Thorburn. Ranzier records an instance in a man who had a chronic empyema for 14 years before his death. Enlargement of the hands, feet, and wrist was noted, especially during the last 5 years of life. At the postmortem examination ulceration of the cartilages and slight excess of synovial fluid were found in the knee and elbow. The articular extremities of the bones were large, as were also the bones of the tarsus and carpus. There was, however, congenital enlargement in this case and also in the patient's father. Bamberger reports 11 cases of swollen joints associated with pulmonary and heart disease. In 5 of 7 in which postmortem examinations were made some periostitis was found near the articular ends of the bones. In a case reported by Thérèse there was osteoperiostitis with condensing and rarefying ostitis and great proliferation of the medullary elements. G. also considers the confused relationship of osteo-arthropathy and acromegaly, and reports a number of cases under his own observation, some of which he holds are certain cases and some doubtful. Two of his cases, in which marked clubbing of the fingers was observed, showed no decided change in the bones of the fingers, and 1 of them no change at all. He is convinced that there are at least two conditions included under the title osteo-arthropathie hypertrophiante pneumonique, and that those which he has met with are examples of the form associated with chronic septic suppuration complicated with clubbing of the fingers. The latter, he thinks, has nothing whatever to do with the disease. [The author, it seems to us, underestimates the bony changes and overestimates the part played by the soft tissues in producing the deformity of the ends of the fingers, etc.]

Walton [1] reviews the subject of osteo-arthropathy and abstracts 65 cases reported in the literature. He separates 3 groups : (1) typical osteo-arthropathy with bone-changes and a peculiar form of club-fingers ; (2) cases in which only the clubbed fingers have been noted ; (3) mixed cases, embracing those in which the enlargement of the extremities appears to have been primary and others of uncertain nature, in which insufficient details prevent proper classification. He notes, as the characteristics of the typical cases, a history of previous thoracic disease with peculiar clubbing of the ends of the fingers and toes and bony enlargements mainly of the articular ends of the long bones, effusion and other changes near the joints, these being roughly symmetrical ; then hypertrophy of the adjacent soft parts, and other less frequent features, including dermal, vascular, urinary, and other symptoms. The peculiarities of the fingers are the hypertrophy of the bones and the peculiar clubbing of the ends. The nail is curved in both directions and the root is long and mobile. The body is striated, furled, pink or cyanotic in color, and brittle ; the growth is abnormally rapid. The thumb, middle finger, and great toe are mainly affected. Of the bony changes the most characteristic are those of the phalanges, heads of the metacarpal and metatarsal bones, the lower ends of the radius, ulna, and fibula. The bones about the elbow and knees may be affected, and, less frequently, the outer end of the clavicle, the acromion process of the scapulæ, the ribs, the iliac crests, and the vertebræ. The main changes are referred to the periosteum and the subjacent bone. The disease may be progressive, or there may be paroxysmal changes with stationary intervals. There is no tendency to suppuration or necrosis. Clinically, there is no pain, and the joint-effusions are similarly sluggish. In discussing the cause he notes that the vast majority of cases follow empyema or bronchiectasis, and most of the remainder follow phthisis. It is likely, therefore, that

[1] St. Thomas's Hosp. Rep., vol. xxiv., 1897.

some change in the blood or liquids of the body is the cause, and he concludes that certain poisons of the nature of toxins or ferments, not necessarily identical in different cases, are the direct cause.

Teleky[1] reports 2 cases of hypertrophic osteo-arthropathy. The first of these was a shoemaker, 40 years of age, who had had an attack of dysentery 2 years before his admission to the hospital. The lungs were absolutely negative; the heart slightly hypertrophied; there was slight kyphoskoliosis in the dorsal region; the end-phalanges of the fingers were increased in all diameters; the lower part of the forearm was broader than normal; and the toes were also, though to less extent, enlarged. The subjective symptoms consisted of severe pains in the joints. Specific treatment produced no effect. As the pneumonic element was entirely lacking, Teleky therefore concludes that the dysentery, being a suppurative disease, had some connection with the causation. The second patient was 40 years of age, and suffered from advanced pulmonary tuberculosis and great cachexia; however, about 10 years before his admission to the hospital the end-phalanges of 2 fingers that had been injured became enlarged to such an extent that they interfered with his work. When examined the drumstick alteration of the fingers was very marked, and they were greatly increased in thickness. When examined by the Röntgen rays the bones gave the appearance as if their thickness had been increased by fine exostosis upon the surface. Although the pneumonic element was evident in this case, nevertheless the enlargement seems to have commenced as a result of severe traumatism before the pulmonary disease developed. Based upon these cases and a number of others collected from the literature, the author suggests the following classification of the causes of this condition: (1) diseases in which suppuration and gangrenous decomposition occur in the organism; (2) infectious diseases and chronic intoxications; (3) heart-lesions, especially congenital; (4) malignant tumors; (5) diseases of the nervous system, such as syringomyelia and neuritis; and suggests in the place of the term proposed by Marie that of secondary hyperplastic osteitis. [It seems to us that the author confuses several distinct conditions. Mere clubbing of the fingers does not constitute Marie's disease.]

F. H. Westmacott[2] states that the postmortem examination of cases of hypertrophic pulmonary osteo-arthropathy showed almost universal osseous and articular change. The limb bones were covered with a rough, finely porous layer of subperiosteal bone, specially marked in the long bones and at the attachments of the muscles and fasciæ, and in nearly all cases confined to the diaphyses. The cartilages of the joints were almost invariably eroded, especially at the margins. The viscera showed a general but subdued tuberculosis. The liver and spleen were amyloid. The present case supports the theory of Thorburn that the disease is a mild tuberculous osteoperiostitis.

Guerin and Etienne[3] have examined the condition of the urine in cases of hypertrophic pulmonary osteo-arthropathy for lime, urea, magnesium, and phosphates. There were, from time to time, marked deviations from the normal during the period of examination. The quantity of lime reached double the normal on many days for the period of 4 months, but after that diminished and became less than normal. The quantity of magnesium did not vary markedly. The phosphates were always extremely low and urea was present in minimum normal amounts. The authors believe that this examination justifies the view that in the first period of the disease the bone becomes decalcified. They explain the enlargement of the ends of the bones as being due to second-

[1] Wien. klin. Woch., Feb. 11, 1897.   [2] Brit. Med. Jour., Oct. 3, 1896.
[3] Arch. de Méd. expériment., July, 1896.

ary ossification following the primary process, this period being that in which the lime reaches its minimum excretion.

GOUT.

Etiology and Pathology.—Malfatti[1] subjects the theory of Kolisch, who looked upon bodies of the uric-acid group as of considerable influence in connection with gout, to severe criticism. He denies that the alloxur bodies, or even the total nitrogen, is increased during a gouty attack. In fact, in the only investigation that he was able to make himself the total nitrogen for 24 hours during an interval was 12.33 gm., while during the attack it was but 10.8 gm. Phosphoric acid, however, showed a reduction of from 2.8 to 1.023 gm. As the formation of uric acid in the kidney seems to be exceedingly questionable, the transformation of xanthin bodies into uric acid there seems still less probable. Malfatti then undertook to see what would be the influence of renal extract upon the transformation of the xanthin bases found in the spleen, and his results were negative. He therefore concludes that the only explanation of gout that is at present possible is that it is a process in which the normal metabolism is so changed that the excretion of nitrogen no longer corresponds to the ingestion; but that periodically nitrogen is excreted in excessive quantities and at other times retained in the body. As, however, the slight increase in the body-weight in the latter condition does not permit us to assume the deposition of the nitrogen in the form of albumin, we must always suspect other nitrogenous combinations. In the former condition we must suspect renal insufficiency in relation to these bodies, or rather a congenital or an acquired increase of the normal irritation-point at which these combinations in the circulating blood are excreted.

Rommel[2] also objects to the theory of Kolisch, that the excretion of alloxur bodies is increased in gout. He calls attention to the failure of various investigators to find this condition, and has himself failed to discover it in a typical case of chronic gout. On the other hand, he has found an abnormal amount of the alloxur bodies in the urine of a patient without symptoms of gout, and with the characteristic symptoms of contracted kidney.

A. E. Garrod[3] takes occasion to disagree with both Klemperer and Kolisch in regard to the pathology of gout; holding that, as yet, the only firmly established facts are the excess of uric acid in the blood and the deposition of urates in the tissues.

Laquer,[4] in alluding to recent works upon the excretion of **uric acid and alloxins** in gout and other conditions, calls attention to the fact that the method of Krüger and Wulf, now so commonly relied upon, is often fallacious. In proof of this he cites his recent experiences, which give quite paradoxical figures. The author points out that the alloxins and uric acid are estimated by first determining the alloxin nitrogen in the precipitated alloxins and then the uric-acid nitrogen by the Salkowski-Ludwig method, and subtracting the latter from the former. In his own figures it happened a number of times that the latter figure was greater than the former, showing that some error must exist in the method employed; further, he denies the significance of the excretion of alloxins as indicating pathological processes. [The uncertainty in this and other methods probably accounts for the varying results of different investigators.]

[1] Wien. klin. Woch., Aug. 6, 1896.   [2] Deutsch. Arch. f. klin. Med., H. 1 and 2.
[3] Practitioner, Sept., 1896.   [4] Centralbl. f. innere Med., Oct. 31, 1896.

A. Luff[1] holds that uric acid is not normally present in the blood, but is produced by the kidneys. However, in gouty conditions it may be formed in excess, and then appear in the blood as soluble sodium quadriurite. Gout is probably always preceded by some affection of the kidneys. In regard to the treatment, he does not think that the reaction of the blood increases or decreases the tendency to deposition of the uric acid, but that the solubility is considerably increased by the presence of the saline constituents of vegetables, and diminished by the presence of the saline constituents of meat.

Futcher[2] contributes a paper on the relations of the perinuclear basophilic granules of Neusser and the excretion of alloxins. He believes that the bodies in question probably represent results of karyorrhexis rather than specific products, and he was able to produce them artificially by subjecting pieces of tissue to a temperature of 40° C. He has observed clinically that the number of granules varies very greatly in different diseases, and in the same disease, and often in apparently healthy persons, from time to time. To determine the exact relation between the occurrence of these bodies and the excretion of alloxins he made careful studies of the metabolism in 8 individuals. These studies showed that there is no regular coincidence between the number of perinuclear granules and excessive excretion of the substances named, nor a strict confinement of the occurrence of these granules to cases of alloxin-diathesis. Very abundant granulations were sometimes found with relatively small quantities of alloxins, and the reverse.

Cornillon[3] reports a case of gout that appeared after dislocation of a shoulder-joint, another after sudden muscular effort, and a third 3 months after severe contusion. He believes that the **injury** was the direct cause of the development of the disease.

Symptoms.—A. Haig[4] discusses the effect of certain diets on the excretion of uric acid, showing by tables the relative as well as the actual quantities of uric acid and urea. He still holds that the uric acid taken in the food constitutes the bulk of the uric acid eliminated; and he concludes that the avoidance of animal food containing xanthin-compounds or uric acid, and also tea, coffee, and cocoa, whose alkaloids are similar xanthin-compounds, will gradually eliminate excess of uric acid in the system. The time when this is accomplished may be determined by administering a dose of salicylate of sodium. If any of the excess of uric acid still remain in the system, this drug will cause an immediate great increase of the uric acid as compared with the urea. His rule is that, if any one taking a dose of salicylate of sodium gets as a result an excretion of uric acid greatly above the relation to urea of 1 to 30, such person is not free from uric acid.

C. E. Nammack[5] reports a case of chronic gout and one of rheumatoid arthritis with Röntgen-ray illustrations of the hands of the patients. These show very clearly the essential difference between the two conditions. In gout the joints are surrounded by splint-like deposits of crystals of sodium urate and the bones do not present exostoses.

A. L. Fisk[6] also reports a case of gout, with skiagraph.

W. Wade[7] calls attention to the frequency with which **periarticular neuritis** may be observed in gout, and rather doubts that the attack itself is necessarily due to the deposit of urates in the joints, having observed these deposits in joints that presented no symptoms and found them absent in those that had been repeatedly attacked.

[1] Brit. Med. Jour., Mar. 27, 1897.   [2] Centralbl. f. innere Med., Sept. 26, 1896.
[3] Program. méd., Jan. 29, 1897.   [4] Brit. Med. Jour., Oct. 3, 1896.
[5] Med. Rec., Apr. 24, 1897.   [6] Med. News, Apr. 17, 1897.
                    [7] Brit. Med. Jour., Feb. 27, 1897.

Kittel [1] reports 4 cases of deposition of urates in the soles of the feet, which he looks upon as an irregular form of gout.

Diagnosis.—W. H. Thomson [2] has compared 34 cases of gout with 49 cases of rheumatism. In the former the attack is more apt to be monarticular, the pulse is almost invariably of high tension, tophi can be occasionally observed, and in all cases of inflammation of the joints the points of greatest tenderness to pressure were the condyles or malleoli. In the latter disease the pulse is most frequently of low tension, the heart is commonly affected; a number of cases exhibit tonsillitis or pleurisy, and the first attack is nearly always polyarticular. When the joint is acutely inflamed there is much more superficial tenderness, and at the same time there are points of special sensitiveness, usually situated over the tendons in most immediate relation to the joints. When the hips and shoulders are affected it is exceedingly difficult to make out special points of tenderness in either condition.

Treatment.—Levison [3] agrees with Kolisch that renal degeneration is an important element in the causation of the disease, and he advocates the exclusion of thymus gland, liver, kidney, and pancreas from the diet. Further, he objects to yolks of eggs, as these, according to Kossel, contain notable quantities of paranuclein. He also is favorable to the employment of **electricity,** using a battery of 48 large Leclanché cells, and applying the positive pole connected with a carbon electrode in a 2% solution of lithium chlorid rendered alkaline with lithium carbonate, and the carbon negative electrode in a very weak solution of sodium chlorid. The part of the body treated is placed in the lithium bath and a convenient part, as a hand or a foot, in the salt solution, while a current of 10, 20, or 30 ma. is passed for 30 minutes. In 10 of 15 cases he found useful results, the joints becoming more pliable and the pains subsiding. He believes that the lithium is disassociated by the electric action and carried into the body in available form.

John Fawcett [4] has analyzed the urine in 13 cases of gout, and has studied the effects of **colchicum** and **salicylate of sodium.** The total acid and the daily excretion of urea and uric acid were determined. The amount of uric acid was distinctly subnormal between acute attacks, and decidedly greater during the attacks themselves, though it did not reach the normal average. There was no relation between the amount of urine and the quantity of uric acid, but the acidity of the urine and the quantity of the urea corresponded closely. Colchicum did not increase but rather decreased the uric acid, while salicylate of sodium constantly caused decided increase.

Hans Froehlich [5] does not hold that uric acid is the original cause of gout, but believes that its removal from the affected joints is the most important part of the treatment, either by direct surgical intervention or by subcutaneous injections of weak solutions of sodium bicarbonate into the joints with massage.

M. A. Boyd [6] believes that the clearing of the system of uric acid by alkalies or salicylates leaves the principal part of the work undone, which is the use of suitable remedies to correct the faulty metabolism in whatever system the disease first arose.

Laquer [7] contributes an interesting paper on the metabolism in the course of a milk-diet and under other conditions. These studies show that the administration of **milk** increases the excretion of xanthin-bases and reduces that of uric acid. Increased quantity of liquid (water) in the diet increases the

[1] Berlin. klin. Woch., Apr. 26, 1897.   [2] Am. Jour. Med. Sci., Aug., 1896.
[3] St. Petersburg. med. Woch., No. 1-2, 1897.   [4] Guy's Hosp. Rep., vol. lii., 1896.
[5] Jour. Am. Med. Assoc., Jan. 30, 1897.   [6] Lancet. Aug. 8, 1896.
[7] Berlin. klin. Woch., Sept. 7, 1896.

alloxin bodies (uric acid and xanthin-bases) in healthy individuals. Fat milk, according to Gärtner's formula, is recommended as a suitable diet for all cases of gout. [Salkowski points out that this formula furnishes no advantages over ordinary milk.]

G. Harley[1] discusses the relations of **sugar and champagne** to gout. He denies the importance of sugar, and calls attention to the fact that those accustomed to a saccharine diet have no special tendency to gouty arthritis, and that the urine of herbivorous animals, in whose diet sugar plays an important part, is alkaline in reaction. His own son, a subject of gout, took at one time 400 gm. of sugar daily until he suffered with total anorexia, and on another occasion 525 gm. in 24 hours, without producing any gouty manifestations. The relation of champagne to gout is difficult to determine, as the constituents of various preparations vary greatly. Of its constituents, sugar is, according to his view, the least and acetic acid the most harmful. [These views are so at variance with accepted belief that far greater proof than the author adduces will be required to gain for them any general credence.]

T. J. Mays[2] recommends the use of **salicylate of sodium** in the treatment of certain forms of **hemoptysis** that he holds are due to a rheumatic or gouty diathesis. This form has the following characteristics: the patient generally seems in fair health, and is usually seized while at work with sudden hemorrhage that tends to recur. There is neither history nor signs of phthisis, alcoholism, or syphilis; and a rheumatic or gouty history is frequently obtainable. The author cites 2 cases of this description benefited by salicylate treatment. He is particular to state that he does not advise the salicylates in every case of hemoptysis, nor exclusively in any.

GLYCOSURIA.

Strümpell[3] contributes a study of **dietetic glycosuria.** He points out that as far as our knowledge of carbohydrate metabolism is concerned there is one important process, that of oxidation of the saccharine bodies, and providing the amount of carbohydrate food is sufficiently great this oxidation will fail to be adequate and sugar will appear in the urine. He has administered varying quantities of glucose to persons suffering with nutritional diseases, and has found that in ordinary cases of marantic conditions, such as in the severe anemias, moderate quantities of sugar (100 to 150 gm.) did not cause glycosuria. This may be due to the slow absorption of the sugar in such cases. In cirrhosis of the liver and in catarrhal jaundice the result was not uniform; and in 2 patients with chronic gout no glycosuria was produced. He was interested to study the effect in patients suffering with progressive muscle-atrophy, on account of the part supposed to be played by the muscles in carbohydrate metabolism. In 3 cases, however, no glycosuria was produced. The most positive results were obtained by him in alcoholics, particularly habitual and excessive beer-drinkers. In such he was able almost regularly to obtain striking results, and he is disposed to rank beer-drinking as an important cause of glycosuria. It was sometimes possible to demonstrate sugar after excessive indulgence in beer without the use of glucose in the diet; but it was not possible to produce glycosuria after copious meals of other starchy foods, such as bread, doubtless because of slower absorption.

L. C. Wadsworth[4] reports **a case** of a man of 25, who accidentally discovered the presence of sugar in his urine. He had no symptoms whatever

1 Lancet, Aug. 1, 1896.
3 Berlin. klin. Woch., Nov. 16, 1896.
2 Phila. Polyclinic., Oct 24, 1896.
4 Med. Rec., May 29, 1897.

of diabetes. He was the oldest of 11 children, and examination of specimens from the other 10 showed high specific gravity and the presence of more or less sugar in all. They were all healthy and passed a normal quantity of urine. The patient passed about 10% of sugar a day, but this quantity could be some-what reduced by an exclusive milk-diet.

Mossé[1] has repeated the work of Seegen, who found that the venous blood coming from the liver contains as much as 100% more sugar than the portal blood. In order to avoid post-operative changes he received the hepatic blood through a catheter inserted into the jugular vein and pushed downward into one of the hepatic veins. He compared this with the blood of the arteries, which Seegen found to contain the same proportion of sugar as the portal blood. The average of 7 experiments was: arterial blood 0.093% of sugar, and the hepatic blood 0.107%, an excess in the latter of 0.014%. This difference is only about ⅓ of that found by Seegen, and the author concludes that the **formation of sugar in the liver** is not so great as that author believed.

Neugebauer[2] reports a case of **incarcerated inguinal hernia** in which the urine was examined just before the operation and found to contain a considerable quantity of sugar. The operation was nevertheless performed, and the intestine, which was not in the least gangrenous, returned to the abdominal cavity. The urine passed the same night again contained sugar. When questioned regarding his previous life the patient absolutely denied any symptoms that pointed to diabetes, and, in fact, all further examinations of the urine proved negative. As no similar case of glycosuria as a result of intestinal obstruction had been recorded, the author undertook some experiments, using dogs, guinea-pigs, and human beings, and reached the conclusion that incarceration or ligature of the duodenum or jejunum, or incarceration of hernias in which the greater part of the small intestine is included may cause a temporary glycosuria, which disappears a few hours after the obstruction is removed. In conclusion, he reports another case which was almost identical with the first one, sugar being found just before the operation and continuing present for little more than a day afterward, when it entirely disappeared. [Disturbances of abdominal circulation and of intestinal absorption doubtless play a part in these cases.]

Loeb[3] reports several cases illustrating the **method of onset** of diabetes mellitus, which show that small amounts of sugar may appear in the urine for some time—even years—before the appearance of any definite symptoms. He does not believe that such cases invariably lead to diabetes.

DIABETES.

Etiology.—Senator[4] analyzed 770 cases of diabetes which came under his observation to determine its **frequency in married couples**. He found this coincidence in man and wife in 9 couples—viz., in 1.19% of the cases. Three of the cases were markedly disposed by hereditary influence, and he omits these; in 4 others the time that elapsed from the date of possible transmission to the occurrence of the disease was so long that it was difficult to assume a causal relation. In 1 case, for example, the husband had been dead 5 or 6 years when the disease occurred in the wife. There are, therefore, only 2 cases in which the disease arose without obvious causes, and this number is so small that he prefers to regard the coincidence as purely acci-

[1] Pflüger's Archiv, Bd. lxiii., p. 613.
[2] Wien. klin. Woch., Sept. 10, 1896.
[3] Centralbl. f. innere Med., Nov. 21, 1896.
[4] Berlin. klin. Woch., No. 30, 1896.

dental. [This analysis agrees very well with that of Opler and Külz; see *Year-Book*, 1897.]

H. A. Hare[1] has studied the **statistics of diabetes,** and finds that the disease is apparently increasing very rapidly in frequency. [It must be remembered, however, that much more attention is paid to urinary analysis at the present time than was paid to it 20 years ago.]

Pathology.—James[2] has studied the **blood** in 13 cases of diabetes. The number of red cells was over 6,000,000 in 5, 5,000,000 in 5, 4,000,000 in 2, and 3,000,000 in 1. The quantity of hemoglobin was over 100% in 3, 80% in 8, and 50% in 2. The specific gravity was estimated according to the method of Roy, and was found to be only 1054 to 1060—*i. e.*, about normal. This last fact is against the view that there is a concentration of the blood due to polyuria. The condition of the blood maintains itself, according to the author, until the general strength of the constitution begins to weaken, when the character of the blood deteriorates. His own theory is that the blood of the diabetic patient, as also the digestive power of the stomach, increases in order that the great mass of the oxidizable material may be disposed of by increased oxidating power of the blood.

Kalmus[3] reports 3 cases of diabetes mellitus, in 2 of which there were remarkably extensive degenerations in the posterior columns of the **spinal cord,** particularly in the columns of Goll.

Teubaum[4] has found, as a result of investigation upon 12 cases of diabetes, that the amount of **calcium** excreted in the urine is in great excess in the severer forms, but only slightly increased in those that are milder. He believes that this is due to the increased amount of food ingested, although, in certain cases where the quantity excreted is in great excess he is inclined to consider that it represents, in part at least, the disintegration of the body albumin.

Symptoms.—Triboulet[5] notes that there are comparatively few accurate observations upon the liver in diabetes, and the reports of the findings are at variance. As **hepatic symptoms** are frequent, such as tenderness, increase of size, and functional disturbances, he holds that further observations are required to establish the exact pathology.

A. B. Elliott[6] classifies the causes of **albuminuria** in diabetes mellitus as follows: irritation by the sugar during its excretion, suppurative conditions of the urinary passages, increased ingestion of albuminoid foods, and increased liability of diabetics to various morbid changes the result of disassimilation and coexisting nephritis.

Rendu and De Massary[7] report a case of acute diabetes complicated by pigmentation of all the tissues excepting the voluntary muscles and the semilunar ganglion. The pigment was of a yellow ochre color and contained iron. No pigment-emboli were found in any part of the body. A diagnosis was made of **bronzed diabetes.**

Diagnosis.—R. T. Williamson[8] describes a method of determining the existence of diabetes by **testing a drop of the blood.** As the chemical examination requires a large quantity of blood, the author was led to study the reaction with anilin dyes, and found that methyl-blue was very sensitive. His method is as follows: a narrow test-tube is well cleaned and at the bottom are placed 40 c.c. of water, using Gowers' hemoglobinometer pipette for this

[1] Med. News, June 12, 1897.
[2] Edinb. Med. Jour., Sept., 1896.
[3] Zeit. f. klin. Med., vol. 30, H. 5 and 6.
[4] Zeit. f. Biol., 1896, p. 379.
[5] Rev. de Méd., No. 2, 1896.
[6] Jour. Am. Med. Assoc., Dec. 26, 1896.
[7] Presse méd., No. 11, 1897.
[8] Brit. Med. Jour., Sept. 19, 1896.

purpose; the finger is cleansed and pricked, and a large drop is drawn into th small capillary hemoglobinometer tube to the 20 c.c. mark. The blood i then mixed with the water in the test-tube, and 1 c.c. of a 1 to 6000 aqueou. methyl-blue solution is added; finally, 40 c.c. of liquor potassæ are added and the tube well shaken. A control-test is made with normal blood. The fluid in each tube is now deep blue in color. Both tubes are then placed in a beaker containing water, and this is heated until it boils and continued at this point for 4 minutes, at the end of which time the tube containing diabetic blood changes to a dirty yellow. Shaking must be avoided. He has made over 30 examinations in 6 cases of diabetes, and has found that the reaction was characteristic. In 4 the disease was severe, and a solution of methyl-blue of double strength (1 to 3000) was decolorized. In a large number of normal cases the reaction was not obtained. The author believes this reaction is dependent upon the reducing power of the sugar. If this were the case, larger quantities of normal blood should give the reaction, and he has found that 60 c.c. of normal blood plus 1 c.c. of methyl-blue plus 4 c.c. of liquor potassæ react. [If this reaction be due to the cause stated, it will probably be found in other conditions, such as carcinoma, in which increase of sugar occurs in the blood. Also, it is likely that other reducing agents will give the reaction and interfere with the usefulness of the test.]

Bremer[1] has studied the **color-reactions of normal and diabetic urine,** finding that both dissolve eosin very well, but that normal urine does not dissolve gentian-violet or only very imperfectly. Diabetic urine, on the other hand, dissolves the latter substance very poorly and slowly, whether it contains sugar or not. The solution of gentian-violet does not mix easily with a solution of eosin, and this gives rise to certain peculiar appearances in the liquid.

Lepine and Lyonnet[2] have found the **reaction of the red blood-corpuscles** described by Bremer as occurring in diabetes in a case of this disease and also in a case of leukemia, and attribute it to the reduced alkalinity in the 2 cases examined. There is nothing to substantiate the view of Bremer that diabetes is based upon disease of the red blood-corpuscles. [We have also obtained this reaction in normal blood that had been carelessly fixed.]

Treatment.—Samuel West[3] contributes a further article on the value ·of **uranium nitrate** in the treatment of diabetes. One of his previous cases declared that the remedy made her ill; and although he does not feel assured that this was the case, he does not deny its possibility. He then reports 5 new cases in which the remedy was more or less successful. The first, a young woman of 22, had suffered with the disease for 2 years; the drug was taken without any disturbance. The amount of the urine remained the same, but the percentage of sugar fell from 6% to just above 4%, and lost its previously marked fluctuations. In the second case, in a woman of 44, the quantity of sugar was greatly reduced and the fluctuations disappeared. The same was true of the third case, and in this it was noted that the quantity and specific gravity were but little affected. In the fourth case, under the combined action of the drug and diet, the quantity was reduced by about 1 pint in 24 hours. The specific gravity remained the same and the percentage of sugar fell slightly. In the last case the drug had no good effect and dyspepsia was produced by its use. He concludes that this drug is of considerable value, though it cannot be relied upon to produce equally good results in all cases.

J. Gibbs Blake[4] has tried **phloridzin** as a remedy for glycosuria. He recalls

---

[1] N. Y. Med. Jour., Mar. 13, 1896.   [2] Lyon méd., No. 23, 1896.
[3] Brit. Med. Jour., Sept. 19, 1896.   [4] Birmingham Med. Rev., July, 1896.

that nitrate of uranium, which has lately been lauded in diabetes, was long since known to be capable of producing artificial glycosuria. This led him to think that phloridzin, which is capable of causing glycosuria, might prove an efficient remedy. He has tried it in several cases and found it useful, especially in middle-aged persons, finding that in children and phthisical subjects, like uranium nitrate, it had little advantage.

D'Arsonval and Charrin [1] have employed **currents of high frequency** in a case of diabetes, with the result that after 1½ months of treatment the sugar had decreased from 622 to 186, and the volume of urine from 12 to 8 l. per day. In another case the glucose was decreased from 144 to 57, and the patient presented considerable improvement in all his physical signs.

Diet.—Edward L. Munson [2] reports a case of diabetes whose urine before diet failed to give the reaction for diacetic acid, but this substance appeared within 48 hours after the withdrawal of carbohydrates. His condition rapidly grew worse and there was considerable increase in the amount of ammonia present in the urine. Finally, it was decided to permit him to partake of carbohydrates, whereupon he improved very remarkably, although there was a slight increase in the amount of sugar excreted. The author believes that sugar is always present in the blood and is not obtained exclusively from carbohydrates. As the diabetic patients are still able to burn sugar, it is necessary to permit them at least as much as would be given a healthy person, and, if given, it prevents altered metabolism of the albuminous bodies and the formation of toxic substances. This sugar is absorbed in the same way as if it were ingested in a healthy organism. More sugar, however, is excreted because the isomeric albuminous sugar, which would otherwise be burnt up, is not needed, and is excreted as a waste product.

Chas. W. Purdy [3] objects to a too exclusive milk-diet in diabetes, particularly when skimmed milk is employed. He also prefers a limited quantity of table-bread to any of the so-called nonstarchy substitutes.

Renzi and Reale [4] have investigated the value of levulose in supplying the place of dextrose in the diet of diabetic patients. They find that as much as 82 gm. per day are completely burned in the organism and to a considerable extent economize albumin.

OSTEOMALACIA.

Hoffmann [5] has investigated the urine of 2 cases of osteomalacia in order to see whether the theory that the solution of the bone-salts is due to the presence of lactic acid in the blood could be inferred from the presence of this substance in the urine. In one case 15 l. and the other 20 l. were tested; neither contained any traces of lactic acid.

Senator [6] reports a case of osteomalacia to which he gave thyroid gland and oöphorin. Under both substances the amount of calcium excreted was considerably increased, but the patient showed marked improvement.

Seegleken [7] reports a case of **multiple myeloma** occurring in a man of 61. He had had rheumatism and had suffered a severe injury to the head. The disease commenced with deep-seated pains in the neck and breast. During its progress the sternum sank inward and the spinal column became kyphotic. The cardiac impulse was vigorous; there was a systolic murmur at the pul-

---

[1] Compt. rend. de la Soc. de Biol., July 10, 1896.
[2] Jour. Am. Med. Assoc., May 8, 15, 22, 1897.
[3] Ibid., Dec. 19, 1896.   [4] Wien. klin. Woch., Feb. 27, 1897.
[5] Centralbl. f. innere Med., No. 14, 1897.   [6] Berlin. klin. Woch., Feb. 8, 1897.
[7] Deutsch. Arch. f. klin. Med., vol. lviii. H. 2, 3.

monary cartilage, but otherwise all the organs were normal. The urine contained the peculiar albumose that has been described in similar conditions by Bence-Jones. At the autopsy numerous soft vascular tumors were found in the skeleton, which in places had destroyed large portions of the osseous tissue.

DISEASES OF THE BLOOD.

General Considerations concerning the Blood.—Knopfelmacher[1] has examined the blood of the newborn, particularly to determine its relations to infantile jaundice. He determined that the red corpuscles bear no etiologic relation to icterus neonatorum. The number of erythrocytes during the first week of life is independent of the occurrence of jaundice. The fluctuations in particular are more dependent upon the changes in the volume of plasma. The "resistance" of the red corpuscles is the same at the time of birth as in the adult, and it is not altered in consequence of jaundice. He could find only evidences of rapid formation of corpuscles, never any indications of destruction.

Epstein[2] describes the changes in the blood in a case of carcinoma with **metastatic involvement of the bone-marrow.** The patient was a woman who had suffered with mammary carcinoma and extensive metastasis; the proportion of white to red cells in the cover-glass preparations was from 1 to 25 to 1 to 40; the hemoglobin was 19 % and there was marked reduction of the red corpuscles. The latter were exceedingly irregular in size and many of them contained nuclei. Of the latter there were normoblasts and megaloblasts, often with irregular clover-leaf and rosette-formed nuclei or with nuclear fragmentation. Polychromaphilia of the nucleated and of the non-nucleated cells was detected, and the white corpuscles, especially the large mononuclear forms, for the most part contained neutrophile granules and were increased in number. Myelocytes corresponding to Cornil's description and a few eosinophile cells were found. The author concludes that the involvement of the marrow was shown by the great number of the "*markzellen*" and the enormous number of nucleated red corpuscles, especially the megaloblasts. He points out, however, that it is impossible to determine the nature of the changes in the marrow from the character of the blood, since marrow-changes are common in various conditions and the blood may or may not be altered.

Methods of Examination.—Rabl[3] describes a method of **staining the blood-plates.** This consists essentially of the method of Heidenhain for centrosomes. The preparation of blood dried in air is fixed for $\frac{1}{4}$ to $\frac{1}{2}$ hour in a saturated solution of corrosive sublimate in $\frac{3}{4}$ % NaCl, then washed and placed in a solution of chlorid of iron for 1 hour, again washed and stained for $\frac{1}{2}$ to 1 hour in a saturated aqueous solution of hematoxylin. After all the cells have become stained a bluish-black the preparation is placed a second time in an iron solution; after $\frac{1}{4}$ or 1 minute the preparation becomes yellowish-gray in color and is ready to be washed, dried, and mounted. The red corpuscles are wholly decolorized. The blood-plates are dark bluish-black, and the leukocytes are somewhat similarly stained.

Zuntz,[4] in investigating **Hammerschlag's method** for determining the specific gravity of blood, notes that blood shaken in a mixture of chloroform and benzol exerts a powerful attraction upon the latter, absorbing it and therefore becoming lighter. As, however, this absorption occurs slowly, it does not necessarily interfere seriously with the method. He suggests, however, that

[1] Wien. klin. Woch., No. 43, 1896.
[2] Zeit. f. klin. Med., Bd. 30, H. 1, 2.
[3] Wien. klin. Woch., No. 40, 1896.
[4] Pflüger's Arch., Mar. 31, 1897.

after the correction a new drop of blood should always be used in order to test the accuracy of the solution. He has been unable to replace the benzol with any of a variety of substances with which he experimented. [Used in this way Hammerschlag's method has given fairly accurate results in our hands, though it is somewhat tedious and in no way comparable with the pyknometer method in accuracy. The difficulty with the latter is that accurate chemical balances are indispensable.]

Gryn's [1] reaches certain conclusions regarding the **estimation of the volume** of corpuscles and serum in a study of osmosis and diffusion in regard to the red corpuscles. Then he considers the clinical method to determine the volume of the corpuscles by centrifugation, and finds that the same amount of sediment may be determined repeatedly in the same blood when accurately isotonic solutions are employed for dilution. He recommends for human blood a solution of NaCl of 0.84 to 0.88 % strength. To this crystalline ammonium oxalate or a solution of sodium oxalate is added to prevent coagulation. The solutions recommended for diluting by Hedin, Daland, and others should not be used, as they change the volume of the corpuscle.

Berend [2] describes a new method of **estimating the alkalinity** of the blood. He draws 0.1 c.c. of blood into a specially prepared pipette and then 5 c.c. of 1 % solution of NaCl; the mixture is centrifugated and the diluted serum colored blue with litmus. It is then treated with acid solution in excess and titrated with alkali back to the neutral point. The corpuscles in the centrifugated sediment are first treated with 10 c.c. of neutral water and poured into a porcelain dish; the tube is washed with 5 c.c. of water and litmus added until a bluish-green opaque solution is formed; excess of acid is then added and the mixture is titrated back with alkali until the red color disappears and the opaque condition of the mixture is restored. In this way the total alkalinity of the serum and of the corpuscles is determined. He has studied the blood of 29 children with this method and finds that the normal in infants lies between 0.34 and 0.44. The alkalinity decreases in the first few days of life, and sometimes subsequent elevation occurs. In adults the figures are from 0.46 to 0.50.

Clinical Method.—J. H. Ford [3] recommends the following method of his own for the discovery of the **total quantity of blood** in the body: venesection is performed, a definite quantity of blood removed, and its specific gravity determined; then a similar quantity of normal salt solution of known specific gravity is injected into the vein. After 5 minutes the same quantity of blood is drawn again and the specific gravity again determined. The mass of blood is determined from these facts by simple calculation. [While this method seems perfectly simple and has been occasionally considered by previous writers, it is subject to so many fallacies that we should scarcely deem it reliable. It must be remembered that the abstraction of blood in sufficient quantity to make substitution of salt solution practically useful in the determination brings about changes in the vasomotor system and probably in the lymph-stream that would tend to vitiate the results. It is still uncertain whether the withdrawal of blood quickly determines the inflow of lymph into the circulation or not, but this is at least probable. Further, it may be that the altered blood after addition of saline solution rapidly discharges part of its fluid element to equalize the specific gravity.]

The Leukocytes.—Clarisse [4] has studied the modifications that take place in the **number of leukocytes** produced by massive injections of saline

---

[1] Pflüger's Archiv, Bd. 63, p. 86. [2] Zeit. f. Heilk., Bd. 17, H. 2-3.
[3] N. Y. Med. Jour., Jan. 18, 1896. [4] Compt. rend. de la Soc. de Biol., July 24, 1896.

solutions **in febrile conditions.** In one case of general streptococcus infection they were ordinarily reduced about $\frac{1}{2}$, although there were a rapid reaction and increase in temperature after each injection. In another case of a man suffering from a phlegmonous inflammation of the arm the leukocytes were decreased from 26,000 to 11,000 per mg.; in the third case, one of intense puerperal infection, the reduction was again $\frac{1}{2}$. In all cases, after the primary reaction there were a rapid fall of the temperature and a temporary improvement in the general condition of the patient. The author refrains from drawing any conclusions.

Burian and Schur[1] have made a number of experiments upon **digestive hyperleukocytosis,** with the usual result that they find it somewhat variable. At the same time they estimated the amount of nitrogen in the urine, and found that it was distinctly increased for some hours after the ingestion of considerable quantities of albumin, and that this increase did not necessarily bear a close relation to the degree of leukocytosis. They therefore conclude that the absence of the digestive hyperleukocytosis is not of itself a symptom of imperfect resorption. In an endeavor to discover the nature of this leukocytosis they start with the observation that more lymphocytes are found in the radicles of the portal vein than in the arteries leading to the digestive tract, and infer from this that the lymph-glands of the intestines and mesentery have an active part in the increase in the leukocytes, assuming that their action is one of protection to the organism, and that the leukocytosis is simply the expression of their effort to destroy digestive substances that are attempting to penetrate into the tissue. In cachectic states, after the introduction of nourishment, there is hypo- instead of hyperleukocytosis, and they report 3 cases of gastric carcinoma in which this condition was very marked.

G. L. Gulland[2] holds that it is impossible to devise a thoroughly satisfactory classification of the leukocytes, as the different forms are all variations of one body at different stages and no sharp dividing-line can be drawn. It is convenient to distinguish hyaline cells (without granulations), acidophile and basophile leukocytes, all 3 being derivatives of the lymphocyte. The neutrophile and amphophile cells he places among the acidophile, as do Kanthack and Hardy. He holds that the granulations of the leukocytes are not products of the cellular protoplasma, as Ehrlich maintained, but only microsomes. [The paper is one of great value, but cannot be more extensively noted in this place.]

R. J. M. Buchannan[3] believes with other observers that in their mature stage any one leukocyte exhibits only one form of specific granules. It is not improbable, however, that the cells may at one period of their existence contain oxyphile and at another basophile granules. In abnormal instances a deviation may occur and both stages may be represented in the cells at one time. His observations on leukemia have persuaded him that this is a not infrequent occurrence. He noted among cells identical with the large uninucleated marrow-cells some in which only fine basophile granules were brought out by staining with methylen-blue and eosin (the stains being used separately) and others in which both forms of granules, oxyphile and basophile, occurred, the specimens being stained with a mixture of methylen-blue and eosin, and then further stained with methylen-blue. [One of the editors has found similar results not only in leukemia, but in other conditions. It is necessary to call attention to the fact that the author is in error in regard to the novelty of this view. Arnold, among others, called attention to the occurrence of different forms of granules in one cell some time since. We have found that staining with methylen-

---

[1] Wien. klin. Woch., Feb. 11, 1897.   [2] Jour. of Physiol., 1896.
[3] Liverpool Med.-Chir. Jour., July, 1896.

blue and eosin, or with strong methylen-blue, is prone to produce results different from those we have seen in specimens stained with Ehrlich's triple mixture and with other combinations. Even the granules which take up the Ehrlich triple neutral stain very well (the polymorphous leukocytes) may be intensely and sharply stained with methylen-blue, provided this acts sufficiently long upon the specimen. In using Chenzinsky's mixture, and heating the specimen in the oven for some hours, as was done by Canon, the frequency of this result is striking.]

Gumprecht [1] discusses the subject of **leukocytic degenerations** in leukemia and in severe anemias. The author's paper, which was read before the German Society for Internal Medicine at the meeting of 1896, has already been briefly referred to (*Year-Book*, 1897). The full paper is now published. He has studied the question from the side of the morphology of the leukocytes as bearing upon the chemical changes in leukocytic destruction, and points out that in most cases of leukemia there is increase in excretion of uric acid and the alloxins, and that there is a close relationship between the destruction of cells in the blood and the excretion of uric acid. Morphological evidences of cellular destruction are recognized in the blood and elsewhere, and 2 forms in particular may be described, known as hyperchromatosis and hypochromatosis. The author's investigations show that lymphocytes of different origin (thymus glands, lymph-glands, etc.) degenerated outside the body, or when subjected to heat exhibit hypochromatosis. The circumference of the nucleus becomes irregular, its structure is lost, and the chromatin gradually disappears. The same type of degeneration is seen in the leukocytes in certain severe anemias, especially in leukemia. In the acute forms of the latter disease the number of such degenerated cells is very great and is an indication of the nuclein destruction. Practically the same morphological changes are seen in the lymphocytes and in the myelocytes as are seen in the artificially degenerated cells. In normal blood the evidences of degeneration are slight.

Kuhnau [2] has studied the **effect of the dissolution of the blood upon the leukocytes,** and concludes that there are marked leukocytosis, increase in the excretion of uric acid and xanthin-bases, and increase at first in the excretion of phosphoric acid, followed by marked diminution; and an increase ultimately in the excretion of the chlorids, which appear to be affected inversely as the phosphoric acid. The increase of the alloxur bodies is caused chiefly by the disintegration of the leukocytes. The leukocytosis is due to the direct leukotactic action of the poison in the blood, to the liberated nuclein substances, and to the fragments of blood-cells in the circulation.

Uhlman [3] has studied the effect of certain substances upon the white corpuscles by placing mica disks impregnated with toxic substances in the anterior chamber of the eye of rabbits. The leukocytes find their way into the crevices, and after the experiment is finished the disks are split and fixed in concentrated sublimate or 1% osmic acid and stained. Various forms of nuclear or protoplasmic changes were discovered. Among others change of shape, fatty degeneration, swelling and vacuolation, and fragmentation of the protoplasm, and indefiniteness of contour, nuclear destruction, or increase or decrease of size of the nuclei. The author did not determine any specific change for individual poisons.

M. L. Perry [4] has studied the blood of 10 insane patients during the administration of thyroid gland. The number of red and white corpuscles was little

---

[1] Deutsch. Arch. f. klin. Med., Bd. 57, H. 5-6.   [2] Deutsch. med. Woch., June 1, 1897.
[3] Ziegler's Beiträge zur path. Anat., Bd. 19, H. 3.   [4] Med. Rec., Aug. 27, 1896.

influenced.   The **differential count** of leukocytes, however, showed increase in the mononuclear forms (lymphocytes) at the expense of the polymorphous forms.   The increase began about the 3d day and lasted several days after the administration of the remedy had ceased.   It was proportional to the amount of thyroid extract given and constituted about 10 to 20 % of the whole number of leukocytes.   At the height of the administration the lymphocytes seemed smaller than normal, and their nuclei stained more deeply than before the administration.

The Erythrocytes.—Lafon[1] has examined the **relation of the red blood-corpuscles to the body-weight** in a number of persons with the uniform result : that with the decline of the body-weight the number of red corpuscles and the quantity of hemoglobin decreased, and with the increase of the body-weight the corpuscles and hemoglobin increased, while the leukocytes decreased proportionately.   An increase of 500 gm. of body-weight indicated an increase of 200,000 red corpuscles; an increase of 1500 gm. an increase of 1,500,000, and 8 kilos increase almost 20,000 more corpuscles. The hemoglobin increased in these instances from 1 to 2 or 5 %.   [It is impossible to establish so simple a relationship as the author attempts.   So much depends upon quantities of serum or plasma, upon conditions of the circulation, etc., that any direct relation of mere weight or strength to the condition of blood cannot be determined.]

Conditions affecting Constitution of the Blood.—Breitenstein,[2] in a study of the **relation of cold to the circulation** of healthy persons and those suffering with fever, alludes particularly to the condition of the blood.   In 26 subjects suffering with typhoid fever he found after cool baths (22° C., 10 min.) that the red corpuscles increased at the least 50,000 per c.mm., and that with corresponding increase in the hemoglobin measure a similar, though less pronounced, result was obtained in 11 healthy persons. The increase of corpuscles bore no relation to the fall of temperature in these cases ; and antipyretic remedies, such as antipyrin, caused no such result.   No relation could be found between the changes in the blood and the alterations in blood-pressure, respiration, and pulse-rate.   The apparent explanation was that the change in the number of red corpuscles is due to a transfer of the corpuscles previously massed in some part of the circulation into the peripheral circulation in consequence of the increased blood-pressure.   After the bath this view was confirmed by experiments upon rabbits.   When these animals were heated the erythrocytes in the peripheral circulation decreased and were found to be massed in the liver.   This condition corresponds closely with that observed in typhoid fever.

Löwy[3] has studied the **effect of heat** upon the constitution of the blood. He placed rabbits in an incubator and maintained them at a temperature of 30° to 36° C. for 24 hours, when the blood was found to have lost in sp. gr. and solid residue, while the serum had increased in solid residue.   This result was rather surprising in view of the loss of water which the entire organism must suffer under the conditions of the experiment.   He examined portions of muscle in order to determine the loss of water, but found no uniform results, though in the majority there was some loss.   In 11 cases the average normal solid residue in the blood was 16.88 % and the average after heating 15.43 %.   Omitting 1 case in which the estimation was doubtful, the average after heating was 16.14 %.   The sp. gr. in 3 cases declined respectively 6.0, 0.5, and 1.8 points, while the serum in the same cases increased respect-

[1] Compt. rend. de la Soc. de Biol., No. 18, 1896.
[2] Arch. f. exper. Pharmakol., Bd. 37, p. 253.   [3] Berlin. klin. Woch., Oct. 12, 1896.

ively 3.5, 2.75, and 6.9 points. It is therefore evident that the sp. gr. of the entire blood did not suffer in consequence of dilution simply. The author concludes that it is due to the retention of the corpuscles in the smaller vessels or capillaries, and to prove this shows that the number of corpuscles in the blood taken from the ear of a rabbit at parts removed from the large blood-vessels increases after heating. He does not believe that any exchange of water by evaporation through the lungs, or any noteworthy addition of serum from the lymphatic channels occurs in these cases on account of the condition of the serum of the blood, as well as from the fact that practically the same results are obtained by heating the animals for from half a minute to 15 minutes at 60° to 70° C.

Grawitz[1] replies that his previously published explanation of the occurrence of diminished concentration of the blood in animals subjected to heat—viz. that it is due to increased influx of lymph into the circulation—is unaffected by Löwy's observations. He points out that the solid residue of the serum in the experiments of the latter increased only slightly, from 6.88 to 7.06 %. He holds that this proves his own point, since the loss of water by evaporation must have produced greater thickening of the serum if there were no additions of lymph to the blood-stream. [It is evident that Grawitz does not deny the possibility of disturbances of circulation and peripheral corpuscular congestion, though he maintains also and especially the addition to the circulating blood of lymph. This view seems to us to correspond very accurately with the probabilities, and we are therefore disposed to accept it as likely.]

Eger[2] contributes an interesting paper on the **regeneration of blood after hemorrhage.** His experiments were performed on dogs. He summarizes his results as follows : the animal organism reproduces the blood after the loss of $\frac{1}{3}$ of its total bulk very slowly and imperfectly, and sometimes not at all, when the diet is comparatively poor in iron. The addition of inorganic preparations of iron increases the rapidity of regeneration, but is not as satisfactory as a diet containing a sufficient quantity of iron in combination (meat). Even in the cases of the latter diet, however, the addition of iron in inorganic or organic form hastens regeneration. After a severe loss of blood, therefore, he holds that milk-diet is contraindicated, and that the ordinary diet and iron salts should be administered. He studied the changes in the sp. gr. and dry residue of the blood and the serum after and before hemorrhage, and discovered that in severe traumatic anemia the sp. gr. (and therefore the albumin) of the latter corresponds with the decrease in the number of blood-corpuscles and hemoglobin. He does not, therefore, confirm the view of v. Jaksch and others, that the serum maintains itself at practically a constant condition, despite the change in sp. gr. of the blood as a whole.

Tarchetti[3] has studied the **effects of hemorrhage** upon the constitution of the blood. He found that in dogs, after considerable venesection, producing acute anemia, the hemoglobin-value of the corpuscles is unaltered ; when a subacute or chronic anemia is produced by repeated hemorrhages, each small in amount, the hemoglobin of the corpuscles is relatively deficient, and this persists after the number of corpuscles has returned to the normal ; and even after it has become greater than the original number. He explains these effects by assuming that the production of hemoglobin is independent of that of the red corpuscles. The tendency of the organism is to reproduce red corpuscles more quickly than hemoglobin, and the increased number of corpuscles

[1] Berlin. klin. Woch., Nov. 9, 1896.   [2] Zeit. f. klin. Med., Bd. 32, H. 3-4.
[3] Arch. fer la Scienze Mediche, No. 1, 1896.

is, perhaps, in a measure, a compensation for the tardy development of hemoglobin. He explains the reduction in hemoglobin-value by the assumption that youthful, often nucleated, and hemoglobin-poor red corpuscles of the marrow are cast into the circulation in the process of regeneration.

Eubank and Hall[1] report a series of experiments upon the regeneration of the blood. Dogs were bled and at the same time a slightly excessive amount of artificial serum was injected. This increased the rapidity of the regeneration. The regenerative processes were more rapid in the third and fourth than in the first and second weeks, and once started they carried the blood into a condition in which the corpuscles and hemoglobin were in excess of the normal. The amount of hemoglobin per volume of red corpuscles was not constant, and during the regenerative period the hematocrit ordinarily gave higher readings than the hemocytometer, the differences being due to increase in the diameter of the red blood-cells as determined by the micrometer.

Limbeck[2] discusses the effect of biliary salts upon the blood. He noted some years ago that the **isotonicity** of the corpuscles was regularly less in icterus than in health, being 0.38 % or less, instead of 0.46 or 0.48 % as in health. The explanation of this was that the more fragile corpuscles had been destroyed by the biliary salts, leaving the more resisting in the circulating blood. He found the hypertonicity of the serum somewhat reduced, which led him to investigate the volume of the corpuscles, as Köppe has recently shown that this bears a certain relation to the tonicity of the serum. In each of 3 cases he found a rather notable increase in the volume of the corpuscles and decrease in that of the serum, and he found that a similar increase of corpuscular volume could be produced artificially by addition of biliary salts to horse's blood. He was unable to produce, artificially, any change in the isotonic relations of the corpuscles; and he concludes, with Hamburger, that the isotonicity of the corpuscles is independent of the condition of the serum. Finally, he inclines to believe with F. Hoppe-Seyler that the hemoglobin of the corpuscles is in some form of actual combination with the stroma of the corpuscles, and that the influences which cause changes of tonicity affect this combination in one direction or another.

Camus and Gley[3] have found that the **injection of peptone** into the blood produces considerable increase in the number of red blood-corpuscles and the amount of hemoglobin. As there is no hemoglobinuria, they believe this to be due to diminution of the plasma.

Strauss[4] has studied the **alkalinity of blood** from the median vein after the method of Löwy. The measure of the alkalinity in healthy persons was found between 320 and 325 mg. of NaHO; the figures, however, varied somewhat in individuals, and he therefore assumes that alkalinity is abnormally high when it is above 400 and abnormally low when it is below 250. There are no great variations at different times of the day in consequence of food or exercise, although small differences may be determined. In cases of gastritis with subacidity or hyperacidity no decided differences were found. In febrile cases there was normal alkalinity in a number of cases and decided increase in some, but never any reduction. An attempt to alter the alkalinity experimentally showed that the blood of man offers considerable resistance to such procedures as compared with that of herbivorous animals. Alkalies are quickly eliminated through the kidneys, and the acids are soon combined with ammonium and eliminated in that form.

---

[1] Jour. Exper. Med., Nov., 1896. [2] Centralbl. f. innere Med., Aug. 15, 1896.
[3] Compt. rend. de la Soc. de Biol., July 24, 1896.
[4] Zeit. f. klin. Med., Bd. 30, H. 3 and 4.

Caro[1] has studied the **variations in the alkalinity** of the blood and their relation to leukocytosis. After injections of spermin, tuberculin, and pilocarpin there are moderate and temporary alterations in the alkalinity, usually increase and then reduction. The amount and duration of these changes are so slight, however, that it is difficult to explain their occurrence. He could find in men no such relation between alkalinity of the blood and the number of white corpuscles as Löwy and Richter claim for rabbits.

Ehrlich and Lindenthal[2] describe a case of **"nitrobenzol"-poisoning** with certain peculiar features in the blood. The patient, a woman of 50, had stupor, cyanosis, and collapse. Artificial respiration restored her to a certain extent, and she gained in strength; but, finally, after the development of jaundice, death occurred in coma on the 17th day of the disease. The blood was dark colored and showed the spectroscopic peculiarities of methemoglobin. There were distinct poikilocytosis and many nucleated red corpuscles and leukocytosis. At first the nucleated red corpuscles were of both kinds, normoblasts and megaloblasts, but as the case progressed the latter predominated. They noted with particular interest certain clover-leaf-shaped nuclei in large red corpuscles. The fact that these took on a polychromatophilic stain led them to regard these corpuscles as degenerative. Altogether, the blood resembled that of pernicious anemia.

Abnormal Constituents.—H. F. Müller[3] describes certain very small, colorless, sometimes light-colored, sometimes dark, strongly refractive bodies, showing active molecular movements in the fresh preparations. They are not colored dark with osmic acid, and therefore do not contain fat. Acetic acid does not dissolve them, and they are independent of fibrin-formation, as they are invariably outside of the fibrin network. He has found them in all normal specimens of blood, although in different quantities in different persons and at different times. They are sometimes present in enormous numbers, and they seem to be decreased in states of hunger or cachexia. The author does not decide as to their exact significance, but terms them hemokoniæ. [We have frequently observed these bodies and have concluded that they are minute fragments of red corpuscles. They find almost exact analogues in artificial fragments produced by heat and other destructive agencies.]

Winterberg[4] investigated the presence of **ammonia in human blood.** In a normal dog he was able to demonstrate a considerable quantity. In a dog from which the kidneys had been extirpated it was not altered. In 2 patients, one suffering from uremia and the other from chronic nephritis without uremia, the amount of ammonia was only slightly increased in the second. He concludes that normal human blood contains preformed ammonia to about the amount of 1 mg. in 100 c.c. In fever this quantity varies considerably; usually it is increased, but not infrequently notably diminished. It is not increased in chronic disease of the liver or in acute yellow atrophy, and we cannot conclude that uremia is due to poisoning with carbaminic acid; he therefore holds that ammonianemia as a pathological condition does not exist. [See also Fever.]

ANEMIA.

General Considerations.—F. Taylor[5] opened a discussion on **anemia** with a general consideration of the causes, varieties, and pathology, devoting particular attention to chlorosis, pernicious anemia, and splenic anemia. He

[1] Zeit. f. klin. Med., Bd, 30, H. 3 and 4. [2] Ibid., H. 5 and 6.
[3] Centralbl. f. Allg. Path. u. path. Anat., p. 529, 1896.
[4] Wien. klin. Woch., Apr. 8, 1897. [5] Brit. Med. Jour., Sept. 9, 1896.

defined anemia as an abnormal pallor of the tissues due to diminution in the quantity or some defect in the solid constituents of the blood, an essential condition being the diminution in the total quantity of hemoglobin. The diminution in the number of leukocytes is not essential, and he therefore omits this from the definition. Speaking of secondary anemias, he notes that though we recognize the occurrence of anemia after various diseases, we do not know all the links in the chain of causation—for example, between the deposition of tubercle or the growth of cancer and the want of hemoglobin or corpuscles. [The definition of anemia given by the author seems to us too restricted. It is true that distinct changes in number and character of leukocytes indicative of anemia are unknown, but it is altogether likely that changes in these as well as in the plasma are a part of anemia as much as the better known changes in the erythrocytes.]

Diebala[1] contributes an elaborate study on the relations existing between the quantity of **hemoglobin and the specific gravity of the blood in anemia.** The specific gravity was estimated by the benzol-chloroform method; the hemoglobin by Fleischl's instrument. He concludes from these studies that the former is in great measure dependent upon the latter, though it may vary as much as 13.5 parts per thousand, with similar hemoglobin quantity. A difference of 10% in hemoglobin indicates, on an average, a difference of 4.6 per thousand in specific gravity. With equal quantities of hemoglobin the specific gravity of the blood of women is 2 to 2.5 parts lower than the blood of men, both in physiologic and pathologic conditions. The variability in the specific gravity is greater in cases in which there is considerable hemoglobin than in those in which anemia is marked. The specific gravity in nephritis is from 4 to 5 points lower than in other conditions, this being due to hydremia of the plasma. The specific gravity in leukemia is greater than the hemoglobin would indicate, this disproportion being according to the number of leukocytes. In chlorosis the specific gravity is about 2.5 parts higher than in secondary anemias; but this peculiarity of the blood rapidly disappears during regeneration. In cases of pernicious anemia, in which the number of the red corpuscles is decreased greatly in comparison with the quantity of hemoglobin, the specific gravity is generally about 2 parts lower than in the secondary anemias; this peculiarity also disappears during regeneration of the blood. From these facts he concludes that the number of the red corpuscles (their stroma) exercises a positive influence on the specific gravity, so that in spite of equal quantities of hemoglobin there may be a difference due to this factor of 4 to 5 parts per thousand.

Moraczewska[2] has examined the blood in 34 cases of **chronic disease associated with anemia.** In pernicious anemia she found a marked reduction in alkalinity, and high specific weight, due to the presence of an increased quantity of the mineral salts. The blood contained an excess of nitrogen. In chlorosis there were similar changes, excepting in regard to the red blood-corpuscles. The anemias due to carcinoma showed increased alkalinity, diminished specific weight, and, relatively, a considerable number of red blood-cells that stained faintly.

R. Schmidt[3] has observed that in severe chronic anemic conditions the excretion of the alloxur bodies is increased if a large quantity of albumin, poor in nuclein, is added to the nourishment. At the same time there are an increase in the neutral sulphates and a diminution in the earthy phosphates.

[1] Deutsch. Arch. f. klin Med., Bd. lvii., H. 3 and 4.
[2] Virchow's Archiv, vol. cxliv., p. 127.
[3] Wien. klin. Woch., June 10, 1897.

Mann[1] has given 22 male patients of anemic appearance a dram of extract of bone-marrow, 3 times daily. The average increase of red corpuscles was 1,360,000, and the average increase in hemoglobin $12\frac{1}{2}\%$. There was usually a decrease in the number of leukocytes in cases with leukocytosis.

CHLOROSIS.

Etiology.—Taylor[2] discusses the nature and causation of chlorosis. Referring to certain published cases of chlorosis in males, he states that the mere fact of greater decrease in hemoglobin than in corpuscles does not suffice to constitute true chlorosis. " I must allow, however," he says, " that if there is no distinctive feature in the blood, it is difficult to know what we are to regard as the characteristic of the disease." Among the more likely theories are the mechanical action of the corset, causing ulcerations and hemorrhages from the stomach or by forcing the stomach into an abnormal position, and the supposed extraordinary demand that puberty makes upon the blood-forming organs. He does not venture upon positive conclusions as to these or other supposed causes. [We note that the author's comment upon certain published cases of supposed male chlorosis are the same as our own in reviewing this publication in the *Year-Book* for 1897.]

Biernacki[3] discusses the nature of chlorosis, and is led to doubt whether reduction in hemoglobin is an essential element from the fact that considerable alteration in the blood may take place without the malaise experienced by chlorotic patients, and undoubted cases of chlorosis have been reported in which this reduction did not occur. He holds that more important blood-changes are hydremia and the diminution of potassium and of phosphoric acid. C. E. Simon[4] discusses various problems connected with chlorosis, and has studied its etiology and treatment. He refers to the view of certain observers that visceral descent or **splanchnoptosis** is a factor of importance, and then analyzes a number of cases in which this point was studied. He found that it was associated with anemia in a fairly large proportion of 39 individuals, and this was true, more particularly, of nephroptosis. There was, however, a considerable number in which the amount of hemoglobin was practically normal and yet the descent of the viscera was striking. [The author does not state the method by which he determined the presence of nephroptosis in so large a proportion of the individuals examined.] In a second group of 25 cases he investigated the results of simple gastric atony and anemia, finding that there was no definite relation. He concludes that neither atony nor splanchnoptosis has any part in the causation of chlorosis. [We must, however, call attention to the fact that his method of excluding these factors is not entirely logical; it has not been held for example, even by enthusiasts, that atony or splanchnoptosis invariably causes chlorosis.] The examinations of the stomach-contents and of the urine are interesting. In $\frac{1}{3}$ of his cases the amount of HCl was normal, in $\frac{3}{10}$ excessive, in $\frac{1}{6}$ deficient, and in $\frac{1}{3}$ HCl was absent. Indicanuria beyond the normal was found in a minority of the cases (9 in 31). The author finally concludes that as none of the etiological factors usually referred to is entirely satisfactory, in the great majority of cases chlorosis is essentially a disease of malnutrition; the result of abnormal feeding in early childhood. As a groundwork of this view, he defines chlorosis as an anemic condition or simple anemia in which the percentage of hemoglobin is lower than 70, and the number of corpuscles approximately

[1] Am. Jour. Insan., Jan., 1897.
[2] Brit. Med. Jour., Sept. 9, 1896.
[3] Wien. med. Woch., Feb. 2, 1897.
[4] Am. Jour. Med. Sci., Apr., 1897.

normal. [This view seems to us to express a great fallacy in the author's work. Nothing is more certain than that chloranemia and chlorosis are independent and separable conditions, and rather than adopt the view of the author that the term chlorosis should be displaced because it refers to but one of the symptoms, we would hold that this term, or a similar one, should be retained for that very reason. There is too great a disposition to diagnose chlorosis from the condition of the blood. Hemotologists are united in declaring that this cannot lead to satisfactory results. The blood examination must be considered together with the clinical symptoms.] Next the author refers to the question of treatment, and alludes particularly to cases in which iron does not relieve the condition. He recommends extract of boue-marrow or the marrow itself as a valuable article of diet, and suggests that it may have a specific action as well. Suitable diet is always essential.

Schroth[1] studied 44 cases of chlorosis, and was unable to determine any secretory or motor disturbances of the stomach, and he believes that the occurrence of a certain amount of gastro- or enteroptosis is of no significance. His own view is rather that chlorosis results from reflex nervous impressions, originating in disturbances of the genital organs.

Pathology.—Hayem[2] presented specimens from a case of chlorosis before the Société méd. des Hôpitaux; the patient died from the effects of sudden emotion while under treatment for chlorosis. She had previously had phlebitis in the left leg. When she came under observation she had the usual signs of chlorosis, with small pulse and strong, irregular action of the heart. There were a thrill at the apex and a bruit sometimes resembling a friction-sound, sometimes a valvular murmur; there was an additional bruit at times, giving the rhythm of *bruit de galop*. Change of position did not moderate the sounds. Postmortem the pulmonary artery was found entirely obstructed by clots, some old and adherent, others more recent and extending from the heart upward. The heart itself was small, and there were numerous papillary cauliflower vegetations in the right ventricle and on the intraventricular septum. Near the infundibulum was a large clot partly adherent, portions of which were encrusted with calcareous deposits and covered by prolongations of the endocardium; the extremity of this clot was also covered with debris of recent formation, like that in the pulmonary artery. He believed that the phlebitis had been accompanied by endocarditis, then by obstruction of the pulmonary artery of a slowly developing form. There was no pulmonary embolism, but the lungs were collapsed, infiltrated, and suffused with blood.

J. O. Affleck,[3] in discussing Taylor's review of anemia, alludes to a fatal case of extreme chlorosis in a girl of 17, who died of acute pneumonia, in which postmortem examination was obtained. The aorta was found to be extremely small, and the pathologist compared it to the size of a normal innominate artery. No other details were given.

Talma[4] discusses the **relations of the conus arteriosus** to chlorosis, and the significance of murmurs heard over the base of the heart. The conus, which in normal conditions contains more blood than the remaining portions of the right ventricle, is, according to his observations, particularly dilated in chlorosis. The distention occurs in a direction upward and to the left, and alters the cardiac dulness so that the upper border on the left side is found in the third, or even in the second or first interspace, in consequence of the displacement of the root of the pulmonary artery. The pulmonary sounds are

[1] Ann. der Stadt. Allg. Krankenhaus. zu München, ii., 3, 1896.
[2] L'Union méd., No. 12, 1896.   [3] Brit. Med. Jour., p. 726, Sept. 19, 1896.
[4] Berlin. klin. Woch., No. 44, 1896.

heard with greatest intensity pretty far to the left of the sternum. Frequently systolic murmurs are heard over the dilated conus, and the author believes it possible to distinguish whether these are produced in the dilated conus or in the position of greatest intensity. In the latter case the pulmonary artery by the position of greatest intensity. In the latter case the murmur is heard further to the left and above. Finally, he contends that this enlargement of the conus forms a sign of much diagnostic value, occurring most regularly in chlorosis, although it occurs in cases of cardiac weakness due to intoxications and in myocarditis. [This paper seems to us one of considerable importance, and the subject presented is worthy more extensive study.]

Ventriui[1] has studied the **resistive powers of the red blood-cells** in 2 cases of chlorosis and found them diminished. After subcutaneous injection of iron salts, however, he found them considerably increased, and this appeared to be more or less constant. In 2 cases of anemia the iron salts did not appear to have this beneficial effect.

Symptoms.—Gilbert and Garnier[2] carefully studied the **venous murmur** in a case of chlorosis. They found that it was heard best along the line which corresponds exactly to that of the superior vena cava, and concluded that it arose from disturbance of this vessel. As the murmur was distinctly increased by rotation of the head to the left, they assumed that it was due to pressure which might have been exerted by the sterno-mastoid muscle upon the internal jugular vein or by the clavicle upon the brachiocephalic trunk. This particular venous murmur has not previously been recognized.

Treatment.—Spillmann and Etienne[3] have employed *ovariin* and fresh and dried **ovarian tissue** in the treatment of chlorosis. In 2 of 6 cases they observed marked improvement. The treatment, however, sometimes caused increased rapidity of pulse, elevation of temperature with pain in the abdomen and kidneys, headache, and vague myalgias.

J. L. Corish[4] reports 3 cases of chlorosis which were treated by **inhalations of oxygen** under pressure, in addition to iron and arsenic. In all improvement occurred. He believes that chlorosis may be due in part to absence of oxygen in the blood-corpuscles without much diminution in the amount of iron.

PERNICIOUS ANEMIA.

Etiology.—Taylor[5] holds that it is too great a restriction of the term pernicious anemia to apply it only to apparently idiopathic cases. It ought to include, or at any rate we must recognize as very obscure, those cases in which a temporary cause is followed by persistent anemia. For example, continuous loss of blood may be expected to cause severe anemia, but that pregnancy, a course of lactation, or a single hemorrhage should leave behind anemia which persists or progresses long after the complete cessation of the ordinary phenomena of the confessed cause, requires as much explanation as those cases in which the anemia has appeared to be entirely spontaneous. In reviewing the opposing views of Hunter and Stockman, he rather sides with Hunter, and very properly points out that if the symptoms of the disease result, as Stockman states, from innumerable small hemorrhages due to primary disease of the vessel-walls, it remains to be shown by that author what caused this vascular disorder to arise.

J. B. Herrick[6] discusses the relations of **shock** to pernicious anemia in connection with a report of one of his cases. The patient, a woman of 63, of good

---

[1] Gaz. med. di Torino, No. 52, 1896. [2] Compt. rend. de la Soc. de Biol., May 7, 1897.
[3] Therap. Woch., No. 50, 1896. [4] N. Y. Med. Jour., Feb. 13, 1897.
[5] Brit. Med. Jour., Sept. 9, 1896. [6] Alienist and Neurol., July, 1896.

appearance, and weighing 137 pounds, was an active practitioner of medicine. Her family history was good. She was married and had 5 children. She fell on a sidewalk, hurting her back and left side extensively. After this she became physically and mentally weaker. Soon her legs began to swell, dizziness and faintness developed, pallor was noted, and she was confined to bed a large part of the time. She was suspected of malingering, but this could scarcely be proved. Later physical examination showed signs of pernicious anemia, numerous retinal hemorrhages, cardiac murmurs; the blood was pale, the corpuscles varying greatly in size, a few containing nuclei—most of these being normoblasts. The leukocytes were increased relatively, and there were many lymphocytes. Red corpuscles 666,000; hemoglobin 25%; the temperature varied from 97° to 102°. The patient later passed from observation. In discussing this case the author shows that there was no distinct organic lesion discoverable, and refers to shock as the possible cause. He alludes to the papers of Curtin, Musser, and others, and concludes that shock or injury to the nervous system may have a predisposing causal relation. In the discussion of the paper Musser referred to 2 recent cases under his care in which pernicious anemia was secondary to, if not due to, nervous influence.

Ralph Stockman [1] reports a case of pernicious anemia occurring in a pregnant woman. 2 months prior to delivery she began to grow weak and pale and was greatly troubled with distention of the abdomen. Physical examination of the heart, lungs, and liver was negative, and the blood showed red blood-corpuscles 1,680,000, hemoglobin 24%; subsequently, red blood-corpuscles 920,000, hemoglobin 20%. The patient died. At the autopsy dilatation of the stomach and enormous distention of the ascending and descending colon were observed. The transverse colon and rectum were normal and there was no obstruction. A suspicion had been entertained before death that the case was one of malignant obstruction of the large intestine. There was no excess of iron in the liver or spleen. The patient did not suffer unusual loss of blood at time of labor. [A case under our own care showed a similar relation of **intestinal disease** to pernicious anemia. The patient recovered almost completely, but is now under our care again with even more typical symptoms.]

Ransom,[2] in discussing his pathologic observations in 18 cases of pernicious anemia, comes to the following among other conclusions: that there is always **hemolysis,** and often evidences of **absorption of the hemolytic poison** from the alimentary canal. In some cases the poison may arise elsewhere, as from the uterus or from other situations in various infections. Increase of iron pigment is usually found in the liver, spleen, and kidneys, but may be absent in any one of these. It may also be found in the lymphoid tissues of the intestines, more especially in the colon, where it is in process of excretion. It is probably brought to the organs in a soluble form other than hemoglobin. Hemolysis by itself probably rarely causes pernicious anemia. Insufficient hemogenesis must be superadded. In some cases abnormal hemogenesis is the initial phenomena, the corpuscles being too fragile to resist the normal hemolytic influences of the system. He could find no evidence that multiple small internal hemorrhages could cause pernicious anemia. [These views coincide very accurately in most respects with our own opinion. One of the editors particularly has insisted upon the necessity of assuming that a reduced power of hemogenesis must play an important part in the development of the disease. We cannot, however, agree that there is decided evidence in favor of the view that the hemogenetic deficiency is ever primarily operative.]

[1] Edinb. Hosp. Rep., vol. iv., 1896.   [2] Brit. Med. Jour., Dec., 1896.

Wharton Sinkler and A. A. Eshner[1] report **3 cases** of profound anemia occurring **in one family**—the father and 2 daughters—with development of the symptoms of posterior spinal sclerosis and a fatal termination in 1 case. Briefly they were as follows : (Case 1) A salesgirl of 16, presented herself at the clinic with the history that her father had died of locomotor ataxia and pernicious anemia at 45. She had been weak and often ill, but her habits, mode of eating, and daily life accounted for this. She had cardiac palpitation, pain in the chest, numbness and cramps, and frequently staggered in walking. Cough with considerable expectoration was present. She had suffered with chills, flushes, dyspnea, and headaches. Her blood was examined and showed 3,000,000 red corpuscles and 20 % of hemoglobin. Under treatment with arsenic and iron she improved and was discharged practically well. A sister (Case 2) presented herself complaining of vertigo, nausea, and weakness when in the erect posture ; anorexia, constipation, and shortness of breath. She ascribed these symptoms to grippe, with which she had suffered nearly 2 months earlier. She was anemic in appearance, but no blood-examination is recorded. She improved greatly under arsenic and iron. The father of these 2 patients (Case 3) had been treated at the infirmary previously. He was then 41 years of age ; a laborer. His only children were the 2 girls and a brother. His wife had had several miscarriages. He had suffered with great derangement of the digestion for 8 years, vomiting sometimes thrice daily. He had had a sudden attack, like a " giving way " in the back, while wheeling a barrow 4 years previously, and for a time was unable to straighten himself ; he seemed to recover perfectly. His subsequent trouble began with a feeling of numbness in the legs and later distinct ataxia developed. The patient was pale, presenting a somewhat muddy tint. His blood-examination showed at first 2,700,000 red blood-corpuscles and from 27 to 35 % hemoglobin ; later about the same figures ; and, finally, 4,475,000 blood-corpuscles with from 60 to 80 % hemoglobin. Subsequently it again declined, and there was poikilocytosis with irregularity in size, but no nucleated red corpuscles. He was in bed for the anemia, but recovered and returned to work. He then had a relapse, and finally died in the second attack. The case is of interest, as being one of somewhat irregular ataxia associated with anemia. The authors are disposed to rank it as a case of ataxia secondary to anemia. The cord has not yet been studied. [The exact nature of these cases is uncertain.]

Pathology.—R. F. Ruttan and J. G. Adams[2] have studied the composition of the **blood-serum** in a case of **pernicious anemia.** The blood was obtained postmortem from the distended right heart 5 hours after death. As the temperature of the room was near zero, it may be assumed that but little change took place. The case was typical, and gastric lesions were discovered postmortem (gastritis polyposa). The serum was clear, almost colorless, and had a sp. gr. of 1026. It contained only 5.2 % of proteids by weight. Of these, 2.3 % was globulins precipitated by saturation with magnesium sulfate and 2.9 % was serumalbumin. There was 0.875 % of ash. The total proteid was about 40 % below the average normal quantity. The normal ratio of globulin and serumalbumin was considerably altered, while the amount of ash was about 12 times the normal. Analysis of the liver for iron showed 0.2433 % by weight calculated for the fresh, undried tissue and 0.72 % in the dried tissue. These represent a great increase.

Venous Disturbances.—Petren[3] records 9 cases of pernicious anemia in which the **spinal cord was found more or less diseased.** Two

---

[1] Am. Jour. Med. Sci., Sept., 1896.   [2] Brit. Med. Jour., Dec. 12, 1896.
[3] Nord. Med. Arkiv, No. 7, 1896.

showed spinal symptoms during life. In the first, disturbances of sensibility, paresis, ataxia, loss of knee-jerk, and finally incontinence of urine developed. Anemia had existed 6 months and spinal symptoms for 2 months. The spinal cord showed degenerations of the posterior columns and swelling of the glia-cells, but never of the axis-cylinders. These changes were found in all parts of the cord except the dorsal region. In the second case the patient was attacked with paresis of the legs 3 years before death and 25 years after a specific infection, which, however, had never given rise to any symptoms. Two days before his death he was examined and the characteristics of severe pernicious anemia with paraplegia were discovered. There was complete degeneration of the column of Goll and moderate degeneration of those of Burdach that did not reach the lower half of the lumbar cord. The author does not deny the probably syphilitic nature of this case. Taking the entire 9 cases, it may be noted that hyaline degeneration of the blood-vessels in the white matter of the cord was found in 4, while small hemorrhages or focal sclerosis secondary to hemorrhages were found scattered throughout the cord in the other 5.

R. C. Cabot[1] contributes a careful study of 50 cases of pernicious anemia. Of these, 8 came to autopsy and the others were recognized by the clinical features. He defines pernicious anemia as a profound and almost invariably fatal anemia without adequate known cause, characterized by an extreme diminution in the number of red blood-cells and usually by other changes in the blood as well as by the absence of emaciation and a tendency to spontaneous temporary improvement followed by relapse. In regard to the etiology, 3 of the 17 female patients dated their symptoms from the time of the menopause. Atrophy of the gastric tubules was not found in any of the autopsies. Hemorrhage occurred in 17 cases; in 12 after symptoms of profound anemia; and in 5 before that time. Symptoms affecting the nervous system especially were found in 20 cases; paresthesia of the extremities in 2; numbness in 8, of which 5 also showed motor weakness and pain or tenderness along the nerves; the knee-jerks were absent in 4, and in 1 of these there were shooting-pains; 1 case had blurred sight and marked constipation; 1 case had atrophy, weakness, and numbness of the left arm and leg, and tremor of the left hand was noted; in another, a spastic gait with increased reflexes and clonus; 2 cases had total paralysis of all the extremities and loss of control of the sphincters toward the end of the disease. Aphasia was found in 2, 1 of which had suffered sudden coma sometime previously. Sudden inability to swallow, with paresis of the arm and leg on one side and drawing of the veins on the opposite side, occurred in 1 case. Regarding the urine, the author notes that the sp. gr. was low, averaging 1015, and the color high in but 3 of the cases. The red blood-corpuscles are usually about 1,000,000. Partial improvements are frequent, and in these the corpuscles increase somewhat, but not as much as the symptoms would indicate. The white corpuscles are usually diminished or normal in number, and the hemoglobin was apparently higher than the corpuscles in 13 cases, and lower than the corpuscles in the rest, as in secondary anemias. The last point, however, the author regards as of little value, as an estimation of hemoglobin by Fleischl's apparatus is inaccurate. Regarding the red corpuscles, he lays particular stress upon the occurrence of large megaloblasts as well as upon various other forms of huge cells which he distinguishes from normoblasts. Altogether he recognizes 9 types of nucleated red corpuscles. The differential count of the leukocytes shows the lymphocytes relatively in excess, and the almost invariable presence of a small percentage of myelocytes. [We are surprised at the proportion of cases in which marked nervous symptoms occurred.

[1] Boston M. and S. Jour., July 30, 1896.

It would have been interesting to know to what extent arsenic (used in the treatment) could be regarded as having caused these symptoms. Some of them could easily have been so caused. The discussion of the blood-condition is thorough, but we cannot admit the advisability of distinguishing a large number of forms of nucleated corpuscles. The matter of morphology is already overdone by many writers.]

Colquhoun [1] describes a case of pernicious anemia in which **spinal symptoms** were observed. At first there were loss of knee-jerks, pain in the muscles of the calf, and loss of coordination. The author regarded these symptoms as due to arsenical neuritis, but subsequently the reflexes became much exaggerated and another explanation seemed necessary. The condition resembled that seen in mixed sclerosis (posterior and lateral) of the cord, and though arsenic may be the cause of these lesions, the author notes that he has frequently given large and continuous doses without such results.

Teichmüller [2] reports a case of pernicious anemia with nervous symptoms—paresthesia and increased knee-jerk. The patient had arteriosclerosis and evidence of chronic enteritis. Postmortem small hemorrhages were found in the corpora quadrigemina and in the corpora striata. Microscopic examination discovered changes in the posterior columns of the cord, as well as hemorrhages in the gray and white matter, with degeneration in the anterior lateral columns of the cord. The author regards the changes in the gray matter as the most important.

Treatment.—Delmis [3] states that the **pernicious anemia of pregnancy** differs from ordinary anemia only by the greater intensity of the symptoms. Treatment with iodid of iron is generally successful, even in severe cases. He gives from 1 to 2 tablespoonfuls of a syrup of iodid of iron with each meal and increases in the later stages. The food should be nutritious. If the treatment is begun early, especially in primiparæ, as soon as symptoms develop, the severer grades may be prevented. Even in multiparæ, who had previously suffered with anemia, the subsequent pregnancy was freed from any complications by this treatment.

H. A. Hare,[4] in describing a series of cases of leukemia and pernicious anemia, details 1 in which the patient improved markedly under the use of **arsenic and iron sulfate,** the red corpuscles increasing from 886,000 to 4,360,000 during one period of the treatment. The last-named figure was found at the last visit, and the author regards the case as cured. The patient had previously improved greatly several times and subsequently relapsed, but the amelioration after the last attack was more prolonged. [Although it seems scarcely proper to speak of the case as one of cured pernicious anemia, the improvement in the blood is certainly remarkable.]

J. M. Clarke [5] reports a case of anemia with a blood-count of 810,000 and hemoglobin 31%. Arsenic having failed to give any beneficial effect, transfusion of blood in solution of phosphate of sodium was employed. Several days later this was followed by hematuria, which recurred again after a second transfusion. **Inhalations of oxygen** had been systematically employed from the beginning. At the autopsy the lesions of pernicious anemia were found. Three cases of profound anemia are also reported in which oxygen inhalations were employed, apparently with great benefit, all the patients making a good recovery.

[1] New Zealand Med. Jour., Oct.. 1896.   [2] Deutsch. Zeit. f. Nervenh., Bd. 8, H. 5 and 6.
[3] Gaz. des Hôpitaux, No. 48, 1896.   [4] Med. News, Mar. 27, 1897.
[5] Bristol Med.-Chir. Jour., Dec., 1896.

LEUKEMIA.

Etiology.—Bonvicini [1] found that the organs of a dog that had died of leukemia contained a diplococcus that, when inoculated into dogs, produced swelling of the lymphatic glands, and when injected into mice, guinea-pigs, and cats produced typical leukemia. [Similar reports have been made before, but the matter is by no means so easily determined.]

Pathology.—C. F. Martin and G. H. Matthewson [2] discuss the relation between **leukemia and pseudoleukemia,** and contend that these diseases are closely allied and often not to be distinguished readily by the conditions of the blood. They refer particularly to a case in which there were purpuric spots, and hemorrhages from the stomach, gums, and intestines in a patient who had previously suffered with malaise, enlargement of the spleen, and some fever; the leukocytes were increased (1 to 10), and chiefly of the mononuclear variety. Within a week the patient died, having developed nodules in the skin, high fever, and great weakness. Shortly before death mononuclear leukocytosis was more marked, and a diagnosis of leukemia was made. The necropsy showed primary sarcoma of the cervix uteri and secondary nodules. In a second case, admitted for hemorrhage from the stomach and purpuric spots, the disease ran a rapid course of 2 weeks, terminating fatally. The ratio of white to red cells was 1 to 21, the leukocytes being chiefly lymphocytes. From the knowledge of the last case and from the published records of Fagge, they made a diagnosis of sarcomatosis, and the autopsy revealed such lesions. In another patient, a girl of 11, admitted to the hospital on account of marked hematemesis, there were great anemia, enlargement of the spleen, and the ratio of white cells to red probably " between that usually seen in leukemia and in leukocytosis." After a few days the patient died, and presented the typical lesions of leukemia or Hodgkin's disease. They conclude, therefore, that an enormous increase of white cells is not in itself diagnostic of leukemia. They then study the nature of the leukocytosis that occurs in leukemia, and develop the fact that in Hodgkin's disease there may be considerable leukocytosis and that small mononuclear elements are prone to be numerous. They finally report a case of lymphatic leukemia illustrative of the difficulties of distinguishing the diseases. In this case the leukocytes at first numbered only about 24,000 per c.mm.; subsequently they increased to 60,000; and fluctuations were noted ranging between the last figure and 17,000. The authors state that myelocytes were not present. A point of interest in this case was the fact that the patient had suffered an injury to the month with inflammation and swelling, and the general disease followed this condition. [All writers in recent years agree that no sharp dividing-line may be drawn between leukemia and Hodgkin's disease, and it is a matter of regret that so frequently irrelevant statements are incorporated in the discussions, and badly observed cases are ranged by the side of those carefully worked out. We note, for example, in the present author's paper allusion to cases of Litten and others in which the transformation of pernicious anemia into leukemia was said to be observed. The occurrence of terminal leukocytosis in pernicious anemia and other severe anemias is now so well known that such cases (observed many years since) ought not to be included among others well studied as instancing transformations of one disease into another. Thus, too many of the cases of supposed transformation of Hodgkin's disease into leukemia are probably of the same sort, but there are other instances in which actual and positive transformation has occurred. Some authors state positively that cer-

[1] Bologna, 1896.   [2] Brit. Med. Jour., Dec. 5 and 12, 1896.

tain cases were instances of diffuse sarcoma, though previously regarded as leukemia, ignoring the great difficulty and the practical impossibility in some cases of distinguishing the lesion of leukemia from lymphosarcoma. We agree with the conclusions of the authors that there is no line of demarcation between these diseases, and we hold them to be similar or identical in their pathology; but we cannot agree that there is very frequently difficulty in establishing a diagnosis of the clinical picture of the one or the other disorder.]

Benda[1] examined 7 cases of **acute leukemia** postmortem, and found hemorrhages into the organs and swelling of the lymph-glands. The spleen was neither as large nor as soft as in acute infectious diseases. The blood invariably showed great increase in the mononuclear elements. The cause of the hemorrhage appears to be a disease of the walls of the veins.

Vanderwey[2] has studied **metabolism** in 2 cases of leukemia. In the first, which was examined at 4 different periods, there was always abnormal tissue-destruction, despite the fact that the diet was satisfactory. In the 2d case, during 7 days, the nitrogenous balance was maintained despite the existence of fever. In the 1st case the amount of tissue-destruction seemed in a measure parallel with the elevation of the temperature; still this rule was not absolute. There was a constant excess of uric acid in the urine, the greatest quantities occurring at the acme of the febrile paroxysm; and, although no constant relation could be made out between the amount of uric acid and the amount of nitrogen excreted, still both of these increased at the same times, and this increase was accompanied by increase in the quantity of urine. In this respect he substantiates the results of Jacob and Salkowski.

Symptoms.—R. J. M. Buchannan[3] reports 6 cases of leukemia and recognizes 2 divisions of the disease: (*a*) characterized by predominating increase of small uninuclear lymphocytes of gradually increasing size and accretion of basophile granulations; (*b*) splenomyelogenous, with large uninucleated myelocytes and atypical oxyphile and basophile cells, and, as a special feature, no increase of lymphocytes. Mixed forms occur probably in all cases. So long as the abnormal elements are found in the blood, no matter if the number of leukocytes returns to normal under treatment, a relapse invariably occurs. The primary factor giving rise to one or other form of the disease still remains unknown, but the peculiarities shown by the persistent multiplication of a certain class of cell strongly favor the idea that the result is a proliferation of cellular elements analogous to the growth of certain tumors.

Von Hayek[4] reports a case of leukemia that was under observation for $3\frac{1}{2}$ months. During the whole period there was a **daily rise of temperature** followed by a gradual fall. The highest point was usually reached late in the afternoon, and was frequently accompanied by chill. Night-sweats were almost constant. The proportion of leukocytes to red blood-corpuscles was about 1 to 5, the leukocytosis being less in the morning and greater in the afternoon. The differential count was, polynuclear, 29%; transitional, 21%; large mononuclear, 42%; myelocytes, 1%; and lymphocytes, 7%; 3% of the cells showed eosinophile granulations. There was no ground for suspecting the presence of malaria, tuberculosis, or a local focus of suppuration. At the autopsy a diagnosis of uncomplicated leukemia was fully sustained.

Sharon and Gratia[5] report a case of **splenic leukemia** occurring in a

[1] Centralb. f. innere Med., June 26, 1897.
[2] Deutsch. Arch. f. klin. Med., vol. lvii., H. 3 and 4.
[3] Jour. Path., Bd. 4, No. 2.　　　　　　　　　　[4] Wien. klin. Woch., May 20, 1897.
[5] Bull. de la Soc. roy. des Sci. med. et nat. de Bruxelles, No. 7, 1896.

girl of 8 years, who had been under observation with an abdominal tumor for 6 years. The child was brought for operation, but examination showed that enlargement was due to a hypertrophied spleen. The liver was also increased in size. The subcutaneous veins were dilated, but there was no marked ascites. The blood showed 1 white to 5 red corpuscles. Subsequently it became worse, and death took place with symptoms of dyspnea.

J. Craig[1] describes a case of **lymphatic leukemia.** The patient, a lad of 19, died after an illness of about 2 months. There were universal enlargement of the lymphatic glands, bleeding from the nose, persistent diarrhea, severe pain in the stomach, priapism, and marked increase in the number of white blood-corpuscles, the small lymphocytes being especially increased. The autopsy showed great involvement of the lymphatic glands in all parts of the body, and also some enlargement of the spleen and liver. The condition of the bone-marrow was not noted.

H. A. Hare[2] reports a number of cases of diseases of the blood, including one which he describes as "lymphatic leukemia or lymphatic anemia." The patient, a barber aged 24, was a man of good habits, who had been well until 7 years previous, when he had an attack of grip that confined him to bed for 4 weeks, during which he was sometimes delirious. He had a severe attack of double pneumonia 2 or 3 years before, and later in the same year fell down a declivity and suffered considerable injury to the head and neck. The next year he first came under observation, complaining that some time previously he had felt a severe pain beneath the clavicle. This persisted for 3 days and then descended to the left hypochondriac region. Profuse sweating with rapid pulse and moderate fever was noted, and he states that he was unconscious for 3 days. He began to lose weight and remained in bed for a month. He then began to improve, but the pain continued and there was a feeling of weight in the left side. On admission to the hospital he was noticeably pale, and the temperature was 102.4°. A large spleen occupied the left side of the abdomen. There were retinal hemorrhages and subsequently hematuria. Anemic murmurs were heard in the neck. Examinations of the blood at various times showed from 1,000,000 to 2,800,000 red corpuscles, and from 14 to 48% hemoglobin. The leukocytes varied from 4000 to 9000, and the differential count showed 84% of lymphocytes, 4% of mononuclear cells, 8% of polymorphous cells, and 3% of eosinophiles. The author states that the large proportion of the lymphocytes would apparently place it under the head of lymphatic leukemia, though there was an entire absence of enlargement of the lymphatic glands and no leukocytosis. [The excessive number of lymphocytes in this case cannot be given the importance the author attributes to it. Lymphocytosis is a condition so frequently observed in various diseases or abnormal states, particularly in cachectic or anemic persons, that its significance is doubtful. The case cannot, by any possibility, be spoken of as leukemia from the facts presented in the paper. The further progress of the case might however justify the diagnosis.]

Fränkel[3] states that as the **hemorrhagic diathesis** is one of the characteristics of **acute leukemia,** the latter is frequently mistaken for purpura hemorrhagica when the blood-examination is not carefully made. The condition of the blood is characteristic. There is an increase exclusively in the mononuclear leukocytes with the absence of Ehrlich's neutrophile granulations; it can, therefore, be spoken of as an acute lymphocythemia. He reports a case with peripheral facial paralysis following leukemic neuritis. The proportion of white

[1] Dublin Jour. Med. Sci., Sept. 1, 1897.   [2] Med. News, Mar. 27, 1897.
[3] Centralbl. f. innere Med., June 26, 1897.

to red cells was 1 to 94. Magnus Levy investigated the urine and found that 12 gm. of uric acid were excreted per day.

Complications.—Ebstein[1] describes a case of leukemia in a woman of 76, with hoarseness and cough. Later, symptoms of laryngeal obstruction developed and tracheotomy was required. The cause of the obstruction was found during life to be infiltration of the epiglottis on its laryngeal surface, of the false cords, and of the mucous membrane below the cords. The color of the mucous membrane was a pale grayish-red. The absence of any sign of ulceration and the general condition of the patient led to the diagnosis of leukemic infiltration, and this was confirmed by the histological examination postmortem. The epithelium was healthy, but immediately beneath it there was an irregular cellular infiltration containing a large proportion of eosinophile cells. It is of some interest to note that Charcot-Leyden crystals were found in the glands in the mucous membrane.

Mager[2] describes a case in which a diagnosis of leukemic **infiltration of the larynx** was made by Schrötter. The patient, a man of 58, presented the leukemic characters of blood, the ratio of white to red corpuscles being 1 to 4. At first the larynx showed only signs of acute catarrh, but 3 weeks later there were diffuse redness and infiltration, especially over the right arytenoid cartilage. After a few days there was irregular elevation of the posterior surface of the right arytenoid cartilage and a nodule on the middle of the aryepiglottic fold. Tracheotomy was performed on account of dyspnea, but death occurred 8 days later. At the autopsy there was found perichondritis of the arytenoid cartilage in addition to the leukemic infiltration. The periosteum in the right half of the larynx was evidently partly infiltrated by the leukemic and partly by a simple inflammatory process. In the left half the infiltration was purely leukemic.

Marjschler[3] reports a case of leukemia occurring in a man 61 years of age. Upon admission to the hospital the erythrocytes were 3,450,000, the leukocytes 96,000, the hemoglobin 50%. The differential count of the leukocytes showed 82% mononuclear and only 15% polynuclear forms. The lymph-glands were everywhere considerably enlarged and the spleen extended 3 fingers' breadth below the border of the ribs. The course of the disease was not unusual. At one period hematuria occurred, and some 2 months after admission a tumor could be detected beneath the edge of the liver. Some time later a fragment of tissue was passed in the urine that was diagnosed as coming from a neoplasm. During the latter period there was considerable change in the character of the leukocytes: they became progressively less numerous till, toward the end, they sank to 72,000. The polynuclear forms increased rapidly, the myelocytes of Ehrlich appeared, and the mononuclear forms diminished. At the last differential count the mononuclear were 40%, the polynuclear 57%, and the myelocytes 0.16%. At the autopsy a perithelioma carcinomatodes supraglandulare was found in the right kidney, with extension into the ureter. Neither the lymph-glands nor the spleen showed any traces of malignant new growth, but only typical changes of leukemic infiltration. Hitherto but 2 cases of the **coexistence of carcinoma and leukemia** have been described, in neither of which are there any definite statements as to the influence of malignant growth upon the course of the disease. It has, however, been observed in cases of leukemia complicated by various septic processes that considerable improvement, at least in the lenkocytosis, occurs as the infection develops. Marischler is inclined to believe that

[1] Wien. klin. Woch., No. 22, 1896.   [2] Ibid., No. 26, 1896.
[3] Ibid., July 23, 1896.

in the present case improvement took place, but was manifested more by a change in the character of the leukocytes than by any great diminution in their number. [From the description of the tumor, and the fact that it extended without giving rise to metastasis, we are inclined to regard it as an endothelioma, a form of neoplasm that is not especially malignant nor apt to give rise to general symptoms.]

Thorsch [1] discusses the **effect of acute infectious diseases** upon leukemia. A patient under treatment for lienolymphatic leukemia died in consequence of an intercurrent migratory croupous pneumonia. There was at first a rapid decrease in size of the lymphatic glands, the spleen, and the liver, and a striking decline in the number of leukocytes. These had been steadily increasing in number before the pneumonia began, but rapidly sank to 43,500 afterward. When it was fully developed, however, the number of leukocytes again increased and by the time the fatal termination occurred had become greater than originally.

SPLENIC ANEMIA.

Taylor [2] holds that splenic anemia, as described by Banti and Bruhl, is a distinct disease. He refers to the case of a little girl who began to be ill at 9 years of age, and came under his observation at 13. There was paroxysmal pain in the left side recurring at intervals. A swelling was noticed in the left side of the abdomen, and a year later she began to grow pale. There were no hemorrhages, but when first seen she was thin and very anemic, and the spleen extended almost to the iliac crest. The red corpuscles numbered 2,700,000, but there was no leukocytosis, no malarial plasmodia could be found, and there were no retinal hemorrhages. Hemoglobin was greatly diminished. Treatment was unavailing; at one time there were indications of a splenic infarct—tenderness, pain, and palpable and audible friction. She died 3 months later. The author excludes amyloid disease and tumors. He points out that, pathologically, the chief change is in the spleen, which is greatly enlarged and presents sclerotic or fibroid change with atrophy of the Malpighian bodies and considerable thickening of the trabeculæ; changes that differ from those observed in the splenic form of Hodgkin's disease. Finally, he cites without particular comment a case of Dr. Coupland, in which a diagnosis was made and the spleen removed. Death occurred some years later, and at the autopsy extensive syphilitic disease of the liver was found. This case he includes by way of illustrating certain pitfalls in the diagnosis. [The paper merely expresses a personal view without any attempt at its elaborate defence. For ourselves we see no reason as yet to admit the existence of a distinct disease—splenic anemia. The cases are, many of them, instances of secondary anemia with splenic enlargement, and some no doubt have been cases of splenic Hodgkin's disease.]

Terrile [3] discusses a case of **idiopathic enlargement of the spleen.** The organ extended from the fifth rib to the iliac fossa. The patient was cachectic in a high grade, but presented no other symptoms, excepting a moderate enlargement of the liver and a soft blowing murmur at the apex, and the reduction of the red blood-corpuscles, which was very striking and suggested pernicious anemia. There was no etiological factor to account for the condition. There was no leukemia, swelling of the glands, pseudoleukemia, nor cirrhosis of the liver. The condition persisted for several years. He holds that cases

[1] Wien. klin. Woch., No. 20, 1896.   [2] Brit. Med. Jour., Sept. 9, 1896.
[3] Gaz. degli Osped. e delle Clin., No. 86, 1896.

of this kind are not rare, and that they lead to cachexia by the formation of a distinct toxic principle. The best treatment is operative interference. [We cannot agree with the author in so readily excluding pseudoleukemia, though the limitations of this disease remain to be established. The anemia and distinct disease of the spleen in this case would warrant its classification as one of splenic Hodgkin's disease, as far as we are able to classify such cases. This course would at least seem to be more justifiable than to consider the case as one of a special and obscure disease.]

PSEUDOLEUKEMIA.

Pathology.—Dietrich[1] discusses the uncertainty regarding the nature of pseudoleukemia and its relation to tuberculosis, and concludes that combinations of malignant lymphoma and ganglionar tuberculosis exist, and that there are cases in which a differential diagnosis is almost impossible. Necrosis of the gland is not of itself sufficient indication of tuberculous infection, but the presence of numerous eosinophile cells is more significant. (See also *Leukemia*.)

Jolles[2] has examined the urine from a case of pseudoleukemia and was able to determine the presence of **nucleohiston,** which he was convinced is identical with the albuminous bodies that are precipitable by acetic acid.

G. D. Robins and J. F. Argue[3] record a case of " **so-called acute Hodgkin's disease.**" The history was as follows: a young man of 19 was well until July 1, when he noticed great weakness after his work, headache, giddiness, anorexia, pallor, slight bleeding from the gums, and a vesiculopustular eruption on the skin of the hands and face. July 15, he first noticed swelling under the jaw which grew rapidly worse; mental stupor increased, and on August 3 there was marked epistaxis. He was admitted to the hospital and found to be dull and apathetic, with slight edema of the lower extremities and pronounced pemphigus of the hands and face. The left leg showed signs of old infantile palsy. All the lymph-glands of the neck, occipital region, axilla, epitrochlear region, and groin were distinctly enlarged, movable, and slightly tender. The skin over the glands nowhere showed signs of inflammation. The temperature was $102\frac{3}{5}°$ and the pulse and respirations rapid. The spleen was distinctly palpable below the ribs, but not greatly enlarged. The liver was not palpable. The blood showed 3,160,000 red corpuscles, 8000 white corpuscles, and 42 % of hemoglobin. The retina was edematous and a few hemorrhages were found in the outer granular layer. Subsequently the temperature declined to normal, but immediately rose again and continued intermittent. At the same time the leukocytes increased to 66,600 per c.mm., the red cells at this time numbering 2,000,000. Stained specimens showed the leukocytes to be mainly lymphocytic. There was again a decline in the number, until the day before death the leukocytes were 14,000. The authors state that at no time during the leukocytosis was the uric acid increased in the urine, but a distinct increase occurred in the week following the subsidence of the leukocytosis. This opinion seems to be based upon the character of the urinary sediment, and is therefore of no value. [The authors refer to the similarity of this case to one recorded in Ebstein's monograph. We would point out, however, that they ignore the possible significance of the pemphigoid disease. There was here undoubtedly a form of infection in which glandular enlargement may occur. We are far from ready to accept the diagnosis "acute Hodgkin's disease" so frequently proposed, and furthermore agree with the

---

[1] Beiträge z. klin. Chir., vol. xvi., p. 377.   [2] Wien. klin. Woch., May 29, 1897.
[3] Montreal Med. Jour., Oct., 1896.

authors in deprecating hasty changes of diagnosis from leukemia to Hodgkin's disease according as the number of leukocytes suffers temporary increase or decrease. We should, therefore, look upon this case as one of obscure infection with skin-eruption and glandular enlargement, and regret that accurate bacteriologic examinations of the blood were not undertaken.]

Revilliod[1] reports an interesting ease of obscure **abdominal tumor.** The patient, a man of 38 and strongly built, entered the hospital on account of rheumatic pains. A tumor was found in the left hypochondrium and epigastrium, reaching to the umbilicus. This was hard, uneven, and did not move with the respirations. The liver was somewhat enlarged. The examination of blood showed 4,000,000 red corpuscles, 9000 leukocytes, and 60% of hemoglobin. The urine contained no sugar. A left-sided pleurisy occurred and 3000 c.c. of opaque, reddish liquid were withdrawn. The patient died, and at the autopsy a tumor weighing 11 lbs. was found. This consisted of a conglomeration of enlarged lymphatic glands, in the center of which was a hyperplastie spleen. The mesentery was studded with enlarged glands and the thoracic duet was surrounded by them. [There was no disease of the other organs. The nature of this case is very doubtful. It does not seem to have been one of Hodgkin's disease, but may be considered in connection with that affection.]

Stein[2] reports a case of splenic and glandular enlargement without leukocytosis. A diagnosis of pseudoleukemia was made, but the patient failed to improve under arsenic or after extirpation of the spleen. Syphilis was then suspected and rapid recovery ensued under mixed treatment.

THE HEMORRHAGIC DISEASES.

J. N. Matthews[3] records a case of **purpura hæmorrhagica** presenting certain interesting features. The patient, a girl of 13, was extremely pale with tense pulse and rapid respirations. Several purpuric spots appeared on the legs and arms. Her temperature was 101°. Later there was severe epistaxis, blood appeared in the urine and in the bowel-movements, spots were found on the gums and in one of the nostrils, and there were retinal hemorrhages. Successive crops of spots appeared, these being flat or raised and indurated, and a few being elevated in the centre and having a ring of purpuric discoloration around them. Five days later the tongue was thickly coated, and the patient was attacked with hematemesis. Eight days after she was first seen the symptoms were those of typhoid fever, and she continued under treatment for this at the time of the report, about a month after she first came under observation. [This case presents features of a ease of typhoid fever beginning with hemorrhagic manifestations. It is, however, one of unusual character.]

W. Steer[4] records a ease of purpura of some interest. The patient, a lad of 14, had always been healthy; the present attack began with the eruption of a number of small purple spots on the front of his legs. Three days later the rash appeared on his wrists, his elbows and knees became tender, and he had muscular pains. Blood appeared in the bowel-movements, and vomiting of greenish liquid was observed. No cause could be discovered for the illness. On admission the symptoms were about the same, but in addition the purpuric spots were found on the mucous membranes. The gums were healthy in appearance. There was some tenderness of the abdomen, especially near the stomach and spleen. He improved, but twice after slight relaxations in diet

---

[1] Rev. Méd. de la Suisse romaine, No. 9, 1896.   [2] Wien. klin. Woch., June 5, 1897.
[3] Brit. Med. Jour., Sept., 1896.   [4] Ibid., Sept. 26, 1896.

relapses with moderate fever occurred. The usual drugs administered in purpura were without effect, but iodoform in pills of 1 gr. each given 3 times daily seemed to be beneficial. The boy made a good recovery.

E. Apert[1] believes that the eruption of purpura is due to 3 conditions : lesions of the arteries, influence of the nervous system, and the action of microbes. He describes the various lesions that are associated with purpura in the internal organs, and finally divides the disease into 4 groups : exanthematic (or rheumatoid) purpura, infectious purpura, Werlhoff's disease, and secondary purpura.

J. Clifford Perry[2] reports a case of **hemophilia** in a man of 20 who was incised for alveolar abscess. The incision was only $\frac{1}{8}$ of an inch long through the mucous membrane. The bleeding was profuse and continued in spite of styptics and pressure. It was then learned that the patient was one of a family of bleeders, two brothers having died from hemorrhage in infancy from very trivial injuries. He himself had on several occasions bled until he fainted. When this history was obtained the patient was given chlorid of calcium in doses of 1.3 gm., and in a few hours the effect was said to be marvellous. The blood, which had shown no signs of clotting, began to form a firm clot and the hemorrhage was completely arrested. The remedy was continued for 3 days. [While it seems likely that the remedy was of use in this case, it must be remembered that after loss of large quantities of blood the coagulability is normally much increased.]

Hutschneker[3] reports 4 cases of hemophilia, being all the male children of a family of 7. There was no history of hemophilia in the ancestors.

ADDISON'S DISEASE.

Pathology.—Rispal[4] observed a case of Addison's disease in a man of 24 that lasted about 10 months. At the autopsy no tuberculous lesions were found. The suprarenal capsules were absent. There was no lesion of the abdominal sympathetic ganglion.

B. Bramwell[5] reports 3 cases of Addison's disease. The 1st, a man of 50, suffered with weakness and emaciation after an attack of influenza he had had 3 months before. He suffered with extreme debility and cardiac asthenia, and with marked and rapid emaciation. His face, neck, and the backs of his hands were darker than normal, but no darker than might be expected from the exposure to which the man had been subjected. There was a distinct pigmented patch on the inner side of the left cheek. At the autopsy there was found extensive tuberculosis of the peritoneum, the membrane was studded with recent miliary tubercles, and the suprarenal capsules were decidedly enlarged and extensively diseased, being typical examples of fibrocaseous change. In connection with this case the author refers to certain of the more important symptoms of the disease; among others, to extreme asthenia, to the pigmented patches on the mucous membrane of the mouth, and emaciation. He notes that a few cases have been reported in which pigmentation identical with that of Addison's disease was found in other conditions, always, as far as he knows, cases of phthisis or tuberculous diseases. He notes that some authorities have held that emaciation is a point against the diagnosis of Addison's disease, but to maintain his own view he quotes the 2d case of his series, which occurred in a man of 36, who had progressive weakness during 6

---

[1] Gaz. hebdom. de Méd. et Chir., May 23, 1897. [2] Jour. Am. Med. Assoc., Mar. 13, 1897.
[3] Wien. med. Woch., May 1, 1897. [4] Sem. méd., 343, 1896.
[5] Brit. Med. Jour., 2 and 9, 1897.

months. There was distinct anemia, and the corpuscles numbered 3,500,000. They were normally shaped and formed rouleaux in the ordinary manner; there was no leukocytosis. The patient had lost 45 pounds in weight. The only pigmentation visible was found over the spines of some of the dorsal vertebræ. There was a brown discoloration on the inner side of the left cheek. Postmortem the only lesion found was a simple cirrhosis and atrophy of the suprarenal bodies. The 3d case was a man of 37, whose illness was said to have commenced 2 years before, following an attack of influenza. He was extremely weak but not much emaciated. He was much pitted by small-pox, which he had had 30 years before. The skin of the face was dark yellow and the smallpox pits were much more deeply pigmented than other parts— in places they were almost black. There were numerous pigmented patches on the lower lip and on the buccal mucous membrane. The examination of the blood showed 5,600,000 red corpuscles, 85 % hemoglobin, and no leuko-cytosis. The patient passed from observation and subsequently died. The organs were removed by the physician in charge and sent to the author. Above the kidneys were found masses of fat, and in the center of that over the left kidney was seen a brownish streak, suggesting the outline of the suprarenal capsule. Microscopically no evidence could be found of suprarenal structure, and the physician who made the autopsy stated that he was certain the glands had not been left in place. [It seems to us rather questionable to regard the suprarenal capsules in this case absent or completely degenerated upon the evidence offered.] Finally, the author, in discussing the diagnosis and the nature of the disease, states that 3 factors are necessary to establish its pres-ence : (1) the occurrence of characteristic weakness, vomiting, abdominal pain, etc. ; (2) pigmentation of the skin and mucous membranes; (3) the absence of any local disease other than the lesions of the suprarenal capsules. He is inclined to favor the glandular theory of the disease, holding that disturbed secretion or function of the gland accounts for its presence. Regarding the treatment, the beneficial effect reported in his last case after the administration of suprarenal extract is noteworthy.

J. S. Berry[1] reports a case of Addison's disease that occurred in a girl of 13. As an infant she had suffered from rickets and diarrhea and had always been very delicate; 2 years before admission it was noticed that her skin was becoming darker; this, however, disappeared. A year later she suffered from symptoms of gastric disturbance, and in a short time the pigmentation reap-peared and progressed until all parts of the surface of the body were of a brownish color. Upon admission there were obstinate vomiting, emaciation, and great weakness. In spite of energetic treatment with suprarenal bodies, · she grew rapidly worse and died. Tuberculosis of both suprarenal bodies was found at the autopsy.

Treatment.—Saveno[2] reports 2 cases of Addison's disease, the first of which was remarkable for the extensive distribution of the pigment ; in the second, which had occurred late in life, the pigment was not so well developed. Both showed great improvement without treatment when placed under favor-able hygienic conditions.

Miliam[3] reports a case of Addison's disease in which there occurred an abundant papular eruption associated with intense pruritus. Extract of supra-renal capsules produced considerable improvement.

Cervellini[4] reports a case of Addison's disease occurring in a young peasant about 22, complicated with tuberculosis of the testicle. The extirpation of this

---

[1] Lancet, June 19, 1897.   [2] Ital. de clin. Med., Punt 1, 1896.
[3] Gaz. hebdom. de Méd. et Chir., June 6, 1897.   [4] Riforma Med., No. 154, 1896.

organ and an exploratory incision into the abdomen, together with iodid of potassium and a strict albuminous diet, led apparently to a complete cure. The author suggests laparotomy in future cases of Addison's disease. [The case is of interest, although the diagnosis must remain to a certain extent doubtful.]

DISEASES OF THE PERICARDIUM.

W. Ewart[1] ascribes the **dorsal area of dulness** occurring in pericardial effusion to some condition diminishing the normal resonance over the region of the liver. As it is normally present in childhood and abnormally present in some wasted adults, it cannot be due to the effusion.

Perez[2] describes a new auscultatory sign which he discovered in a patient subject to attacks of mediastino-pericarditis. When the patient raised either arm from his side to a vertical position over the head, or lowered it again from that position, most remarkable sounds were audible over the whole length of the sternum. As these were independent of any friction-sounds synchronous with the heart-action or breathing, they were ascribed to dragging upon adhesions surrounding the great vessels external to the pericardium, in consequence of the traction by the vessels of the arms.

G. G. Sears[3] reports the statistics of **100 cases** of pericarditis. Of these, 54 were dry, 41 serous, 4 hemorrhagic, and 5 purulent. Seventy-four were males and 26 females. The great majority were persons in early adult life. Occupation seemed to have little influence. The majority of the cases occurred in January. Thirty-four had previously suffered from heart-disease and still showed valvular lesions. The temperature was usually low, rarely reaching 103°, although in 1 case, complicated by pneumonia, 107.4° was recorded. Acute rheumatism was the cause in 51 cases; pneumonia in 18; chronic nephritis in 7; pleurisy in 5; chronic rheumatism in 2; gonorrhea in 2; and various causes in the others, 9 cases being classed as idiopathic. Forty-three cases died and 4 were discharged unrelieved. The etiology seems to have much influence upon the prognosis, only 5 of the cases occurring in the course of acute rheumatism being fatal.

Acute Pericarditis.—[The question of surgical interference in purulent pericarditis seems to have been settled in the affirmative. The following cases are instances of the success that may attend this method of treatment:]

G. B. Shattuck and C. B. Porter[4] report a case of **purulent pericarditis** following pneumonia in which, after aspiration, and then free incision of the pericardial sac, recovery ensued. The pneumococcus was found in the pus. The authors have collected 24 cases of this condition, with 8 recoveries and 16 deaths. Frank W. Garber[5] reports a case following punctured wound of the chest. As the symptoms became very severe and all the signs of collection of pus in the pericardial sac were present, operation was decided upon and the sac opened and drained. Recovery was uneventful.

T. L. Coley[6] reports a case of **malignant endopericarditis** with recovery. The diagnosis was made from the existence of soft blowing murmurs, extreme prostration, and hectic temperature. There were gastric irritability and considerable delirium. Bacteriologic examinations of the blood were negative. There was no leukocytosis and neither symptoms of infarcts nor abscesses. [The diagnosis, therefore, is at least doubtful.] Recovery finally occurred after an illness of 6 months.

[1] Brit. Med. Jour., Jan. 23, 1897.   [2] Ibid., Dec. 19, 1896.
[3] Boston M. and S. Jour., Apr. 22, 1897.   [4] Ibid., May 6, 1897.
[5] Jour. Am. Med. Assoc., June 26, 1897.   [6] Med. Rec., Jan. 2, 1897.

L. Dickinson [1] contributes a study of **adherent pericardium** as the cause of fatal enlargement of the heart. He limits the term to complete obliteration of the pericardial sac by organized tissue. There may be no alteration of the heart nor even atrophy or arrested growth, although in most cases the heart is enlarged. In many cases diseases of the cardiac valves or muscle, the kidneys, or lungs may explain the enlargement, but in some there is no such explanation. The author refers to cases of the latter kind, of which he has observed 9 fatal instances during 3 years. The ages ranged from 8 to 21 years, the average being slightly over 15. During the same period adherent pericardium was found in 28 other patients dead of various diseases, in no instance, however, presenting the great enlargement referable to simple adhesion. The ages were mostly over 15 years and averaged upward of 36. In 12 cases the history of the initial trouble could be obtained, and the pericarditis was known to have occurred at an age later than that of puberty. In 5 cases it occurred in childhood, and 4 of these had advanced valvular disease and died at early ages with great enlargement of the heart, for which the adhesion was only partly responsible. The fifth is the solitary case in which adhesion, certainly contracted in childhood, proved harmless. Pericardial adhesion contracted in adult life is comparatively unimportant. In children it generally causes early death, and is associated with great enlargement of the heart. Pericarditis in children, if the very young be excluded, is almost always rheumatic and accompanied by endocarditis. Much fluid effusion is exceptional, and death results in the acute stages from failure of the cardiac muscle and dilatation of the ventricles. In the cases that recover from the acute attack enfeeblement and dilatation of the heart are often severe and prolonged. Hypertrophy may follow, but compensation is never attained. The right heart suffers more than the left, as was evidenced by the fact that dropsy occurred in 7 and nutmeg livers in 2 of his cases. · This failure of the right heart was not due to backward pressure from the left, for there was no congestion of the lungs in 5 cases, and in only 4 well-marked congestion or pulmonary apoplexy, indicating primary disturbances of the left ventricle. Regarding the relations of the mitral valve and the ventricle, it was noted that the valvular disease was gradual and of the kind that would ultimately develop into stenosis, although this had not actually occurred in any case, being antagonized by the tendency to regurgitation from dilatation of the mitral orifice by the traction of the pericardium. The diagnosis is made from the combination of symptoms and physical signs. Systolic retraction of the lower ribs is practically pathognomonic, but rarely observed. One of the most characteristic indications in the rapid progress of the cases to this fatal end is the failure of the remedies ordinarily useful in cardiac diseases.

Pick [2] describes a form of ascites suggesting ordinary cirrhosis of the liver, but due to pericarditis. He describes 3 cases, and terms the condition **pericarditic pseudocirrhosis of the liver.** The disturbance of circulation in the liver due to pericarditis leads to hyperplasia of the connective tissue surrounding the portal blood-vessels and ascites results. Clinically, the cases resemble mixed forms of cirrhosis of the liver, with enlargement and marked ascites, but no icterus. He distinguishes the conditions by the absence of any etiological factor pointing to cirrhosis, the pre-existence of symptoms pointing to pericarditis, and previous edema of the feet A certain diagnosis is only possible when a careful examination of the heart has been made.

Ewart [3] suggests that pericarditis may arise gradually without severe symp-

[1] Am. Jour. Med., Sci., Dec., 1896.   [2] Zeit. f. klin. Med., Bd. 29, H. 5 and 6.
[3] Lancet, Nov. 21, 1896.

toms. He noticed the fact that bands of adhesion, etc., may be found post-mortem in cases in which there was no history pointing to pericarditis. He reports 3 cases (nephritis, valvular disease, acute rheumatism) in which peri-cardial effusion came on without notable symptoms, persisted a few days, and then disappeared. Diagnosis was only made by careful examination. He concludes that effusions may take place independently of acute pericarditis, and if moderate may be reabsorbed without manifesting marked symptoms. In some cases subacute inflammatory processes may be present; more often the effusion is passive or mechanical.

DISEASES OF THE HEART.

Methods of Examination.—H. C. Thomson [1] advises the use of **the fluoroscope** for the estimation of the size and shape of the heart, and has found it highly satisfactory. A permanent tracing is easily made by holding a sheet of paper over the fluorescent screen and tracing upon it with a metallic pencil. A metal button may be used to mark the position of the nipple and the ribs may be traced so as to aid further in establishing the relations. [We have also used this method and have been enabled to study the outline of nor-mal as well as pathological hearts. Occasionally we were deceived by the fact that the shadow thrown upon the screen was larger than the heart itself; but the outline determined by the use of rays as nearly perpendicular as possible usually agreed very closely with that obtained by careful percussion. For the reason given above radiographs were not as satisfactory as the screen. The following author has apparently had a similar experience, but assigns a differ-ent reason :]

F. H. Williams [2] contributes a paper on the study of **internal diseases,** and especially the determination of the outlines of the heart by means of the fluoro-scope. The heart may be more or less well seen. The ventricles are distinct, as a rule, and in favorable conditions also the auricles ; but it is difficult to dis-tinguish the left from the pulmonary artery. The constant movements of the heart and diaphragm interfere with radiography, and therefore render fluoro-scopy of more value. The position of the heart, as a rule, makes it impossible to see more than a certain portion of its outline, but by contracting the dia-phragm a better result is obtained, the abdominal organs then being depressed and the heart exposed surrounded only by the lungs. Several cases, in which the outlines as determined by percussion and those found by fluoroscopy are con-trasted, show that the fluoroscope gives a wider area than percussion. Consoli-dation of the lungs obscures the cardiac outlines and the border contiguous with the liver is normally not easily determined. Fluid in the pericardial or pleural sacs and various diseases of the lungs causing consolidation may be readily detected. Sometimes areas of consolidation not readily detected by physical examination are discovered. He has found fluids withdrawn from the body less permeable to the rays than water.

C. F. Disen [3] marks a normal outline of the heart upon the chest by means of a copper wire, then puts a fluoroscopic screen at the back of the patient, and is able to recognize whether the shadow of the heart is within the wire or extends beyond, in which case he assumes hypertrophy.

Auscultatory Percussion.—W. D. Herringham [4] has studied the value of direct and auscultatory percussion upon the cadaver. He found that the former method gave strikingly accurate results, as tested by inserting pins into

[1] Lancet, Oct. 10, 1896.
[2] Boston M. and S. Jour., Oct. 1, 1896.
[3] Med. Rec., Jan. 9, 1897.
[4] Brit. Med. Jour., Sept. 19, 1896.

the body and determining their position when the sternum was removed. Auscultatory percussion was fairly accurate, but had a number of drawbacks. He confirms Dr. Herschell's statement regarding the area of about 1½ in. around the stethoscope in which the vibrations transmitted in the skin interfere with the vibrations dependent upon deeper structures. Beyond this "useless area" good results may be obtained for a certain distance, but as the distance is increased the note is decreased and cannot well be judged. The stethoscope must be on a resonant area. In percussing the heart, for example, it must be placed over the lung. The method deprives us of aid which the feeling of the fingers gives in percussion; the note is very different if obtained over the rib or over an interspace. Finally, the note over the sternum is so shrill as to make the discrimination of changes of pitch impossible within 3 in. of the stethoscope. [We are surprised at some of these results. They do not accord in the slightest with our experience. The statement regarding the necessity of placing the stethoscope over a resonant structure is as far as possible from the fact. We never follow this rule. It may be said here that some experience with this method is necessary, and that those who would put it to the test should first acquaint themselves with its limitations by a certain amount of practice. It is striking that those who have proclaimed most loudly against its value are those who have, without previous experience, entered upon an investigation of its defects.]

P. W. Williams[1] states that he has followed the method of auscultatory percussion detailed by Jackson, of New York, and has come to the conclusion that though it is not an absolutely accurate method to determine the deep cardiac dulness, it is more accurate than any other. He points out, however, that the area of cardiac dulness does not absolutely determine the size of the organ, since the relations of the curved surface of the heart to the curve of the thorax cause apparent differences in size that may not be real. He has practised the method on living subjects and also on 12 cadavers, controlling the results by the insertion of pins into the chest-walls. [It is striking that the author's results vary so greatly from those of Herringham in regard to the test on the cadaver. We can only explain the difference by the assumption mentioned in commenting upon Herringham's paper, that greater experience leads to more satisfactory results.]

A. Stengel[2] advocates very strongly auscultatory percussion in diagnosis. He prefers the simplest method of placing the stethoscope directly over the organ to be outlined. It is important to percuss always with strokes of the same force. He warns against mistaking the change of note which occurs as a result of the approximation of the pleximeter to the stethoscope, and is due to vibrations in the chest-wall, from the more characteristic change which occurs only at the edge of the organ, no matter in what part of its area the stethoscope may be placed. The most satisfactory application is to the heart, the point of election for the stethoscope being near the apex. Over the lung it is chiefly valuable for delimiting areas of consolidation; applied to the stomach, it is most useful in connection with inflation. It is also possible to determine the size and position of the colon, of the liver, of the spleen, and, under possibly favorable circumstances, of the kidneys.

Holowinski[3] has devised a method for the **graphic representation of the cardiac sounds** by means of 2 small glass plates upon the diaphragm of a telephone. Between these Newtonian lines appear and vary with the

---

[1] Brit. Med. Jour., Sept. 19. 1896.   [2] Boston M. and S. Jour., Apr. 15, 1897.
[3] Zeit. f. klin. Med., vol. xxxi., p. 201.

vibrations produced by the heart-sounds; by means of a special apparatus it is possible to photograph these changes.

General Symptomatology.—T. Fisher[1] contributes a brief study of the **bruit de galop** and its causation. He shows by sphygmographic and cardiographic tracings that there is in this condition a rise of the lever, indicating a wave, preceding the ordinary impulse, followed by a recession, and then by the regular impulse. This was shown in one case on several occasions when the bruit was present, and could not be demonstrated when the latter was temporarily absent. In seeking for an explanation of this phenomenon he considers several of the theories that have been held regarding the bruit. Potain and others have attributed it to the distention of the left ventricle during the inflow of blood from the auricle. This fails to explain the recession of the wave. "One would suppose," says Fisher, "that the ventricle would remain distended and keep the chest-wall raised until the commencement of the ventricular systole, when a further rise would occur." Dr. Sansom suggests that the first inrushing of the blood strikes the apex, but that afterward a considerable quantity rebounds toward the base behind the great anterior mitral flap. Fisher believes that some such movement of the blood does take place, but doubts the explanation. His own explanation is—the region of the base of the heart being strengthened by the contractions of the papillary muscles and chordæ during the auricular systole, distention occurs at the relatively unprotected apex; afterward, when the necessity for contraction is relieved and the outward pressure upon the mitral flap has ceased, the intraventricular pressure is left to distend the heart as it will. In consequence of this there is displacement of the blood in the direction of the base, tending to throw the mitral flaps together, and there is simultaneous recession of the apex. The author's theory agrees closely with Sansom's, although not in his explanation of the recession. He points out that clinically the bruit occurs most frequently when the muscle of the heart suffers without valvular disease. In hearts recovering from poisoning by toxins, in dilated hearts associated with arterial disease, interstitial nephritis, overwork, or alcoholism the bruit is common; and it may occur in severe cases of anemia. In all such cases there is impairment of the power of the heart-muscle. As regards prognosis, he holds that the sign is one of importance, dependent upon the nature of the heart-failure with which it is associated. In cases of hypertrophy without valvular disease he has seen it come and go without much reference to the general condition. In one instance it was the only abnormal sign present, when sudden death overtook a patient who had not been considered seriously ill.

Braun[2] discusses the significance of the **cardiac impulse** transmitted by the thoracic wall. He had the opportunity to observe for some time a patient who, as the result of a gunshot-wound, had had the left 4th, 5th, and 6th ribs excised between the parasternal line and the sternum on the left side, leaving nothing but the transparent pericardium between the heart and the observer. The following cardiac phenomena were observed: the wave commenced at the base with a slight dilatation of the muscular wall and then contraction. This was transmitted downward, and as it reached the apex became associated with the upward movement of that part of the heart. The movement of the apex was very sudden, and corresponded apparently to the 2d part of the wave: as it was thrust upward, it was also observed that the heart underwent a spiral rotatory movement from the left forward and then upward. Braun therefore holds that the apex-beat is caused solely by the systolic change of form of the heart-muscle, and is an expression of the cardiac movement against

[1] Am. Jour. Med. Sci., Sept., 1896.   [2] Wien. klin. Woch., Nov. 28, 1896.

9

the wall of the thorax.   In Braun's case, however, pericardial adhesions were
formed before death occurred and resulted in a change of movement, so that,
instead of showing wave-like contraction, a systole of the heart represented a
simultaneous contraction of all the portions.

J. D. Steele[1] contributes a study of the distribution and etiology of **cardiac
hydrothorax.**   He notes that authors with few exceptions make the statement that in heart-disease the effusion is always bilateral, though some assert
that there is apt to be more fluid on one side than the other, and a few mention the right side as the one more frequently affected.   His attention having
been called to the disproportion in fluid on the 2 sides, he undertook to ana-
lize all the records of autopsies based upon the notes of 1652 cases reported
in the *Middlesex Hospital Reports* for the 6 years ending 1896, and upon
775 cases at the Philadelphia Hospital (Blockley) from March, 1893, to September, 1896.   The total number of autopsies was 2427.   He selected only
cases in which the hypertrophied heart weighed at least 400 gm. in the adult
male and 370 gm. in the adult female, so as to exclude cases of dilatation secondary to some acute disease and dropsies occurring in the last hours of life.
Cases in which complicating conditions such as aneurysm, pleurisy, etc., occurred were also excluded.   He found :

```
Total number of cardiac cases in which requirements were fulfilled . . . . . . .173
Total number of cases of hydrothorax . . . . . . . . . . . . . . . . . . 75
Bilateral equal hydrothorax . . . . . . . . . . . . . . . . . . . . 22 or 30%
Bilateral unequal hydrothorax . . . . . . . . . . . . . . . . . . . 40 or 53%
      "           "           "      . . . . . . . . . . . . right greater  31 or 77%
      "           "           "      . . . . . . . . . . . . left      "     9 or 23%
Unilateral hydrothorax . . . . . . . . . . . . . . . right    "    10 or 77%
      "           "        . . . . . . . . . . . . . . . left    "     3 or 23%
```

It will be noted that the effusion was unequal in 70% of the cases.   Equal
bilateral hydrothorax was very much oftener associated with general dropsy
than was the unequal form.   He then details 4 cases and abstracts 2 others
from the literature, and proceeds to consider the pathogenesis and especially
the theory of Villani, that right-sided hydrothorax is dependent upon beginning interstitial hepatitis which causes distention of the capsule of the liver
and a low grade of inflammation of this coat extending also through the diaphragm to the pleura or upon a similar sequence of pathological events following congestion of the liver.   Swelling of the liver does not explain left-
sided effusions and does not seem applicable to cases in which the effusions
have been excessive.   The author himself, though accepting this explanation
as plausible in some cases, looks with greater favor upon the theory that low-
grade inflammation of the pleura once established will prevent a reabsorption
of the fluid exudate in the affected side and thus occasion a unilateral collection.   The study of the anatomical relations at the root of the lungs was carefully made ; the results that may follow from pressure exerted by the dilated
auricles are given as follows : pressure of the dilated left auricle and vena cava
upon the root of the lung may cause : 1, obstruction of the venous circulation
of the right pleura through the azygos vein and its branches and to a less
extent through the bronchial veins ; 2, obstruction of the lymphatic vessels
supplying the visceral layer of the pleura.   Pressure of the dilated left auricle may cause : 1, obstruction of circulation of the bronchial veins and lymphatics of the left lung ; 2, obstruction of the left superior intercostal vein and
vena azygos minor.   In 16 of the 35 cases of the unequal right-sided bilateral
hydrothorax dilatation of the right auricle is specially mentioned, and in 2 of

---

[1] Univ. Med. Mag., May, 1897.

the 5 cases of unequal left-sided hydrothorax the left auricle was stated to have been particularly dilated. He concludes, then, that this mechanical theory is the one most generally applicable.

A. H. Smith[1] calls attention to the presence of **anemia in heart-disease** as a result of the combined action of rheumatism and the salicylates. Clinically it can be recognized by the pallor, hemic murmurs, the venous bruit, and the examination of the blood. He has had the greatest success from the treatment with rectal injections of defibrinated blood.

Acute Endocarditis.—[The evidence in favor of direct infection of the endocardium by the gonococcus appears to be increasing, although in some cases it is unquestionable that post-gonorrheal endocarditis is due to other microorganisms.] Keller[2] records a case of **malignant endocarditis following gonorrhea.** The patient, a man of 25, had gonorrhea followed by rheumatism after an interval of 4 weeks. Two months later he entered the hospital and then had endocarditis of the pulmonary valve with intermittent fever and enlargement of the spleen. Three weeks later hemorrhagic nephritis developed. The heart gradually weakened, and dyspnea developed; pericarditis occurred, followed by death 6 months after the beginning of the attack of gonorrhea. Postmortem verrucose and ulcerative endocarditis of the pulmonary leaflets, thrombosis of the left ventricle, infarcts in the kidneys and spleen, and emboli in the pulmonary arteries with hemorrhagic nephritis were the lesions found. The patient had leukocytosis and considerable anemia. Bacteriologic examination of the blood from the right ventricle was negative, but abundant streptococci were obtained from the pericardial fluid, from the endocardial vegetations, and elsewhere. Diplococci (staining by Gram's method) were found with the streptococci in the kidneys. Gonococci could not be demonstrated. The author believes that the urethral disease furnished a portal of entrance for the streptococci.

Alfred Stengel[3] reports a case of endocarditis occurring in a woman of 20 years of age. She had suffered from gonorrhea, and shortly before admission to the hospital had shown symptoms of acute general infection. There were dyspnea, considerable enlargement of the heart, and, at the apex, a loud presystolic followed by a systolic murmur, and a systolic murmur in the aortic region. Death occurred 7 weeks from the onset. At the autopsy a congenital lesion of the mitral valve was found, and the wall of the left auricle showed both old and recent endocarditis. Bacteriologically, the vegetation from the aortic wall showed diplococci that in all respects resembled microscopically the gonococcus. No growth was obtained upon agar and ordinary serum culture-tubes. The author is inclined to regard the case as one of gonorrheal origin, although he admits that the evidence is not conclusive. He collects 13 other cases in which careful clinical and bacteriologic studies have been made, in only one of which characteristic cultures were obtained from the vegetations. These cases were all characterized by the symptoms of malignant endocarditis, the aortic valve being the most frequent seat of the disease.

Wieghein,[4] in the Berliner Verein. f. in. Med., presented the specimens of a case of acute endocarditis secondary to gonorrhea. Cultures from the vegetations on blood-serum were negative, but microscopically organisms were found in them that corresponded exactly to gonococci. [It is generally admitted now that other cocci occur that cannot be distinguished either morphologically or by their staining reaction from gonococci. The only positive tests

---

[1] Med. Rec., Dec. 12, 1896.   [2] Deutsch. Arch. f. klin. Med., Bd. lvii., H. 3 and 4.
[3] Univ. Med. Mag., Mar., 1897.   [4] Centralbl. f. innere Med., Apr. 17, 1897.

are either inoculation or the culture. The absence of growths in culture-tubes is important.]

Hitchmann and Michel [1] describe a case in which a chill, fever, and evidences of acute endocarditis developed a few hours after dilatation of a urethral stricture. Jaundice, hemorrhage, and death followed, and at post-mortem ulcerative endocarditis with pyemic abscesses was discovered. The bacillus coli communis was demonstrated in all of the secondary lesions. The authors conclude that the **infection** occurred primarily from **the urethral mucous membrane.**

Geo. Dock [2] reports a case of endocarditis due to **infection with the staphylococcus aureus,** with rhythmic paroxysms of fever simulating exactly the double quotidian type. [See *Year-Book* for 1897.]

Edmond Gladmon [3] reports a case of malignant endocarditis coming on apparently as the sequel of a series of attacks described as **bilious** that consisted of sudden vertigo followed by vomiting and violent pain, either centering solely in the umbilicus or radiating to the liver. These attacks usually lasted about a week and occurred irregularly for 5 years before his death. The case finally developed severe pyemic symptoms. At the autopsy there were large, irregular vegetations upon the sclerotic endocardium, containing the diplococcus lanceolatus, metastatic abscesses of the spleen and kidney, and fatty infiltration of the liver; the intestines were normal.

Jas. W. Walker [4] reports **a case of acute vegetative endocarditis,** confirmed by autopsy, in which during the early period of the disease the symptoms closely resembled typhoid fever, and there was nothing to call attention to the heart. Murmurs were absent throughout.

Reichel [5] believes that recent **rheumatic endocarditis** occurs more frequently than the older authors admit; that is, in from 60 to 70% of all cases of acute articular rheumatism. Its diagnosis is quite impossible when it is restricted to the cavities of the heart. Ordinarily it presents the following clinical picture: a rough murmur appears at the apex covering the systolic tone and the apex deviates to the left. Then there is accentuation of the second aortic sound, which subsequently yields to a greater accentuation of the second pulmonic. This develops into a mitral insufficiency. If stenosis occurs, the earliest symptom is diminution.in the strength of the pulse, with accentuation of the systolic tone at the apex. Aortic regurgitation is sometimes indicated by the presence of a presystolic murmur. In those mild forms of endocarditis that occur in the course of gonorrheal rheumatism the symptoms are essentially the same.

W. M. Gibson [6] calls attention to a febrile form of **endocarditis in the aged,** which he claims is frequently overlooked. It usually occurs in patients already suffering from valvular lesions, in the course of articular rheumatism or other infectious diseases. He holds that in old patients suffering from such valvular disease fever, even if transitory, should arouse suspicion of acute endocarditis.

H. Sainsbury [7] records a case of ulcerative endocarditis in a lad of 13. On July 1, **streptococci** were found in the blood. There was a variable temperature from 100° to 104.4°, vomiting, cough, and bloody sputum. The spleen was slightly enlarged, the abdomen tender, and a symmetrical erythematous rash developed on the buttocks, spreading over the rest of the body.

[1] Wien. klin. Woch., No. 18, 1896.   [2] N. Y. Med. Jour., Jan. 30, 1897.
[3] Med. Rec., Sept. 26, 1896.   [4] Jour. Am. Med. Assoc., Apr. 3, 1897.
[5] Wien. med. Woch., Apr. 10, 1897.   [6] Internat. Med. Mag., Sept., 1896.
[7] Lancet, Oct. 17, 1896.

On August 17, 20 c.c. of **antistreptococcic serum** were injected; the temperature was 99.8°; there was no reaction. On the 18th, 20th, 22d, and on the 25th, 10 c.c. were administered, and there was great improvement. On the 31st the patient was up and walking in the ward. The area of cardiac dulness had become normal, and the heart's apex was well within the nipple-line. On September 1, again 10 c.c. were injected, and there was local and general reaction. After this the patient became normal in every way and was discharged soon after apparently cured. [The results of the employment of antistreptococcic serum, experimentally as well as clinically, are so conflicting that it is difficult to decide as to its value. It seems questionable in the present case whether the treatment was beneficial.]

CHRONIC VALVULAR DISEASE.

J. K. Crook [1] reports the **statistics** of 503 cases of heart-disease. Of these, 277 were functional disorders and 226 organic diseases. The latter were classified as follows: mitral regurgitation, 60; mitral stenosis, 35; aortic regurgitation, 7; aortic stenosis, 36; tricuspid regurgitation, 6; pulmonary stenosis, 1; double combined lesions, 46; lesions of double character, 7; simple hypertrophy, 10; and other conditions, 15. Functional diseases predominated in females and organic diseases in males. [The very large proportion of cases of aortic stenosis does not correspond with the results of the autopsy-room. A systolic murmur at the base does not necessarily or even usually imply a narrowing of the ostium.]

Symptomatology.—Kasem-Beck [2] refers to the significance of the **presystolic murmur** at the apex of the heart. He points out that numerous cases have recently been reported in which this murmur was detected and the autopsies showed no narrowing of the mitral orifice, although in some aortic narrowing was discovered. In 16 cases out of 19 the symptoms of aortic insufficiency and mitral stenosis coexisted during life, but the autopsy showed no stenosis. In another group of cases neither valve was found diseased, but adhesive pericarditis existed, and a few instances are recorded in which there was merely dilatation of the left ventricle. Picot has recorded cases in which a presystolic murmur was heard at the apex in hysterical patients, and holds that it is due to contractions of the papillary muscles. After this introduction the author refers to the case of a man of 63 who entered the hospital complaining of severe pains in the breast extending to both arms and severe dyspnea. Positive pulsation was found in the veins of both sides of the neck; the left and right ventricles were hypertrophied; the peripheral arteries were sclerotic; there was a loud presystolic murmur with a muffled first sound at the apex, while the second sound was loud. Auscultation over the tricuspid area discovered no murmur. The second sound was accentuated over the pulmonary region. Stenosis of the mitral orifice was supposed to be present, but the autopsy showed no narrowing at all. There was found near the apex of the heart an aneurysmal dilatation the size of a small apple. The author believes that the presystolic murmur was due to diversion of the stream of blood into this cavity. Although both auriculo-ventricular orifices were dilated, no systolic murmur was discoverable. Finally, he believes with Skoda that a strong pulsation in the intercostal space at the apex and a small pulse at the wrist are sure signs of aneurysm of the left ventricle. [While we cannot agree with the last statement of the author's, the report is of interest in furnishing another instance of presystolic murmur without mitral stenosis. Authors who

[1] N. Y. Med. Jour., June 19, 1897.   [2] Centralbl. f. innere Med., Feb. 13, 1897.

have reported such cases appear to us to have laid too little stress upon the character of the first sound. We have repeatedly distinguished Flint's murmur from the murmur of mitral stenosis by the weakness of the first sound in conjunction with other evidence.]

Leube[1] discusses the diagnosis of **systolic heart-murmurs** and gives the following summary of the principles to be observed in their examination. First, an accidental murmur is present if the area of cardiac dulness is normal, the second pulmonary sound not accentuated, and the murmur heard either only in the pulmonary area or also at the apex of the heart. If the murmur is accompanied by a heart-sound, it is to be assumed that it is due to a transient dilatation of the pulmonary arteries resulting from the diminished tone of the vessel-wall. If not so accompanied, it is due to a diminution of blood-pressure in the large vessels. The diagnosis is slightly more difficult if the area of cardiac dulness is slightly enlarged and the pulmonary second sound is accentuated. Under these circumstances an acute endocarditis with secondary acute mitral insufficiency is to be diagnosed, if the enlargement of the cardiac area is only slight and chiefly toward the left, and there are fever and the presence of some infectious disease. Should, under these circumstances, the right ventricle also show increase in size, it must be assumed that there is some weakness of the heart-muscle, and that therefore, in addition to the endocarditis, a myocarditis is also present. A relatively subacute or chronic insufficiency of the mitral valve is to be diagnosed if there are considerable enlargement of the area of cardiac dulness over both sides and accentuation of the second sound in the pulmonic area. If the murmur is purely systolic, of moderate intensity, and not always of the same force, whilst at the same time the cardiac impulse is weak and the second tone only moderately accentuated, with a relatively small or even irregular pulse, the insufficiency of the mitral valve is probably relative or functional. This condition occurs in anemia, in cases with enfeebled heart-muscle, or of excessive dilatation of the left ventricle, and also if there are myocarditic changes in the muscles controlling the valves. A constant loud systolic murmur with a relatively small cardiac impulse, and a relatively good pulse with great accentuation of the second pulmonary sound, indicate the presence of mitral insufficiency resulting from chronic endocarditis. The intensity of the second pulmonic sound depends upon a variety of conditions, such as the perfection of compensation obtained by the hypertrophy of the right ventricle or the duration of the diastolic pause. In these cases the diagnosis is often rendered more certain by the discovery of a presystolic murmur in addition to the systolic one, a combination that occurs in no other condition. The distinction between endocarditic and relative mitral insufficiencies is more difficult when compensation is lost. Under these circumstances, however, the clinical picture is of much value, for the relative insufficiencies occurring in the course of anemia present incomparably milder symptoms. If, however, the relative mitral insufficiency with loss of compensation is due to myocarditic changes, the differential diagnosis from a pure mitral insufficiency due to endocarditis is impossible. This, however, is rarely the case, as an insufficiency due to endocarditis is almost invariably accompanied by more or less stenosis. As a result, in addition to the systolic there is almost always a presystolic murmur, which enables one to make the differential diagnosis.

Heitler[2] discusses the **localization of the mitral systolic murmur,** and declares that it may be heard simultaneously in various portions of the cardiac area with equal intensity. Thus, it may be loud at the apex, diminish

[1] Deutsch. Arch. f. klin. Med., Nov. 5, 1896.   [2] Wien. klin. Woch., Feb. 18, 1897.

toward the base, and reappear in the aortic region with full intensity. Various modifications of the generally accepted rule often occur. Sometimes the murmur is loudest at the apex, diminishing in intensity in all directions; at other times a similar condition exists, excepting that it reappears at distant points, where it may be heard even more loudly than at the apex. Usually when it does reappear it is found at the left border of the sternum; sometimes, however, it is quite weak at the apex, being loudest in the parasternal line. In general, it may be said that systolic mitral murmurs may be heard most loudly at almost any point in the area lying to the left of the left border of the sternum and below the second intercostal space. The intensity of the murmur depends to a large extent upon the energy of the heart's action and varies considerably from time to time. This alteration may be qualitative as well as quantitative, so that the whole character of the murmur becomes different. He then considers the **tricuspid murmurs.** These, when systolic, have a peculiar acoustic character and are heard in a definite area; they are usually faint, delicate, and breathing, and only exceptionally rough, superficial, and short. Usually they are higher in pitch than the corresponding mitral murmurs. The area in which they are best heard varies in height and breadth according to the intensity of the murmur. Loud murmurs may be heard over any part of the sternum up to the first intercostal space, with the maximum intensity usually between the levels of the 3d and 5th ribs. Usually they are somewhat louder in the left half of the sternum than in the right. The murmur is transmitted to the right, sometimes more strongly to the left, as far as 6 cm. from the median line. On the right side transmission is rarer, and it is very unusual for the murmurs to be heard more than 3 cm. from the edge of the sternum. The differential diagnosis between tricuspid murmurs and mitral murmurs is usually easy, and is to be made by a consideration of the acoustic character and the points of the greatest intensity and areas of transmission.

T. Fisher [1] emphasizes the importance of careful **discrimination** as to the existence of mitral regurgitation when systolic murmurs are heard over the heart, even in cases of rheumatism. Many of these murmurs disappear spontaneously under the influence of rest, and it is likely that they are the expression of moderate dilatation of the left ventricle and similar to the murmurs heard over the pulmonary area when the right ventricle is dilated.

Mitral Stenosis.—R. G. Curtin [2] describes cases which he regards as instances of moderate **congenital narrowing of the mitral orifice** manifested by irritability of the heart with "dwarfed life." The first case, a young woman, had blue lips and extremities, and was regarded as a case of vasomotor and trophic affections of the fingers. A year later he observed similar cases in 3 young boys. In all of these the symptoms were rapid, irritable heart, suffused face, shortness of breath, loss of strength and appetite, and a murmur over the heart. On inquiry he found that the boys had previously led quiet lives, were easily fatigued, and even in early childhood had been unable to cope with their fellows in active play. Their subsequent occupation, as "eash-boys" in a large store, led to the development of the symptoms. He then details 6 additional eases, calling attention to the inability of the affected persons to engage in active work or play, and the tendency to lung and pleural trouble of a chronic kind, with hemoptysis and night-sweats. The lesions in the lung and pleura were generally on the left side. In the severer eases auricular pulsation was marked, and a murmur could be developed in all of them that was heard above and outside the usual apex-region, and either presystolic or

---

[1] Lancet, July 18, 1896.　　　　　　　　　　[2] Tr. Am. Climat. Assoc., 1896.

in the early part of systole. It was not transmitted except when conveyed by a consolidated lung. Accentuation of the pulmonary second sound was generally present. Most of the patients were boys and growing men. Post-mortem examinations were obtained in 3 cases, but with negative results in all so far as the size of the mitral orifice was concerned. The difficulty in this was to determine the normal size of the orifice for a heart of given size. In all cases the endocardium was healthy, but the left auricles were hypertrophied and dilated. The author concludes from the clinical symptoms and physical signs that a moderate amount of mitral stenosis exists in these cases, and that the orifice permits sufficient blood to pass during the quiet state, but not enough when the heart becomes more active. The most suitable treatment consists in hygienic regulations.

Samways[1] maintains that hypertrophy of the **left auricle in mitral stenosis** predominates over dilatation until the failure of compensation. He explains the competence of the relatively weak auricle as compared with the ventricle upon the ground that a hollow sphere of small size requires a much greater pressure to bring on dilatation than one of larger size. He believes that the contraction of the auricle encroaches upon the ventricular contraction and this prevents regurgitation. In the later stage, when the auricle fails, a murmur of valvular incompetency develops.

H. D. Rolleston and W. L. Dickinson[2] report 3 cases of what they term **"relative mitral stenosis."** In these the mitral valves presented the usual appearance of stenosis, but the orifice and leaflets were of such a size that there was not actual obstruction. Clinically, there were a mitral regurgitant murmur and frequently a more or less characteristic presystolic murmur. They do not believe that the condition was due to subsequent dilatation of the ventricle in cases of mitral stenosis, thinking that it is hardly probable that the valve having attained so high a grade of rigidity could subsequently become so much dilated. Their view is that the valve, while tending to stenosis, has been held open by the primary dilatation of the ventricle. Most of the cases of relative stenosis are found in cases of adherent pericardium in young persons arising from rheumatic pericarditis, dilatation of the ventricle and mitral endocarditis occurring simultaneously. Other cases are instances of aortic regurgitation, the dilatation of the ventricle having prevented the usual contractions of mitral stenosis.

Wm. Osler[3] reports a case of mitral stenosis with signs of cardiac insufficiency. Death occurred suddenly. At the autopsy the mitral orifice was found to admit the tip of one finger, and in the left auricle there was a firm **ball-thrombus** unattached to the walls, but occupying a funnel-shaped space leading to the mitral orifice. It was ovoid and about 3 cm. long. [We have seen two specimens of this condition, in one of which the ball was perfectly round; in the other, attached by a pedicle to the wall of the auricle.]

A. A. Eshner[4] reports a case that at first presented the symptoms of mitral stenosis, but, after taking digitalis, developed a diastolic murmur of booming character transmitted toward the axilla. Still later there was also a systolic murmur at the apex; nevertheless he regards the case as one of typical mitral stenosis.

Cheverau[5] describes a form of mitral stenosis that he believes to be due to **spasm of the papillary muscles,** resulting directly from nervous influence. This occurs particularly in hysterical or saturnine persons, and is charac-

[1] Thèse de Paris, 1896.   [2] Lancet, Mar. 6, 1867.
[3] Montreal Med. Jour., Mar., 1897.   [4] Phila. Polyclinic, Dec. 19, 1896.
                         [5] Sem. méd., 1896, p. 288.

terized by the presence of a harsh fremissement and a presystolic murmur, but without the other phenomena characteristic of mitral stenosis. The pathognomonic sign is the extreme variability, with a transient or final disappearance of all the abnormal auscultatory phenomena. The duration is naturally nucertain. The only complication that it can produce is pulmonary congestion, and even this never reaches a serious grade. Treatment should be directed wholly to the nervous condition, sedatives, such as bromid of potassium, having been found most useful.

Servin[1] has recently studied the question of **heredity in mitral disease.** He holds that it is not unusual for the parents to transmit visceral peculiarities, and that the heart is especially liable. Pure mitral stenosis often seems rather a variation of structure than an actual disease, and he notes that its transmission has been actually observed, and that it constitutes at times a real family affection. He holds, therefore, that when one of the parents suffers with mitral stenosis the children should be carefully examined, so as to institute proper hygienic measures.

Mitral Regurgitation.—Theodore Fisher[2] discusses the frequency and seriousness of mitral regurgitation due to valvular disease, which appears to be much more frequent at the bedside than it is postmortem. Mere thickening of the flaps may be frequently discovered, but actual contractions are very rare. It is not likely that the small, bead-like vegetations seen in early endocarditis interfere with the competency of the valve. A slight degree of ventricular dilatation may occur in many cases, and this may be sufficient, in attacks of rheumatism, to cause a systolic murmur at the apex. The frequency of a systolic murmur audible over the pulmonary area is of importance in this connection. Foxwell ascribes this to the dilatation of the conus arteriosus of the right ventricle, and Fisher has observed a case during life and postmortem of striking character. "We have then," he states, "a systolic murmur audible over the pulmonary area occurring in attacks of rheumatism, but we have reason to believe that this is sometimes due to dilatation of the right side of the heart;" similarly we may suppose that dilatation of the left side occurs. In Dr. Caten's recent paper he alludes to the disappearance of murmurs in patients who were kept in bed for a considerable length of time, and attributes it to the cure of the endocarditis. Fisher believes it due to the subsidence of the dilatation. Referring to his postmortem experiences and to other records, he finds that death due to uncomplicated mitral regurgitation is rare. The records of the Bristol Royal Infirmary for 20 years showed only 11 cases. The records of Guy's Hospital for 10 years showed only 5 cases. In these statistics he excludes cases in which there were other lesions, such as general adhesions of the pericardium and aortic valve-disease. When the mitral valves suffer acute endocarditis stenosis is almost invariably the result. The usual explanation of the regurgitant murmurs then is dilatation of the ventricle. [We heartily endorse these views. In a very considerable postmortem experience we have rarely found pure mitral regurgitation due to valve-disease, but have repeatedly seen a dilated ventricle (and, therefore, presumably mitral leakage) in cases in which there were the usual indications of acute rheumatic or infectious endocarditis.]

E. H. Starling[3] states that mere perforation of the mitral and tricuspid valves in a heart otherwise normal may give rise to very little disturbance of the circulation or in the conditions of the heart itself, because of the sphincter-like action of the circular band of fibres surrounding the orifices. If, however,

[1] Jour. de Méd., Sept., 10, 1896.   [2] Lancet, Oct. 18, 1896.
[3] Ibid., Feb. 27, 1897.

the muscle becomes feebler, these relax and regurgitation develops. He performed a number of experiments in order to determine the effect of cardiac insufficiency upon the blood-current, and found that the number of corpuscles was usually increased to a greater extent than the hemoglobin. This, in connection with the fact pointed out by Lloyd Jones, that in failure of compensation there is marked diminution in the specific gravity of the blood, leads him to believe that in heart-disease there is not a condition of plethora, hydremic or otherwise, but that the lowering of specific gravity is due to the diminution of the solids of the plasma—that is to say, hydremia without plethora. [This view is not shared by others and certainly needs further demonstration.]

A. O. J. Kelly[1] mentions the case of a man in whom there was distinct Corrigan pulse, but no diastolic murmur. The diagnosis of **aortic insufficiency** was confirmed at the autopsy.

Pulmonary Stenosis.—[See also the section upon Tuberculosis.] Henry Hun[2] reports a case of **pulmonary stenosis complicated with pulmonary tuberculosis.** At the autopsy the pulmonary leaflets were found united, leaving a small triangular opening. The right ventricle was hypertrophied. The ductus arteriosus was not examined. There was extensive caseous tuberculosis of both lungs. Hun regards the lesion as of inflammatory nature, occurring during fetal life. R. H. Babcock[3] reports an interesting case of pulmonary stenosis complicated with pulmonary tuberculosis, which was recognized during life from the presence of a loud, harsh systolic murmur, best heard in the second intercostal space to the left of the sternum. At the autopsy the pulmonary artery was found occluded by a smooth membrane without ridges in the form of a truncated cone, with a small hole at the top. The right ventricle and right auricle were both hypertrophied and dilated ; the ductus arteriosus was not examined.

Robt. B. Preble[4] reports a case of **relative insufficiency of the pulmonary leaflets.** Both sides of the heart were enlarged ; there were a systolic murmur and a presystolic thrill at the apex, and 2 diastolic murmurs at the base, 1 transmitted toward the apex, the other along the sternum. Both second sounds were absent. At the autopsy aortic and mitral insufficiency were found and the pulmonary valves were insufficient by the hydrostatic test ; they showed no pathologic alteration.

J. B. Herrick[5] reports 3 cases of **tricuspid stenosis.** All showed associated mitral stenosis, and in 1 there was also aortic regurgitation. The patients were all females in early adult life ; 2 gave rheumatic histories and the other rheumatic antecedents. None of them presented symptoms of heart-disease until after puberty. Forty cases collected since 1868 are abstracted in this paper.

J. Mackenzie[6] has taken tracings of the jugular pulse during **tricuspid regurgitation,** and finds that it consists of a low wave due to auricular contraction, a fall due to auricular diastole, a very high wave due to the ventricular systole, and finally a 2d fall due to the diastole of the ventricle. In cases of debility these waves are similar in order but less pronounced. In cases of hypertrophy of the right ventricle and dilatation of the auricle the auricular wave disappears and the ventricular wave becomes higher. If, however, tricuspid stenosis exists at the same time, then the auricle is to a certain extent protected, although the hypertrophy of the right ventricle still produces a high ventricular wave, so that we have a diminished auricular and an ex-

[1] Med. News, July, 1896.   [2] Albany Med. Ann., Feb., 1897.
[3] Medicine, May, 1897.   [4] Jour. Am. Med. Assoc., May 29, 1897.
[5] Boston M. and S. Jour., Mar. 18, 1897.   [6] Brit. Med. Jour., May 8, 1897.

aggerated ventricular wave in the tracings. As in these conditions pulsation of the liver almost invariably occurs, and as it fails to occur in slight conditions of tricuspid regurgitation without dilatation of the ventricle, a tracing taken from the pulsating liver with an auricular wave is probably pathognomonic of tricuspid stenosis. Mackenzie has examined 7 cases of this condition, 5 of which have been confirmed by postmortem examination, and in all he has found this form of tracing.

CONGENITAL LESIONS OF THE HEART.

Josephine E. Young[1] reports a case in which the finger-ends were clubbed, the heart enlarged, and a loud systolic murmur was heard over the whole precordia. There was no cyanosis, and the patient died from heart-failure in the course of an attack of acute erysipelas. At the autopsy stenosis of the conus pulmonalis was found about 4 cm. below the upper margin of the semilunar valves. The foramen ovale was patulous, and there was a defect in the ventricular septum more than 2 cm. in diameter. There was recent vegetative endocarditis of the pulmonary tricuspid valves.

W. Moore[2] also describes a case. The patient came under observation at the age of 8 and remained alive until 13. She was fairly well developed, but had marked cyanosis and clubbing of the fingers and toes. There was a confusion of bruits over her heart. At times she would suffer with pyrexia and cough, and sometimes had severe hemoptyses. She was transferred to the consumptive wing of the hospital and died of tubercular meningitis. The heart showed an aperture in the ventricular septum and the aorta entered just above this point, so that it communicated equally with both ventricles. The opening of the pulmonary artery was considerably contracted. The foramen ovale was open. The lungs contained fresh tubercles.

Rheiner[3] reports 2 cases of extreme malformation of the heart. The first seemed a healthy infant, but was attacked with bronchitis. A loud double cardiac murmur was heard and the child died after 8 months. The septum between the ventricle was deficient, and the aorta sprang from the right ventricle. The pulmonary artery was stenosed. The 2d patient, a girl of 5, almost an idiot, and suffering with caries of the temporal bone, became cyanosed and died of purulent meningitis at the age of 5. The heart-sounds were very puzzling, but she had been in a fairly good condition. The autopsy showed extreme pulmonary stenosis; the pulmonary valves showed hardly any division and the septum between the ventricles was deficient.

F. A. Packard[4] reports a most interesting instance of **imperfect closure of the auricular and ventricular septa** in a man who died at the age of 50 from abscess of the brain. The patient was a sailor, and came under observation with a history of having suddenly lost consciousness and having remained in a semiconscious condition for 10 minutes. There was localized convulsion of the right side and later a numb feeling of the entire right side. Physical examination discovered a blowing systolic murmur over the heart with enlargement of the organ. The lungs were negative. The postmortem examination showed a collection of pus beneath the pia, covering the lower surface of the cerebellum, and there was a large abscess in the parietal lobe of the left brain and extending into the ventricles. The basal nuclei were softened. The heart was filled with agonal and antemortem clots. It was globular, the apex being made up of the right ventricle. The right auricle was dilated. The

[1] Medicine, June, 1897.　　[2] Intercol. Med. Jour. Austral., Oct. 20, 1896.
[3] Virchow's Archiv, Dec., 1896.　　[4] Med. News, Aug. 29, 1896.

muscle-substance of all the chambers was a deep brown, and the weight of the organ, free from clots, 15 oz. The endocardium of the auricles was smooth and the foramen ovale patulous. Immediately below it there was a deficiency in the septum ; and there was a deficiency in the ventricular septum, the unde- fended space being closed merely by the posterior tricuspid and anterior mitral leaflets. The aortic and pulmonary orifices and the endocardium were normal. The author reviews the opinions of pathologists regarding the development of malformations of this kind, and particularly remarks upon the great lack of development of the auricular septum, the smallness of the left and the great hypertrophy of the right side of the heart, and the peculiar arrangement of the anterior mitral leaflets and of the chordæ tendineæ, the latter springing for the most part from a single papillary muscle. Clinically, the case is of interest from the lack of symptoms despite the arduous duties of the patient, and from the occurrence of cerebral abscess, the only cause of which, as far as could be discovered, being a slightly diseased vermiform appendix.

Geronzi[1] reports **an extraordinary anomaly** occurring in a woman of 23. Her previous history was that she had always been slow in her movements, easily fatigued, and of impaired intellect; her color was pale without cyanosis and without edema of the face; but there was moderate swelling of the lower extremities. The area of cardiac dulness was greatly increased ; there was gallop rhythm, and a murmur that resembled a peri- cardial friction-sound could be heard over the whole heart. There was

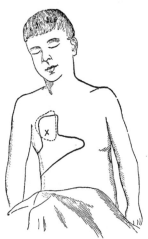

FIG. 2.—Dr. Maclennan's case of dex- trocardia (Brit. Med. Jour., Oct. 31, 1896).

also considerable effusion into the left pleural cavity. A diagnosis of pericarditis was made. Death occurred shortly afterward as a result of anuria from a renal calculus. At the au- topsy complete absence of the interauricular septum was found. The right ventricle was enormously hypertrophied, the left appearing to be merely an appendix to it. The opening of the pulmonary artery was 10 mm. in diameter, of the aorta 5 mm. The mitral orifice was very narrow and slightly stenosed ; the tricuspid orifice very wide. The author explains the absence of cyanosis, in spite of the mixture of arterial and venous blood in the auricle, by the fact that the enormously enlarged right ventricle and pulmonary artery and the narrowness of the aorta in a way compensated the congenital anomaly.

Futran[2] reports an interesting case that presented the symptoms of cardiac insuf- ficiency and signs of cardiac dilatation and mitral regurgitation. There was marked centrifugal pulsation in the veins of the neck, although both sounds in the tricuspid area were clear and sharp. A diagnosis was therefore made of **patulous foramen ovale.**

W. Maclennan[3] describes a case of **dextrocardia** without displacement of other viscera in a lad of 15. The left lung was emphysematous and the left chest somewhat more voluminous than the right, the clavicle being noticeably

[1] Riforma med., Nos. 203 and 204, 1896.   [2] Berlin. klin. Woch., Feb. 8, 1897.
[3] Brit. Med. Jour., Oct. 31, 1896.

elevated on that side. The entrance of air seemed somewhat impeded on the right and the percussion slightly duller than normal. Probably this was due to pressure of the displaced organ upon the right bronchus.

Vehsemeyer [1] reports a case of dextrocardia complicated with chronic pneumonia of the left lung. The great vessels and the abdominal organs did not share in the transposition. Anschutz was able to take a satisfactory radiograph of the condition.

Ferrind [2] reports a **curious case** of cardiac disease. At each pulsation of the heart the left side of the thorax was elevated, the greatest elevation being observed in the 4th to 6th intercostal spaces. These pulsations were very vigorous and accompanied by a fremissement which could be felt as far as the right clavicle. The apex was in the 6th intercostal space to the left of the mammary line. The area of dulness was greatly increased. At the base systolic and diastolic murmurs were heard. In the 4th and 5th intercostal spaces there was a kind of mesosystolic rubbing, somewhat rougher in quality than a murmur. The arteries of the neck showed typical Corrigan pulsation, but in the lower limbs this condition was much less marked. A systolic murmur was heard in the femoral. In view of the history, which pointed to a congenital cardiac lesion, and the peculiar symptoms, Ferrind felt compelled to make a diagnosis of **congenital stricture of the aorta** at the end of the transverse portion of the arch.

Lytten [3] presented a patient of 22 years, suffering from a congenital lesion of the heart, with marked **drum-stick fingers.** A radiograph showed that the thickening was due entirely to hypertrophy of the soft parts.

Diseases of the Myocardium.—De Domenicis [4] holds that the so-called **idiopathic hypertrophy** of the heart is undoubtedly due to increased activity with corresponding increase in the amount of nutrition absorbed, and that this increased activity may be due to a variety of irritating influences acting directly upon the heart-muscle.

Wm. C. Krauss [5] discusses **the danger of bicycling** and reports a case of acute cardiac dilatation due to this cause. The patient was not accustomed to the exercise, and collapsed after riding 8 miles. Physical examination some weeks later showed a heart extremely dilated but with no murmurs. The pulse varied from 130 to 150 per minute.

R. Van Santvoord [6] reports a case that he regards as **traumatic myocarditis** occurring in a man of 24, who, after a severe concussion, had an irregular, feeble pulse of about 106 per minute, which continued for several days, when death occurred from edema of the lungs. [Unfortunately no autopsy is reported.]

Cardiac Syphilis.—S. Phillips [7] discusses syphilis of the heart-wall, reporting first a case of his own that was suddenly attacked with pain in the precordial region. This was relieved by morphin, but 18 days later the patient suddenly died while reading a newspaper. At the autopsy a gumma was found in the left ventricle. The author collected 25 cases of this condition, in all of which the diagnosis was confirmed by autopsy, and then reports 14 cases without autopsies of his own, dividing them into those suffering from severe angina without physical signs of cardiac disease; those suffering from dilatation of the heart, only distinguished from similar conditions due to other causes by the more pronounced symptoms; those in which there is gradual, progressive loss of

[1] Deutsch. med. Woch., Mar. 18, 1897.   [2] Sem. méd., 1896, p. 381.
[3] Deutsch. med. Woch., Mar. 18, 1897.   [4] Wien. klin. Woch., May 22, 1897.
[5] Jour. Am. Med. Assoc., Oct. 10, 1896.   [6] Med. Rec., Aug. 11, 896.
                    [7] Lancet, Jan. 23, 1897.

cardiac power without dilatation of the left ventricle, which he ascribes to diffuse fibroid change ; and, finally, cases with hypertrophy of the heart not apparently due to valvular disease. He also reports 1 case in which a gummatons growth had evidently preceded the development of cardiac aneurysm. In regard to diagnosis the most important element is, of course, evidence of syphilitic infection. Gumma of the left ventricle may be suspected in any individual with such syphilitic antecedents if there occur signs of derangement of the left ventricle with symptoms of defective or embarrassed action, especially angina pectoris, tachycardia, or syncopal or epileptiform attacks ; in the right ventricle when dyspnea otherwise unaccounted for occurs. Syphilitic disease is also indicated by extreme feebleness of the heart without dilatation or hypertrophy and without ascertainable cause. In regard to treatment, Phillips believes that it is probable that gummata or even extensive fibroid change may be relieved by mercury and potassium iodid. [The author is too prone to make the diagnosis of syphilis, according to our view. Accepting his points for diagnosis, we should probably be led to regard myocardial syphilis as a very common disease, which is not the case.]

F. Coggelshall [1] reports a case of cardiac syphilis occurring in a man who in youth had been extremely dissipated, and later had indulged to excess in physical exercise and hard study. The attacks at first resembled syncope, the patient becoming slightly cyanosed, pulseless, and very weak, but not unconscious. Later they became more epileptic in type and accompanied by signs of cardiac failure, particularly extreme bradycardia, the pulse being only 15 to 20 per minute. These attacks occurred several times a day, but the patient reacted well to stimulation. The physical signs during these attacks consisted of a loud, rough murmur heard all over the cardiac area, but most distinctly at the base, that replaced both sounds. The presence of a large thrombosis in the right ventricle was suspected. At the autopsy, however, syphilitic myocarditis was found.

Rosenthal [2] reports a case of syphilitic myocarditis. The patient after numerous relapses appeared to be cured of the specific disease ; he then commenced to exercise and used alcohol to excess. On one occasion, after a severe bicycle ride, he had a feeling of oppression in the region of the heart and dyspnea. This continued until he came under treatment. He was then found to have a rapid pulse, arrhythmia, and a split second sound at the base. The aortic second tone was accentuated ; the area of cardiac dulness extended somewhat to the right. Treatment with tincture of iodin and strophanthus caused rapid improvement in the subjective symptoms ; a systolic murmur developed over the pulmonary artery, and occasionally one could be heard in the mitral region. The arrhythmia continued. The author believes that the strain to which the heart-muscle was subjected caused it to be particularly selected by the poison in the system.

Aneurysm of the Heart.—A. N. Davis [3] describes a case of aneurysm of the heart in a woman of 57 who had been insane for a number of years. Four months before her death dyspnea, pain in the heart-region, moderate cough, hemoptysis, and night-sweats developed. At the autopsy an aneurysm of the left ventricle was found on the anterior wall of the heart, and hemorrhagic infiltration of the heart-muscle.

T. S. Short [4] reports a case of aneurysm of the ventricular septum that during life caused profound dyspnea unless the patient occupied the recumbent position. Murmurs were occasionally heard, both systolic and presystolic in time,

[1] Boston M. and S. Jour., Dec. 10, 1896.   [2] Deutsch. med. Woch., Apr. 1, 1897.
[3] Lancet, Aug. 8, 1896.   [4] Brit. Med. Jour., May 8, 1897.

but were inconstant. At the autopsy the aneurysm was found projecting into the cavity of the right ventricle and partially occluding the pulmonary orifice.

Cardiac Tumors.—Kayserlink[1] reports a case of tumor of the heart. The patient was emaciated, the heart was enlarged, and there was decided fremitus beside the apex-beat and over the base of the heart. Tenderness on pressure was observed posteriorly, and there was severe pain in the breast and arm. Paraplegia developed suddenly and was followed by cystitis and decubitus. The patient succumbed. Postmortem there was found a pericardial effusion, a tumor of the auricles, and a tumor, probably primary, in the hilum of the left lung. This extended along the bronchi into the lung. There were metastases in the second and third dorsal vertebræ, the collapse of which had caused the paraplegia. The tumor was a lymphosarcoma. Leroux and Meslay[2] report a case of multiple sarcomata of the heart secondary to orbital sarcoma. The heart's action had been rapid and irregular, but there had been no murmurs.

Rupture of the Heart.—F. O. Simpson[3] describes a case of rupture of the heart in a man of 62, a senile dement. The patient had regular but slow action of the heart and atheroma of the vessels. One day while sitting quietly in a chair he suddenly became unconscious and very pale; his radial pulse could not be felt, and the sounds of the heart were inaudible; the breathing was frequent, and death followed in about 25 minutes. At the autopsy the pericardial sac contained 210 gm. of blood-clot. The heart weighed 370 gm. There was a rupture of the posterior wall of the ventricle about 1 cm. in length. The myocardium was markedly degenerated. A. N. Kelynack[4] also reports a case. The patient, a man of 68, was brought to the hospital unconscious. He had worked all day but felt unwell. In the evening he went into the back yard and was shortly afterward found unconscious. During the 6 months previous he had had 2 or 3 fainting attacks; his memory had been deficient, and he acted strangely. On admission there was no paralysis, tremor, or rigidity; the pupils were equal and reactive. He began to recover in about 5 minutes, and soon was able to speak, although dazed, and was able to walk feebly. He slept all night, and the next morning felt quite well. About midnight the next night he became restless and insisted on getting out of bed. The next morning he was apparently well, but about midday had an epileptiform attack with spasms of the right hand and arm and with traction of the mouth toward the left side; breathing was stertorous, then irregular, and he died in 10 or 15 minutes. Just before death the heart-sounds could not be heard. The autopsy showed a rupture of the heart along the postero-external border of the left ventricle. The heart-muscle was softened at this point, and the ventricular wall was soft and flabby; the coronary arteries were extremely atheromatous. There was no focal lesion in the brain. The case is of interest as showing that death may not be instantaneous and that cerebral symptoms may complicate the clinical history. W. Groom[5] reports a case occurring in a boy of 16 a month after an injury. The rupture took place in the right ventricle, which at this point consisted only of epicardium.

Bernstein[6] has collected about 121 cases of cardiac diseases ascribed to traumatic injuries or contusions, and points out that there is no specific traumatic heart-disease. He gives the details of 13 cases of his own, in only 1 of which was the contusion directly over the heart. Nervous disturbances were relatively uncommon. The only positively ascertained immediate results are rup-

---

[1] Centralbl. f. innere Med., No. 32, 1896.   [2] Bull. de la Soc. anat. de Paris, Oct., 1896.
[3] Brit. Med. Jour., Dec. 12, 1896.   [4] Lancet, July 18, 1896.
[5] Lancet, May 1, 1897.   [6] Zeit. f. klin. Med., Bd. xxix., H. 5 and 6.

ture of the heart-muscle or valves. In the former case some disease of the muscle has usually preexisted, while in the latter case healthy segments and those of the right heart particularly are affected. The clinical effects of these injuries, as a rule, do not manifest themselves until some time after the injury, probably on account of the reserve power of the organ. The inflammatory lesions of the endocardium are prone to become chronic, while in traumatic pericarditis both acute and chronic forms are met with. Acute endocarditis may be simple or septic in character; traumatic pericarditis may be benign or purulent. The author could find no instance of isolated traumatic myocarditis.

James Jamieson [1] reports the case of a young butcher who was suddenly subjected to severe strain and immediately felt as if something had given way in his chest, and was seized with pain in the region of the heart. Upon admission there were some cyanosis and the signs of cardiac dilatation; on auscultation a double murmur was heard at the aortic region, and an inconstant mitral systolic murmur. He improved upon digitalis, but died suddenly after eating. At the autopsy it was found that the partition between 2 of the segments of the aortic valves was partially torn away from the wall, throwing the 2 pouches into one. The valves were otherwise normal. The author believes that the septum was suddenly ruptured.

W. J. Hanna [2] describes the case of a criminal who stabbed himself in the region of the heart with a sharpened wire. There were pain of moderate severity and dyspnea, but no very marked symptoms for $29\frac{1}{2}$ hours, when the patient was hanged. The autopsy showed the left ventricle **completely penetrated** and 12 oz. of blood in the pericardial sac.

Treatment of Cardiac Disease.—[The Schott method for the treatment of heart-disease is still exciting considerable discussion. In general, the evidence is favorable, although warnings against its indiscriminate use are not lacking.] H. N. Heineman [3] describes the **Schott method.** He lays particular stress upon the local effects of carbon dioxid, holding that its action is to dilate the capillaries in the skin and prevent cooling of the surface, having observed that when the bubbles are brushed away from any portion of the skin it remains white and is subjectively cold. He believes that the salts in the bath are absorbed as far at least as the cutaneous nerves, upon which they act and cause the reflex stimulation. The artificial baths are slightly inferior to the natural baths at Bad Nauheim. Usually the first bath consists of a 1 or 2% solution of NaCl, to which a $\frac{1}{2}$% solution of $CaCl_2$ is added; subsequently the bath may be made stronger and carbonated by the addition of Na_2CO_3 and HCl. The movements must be adapted to the peculiarities of the patient. When interruption of the heart-beat occurs exercise should be at once suspended. Outside of Nauheim, it is well to use also the ordinary methods of treatment. In conclusion, he reports 12 cases, all of which were greatly improved.

Alex. Morison [4] commends the Schott method very highly. He uses Potain's method for indicating the size of the heart, which is as follows: the greatest height of the cardiac area is multiplied by the greatest breadth and the product by an empirical coefficient, 0.83; the result in sq. cm. is approximate if the figure obtained does not depart far from the usual outlines. In one of the cases under Dr. Schott's treatment the measurements were reduced from 22 by 12 cm. to 17 by 9 cm. Using the formula, from 219.1 cm. to 126.9 after. Such a shrinking of the cardiac area or encroachment of the lung can only be temporary, but a repetition of the treatment is sufficient to establish permanency.

[1] Intercol. Med. Jour. Austral., Nov. 10, 1896.   [2] Occidental Med. Times, July, 1896.
[3] Med. Rec., Dec. 12, 1896.   [4] Practitioner, Sept., 1896.

Schott[1] has employed **the Röntgen rays** for the determination of the alterations produced in the size of the heart by his methods. As the tube always occupied a definite position with relation to the patient, it was possible to apply mensuration to the results; thus, in a boy of $8\frac{1}{2}$ years suffering from mitral insufficiency the breadth of the heart at the 3d rib before gymnastics was 9.7 cm.; after, 8.8 cm. It is not possible to determine variations in the vertical diameter of the heart. The effect of the baths was the same. In a 14 year old girl the greatest diameter diminished 0.8 cm.

George Herschell[2] is still uncertain of the value of the baths in use at Nauheim and elsewhere, but admits freely the utility of resisted movements. He prefers mechanical resistance, especially an apparatus consisting of rubber cords with handles attached somewhat in the manner of pulley-weights. He warns against careless use of this treatment, and urges that the pulse and sphygmographic tracings be taken before, during, and after the exercise; that the rate of the respirations be noted, and the area of cardiac dulness and the apex be carefully observed.

S. Solis Cohen and C. West[3] report a case of cardiac dilatation occurring in a woman of 58 years with, apparently, considerable myocarditis, treated by the **Schott method** of passive movements. As a result, the apex receded from 1 in. to the left to the right of the nipple-line, and from the 6th to the 5th interspace. The pulse diminished from 96 to 58. Contraindications are advanced arteriosclerosis, degeneration of the myocardium, and aneurysm.

H. N. Heineman[4] reports 4 cases of stenocardia in which the Schott method was employed with excellent results.

J. W. Bell[5] suggests the use of **saline baths** of suitable temperature for the purpose of freeing the peripheral circulation and thus relieving the venous engorgement due to an insufficient senile heart.

T. G. Stewart[6] opened a discussion on the treatment of "cardiac failure" before the British Medical Association, with a general consideration of the various plans of treatment. The most important elements are **rest,** particularly serviceable in individuals accustomed to severe physical exertion, and diet. Some patients require increased allowance of food, some a diminution, while some require alteration in the quality. In patients who have been underfed, or in hospitals or institutions of other kinds, a more liberal amount of meat than is the rule may be advised. Alcohol in moderate doses is useful, but excess, even though slight, and forms that disturb the stomach must not be employed.

He then considers the effects of **exercise,** and, first, passive exercise. He has practised the method of Ling in a number of cases, and concludes that the area of cardiac dulness perceptibly diminishes during each administration, and that the sounds and action of the heart and pulse correspondingly improve. The patient experiences subjective improvement, which may pass off in a few hours completely or incompletely. Repeated applications may give permanent improvement. Occasionally these exercises are not well borne.

He next refers to the "**resisted movements**" of Schott. His experience with this method leads him to the following conclusions: that in a large proportion of cases there is immediate improvement in the condition of the heart as shown by percussion or auscultation, the sounds becoming more distinct and the area of dulness diminishing; in many cases the rhythm of the pulse improves and the beat becomes stronger; the results are temporary, but

[1] Deutsch. med. Woch., Apr. 1, 1897.   [2] Lancet, Aug. 15, 1896.
[3] Phila. Polyclinic, Mar. 6, 1897.   [4] Med. News, Jan. 9, 1897.
[5] Ibid., Sept. 26, 1896.   [6] Brit. Med. Jour., Sept. 19, 1896.

10

the heart rarely goes back to its original condition; while repeated treatment leads to gradual and lasting improvement. The author refers to a number of cases. He points out that in this treatment the blood-vessels of the muscles dilate during contraction; this leads to lessening of the peripheral resistance and increased inflow of blood by contraction of the veins. In spite of the latter, however, the amount of blood in the heart is diminished because of the arterial dilatation. Excess of muscular work would lead to an inordinate inflow of blood into the heart and its work would be increased.

The Schott method is so conducted as always to fall short of this point. He believes that it is not impossible that increased proportions of CO_2 in the blood may be one result of the method and may contribute to peripheral dilatation of the vessels through the vasomotor system. He concludes that the Schott method is best suited to cases in which there remains a certain power of the heart, while the mere passive exercises of massage are applicable to weaker conditions of the organ. The **method of Oertel** of climbing heights is not widely applicable.

He has experimented with artificial baths, finding as follows: baths of ordinary Edinburgh water at a temperature of 95° led to no change in the size of the heart after 15 min., either in normal cases or in cases with dilated heart. Practically the same results were obtained with saline baths. When, however, large quantities of carbonic acid gas were disengaged in the saline bath peripheral reddening and diminution in size of the heart were noted. The author points out that, as a rule, diminution of peripheral resistance should be followed by a quickened action of the heart and fall of arterial pressure, and not by a slower rate of beat, as is the case. He suggests, as an explanation, that the heart has been previously acting irregularly and too quickly, in consequence of its unfitness to meet the demands upon it; but he does not deny that the carbonic acid and the baths in general may have some direct influence upon the nerves of the skin. Finally, he concludes that none of these methods is entitled to displace the **older methods of treatment**—rest, diet, and medicine. In this opinion he believes Dr. Schott concurs. The methods of treatment referred to are valuable auxiliaries, and may allow us to dispense with remedies that are not well borne.

In the discussion which followed a number of gentlemen participated, including Leith, Saundby, Byrom Bramwell, Thorne, Morison, Savill, and Fisher. The opinion was quite general that the mechanical methods of treatment afford decided advantages.

J. Neumann [1] believes that **sodium iodid** is useful in certain cases of chronic insufficiency that are not adapted to the method of Schott or Oertel. He usually prescribes it in combination with the infusion of digitalis.

Hirschfeld,[2] in discussing the question of **diet in cardiac disease,** states his belief that the former custom of administering small quantities of food during stages of broken compensation in heart-disease is more or less well founded. Reduction in the amount of nutrition does not prevent proper cardiac nourishment, as Timofejeff saw hypertrophy develop in dogs after artificial valvular defects had been established, in spite of starvation diet. Moreover, the periodical consumption of food places a certain amount of strain on the heart, especially the consumption of liquids, as Oertel taught; it requires considerable cardiac activity to supply blood for the functions of the glands concerned in active digestion, and the mere mechanical problem imposed by the periodical distention of the stomach may have further unfavorable influence. The best results with milk-diet have been obtained by those who used

[1] Brit. Med. Jour., May 3, 1897.   [2] Berlin. klin. Woch., Aug. 17, 1896.

very small quantities (600 to 800 c.c.) of milk per day. When the quantity was increased the cases did badly. He holds that the diuresis resulting in these cases is not due to the milk-diet, because the addition of other food or of milk at once stops the beneficial action. He himself has made some 20 experiments with reduction of the diet, some of which have been previously published. Of the first 5 cases 3 showed very positive results. Later he sometimes obtained useful results, but none so convincing. It seemed desirable, therefore, to determine in what cases this reduced diet is specially useful. One of the first results is the reduced demand for liquid, and a beneficial result may therefore be expected when there is only a moderate grade of edema and when disturbances of compensation have not existed too long a time. Another consideration of importance is that the appetite of the patient shall have been previously satisfactory. Under these circumstances a sudden reduction of diet brings about the most striking results. The amount of nutriment irrespective of its quantity exercises a powerful influence, for in cases in which the same amount of food was introduced at different times, but with varying quantities of nutriment contained therein, he found the edema and dyspnea increased as soon as the nutriment was increased. He therefore opposes Oertel's view that an abundant or rich diet should be given to patients emaciated or reduced in vitality. As soon as compensation has failed it is advisable to reduce the diet. The nutrition may be improved after compensation has been restored. [This paper undoubtedly contains much that is true. The author does not deny—in fact, asserts—the importance of mere quantitative reduction of diet, but he gives this a place inferior to qualitative reduction. We should be less disposed to view the latter so favorably, though he is undoubtedly correct in asserting that cases of beginning failure of compensation with slight edema may be placed on reduced diet with advantage.]

Molderescu [1] advises the use of **calomel** in the treatment of cardiac diseases; he administers as much as 8 to 10 gr. divided into 6 doses, especially in cases in which there is a comparatively moderate valvular lesion, with marked dyspnea, hypertrophy, dilatation, albuminuria, or dropsies. After a few doses diuresis is usually established, and by the 2d or 3d day copious action of the bowels. As a rule, it is better to administer somewhat small doses for long periods of time, and in order to prevent salivation he employs a mouthwash composed of chlorate of potash and tannic acid. Out of 170 cases of grave cardiac disorder treated in this manner, 14 died, 2 of pneumonia, after the heart-symptoms had been relieved, 3 before the treatment had been sufficiently under way; the 9 others were persons of advanced years in whom the disease was well established. [One of the editors, in a communication a year or two since, recommended this remedy as of particular value in certain forms of combined renal and cardiac disease. He did not find continuous use of the remedy advisable, and obtained results only when considerable doses were administered. The effect was most striking when opium was used coincidently to prevent purgation. It does not seem likely to us that Molderescu's view, that the beneficial effect is due to relief of the congestion of the liver, is well founded. Copious diuresis is the most evident and doubtless the most desirable result.]

G. R. Lockwood [2] reports 9 cases of cardiac disease in which removal of all forms of nasal obstruction caused the cardiac symptoms to disappear.

Arnold Lorand [3] urges that patients suffering from valvular heart-disease be sent, if possible, to **warm climates.**

Jaccoud [4] believes that when perfect compensation exists it is not necessary

---

[1] Rev. de Thérap. médico-chir., June 1, 1896. [2] N. Y. Med. Jour., Jan. 16, 1897.
[3] Med. Rec., July 18, 1896. [4] Sem. méd., p. 357, 1896.

to forbid **marriage in heart-disease,** having observed a case in which a woman had 4 children without noticeable increase of a mitral lesion. After the 6th child, however, compensation was lost.

Cardiac Neuroses.—Van der Velde[1] reports some experiments upon normal individuals in regard to their ability to increase the **frequency of the cardiac contraction.** He found that by concentration of the attention it was possible to increase the rate on an average 20 beats per minute in all of the persons investigated, including himself; and he believes that this ability is probably shared by all to a greater or less extent. The cause, he considers, is due entirely to an effort of the will.

Kish[2] describes a nervous cardiac disturbance that occurs among the officers of the German Army. It consists of repeated attacks of **palpitation,** accompanied by a feeling of oppression and anxiety. Often there is some uncertainty in the gait, and dizziness and even unconsciousness. In the interval the pulse is usually rapid, from 80 to 100 per minute, and the arteries soft and less elastic than normal. As all the other conditions can be excluded he believes that the cause is some psychical influence.

T. Henderson[3] reports a case of paroxysmal **tachycardia** which developed after a period of severe labor and anxiety. The heart was not enlarged and the sounds were clear and normal. The ordinary rate was about 80. At times it would commence suddenly to pulsate with such rapidity as to cause vibration of the precordia. The pulse apparently exceeded 200 per minute.

J. W. Ogle[4] reports 4 cases of **bradycardia,** in all of which fibrous deposits were found in the myocardium. He believes that these morbid deposits act as foreign bodies and impede the action of the intracardiac ganglia. Two of these cases had epilepsy.

P. A. Dewar[5] reports 2 cases of **slow pulse.** The first, a man of 63, had always been active, both mentally and physically; he had suffered from acute rheumatism, but made apparently a good recovery. For 2 years he had been pale, weak, and suffered from sighing respiration, and his pulse had averaged about 20 beats per minute, although the heart's action was strong and regular. The lowest rate recorded was 16 and the highest 36. Ultimately, he had attacks of what seemed to be petit mal, and convulsive seizures in which he bit his tongue. After this the heart became weak, rapid, and irregular. The second case was a man, apparently healthy, strong, and active. Nevertheless his pulse was irregular and running 20 to 25 per minute. From time to time he suffered from attacks of loss of consciousness, which, under bromids, became rarer.

W. E. Risdon[6] reports a case of a man of 38 years who was suddenly seized with **faintness.** In the recumbent posture he recovered, but on attempting to stand he became pulseless and deeply unconscious for 2 hours. Then the heart recovered somewhat, beating from 24 to 30 times per minute. This was followed by intermissions and progressive cardiac failure. Death occurred 3 days later. At the autopsy a few streaks of fat were found at the apex of the heart, but otherwise it was normal.

Lewin[7] states that in acute **lead-poisoning,** particularly that due to lead acetate, the pulse is sometimes small and very rapid. He has collected 5 cases in which this occurred, and 10 cases in which there was bradycardia; in 1

---

[1] Pflüger's Archiv, vol. lxvi., p 232.   [2] Berlin. klin. Woch., Feb. 1, 1897.
[3] Brit. Med. Jour., July 18, 1896.   [4] Lancet, Jan. 30, 1897.
[5] Canad. Jour. M. and S., Jan., 1897.   [6] Lancet, Mar. 29, 1897.
          [7] Deutsch. med. Woch., Mar. 18, 1897.

case the pulse dropped to 15 beats per minute. In 1 case it was unaltered by the poison.

D. Drummond[1] reports 6 cases of **functional murmurs,** and concludes that these murmurs occur in highly neurotic people and are associated with violently acting ventricles independent of the lung conditions, or may be intimately connected with respiratory and structural alterations in the lung. They are not limited to any cardiac area or period, and usually alter under the influence of rest, position, or respiratory movement.

Melo[2] discusses the **nervous disturbances,** such as hysteria, neurasthenia, epilepsy, and even insanity, that occur **in the course of uncompensated heart-disease.** He considers that the valvular lesions act either as predisposing or exciting causes, particularly in persons with a hereditary predisposition, as all these cases are of the clinical type of the hereditary neuropathies.

A. A. Smith[3] exhibited a patient in clinic with valvular heart-disease. Upon one occasion she became excited and had palpitation and evidence of want of heart-compensation. The **temperature** was taken and found to be at least 112°, the limit of the thermometer. The observation was repeated in the rectum with several thermometers and confirmed. The following morning it had fallen to 104.6°, but in the evening rose again to 108°. The patient exhibited many symptoms of hysteria.

ANGINA PECTORIS.

Wm. Osler[4] looks upon angina pectoris not as a disease, but as a syndrome, characterized by a heart-pain and the fear of impending death. He recognizes the following abnormal cardiac sensations : consciousness of the heart's action— that is, palpitation and a sense of tension in the chest ; pain of almost any variety and intensity, and a peculiar condition which consists of a sense of imminent dissolution (*angor animi*). He recognizes 2 forms—angina pectoris vera and angina pectoris notha—which he subdivides into hysterical, vasomotor, and toxic forms. It is not clearly understood how the common lesion, some obstruction of the coronary circulation, causes the disease. It is certain that gradually developing obstruction may not lead to serious symptoms. Osler recognizes 4 groups of the disease : 1st, sudden death without other manifestations of angina pectoris ; 2d, death in the first well-marked paroxysm ; 3d, recurring attacks extending over a period of months or years ; 4th, rapidly repeated attacks over a period of days or weeks with rapid development of a state of cardiac asystole (*l' état de mal. angineux*). In further discussing the symptomatology, he calls attention to 4 interesting conditions, closely allied to true angina, that may either develop in the course of an attack or occur spontaneously in the subjects of heart-disease or arteriosclerosis. These are syncope anginosa—that is, a tendency to faint during the attack, although this is not common ; 2d, Adam-Stokes' syndrome, characterized by permanent slowness of the heart and vertigo or syncope ; 3d, angina pectoris sine dolore ; and 4th, cardiac asthma. He next takes up pseudo-angina, which has 3 characteristic features : it occurs chiefly in women, in younger persons, and does not cause death. There are 3 main types—the neurotic (occurring usually in hysteria), the neurasthenic, and the toxic (most commonly observed among tobacco-smokers). In attempting to explain the nature of the lesions he calls attention to the remarkable phenomena known as intermittent claudication, a condition apparently due to the blocking of the main artery and the insufficiency

[1] Lancet, Apr. 6, 1897.　　　　　　　　　　[2] Thèse de Paris, 1896.
[3] Med. News, Dec. 19, 1896.　　　　　　　[4] N. Y. Med. Jour., Aug. 8, 1896.

of the collateral circulation to meet the unusual demands. In explanation of the pain he offers 4 theories : (*a*) a cramp of the heart-muscles ; (*b*) distention and stretching of the cardiac wall ; (*c*) arterial pain ; (*d*) neuralgic or neuritic pain. [It is impossible, with the limit of space at our disposal, to do justice to this remarkable series of lectures.]

D. W. C. Hood[1] states that the following clinical groups may present symptoms of anginoid character : 1, acute dilatation of the heart due to sudden, prolonged effort ; 2, chronic dilatation of the heart due to slow degeneration ; 3, dyspneal angina sine dolore ; 4, neurotic—functional and organic ; 5, gouty ; 6, reflex—stomach, tobacco ; 7, asthmatic—right-sided heart-disease ; 8, renal ; 9, pseudo-angina, fictitious angina—neuralgic, anemic, climacteric, alcoholic, etc. This classification, he admits, is artificial and purely clinical. In cases of angina sine dolore the patient frequently describes his symptoms as arising from dyspepsia, and the fact that discharge of flatus often gives relief seems to add confirmation. The author, therefore, advises that attention should be paid to flatulent discomfort after food or exertion, occurring in persons in advanced middle life.

Grocco[2] distinguishes **2 forms** of angina pectoris—the neurotic and the arteriosclerotic. He has observed 3 cases of the former type with distinct lesions of the nerves at the base of the heart, consisting of interstitial neuritis and degeneration. In the arteriosclerotic forms myocardial degenerations are of great importance ; but even in these cases he holds that the nervous mechanism within the heart may be the part that suffers first.

John Maddin[3] reports 5 cases of angina pectoris, in none of which was it possible to detect by physical examination any organic disease of the heart. He looks upon these as the true **idiopathic form.**

H. L. Elsner[4] reports the case of a patient of 46 who suffered from shortness of breath after exertion and attacks of angina pectoris, although repeated examinations by various physicians failed to detect signs of cardiac disease. Death occurred in the course of one of the anginoid crises. An autopsy could not be obtained. The author regards the case as one of **myocarditis,** probably specific in nature.

Treatment.—Schott[5] recommends **nitroglycerin** as the most reliable symptomatic remedy for angina. The action is most satisfactory in cases in which the symptom is due to spasm, and next in efficiency in cases in which there are associated lesions of the aorta. It is less reliable when there is myocarditis or fatty degeneration of the heart. He advises administration in liquid form, as the tablets frequently prove inefficient. He claims that the doses should be larger than those usually administered.

Vierordt[6] recommends the employment of **sodium iodid** in cases of angina pectoris, particularly those in which there is distinct cardiac weakness or the presence of albuminuria.

Ostwick[7] has employed **hyoscin** in a case of angina pectoris that he believed to be of neurotic origin, with excellent results.

EXOPHTHALMIC GOITER.

J. Dreschfeld[8] discusses Graves' disease, reporting 40 cases. He found that the most frequent symptoms, in addition to those peculiar to the dis-

[1] Lancet, Sept. 26, 1896.   [2] Settimana Med., Nos. 1 and 2, 1896.
[3] Jour. Am. Med. Assoc., June, 1896.   [4] Med. News, Sept. 5, 1896.
[5] Therap. Monatsh., Oct., 1896.   [6] Centralbl. f. innere Med., June 26, 1897.
[7] Med. Rec., May, 1897.   [8] Practitioner, Aug., 1896.

ease, are tremor, muscular cramps, localized atrophies, and alteration of the reflexes. The 3 latter symptoms he was unable to observe in any of his own cases; however, he noted that psychical disturbances are chiefly depressing in nature, although occasionally the patient is irritated. In one case he observed epileptic convulsions. Profuse perspiration was present in all, but most marked in those where there were tachycardia, pyrexia, and emaciation. In 7 cases he observed pigmentation of the skin, and in 6 the areas of pigment were placed symmetrically. In 7 cases there was persistent vomiting, invariably associated with and probably due to acetonuria. Diarrhea was present in 10 cases and paroxysmal dyspnea occasionally. In 1 case there was marked polyuria, in another swelling of the lymph-glands. Dreschfeld has been able to confirm the observation of Charcot, that patients usually improve markedly after delivery, if allowed to go to full term. In regard to the treatment, he doubts whether the benefit derived from surgical interference justifies the danger of the operation, the total mortality being at present 12 %. He also is skeptical of the value of thyroid-feeding. He is more favorable, although he has never employed it himself, to the injection of the blood-serum of dogs whose thyroid glands have been removed.

Lemke [1] regards tachycardia and tremor as the most significant symptoms of Graves' disease. He holds that it results from some form of **specific muscle-poison** produced by the thyroid gland.

R. G. Curtin [2] believes that Graves' disease is hereditary, and that, therefore, the **marriage** of those suffering from it should be discouraged.

J. A. Booth [3] reports a case of exophthalmic goiter presenting the unusual symptom of edema of the eyelids. After the removal of one lobe of the thyroid gland there was marked improvement in all the symptoms excepting this.

Treatment.—[This disease has, for some reason, appeared more suitable for organotherapy than almost any other. As a result, various organs have been utilized with more or less doubtful results.] H. Mackenzie [4] has collected the reports of 15 cases of exophthalmic goiter treated by large doses of **thymus gland.** In 14 of these there was very considerable improvement. To these he adds 20 cases of his own: 1 died; in 6 no improvement was observed; in 13 there was some improvement. However, the effect produced upon the most important symptoms does not lead him to believe that the gland has any great value. The pulse was not altered in 12 cases; it was increased in 2; it was diminished in 6, but in 5 of these only slightly. In only 3 cases was there any material diminution in the size of the thyroid gland; in 2 it increased; in 1 only there was diminution in the exophthalmos. Comparison with the notes of 20 cases treated by other methods shows that the thymus has little, if any, advantage over them. A. Maude [5] reports 4 cases of exophthalmic goiter treated with tabloids of thymus gland. All were extreme cases with typical symptoms; 3 of them presented considerable psychical alteration, and all had been treated by the ordinary methods without result. All showed remarkable improvement under the thymus treatment, but without much reduction of the size of the gland. Particularly the rapidity of the heart's action and the tremor were much diminished. R. M. Whitefoot [6] reports a case of exophthalmic goiter occurring in a girl of 18 years, with a neurotic family history. There were all the characteristic symptoms, and in addition profuse menstruation. Treatment with extract of **thyroid gland** produced decrease in the size of the tumor, reduction of the eyeballs, and a greater regularity in the action of

[1] Münch. med. Woch., No. 15, 1896.   [2] Internat. Clin., vol. iv., series 6, 1897.
[3] Med. Rec., July 11, 1896.   [4] Am. Jour. Med. Sci., Feb., 1897.
[5] Lancet, July 18, 1896.   [6] Med. News, Oct. 3, 1896.

the heart, but at the same time the patient became melancholic and emaciated. On account of loss of appetite and nausea treatment was suspended at various times, but at the end of 60 days she had become apparently entirely well.

H. C. Wood,[1] in a paper on the functions and therapeutics of the ductless glands, refers to a case of exophthalmic goiter under his care, in which suppurative splenitis developed without apparent cause. The abscess discharged and there was a period of many months of severe sepsis, followed by recovery. In the second or third week of the splenitis the thyroid gland began to decrease in size, and eventually there was permanent cure. This case led him to use **splenic extract** in cases of Graves' disease. He has found, however, that doses sufficiently large to produce effects are apt to derange digestion, and hypodermically great irritation and even abscesses are caused by the extract. In one of his cases, which could be followed systematically in the hospital, the patient insisted that she had recovered after some weeks and refused to stay longer, although there was still some enlargement of the thyroid gland. In another case there was violent gastric irritation, and the remedy was therefore administered hypodermically; improvement soon manifested itself and continued until the enlargement of the gland entirely disappeared. The other symptoms had somewhat improved. [The evidence in favor of this treatment is certainly slight, and the possible elements that may have contributed to the spontaneous improvement in his first case after the development of splenitis are many. The most immediate suggestion is that the infection may have been instrumental.]

A. Carless[2] discusses the treatment of exophthalmic goiter. Of all the methods hitherto suggested, he is inclined to consider **phosphate of sodium**, suggested by Trachewsky, as the most likely to be of value. He admits that thyroid extract may be of use, but points out that in some cases, at least, it predisposes to heart-failure. He also mentions, without criticism, the use of thymus extract and the serum of myxedematous dogs. Finally, after discussing the operative methods, which he regards as dangerous, he mentions section of the cervical sympathetic as suggested by Jaboulay, a method too recent to have given definite results.

Tricomi[3] reports 3 cases of Graves' disease in which **removal of part of the gland** resulted in benefit. These cases were typical and the goiter was very prominent. Palpitation, exophthalmos, frequent pulse, tremor, etc., were present, but Graefe's sign was absent. After operation the symptoms disappeared in 2 cases, and in the third there was noteworthy improvement. Two cases had begun after influenza.

Matthes[4] has examined the **nitrogen-balance** in cases of exophthalmic goiter before and after strumectomy. Before the operation it was found that the excretion was in excess of the ingestion, although it was possible by the introduction of large quantities of albumin and calories to obtain a balance. After the operation the bodyweight increased, and disintegration of the albumin was diminished to 25 % of the nitrogenous metabolism. When the gland that had been extirpated was fed to the patient, it was found that the amount of nitrogen excreted increased. [These results are important, because they indicate that partial removal of the thyroid gland may have an important effect upon the general nutrition, whether it improves the so-called cardinal symptoms or not.

Jaboulay[5] describes a case of Graves' disease in which the right lobe of

[1] Am. Jour. Med. Sci., May, 1897.   [2] Practitioner, Nov., 1896.
[3] Il. Policlinico, Nov. 15, 1896.   [4] Centralbl. f. innere Med., June 26, 1897.
[5] Lyon méd., No. 12, 1896.

the thyroid gland was removed; later the left one, this having become hypertrophied; the middle lobe then enlarged, and a third operation was undertaken, the sympathetic nerve between the upper and middle cervical ganglia being removed. The palpitations, tremor, and exophthalmos diminished, but the former returned after 3 months.

DISEASES OF THE ARTERIES.

Litten [1] discusses the physical signs of **pseudo-aortic insufficiency** and atheroma of the abdominal aorta. The former is characterized by a thrill in the carotids when they are lightly pressed upon, and considerable accentuation of the aortic second sound without a diastolic murmur. Atheroma of the abdominal aorta is also to be recognized by this abnormal development of an arterial thrill, associated with pains in the abdomen, particularly at night, that do not extend toward the spinal column. Palpation also reveals more or less enlargement of the aorta, and if the wall of the latter contains calcareous plates they may sometimes be felt crackling under strong pressure.

Gerhart [2] reports a case exhibiting **pulsus paradoxus** on one side of the body with unequal pulses of the arteries of the two arms. The patient was a woman of 66, who had for years suffered with ulcers of the legs and who had had a fracture of both bones of the forearm a few years before. In December, 1895, she suffered with dyspnea, fever, swelling of the feet, and diminution of the daily quantity of urine. On admission to the hospital it was found that she had bronchitis and mitral regurgitation. The pulse was irregular, from 80 to 90. There was a sharp blowing systolic murmur at the apex, and occasionally a diastolic murmur suggesting stenosis. She had moderate ascites, edema of the feet, and albuminuria with hyaline and granular casts. The left pulse was strikingly smaller than the right, not only in the radial, but also in the brachial and carotid arteries. The femoral pulses were equal. The arteries were thin-walled and soft. The pulse was irregular and showed irregular after-waves. In the left radial artery the beats became smaller and nearly impalpable during the height of inspiration. Counted at different times by different trained observers, the right and left radial arteries showed as follows: right 84, left 57; right 69, left 64; right 73, left 69; right 72, left 64. The brachial arteries showed: right 88, left 84. The carotids: right 84, left 76, the heart-beats at the same time being 86; at another time right 83, left 79, heart-beats 79. The sphygmogram showed these differences, and also the diminution of the pulse during inspiration. The cause of this condition is doubtful. The fracture of the forearm would not, of course, explain the difference in the brachial and carotid pulses. The author further alludes to a case of Heubner, in which a woman of 52, with fatty heart and atheroma of the aorta, had inequality of the pulse, the left being stronger in the radial, brachial, and subclavian arteries. The autopsy showed a thrombus in the subclavian artery. The fact that the pulse occasionally failed in the right radial must have led to irregularity in rate on the two sides. He also alludes to a case of Mainzeu in a man of 27, with a large left-sided pleural effusion. The pulse ceased with inspiration, this condition disappearing after aspiration and reappearing with subsequent collections of the fluid. The left pulse was always weaker than the right. He also reports [3] a second case of this condition. The patient was a woman of 69, who had had an attack of apoplexy with subsequent paresis of the right leg. The left radial showed a smaller and

---

[1] Wien. klin. Woch., Sept. 26, 1896.   [2] Berlin. klin. Woch., Jan. 4, 1897.
[3] Ibid., Apr. 5, 1897.

more irregular pulse than the right. When counted, the rate was l. 92, r. 112. A later observation gave a pulse-rate of r. 52, l. 42. Death occurred shortly after this. At the autopsy there were found recent purulent pleuritis and pericarditis. The aorta was normal, but the right subclavian artery was 2 cm., the left 0.8 cm. in diameter. [We have recently observed a case of this condition; the patient was a woman, about 70 years old, with the signs of atheroma of the aorta. The action of the heart was irregular, but there was usually a difference of 4 or 5 beats, the left pulse being the slower. The radials were apparently of the same size.]

Schlesinger[1] reports several cases that presented peculiar **venous phenomena.** These consisted essentially in prominence of the superficial veins, the walls becoming, apparently, very thick and resistant, and feeling like hard cords. All these changes disappeared at times, so that the veins were no longer palpable and appeared as fine blue lines beneath the skin. An extirpated portion of one of these veins showed that the walls were perfectly normal. The only explanation that he is able to offer is, that the thickening was probably due to the swelling of the endothelial lining. All the cases hitherto observed have been in very cachectic individuals.

T. D. Savill[2] reports 2 cases of what he regards as **idiopathic arterial hypermyotrophy.** The arteries in this condition show great increase in thickness, due almost entirely to hypertrophy of the middle coat. In one of his cases he found also atheromatous patches. The symptoms may be in abeyance for a long time if the compensation of the heart is sufficient. The characteristic thickening of the peripheral vessels can, however, be determined early. It is readily distinguished from the atheroma by the absence of bead-like inequalities. The characteristic of the pulse in the present disease is its constant high tension. Vertigo was a striking symptom in both the cases reported. Paroxysmal dizziness, headache, occasional hemorrhage, tendency to gangrene of the extremities, and angina pectoris are noted as symptoms. The urine presents no characteristic change, but is increased slightly, and the sp. gr. is usually a little too low. [In reading the description of these cases we see no reason for regarding them as other than instances of general diffuse arteriosclerosis. In one of them, indeed, there was associated nodular atheroma. It is surprising that the author does not take into consideration in his discussion the possibility of diffuse sclerosis. It has been often pointed out that the hypertrophy of the media may be in excess of the seeming thickening of intima or adventitia in this disease.]

Graf[3] describes a case of **arteritis nodosa,** with interesting clinical symptoms. The patient, a laborer of 39, suffered with gastralgic pains, and later with swelling of the liver and jaundice. After a few months symptoms of cardiac weakness developed, including rapid, small pulse, increasing edema, and later albuminuria. From the very beginning of the illness the patient was cachectic, and later cachectic leukocytosis was observed. The patient died 3½ months after the onset, and the characteristic lesions of Kussmaul's disease with multiple aneurysms were discovered. The changes were most marked in the arteries of the heart, spleen, liver, mesentery, and kidneys. The aorta and the large vessels were intact. There was no evidence of a specific taint in this case; but though the same was true of 8 others reported in literature, the author still inclines to the belief that this factor must be taken into consideration.

B. Bramwell[4] reports an unusual case of **ossification of the arteries** occurring in a man 25 years of age. He suffered from extreme asthenia, car-

[1] Wien. klin. Woch., Dec. 24, 1896.   [2] Brit. Med. Jour., Jan. 23, 1897.
[3] Ziegler's Beiträge zur path. Anat., Bd. 19, p. 181.   [4] Edinb. Hosp. Rep., vol. iv., 1896.

diac debility, anemia, pigmentation of the skin, subcutaneous swellings, rigid arteries, polyuria, the urine containing phosphates and a small quantity of albumin. The rigidity of the arteries rapidly increased until they ceased to transmit pulsation. At the autopsy the heart was found to be in an extreme degree of calcareous degeneration, many of the muscular fibers being entirely ossified. Similar calcareous changes were seen in the left kidney, the right being almost entirely destroyed as a result of some earlier condition. There was no good reason for the condition, but it was supposed that the hardships to which the patient had been previously exposed had caused the blood to become loaded with calcareous salts, which were rapidly deposited in the vessels and kidneys. The fact that the patient was able to engage in laborious exercise until 3 months before his death seemed to indicate that the process was acute.

W. Bell[1] describes a case of **thrombosis of the abdominal aorta.** The patient, a man of 30, was suddenly seized with intense pain in the back and abdomen while walking along the street. He became powerless and fell to the ground. There were absolute paralysis of both legs and anesthesia and analgesia as high as the lower third of the thighs. There was hyperesthesia for 2 inches above the anesthetic area. The reflexes were absent; the sphincters were paralyzed. The legs became cold and finally gangrenous. The patient died in collapse. Autopsy showed no visible disease of the lumbar cord or canda equina. The aorta and both iliacs contained a firm white coagulum from a point about $\frac{3}{4}$ in. above the bifurcation to 1 in. below in the left and $\frac{7}{8}$ in. below it in the right iliac. No change was found in the coats of the arteries. The author believes that the symptoms were caused by the sudden occlusion of the lowest lumbar arteries which supply the lumbar cord. Charrier and Apert[2] report the case of a woman, 51 years old, who had suffered for 20 years from mitral obstruction. She was suddenly attacked with severe pain in the left leg followed by symptoms of embolism in the iliac artery; 6 days later the same symptoms occurred in the right leg, but disappeared within a short time; 3 weeks later there was an attack of right hemiplegia, and shortly afterward the left foot became gangrenous. At the autopsy there was found complete thrombosis of the aorta, beginning just below the inferior mesenteric artery, and embolism with great softening of the left cerebral hemisphere.

A. Burton[3] and J. B. Bradbury[4] report together 3 cases suffering from high arterial tension that were greatly benefited by the administration of **erythroltetranitrate.**

Rumf[5] holds that an **exclusive milk-diet** is by no means appropriate for patients suffering from calcareous infiltration of the arteries. He has made some experiments, and found that the amount of calcium introduced with a sufficient quantity of milk to nourish an adult is in excess of that excreted. He has endeavored, therefore, to find a diet that will nourish the patient, and, at the same time, introduce a minimum quantity of calcium, and recommends the following formula: meat 250 gm. and 100 gm. each of bread, fish, potatoes, and apples. The next indication to be met is to provide for the increased excretion. This can be, to a certain extent, accomplished by diuretics composed of the salts of vegetable acids, particularly lactic and citric acids. The quantitative estimation of the amount of calcium excreted under this medicament showed that it was considerably increased. In conclusion, he reports 3 cases treated according to these principles in which, as long as the treatment and diet were continued, almost complete health existed.

---

[1] Brit. Med. Jour., Oct. 24, 1896.   [2] Bull. de la Soc. anat. de Paris, Nov., 1896.
[3] Brit. Med. Jour. Apr. 3, 1897.   [4] Ibid., Apr. 10, 1897.
[5] Berlin. klin. Woch., Mar. 29, 1897.

Aneurysms.—Mir[1] in 436 autopsies observed 19 cases of **rupture of aortic aneurysms.** 5 of these were in the ascending aorta, 5 in the transverse aorta, and 9 in the descending aorta, which proves that the more freely the aneurysm can develop the more likely it is to rupture; as, for example, an aneurysm occurring in the pericardial cavity. He finds the chief lesion to be disease of the media, which may be the result of traumatism or of simple or specific inflammations.

Buberl[2] reports 2 cases of aortic aneurysm, neither of which produced symptoms of much distress until rupture occurred. The 1st patient, 12 days before his death, had a sticking pain in the right side and coughed up about 200 c.c. of blood. This was repeated twice. At the autopsy it was found that it had ruptured into the tissue of the lung which formed part of its wall. The 2d case presented an enormous swelling of the anterior part of the neck, which apparently consisted of blood, due to rupture of a large thoracic aneurysm. This had lasted for about 4 weeks and caused considerable dyspnea. At the autopsy an aneurysm of the aorta was found that had ruptured into the posterior mediastinum, causing infiltration in this region and extending upward.

Fränkel[3] reports a case of double aortic aneurysm, one commencing above the semilunar valve and extending to a point where the arch crosses the left bronchus, the other commencing immediately beyond, so that the 2 embraced the bronchus, and at each systolic pulsation drew it downward, thus giving rise to a tracheal tugging.

A. McPhedran[4] reports a case of aneurysm of the aorta that communicated with the left auricle. The patient had always been fond of violent exercise, and on one occasion, after severe exposure, was taken with a chill followed by, persistent shortness of breath. There were extensive precordial impulse, irregular, tumultuous cardiac action, and considerable edema. A loud systolic murmur was heard over the whole cardiac region and beyond, and even in the back. Treatment was without effect. At postmortem examination 3 small aneurysms were found in the aorta just above the sinuses of Valsalva. One of these communicated with the left auricle by an opening 4 mm. in length.

Otto Lerch[5] reports a case of aneurysm of the descending aorta that pressed upon the esophagus and partially occluded and eroded the bodies of the 3d, 4th, and 5th dorsal vertebræ. Death finally occurred from hemorrhage. The aneurysm ruptured into the esophagus, and the first hemorrhage occurred 3 weeks before death. Great relief was given, curiously enough, by the passage of the esophageal sound.

J. H. Musser and J. D. Steele[6] report a case in which a negro was suddenly prostrated with pain in the left iliac region, extending to the right hypochondriac. There were constipation and frequent hiccough; at times the patient was delirious. Upon admission he was in collapse, the abdomen scaphoid and excessively tender, and there was great emaciation. At the autopsy a saccular aneurysm was found springing from the abdominal aorta, from which the thrombus extended into the right renal artery. The left kidney was in a condition of acute inflammation and showed hyaline and fatty degeneration. Benedict[7] reports a case of thoracic aneurysm which, on account of the presence of goiter, had been treated as a case of Graves' disease. The proper diagnosis was first made when the Röntgen rays were employed.

---

[1] Rev. de la Soc. med. Argentina, 1896.   [2] Wien. klin. Woch., Apr. 24, 1897.
[3] Deutsch. med. Woch., Mar. 18, 1897.   [4] Canad. Pract., Aug., 1896.
[5] New Orl. M. and S. Jour., Mar., 1897.   [6] Internat. Med. Mag., Sept., 1896.
          [7] Wien. med. Woch., Dec. 19, 1896.

Fränkel[1] considers particularly the **pulmonary complications** of aortic aneurysm. He notes 4 groups: 1, fibrinous pneumonia; 2, indurative pneumonia; 3, gangrene of the lung; 4, tuberculosis. All of these are dependent more or less upon mechanical causes—that is, the pressure upon the main bronchus. At the point of greatest pressure necrotic ulceration occurs, and the excretion from this, flowing into the lungs, causes inflammation or coincident infection of tuberculous processes there. One of the points in favor of this mechanical theory is the greater frequency of inflammation in the left lung. In 2 of 30 cases he saw perforation into the vena cava superior. The clinical history of these cases was a feeling of constriction in the neck, followed by cyanosis and edema of the face and upper parts of the body. Autopsy was obtained in only one case. Syphilis was present in 36% of his cases, and in the arteriosclerotic plates of these, instead of finding calcium salts, he discovered granulation-tissue, sometimes with giant cells.

DISEASES OF THE RESPIRATORY TRACT.

General Considerations.—G. W. Fitz[2] made careful estimates of the ratio between **thoracic and abdominal respiratory movements.** His conclusions are as follows: (1) children of the two sexes differ very little in the character of their respiratory movements; (2) there is little difference between adults and children of either sex; (3) childbearing does not permanently affect respiration; (4) in the unrestricted individual the chest contributes the same bulk of air as does the abdomen, but constricting dress causes preponderance of the thoracic movement.

Francois-Franck[3] contributes a study of the **relation of the nervous system to the pulmonary circulation.** Irritation of the sympathetic causes an increase of pressure in the pulmonary artery and a decrease in the aorta, not due, as was formerly supposed, to different activity of the cardiac chambers under the influence of sympathetic stimulation, but, according to his studies, to active contractions of the pulmonary artery. In case of excessive pressure in the aortic system this mechanism may be of practical advantage. Sensory impressions in such cases may serve to contract the pulmonary artery and thus to limit the quantity of blood reaching the left heart and the aorta.

Osteoarthropathy.—J. S. Billings, Jr.,[4] reports a case of asthma with symmetrical enlargement of the arms, and nodular swellings over the parietal bones. The blood showed slight leukocytosis, and the differential count revealed more than 50% of eosinophile cells. Curschmann's spirals were present in the sputum. Although there were neither signs nor history of syphilis, the patient was put upon mixed treatment, with immediate benefit: reduction in the swelling of the arms, disappearance of the swellings on the parietal bones, and great reduction in the number of eosinophile cells.

Diseases of the Bronchi.—**Symptoms.**—Aufrecht[5] discusses a new **symptom of tracheal stenosis** that he was able to observe in 3 cases; 2 of mediastinal carcinoma and the other of a syphilitic gummatous swelling situated on the lower portion of the trachea and occupying the left half of the wall. The symptom was elicited by placing the stethoscope upon the trachea just above the jugulum sterni, when a rough bronchial breathing, which is normally heard through the whole period of inspiration and expiration, was

[1] Centralbl. f. innere Med., Nov. 14, 1896.   [2] Jour. Exper. Med., Nov., 1896.
[3] Bull. de l'Acad. de Méd., No. 6, 1896.   [4] N. Y. Med. Jour., May 22, 1897.
[5] Centralbl. f. innere Med., Jan. 9, 1897.

replaced by a brief, faint, soft breathing, or else was completely interrupted for a moment. He explains this as follows : when under normal conditions the air passes from the narrow glottis into the wide trachea eddies are formed just beyond the constricted opening that produce bronchial breathing-sounds. Before it produces these a certain rapidity of the current is necessary, which, under normal circumstances, is assured by the practically uniform size of the trachea. If this, however, is narrowed in one place, so that its lumen is only as wide as that of the glottis, the eddies of the air upon leaving the glottis are weaker, and produce a modification in the breathing that may be used as a diagnostic symptom. The same author [1] reports a case of severe dyspnea that preceded and was accompanied by a peculiar symptom—that is, the disappearance of the respiratory murmur over the trachea. A diagnosis was made of obstruction of both main bronchi, and at the autopsy a tumor was found at the bifurcation of the trachea that caused this condition.

Bronchitis.—Cassaet [2] describes a form of acute bronchitis, accompanied by rapid emaciation, fever, and green and bloody expectoration, in which he is unable to find tubercle-hacilli, and often finds virulent forms of streptococci. He suggests that it is frequently confounded with pulmonary tuberculosis.

Fernet and Lorraine [3] report the case of a man of 56 who was taken ill with bronchitis and at the same time had a swelling of the left sternoclavicular and the right shoulder-joint. After 3 days the fever subsided and he improved ; but 2 days later chills and fever occurred with marked sweating and unconsciousness, and death followed in sequence. The autopsy showed suppurative meningitis of the base, and of the upper part of the spinal canal. There was congestion of the lungs without pneumonic foci. The sternoclavicular joint was swollen, and the serous liquid as well as the pus in the meninges contained pneumococci.

Klein [4] reports a case of **fibrinous bronchitis** occurring in a girl of 19. The bronchial casts were sometimes enormous, producing marked obstruction, which was only relieved by their expectoration. In one case the total length exceeded 20 cm. In addition the sputum contained a large number of tubercle-bacilli. At the autopsy there were found chronic tuberculosis of the bronchial lymph-glands and lobular pneumonia in both lungs, with cheesy necrosis of the exudate, and, in addition, recent miliary tuberculosis. The bacteriologic examination revealed also the presence of typical pneumococci. The chemical analysis of the bronchial cast showed the presence of globulin, albumin, and, in much larger proportion, mucin ; and it consisted, not of fibrin, as had been supposed, but of mucin. This opinion was strengthened by the fact that the other shreds were not colored by the Weigert method.

J. W. Brannan [5] reports a case of fibrinous bronchitis occurring in a neurotic patient with rheumatic family history. The attacks came on suddenly with great dyspnea, that was relieved by the expulsion of bronchial casts. She had previously had attacks of angioneurotic edema.

Treatment.—Brunet [6] has treated 5 cases of chronic bronchitis and emphysema with injections of **glycerin extracts of pulmonary tissue.** All the cases showed diminution and increased fluidity of expectoration, improvement in the physical signs, and considerable amelioration of the other symptoms. [There seems to be no reasonable basis for this treatment, a large part of the symptoms produced by these conditions being due to purely mechanical causes.]

---

[1] Deutsch. Arch. f. klin. Med., June 1, 1897.   [2] Sem. méd., 1896, p. 343.
[3] Gaz. des Hôpitaux, No. 40, 1896.   [4] Wien. klin. Woch., July 23, 1896.
[5] Med. News, Aug. 15, 1896.   [6] Gaz. hebdom. de Med. et Chir., Apr. 1, 1897.

J. L. Barton[1] advocates the treatment of bronchitis, particularly when associated with incipient tuberculosis, by **intratracheal injection** of appropriate solutions.

Fronz[2] reports 3 cases of **bronchial tuberculosis ;** the first 2 were admitted to the hospital with symptoms of severe expiratory dyspnea. Tracheotomy was performed and caseous masses representing broken-down bronchial glands, which had acted as foreign bodies in the bronchi, were discharged through the tube. The first patient recovered, but subsequently developed signs of pulmonary phthisis. The second died as a result of reobstruction by another caseous gland. The third patient presented paroxysmal hemoptysis, which, at the autopsy, was found to proceed from a small aneurysm of a branch of the pulmonary artery that had ruptured into a caseous bronchial gland. The author believes that early diagnosis in these cases is important, as tubercular lymph-glands can be cured by energetic mercurial inunction.

Buberl[3] reports the case of a **foreign body** (fragment of pipe-stem) in the right bronchus which caused death by ulceration and perforation into the right pulmonary artery. The immediate cause of death was a profuse hemorrhage resulting from this condition, which had not been suspected during life, either by the patient or by the physician. Upon admission to the hospital there was a history of cough with considerable expectoration and occasional hemoptysis, and consolidation of the lower half of the right lung. Hector Mackenzie[4] refers to an extraordinary case in which a half sovereign remained in the left bronchus for 24 years. The coin lay in the axis of the left bronchus, with its edge close to the septum of the first branch, in such a position that the air could pass freely. He also refers to a case cited in the monograph of Gross, in which a piece of bone was said to have been expelled from the bronchus 60 years after its reception ; and adds that Durham refers to 28 cases of spontaneous expulsion followed by recovery in which the interval varied from 1 to 17 years. Godlee has reported 5 cases in which bronchiectasis resulted. In one of the author's cases the patient had symptoms of bronchiectasis for 2 years and finally died, the autopsy showing a piece of bone impacted in the bronchus. No history of the lodgement could be obtained ; in another, multiple abscesses and consolidation of the lung followed the lodgement of a clove in the bronchus.

Diseases of the Lungs.—A. E. Tussey[5] speaks of the importance of studying the **prolongation of the expiratory murmur** in pulmonary disease. He believes that when not due to asthma or emphysema it always indicates partial infiltration of the air-cells, and often precedes impaired percussion and resonance.

PNEUMONIA.

General Considerations.—C. F. Folsom[6] contributes a **statistical study** of the prevalence and fatality of pneumonia. Since 1852 the death-rate from pulmonary consumption and from infectious diseases as a whole has decreased greatly ; but in the case of pneumonia it has increased. In 1852 it was less fatal than typhoid fever, in 1856 their lines crossed, and in the last few years the average death-rate from pneumonia has been more than 5 times as great. It is possible that the great increase in mortality from pneumonia is due to a lowered general standard of vitality and habits in the community

[1] Med. Rec., Aug., 1896.
[2] Jahrb. f. Kinderh., vol. 44, H. 1.
[3] Wien. med. Woch., Aug. 22, 1896.
[4] Practitioner, Oct., 1896.
[5] Am. Med. and Surg. Bull., Sept. 5, 1896.
[6] Boston M. and S. Jour., Dec. 16, 1896.

and more accurate diagnosis and better registration. [It seems to us that the question of registration is a most important one in this connection. The diagnosis, for example, of typhoid fever is much more frequently accurate at the present time than formerly, and many cases previously registered as typhoid are thus eliminated. In the case of pneumonia, a more generally fatal disease, a reverse effect upon the statistics would occur.] Tracing the frequency of pneumonia in different months of the year, he finds that the curve follows very closely that of scarlet fever and diphtheria. In all respects, then, pneumonia may be classed with the infectious diseases, and he urges compulsory registration.

Connolly[1] reports an **epidemic of pneumonia** that occurred during 1896 in Brisbane, Australia. Altogether he had 26 cases in private practice and 55 in the hospital. The death-rate from this disease during the year was the largest that has ever been known. The cases all presented the initial chill; none showed any marked expectoration, although what there was was usually rusty, and nearly all had hyperpyrexia. One case exhibited a distinctly maniacal phase with delusions of persecution, which disappeared with the crisis.

W. J. Tyson[2] recognizes the following **clinical types** of pneumonia as probably distinct: pneumonia of influenza, septic pneumonia, epidemic pneumonia, asthenic pneumonia, pneumonia of the aged, and alcoholic pneumonia.

Etiology.—A. D. Heath[3] reports 3 cases of pneumonia in the same house, the 2d and 3d apparently arising as the result of **contagious contact** with the 1st. The disease was not prevalent in that district at the time.

Kohn[4] refers to his **bacteriologic studies of pneumonia,** partienlarly of the blood taken from a vein of the arm. In 32 cases of acute pneumonia 18 gave negative results, and these all recovered. In 7 cases he found pneumococci; these cases died. Five cases in which the result was negative died, 2 of them in consequence of empyema due to staphylococci. He refers to 2 further cases in which pneumococci were found in the blood, which recovered, but only after general pyemic and metastatic abscesses. He concludes that the presence of pneumococci in the blood of pneumonia is most unfavorable in prognostic significance, and holds that there is a distinct **pneumococcus sepsis** which has to be reckoned as one of the causes of death in addition to those usually recognized. Weismayr[5] has collected 39 cases of croupous pneumonia in which bacteriologic investigations were made. Thirty-four were associated with the Fränkel-Weichselbaum diplococcus, only 5 showed critical fall of temperature, and only 3 were fatal. Two cases were due to a mixed infection with staphylococcus and streptococcus. Both were remarkable for the persistence of the signs of infiltration. Three were cases of pure streptococcus infection, all of prolonged course. The presence of streptococcus, therefore, should lead one to expect deferred resolution.

Caprara[6] has found that both the vitality and virulence of the **Frankel-Weichselbaum pneumococcus** are excellently conserved in milk. In one of his experiments a culture in milk that was kept at 15° C. for 14 days showed no diminution of virulence.

Fränkel,[7] in Vereine f. innere Medicin of Berlin, presented cultures from a case of pneumonia. The first was made 4 days before death, 1 c.c. of blood

[1] Australian Med. Gaz., Sept. 21, 1896.   [2] Lancet, June 26, 1897.
[3] Brit. Med. Jour., Apr. 10, 1897.   [4] Berlin. klin. Woch., Dec. 14, 1896.
[5] Zeit. f. klin. Med., vol. xxxii.   [6] Riforma med., Nos. 187 and 188, 1896.
[7] Deutsch. med. Woch., Mar. 18, 1897.

giving 300 colonies of pneumococci; the 2d, a day before death, giving about 100 colonies, showing a distinct diminution of the number of organisms in the circulation. Neither culture proved to be as virulent as the cultures obtained from the sputum and, at the autopsy, from the pulmonary tissue, showing that the blood in some measure exerted its bactericidal qualities and that the presence of the organisms in it cannot be supposed to have been the cause of death.

Bruhl [1] reports a case which began suddenly with the symptoms of acute pneumonia. On the 8th day, however, there was an abundant roseolar eruption, followed by the symptoms of typhoid fever, complicated by intestinal hemorrhage and ruptured intestine; the **bacillus of Eberth** was recognized in the pus of the peritoneum. In order to determine whether the pulmonary complication was due to the typhoid bacillus punctures were made, and these organisms were found in pure culture in the fluid obtained from the lung. The author reports a second case of the same disease which presented a picture of acute tuberculosis so predominant were the symptoms in the lungs.

Symptoms and Complications.—Dunin and St. Nowaczek [2] have examined systematically the amount of **uric acid secreted in** 5 cases of **croupous pneumonia,** in order to discover whether it bore any relation to the leukocytosis. They found a moderate increase for a few days before the crisis and a pronounced increase immediately afterward, so that sometimes 3 times as much was excreted as during the febrile stage. This enormous increase continued for from 2 to 4 days and then gradually decreased, reaching the normal point in about a week. This increase bore apparently no relation whatever to the polyuria.

Zuber [3] refers to **lesions accidentally provoked** in the course of pneumonia. The microorganism of pneumonia may cause various metastatic lesions, whose localization is probably dependent upon abnormal states of the organs or tissue in question. He mentions a case of osteitis in consequence of an old fracture, 1 in connection with osteomyelitis, and 1 of a suppurative arthritis occurring in a gouty joint. In the same connection it is interesting to recall that abscesses containing the pneumococcus not rarely develop in consequence of hypodermic injections of irritating substances.

Lemoine [4] finds that beside the ordinary pleurisy which may follow pneumonia, the so-called metapneumonic pleurisy, there is another in which effusion comes on with hepatization or immediately after the latter. He calls this parapneumonic, and holds that the effusion in this case is apt to remain serous, and has been found to contain no microorganisms, especially no pneumococci. He believes, however, that it is due to the latter organisms, which for some reason are incapable of producing suppuration. The physical indications of these forms are those of pleurisy added to pneumonia. The effusion may disappear before the crisis, or may persist for some time, the processes, pulmonary and pleural, being independent. He suggests that aspirations should be performed.

H. P. Bowditch [5] reports 4 cases of pneumonia with **pleural effusion.** All showed flatness, but over the dull area there was heard a loud, persistent bronchial respiration; tentative aspirations in each case showed the presence of fluid, and after this was removed the bronchial respiration disappeared.

Vogelius [6] reports 2 cases of acute lobar **pneumonia,** complicated by

[1] Gaz. hebdom. de Med. et Chir., No. 9, 1897.
[2] Zeit. f. klin. Med., vol. xxxiii., 1 and 2. [3] Thèse de Paris, Steinheil, 1896.
[4] Jour. de Méd., Oct. 10, 1896. [5] Boston M. and S. Jour., Apr. 2, 1897.
[6] Arch. de Méd. expér. et d'Anat. path., Bd. viii., No. 2.

11

arthritis, in which the pneumococcus was found in the exudate of the joint. He has collected 11 similar cases from the literature. In the majority of these the complication became apparent within 5 days after the onset of the pneumonia, but in 1, not until the eleventh day. The exudate was purulent in 6 cases, seropurulent in 2, and serofibrinous in 1. In the other 2 the nature is not mentioned. Considerable destruction of the joint occurred in 4 cases.

Banti[1] studied the bacteriology of a number of cases of pneumonia in which **icterus** was present. He found that the diplococcus present was strongly pathogenic for dogs. When injected it gave rise to the appearance of urobilin and bilirubin, as well as to a considerable quantity of hemoglobin in the urine. In rabbits marked hemoglobinuria occurred in all cases. This tendency to produce hemoglobinuria disappeared after a number of reinoculations. He concludes that the icterus of pneumonia is due to an accidental hemolytic action of the diplococcus, and is therefore hemogenic.

Widal[2] refers to a case of **suppurative hygroma** beneath the deltoid muscle in a case of pneumonia. At the end of 3 weeks he could not find any bacteria. The seat of metapneumonic suppuration is classic, the predilection of the pneumococcus for the serous membranes of the shoulder-girdle being well known. At the second puncture in his case, 20 days after the first, there was only serofibrinous liquid, and recovery soon ensued. The pneumococci (assuming that these were present at first) therefore survived only a short time in the diseased joint.

J. L. Spruill[3] reports a case of pneumonia which, on the fifth day, began to show signs of heart-failure, progressing to death in the course of an hour. At the autopsy a large **fatty tumor** was found in the right auricle firmly attached to its walls.

Galliard[4] records a case of pneumonia in the course of which severe vomiting and diarrhea occurred, leading to almost complete collapse. In consideration of the pathogenicity of the pneumococcus he believes that it is fair to call this condition a **pneumoenteritis.** The question arises how the organisms reached the intestinal tract. It seems unlikely that they could have passed through the stomach and maintained their vitality after having been exposed to the gastric juice, and it is altogether more probable that the inflammation of the mucous membranes represents an effort at their elimination from the body.

French[5] reports a case of pneumonia occurring in a man of 75, in which, on the eighth day of the disease, persistent **hiccough** set in, some of the paroxysms lasting as long as 14 hours without a break. Recovery eventually ensued.

Prognosis.—Wm. Osler,[6] in discussing the prognosis of pneumonia, refers to the uniformity of mortality in the various statistics. Of 124 cases in the Johns Hopkins Hospital, 37 died, a mortality of 29.8. He holds that, apart from certain complications, the death-rate occurs as a result of toxemia or mechanical interference with respiration and circulation, and he dwells particularly upon the danger of toxemia. This may develop early, and from the very first there may be cerebral symptoms; the latter sometimes quite out of proportion to the extent of disease in the lung. Other cases may be observed in which a large part of the lung is involved and scarcely any toxemia occurs. Many of the cases with decided intoxication show variations from the typical

[1] Centralbl. f. Bakt. u. Inf., Dec. 10, 1896.
[2] Gaz. hebdom. de Méd. et de Chir., No. 30, 1896.   [3] Med. Rec., l. 355, 1896.
[4] Sem. méd., p. 337, 1896.   [5] Virginia Med. Semi-monthly, Mar. 12, 1897.
[6] Am. Jour. Med. Sci., Jan., 1897.

course of the disease. Thus, there may be no cough nor expectoration, very slight fever, and no leukocytosis. Two cases are then detailed : one the case of an able-bodied man of 28, who became delirious and finally quite insane while on a train. He was afterward put in a straight-jacket, having made an attempt at suicide. There was no cough and little fever, but he complained of pain in the side. Physical signs were quite well developed; the patient improved somewhat, but subsequently died suddenly. The second case occurred in a man of 66, who complained of a slight chill and then of pain in the back with aching in the joints and legs. There was no cough nor shortness of breath, the fever was slight, delirium was quite marked. Regarding the cases in which sudden and unexpected death occurs, Osler believes that the action of the specific toxins on the heart-center is of greater significance than the effect of fever on the heart-muscle. He details 3 cases in which this termination occurred. In one there was massive pneumonia with blocking of the bronchial tubes and obscuration of the physical signs; death occurred on the sixth day. In the second case there was well-marked pneumonia of the lower left lung and death occurred on the fourth day ; while in the third case cardiac weakness developed almost at once and the patient had 3 attacks of syncope, the last proving fatal on the third day of the disease. The author is not inclined to attribute much importance to mechanical obstruction of respiration and circulation, calling attention to the fact that the obstruction remains the same for some time after the crisis despite a most remarkable change in symptoms (dyspnea and cyanosis). [We can substantiate these statements entirely. Cases of sudden and unexpected termination have frequently occurred in our experience, and in some of these the disease of the heart-muscle has been very trivial. We have also been struck with the very rapid subsidence of all symptoms of cardiac and pulmonary embarrassment after the crisis, despite the persistence of the pulmonary conditions.]

Treatment.—[Considerable attention has been devoted to the production of an effective antipneumococcic serum. The experimental results are satisfactory, but the clinical reports are very conflicting. This may be explained in part, perhaps, by the frequent neglect of clinicians to make a careful bacteriologic diagnosis, and their tendency to use the serum in all cases presenting the physical signs of pulmonary consolidation irrespective of the nature of the process.] De Renzi[1] gives his experience of **serum-therapy** in pneumonia. Seven cases were admitted in the year 1894–95, and 2 of these received serum in addition to the usual alcoholic treatment; all recovered. In 1895–96, 27 cases were admitted ; 13 were treated without serum, of which 3 died, or 23% ; and 14 were treated with serum, of which 2 died, or 14% ; of the 2 fatal cases, one was *in articulo mortis* when admitted, and the other had arterial and renal lesions apart from the pneumonia. The temperature usually dropped from 1° to 3° after the injections, and the latter never gave rise to any bad symptoms. In another paper[2] he gives slightly different figures. He was able to obtain serum from animals that had been rendered immune to the pneumococcus, and injections of this had given very satisfactory results. Of 16 cases only 2 died, 1 was in the death agony when the first injection was made, and the other suffered from a severe cardiac lesion.

A. Cooke[3] reports 2 cases of acute lobar pneumonia treated with antipneumococcic serum. The first patient was injected on the sixth day of the disease ; the following day there was slight improvement with a fall of temperature ;

---

[1] Supplem. Il. Policlinico, Oct. 31, 1896.
[2] Gaz. degli Osped. e delle Clin., No. 140, 1896.   [3] Brit. Med. Jour., May 22, 1897.

subsequently she again passed into a febrile state, which was diagnosed as typhoid. Distinct crisis was not caused by the serum. The second patient was injected on the fourth day of the disease. Convalescence did not set in until the tenth day, the serum having apparently had no influence upon the febrile course. [No effort was made to find the pneumococcus.] Spurrell[1] reports a case of pneumonia which, on the third day of the disease, was given 660 units of pneumonia antitoxin. On the same day a second injection of the same strength was given; this was repeated on successive days 8 times. Nevertheless, death occurred on the tenth day, the only result observed from the injections being a slight fall of temperature, although occasionally a slight rise occurred. C. J. Harnett[2] reports a case of alcoholic pneumonia that on the sixth day of the disease was injected with antipneumococcic serum. The next day the patient was distinctly worse; vigorous stimulation, however, had good effect, and he ultimately recovered. Washbourne[3] Immunized a pony against the pneumococcus by the usual method, then bled the animal, and tested the protective properties of its serum, which he found to be considerable. He reports a case treated with this serum in which, on the eighth day of the disease, 660 units were injected; 2 hours later the temperature fell 3°, but soon rose again. Another injection was made a day later, and the condition of the patient was much improved. He reports another case in which, after numerous injections of 660 units of serum, great improvement occurred on the sixth day. Defervescence took place by lysis. Denys[4] has performed a number of experiments with the serum of animals immunized against the pneumococcus. Serum procured from a horse that had been treated in this manner showed both preventive and curative action. It seems also to have an antitoxic action; causing reduction of temperature in an animal that had been inoculated with toxin 7 days before, and preventing a rise of temperature when mixed with toxin in vitrio and then inoculated. Auld[5] has inoculated animals with the toxin of virulent cultures of the diplococcus pneumoniæ. If sufficient toxin was injected to raise the temperature to 105°, it was possible to produce immunity to the living organism, and the serum of the animals so treated was found to confer immunity upon animals into which it was injected.

E. H. Martin[6] has employed **fowl serum** in pneumonia, reasoning that it must contain some antipneumonic element. Fresh blood was administered by the mouth, and his results, although as yet inconclusive, are encouraging.

Davis[7] has used **nucleinic acid** in a number of cases of pneumonia; but although the results were favorable he cannot ascribe a distinctly beneficial action to it in any case.

Barth[8] reports 2 cases of severe pneumonia treated by large doses of **digitalis** with prompt beneficial effect. He believes that all cases that are severe, or where treatment with baths is contraindicated, should be treated in this way. Particularly is it to be employed when the intensity of the fever, dyspnea, and frequency and softness of the pulse lead one to suspect cardiac weakness.

Gingoet and Degui[9] report 10 cases of pneumonia treated by **digitalin,** with 10 recoveries, 2 of which were unexpected on account of the severity of the symptoms. The authors believe that digitalin exercises a specific action upon the disease, even going to the length of suggesting that it be employed

[1] Brit. Med. Jour., Apr. 17, 1897.　　　　　[2] Ibid., May 22, 1897.
[3] Ibid., Feb. 27, 1897.　　　　　　　　　　　[4] Sem. méd., p. 311, 1896.
[5] Brit. Med. Jour., Mar. 27, 1897.　　　　　[6] Med. Rec., Mar. 20, 1897.
[7] Jour. Am. Med. Assoc., Apr. 10, 1897.　　[8] Sem. méd., p. 281, 1896.
　　　　　　　　[9] Rev. de Méd., Mar. 10, 1897.

for the purpose of making a differential diagnosis between pneumonia, pulmonary tuberculosis, and typhoid fever.

Folsom[1] believes that the medical profession is too prone to rely upon medicinal treatment for pneumonia. He has used **cold sponge-baths** and occasionally applications of ice during the last 3 years, in all cases except those *in extremis*. The greatest number of baths in a single case was 25 and the effect was invariably pleasant.

R. W. Amidon[2] claims that the mortality of pneumonia has increased 10% in 50 years. He thinks that this is due to the neglect of **venesection** in the treatment of the disease, and cites 2 cases, in both of which great relief was afforded by spontaneous hemorrhage.

Shech,[3] in discussing **asthma** and **emphysema**, holds that bronchial spasm comes first, bronchitis second, and overdistention of the lungs last. The latter disappears more or less rapidly in nasal cases, and there is no true emphysema. Cases of this kind may be regarded as emphysematous for a long time, and finally after removal of polypi, etc., the condition may greatly improve. Long continuance, however, leads to true emphysema.

Huchard[4] believes that 3 elements are concerned in the causation of **pulmonary edema**—acute insufficiency of the right ventricle, disturbance of cardiopulmonic innervation, and impermeability of the kidneys with consecutive intoxication. In order to meet the first indication venesection should be employed; to meet the second strychnin; and to meet the third milk-diet and diuretics.

A. McPhedran[5] reports a case of **gangrene of the lung** coming on after an attack of uremia. The breath was offensive, sputum dark, and there were frequent hemorrhages of varying amounts. There were moderate fever and emaciation. The physical signs consisted of restricted respiratory movements and increased percussion-dulness over the apex of the left lung, including rales and bronchial breathing. The symptoms improved, only to recur for several months. Finally permanent recovery ensued. In regard to the etiology of this condition, the author suggests the inhalation of a foreign body during the comatose state, or sclerosis of the pulmonary arteries with resulting thrombosis.

G. E. Bushnell[6] reports 2 cases of **subpleural pulmonary abscess.** He calls attention to the fact that there has been much discordance between the observations of pathologists and clinicians, the former finding what seems irreparable destruction of the lung-tissue; the latter reporting cases which terminate in quick recovery. The diagnosis in cases which recover is often very doubtful, and the disease, when present, is frequently unrecognized. The first case, a young man in previously good health, suffered with mild bronchial catarrh and then with croupous pneumonia of the lower left lobe. Subsequently his condition became much depressed and an area of dulness with absent breath-sounds was discovered in the lateral and posterior parts of the lower left lobe. An aspirator-needle was introduced several times, and later an incision was made which showed the lung to be retracted. The pus was obtained only by inserting the needle into the lung. Subsequently the collection reaccumulated, but finally discharged through the bronchus and the patient recovered. The second case was less clearly one of intrapulmonary abscess. In discussing its nature the author points out that localized empyema, which is frequently the diagnosis made, would not heal so quickly after dis-

[1] Boston M. and S. Jour., Dec. 16, 1896.   [2] Med. News, Mar. 6, 1897.
[3] Münch. med. Woch., Aug. 18, 1896.   [4] Bull. de l'Acad. de Méd., Apr. 27, 1897.
[5] Am. Med. and Surg. Bull., Aug. 29, 1896.   [6] Am. Jour. Med. Sci., Oct., 1896.

charge of the pus. [In his first case ordinary saccular empyema was easily eliminated, but the author does not consider the likelihood of this case having been one of interlobar empyema. This condition could very readily have produced the symptoms, although it must be confessed that there are no special reasons for regarding the case as one of such nature rather than one of true abscess of the lung. The second case, it seems to us, was more doubtful in character.] A diagnosis between abscess and empyema may be made by microscopic examination of the aspirated pus, the discovery of elastic tissue in the latter pointing to abscess of the lung itself. Among his other conclusions are: 1, pulmonary abscesses affect the connective tissue, and the most favorable and common form is a subpleural abscess; 2, these may attain to large sizes without the corresponding destruction of pulmonary tissue, since the individual pulmonary lobules retract before the suppurative process, as the whole lung retracts before the pleural effusion; 3, the disease is more common than supposed and is generally mistaken for empyema.

Zagari [1] has studied 7 cases of **malignant intrathoracic tumors,** and has endeavored to obtain a more or less uniform clinical picture of this condition. He gives the following symptoms, the presence of a number of which should lead to a suspicion at least of the true nature of the disease: **1,** gradual commencement; 2, pronounced general weakness; 3, absence of fever; 4, constant and increasing pain; 5, swelling of the glands chiefly upon one side, and eventually distention of the veins on the breast-wall; 6, increase of local sweating upon one side of the chest; 7, dyspnea and feeling of oppression such as occur in hydrothorax; 8, irregularity in thoracic expansion, especially in the upper portion; 9, neither bulging nor widening of the intercostal spaces; 10, absolute dulness, particularly noteworthy when in the upper and anterior parts of the thorax, and in juxtaposition to clear pulmonary resonance; 11, dulness over the sternum and near it, indicating dislocation of the mediastinum toward the healthy side, with the peculiarity that this dislocation is irregular; 12, Skoda's murmur over the clavicle and sternum; 13, bronchial respiration; 14, persistence of physical signs after the evacuation of a considerable quantity of liquid; 15, the character of liquid (fibrinous, of high sp. gr., hemorrhagic, and containing characteristic cells); 16, the sensation of a thick, compact tissue resisting the needle when exploratory puncture is made; 17, unsuccessful puncture before the rapid formation of an exudate; 18, slight dislocation of the heart and liver, such as would occur in large collections of liquid. [We have found it more satisfactory to consider the symptoms according to the location of the tumor in the thorax.]

Hampeln [2] discusses the diagnosis of **carcinoma of the lung.** He points out that it is an error to regard this diagnosis as of extraordinary difficulty, the prevalence of this view preventing the more frequent recognition of the condition. Sometimes the symptoms are practically wanting, as in other diseases; but when they are well developed the disease is easily recognized. Among the important indications are consolidation of one lung with increase of the thorax on the affected side, or retraction of the same side; bronchial irritation, cough, and expectoration; pleurisy, with fibrinous, serous, hemorrhagic, purulent, or putrid exudate; symptoms of pressure upon the nerves or veins, and finally cachexia. He then turns his attention particularly to the character of the expectoration, which he believes to be highly significant. The discovery of signs of consolidation of the lung of progressive character, and only a moderate catarrh of the bronchi with scanty expectoration may lead to suspicion; but hemorrhagic sputa is more significant. The color and

[1] Naples, 1896.   [2] Zeit. f. klin. Med., Bd. 32, H. 3 and 4.

character of this are not of great importance, but its duration may be. He refers to a case in which it persisted for 2 months, and to one reported by Israel, in which the duration was 9 months. There is never abundant hemoptysis. Nine cases are then briefly abstracted to illustrate the frequency of this symptom. One of these he reported a number of years ago in illustration of the diagnostic value of cancer-cells. *A priori* we should expect either particles of carcinoma or individual or aggregated carcinoma cells in the sputa. The former was recorded by Ehrlich in one of his cases, but has not been observed by any other clinician. The author himself lays stress upon the occurrence of large, non-pigmented polyhedral cells, and especially these in association with giant cells. Though these cannot be said to be specific forms of cells, it is true that they occur only when there is a productive growth. They may be found in any form of carcinoma, and do not indicate a particular seat. Thus a squamous epithelioma of the bronchi may present this form of cells, though one might expect a large squamous cell. The situation may be judged of by the occurrence of tissue-particles, but, as was pointed out, this is rarely possible. Betschart[1] reports a case of tumor of the lung in which the diagnosis was established during life by the character of the sputum. This varied in color, being often brownish-red, and microscopically there were discovered small fat-globules, leukocytes, and large numbers of epithelioid cells, more or less aggregated. There were also a number of particles visible to the naked eye of brownish-yellow color and gelatinous appearance, which proved to be carcinomatous on microscopic examination. The diagnosis was confirmed postmortem.

DISEASES OF THE PLEURA.

Pleurisy.—Etiology.—Aschoff[2] reports the results of his observations in 200 cases of serous pleurisy. Forty-one of these were idiopathic; of the remaining 159, 43 were associated with tuberculosis, 16 with rheumatism, 29 with pneumonia, 11 with influenza, and 41 with various other affections of the respiratory or circulatory organs. The effusion was investigated bacteriologically, chiefly microscopically or by smearing 3 drops upon agar. In 193 case the result was negative. Of the 7 positive results, 1 showed tubercle-bacilli, 1 pyogenic bacteria, 1 pneumococci, 1 streptococci, and 2, not associated with pulmonary disease, gave also pneumococci and streptococci; finally, 1 following gangrene of the lung also showed streptococci; the last 5 cases all developed pyopericardium. The exudate from 57 cases was injected into guinea-pigs in order to test whether tubercle-bacilli were present or not. Of these, 25 were associated with tuberculosis, and 12 apparently idiopathic; of the former group, 68% of the animals became tuberculous, and of the latter group 75%, from which the author concludes that the majority of the cases of idiopathic serous pleurisy are tubercular.

Peron[3] states that the tubercle-bacilli are transported to the parietal layer of the pleura enclosed in leukocytes, and that they may almost invariably be found in the acute serofibrinous form of tubercular pleurisy, either in the liquid or in the false membrane.

Chauffard[4] reports a case of pneumothorax due to simple alveolar rupture, and not to tuberculosis. Tuberculin prepared by Roux was injected at intervals of 4 days, and there was not the slightest reaction, while the control in a known tuberculous patient was followed by a decided reaction. The pneumothorax subsided and recovery was complete in 4 weeks.

[1] Virchow's Archiv, Bd. 143, H. 1.   [2] Zeit. f. klin. Med., Bd. 29, 1896.
[3] Bull. de l'Acad. de Méd., Oct. 27, 1896.   [4] Sem. méd., Feb. 12, 1897.

G. G. Sears [1] reports the results of the study of 30 cases of **hemorrhagic pleurisy** as follows: it may be either a primary affection or a complication of other diseases; tuberculosis is the most frequent single cause, but it is not necessary to suppose every ease of hemorrhagic pleurisy to be of this nature. The next most important cause is the pneumococcus. Predisposing conditions are advanced age, alcoholism, and the presence of severe constitutional disease, particularly nephritis and rheumatism. Prognosis naturally depends largely upon the nature of the ease, and unless it appears as a complication in the later stages of some other disease the hemorrhagic effusion may be expected to run a favorable course. Sometimes the case will terminate in empyema, and occasionally the recurrence of the liquid after aspiration will be so rapid as seriously to deplete the patient.

Pathology and Symptoms.—Auche and Carrière [2] have examined the liquid found in **hemorrhagic pleurisy** and found leukocytosis. Often the number of oxyphilic leukocytes is greater than normal.

Koll [3] reports a series of eases of pleuritis that ran their course without the appearance of a liquid exudate and were particularly characterized by physical signs in the anterior pleural sinuses. Altogether about 30 cases were observed in the course of 9 months. The majority of these commenced suddenly with the characteristics of an acute infectious disease; 2, however, commenced more slowly, and 2 were associated with rheumatic phenomena in other parts of the body. The subjective symptoms were those of an acute or chronic affection of the stomach; diffuse or circumscribed pain in the gastric region often commencing abruptly and increased by taking food and pressure. The patients also complained of discomfort in the cardiac region, and in nearly all cases there was tachycardia. At the beginning there was always a chill and afterward moderate continued fever. The temperature rarely exceeded 38.5°. The physical sign consisted of a fine, soft friction-sound, heard best in the region of the pleural sinus, and sometimes extending along the lateral inferior boundary of the lung. Frequently this was also heard in the middle of the sternum; occasionally it was continued when the respiration was stopped, and was then synchronous with the heart-beat. In 2 cases the symptoms of perisplenitis developed, and in 1 those of perihepatitis; these attacks coming on after the pleurisy had subsided. The course was usually long. No influence was noticed from salicylic acid or phenacetin. In only 7 cases was the cure complete when they were discharged from the hospital. Although this disease has much in common with diaphragmatic pleuritis, nevertheless the author believes that the primary condition consists of an inflammation of the pleura in the localities mentioned, and prefers to call it **sinus pleuritis.**

C. H. Goodrich [4] reports 10 eases of **pleurisy with effusion.** In 3 of these the general health of the patients had been excellent; 2 had suffered from pneumonia and 1 from acute articular rheumatism. Two of the cases had been preceded by acute bronchitis and 3 by lobar pneumonia; 1 case had all the physical signs of apical tuberculosis. Three eases commenced with chill, 6 with pain, and 1 gradually. In only 1 case was there much sweating, and in this it was excessive; in 4 cases bronchial breathing was persistent and indeed unusually loud below the level of the effusion. One case died, death being due to pneumonia.

Hervouet [5] objects to the theory that the **bronchial breathing** occurring

[1] Boston M. and S. Jour., Sept. 17, 1896.   [2] Sem. méd., p. 344, 1896.
[3] Deutsch. Arch. f. klin. Med., Dec. 18, 1896.   [4] Am. Med. and Surg. Bull., Aug. 29, 1896.
                    [5] Sem. méd., p. 343, 1896.

in pleurisy is due to compression of the lung on the ground that it should always occur in this condition, whereas it is quite inconstant. He prefers to consider it as an indication of a separate pulmonary disease, such as tuberculosis or pneumonia.

Langenhagen[1] observed severe pain accompanying eructations of gas in a patient suffering from diaphragmatic tubercular pleurisy. This he believes to be due to the vibrations set up in the diaphragm as a result of a sudden dilatation of the cardiac orifice.

Treatment.—Neumann[2] has used the alkaline waters of the Werzberg spring in 3 cases of pleurisy, 2 tubercular and 1 syphilitic. The effects were absorption of the exudate, polyuria, and stimulation of the appetite.

Macalister[3] contributes an experimental investigation regarding the effect of **thoracic effusions.** He cites a case in a child 5 years of age of rapidly developed empyema, with the physical signs of a large effusion, though the amount of liquid was very small. Only 10 oz. escaped from the chest when this was opened, but the percussion-note was absolutely dull from base to apex and the dyspnea was terrible. To elucidate the effects of rapid effusion he inserted a rubber bag into the pleura of a dog and allowed water to flow in through a tube. The most important result of this experiment was the discovery that the diaphragm quickly showed a central bulging of the cupola on the affected side, and this bulging became extreme when the quantity of liquid was much. This bulging explained the early interference with respiration and also the fact that toward the end, when the pleural effusion is excessive, contractions of the diaphragm may actually interfere with inspiration, rather than aid the latter. The diminished breath-sounds over the pleural effusion, he holds, are explained by the lessened amount of inspiration due to diaphragmatic interference, as well as to the difficulty of conduction of sound through the fluid. Next he studied the effect of pleural effusion in producing displacements of the heart and other organs, citing in the first place the theory of Powell, "that this displacement is due to the traction of the elastic lung on the healthy side." Against this view he first notes that liquid is frequently ejected forcibly from the empyema when an incision is made, thus indicating pressure; and quotes a case of his own in which a double empyema existed and in which the position of the heart changed from side to side, according as one or the other side contained most fluid. He experimented upon a cadaver, by inserting a needle directly into the apex of the heart in a perpendicular direction and then injecting liquid into the left pleura. After the first 5 to 9 oz. of liquid had been introduced the heart moved horizontally toward the middle line, and continued to move in the same direction until 29 oz. had been introduced; the motion then began to be somewhat downward, and when 56 oz. had been inserted into the cavity the needle pointed toward the left axilla. A second needle was inserted into the left lobe of the liver, when the heart began to move downward. The second needle began to rotate in a way indicating that the left lobe of the liver was also travelling downward. The right side of the chest was bulging at this time, and on dissection the right pleura was found distended and partly covering the pericardium. He concludes from this experiment and from others upon dogs that the displacement of the heart is purely mechanical.

Senator[4] describes a case of chylous ascites and chylothorax. This occurred in a woman of 47 in whom ascites was found as well as effusion in both pleural cavities. On aspiration a milky liquid was obtained, of alkaline reaction, and

[1] Sem. méd., p. 344, 1896.
[2] Deutsch. med. Woch., Jan. 28, 1897.
[3] Liverpool Med.-Chir. Jour., July, 1896.
[4] Charité Annalen, Jahrg. 20.

sp. gr. 1015.5; poor in albumin; there was no sugar. The microscopic examination showed fine granular particles, a few leukocytes, and a few round cells containing fat-granules. The fat obtained by extracting with ether melted between 27° and 31° C. After administration of olive oil and a second puncture of the abdomen and the pleura the liquid was found remarkably yellow, and seemed to contain more fat, the melting-point of this being reduced to 17° and 18° C. The sp. gr. of the liquid was 1011.5. A diagnosis of carcinoma of the pelvic and abdominal organs and of the thoracic duct was made and confirmed postmortem. Primary carcinoma of the ovaries and metastasis involving the mesenteric lymph-glands and the thoracic duct were discovered. Thrombosis of the lacteals of the mesentery and the intestines was found.

Sackur[1] examined rabbits and dogs in which he had produced an artificial pneumothorax and found that the blood-pressure was not reduced; and concluded that the stimulation of the respiratory centre could not be due to an inadequate supply of blood. He then examined the blood in the carotid artery and found that the quantity of oxygen it contained was only half the normal, and he believes that this diminution of oxygen accounts for the increased respiratory activity.

Samuel West[2] discusses the **prognosis of pneumothorax.** He collected altogether 160 cases of the disease, of which 104 died, giving a mortality of $62\frac{1}{2}$%. It is, however, to be observed that the mortality in those cases in which the pneumothorax developed in the hospital was much higher (77%) than in those admitted some time after the condition had been established (33%). This West explains by the fact that the proportion of deaths is much greater during the first week than at any subsequent period. Of 39 cases in which the duration was exactly known, 10 patients died on the first day of the disease, 2 within $\frac{1}{2}$ hour, and the other 8 within a few hours; 8 more died within the first week and 3 during the second week; finally, 6 died during the second fortnight. Death is due to 3 causes, either rapid suffocation or shock within a very short period after the rupture; or as a result of effusion; or as a result of the diseased-process which produced the pneumothorax, usually phthisis. The prognosis, therefore, even as regards the immediate risk of life, is rather doubtful. It depends upon, 1st, the urgency of the symptoms—that is to say, the amount of dyspnea and cyanosis; 2d, the condition of the opposite lung, the development of rales being a very bad omen; 3d, the ability of the right heart to overcome the increased resistance in the pulmonary circulation, any sign of dilatation being unfavorable; 4th, the general strength of the patient, particularly the development of the respiratory muscles; 5th, the nature of the disease which has led to the pneumothorax. As regards the duration of life, the prognosis of course depends upon the condition of the patient and the nature of the disease. Recovery is rare; it does, however, occur and may be apparently complete and permanent. The most favorable cases are those in which there is no pulmonary disease and in which no effusion has taken place. If the effusion does occur, but is purely serous in character; the prognosis is also good. When, however, it is purulent, the chances for recovery are reduced. Even cases occurring in the course of phthisis, however, do sometimes recover. He then reports in detail 11 cases in which recovery took place, although 2 subsequently died of phthisis.

Benda[3] observed a case of **primary " carcinoma of the pleura "** in a man of 54, who had been ill for 2 years. On admission pleural effusion was discovered; 3 liters of liquid were removed; aspiration was repeated 16

---

[1] Zeit. f. klin. Med., Bd. 29, 1896.   [2] Lancet, May 8, 1897.
[3] Berlin. klin. Woch., Mar. 1, 1897.

times, the exudate remaining clear. Finally, resection of a rib was undertaken and a tumor was discovered on the pleura. Exudate reaccumulated, pyemic symptoms developed, and the patient died after metastatic abscesses had formed. Postmortem numerous small nodules were found distributed over the left pleura, the latter being normal in very few places. The microscopic examination showed the characteristics of endothelioma. The author refers to multiple nodules of primary eruption and the failure of metastasis as characteristic peculiarities. Among the clinical characteristics he cites the marked hemorrhagic character of the exudate, which may, however, be absent, and the decided pain after aspiration resulting from the inability of the lung to expand.

DISEASES OF THE MEDIASTINUM.

Kiserling[1] presented to the Berlin Med. Society the specimens of a **mediastinal tumor** that Leyden had diagnosed as an aneurysm during life. The clinical symptoms had been : severe pain at the level of the nipples and over the vertebral column ; increase in the area of cardiac dulness, especially toward the right side ; and a double impulse at the apex. Later, the symptoms of total paraplegia appeared, and at the same time the painful symptoms vanished. At the autopsy a grayish-white solid tumor was found upon the posterior surface of the heart, which had invaded the posterior wall of the left auricle and partially that of the right. A second tumor was found at the hilus of the left lung and extended along the principal bronchus and invaded the bronchial glands. Finally, the second dorsal vertebra had also been invaded by the tumorous process and had been destroyed, with the production of pressure upon the spinal cord at this point. The tumor proved to be a lymphosarcoma.

H. D. Rolleston[2] reports a case of tumor of the anterior mediastinum. The patient was admitted with swelling of the face, neck, and left arm ; dulness beneath the sternum and to the left, with bronchial breathing at the root of the left lung and dilatation of cutaneous veins. Later, signs of pleural effusion developed, and 40 oz. of blood-stained fluid were withdrawn, as was proved subsequently, from the pericardial cavity. At the autopsy a large tumor was found occupying the anterior and superior mediastinum and covering the upper half of the pericardium, to which it was firmly adherent. On microscopical section it was found to consist of a cortical part containing fibrous and unstriped muscle-tissue and small cysts lined with mucous glands, and a central part containing sarcoma-cells and spots of hemorrhage, and in which were also found numerous islands of almost normal cartilage. The author concludes that it was a sarcoma arising from the thyroid gland and resembling parotid tumor.

DISEASES OF THE MOUTH AND PHARYNX.

Futterer[3] reports 2 cases of **salivary calculi**: the first occurred in the submaxillary gland in a man subject to biliary colic. The first symptom was a transient swelling of the gland that was repeated for 4 years, when permanent swelling with inflammatory symptoms rendered an operation necessary. The calculus was composed of potassium and sodium phosphates with traces of xanthin and hypoxanthin. The second occurred in Wharton's duct in a

[1] Sem. méd., 1896, p. 277. [2] Jour. Path. and Bact., vol. 4, No. 2.
[3] Medicine, July, 1896.

patient aged 50, who had frequently noticed a small lump after partaking of sour food. Stomatitis developed 2 months before the operation, when the lump had been continuously present for some time. Occasionally, however, the swelling would grow acutely worse, and at rare intervals disappeared spontaneously. Fütterer also reports a case in the practice of Dr. Verity, in which the calculus, in the duct of the sublingual gland, had given rise to suppuration. He then described the symptoms of calculi of the salivary glands as follows: rarely, well-marked severe pains in the initial stages, then transient swellings when eating or during attacks of stomatitis, and, finally, suppuration, which may recur several times or become extremely chronic. The treatment is always operative.

Stoos[1] has investigated the etiology of **aphthous stomatitis** and thrush. In 15 cases of the former condition he found regularly, besides other bacteria, a large diplo-streptococcus that stained well by Gram's method and formed clusters. As he has never found this in healthy persons or in other diseases, he is inclined to regard it as pathogenic. In thrush he has invariably found staphylococci and streptococci in addition to the ordinary organisms, and believes that these play an important part in preparing the mucous membrane for subsequent infection, setting up a preliminary erythematous stomatitis.

Stoos[2] has found various bacteria in **ordinary angina,** all of which, however, occurred in health. He concludes that angina is a form of auto-infection, in which the streptococci play a most important part. Staphylococci and pneumococci are less frequent. The micrococcus tetragenes, Friedländer's bacillus, and the coccus conglomeratus are doubtful in action; while the leptothrix is very uncertain. There are no distinct clinical types, but the severest cases are those in which the streptococci occur.

Blumenau[3] describes a case of **primary gangrene of the pharynx.** The patient, a man of 22, had suffered with catarrhal jaundice, following which pharyngitis and laryngitis developed. Two weeks afterward gangrene began in the form of rounded spots of dirty black color on the right tonsil, eventually destroying the whole tonsil, the right half of the soft palate, and nearly the entire root of the tongue. The process then extended toward the epiglottis. There were horrible fetor and repeated small hemorrhages from the ulcerated tonsillar artery. Death occurred in 2 weeks, and at the autopsy numerous hemorrhages were found in the pia, pericardium, endocardium, pleura, and lungs. The author doubts an etiological relation of the jaundice to the gangrene. Bacteriologic examinations were not made.

DISEASES OF THE ESOPHAGUS.

Störk[4] describes his **esophagoscope.** This consists of a stiff tube with a number of joints at the lower end, that may be introduced like a bougie. A solution of gum arabic is employed to make the operation more easy. The patient sits, with his head bent backward, upon a low stool, and the tube is introduced like a sound until it meets with resistance. An accurately fitting mandarin is then withdrawn and the inspection made with the aid of a reflector.

Rumpel[5] reports a case of **fusiform dilatation** of the esophagus, in which the diagnosis was made during life from the following signs: the patient, a tailor 25 years old, had suffered with gradually increasing vomiting

[1] Mittheil. aus klin. u. Med. Institut. der Schweiz, R. iii. H. 1.   [2] Ibid.
[3] Deutsch. med. Woch., No. 26, 1896.   [4] Wien. klin. Woch., No. 28, 1896.
[5] Münch. med. Woch., Nos. 15 and 16, 1897.

for 2 years. If the stomach-sound was passed shortly after a meal, the following phenomena were observed : in the upper portion of the esophagus it passed easily without obstruction ; then the end appeared to enter a free space, and at the same time a considerable quantity of liquid material was expelled that could be proved to consist only of the contents of the esophagus. A little further on it encountered distinct resistance at a distance of about 49 cm. from the teeth, which was only overcome with difficulty and the causation of considerable pain. The sound then entered the stomach and the normal stomach-contents were expelled. The lesion could not have been a bend in the esophagus, as this would have been increased after the taking of food ; on the contrary, it was then easier to pass the sound. An interesting experiment was now performed—a small tube was introduced into the stomach ; alongside of this a still smaller tube was passed for 40 cm., and through the latter 300 c.c. of water were poured, all of which could be subsequently recovered by sinking the funnel, and none of which apparently entered the stomach. In order to determine now whether the second sound entered a sac or simply a dilatation of the esophagus, holes were cut in the first one, and it was found that the liquid flowed through these into the stomach, proving that a saecular dilatation did not exist. The author believes that this condition is due to the spastic contraction of the lower portion of the esophagus, and in the present instance treated the condition by feeding exclusively through the stomach-tube. He believes, however, that it might be possible to adopt surgical measures. Finally, he states that by means of an emulsion of bismuth subnitrate introduced into the esophagus it was possible to see the enlargement with the fluoroscope. He has collected 20 cases of this condition from medical literature, none of which were diagnosed during life.

Danel[1] has reported an interesting case of **tuberculous esophagitis.** The patient, a woman of 76, came under observation with the signs of pulmonary tuberculosis and bronchopneumonia in the lower part of the left lung, and several areas of superficial ulceration in the submaxillary regions. The patient died, and postmortem there was discovered ulceration of the posterior wall of the esophagus ·for a distance of nearly 4 in., involving the mucous membrane. The margins contained numerous granulations that also involved the anterior wall. A communication between one of the peribronchial lymphatic glands and the esophagus was found opposite the right bronchus. The. stomach was enlarged and contained a number of granulations, probably tuberculous. The glands of the neck were tuberculous. [The disease of the esophagus in this case evidently was secondary to that of the lymphatic glands.]

Berger[2] describes a case of stenosis of the esophagus near the cardiac end in a man of 55 without definite specific history. There was considerable loss of weight after a year's duration. The long continuance of the disease and the absence of cachexia suggested a **syphilitic origin** and KI was prescribed. In a month it was possible to pass a sound into the stomach, whereas there had been before complete obstruction. The author excluded an ulcerating carcinoma.

Poncet[3] reports a case of **esophageal actinomycosis.** A woman of 28 was suddenly seized with paroxysmal cough, and a few days later was found to suffer with inability to swallow properly, each attempt being followed by violent coughing and threatened asphyxia. Esophagotomy was performed and a tracheal perforation closed with ligatures. After 48 hours the

¹ Jour. des Sci. méd. de Lille, No. 22, 1896.   ² Deutsch. med. Woch., No. 32, 1896.
⁴ Bull. de l'Acad. de Méd., No. 15, 1896.

patient could swallow without difficulty. The ray-fungi were found in the sputa.

F. Savery and F. Semon [1] describe a case of complete bilateral **paralysis of the recurrent laryngeal nerve,** due to **carcinoma of the esophagus.** The patient, a man of 54,. had the usual symptoms (aphonia and dyspnea) and difficulty in swallowing when sitting in an upright position. He could swallow readily in the horizontal position, upon one side, or with the head hanging over the edge of the bed, as in cases of diseases of the larynx and epiglottis. [The occurrence of laryngeal symptoms due to involvement of the recurrent laryngeal nerve has been studied by MacKenzie and others; but bilateral palsy is extremely rare, and the condition is, in general, too rarely considered.]

Galliard [2] reports a patient whose repasts were frequently interrupted by severe coughs with expectoration of portions of food. A diagnosis was made of a fistula connecting the esophagus and a bronchus. At the autopsy a huge **carcinoma** was found, occupying the lower portion of the esophagus, with a fistula leading to the postero-inferior portion of the right lung.

DISEASES OF THE STOMACH.

Methods of Examination.—Haan [3] has tested the value of different varieties of bread and tea when employed in the test-meal of Ewald, and finds that they exert considerable influence upon the results. The best bread is one composed of gluten and poor in starch. Tea is modified in various ways—by the temperature at which the mixture is given and the concentration of the infusion.

De Niet [4] discusses the diagnosis of gastric malpositions. For general purposes he prefers **distention** of the stomach **with CO_2,** as the inflation with air requires the introduction of a tube. Theoretically, 5 gm. of tartaric acid and 6 gm. of sodium bicarbonate produce 2 l. of CO_2 at the temperature of the body. The determination of the lower border of the stomach is always made with reference to the normal position of the umbilicus—*i. e.,* a point midway between the ensiform process and the pubis. He examined only women, 58 in all. In 13 he found gastroptosis, in 11 subvertical position, in 17 a combination of these conditions; in 11, normal relations; while in 6 the exact condition could not be well determined. In every case he determined Rosenheim's line (the greatest diagonal measurement), the height and the breadth of the organ, and the position of the pylorus. Among 11 normal cases some laced very tightly, so that the author cannot agree with Meinert, who holds that after one and a half year of lacing enteroptosis invariably develops. In speaking of gastrodiaphany the author states that this method is unreliable. [The introduction of a tube is not usually a matter of difficulty, and it has been our experience that inflation by this method gives more trustworthy results.]

Schmilinsky [5] has tried **Boas's method of outlining the stomach** by means of palpation and a sound. He found it succeeded in 97 out of 100 cases. Besides determining the situation of the greater curvature, it was also of value in localizing gastric tumors and in excluding tumors that were not adherent to the stomach.

Meltzing [6] has used the magnetic needle in connection with gastrodiaphany

[1] Lancet, Sept. 19, 1896.
[3] Compt. rend. de la Soc. de Biol., May 28, 1897.
[5] Arch. f. Verdauungskrank., Bd. 3, p. 3.
[2] Sem. méd., 1896, p. 285.
[4] Diss., Leyden, 1896.
[6] Ibid., Bd. 2, H. 4, Dec., 1896.

to demonstrate the reliability of **illumination** as a method of diagnosis in gastric diseases. He introduced a magnetic sound into the stomach and then, with the aid of a balanced magnetic needle, determined the position of its tip. The only error possible in this method, he holds, is that the sound introduced may depress the greater curvature of the stomach; but its delicate construction renders this unlikely. The instrument had previously been described by Martins. The results obtained by this method, in the empty and in the distended stomach, have corresponded with the results obtained by illumination, the difference being scarcely the breadth of a finger. Illumination has the advantage of showing the character of the entire wall of the stomach. He holds that the conditions during life are very different from those that exist in the cadaver; and, therefore, that Luschka's figures, based upon postmortem examination, do not contradict his own. Change of position and change of contents exercise a decided influence upon the position of the organ. [Confirmation of the work of Martius and Meltzing with the magnetic sound is necessary in order to decide its value as an aid to illumination. Other authors, using the ordinary method for control, have reached very different conclusions regarding the value of illumination, and this newly suggested method of confirmation may prove equally unsatisfactory.]

Lindemann [1] has been able to demonstrate the outline of the stomach by means of the **Röntgen** rays. He introduced a flexible sound containing a metal mandril and laid the patient prone upon the plate. He believes the sound passes closely along the greater curvature and that the pictures are quite accurate.

Hemmeter [2] describes his experiments to perform **duodenal intubation.** He distends the stomach with the aid of a rubber bulb and then passes a somewhat curved tube along the lesser curvature through the pylorus. [The technical difficulties in the application of this procedure appear so great that it is not likely to be of much practical service.]

Oppler [3] objects to Hammerschlag's quantitative pepsin-estimation for exact work. By more careful methods he found that **pepsin digestion** never failed entirely in 26 cases that he examined, and that its extent was directly proportionate to the amount of HCl and the activity of the curdling ferment. He therefore concludes that variation in pepsin-secretion is not pathognomonic of any condition. [This is the most careful work that has been done upon this subject, but needs confirmation before it can be unreservedly accepted.]

J. Friedenwald [4] contributes an interesting paper upon **the relations of saliva to gastric digestion,** and cites particularly the experiments of Biernacki. This author concludes that the saliva exercises some sanitary influence upon the digestive processes in the stomach, this influence being exerted locally when the food is being swallowed. The same beneficial effect was not obtained from the saliva when it was introduced into the stomach after the test-meal had been administered, and it was not due to ptyalin or to sulphocyanid of potassium. He concluded that the beneficial effect of saliva is dependent upon its alkalinity, and that the starchy alkaline breakfast is in some way converted into a less alkaline condition by the action of the saliva. Friedenwald repeated these experiments in several healthy and diseased cases, and was able to confirm the results. He found that there was always a greater quantity of gastric contents in the cases in which the saliva was not swallowed than in those in which it was, and the acidity and free HCl

[1] Deutsch. med. Woch., Apr. 22, 1897. [2] Arch. f. Verdauungskrank., ii, 1, 1896.
[3] Ibid., vol. i, No. 1. [4] Internat. Med. Mag., Aug., 1896.

were always greater when the saliva was swallowed than when it was not. No especial difference could be noted in normal cases in pepsin digestion. The rennet activity, however, seems more pronounced when the saliva has mingled with the special test-meal than when it has not been swallowed. In pathological conditions the stimulation of the pepsin and rennet ferments when the saliva is allowed to mingle with the food is more striking. He determined that the mere act of mastication did not exercise the beneficial influence, and, further, that the saliva swallowed after the food exercised a much feebler influence than that swallowed with the food. The effect, he holds, is produced entirely while the food is passing through the month. The author differs from Biernacki regarding the influence exerted by the saliva upon the reaction of the food. Biernacki concluded, from the fact that an alkaline solution previously colored by phenolphthalein lost its color in the month, that the saliva has the power to reduce the alkalinity. Friedenwald maintains that this is due rather to the presence of CO_2, from the fact that he was able to restore the color by boiling, and from the fact that the gases evolved caused turbidity in calcium solutions. He then cites experiments showing that a neutral or slightly acid reaction of the food stimulates greater gastric digestion than alkaline food, and points out that bicarbonate of sodium exerts a more beneficial influence than ordinary sodium hydrate, probably in consequence of liberation by the former of CO_2 when the salt combines with HCl. He is led to suspect that the saliva exerts a beneficial effect in part from the swallowing of carbon dioxid.

Changes in Form and Position.—Bial[1] considers the subject of vertical displacement of the stomach in the male sex. To determine the exact relations he has investigated the position of the stomach and the character of digestion in 50 men of various ages, using inflation with air to determine the position of the stomach, and incidentally placing himself on the side of Meinert and others, who have found this method most useful, and against Martins. He has studied barticularly cases of narrow thorax due to rachitis and other causes, and cases of phthisis and of emphysema, and found that dislocation of the stomach in such individuals is very frequent, but not invariable. His figures show gastroptosis in 12 of 18 cases of malformation of the thorax, and in 18 of 26 cases of emphysema of the lungs. In 17 of 36 patients presenting this condition no disturbances of digestion were discoverable. In a few cases he found typical manifestations of nervous dyspepsia, some of which, however, were ascribable to disturbed secretion, probably the result of displacement. Finally, he concludes that the displacement alone does not explain the occurrence of the severe symptoms in women, these being in greater measure due to a general neurotic organization.

Kutter and Dyer[2] believe that gastroptosis is more frequently the result of tension from below due to the weight of the retained stomach-contents bearing upon the relaxed walls of the organ, than of pressure from above. The nervous and general conditions that are associated with it are probably more frequently its cause than result. In all cases of this condition there appears to be a considerable reduction in the hemoglobin of the blood, 38 cases that they counted giving an average of 77.2%. In criticism of Bial's paper (vide supra) they state that they cannot agree with his conclusions that gastroptosis is less frequently productive of symptoms in men than in women.

Wm. Pepper and Alfred Stengel[3] contribute a discussion of the diagnosis of **dilatation of the stomach.** They first insist that atony cannot be sharply

---

[1] Berlin. klin. Woch., Dec. 14, 1896.   [2] Ibid., May 17, 1897.
[3] Am. Jour. Med. Sci., Jan., 1897.

separated from dilatation, as there is of necessity a certain amount of dilatation with even the least grades of atony. In the second place, they point out that the normal size of the organ is difficult to determine, and that cases of so-called megalogastria may be met with. To determine the limits of gastric capacity they made studies at the postmortem table, filling the stomach with water under a vertical pressure of about 25 cm., and found wide variations. The smallest organ held only 500 c.c., and was found in a boy of 19, 1.73 m. in height, who had died of pulmonary pthisis. The stomach held but 500 c.c. The largest stomach held 2600 c.c., and was found in a woman of 29, of rather delicate construction, and 1.55 m. in height. A number of cases exceeded 1680 c.c., the maximum figure found by Ziemssen. After reviewing the principal etiologic factors in dilatation the authors discuss the physical signs. Attention is called to the depression frequently seen in the epigastrium, the distention of the abdomen being in the lower regions. Auscultation discovers splashing sounds, but these are comparatively valueless. Percussion, as ordinarily practised, is unreliable; but the method of auscultatory percussion has given them very satisfactory results. By far the most useful method is inflation, which they invariably practise with the aid of a stomach-tube and a rubber bulb. The effervescing powders are unreliable and unsafe in comparison. The motor power is best estimated by determining the presence or absence of food-particles in the stomach at long intervals after administration of the test-meals. If any particles remain 7 hours after a meal of meat, soup, and bread, atony may be assumed to exist. The differential diagnosis between megalogastria and dilatation, between gastroptosis and gastrectasia, and between atonic and obstructive dilatation is detailed, and finally that between malignant and nonmalignant obstruction at the pylorus. Of particular interest is the differentiation of gastroptosis, and the authors lay particular stress upon the determination of the position of the lesser curvature of the stomach. If this is displaced downward in equal proportion with the displacement of the greater curvature, there is probably more dislocation than enlargement, and the method of inflation finds its greatest usefulness in making the determination easy. A number of cases and diagrams are included in the report to illustrate the position of the stomach in different conditions and the reliability of different methods in differentiating these conditions.

Rosenstein[1] reports the case of a young man that 7 years before the observation had presented the symptoms of a gastric ulcer; 5 years later he had hematemesis, and then presented the appearance of a case of pneumothorax; it was, however, noticed that the metallic signs were very inconstant, and independent of the expiratory movement. At the autopsy it was found that the enlarged stomach had pressed the diaphragm upward as high as the 1st rib, thus giving rise to the symptoms.

Gastritis.—Chanutin[2] reports a case of **phlegmonous gastritis,** and tabulates the following as the most characteristic symptoms : chills, high temperature, frequent sweats, rapid pulse, and typhoid state; vomiting of bilious matters, the presence of pus-corpuscles in the vomita, or pure pus ; burning or stabbing pains in the region of the stomach ; constipation and sometimes diarrhea; tenderness in the region of the stomach and sometimes presence of swelling. His own case occurred in a woman of 26, and began with nausea, vomiting, and transient diarrhea, followed by pain in the region of the stomach and frequent vomiting ; irregular chills with marked fever developed, and the vomita became purulent and fetid. Finally, pure blood was ejected; the

[1] Arch. f. Verdauungskrank., vol. ii., H. 3.
[2] Vratch, Nos. 32 to 36, 1895 ; Centralbl. f. innere med., No. 40, 1896.

abdomen was depressed and the region of the stomach extremely tender. Pressure on the epigastrium caused nausea and vomiting. The spleen was enlarged ; microscopically pus-corpuscles were found in the vomita, and an almost pure culture of staphylococcus, with a few streptococci, was obtained. The contents were at first alkaline and later acid, and only once contained free HCl. The stomach could retain only ice pills.. The patient gradually recovered.

Dorbeck [1] reports a second case from the same hospital in a woman of 63 who suffered with headache, chills and fever, coryza, cough, and pain in the limbs. The tongue was coated, the tonsils swollen, and there was herpes on the nose. There was no vomiting nor diarrhea; the lungs and heart were negative; the spleen was a little enlarged; the abdomen was slightly thickened. The temperature was 104° and the pulse and respirations rapid. On the third day bronchitis and diarrhea developed, the abdomen became distended, and the patient died. Autopsy showed superficial ulceration of the mucous membrane of the right side of the stomach, with extensive thickening of the deeper layers. The mucosa was partly detached by purulent collections and the infiltration extended as far as the peritoneum. The pus in the submucosa contained many streptococci. [Even with the symptoms present in the first case, the existence of a gastric phlegmon could hardly be established, particularly as considerable quantities of pus may be found in the vomita in other conditions.]

Roux [2] refers to a case of **febrile gastritis followed by paralysis.** The patient, a soldier of 22, presented paralysis of the upper and lower extremities, without noteworthy sensory manifestations, suggesting a lesion of the anterior horns of the cord. The whole course of the disease had analogy with the spinal paralysis of Duchenne-Aran. The cause of the paralysis was undoubtedly the gastric disturbance and the overwork and fatigue incurred about the same time. [Spinal muscular atrophy has occasionally developed after an acute disease, but the etiological relation of the latter has not been established beyond doubt.]

Thiemich [3] has studied **32 cases of gastroenteritis** in children and has found lesions of the liver in a large proportion. In 9 cases there was no change, in 20 moderate and focal, and in 3 high grade and diffuse fatty degeneration. The changes in the nuclei of the cells led to the conclusion that it was a true fatty degeneration. The periportal accumulation of fat, such as is characteristic of ordinary infiltration, is explained by the view that the poison is most active at the point where it first comes in contact with the liver-structure after leaving the blood coming from the gastrointestinal tract. [While the author's paper is not entirely convincing that the changes noted are of peculiar type, or directly related to the gastrointestinal disease, it is suggestive in indicating the existence of a general toxic condition. This is, of course, particularly true of children, but plays an important part in the intestinal disturbances of adults as well.]

Functional and Neurotic Disturbances.—Schreiber [4] defends his previously expressed view that **chronic gastrosuccorrhea** is not an independent disease, but rather a symptomatic condition occurring in the course of certain diseases of the stomach ; notably atony and dilatation. He states his own view regarding Reichmann's disease, and proposes, instead of gastrectasia, the term *Stauungsmagen* to indicate the retention of food. As there is always some remnant of food retained in such a stomach and there is

[1] Vratch, Nos. 32 to 36, 1895 ; Centralbl. f. innere med., No. 40, 1896.
[2] Gaz. hebdom. de Méd. et de Chir., No. 67, 1896.   [3] Ziegler's Beiträge, Bd. 20, H. 1.
[4] Arch. f. Verdauungskrank., Bd. 2, H. 4, Dec., 1896.

constant or permanent digestion, the term *Stauungsmagen with permanent digestion*, or permanent digesting stomach, vould seem to be justified. Chronic gastrosuccorrhea, he believes, is a frequent condition, and is usually supposed to occur either pure and uncomplicated or complicated vith gastrectasia. The uncomplicated cases do not differ in any notable particular from the cases of gastrectasia, and it is possible to relieve the increased gastric secretion by relieving the gastrectasia. He points out that the exclusion of gastrectasia in the so-called typical cases of gastrosuccorrhea by authors vho admit the existence of such a distinct disease rests upon very poor foundation, such as existence of sarcinæ in the dilated organ or the like. He has demonstrated that abstinence from food for the period of 48 hours after careful and systematic lavage had been practised for some time, vith rectal feeding, leads to the disappearance of the symptoms. He alludes to a case in vhich the gastrosuccorrhea disappeared promptly after gastroenterostomy had been performed.

Dauber [1] reports a case vith symptoms of gastritis and continuous excessive secretion of mucus, and proposes the term " **gastrosuccorrhea mucosa.**"

Martius [2] discusses **achylia gastrica,** which, according to him, is not a disease but merely a symptom, and is characterized by the total absence of ferments of the gastric juice. It occurs in gastric carcinoma, in acute and chronic gastric catarrh, in atrophy of the gastric mucous membrane, and in gastric neuroses. He has examined 17 cases, vhich he divides into 2 groups: those in vhich the symptoms of progressive pernicious anemia are present, and those in vhich health is apparently unimpaired. All shov the characteristic change in stomach-contents—that is, after a test-meal neither ferments nor HCl vere secreted, nor vere there any signs of decomposition of the stomach-contents. In the 2d group the motor functions of the stomach are normal and the intestinal digestion and absorption are perfect. The 1st group appears to be invariably associated vith some severe general condition, such as tuberculosis.

Rosenheim [3] discusses **motor insufficiency of the stomach,** by vhich term he implies all injuries to the motility of the stomach, vhether considerable or slight, and whether they occur in a small, normal, or enlarged organ. This condition may arise acutely or suddenly, vhilst in the interval the stomach is entirely normal. Diagnosis can usually be made vithout difficulty by the use of the sound. The most important feature, however, is the discovery of the etiology of the condition. There is by no means invariably stenosis of the pylorus, and Rosenheim reports 2 interesting cases in vhich diminished contractility and secretive pover occurred as manifestations of tabetic crises. Traumatism also is a not infrequent cause, acting either reflexly or else by producing a perigastritis. Another is ventral hernia. Nevertheless, vhen ventral hernia exists it must not be rashly concluded that it is the cause of gastric disturbance. Prognosis is not invariably unfavorable, even in the severer forms, for almost complete cure can, as a last resort, be secured by gastroenterostomy.

Max Einhorn [4] reports a number of cases illustrative of the fact that chemical derangements of the gastric secretion are frequently the cause of either diarrhea or constipation, these latter conditions disappearing as soon as the gastric disturbances are corrected.

Sutherland [5] has described a case of **gastric flatulence** of a peculiar

[1] Arch. f. Verdauungskrank., Bd. 2, H. 4, Dec., 1896.
[2] Wien. klin. Woch., June 3, 1897.   [3] Berlin. klin. Woch., Mar. 15, 1897.
[4] Med. Rec., Feb. 27, 1897.   [5] Lancet, Aug. 1, 1896.

type. The patient, a man of 51 years, began to suffer in 1871 with gastric pain, heartburn, and flatulence, the result of drinking ice-water immediately after exercise. He lost in weight and strength and frequently suffered with acidity. He would stay awake a large part of the night, tormented by eructation. It was found that he had some dilatation of the stomach, and on examination during an attack of eructation this was discovered to be spurious, the air being taken into the esophagus by a swallowing effort, with the muscles of the neck tightly fixed, and then regurgitated. It was explained to him that this eructation really did not come from the stomach and that he could control it by effort. He succeeded in this on the very first trial, and from this time rapidly improved until the habit was completely cured.

Boas,[1] in discussing **dyspeptic asthma**, alludes to 12 cases of his own. In some of these he found diseases of the lungs or heart, in others gastrointestinal disease, especially cases of excessive HCl with atony of the walls of the stomach. The nature of the attacks is obscure, but the author found in some of his cases that the diaphragm was elevated above its normal position. He opposes the theory of autointoxication, stating that his own examinations have not shown any evidence of this.

Rosenbach[2] contributes an elaborate paper on the **dyspepsia of emotion.** The symptoms in general are somewhat as follows: after a severe emotional disturbance, especially in nervous, anemic persons, either at once or in a short time, there are mild or severe digestive disturbances, complete loss of appetite, alternating attacks of increased salivary secretion and dryness, a feeling of constriction in the neck, and sense of pressure in the epigastrium and the abdomen. These patients, as a rule, are able voluntarily to distend their bellies. Dyspnea and sighing respiration with a feeling of constriction beneath the sternum are frequent, and eructation, often associated with air-swallowing, may be observed. Peristaltic activity and noisy borborygmi are frequent. Colicky pains and alternating constipation and nervous diarrhea are significant. The anorexia may be interrupted by periods of excessive appetite, the acid foods being specially craved. Insufficient food taken by these patients leads to exaggeration of the symptoms, and especially of the subjective sensations. The digestive process itself is normal, and examination of the stomach-contents or of the vomited matters discovers no evidences of organic disease. The prognosis depends upon the nature and removability of the cause. Under proper conditions the outlook is favorable. Warm applications, the drinking of moderate quantities of warm water, and the insistence upon a proper diet are important, and small doses of sedatives with small quantities of brandy are advisable.

Mathieu[3] refers to a group of symptoms met with in **hysteria** suggesting genuine **hematemesis.** There is usually vomiting of bloody fluid at night, after a feeling of distress and burning beneath the sternum and in the epigastric region. The quantity is usually about 100 c.c. and the fluid presents the appearance of raspberry syrup. It does not contain clots, traces of food are seldom found, and it grows darker on standing. These attacks occur monthly in certain women, who show typical hysterical symptoms with vague dyspeptic manifestations. The vomiting is rarely preceded by nausea. The stomach is distended with gas, and a point of tenderness is found to the right of the middle line about the position of the pylorus. The attacks may occur daily, or may be longer in duration with intermissions of several days. The vomited matters tend to separate into layers, the lower being composed of mucus

[1] Berlin. klin. Woch., No. 39, 1896.   [2] Ibid., Jan. 25, 1897.
[3] Gaz. des Hôpitaux, Nov. 16, 1896

and corpuscles with detritus, the upper of clear liquid. On testing it is found that saliva is present, the starchy digestion being demonstrable. The sources of blood in these cases is doubtful, though it could be traced to denuded mucous membrane in the mouth in several cases.

Treatment of Chronic Gastric Disease.—Sawyer[1] advocates the use of **arsenic** in the treatment of gastralgia. He accepts the classification of Romberg, who distinguished two forms, *gastrodynia neuralgica*, which he holds to be hyperesthesia of the gastric branches of the vagus, and *neuralgia cœliaca*, which he attributed to hyperesthesia of the solar plexus. Clinical experiences show that this distinction is of doubtful use, treatment being the same. He gives arsenic in pill-form (arsenious acid gr. $\frac{1}{24}$) with 2 or 3 gr. of a vegetable extract such as gentian, 3 times daily between meals. The medicine should be continued for some weeks. In severe cases he also uses counterirritation over the epigastrium. A full and varied diet is better than restricted food.

Storck[2] employs **formalin** as an irrigating solution of a strength of 1 : 1000 in chronic gastric disease with marked fermentation.

Max Einhorn[3] contributes an experimental paper upon the **effect of electrical currents upon the contractions of the stomach.** Meltzer found that direct and indirect faradization of the stomach in animals demonstrated an inordinate resistance on the part of its mucous membrane to the passage of electrical currents. Einhorn found that by placing one electrode upon the serous coat and the other in the stomach contractions were readily elicited. The same occurred when one electrode was placed on an adjacent part of the body and the other in the stomach. Both poles being placed in the stomach, peristaltic contractions could be produced, though not active ones. He claims to have proved by direct experiment that the mucous membrane is a good conductor. In a patient with one electrode in the stomach and one upon the skin over the epigastrium the resistance measured by Wheatstone's apparatus was 6800 ohms. When the electrode was taken from within the stomach and placed upon the back the resistance became 22,000 ohms, proving the ready transmission through the mucous membrane. [While these experiments are somewhat crude the conclusions seem to us entirely justified.]

Salomon[4] subjects **Rosenheim's stomach-sound** to a severe criticism, finding that it does not under ordinary pressure project fine streams laterally against the walls of the stomach. He suggests as improvements diminution in the size of the central hole and reduction of the number of side holes from 24 to 9, making the lumen slightly less and giving them an upward direction. With these changes he finds that it is a most satisfactory instrument.

Lauenstein[5] reports a case of hour-glass deformity of the stomach, in which **gastroanastomosis** was performed. The patient, a woman of 43, had suffered with vomiting, cardialgia, constipation, hematemesis, and loss of flesh. Examination with the stomach-tube detected reduction in the size of the organ. Operation was undertaken and hour-glass deformity was discovered. The lesser curvature was adherent to the under surface of the liver and a constriction appeared at this point. Marked improvement followed the operation.

Gastric Ulcer.—F. Page,[6] C. F. Dent,[7] and R. F. Jovers[8] each report a case of **perforated gastric ulcer,** in which **laparotomy** was performed

[1] Lancet, July, 1896.   [2] New Orl. M. and S. Jour., Mar., 1897.
[3] N. Y. Med. Jour., Dec. 12, 1896; Arch. f. Verdauungskrank., Bd. 2, H. 4, Dec., 1896.
[4] Berlin. klin. Woch., Aug. 3, 1896.   [5] Münch. med. Woch., No. 21, 1896.
[6] Lancet, May 23, 1896.   [7] Ibid., June 20, 1896.   [8] Ibid.

and recovery ensued. Further cases are reported by A. Thomson[1] and W. H. Bennett.[2] In all there were 6 cases, 5 of which recovered. The 6th case died of pneumonia on the seventh day. The patients were 3 women, between 19 and 27, and 3 men, between 32 and 44. The ulcer occupied the anterior wall of the stomach in each case, and there was generally considerable extravasation of the gastric contents into the peritoneal cavity at the time of the operation. The symptoms previous to the rupture were sometimes uncertain, as in the case of Bennett's, in which the clinical history was very indefinite for weeks, and at last resembled that of intestinal obstruction. Operation was undertaken in 5 of the cases between $3\frac{1}{2}$ and 7 hours after severe pains indicated a rupture; in one case it was 24 hours after rupture. Thomson refers to the fact that hemorrhages into the gastrointestinal tract, without the external appearance of blood, in the course of gastric ulcer, may cause symptoms of perforation, and he refers to a case in which perforation of gastric ulcer was suspected and in which he made an incision, only to find a healthy peritoneal wall.

Kuttner[3] reports a case of gastric ulcer in which pain in the epigastrium came on acutely and was associated with obstinate constipation. Enemata of oil relieved both symptoms temporarily; but the pain recurring, associated with resistance in the epigastric region, operation was performed, and an abscess was found in the liver, through which gastric contents were discharged. At the autopsy an ulcer was found on the posterior wall of the stomach, perforating into the liver.

H. M. Lyman[4] reports a case of gastric ulcer that presented subjective symptoms for 3 years. 6 months before admission the patient had vomited mucus streaked with blood. Finally, there was intense hemorrhage lasting for nearly 24 hours and causing a profound anemia.

Treatment.—Ratjen[5] adopts **absolute withdrawal of all nourishment by the mouth** with absolute rest in bed for a period of 10 days for the cure of gastric ulcer. In 55 cases in which this was tried the cure seemed to be complete; for the purpose of quenching thirst water and a few indifferent teas were employed, and no drugs given excepting sometimes a little cognac.

Hirsch[6] reports a case of gastric ulcer that for 2 years had not produced any symptoms and then, immediately after a severe fright, led to erosion of a vessel and fatal hemorrhage. He discusses the indications for **operative procedure** in such cases, and suggests that possibly it would be easier to discover the ulcer if the operation was performed during the hemorrhage; in general, he believes that operative interference is justifiable when, in spite of strictest rest and diet, there are continually recurring hemorrhages, which, by their quantity and severity, present a serious menace to the life of the patient.

Carcinoma of the Stomach.—Diagnosis.—Czygan[7] believes that **the presence of HCl** and the **condition of the ferments** in the gastric juice are of great importance in the differential diagnosis between carcinoma of the pylorus and of the duodenum. In the latter condition he usually finds hyperacidity and sometimes, as in the case he reports, the absence of leucin, tyrosin, and bile from the stomach-contents. When bile is absent he considers that it indicates the location of the neoplasm between the pylorus and the ductus choledochus.

[1] Lancet, July 4, 1896.   [2] Ibid., Aug., 1896.
[3] Brit. Med. Jour., May 29, 1897.   [4] Jour. Am. Med. Assoc., Mar. 13, 1897.
[5] Deutsch. med. Woch., Dec. 27, 1896.   [6] Berlin. klin. Woch., Sept. 26, 1896.
                    [7] Arch. f. Verdauungskrank., vol. 3, No. 1.

A. Hammerschlag[1] discusses the diagnosis of **cancer of the stomach,** based upon the examination of 42 cases. If there is absence of free HCl for a period of several weeks, if the albumin digestion is reduced below 15 %, if much lactic acid is present and numerous long bacilli, and if no improvement occurs in the period of observation, cancer may be assumed with considerable likelihood even if cachexia and tumor are not developed. Neither deficient HCl, nor marked loss of peptonizing power is peculiar to cancer ; nor is the presence of lactic acid distinctive. The demonstration of intense lactic-acid formation as a constant symptom warrants the belief that the peptic glands are largely atrophic, and that motor insufficiency of the organ exists. This combination is seen more frequently and earlier in carcinoma than in any other condition.

W. C. Weber[2] discusses the possibility of the early diagnosis of carcinoma of the stomach, and concludes that although it cannot be made positively, nevertheless the continued absence of HCl and the presence of lactic acid, and the condition of the blood, taken in connection with the symptoms of gastric disturbance, enable one to reach a conclusion with reasonable certainty, at least at a period when operative interference is still possible. [It must not be forgotten that all cases of gastric carcinoma are not amenable to operation even in the earliest stages.]

A. L. Benedict[3] holds that the apparent **presence of a tumor** in the abdomen in the region of the pylorus is not always indicative of carcinoma, since the size of the tumor seems to increase with the thickness of the abdominal wall. He is not convinced that the slow absorption of KI is of much significance, having in a number of experiments found that in the same individual, under apparently similar conditions, the time at which it appeared in the saliva was exceedingly variable. Furthermore, he disputes the importance, as a sign of carcinoma, of the diminution of the daily quantity of urea excreted.

Huber[4] reviews the subject of carcinoma of the stomach. Without the presence of a palpable tumor, the diagnosis can scarcely extend beyond a probability. The objective and subjective symptoms, particularly the vomiting of coffee-ground material, which is highly suggestive, are of some value. The absence of free HCl is usual, but the occurrence of this sign in other diseases robs it of value. The presence of lactic acid is of greater significance, and a specially high degree of lactic-acid reaction is highly suggestive. Another sign is the prolonged retention of food in the stomach, which occurs not only when the pylorus is affected, but also when the body of the organ is involved.

Reineboth[5] refers to the **diagnosis of carcinoma** of the stomach **by examination of the fragments of the tissue** obtained in the vomita or in the washings after lavage. Cancer-cells cannot be recognized as such, and the diagnosis therefore rests upon the recognition of groups of cells ; but even cancerous acini or cancer-nests cannot be distinguished offhand from similar aggregations of cells of noncancerous origin. In some cases it is necessary, in order to be certain, to discover other suspicious signs, such as the existence of tumor. If a distinct mass can be felt and then cell-nests are found, the diagnosis is fairly certain ; but cells frequently show considerable alteration due to the action of the gastric juice and of necrosis. He has examined the washings of 28 cases for considerable periods of time. Four of these were cases of old ulcer ; 10 were cases of chronic gastritis and nervous disorders ; 6 were doubtful cases of chronic gastritis and old ulcer or

[1] Arch. f. Verdauungskrank., Bd. 2, H. 1 and 2.   [2] Jour. Am. Med. Assoc., July 11, 1896.
[3] Internat. Med. Mag., Apr., 1897.   [4] Correspondencebl. f. Schw. Aerzte Sept. 15, 1896.
[5] Deutsch. Arch. f. klin. Med., Bd. 58, H. 1, 1896.

cancer; and 8 were cases of pyloric cancer. Of the latter 8, suspicious particles were found in 4, and the same occurred in 1 of the 6 cases in which the diagnosis was somewhat in doubt. The author then details briefly the clinical features of these 5 cases, and concludes that in the 1st the diagnosis was absolute; in the 2d almost so; in the 3d peculiar tubular formations were found in the tissue-particles, but without the existence of a distinct tumor it could not be positively asserted that the case was one of cancer; in the 4th case the diagnosis was negative; and in the 5th case doubtful. In the 5 cases in which fragments were found, 4 of which had pyloric stenosis, the microscopic examination established an undoubted diagnosis of cancer in 2. In 1 of these no cancer could be felt, while in the 2d the diagnosis was made in spite of temporary improvement (gained 15 pounds in $1\frac{1}{2}$ weeks), such as is rarely seen in

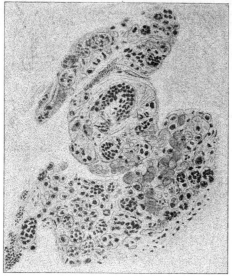

Fig. 3.—Fragment of carcinomatous tissue found in stomach-washings (Deutsch. Arch. f. klin. Med., Bd. 58, H 1, 1896).

cancer. He reproduces some of the drawings made from the microscopic examinations. [It is gratifying to note the author's care in drawing deductions from the microscopic appearances, as contrasted with the reckless manner in which some observers have claimed to be able to distinguish various diseases and even stages of disease in this way.]

W. O'Neill[1] records a very interesting case of **hematemesis,** in which considerable quantities of **tumor-substance were vomited.** The patient, a man of 60, much emaciated and extremely anemic, was almost syncopal. There were pain and tenderness in the epigastric region and the stomach was found to be enlarged. The patient had vomited twice the morning he came under observation. The vomita consisted of blood, mucus, and numerous bits of carcinomatous tissue of the colloid kind. There were 3 portions of this so large that the man's wife said she had pulled them out of his throat to prevent

[1] Lancet, Oct. 3, 1896.

him choking. The quantity of vomited matter was from 8 to 10 oz. On careful examination there was found one portion in the shape of a ring and darker and harder than the remaining parts; this was apparently from the pyloric end of the organ. It is very likely from the appearance of the masses that the carcinoma was of polypoid character. The patient improved very much after he recovered from the immediate effects of the loss of blood.

Symptoms.—Brosch[1] reports a case with the symptoms of obstinate constipation and rending pains in the region of the stomach. There were melena and hematemesis, and a rough, hard, resistent surface apparently connected with the pylorus could be felt in the epigastrium. The stomach was not dilated and free HCl was present. At the operation metastases were found in the abdominal cavity. The autopsy showed a carcinoma upon the posterior surface of the stomach and two annular stenoses of the intestines produced by secondary carcinomata.

Powell[2] describes a case of **infiltrating carcinoma** of the stomach. The patient, a woman of 34, who had always been somewhat dyspeptic, said her illness dated from an attack of influenza 2 months previously. She first suffered with pain, and 5 months later vomiting, eructations, and constipation set in. There was no hematemesis. She discovered a lump in the epigastric region, which, however, remained about the same in size for 6 months, although it underwent temporary variations; she had lost some flesh, and on admission was thin but not emaciated. On physical examination an elongated, somewhat kidney-shaped swelling was found about $\frac{1}{3}$ of the way down below the ensiform cartilage toward the umbilicus. It was 3 in. in length and extended to the left cartilages, being lost beneath the costal margin on that side. On the right side it had a rounded border in the parasternal line. The tumor was movable to some extent, and from time to time it could be felt to harden as if by intrinsic contraction; it descended somewhat with inspiration. The stomach-outline was about normal. No splash could be elicited. It was clear that it was not connected with the liver. The spleen appeared normal, though a small mass felt on deep inspiration below the ribs, and more or less in touch with the tumor, might be either the spleen or an offshoot. Displaced kidney was excluded on account of its superficial position and location anterior to the transverse colon. The position and characteristics of the tumor were compatible with the diagnosis of an omental mass, but the peculiarity that the tumor varied in hardness led to the diagnosis that it was a thickened stomach. The duration of the symptoms and the absence of extension of the tumor or involvement of other organs were against the idea of malignancy. An exploratory incision was made, which showed that the mass was a hypertrophied wall of the stomach, the pylorus itself being healthy. The patient reacted well from the operation but subsequently died, and the autopsy showed the stomach contracted, pinkish-white in color, and opaque. The pylorus admitted the middle finger; the stomach-wall was greatly thickened; there was diffuse cartilaginous infiltration beneath the mucosa. The process was most marked in the pyloric third, although the whole stomach was involved. Accurate analyses of the stomach-contents had not been made, but the vomita did not react with congo paper. [Cases of this kind are of great interest from a diagnostic standpoint, and it is regrettable that accurate studies of the gastric secretions and functions were not attempted. In spite of these, however, a strong suspicion of malignancy was justified by the evident massive thickening of the walls of the stomach. It is to be remembered that many of the older cases in literature of cirrhosis of the stomach were probably instances of such infiltrating carcinoma.]

---

[1] Deutsch. Arch. f. klin. Med., Dec. 18, 1896.   [2] Practitioner, Feb., 1897.

Bouveret[1] describes a case of carcinoma of the pylorus in which a **fistula into the colon** was established. The existence of the latter could be determined by the following points: for 3 months there was permanent diarrhea, uninfluenced by medicines; the evacuations invariably followed 10 or 15 minutes after the patient took food; in spite of marked nausea and attempt at vomiting the patient was able to vomit only once, just before death. The vomited material showed the same constitution as the dejections, which had none of the fecal characteristics, but a marked odor of butyric acid; HCl was never found free or combined. The condition of the nutrition of the patient was such that there was evidence of communication with the ascending colon and therefore a moderate preservation of the digestive activity and absorption.

Septic Infection.—Herard[2] discusses the various forms of sepsis that may occur in cancer of the stomach. The principal entrance is through the portal system, giving rise to an adhesive or suppurative pylephlebitis, the latter being distinguished by a greater severity of the symptoms. Once the organisms have passed the portal capillaries they may produce all the characteristic symptoms of pyemia. These infections often have considerable influence upon the development of the cachexia.

De Besse[3] has studied septic infection occurring in gastric carcinoma. This may remain localized either in the cancer or in its neighborhood, or may be transmitted by the lymph-channels to distant organs, such as the pleura or pericardium, or by the portal vein to the liver, or it may give rise to septicemia or even pyemia; these usually occurring as secondary to suppurative pylephlebitis. He believes that this septic infection has much to do with the development of the cachexia.

Geo. Dock[4] reports a case of primary carcinoma of the stomach which developed in a farmer 18 years of age. At the autopsy, which occurred 2 years later; large masses of carcinomatous lymph-nodules were found surrounding the cardiac orifice, and there was metastasis to the mesentery and liver.

Boas[5] discusses a case of **pyloric tumor** of unusual interest. The patient, a laborer of 56, had suffered with disturbances of the stomach since the latter end of 1895. He had suffered considerable loss of weight, but was not cachectic. No physical alterations could be observed in the stomach, but there were always remnants of food and an intensely acid reaction. There was no free HCl, but lactic acid; no sarcinæ, but long, thread-like bacilli. After these conditions had been determined a number of times a diagnosis of carcinoma was made and laparotomy was performed. A tumor was found compressing the pylorus and removed. On examination this proved to be an adenosarcoma. The man subsequently improved sufficiently to return to work, and at the time of the report presented a healthy appearance.

Pyloric Stenosis.—A. S. Hotaling[6] reports a case that had presented symptoms of gastric disturbance. Upon examination the stomach was found to be greatly dilated with a thickened mass at the pyloric end. At the autopsy an old ulcer was found situated on the posterior wall near the pylorus which had been involved in the cicatricial contraction.

Clay[7] reports a case of obstruction of the pyloric end of the stomach, due to kinking brought about by adhesions following suppuration of the gallbladder. The patient, aged 42, was admitted complaining of vomiting of 2 months' duration. Two years before he had a swelling in the right side, a

[1] Lyon méd., Nos. 9 and 10, 1896.   [2] Gaz. hebdom. de Méd. et Chir., Nov. 15, 1896.
[3] Gaz. des Hôpitaux, Nov. 5, 1896.   [4] Am. Jour. Med. Sci., June, 1897.
[5] Berlin. klin. Woch., Jan. 18, 1897.   [6] Med. Rec., Mar. 20, 1897.
[7] Brit. Med. Jour., Jan. 23, 1897.

little below the region of the gall-bladder, that he was told was an abscess. It ruptured into the bowel and he was apparently cured. Two months before admission he began to vomit fluid of a brownish color, often as much as 2 quarts at a time. There was no pain. Operation was undertaken, but the patient died. At the autopsy the stomach was found to be dilated, and the pyloric end, the colon, and gall-bladder matted together by adhesions. The gall-bladder was full of stones and pus, and a band of adhesions passed between it and the pylorus, so that the latter was drawn up and produced a kink. There was a small opening from the pylorus into the gall-bladder and another sinus passed from the latter downward into the duodenum. There was no other cause of stenosis of the pylorus or of the dilatation of the stomach.

Hayem[1] believes that it is possible in some cases to distinguish between pyloric stenosis and partial subpyloric stenosis or stenosis of the duodenum below the ampulla of Vater. The chief symptom of either condition is the presence of liquid in the stomach in the morning before breakfast. If this liquid is abundant and contains masses of food, the stricture is at the pylorus; if it is scanty and contains bile with no masses of food that can be recognized without the aid of the microscope, it is probably subpyloric. The treatment is entirely surgical; but, as in some cases there is a tendency to spontaneous cure, operation should not be too hastily advised. In the discussion of this paper Robin[2] stated that a large number of the cases of apparent pyloric stenosis were due to pyloric spasm and yielded readily to medicinal treatment; reporting, in support of his statement, 5 cases, in all of which a diagnosis of Reichmann's disease had been made, that recovered without operation. [The differential diagnosis of the two conditions is not as easy as Hayem seems to imply. The number of cases that he studied was too small to establish general points of diagnosis. Neither the presence of considerable liquid, nor of fluid in large masses, is sufficient to exclude subpyloric conditions.]

Finkelstein[3] describes the features of **congenital pyloric stenosis.** The condition was described by Landerer in 1879 and later by R. Maier, who constructed the clinical history from 31 cases. Finkelstein described 10 cases with postmortem examinations in 7. In the other 3 cases the patients survived. The fatal cases lasted from 30 days to 2 years, the symptoms in some of the cases not appearing until a short time after birth. Later, marked gastric symptoms (vomiting—the vomita being without bile—scanty stools, dilatation of the stomach with fermentation) made their appearance. In moderate cases of stenosis there may be merely the indications of a simple chronic gastritis. In one of his cases the thickened pylorus could be felt. This is due to hypertrophy of the longitudinal muscle-fibres and is strictly limited above and below the pylorus.

DISEASES OF THE INTESTINAL TRACT.

Hohigmann[4] has studied the **absorptive power of the small intestine** in a case with a fistula in the lower ileum. Fat was almost completely absorbed, but albumin was only partially utilized; the amount of nitrogenous excretion, especially in the urine, was greatly diminished, as if the organism had endeavored to replace the nitrogen lost in the intestine by withholding that normally excreted, and the same was true of the calcium salts. Experiments were then made to test the amount of iron that could be absorbed by the in-

[1] Bull. de l'Acad. de Méd., May 13, 1897. [2] Ibid., May 27, 1897.
[3] Jahr. f. Kinderh., Bd. xliii., No. 1. [4] Arch. f. Verdauungskrank., Bd. 2, H. 3.

testinal tract, and it was found that 81.3 % of a normal therapeutic dose of ferric citrate was absorbed in 2 days. The patient, however, was suffering from extreme anemia, which possibly favored this process. [The observation in regard to iron is strong proof of its value in anemic conditions, a fact that has been doubted by some modern clinicians.]

Schmidt[1] discusses the **excretion of mucus** from the bowel. The substance to which Hoppe-Seyler called attention that can be extracted with water or alkaline liquid, and precipitated by acetic acid, is not mucin; nor are the hyaline mucous particles and yellowish mucous bodies of Nothnagel mucin. The membranes of mucous or membranous colitis are mainly composed of true mucin, but they contain also a notable quantity of fat or soapy material. Fibrin has never been demonstrated. The degenerated cells observed with the microscope are epithelial or round cells impregnated with soap. The diagnosis of ulcerous process may be established more certainly by scanty mucus than by an abundance of round cells. To determine the origin of the mucus is difficult; at the most, we may say that the occurrence of cells partly digested points to the small intestine as the probable seat of origin. Unless there is rapid peristalsis the mucous particles of the small intestine never remain undissolved and are not, therefore, recognized in the stools.

Constipation and Fecal Impaction.—Gersuny[2] describes a new symptom that he believes is pathognomonic of fecal tumors. It consists in a peculiar feeling of separation of the intestinal wall from the tumor if one presses firmly upon it with the finger, and then, still keeping the finger in contact with the abdominal wall, relaxes the pressure. This he calls the *Klebesymptom*. The conditions that must exist before it can be elicited consist of a certain degree of dryness of the intestinal mucous membrane and of impressionability of the surface of the tumor. If the latter is too hard, it can only be elicited after some method has been used which serves to soften it, such as an oil clysma, and it is of course necessary that the intestine should be distended with gas. He reports the first case in which he was able to discover these symptoms. The diagnosis had been made of a tumor, probably of the adnexa, and laparotomy had been performed; it was while the enormously distended colon was exposed to view that palpation revealed this peculiar sign, and after the wound had healed it was readily elicited through the abdominal wall. He also gives briefly the histories of 2 similar cases in both of which it was also present.

Oliver[3] records an interesting case of **obstinate constipation** with impaction lasting 2 months. The patient, a woman of 53, had suffered for 2 years with indigestion and flatulence, and for a year with constipation. During the first months of 1895, however, she had to take laxatives freely. Gradually the constipation grew worse, and during the last 8 weeks prior to her admission she had had no movement. She was emaciated, sharp-featured, mentally dull, melancholic, and very obstinate. Her emaciation suggested cancer, but no physical signs could be determined. The abdomen was flat and even, except in the iliac fossæ, where there was some bulging. Occasionally peristaltic waves could be seen, and masses could be felt along the descending colon that were easily recognized as fecal in character. Similar masses were observed in the cecum. The patient was etherized and with difficulty the impaction removed. Later copious enemata and purges cleared the bowel. Her mental stupor disappeared or improved greatly as soon as the bowel was relieved; she gained 6 pounds in 1 week, and was apparently entirely cured.

[1] Zeit. f. klin. Med., Bd. 32. II. 3 and 4.   [2] Wien. klin. Woch, Oct. 1, 1896.
[3] Brit. Med. Jour., Sept. 26, 1896.

[We have recently seen 2 cases of very obstinate constipation in young men presenting the symptoms of lassitude and melancholia with a great desire to sleep, both of whom returned to their normal mental condition when the constipation was relieved.]

Max Einhorn[1] states that the most important prophylactic measure in the treatment of habitual constipation is to abstain from administering cathartics during slight transient disturbances of the digestion, and when constipation exists to employ careful hygienic measures, increasing the amount of the vegetables and fats, diminishing mental anxiety and establishing regular habits. Cathartics should be given only infrequently, and then as sparingly as possible.

Intestinal Obstruction.—Herz[2] reviews the subject of **stenosis of the duodenum** and reports 4 cases of his own. Stenosis above the papilla of the bile-duct is scarcely to be distinguished from pyloric stenosis. When the stenosis is below the papilla the symptoms of greater significance are the presence of bile in the stomach and, in some cases, the dilatation of this organ. The absence of dilatation in some cases is remarkable, and is probably ascribable to congenital peculiarities. Whether dilated or not, the stomach is rarely empty, but contains liquid with admixture of bile or saliva. [*Vide* Hayem, under Pyloric Stenosis.]

Wilkinson[3] records a case of intestinal **obstruction due to impaction of a gall-stone;** the patient was a stout woman of 63. On the 4th day of her third attack of biliary colic she was seized with stercoraceous vomiting and general abdominal pain, with tympany and thready pulse. A diagnosis of impacted gall-stone was made and it was decided to use expectant measures. After various fluctuations the stone was discharged 11 weeks after the onset of the first symptoms. It was the size of a pigeon's egg, was faceted, and weighed 341½ gr. The patient recovered completely. [It is evident that, as the author states, the stone must have ulcerated its way from the biliary passages to the duodenum. A case of this kind came under our own observation a few years ago. The patient had never suffered from biliary colic, but died of intestinal obstruction. A large cholesterin stone was found blocking the small intestine. The gall-bladder and duodenum were closely united, and fibrous adhesions were found surrounding the junction of the two. There had evidently been a gradual ulceration of the biliary ducts and subsequently adhesive contraction.]

Aeria[4] reports a case of **gall-stone impacted** in the bowel, causing complete intestinal obstruction. Upon admission the patient gave a history of having been vomiting for a few days; the vomita consisted of undigested food apparently mixed with blood and of rather a sour smell. There were frequent scanty liquid evacuations. Both liver and spleen were normal and there was no temperature, although the patient was in profound collapse. The diagnosis was made of cholera and appropriate treatment employed. The symptoms were progressive, however, and death occurred 9 days after admission. At the autopsy the gall-bladder was found adherent to the duodenum, and through the point of adhesion a perforation had occurred. In the ileum 3 feet from the ileocecal valve there was a large gall-stone, 2½ by 2 inches, which had apparently been broken.

Lundy[5] recommends rapid distention of the colon with CO_2 in cases of suspected intussusception. He reports 3 cases in which the symptoms were not conclusive, but which presented all the signs of gastrointestinal obstruc-

---

[1] Post-graduate, Oct., 1896.   [2] Deutsch. med. Woch., Nos. 23 and 24, 1896.
[3] Brit. Med. Jour., Feb. 13, 1897.   [4] Indian Med. Rec., Jan. 1, 1897.
[5] Lancet, June 19, 1897.

tion, obstinate constipation, vomiting, and pain in the abdomen. In one case
an elongated tumor could be felt. The patients during the inflation, which was
sometimes repeated, felt a sudden, sharp pain followed by immediate relief.
All appeared to be permanently cured.

Turck [1] holds that the presence of bacteria and a suitable soil for their
development are indispensable to fermentative processes in the intestines. In
the **treatment of chronic intestinal disease** he considers bran a most
important element, the indigestible particles aiding in the mastication of food.
He also advocates the use in the colon of his various forms of apparatus for
hydrotherapy. Occasionally the gyromele will pass the sigmoid flexure and
enable the physician to make topical applications to the descending colon.
[Radical treatment of this kind is not free from the danger of aggravating the
existing disease. The gyromele is capable of doing great damage.]

Enteroptosis.—Stiller [2] discusses the nature of enteroptosis, and concludes
that it is a congenital anomaly. It is a descent of the atonic and dilated stomach,
of the large intestine, particularly the transverse colon, of the right or both
kidneys, and rarely of the liver or spleen, occurring in early life in consequence of generalized, congenital relaxation, particularly of the ligaments.
It occurs in persons who have a dyspeptic neurasthenia of congenital origin,
with soft muscles, small amount of fatty deposit, and delicate bony organization. One of the certain indications of this condition is **abnormal movability of the 10th rib.** Grasping the point of the 10th rib, which lies
in the mammary line, it is easy to determine whether it is movable or not.
This movability is due to fibrous instead of cartilaginous junction of the rib
with the sternum.

Max Einhorn [3] holds that enteroptosis begins with a prolapse of the intestines, particularly of the right part of the transverse colon, due to relaxation of
the colico-hepatic ligament. Coincident with this descent the mesentery is relaxed, the small intestine with the stomach prolapses, and the liver and right
kidney are dragged downward. The author describes the symptoms of the
disease as first pointed out by Glénard, and then refers to his own experience.
Among 57 male patients with gastric disturbance he found distinct enteroptosis
and movable right kidney in 4 ; among 33 female patients of the same kind,
13 were thus affected. In another series there were 5 cases among 84 males and
19 among 59 females. Although it is his experience that pronounced enteroptosis may exist without symptoms of any kind, he believes with Glenard that
it may as such produce distinct symptoms. [This condition undoubtedly
occurs as a result of a variety of causes.]

Maragliano [4] reports a case of **diaphragmatic hernia** in which the diagnosis was made during life. In but 7 of 266 cases reviewed by Lachner could
a diagnosis be established *intra vitam.* The author succeeded in his own case by
intestinal inflation. The patient was suffering with influenza, when, during a
paroxysm of coughing, the hernia suddenly developed. After the ordinary
measures of diagnosis had been considered the intestines were inflated with a
pump per rectum, and it was found that the abdomen was not increased appre-
ciably, nor the diaphragm displaced upward, but the thorax increased 1 cm.
in volume. Simultaneously with each insufflation a sound was audible in the
fifth intercostal space. He introduced a needle into the left thorax and introduced a certain amount of liquid. This could be made to bubble as the air
entered the intestine. Finally distention of the intestine with liquid caused
an area of dulness in the left thorax where it had been resonant before.

[1] N. Y. Med. Jour., Mar. 13, 1897.   [2] Arch. f. Verdauungskrankh., ii. p. 285, 1896.
[3] Med. News, Sept. 19, 1896.   [4] Gaz. degli Osped. e delle Clin., Feb. 15, 1897.

Appendicitis.—Goluboff[1] holds that appendicitis is a distinct infectious disease, which may occur as an epidemic. The lighter forms are often overlooked and diagnosed as some other condition, thus interfering with recognition of the epidemic character. He gives the following description of the clinical appearance. The cases occur in early adult life and commence with sudden pain in the region of the umbilicus. The tongue is coated; there are malaise and moderate local edema. The condition disappears in the course of 1 to 3 days. [The frequency of appendicitis has seemed to us to depend upon the greater prevalence of intestinal disorders due to influenza; but we cannot agree with the author that there is any epidemicity.]

Rotter,[2] in discussing 213 cases of appendicitis in the St. Hedwig Hospital of Berlin, states that the mortality is not as great as is often assumed, being only 8.9% of all the cases in his experience, and 2.5% of the cases of circumscribed character; among the localized cases 90% recovered spontaneously, and 84% of the total number of cases received during the first 6 days of the attack. The fever is an important basis of classification. He distinguishes: (1) Cases beginning with high fever (40° C.) and decreasing in 3 or 4 days with rapid convalescence. (2) Same onset, but more continuous fever; among 14 cases of this kind all recovered; 3 required operation. (3) Same onset, with temperature remaining elevated longer than the 5th day; these cases show virulent infection and the prognosis is unfavorable; among 11 there were 2 deaths. (4) The temperature declines at first, but rises again; these always indicate large accumulations of pus. (5) General peritonitis; temperature low and often subnormal in severe infection; higher in progressive cases; the pulse indicates the severity of the attack; recovery only after surgical interference.

Smith[3] reports 2 cases of appendicitis. In the 1st the local symptoms were on the left side, and consisted of a swelling in the region of the sigmoid flexure. Subsequently there were marked tympanites and general peritonitis. Death occurred on the 16th day. At the autopsy considerable adhesive peritonitis was found, and the appendix was adherent to the anterior abdominal wall, showing a perforation communicating with an abscess-cavity. The 2d case commenced characteristically and a diagnosis of appendicitis was made. Apparent recovery took place under the influence of morphin. At the end of 3 weeks the parotid gland on the right side became acutely swollen and subsequently that of the left, both suppurating. After these had discharged signs of peritonitis again set in, and the patient died. At the autopsy there was a large collection of pus about the cecum enclosed in adhesions. A small perforation was found at the base of the appendix. He believes that in the 1st case operation was not justifiable on account of the cachectic state of the patient, and in the 2d on account of the apparent recovery before the development of the parotiditis.

MacNaughton[4] describes the case of a child of 11, which during the convalescence from scarlet fever complained of pain in the abdomen. There was constipation but no vomiting. The temperature was 37.8°. No resistance was detected on palpation; expectant treatment was instituted, and on the third day there was some relief. That night vomiting and diarrhea set in; 2 hours later repeated stercoraceous vomiting and collapse. There was no pain. The patient died, and at autopsy ulcer of the vermiform appendix with abscess-formation posteriorly was discovered. There was general peritonitis. There was no perforation of the appendix itself. [This irregularity of the

[1] Berlin. klin Woch., Jan. 24, 1897. [2] Centralbl. f. Chir., Oct. 24, 1896.
[3] Edinb. Med. Jour., Aug., 1896. [4] Brit. Med. Jour., Oct. 24, 1896.

symptoms, and especially the insidiousness of onset, are often met with in appendicitis in childhood.]

Gill [1] reports 2 cases of appendicitis with supposed endocarditis of the pulmonary valve as a complication. There was no autopsy in the fatal case and the other recovered. Pulsation and murmur were detected over the pulmonary area. [These signs, however, are so uncertain that we feel they scarcely justify the deduction.]

Simon Flexner [2] reports the case of a man who had lived in a malarial district and who was suddenly attacked with chills and fever and severe diarrhea. In the blood malarial parasites were found, and in the evacuations a number of amebæ coli. At the autopsy peritonitis was found and cultures from the peritoneal exudate showed the presence of virulent diplococci and bacteria coli communis. The source of the peritonitis was apparently necrosis of the appendix. [The author urges that this extraordinary case demonstrates the importance of thorough bacteriologic and microscopic examination in all cases, both ante- and postmortem.]

Pick [3] insists upon the occurrence of **stercoral typhlitis** as a clinical condition. In discussing appendicitis he states that the importance of colic of the vermiform process has been underestimated, and that it is mainly due to the presence of a foreign body, though it may be purely nervous and without any anatomic lesions. This form of colic resembles biliary, renal, and intestinal colics. The pain may be severe and may occur with great suddenness. It ceases with the discharge of the foreign body. If this result is not attained, the appendix after a time becomes quiescent from paresis; ulceration and perforation of the walls may then occur.

Cholera Morbus.—Pottien [4] has studied the **bacteriology of cholera morbus** very carefully in 3 cases. In one he found the bacterium coli very virulent for mice, and also a capsulated bacillus resembling the bacillus pyocyaneus which produced a green coloring-matter, and which he calls the *bacillus fluorescens liquefaciens.* The same organism was found in the 2 other cases.

Mucous Colitis.—Franke [5] reports a case of mucous colitis in which there were unbearable pain and great reduction of strength, and in which he performed a colotomy. There was remarkable relief; so much, indeed, that the patient refused to have the artificial fistula closed later. He believes the operation is justified in cases of great severity, such as the one he reported, although he would first try the effect of suggestion, as he regards the disease as hysteric in nature.

Mendelson [6] reports 5 cases of mucous colitis. He believes that the disease presents 3 cardinal groups of symptoms : neurasthenia, mucous passages, and abdominal pain. The mucus is usually found lying upon the feces and not intimately mixed with them. Tenesmus is often agonizing. The cause of the disease seems to be exhaustion of the nervous system, and it usually occurs in women from the ages of 20 to 45 years. Treatment consists of the rest-cure and irrigation of the bowel. All of the 5 cases reported improved very much under this *régime.*

Dysentery.—Etiology.—Janowski,[7] having had occasion to observe a number of cases of dysentery in none of which he was able to find the amebæ coli, undertook an investigation of the literature of this subject in

---

[1] Australas. M. Gaz., Sept. 21, 1896.   [2] Bull. Johns Hopkins Hosp., Sept.-Oct., 1896.
[3] Wien. med. Woch., 15-17, 1896.   [4] Zeit. f. Hyg. u. Infektionkr., Bd. xx., H. 1.
[5] Mittheil. aus de Grenzgeb. der Med. u. Chir., 1-3, 1896.   [6] Med. Rec., Jan. 30, 1897.
[7] Centralbl. f. Bakt. Parasit. u. Inf.'kr., Feb. 5, 1897, ff.

order to determine what relation this organism bore to the disease. He concludes that dysentery is etiologically not a simple disease, and in all probability is never produced by the action of a single parasite, but apparently by the combined action upon the organism of several varieties. The cause of the common dysentery of the temperate zones is some bacterial complex; a form exists, however, entirely different from this both clinically and pathologically, the so-called tropical dysentery, and this is apparently the result of association of bacteria with a certain species of ameba.

Celli[1] concludes from the literature concerning the etiology of dysentery that no peculiar bacillus can be cultivated from the fecal evacuations, but that among others the Bacillus coli dysentericus is usually found, and causes experimental dysentery in animals. The infection is due to the toxins produced by this bacteria, which may have a pyogenic, dysenteric action. It is possible to render animals resistant to the two latter actions, but not to the former action, by repeated doses of the toxin.

Galli-Valerio[2] studied a series of cases of epidemic tropical dysentery at Valentina. In addition to the ameba coli, he found in the stools great numbers of short bacilli varying in length from 1 to $2\frac{1}{2}$ μ with rounded ends. They were motile, and, with the exception of failing to give the indol reaction, presented many of the characteristics of the bacterium coli communis. They were also pathogenic, producing signs of general infection in guinea-pigs, and dysentery in dogs, which identifies them with the bacilli coli dysenterica of Celli. He found that it was possible to produce immunity in a dog by repeated inoculation of the bacilli, and that the serum of this dog was able to protect a guinea-pig from their pathogenic action. He therefore supposes that ere long it will be possible to apply serumtherapy to human dysentery.

Masterman[3] reports a case of wandering edema and purpura that preceded an attack of dysentery. The parts affected by the edema were—first, the left leg, then the left arm, then the eyelids. Three days after the first attack purpuric patches appeared upon the edematous limbs. He regards the case as a sort of septic phlebitis, although the veins were not swollen nor tender.

Treatment.—Maberly[4] reports 90 cases of acute and 10 of chronic dysentery, treated with tincture of **monsonia,** a plant indigenous to South Africa. It acted promptly in all cases, relieving tenesmus in a short time, and, in general, causing a prompt cure without any tendency to relapse. One patient died of cancrum oris after the dysentery was cured, and in one a relapse occurred, but this case had been treated with an old tincture. The author believes, after a careful trial of both in tropical countries, that the drug he has introduced is more certain than ipecac and much less dangerous.

Lockwood[5] reports a case of amebic dysentery treated successfully with enemata of **quinin bisulphate.**

Diseases of the Peritoneum.—Alpago-Nevello,[6] in discussing the early **diagnosis of ascites,** suggests that the patient be put in the knee-elbow position, when the liquid accumulating anteriorly dulness can readily be detected about the umbilical region.

A. R. Edwards,[7] after pointing out that the determination of the existence of abdominal effusion is merely a preliminary to the diagnosis of ascites, offers the following scheme: (a) Is the accumulation due to a mechanical agency (increased pressure)? Is it then a hypostatic transudate? (b) Is it due to

[1] Annali d'igiene sperimentale, vol. vi., p. 204, 1896.
[2] Centralbl. f. Bakt. Parasit. u. Inf.'kr., Dec. 19, 1896.   [3] Brit. Med. Jour., Apr. 3, 1897.
[4] Lancet, Feb. 6, 1897.   [5] Mathew's Quarterly Jour., Apr., 1897.
[6] Gaz. Med. di Torrino, No. 21, 1896.   [7] Medicine, Oct., 1896.

increased permeation of the blood-vessel walls? Is it a cachectic hydrops? (c) Is it due to exudate—inflammation? (d) Is the cause some local peritoneal lesion other than inflammation? In the course of the further discussion he refers to the fact that in hepatic cirrhosis edema of the feet may antedate the ascites by an interval of months or even as much as a year and a half; and he cites a case in which there were swelling of the feet and dilated veins over the lower part of the abdomen and the legs without real jaundice, ascites, or splenic tumor. This has been explained by Thierfelder as only apparent, external edema being more easily discovered than the internal accumulation. Bamberger believes that the pars hepatica of the inferior cava is contracted by the shrinking of the liver. Other explanations are contraction of adhesions about the vena cava, pressure, etc. However, the author holds that, in the case cited by himself, none of these causes was operative, but that the great collateral circulation opened communications between the portal veins and the epigastric veins, by which the blood flowed from the liver to the crural veins and produced the edema of the limbs before marked ascites had developed.

Moneret has described an instance in which by the mechanism suggested an overfilled epigastric vein produced edema of the abdominal walls. Under the heading of cachectic ascites the author refers to 3 instances in which it existed in the convalescence of typhoid fever and in which peritonitis was excluded by the absence of all the usual indications. [He does not refer to the cachectic ascites sometimes seen in chronic malaria.] Under the heading of ascites due to diseases of the peritoneum other than peritonitis, he refers to new growths and to uterine fibromata and ovarian cysts.

Schramm[1] records a case of **chylous ascites** due to carcinoma of the thoracic duct. The patient, a woman of 53, came under observation early in Jan., 1896. She had begun to suffer with emaciation and weakness the previous summer; loss of appetite, with pressure after eating, appeared later. Pains in the back and abdomen and tympany developed shortly before her admission. There were great abdominal distention and liquid effusion, though the latter was apparently encysted, in the epigastric, umbilical, and hypogastric regions. The dulness was not movable. Incision into the abdomen showed the presence of marked whitish-yellow fluid, and the patient died within 48 hours. A hard nodular tumor the size of a fist was found at the head of the pancreas, and numerous secondary nodules were distributed in the neighborhood, involving the gall-bladder and liver. The thoracic duct throughout its entire course was thickened in places and at its upper termination was surrounded by enlarged lymphatic glands which compressed the adjacent veins. The duct was obliterated at various points, especially in the neighborhood of the nodules. No rupture was discovered, and the author concludes that the chyle escaped through the diseased walls. The only previously recorded case resembling this was one of Leidhecker's. This author, in addition, collected 5 instances of cancer of the duct without chylous ascites.

Codd[2] reports a case of chylous ascites that occurred in consequence of thrombosis of the left subclavian vein. The patient, a man of 35, suffered from a cardiac lesion and bronchitis. At the autopsy some 2.5 l. of a chyle-like liquid were found in the abdomen, and the upper portion of the ductus thoracicus was enormously dilated, its diameter being 7 mm. A partially organized thrombus was found in the subclavian vein.

Rotmann[3] describes a case of chylous ascites due to gastric carcinoma with compression of the thoracic duct, another case due to carcinoma of the du-

---

[1] Berlin. klin. Woch., Oct. 26, 1896.   [2] Brit. Med. Jour., May 1, 1897.
[3] Arch. f. Verdauungskrank., Bd. 1, p. 416.

odenum, and a case of chylous thorax due to tuberculosis. He has been able to collect 155 other cases from the literature, the majority of which occurred in the peritoneum. He does not regard the presence of sugar as of much value unless it exceeds 0.2 %, as this amount may be present in other exudates.

Obolenski[1] describes a case of **intraperitoneal adhesions** and refers to 20 similar instances recorded in the literature. The cause of the adhesions was gall-stone in 10, ulcer of the stomach in 6, traumatism in 2, swallowing of caustics in 1, and unknown in 1. In his own case the patient, aged 50, had been injured in the region of the stomach 8 years previously; 2 years after this he had suffered with pains over the stomach and became unable to attend to his work. He then improved, but subsequently relapsed. When the pain occurred a tumor developed in the region of the stomach, which disappeared with the pain. He was constipated, but did not suffer with nausea or vomiting. Food increased the pain. The stomach was somewhat increased in size and showed active peristaltic movements. The stomach-contents seemed normal. The absence of a distinct tumor and the normal condition of the secretions of the stomach excluded the diagnosis of cancer or hypertrophy of the pylorus. Operation was undertaken and firm adhesions between the lesser curvature of the stomach and the liver were discovered. Gastroenterostomy was performed and the patient recovered. Finally, the author cites as characteristic features of adhesions of this kind: (1) marked pain; (2) dilatation of the stomach when the pylorus is involved; (3) fixation of the organ at the point of attachment, this being determined by distention with air, by lavage, etc.; (4) normal physiologic properties of the stomach; (5) absence of tumor; (6) the history, pointing to some recognized cause; (7) the fruitlessness of treatment.

Adami[2] discusses 2 interesting cases of **peritoneal and retroperitoneal lipoma.** The first patient, a man of 45, noticed abdominal swelling in Jan., 1892. General emaciation began, but there was no other symptom. Aspiration failed to discover fluid. In May an incision was made and a solid uniform growth was found filling the entire abdomen. It could not be removed, and some time later a softened area developed, and on aspiration 9 pints of pus were removed, and until his death in Feb., 1893, 60 pints were aspirated at various times. There was never any disturbance of bowels and never any pain. Postmortem a large lobulated fatty tumor was found springing from the left renal region and filling the abdomen. The intestines were for the most part to the right of and behind the growth, the descending and transverse colon, however, being front of it. The tumor was easily removed with the left kidney and the spleen, both more or less completely imbedded. Sections showed the features of lipoma with mucous degeneration, and the author regarded it as a retroperitoneal growth. It weighed 41 pounds.

The second specimen is preserved in the Army Medical Museum. It occurred in a man of 60. The abdominal growth was first noted in Feb., 1869, and it increased until Feb., 1871, when the patient died after exposure. There was great emaciation, and the autopsy revealed a mass of irregular character everywhere attached to the abdominal walls, which were infiltrated and distended with serum. The liver, the stomach, and the intestines were compressed. The tumor weighed 41.5 pounds, and sprang from the left renal region, the kidney being flattened and partly imbedded. The descending colon, as in the other case, passed in front of the tumor. Microscopically this was found to

[1] Medicinskoje Obosrenje, No· 9, 1895; Centralbl. f. innere Med., Oct. 10, 1896.
[2] Montreal Med. Jour., Jan. and Feb., 1897.

be a fatty growth with embryonal connective tissue. The author points out that such tumors are rare. He has collected 42 cases from the literature. A large number originated in the region of one or other kidney. The condition is more common in women, and is as frequent on one as the other side. In 1 case it occurred 14 days after birth, but the most frequent age is from 30 to 50. The growth is slow, the average duration being 2 or 3 years from the first appearance until removal or death. Clinically it is of interest to note that the fluid character of the tumor often leads to the suspicion of ascites, and aspiration with negative results has frequently been recorded. In 26 of 42 cases the tumor was removed in part or entirely, with 12 recoveries.

DISEASES OF THE LIVER.

Cirrhosis.—Van Heukelom[1] does not believe that **alcohol** is the immediate cause of cirrhosis of the liver, but rather that it produces a chronic gastritis, as a result of which much fermentation occurs in the stomach and various poisons, among others fat acids, are produced. The resorption of these may possibly give rise to cirrhosis, especially in those that are predisposed to it.

Kelynack[2] found in 5053 pathologic cases 121 of pure hepatic cirrhosis, and of these 28 had also **tuberculous disease.** Doubtful or complicated cases, such as those of chronic heart-disease, were excluded; but it is not stated whether the subjects had been alcoholics or not.

Boix[3] describes the enlargement of the liver that is frequently found in dyspeptics who have the so-called arthritic diathesis. He believes it to be due to the formation in the gastrointestinal tract of substances that are, to a certain extent, toxic, and irritate the liver. These give rise to frequently repeated congestion, that finally becomes permanent, and constitutes **dyspeptic cirrhosis.**

Letulle[4] believes that alcoholic hypertrophic pigmentary cirrhosis should be classed with the similar forms occurring in diabetes, tuberculosis, malaria, etc.

Regaud[5] does not believe that the presence of **hemosiderin** in the liver in cirrhotic conditions is sufficient to justify the creation of an independent morbid condition. He reports, in support of his contention, 3 cases of cirrhosis, due to malaria, alcoholism, and infection, with abundant visceral siderosis.

Gilbert and Grenet[6] report a case of **pigmentary hypertrophic cirrhosis,** due to alcohol, occurring in a coachman of 49. Among the interesting symptoms were the dilatation of the cutaneous veins, frequent epistaxis, and purpuric blotches on the legs. The liver was greatly enlarged; the urine was slightly decreased in quantity, otherwise normal; but after urea had been used as a diuretic albumin appeared. There was moderate ascites, which in the later months of the sickness became very much augmented. At the autopsy the liver was found to weigh 2900 gm. It showed multiple lobular cirrhosis, the fibrous tissue originating from the periportal spaces and extraordinary proliferation of the biliary canals. The pigment was especially marked in the left lobe, and gave all the chemic reactions of iron.

Loeb[7] reports a case of **hypertrophic cirrhosis with icterus,** in

[1] Ziegler's Beiträge, vol. xx., section 2.   [2] Med. Chron., Jan., 1897.
[3] Bull. de l'Acad. de Méd., Oct. 27, 1897.   [4] Ibid., Feb. 7, 1897.
[5] Compt. rend. de la Soc. de Biol., Apr. 16, 1897.   [6] Ibid., Dec. 25, 1896.
[7] Deutsch. Arch. f. klin. Med., June, 1897.

which there were all the classical symptoms and a loud systolic aortic murmur. Death occurred 10 days after the development of severe symptoms, and at the autopsy the liver and spleen were found enlarged, and the cystic duct was obstructed by a gall-stone. The author explains the heart-murmur by the dilatation of the ventricles as a result of alcoholic myocarditis.

Pussinelli[1] reports the case of a man who suffered with mild jaundice in 1887. The following year increase of thirst was noted, and 1.5 to 2% of sugar appeared in the urine. Up to 1892 an annual visit to Carlsbad was followed by cessation of the glycosuria for some months. In 1893, after a shock, swelling of the abdomen and jaundice appeared, and later pronounced ascites, swelling of the feet, and enlargement of the liver and spleen. The abdomen was tapped several times, when the ascites disappeared. The jaundice and enlargement of the liver and spleen gradually diminished, but did not entirely disappear. Sugar and albumin were found in the urine before the ascites, but during its existence disappeared, to reappear 2 weeks after the last tapping. After 2½ years of fair health the patient died with anasarca and albuminuria. The autopsy showed widespread atheroma and sclerotic changes in the liver, especially in the portal areas. There were fresh tubercles in the peritoneum and pleura and recent tuberculosis of the lungs. The spleen was enlarged and the kidneys characteristic of diabetes. The author regards the liver-disease in such cases as a distinct affection. It is characterized by increase of size with little tendency to subsequent contraction, and accompanied by enlargement of the spleen and pigmentation of the skin.

J. M. DaCosta[2] reports a case of **acute yellow atrophy** of the liver. The patient, a young Italian of 16, was admitted to the hospital in a comatose condition, and died 2 hours later. He had lived an irregular life, was intemperate in alcohol and tobacco, and had recently acquired specific urethritis. He had attended the dispensary suffering with general abdominal distention and vomiting after food, constipation, and jaundice, the latter having appeared several days before his admission. On admission he was intensely jaundiced, and had severe dyspnea with convulsive movements and opisthotonos, and the pupils were dilated. The temperature was 102°, the urine was passed involuntarily, and some obtained postmortem was reddish in color, acid, and slightly albuminous. There were no tube-casts, but a crystal of tyrosin was found. The liver-dulness was diminished, though the margin could be felt below the ribs. The spleen was enlarged. There were some rales in the lungs. At the autopsy ecchymoses were found beneath the pericardium and in the mesentery, and small interstitial hemorrhages were found in the lungs. The gall-bladder was empty; the common duct patulous. The liver was small, weighing 28 ounces, and very flabby, its edge thin, and it exhibited yellow streaks, but the substance cut firmly. The brain was edematous, and a hemorrhage was found beneath the ependyma over the optic thalamus. The microscopic examination of the liver showed widespread fatty degeneration of advanced stage, apparently beginning in the periphery of the acini. The cells showed various forms of nuclear and protoplasmic destruction. In some places no traces of liver-substance remained, new connective tissue with round-cell infiltration taking the place. Miliary abscesses were found scattered throughout the connective tissue beneath the acini. There was a tendency to proliferation of the bile-ducts. The author states that he has found the disease rare in Philadelphia, this being the 5th case that he can recall. The disparity between the sexes is not so great as often stated. When persons have previously been addicted to alcohol the liver may be increased in size by ex-

[1] Berlin. klin. Woch., No. 33, 1896.   [2] Univ. Med. Mag., May, 1897.

cess of connective tissue, and thus show no appreciable diminution during the course of acute yellow atrophy, though there may actually be great destruction of liver-cells. Tyrosin is not a pathognomonic indication, but taken in connection with distinct symptoms of the disease it has great significance. Microbi and Raimaldi[1] have discovered virulent bacilli coli and streptococci in the liver and kidneys of a case of acute yellow atrophy of the liver. There were fresh inflammatory proliferations into the interlobular connective tissue, showing that the microorganisms had been present during life.

Clarede[2] reports an instance of **hepatic disease with great hyperthermia.** The patient had been exposed to the vapors of mineral acids. He was slightly icteric; the urine was diminished in quantity and contained albumin and an excess of nitrogenous matters. The stools were decolored and glairy, and the liver was enlarged and tender. The patient was extremely weak, cyanosed, and cold. The temperature was found to be 33.8° C. (92.8° F.). Subsequently it rose to 40° C. (104° F.) and the general condition improved, the urine became more copious, albumin disappeared, and after two months the patient was dismissed cured. The author ascribes the condition to hepatic changes resulting from intoxication with mineral acids.

S. Flexner[3] reports 2 cases of **perforation into the vena cava of amebic abscess of the liver.** The first patient (under the care of Osler) was a man of 51, admitted with chills, fever, and sweating. His illness began two months before, though he had experienced some chilly feelings and sweating 6 weeks previous to that. The liver was distinctly enlarged and tender. No amebæ were found in the stools. He was moderately anemic. An exploratory incision was made, but no abscess discovered. Later exploration through the lower intercostal spaces with needles discovered pus, and a second incision was made. The patient, however, died some days later. An abscess-cavity about 10 cm. in its greatest diameter was found in the liver, and communicated with the inferior cava, which contained a thrombus at the point of perforation. The intestines were free from ulceration, and only a suspicious, puckered area was discovered. The fresh abscess contained living amebæ and various bacteria. Small surrounding foci contained streptococci only. The second patient suffered with similar symptoms, but the liver was apparently not enlarged nor sensitive on deep pressure. The man, however, expectorated blood-tinged sputa of characteristic appearance, and on examination the breath-sounds in the right lung were impaired and there were rales. Amebæ were found in the sputa, as well as crystals supposed to be bilirubin. No amebæ could be discovered in the intestinal mucus. An incision was made into the lower part of the chest, and a large quantity of pus removed. Amebæ were found in the intestinal mucus, obtained with a tube several days after the operation, and 5 days later diarrhea set in and continued until death. At the autopsy a condition was discovered similar to that of the first case. The author calls attention to 2 points of interest: 1st, the existence of the amebic abscess of the liver without a distinct intestinal lesion; 2d, the probability that the intestinal lesion followed the disease of the liver in the second case rather than preceded it. [In the first case, if the intestines were not diseased, the mode of infection is obscure. The history of diarrhea during the previous summer was obtained from the patient after he had been in the hospital some time. It is true, no lesion was found in the second case, but it does not follow that the absence of symptoms excludes the existence of lesions prior to the discovery of the abscess. It is of more im-

[1] Arch. Ital. di Clin. Med., 1896, p. 1.   [2] Sem. méd., No. 35, 1896.
[3] Am. Jour. Med. Sci., May, 1897.

portance that the intestinal lesion had the appearance of acute development, and there is no doubt that, if the ulcer existed previously, it suffered an exacerbation just before death.]

Rendu[1] reports 2 cases of **abscess of the liver following tropical dysentery.** The second presented difficulties of diagnosis on account of the absence of fever and the excellent health of the patient. In fact, the tumor was supposed to be a hydatid cyst, until after the operation. Both abscesses were opened and drained with excellent results.

Roger[2] reports a case of a woman of 30 who came under observation with high fever and pain in the region of the left part of the liver. After several weeks' illness a fluctuating tumor appeared in the epigastrium. An operation was performed, but the patient died 8 days later. On examination several other abscesses were found in the right lobe and an old inflammatory focus in the pelvis. In this region as well as in the pus of the hepatic abscesses pure cultures of streptococcus were found.

C. von Kahlden[3] reports a case of **primary sarcoma** of the liver; the patient was a man 32 years of age, who 5 months before his death had noticed an increase in the size of the abdomen. This continued for 3 months without symptoms, when it was noticed that the feces were black and the urine dark. Later the abdomen increased still further in size and nodules could be felt that altered their position after eating. When admitted to the hospital he was found to have anasarca downward from the 8th rib and marked ascites. The skin showed a slight icteroid discoloration, the thorax was negative, the abdomen was enormously distended, and the hepatic dulness commenced at the upper border of the 5th rib; the lower edge of the liver was irregular and could be felt in the neighborhood of the umbilicus. The surface was rough, showing some hard and some rather soft elevations. Death occurred as a result of edema of the lungs. At the autopsy an enormously enlarged liver was found, that was covered with numerous small or confluent nodules, some white some yellowish in color. In the tissue that was still preserved the acini showed a retracted brown center and a swollen yellow periphery. Microscopically the tumor was found to be a round-celled sarcoma, that apparently sprang from the endothelium of the blood-vessels, although a number of small giant-cells were found with 4 or 5 nuclei. v. Kahlden does not care to call it a giant-cell sarcoma. He finds that the description he has given corresponds closely with the description given by Arnold of his 2 cases, although in these, as well as in the cases of Windrath, the color of the nodules was grayish-red and therefore more characteristic of sarcoma.

B. Bramwell and R. F. C. Leith[4] describe a case of **primary sarcoma** of the liver. The patient was a woman of 25, and presented certain signs pointing to abscess of the liver. The enlargement was considerable, especially in an upward direction. The heart was displaced to the left and upward, and there was tenderness on pressure in the 6th interspace and in the anterior axillary line. At this point the chest was aspirated and bloody liquid removed. A week later incision was made, and 1500 c.c. of blood removed. Death occurred from secondary hemorrhage and exhaustion a month after the first puncture. The liver was considerably enlarged and contained a cystic tumor of angiosarcomatous spindle-cell type. There were small cysts lined with endothelium. The growth had evidently sprung from the connective-tissue surrounding the perivascular lymphatic channels.

[1] Sem. méd., 1896, p. 285.
[2] Presse méd., 1896.
[3] Ziegler's Beiträge, vol. xxi., H. 2, 1897.
[4] Edinb. Med. Jour., Oct., 1896.

Pickler [1] reports a case that had a large liver with pain in the abdomen and delirium. The urine was dark red in color and on standing became darker. It contained some sugar, and upon the addition of Fe_2Cl_6 became black. There was some leukocytosis, many of the leukocytes containing pigment, and there was also some free pigment in the blood. A diagnosis of **melanotic sarcoma of the liver** was confirmed by the autopsy.

Chauffard [2] reports a case presenting a large fluctuating tumor of the liver. This was punctured and 10 c.c. of liquid withdrawn, immediately after which the patient was seized with convulsions and finally died in asphyxia. At the autopsy a **hydatid cyst** was found, it and the liver weighing together 6500 gm.; the liver itself weighed 2600 gm., and histologically showed similarity with the structure of the fetal liver, being compensatorily hypertrophied. All the other organs were normal, and the author is obliged to assume a sort of relative toxicity on the part of the fluid of the cyst, which, in some way, had been excited by the puncture and served to produce death.

Stefanile [3] records a case of **echinococcus cysts** of the liver, treated by the method of Baccelli. This consists of injection into the cyst of 20 c.c. of distilled water containing 0.02 gm. of corrosive sublimate after the withdrawal of 30 c.c. of the liquid. In his own case the volume of the tumor remained the same for about a week and there was moderate fever; then the temperature declined, and the tumor decreased in size, disappearing wholly within 25 or 28 days after the injection. Four months later there was no sign of the tumor or any other symptoms. The author refers to 7 similar cases. The successful results obtained by this method justify the belief that it should be practised in the treatment of echinococcus cysts before a formal operation is undertaken.

F. A. Packard [4] reports an instance of **movable liver** occurring in a man of 40. The patient had had acute rheumatism and typhoid fever. Later he complained of pain in the abdomen, especially in the region of the liver and gall-bladder, which was paroxysmal, always worse in the evening, and sometimes very severe. Five days after its onset he was slightly jaundiced. The stools became light-colored and the urine contained bile-pigment. There were slight fever and distention of the abdomen, and, on physical examination, the liver was found to extend from the upper border of the sixth rib to a point 9 or 10 cm. below the ridge, where the edge could be distinctly felt. There was no splenic enlargement or ascites. The lungs were decidedly emphysematous. Dulness was discovered posteriorly at the base of the chest, and it was suspected that it was caused by subdiaphragmatic abscesses. Operation was contemplated, but the patient died shortly afterward. At the autopsy it was discovered that the right pleural sac contained ½ pint of liquid without evidence of pleurisy. The liver weighed 610 gm., and was found in its normal position under the diaphragm, almost hidden by the costal cartilage; the discovery of a puncture in the convexity in the organ due to an attempt at aspiration during life, allowed it to be placed in the position occupied during life, and showed that this must have been abnormal. Unfortunately, the measurements of the ligaments of the liver, etc., were not obtained. The author cites cases in which the same condition was mistaken for hydronephrosis, typhlitis, and other conditions.

[1] Zeit. f. Heilk., Bd. 17, H. 2 and 3.   [2] Sem. méd., p. 265, 1896.
[3] Riforma Med., No. 76, 1896.   [4] Univ. Med. Mag., Jan., 1897.

DISEASES OF THE BILIARY PASSAGES.

Wm. Osler [1] discusses the **ball-valve gall-stone** in the common duct. His attention was first called to this condition by a patient in the Philadelphia Hospital, who had been admitted a number of times with chills, fever, and jaundice. The attacks had recurred for a period of about 2 years and various diagnoses had been made, such as malaria, hepatic abscess, etc. Finally a diagnosis was made of Charcot's hepatic intermittent fever, probably due to a gall-stone lodged in the common duct. An operation was performed, but no gall-stone was found, and death occurred from peritonitis a few days later. Just beneath the mucous membrane of the duodenum and close to the orifice of the common bile-duct a gall-stone was found which could be pushed to one side. The author subsequently saw 2 similar cases, upon 1 of which he was able to perform an autopsy and to obtain a similar specimen. The other is still suffering from recurrent attacks. Osler lays stress upon the valve-like folds of mucous membrane in the cystic and common duct and upon the sphincter at the orifice of the latter. The fever must bear an important relation to the impaction of the stone, either by reflex irritation or by preventing the escape of toxic ingredients. Of course, in making a diagnosis of this condition it is first necessary to recognize the existence of a stone in the common duct. The exacerbations of jaundice and fever, associated with intense pain, are due to the fact that a gall-stone lodged in the common duct and producing the symptoms in greater or less intensity during the interval, is pushed against the orifice, causing total occlusion. The symptoms, then, of this variety may be given as follows: chronic jaundice, rarely deep and varying in intensity, at times almost or entirely disappearing, to deepen invariably after a paroxysm (the icterus may be of maximum grade and associated with intolerable itching); pain, often a constant sense of discomfort, sometimes only obscure gastric distress, and at others agonizing, griping, and like ordinary liver colic; fever occurring in paroxysms usually preceded by chills and followed by sweats. The chills may be quotidian or tertian in type, or they may recur for weeks on the same day. The spleen is usually enlarged during the febrile paroxysms. Though persisting for months or even years, the general health may be little or not at all affected, and in the intervals between the paroxysms the patient may be able to work as usual. The differential diagnosis is to be made from malaria, abscess of the liver, and suppurative cholangeitis. He gives the records of 10 cases that he has personally seen. Of these, 5 made perfect recovery, 3 died, 1 disappeared, and 1 is still under observation. Treatment may be employed, but Osler does not believe that it is possible to dissolve the stone either with olive oil or sodium phosphate. Surgical interference may be employed and occasionally complete relief may be obtained. As the stone is usually just beneath the mucous membrane of the duodenum it could probably be reached more readily through this organ.

Raimond and Taitout [2] report the case of a patient who at the age of 30 was admitted to the hospital for repeated attacks of **biliary colic** that had commenced after an attack of typhoid fever, 6 years before. The Widal reaction was negative and operation was performed, at which 6 gall-stones were removed. Cultures from the pus of the gall-bladder were found to contain nothing but the bacillus of Eherth. The author did not attempt to explain the absence of the Widal reaction, but maintained that the lithiasis is probably due directly to infection of the biliary tract.

[1] Lancet, May 15, 1897.
[2] Compt. rend. de la Soc. de Biol., Jan. 1, 1896.

Vissering[1] describes a case in which a **gall-stone was discharged through the lung.** There was probably, in the first place, empyema of the gall-bladder following impaction of a stone in the cystic duct. Attachment to the diaphragm occurred and subsequently perforation in the right pleura, then perforation into the lung with abscess-formation, and finally discharge of pus, bile, and gall-stone through the bronchus.

Gilbert, Fournier, and Oudin[2] have skiagraphed biliary calculi and find that those composed of cholesterin produce very faint shadows; those rich in pigment appear darker; nevertheless the results obtained by this method are very doubtful. [Our own experiments coincide with those here referred to.]

Dunin[3] has employed **potassium iodid** in the treatment of biliary colic and has found it very useful in 100 cases. It acts most favorably in instances in which the frequency rather than the severity of the attacks is the important feature; it is especially useful, also, in subjects exhausted by loss of sleep, anorexia, and the use of narcotics. He advises the administration of KI and Carlsbad water. He is in doubt whether it favors the solution of the stone or relaxes the gall-ducts and thus facilitate its expulsion.

Thompson[4] suggests the regular administration of **sodium phosphate** during the intervals of cholelithiasis.

DISEASES OF THE SPLEEN.

Bonardi[5] records the case of a woman in whom **splenectomy** was performed. The patient had been under observation 7 years previously with some enlargement of the spleen, but refused operation. Four years later she suffered with anemia, diarrhea, albuminuria, and had a mitral systolic murmur. There was no alteration in the liver and no ascites. She came under observation again in 1896, complaining of further swelling of the abdomen from ascites, and examination of the blood showed considerable anemia. The urine was highly colored, but contained little urea. The patient improved under a milk-diet and the administration of urea, but paracentesis was finally performed and repeated 12 times, the last fluid being milky, albuminous, sp. gr. 1021, and rich in disintegrated white blood-corpuscles. There was no history of malaria or syphilis, and no abuse of alcohol or food, but the woman had suffered for many years from pellagra.

J. Bland Sutton[6] discusses **wandering spleens** and adds some remarks on splenectomy. Considering the effect of wandering spleen, he shows that the movable organ is liable to congestion, especially when the pedicle is rotated. Complete torsion may lead to atrophy. Traction of the organ upon surrounding structures may be injurious; and among the dangers to life he notices rupture of the stomach or duodenum, intestinal obstruction, and rupture of the spleen itself. He refers to 2 cases in which tumors springing from the pelvis were mistaken for this condition. He has failed to find any evil effect from splenectomy. Patients suffering with wandering spleen are apt to be thin and gaunt, and he has found that this condition persists after the operation.

In discussing the paper Ballance said that one of his cases became extremely emaciated after operation and the blood become considerably impoverished, the leukocytes at the same time being increased. In other cases, too, he has found deterioration of health.

[1] Münch. med. Woch., No. 24, 1896.   [2] Compt. rend. de la Soc. de Biol., May 28, 1897.
[3] Therap. Woch., July 19, 1896.   [4] Med. News, Apr. 24, 1897.
[5] Gaz. degli Osped. e delle Clin., Jan. 3, 1897.
[6] Brit. Med. Jour., Jan. 16, 1897.

DISEASES OF THE PANCREAS.

Simon[1] reports 3 cases of **acute pancreatitis**. The first 2 occurred in stout, middle-aged men, both of whom presented a picture of acute intestinal obstruction with severe abdominal pain. As there was slight icterus but no distention of the abdomen, diagnosis was made of gall-stone impacted in the jejunum. Laparotomy was performed, and at the autopsy both cases presented the signs of severe gastrointestinal catarrh. The head of the pancreas was swollen, softened, and contained fatty exudate. The third case occurred in an elderly woman who was brought into the hospital on the 5th day of the disease, with distention of the abdomen and vomiting. Laparotomy was performed without result, and at the autopsy severe duodenitis with swelling of the pancreas and hemorrhage into the tissues was found. In all 3 cases the bacilli coli communis and an unknown thread-like bacillus were found. As the pancreas was unaffected, the author believes that the infection must have reached it from the intestinal tract.

W. Cayley[2] lectured upon a case of acute pancreatitis. During the first 2 days there were epigastric pains and constipation, then vomiting, and on the 4th day death in collapse. At the autopsy there were fat-necrosis in the abdomen and some sanguinoserous liquid in the peritoneal cavity. The pancreas was enlarged, the lobuli pale red, and the cells in a condition of coagulation-necrosis.

Allina[3] reports a case that was brought into the hospital suffering from severe cramp-like pains in the abdomen, which had been increasing for several days. There had been some vomiting and obstinate constipation. For over a year previous to admission the patient had suffered at frequent intervals from similar attacks. The abdomen was distended and tympanitic with some tenderness just below the umbilicus. In the urine neither sugar, indican, nor albumin was found. In the belief that the condition was one of typhlitis laparotomy was performed, but there were no symptoms whatever of inflammation. On the next day death occurred, and at the autopsy the pancreas was found to be necrosed and hemorrhagic, and there was slight diffuse hemorrhagic peritonitis.

A. C. Hovenden (1)[4] and Stanley (3)[5] report 4 cases of acute pancreatitis. The disease in all cases commenced with severe pain in the umbilical region, vomiting, obstinate constipation, and, toward the end, collapse. At the autopsy the pancreas was found to be increased in size, softened, and reddish, with more or less fat-necrosis in the neighborhood. [It is probable that this disease is much more common than mortality statistics would indicate, the majority of cases being diagnosed as acute intestinal obstruction. In a case that we observed an antemortem diagnosis was made from the fact that the feces were dark and contained a considerable amount of fat; unfortunately, however, the obstinate constipation usually renders this very suggestive symptom unavailable.]

M. MacIntosh[6] reports a case of **glycosuria** for which no adequate cause could be found, but which was evidently associated with considerable gastrointestinal disturbance. At the autopsy it was found that the pancreas had been almost entirely destroyed by a large suppurating cyst.

Chiari[7] discusses the **lesions discoverable postmortem** in the pan-

[1] Lancet, May 15, 1897.
[3] Wien. klin. Woch., Nov. 5, 1896.
[5] Ibid., May 15, 1897.
[2] Brit. Med. Jour., July 4, 1897.
[4] Lancet, Jan. 9, 1897.
[6] Ibid., Oct. 24, 1896.
[7] Zeit. f. Heilk., 1896, Bd. 16, p. 70.

creas. He observed 2 cases in which circumscribed necrotic foci were discovered that were not apparently dependent upon vascular disease or disseminated pancreatitis, and in which bacilli could not be found. In both there were evidences of reactive changes around the necrotic areas, showing that the process must have begun some time before death. He therefore examined the organ in 75 cases, and found in 11 total necrosis of connective tissue, the protoplasm of the cells being homogeneous and the nuclei staining poorly or not at all; in 29 cases there was disseminated necrosis of the acini and connective tissues; in the remaining cases (35) there was no necrosis. He assumes that the condition is one of autointoxication, as neither decomposition nor previous disease could be adduced as the cause.

E. R. Maxon [1] describes the symptoms of **pancreatic carcinoma** as follows: profound cachexia, anorexia, fatty alvine evacuations, and abdominal pains that may extend from the region of the pancreas to the right shoulder.

W. H. White [2] reports 2 cases of **carcinoma of the pancreas.** The first case was extremely cachectic and when examined under anesthesia a hard lump could be felt in the abdominal wall on the right side about on a level with the umbilicus. Secondary nodules rapidly developed and the patient died. At the autopsy a large scirrhus was found occupying almost the whole of the tail of the pancreas. The second patient was brought to the hospital in a state of collapse, vomited blood occasionally, and soon died. At the autopsy a hard, solid carcinomatous growth was found occupying the middle of the pancreas. Neither patient showed any traces of abdominal fat-necrosis.

Picoli [3] reports 2 cases of **sarcoma of the pancreas.** The first patient was a peasant 54 years of age. He had had malaria and was an alcoholic. Four years before his death he was injured in the right hypochondriac region; this was followed by stabbing pains in the region of the liver that were repeated at intervals of 5 or 6 months; 2½ years after this injury he became slightly jaundiced, and this became more and more pronounced at the same time that the pains grew more severe and emaciation gradually developed. Upon admission he was found jaundiced and emaciated, but his digestive functions were apparently intact. The liver and spleen were both slightly enlarged, and there was general enlargement of the lymph-glands. The feces were clay-colored, offensive, and contained a considerable quantity of fat. The urine contained bile-pigment. The psychical functions appeared to be somewhat affected. Later there was some ascites. The cachexia progressed and ultimately terminated in death. At the autopsy a neoplasm was found, which seemed to invade the hilum of the liver, the head of the pancreas, and a portion of the duodenum. Upon section the surface appeared to be grayish, smooth, and homogeneous. Histologically, however, the tumor resembled in most of its characteristics a sarcoma rather than carcinoma. The jaundice was apparently explained by the metastatic mass that had invaded the papilla of Vater and partially occluded the opening of the common bile-duct. The second case was in a laborer, 48 years of age, who had been in excellent health until 3 months before his death, when he suddenly felt severe, stabbing pains in the region of the liver, had anorexia, obstinate constipation, and emaciation. Three weeks later he began to vomit everything, and from time to time there was severe hematemesis. Upon admission it was found that the liver and spleen were considerably enlarged, that there was ascites, and that the liver was exquisitely sensitive. The digestive functions of the stomach were very imperfect. The blood showed marked leukocytosis

[1] N. Y. Med. Jour., Jan. 16, 1897.   [2] Lancet, Sept. 26, 1896.
[3] Ziegler's Beiträge, vol. 21, H. 1, 1897.

(25,000). The cachexia progressed steadily and finally terminated in death. At the autopsy the liver was found to be enlarged and to contain numerous round white nodules. In the pancreas were also several small nodules that appeared to be similar to those in the liver. Histologically it was found that the hepatic neoplasm consisted of a small round-celled sarcoma, and the pancreatic neoplasm, on the other hand, of a giant-celled sarcoma. The author is inclined to regard the growth in the liver as primary, although he admits that a definite decision upon the question is probably impossible. An interesting feature of the cases was the metastasis to the neighboring lymph-glands, particularly in the second case, where this metastasis evidently came from the pancreas on account of the presence of giant cells.

Linossier [1] has investigated the **effect of the presence of HCl upon pancreatic digestion.** He finds that pancreatin is destroyed in 20 seconds when exposed to a solution of 1 : 1000, and if the exposure is continued for a few seconds longer trypsin is also destroyed. As a result therefore of hyperacidity there is often rapid emaciation of the patients. This, however, may be prevented providing there is copious secretion of bile or the pancreatic juice itself is abnormally alkaline. There are therefore 2 classes of cases suffering from hyperacidity: those in which intestinal alkalinity is sufficient or but slightly affected ; and those in which it is insufficient, causing disturbance of intestinal digestion and ultimately profound cachexia.

Zeehuisen [2] has investigated the **digestive activity of various fluids** obtained from cysts or other sources. Among his results are the following : diastatic ferments could be determined in most cases ; no trypsin action was found in the transudates, rich in albumin, in the exudates and cystic liquids, nor in any cyst-contents, poor in albumin, though these liquids easily underwent putrefaction on account of their alkaline reaction. The addition of a few drops of a one-half normal sodium hydrate solution causes no digestive power. Some specimens of urine showed trypsin action after addition of a little alkali, others peptic action after addition of HCl ; still others were negative. Sterilization of the fibrin used to determine the digestive action influences the results very much. These experiments are of value mainly as showing that the discovery of digestive ferments in a liquid should not lead to hasty conclusions in regard to its source. The positive discovery of an emulsifying ferment is conclusive of a pancreatic cyst ; but its absence does not exclude this condition, neither does the absence of trypsin exclude pancreatic cysts, though its presence supports the diagnosis. Diastatic activity is of no significance.

DISORDERS OF THE URINE AND KIDNEY.

Franz [3] experimented on the urine and the urethral secretion in reference to the presence of **bacteria.** In 41 cases the urethral secretion was investigated ; in 21 with positive results and in 13 with negative results. In 52 cases the urine was examined ; in 21 with positive and in 31 with negative results. The patients were selected with reference to their health and general normal condition. The organisms found were chiefly cocci of various kinds, although in one case the bacterium coli was present and in another sarcina alba. His conclusion is that the urethra normally contains bacteria, and all the bacteria found in the urine originate from the urethra ; and, therefore, that any method of bacteriologic investigation of the urine without catheter-

[1] Compt. rend. de la Soc. de Biol., May 7, 1897.
[2] Centralbl. f. innere Med., Oct. 3, 1896.　　[3] Wien. klin. Woch., July 9, 1896.

ization is absolutely worthless. In only 2 cases were organisms found in the urine that were not found in the urethral secretion ; in 1 the bacterium coli, and in the other, a case of myocarditis with passive congestion, streptococci.

Chvostek[1] has utilized the suggestion of Franz and examined the urine bacteriologically in a number of cases, always using the catheter and taking every precaution to prevent accidental contamination. In general results were negative. Whenever, however, fever existed, no matter of what nature, microorganisms were found. In 2 cases the fever was malarial ; in 4 others it was artificially produced by injection of tuberculin. The organism usually found was the staphylococcus albus. It does not seem reasonable to suppose that the fever had rendered the urethra a more favorable culture-bed, so that the possibility of its entrance into the bladder was more likely, but rather that in the febrile state microorganisms remaining latent in the system enter the blood and are excreted by the kidneys. As, however, the organisms found have nothing to do with the fever in any of these cases, it does not seem possible to utilize these investigations for the purpose of determining the etiology of a morbid condition, and that only the recognition of a specific organism, such as that of typhoid fever or tuberculosis, would render it possible to draw any conclusions regarding the nature of the disease, staphylococci appearing to be merely a temporary occurrence in the course of various infectious diseases.

Bunge and Trautenroth[2] have studied the **smegma-bacillus** with special reference to its occurrence in different parts of the body and its distinction from the tubercle-bacillus. Though the occupant particularly of the genito-urinary mucous membranes, it may occur on any part of the surface of the body, wherever sebaceous secretion exists, and has also been found in the mouth, nose, and other mucous cavities. The diagnosis of tuberculosis of these parts must therefore be made with knowledge of this fact, and only after the smegma-bacillus has been excluded. The method of staining they have found most useful is the following : the specimens are spread upon cover-glasses, fixed, and deprived of their fat by extraction with absolute alcohol for at least 3 hours ; then placed in 5% chromic acid solution for 15 minutes ; washed with water, stained in carbol-fuchsin, and decolorized with dilute sulphuric acid solution (3 minutes) and pure nitric acid (1 to 2 minutes) and further by concentrated alcoholic solution of methylen-blue for 5 minutes. This solution decolorizes and counterstains coincidently. This method insures the decolorization of the smegma-bacilli and does not affect the tubercle-bacilli. [We have convinced ourselves that the smegma-bacillus is not always so readily decolorized as the authors contend. There is, however, even in well-stained specimens, a certain difference of appearance from the tubercle-bacillus (the smegma-bacillus is longer, narrower, and stained more yellowish) that may sometimes lead to a suspicion of its nature.]

May[3] reports a case of transverse myelitis occurring in a boy of 16 years. Examination of the urine showed the presence of **dextrose,** and examination with the polarimeter led to the suspicion that **levulose** was also present. A careful chemical examination confirmed this idea, and May states that the following characteristics are sufficient to identify the substance : deviation of the light to the left ; reduction of the metaloxids ; fermentability with yeast-cultures with the formation of alcohol and carbon dioxid ; and formation of phenyldextrosazon. Although dextrose and levulose were excreted by this patient, May is confident that both substances simply pass through the kidneys as such, and that one is not to be looked upon as a derivative of the

---

[1] Wien. klin. Woch., July 23, 1896.   [2] Fortschr. d. Med., Dec. 15, 1896.
[3] Deutsch. Arch. f. klin. Med., vol. lvii., sec. 3 and 4.

other, either as a result of the action of the renal epithelium or of the micro-organisms that might be present in the course of a cystitis, such as existed in the present case.

F. W. Pavy [1] reports a case of **lactosuria** occurring in a woman suffering from slight digestive troubles, who was weaning her child without artificial removal of the milk. Within 2 months lactose had entirely disappeared from the urine even when the patient was given a diet particularly rich in carbohydrates.

McCann [2] has examined the urine of 100 nursing-women and found **lactose** present in all.

Rumpf [3] found that in a series of cases of febrile infectious diseases the amount of **ammonia** was regularly excessive irrespective of the diet. The increased excretion does not come on suddenly, often, indeed, only after some time, and in some cases persists and is particularly notable during convalescence. He estimates the amount of ammonium nitrogen as compared to the total nitrogen in health at 4.87%, and in febrile conditions at 6.7%. Hallervorden [4] also considers this subject, but entirely from a physiological and pathological point of view.

Pfeiffer [5] mentions a patient with gout who, in the course of the disease, had a severe attack of colic, associated with the presence of an enormous quantity of **cystin** in the urine. This was interesting because Baumann was unable to find any diamine in the urine, and he believes that it indicates that they need not invariably occur simultaneously. Two brothers of the patient suffered frequently from renal colic. The urine of his son gave an abundant precipitate of cystin upon addition of acetic acid; the urine of his daughter was negative.

Stange [6] reports a case of **alcaptonuria** that occurred in a young man of 18 years of age. It was noticed that his urine, upon standing, assumed a dark-brown color, and that it contained a substance that reduced copper, but did not ferment in the presence of yeast. The only subjective symptom was extreme dysuria during the period of this attack. His mother reported that when a child he had had a similar attack. The urine contained a small quantity of mucus, a few crystals of uric acid, and numerous crystals of calcium oxalate. Further investigations showed that the reducing substance corresponded very closely to the homogentisic acid, and it was found that the best method of obtaining it in a relatively pure state was to agitate the urine with an equal quantity of ether, which was then separated and distilled, leaving in the bottom of the beaker a dark-brown crystalline mass; this was then further purified, and, finally, a clear, white, needle-like substance obtained. The daily quantity was found to average 5.9 gr., with frequent periods of increase, which could be brought on by giving the patient an exclusive meat-diet. Purgatives had no effect in diminishing the quantity. Stange suggests, although, as he admits, without sufficient clinical warrant, that it is a case of intermittent alcaptonuria. The case differs from those previously reported in the fact that the urine always gave an acid reaction which did not disappear upon long exposure to the air.

Nakarai [7] has examined 250 specimens of urine from 144 patients suffering from 39 different diseases, for the presence of **hematoporphyrin,** using the method of Salkowski. It was found in only 10 cases, 6 suffering from chronic

[1] Lancet, Apr. 17, 1897.
[2] Ibid., Apr. 24, 1897.
[3] Virchow's Archiv, Bd. 143, p. 1.
[4] Ibid., p. 705.
[5] Centr. f. d. krankh. d. Harn. u. Sex. Org., vol. 8, H. 14.
[6] Virchow's Archiv, Oct. 10, 1896.
[7] Deutsch. Arch. f. klin. Med., Mar. 15, 1897.

lead-poisoning, 2 from intestinal tuberculosis with hemorrhage, 1 from rheumatism, and 1 a case of empyema that had used sulphonal for a considerable time. He reaches the following conclusions : that hematoporphyrinuria is a constant symptom in various forms of lead-intoxication, and occurs also in poisoning with sulphonal and sometimes after intestinal hemorrhage, but is in general rare in other diseased conditions.

Strauss[1] finds that 50 gm. per day of Liebig's beef-extract, whilst not producing any subjective symptoms whatever, increase elimination of **uric acid and the alloxur bodies** very considerably, but this increase probably merely represents the excess contained in the extract itself.

Klein[2] reports a case of **fibrinuria** that occurred in a man 52 years of age suffering from nephritis. About a week after admission the urine presented an extraordinary appearance, being filled with white or whitish-gray coagula of various sizes from 1 to 10 cm. in length. In some specimens when the urine was allowed to stand it gradually coagulated, as if it were an ordinary serous fluid. These threads consisted of pure fibrin. The urine showed remarkable decrease in the phosphates, the presence of considerable albumin and globulin, and an alkaline reaction. Regarding the causation of the condition Klein has but little to suggest definitely, although he believes that the factors favoring it were the alkaline reaction of the urine, the large amount of albumin present, and perhaps the diminution of the phosphates during the period when fibrin was present. An interesting feature of the disease was the occurrence of chill and fever in several paroxysms of fibrinuria. After a period of improvement the chills recurred with increasing frequency. Edema and oliguria occurred, followed by death. At the autopsy the kidneys exhibited extreme amyloid degeneration, although it is not stated how this could have had anything to do with the fibrinuria. In addition there was an acute fibrous pericarditis and a tubercular ulcer in the ileum. In the same paper Klein also reports a case of cystitis in the course of which long, fibrous-like threads appeared in the urine which gave the xanthoprotein and biuret reactions, but were not digested by pepsin and free HCl, and were therefore regarded as consisting of a central coagulum of nucleo-albumin surrounded by mucin.

Klemperer[3] distinguishes 2 groups of **renal hemorrhage**: (1) Acute hemorrhage following overexertion, first referred to by Leyden. Klemperer has observed 2 cases. The first was an officer of nearly 50, who had become fatigued by a long horseback-ride, and at the end of this had difficulty in passing urine, which was found to be of a dark-red or black color. The symptom disappeared the next day, and the patient has remained well ever since. The other case was of similar character. (2) Chronic renal hemorrhages, of which he distinguishes renal hemophilia and angioneurotic hemorrhages, constitute the second group. Of the first variety he states that no case has been reported since Senator's. He himself has observed 2 in the clinic of Leyden. The first occurred in a patient whose history pointed to undoubted hemophilia. After a period of several years of freedom the patient had an attack lasting 7 weeks. In the 2d case the hemorrhages had existed during 16 years, and the patient suffered with pain in the region of the right kidney of longer or shorter duration. The existence of casts showed that the hemorrhage was of renal origin in both cases. The use of tepid baths with cold effusions relieved both. Of the angioneurotic form the author has seen 2 cases, the first in a young man of 22, of neuropathic ten-

---

[1] Berlin. klin. Woch., Aug. 10, 1896.   [2] Wien. klin. Woch., July 30, 1896.
[3] Berlin. klin. Woch., Dec. 7, 1896.

dency, in whom the hemorrhage was found, by cystoscopic examination, to come from the left kidney. After nephrectomy there was immediate recovery. The kidney was normal. During the last 7 months he has observed a second case in a nervous man of 37, who suffered with mitral regurgitation, without any evidence that this bore a distinct relation to the renal hemorrhage. For 8 weeks hemorrhage from the kidney had existed, and hydriatic treatment carried on for 3 weeks led to recovery. In the discussion Leyden referred to a further case of hemorrhage after exertion. Mendelsohn referred to 3 cases, in 2 of which traumatism over the kidney was the cause, while in the 3d the excretion of abundant oxalates seemed to indicate another factor. Nitze spoke of 7 cases, all of which were operated on, 5 of them by himself. In 4 the kidney was removed, and in 3 merely an incision was made to the kidney. He holds that renal hemophilia must be carefully distinguished from essential hematuria. The former is only one expression of hemophilia; the latter is a local condition, and must be distinguished from tumors and other local diseases. Senator held that the condition described by him is not merely renal hemorrhage in the course of general hemophilia, but rather a condition of hematuria on the basis of hemophilia without other hemorrhages. He has observed a number of cases of hemorrhage after excessive exertion, and he suggests the following classification : 1, renal hemophilia; 2, essential hematuria ; 3, nephralgie hématurique.

F. R. Ecoles[1] reports 8 cases of **hematuria.** He states that if the bleeding is from the urethra it may ooze between the periods of micturition ; if from the neck of the bladder, it is more particularly noticed at the end of micturition ; if from the bladder, it is usually very abundant, persistent, and more likely to clot, and accompanied by bladder irritability ; if from the kidney, the blood is generally mixed with the urine, although, if the quantity is large, characteristic urethral clots may be found. Of the cases he reports, he believes the 1st and 2d were malignant, the 3d certainly tuberculous, as the urine injected into a rabbit's eye produced characteristic tubercles, and the remainder malarial, although the blood was not examined for the parasite, because in all of these cases quinin produced complete cure. Krauss[2] reports a case of hematuria, at first paroxysmal and later more constant. Frequently fibrous clots were present, and often the first portion of the urine was more deeply colored than the later portion. An operation showed that the condition was caused by numerous small hemorrhoids in the prostatic portion of the urethra.

Klemperer[3] reports 2 cases of **hemoglobinuria.** The first, a man of 28, became suddenly ill with jaundice and hemoglobinuria. The latter lasted 3 days, then the urine became normal. Jaundice and distinct swelling of the spleen continued for 7 days longer and the aspect of the case in general was that of an acute infection. No microorganisms could be found in the blood ; but the patient had eaten blood-sausage the evening before his illness and it is not unlikely that intoxication occurred in this way. The second case occurred in the course of typhoid fever. The patient complained of heat and cold and presented an urticarial eruption.

A. E. Isaacs[4] reports a case of recurrent icteric hemoglobinuria. The attacks commenced with a chill, then vomiting, and, finally, about 24 hours later the development of icterus and passage of dark urine. When the latter was examined by the spectroscope it showed the bands of oxyhemoglobin. Bile was not present. The urine contained a large amount of albumin. No cause is assigned. G. B.

[1] Brit. Med. Jour., June 5, 1897.   [2] Wien. klin. Woch., July 9, 1896.
[3] Charité Annalen, 20, p. 131.   [4] Brit. Med. Jour., Nov. 14, 1896.

14

Sweet[1] reports a case of paroxysmal hemoglobinuria which was apparently caused by sudden exposure to cold water in bathing, and which subsequent examination showed, in his opinion, to be due to cold, as the blood of a ligated finger which had been exposed to freezing was greatly disintegrated and not unlike that found in the urine. The case, however, improved permanently upon the administration of 15 gr. of quinin combined with calcium chlorid, 3 times daily.

Gillespie[2] believes that **albumosuria** is to be explained by excessive production and correspondingly excessive destruction of leukocytes. He supports his theory by the results of his investigations of 2 cases suffering from gout.

Chvostek and Stromayer[3] have extended the observations of Maixner regarding **albumoses in the urine** in cases of gastrointestinal disease. They administered a midday meal of 1 or 2 oz. of "peptone" or somatose, given in warm water or broth, to patients without albuminuria suspected of suffering from gastric or intestinal ulceration. The urine was examined at intervals of 2 or 3 hours for albumose by Devoto's method. In 6 of 9 cases albumosuria to a greater or less extent developed. In these cases, though the symptoms varied greatly, tuberculous ulcers of the intestines were found postmortem. In 3 cases in which similar ulcers existed albumosuria could not be produced, perhaps on account of vomiting or other causes. In 20 individuals without disease of the alimentary tract the administration of these foods failed to cause albumosuria. They conclude that it is impossible in persons whose intestinal tract is normal to produce this symptom, but that a negative result of the test does not exclude ulceration.

Adolph Ott[4] tested 270 specimens of urine in healthy and diseased persons for the presence of **nucleo-albumin,** and obtained cloudiness or precipitate in every case with Almen's solution of tannin. This reaction was not influenced by the degree of acidity of the urine; but in cases of fever, particularly when severe, the amount of these bodies seemed to be increased. At the commencement of febrile albuminurias he was able to note that only nucleo-albumin was present.

Arnozen[5] discusses **cyclic albuminuria** and some allied forms of disease. The nature of the former he believes is that of mild nephritis, which may lead to chronic Bright's disease and uremia, or may terminate favorably, this being the more apt to occur. He then refers to the following: 1, minimal albuminuria—a form in which the quantity of albumin is very small—the nature of this may be very diverse, it has only a clinical importance, and is probably not a pathological quantity; 2, the albuminuria of adolescence; 3, residual albuminuria, a form in which after an attack of nephritis a small amount of albumin may persist; 4, partial albuminuria (albuminurie parcellaire), in which it is assumed that only certain tubules are affected; 5, cicatricial albuminuria—a form described by Bard—in which epithelial desquamation is assumed to be replaced by tissue incapable of restraining the transudation of albumin from the blood; 6, phosphatic albuminuria, in which phosphaturia accompanies the albuminuria.

Kast and Weiss[6] discuss cyclical albuminuria or Pavy's disease, which usually occurs in young subjects. A type somewhat similar to this, but actually very different, is intermittent albuminuria. It is frequently complicated with asthmatic or convulsive attacks, or else is due to malaria. Other types

[1] New Zealand Med. Jour., Oct., 1896.   [2] Lancet, July 6, 1897.
[3] Wien. klin. Woch., No. 47, 1896.   [4] Zeit. f. Heilk., Bd. 16, p. 177.
[5] Gaz. hebdom. de Méd. et de Chir., Aug. 23, 1896.   [6] Berlin. klin. Woch., No. 28, 1896.

of albuminurias are those called albuminuriæ minimæ: of these there are 2 forms. In the first the albumin is constant—that is to say, it is not altered by diet. The other is easily altered by various conditions, such as cold and fatigue.

Albu[1] has invariably found albumin in the urine after long, severe bicycle tours. He is inclined to consider this condition as the result of toxemia rather than of venous congestion, and he is strengthened in this belief by the increased amount of uric acid in the urine and the presence of tube-casts. This albuminuria disappears usually very rapidly.

Halamon[2] discusses the **prognosis of albuminuria,** and considers that it is unfavorable when there is permanent polyuria with considerable albumin; when there is marked diminution in the quantity of urine excreted, whilst the quantity of albumin remains about the same; if the patient is young and shows cardiac hypertrophy and arterial sclerosis, the prognosis is also grave. Albuminuria occurring in the course of other diseases is not always of much significance. If in the course of heart-disease, it is only serious when it persists after compensation has been reestablished. In fever and diabetes, if transient, it is not of grave import.

Nephritis—Etiology.—Macaigue[3] divides **nephritis** due to the **bacillus coli** into 2 groups: (1) that in which infection is from below, and (2) that in which the infection is through the blood, the kidney being affected by "descending nephritis." From the latter he excludes cases in which the bacilli are in the urine merely as a sign of general coli infection, and not as a result of nephritis as the principal condition. He describes 3 cases of descending nephritis of this kind, and notes that autoinfection requires 2 conditions: (1) a breach in the alimentary canal; (2) increased virulence of the bacillus. Diarrhea causes both. The microorganism may enter through any part of the intestinal tract. In one of his cases sore throat was the preliminary lesion. There may be either signs of the ordinary epithelial nephritis with more or less grave symptoms, and with a tendency usually to recover, or suppurative nephritis with pyuria, fever, etc., and more grave prognosis. [The possibility of bacillus coli infection through the mouth would seem to require further proof.]

Pedenko[4] reports a case of acute **nephritis following an infected wound.** The patient, a young man of 20, had a felon on one finger which was not opened until suppuration had extended to the bone. General edema, dyspnea, headache, and great weakness had occurred some days previously. Three weeks after the infection the staphylococcus albus was found in the urine, and the same organism with the aureus and bacilli was found in the pus. As the wound improved the condition of the urine grew better, and finally the bacteria disappeared.

Ebstein and Nicolaier[5] have found that the administration to animals of uric acid, dissolved in alkalies or piperazin, caused severe parenchymatous changes in the kidneys, and a peculiar necrosis of the epithelium of the convoluted tubules and of Henle's loops. They found frequently spheroliths, which dissolved in acids with a production of urates and left an organic remnant. These are, no doubt, derived from cells; they become free when the cells undergo destruction, and are sometimes found abundantly in the urine of animals.

J. J. Thomas[6] calls attention to the frequency with which blood or **albumin**

[1] Berlin. klin. Woch., Mar. 8, 1897.   [2] L'Union méd., No. 36, 1896.
[3] Arch. gén. de Méd., Dec.. 1896.   [4] Presse méd., Dec. 19, 1896.
[5] Virchow's Archiv, Bd. 43, H. 2.   [6] Boston M. and S. Jour., Sept. 3, 1896.

or both have been found in the urine in cases of **infantile scurvy.** Sometimes the disease of the kidneys seems to be the principal disorder. The author then reports a case in which the kidney symptoms were the first and most marked indications. He concludes from his studies that the kidneys are affected in a large proportion of cases, and that the catarrhal nephritis is probably caused by the presence of an irritant in the blood which, by its effect upon the walls of the renal vessels, produces hemorrhages. This condition is interesting mainly as showing another of the conditions which may account for nephritis developing in early life and persisting subsequently.

Bohne [1] has reached the conclusion, after experiments upon mice and guinea-pigs and careful observation upon a number of patients suffering with various diseases, accompanied by coma or conditions similar to that of uremia, that this condition is not improbably due, at least in large part, to the **retention of chlorids in the body.** In the experiments doses of approximately 2 gm. per kg. of body-weight produced distinct motor disturbances, often unilateral, and a condition of stupor. In a patient suffering from carcinoma of the seminal vesicles, who exhibited typical uremic symptoms and finally died in a condition of coma with signs of dyspnea, the average daily excretion of NaCl was less than 3 gm. In other cases it was observed that where the excretion of NaCl was normal the uremic symptoms did not appear; where it was diminished headache, asthma, or edema was nearly always present. In 2 of these cases in which autopsy was obtained it was found that the quantity of chlorids in the liver was greatly increased; Bohne therefore draws the definite conclusion that retention of chlorids in the organism, if not the only cause for the origin of uremic and comatose conditions, is nevertheless the one principally concerned; and he also calls attention to the value of quantitative determination of the chlorids in the urine in order to control, in some measure, the treatment.

N. Tirard [2] discusses the **relation of indigestion to Bright's disease.** Gastric disturbances secondary to renal trouble are, he believes, perhaps a manifestation of the elimination. On the other hand, symptomatic albuminurias frequently occur as a result of errors in diet, or in cases where there is considerable disturbance of the digestive function. He concludes that it is important to test the urine in every case of dyspepsia occurring in middle life.

Pathology and Symptoms.—Pollaci [3] has examined the **sweat-glands** in cases of nephritis in 16 cases, taking portions of the fresh and the hardened tissue from different parts of the body. In the edematous parts of the skin compression of the glands, even to complete atrophy of the lumen and necrosis, was found. In the other portions the lumen of the glands was larger than normal, and cystic formations with a flattened condition of the epithelium were discovered. In parts where the process was most advanced the protoplasm of the cells was granular, and the nuclei either disappeared or refused to take stains. The periglandular connective tissue showed signs of proliferation.

Wooten [4] reports 5 cases of chronic nephritis in which, at some time during their course, albumin was absent from the urine, although the general symptoms of the disease were pronounced. In 2 of these cases casts disappeared as well as albumin.

C. C. Aitken [5] reports a case of chronic **nephritis and uremia associated**

[1] Fortschr. d. Med., Feb 15, 1897.   [2] Lancet, Aug., 1896.
[3] Riforma Med., No. 92, 1896.   [4] Texas Med. Jour., Mar., 1897.
                    [5] Lancet, Sept. 26, 1896.

with Raynaud's disease. The patient, a man of 43, had well-marked gouty diathesis and albuminuria for more than 6 years. Chronic interstitial nephritis was recognized 5 years before. Two years previous to that time the symptoms of Raynaud's disease began and recurred at intervals. Mortification of the digits occurred. The urine frequently contained a small amount of hemoglobin with numerous epithelial and granular casts. The amount of urea was never above 320 gr. daily. Albuminuric retinitis was discovered in each eye, and there were some retinal hemorrhages. Between May 21 and July 2, 1895, there were 7 "uremic convulsive attacks," 5 of which had an apparent close relationship to the crises of the concurring attacks of severe vascular spasm. The patient died of uremic coma. [The author does not consider the possibility of the convulsions having been caused by vasomotor conditions of the brain. Such attacks have been described in pure Raynaud's disease, and must be considered in the present case.]

Haug[1] describes a case of **hemorrhage from the nose and into the ear** in the course of chronic Bright's disease. The patient, an alcoholic, had suffered from weakness of the heart for a year and a half, and 9 months previously had profuse epistaxis. The urine was then nonalbuminous, but recently he had more severe nasal hemorrhages and the urine was found to contain casts and albumin. Severe pains in the ears with deafness and tinnitus due to hemorrhages into the tympanum and membrane followed, and albuminuric retinitis with hemorrhage was discovered. The hemorrhagic manifestations in this case, the author believes, were largely the result of the cardiac condition, although their connection with Bright's disease was also of importance. He holds that blood escapes by diapedesis rather than by hemorrhage, and that the terms albuminuric tympanitis and myringitis are applicable. The condition is probably more common than is supposed.

A. R. Edwards[2] reports 4 cases in which the **differential diagnosis between uremia and meningitis** was extremely difficult. The 1st patient had paralysis of the muscles of the left eye and complete right hemiplegia, excepting the upper branch of the facial. At the autopsy there was some edema of the brain, but no lesions, and a diffuse pyelonephritis. The 2d case presented paralysis of the muscles of the left eye and the lower branch of the right facial. There were hyaline and granular casts, and considerable albumin in the urine. No cerebral lesion was found. The 3d case had no nervous symptoms excepting coma. The urine was heavily loaded with albumin; nevertheless the kidneys were negative, but a profuse, purulent infiltration was found over the base and convexity of the brain. The 4th case presented the symptoms of delirium tremens. The urine was albuminous. Suddenly focal palsies occurred in both eyes, but at the autopsy only the kidneys were diseased. [As a general rule, the focal symptoms of uremia are transient, those of meningitis more permanent; nevertheless we have recently seen a case of tubercular meningitis in which a marked hemiplegia disappeared in the course of a night.]

Clayton[3] reports a case of uremia in which the attack was precipitated by the taking of an ounce of **laudanum** with suicidal intent and exposure to very high temperature. Upon admission the patient had slow respiration, pin-point pupils, and a temperature of 105°. The urine contained a large quantity of albumin and numerous casts. Recovery ensued after several convulsive attacks.

Treatment.—Bettmann[4] has studied the action of **urea** as a diuretic.

[1] Deutsch. med. Woch., Nov. 5, 1896. [2] Am. Jour. Med. Sci., Aug., 1896.
[3] Med. News, July 25, 1896. [4] Berlin. klin. Woch., Dec. 7, 1896.

He treated 12 cases, including 3 of cirrhosis of the liver with marked ascites, 4 of unilateral pleurisy, and 5 of effusion into different serous cavities. He began with 10 gr. 3 times a day and increased this to 20 gr. He found a marked diuretic effect iu only 3 instances. In the first of these the increase of urine occurred after aspiration and might have been ascribed to coincident improvement of the action of the heart. In the 2d and 3d eases there was also improvement after aspiration. The author is inclined to believe that urea may be given with hope of useful results after aspiration, but doubts its efficiency during the existence of ascites. He has never found the decidedly beneficial result claimed for the remedy by Klemperer.

Friedreich [1] has used urea in heart-disease, exudation, and transudation, and also in diseases of the liver. He found that where the kidneys were healthy it exercised a diuretic power. The number of eases is small and the results are not striking; but he attributes the latter fact to the small dose employed.

Lemoine [2] has employed **methylen-blue** in 8 cases of albuminuria. In 5 of these there was rapid diminution; in 3 complete disappearance of the albumin. The diseases represented were subacute and interstitial nephritis, sometimes complicated with renal congestion. All cases treated showed increased diuresis and increased elimination of urea. The doses employed varied from 0.025 to 0.050 gm. per day. No disagreeable result was noticed from its employment, excepting a slight cystitis when impurities were present in the drug. This, however, was readily amenable to treatment. Lemoine concludes that it modifies the functions of the kidneys and is also a diuretic.

Achard and Castaigne [3] recommend methylen-blue for the purpose of testing the permeability of the kidneys. It may be administered either by the mouth, or, as they prefer, subcutaneously, in doses from $\frac{1}{4}$–1 gm. In normal subjects it appears at the end of $\frac{1}{2}$ hour and persists for nearly 2 days. If, however, any lesion of the kidney exist, there is more or less retardation.

Tirard [4] reports a case of dropsy occurring in connection with advanced kidney-disease, in which, other methods having failed, **diuretin** was employed with the result of inducing marked polyuria and reduction of the edema.

Myszinska [5] has treated 10 cases of albuminuria with the tincture of **cantharides.** The first of these, a case of chronic malaria with abundant albumin in the urine, was completely cured. The second, a case of tuberculosis in the stage of cavity-formation, was also cured of the renal conditions. In 3 other cases there was some amelioration, but in 2 cases of saturine arteriosclerosis the patients became rapidly worse. In 2 cases of parenchymatous nephritis there was no effect, and in 1 case of dormant tuberculosis there were an increase in the quantity of albumin and development of fever. Myszinska believes that cantharides is of some benefit, although admitting that the milk-diet which was enforced may also have had considerable influence. [It must be remembered that cantharides is capable of aggravating renal irritation even though given in minute doses.]

Julia [6] reviews the treatment of nephritis by external applications of **pilocarpin.** This method, as employed by Mollière in 1894, consists in the application every morning of inunctions of nitrate of pilocarpin (0.75–1.5 gr.) in 3 oz. of vaselin in the dorso-lumbar region. The surface is subsequently covered with cotton and remains undisturbed during the day. The report embraces 80 eases, some of acute nephritis following cold, some chronic, and

---

[1] Berlin. klin. Woch., No. 17, 1896.   [2] Compt. rend. de la Soc. de Biol., May 7, 1897.
[3] Gaz. hebdom. de Méd. et Chir., May 9, 1897.   [4] Brit. Med. Jour., Mar. 20, 1897.
[5] Gaz. heb. de Méd. et Chir., Feb. 11, 1897.   [6] Lyon méd., Dec. 6, 1896.

some infectious nephritis. The acute cases were generally improved, albumin frequently disappearing from the urine during treatment. There were invariably diaphoresis and diuresis.

Richardiére[1] advocates the use of **artificial serum** in uremia. He bleeds the patient 300 or 400 gm. and immediately introduces 800 gm. of aseptic Hayem's serum, at the temperature of the body, into the cellular tissue. His first case had intense dyspnea, mucous and subcrepitant rales over the chest, and great edema. Under ordinary treatment he grew worse and became distinctly uremic and finally comatose. Serum-injections were practised, and during a few days the patient greatly improved, but relapsed when the treatment was suspended. The treatment was again instituted and no further trouble occurred. In the second case injection was followed by improvement, but relapse occurred in 20 hours. A second injection was followed by profuse diarrhea and then permanent amelioration of the symptoms. The injections are harmless, though painful; they raise the temperature and cause a slowing of the pulse and breathing; the amount of urine increases and there seems to be a tendency to diarrhea, though it is of favorable omen. [This treatment is undoubtedly advisable in many cases. We have practised it in a few with good effect, and commend it from theoretic considerations as well as from practical experience.]

Carrien[2] prefers **hot-air baths** to vapor baths or hot-water baths in the treatment of nephritis. The hot-air bath relieves the kidney by abundant sweating and regulates the metabolic processes. The air is kept at a temperature of 40° C. for 20 minutes. This is repeated every 3 or 4 days. Profuse perspiration, with acceleration of the pulse and elevation of temperature from 1° to 2° C., is observed. The breathing is not embarrassed and, excepting for some palpitation and headache after the first bath, there are no unpleasant symptoms. The day following the bath the urine is usually reduced and the next day there is a marked but transient polyuria. The proportion of albumin decreases progressively. This treatment, he holds, is indicated in acute parenchymatous nephritis and contraindicated when there is coexisting arteriosclerosis, inflammatory skin diseases, or nervous conditions.

Bissman[3] discusses **renal disturbances** occurring in connection **with gastrointestinal disorders.** Most of the patients excrete small quantities of highly concentrated acid urine, although some show the reverse condition. He believes that these conditions are frequently due to lodgement of scybala in the lower bowel, which not only irritate the mucous membrane, but form foci for the development of bacteria.

Auche and Carriere[4] examined the urine in 2 cases of chronic enlargement of the lymphatic glands, one tubercular, the other leukemic, and found that the **urotoxic coefficient** was diminished in both, more markedly in the tubercular.

Ranglaret[5] has studied the effect of **douches and massage** upon the general health. After 8 or 10 consecutive daily applications the body-weight is reduced, this being due to the effect on the general nutrition. The total quantity of urine is slightly diminished, the organic elements being increased. The urinary toxicity is increased even in healthy persons undergoing the treatment.

Cornell[6] reports a case of **enuresis** of 20 years' duration. The only assignable cause was an attack of scarlet fever and a nervous disposition.

[1] L'Union méd., Dec. 5, 1896. [2] Sem. méd., Aug. 15, 1896.
[3] Med. News, Jan. 23, 1897. [4] Compt. rend. de la Soc. de Biol., July 3, 1896.
[5] Ann. d'Hydrologie, Nov., 1896. [6] Physician and Surgeon, Dec., 1896.

Great improvement followed the administration of strychnin and the application of faradic electricity.

Francis[1] reports a case of anuria coming on suddenly in a man that had passed some **calculi,** but who was apparently in good health at the time of the attack. Death occurred on the 10th day from uremia, and at the autopsy calculi were found blocking up the commencement of both ureters. The kidneys showed advanced pyelonephritis.

Geo. Klemperer,[2] in discussing the **treatment of renal calculus,** points out in the first place that firm calculi cannot be dissolved because the uric acid is intimately combined with the organic basis. Stone-formation may, however, be prevented. The deposits of urates and uric acid may be obviated by increasing the amount of water, but, unfortunately, it is impossible to administer sufficient water to accomplish this purpose absolutely. It is necessary to avoid saline and other purges which decrease the amount of urine, and also excessive sweating and exercise. Milk, cheese, egg-albumin, and vegetables are useful, but meat, and particularly organs such as liver and pancreas, are deleterious, as they contain considerable nuclein, which is excreted, in part at least, in the form of uric acid. The acidity of the urine must further be reduced, and this may be accomplished by the administration of remedies like piperazin, lysidin, urotropin, etc., but just as thoroughly by administering sodium bicarbonate. He recommends alkaline waters containing this salt. Finally, he has studied the effect of urea clinically and experimentally, and believes it to be of very great value in the treatment: he prescribes a tablespoonful every 2d hour of a 5 or 10% solution. The remedy has no evil effects, and is useful both for its solvent action and for the increased diuresis which it induces. Mendelsohn[3] believes that the lithium salts are too insoluble to be of much value in the treatment of renal calculi. He therefore prefers persistent but careful administration of the alkalies, with free ingestion of liquids.

CLINICAL INSTRUMENTS.

Egger[4] has investigated the **phonendoscope** of Bianchi. He finds that some overtones are badly conducted or not at all. This explains the disappearance of the metallic sounds and the high tympanic sounds. He holds that Bianchi's contention that the quality of the sound is not altered is incorrect; moist sounds produced immediately beneath the chest-wall may sound metallic. He holds that the phonendoscope may be useful for differentiating murmurs and in distinguishing between endocardial and pericardial sounds. He is skeptical of the value of the instrument in mapping out organs, and with all its advantages does not believe it can replace the ordinary stethoscope. Schaposchnikoff[5] has used the instrument in over 100 cases, and decides that it is very doubtful whether the internal organs can be correctly mapped out by its help, as suggested by the inventor; that the sounds and murmurs are greatly intensified, and therefore their correct interpretation is difficult; and that the sounds produced by the instrument itself interfere with the examination. Pribram[6] finds that the delimitation of organs by stroking toward the staff does not always correspond to the contours obtained by percussion or palpation. He therefore regards the results obtained with that instrument as uncertain. He finds that amplification of the sound causes

---

[1] Boston M. and S. Jour., Apr. 8, 1897.
[2] Berlin. klin. Woch., Aug. 17, 1896.
[3] Ibid., No. 14, 1897.
[4] Münch. med. Woch., Nov. 10, 1896.
[5] Ruskaja. Medzinsk. Gaz., No. 39, 1896.
[6] Prag. med. Woch., No. 33, 1896.

extreme fatigue to the ear. Litten,[1] in describing the phonendoscope constructed by Aufrecht, states that it is not specially advantageous, and in particular he has found that the method of delimiting organs, by drawing an instrument or finger over the skin near the border of the organ, is unsatisfactory. The changes of note detected by the instrument are due to vibrations in the skin and not in the deeper organs. [We have reached exactly the same conclusions.] Schwalbe[2] concludes that sounds which are ordinarily inaudible are readily appreciated by the phonendoscope, and even sounds not heard by other means, such as those of the muscles and joints, etc. Baruch[3] also recommends it, mentioning that the sounds of the heart may be heard in cases of myocarditis, in which they are inaudible with the ordinary stethoscope, and that the patient may be examined thoroughly without disrobing. Manges[4] gives a number of points at which the staff should be placed in order to utilize it to the greatest advantage for outlining organs. These are usually situated over the soft tissue, as the vibrations of bone interfere with the accuracy of the delimitation. However, he has been unable to map out the different ventricles and auricles of the heart, and has also been unable to do very accurate work in connection with the liver and spleen. In regard to the stomach, however, he has confirmed his results by all the other methods and found them to be very accurate. He holds the instrument to be a distinct improvement over the binaural stethoscope.

Chauveau[5] describes a new form of **stethoscope** in which, as he says, the sounds are conveyed to the ear by aërial transmission. It is essentially an ordinary double stethoscope in which the bell is replaced by a heavy metal cup, the open surface of which is covered by a thin disk. Just beneath the point where the 2 branches meet a lateral branch is given off which communicates with the outer air. This, according to Chauveau, permits the sounds to be transmitted to the ear without any interference with their natural timbre.

Zieniec[6] attaches a long tube to the ordinary single stethoscope, preferably of stiff rubber, such as is used for the esophageal sound, and to this an earpiece. He claims that the sounds are clearer and, if the tube is long enough, it is possible to use the instrument in class demonstration. If, however, the distance of the students be considerable, the better method is to employ one of the so-called children's telephones, by which sounds can be transmitted for several meters.

Kingscote[7] describes a **pleximeter** that he has devised, which overcomes the vibrations of the chest-wall and does not hurt the patient. It consists of a wooden cone to which a thick India-rubber ring is attached, so that when this is pressed firmly against the chest the apex of the cone touches a definite point on the skin. The base is struck with a hammer having a bulbous end and a flexible handle.

Max Herr[8] has devised an instrument called the **onychograph,** by which he is able to record the variations in blood-pressure in the capillaries of the tips of the fingers. It consists essentially of the ordinary sphygmograph, which is so arranged that the pelotte can be brought against the finger resting upon a hard surface. The onychogram is extremely variable; it differs from the sphygmogram, the ordinary details being absent. The respiratory influence is best seen when the pulse is failing. Another phenomenon similar to this, but evidently due to nervous influence, is irregularity, variation in size

[1] Centralbl. f. innere Med., Feb. 20, 1897. [2] Deut. med. Woch., No. 31, 1896.
[3] Med. Rec., Oct. 31, 1896. [4] N. Y. Med. Jour., Jan., 1897.
[5] Jour. de Méd. de Paris, Oct. 4, 1896. [6] Wien. med. Woch., Apr., 1897.
[7] Lancet, Dec. 19, 1896. [8] Wien. klin. Woch., Aug. 15, 1896.

occurring several times in a minute. Cyclical conditions are readily observed; the pulse is much smaller when the attention is fixed. The greatest variation occurs in cases of cardiac insufficiency, the movements of the indicator sometimes being so great that they exceed the limits of the paper band. The influence of heat and cold is also very marked. The pulse seems to be increased in icterus, in fever excepting pneumonia, and in insufficiency of the aorta. It is decreased in mitral diseases. In emphysema of the lungs the respiratory variation is absent. In arteriosclerosis the curve is low and blunted. In those cases, however, where the radial is not sclerotic, although there is an atheromatous aorta, the curve is high and steep.

CLINICAL SKIAGRAPHS.

[The application of skiagraphy to internal medicine has been much greater than was at first anticipated, and the results have been very satisfactory, especially in cases of obscure intrathoracic disease.] William Pepper[1] has contributed a very interesting paper upon the diagnostic value of the Röntgen rays in internal medicine, confining his discussion in this paper to the diagnosis of intrathoracic aneurysm. He points out that in many cases this new agency only serves to confirm the diagnosis already established with great confidence by auscultation and percussion. Even in these cases, however, greater precision as to location, size, and form may be obtained with this assistance; and, on the other hand, intrathoracic aneurysms may be of such small size or so situated as to cause few symptoms and to be insusceptible of diagnosis by the ordinary methods, while they are demonstrable by the *x*-rays. Finally, this method serves at times to exclude aneurysm by failing to reveal any increase of the shaded form of the heart and aorta when the symptoms suggest the presence of aneurysm. In 3 cases of suspected aneurysm of the arch of the aorta, under his own care, his associate, Dr. Leonard, practised skiagraphy with surprisingly happy results, confirming the suspicion in two and removing it in the third. The first case was one of certain aneurysm, the physical signs being unequivocal. The patient had previously suffered with aneurysm of the popliteal artery, but after ligation this subsided. The signs of a large aneurysm of the chest were plainly marked. The skiagraph was taken with the patient lying on the plate. A double focusing tube was placed over the middle line of the chest, 18 in. from the plate; exposure was 15 minutes. An impenetrable area was seen in the upper part of the sternal region and to the right of the heart's shadow. The picture is indefinite, but the author states that this is unavoidable, as a longer exposure might cause penetration of the aneurysm by the rays. The second case was also one of marked aneurysm of the thoracic aorta, and the skiagraph fully confirmed this view. In the third case, in which symptoms pointing to aneurysm were present (dulness under the manubrium, paralysis of the vocal cords, tracheal tugging, inequality of pulse, and bruit), the skiagraph failed to show any abnormal opacity corresponding to the dulness on percussion; and the course of the case corresponded with this exclusion of aneurysm. A fourth case of aneurysm of the innominate artery is merely alluded to.

Thompson,[2] in discussing the practical application of Röntgen rays in diseases of the heart and great vessels, reports a case in which aneurysm was suspected, but physical signs were not sufficient for a positive diagnosis. Upon examination with the fluoroscope an indefinite shadow above the heart, to the left, was seen from the front, which, examined from the back, showed the

[1] Univ. Med. Mag., Jan., 1897. [2] Lancet, Dec. 12, 1896.

outline of a large mass just above the heart. Subsequently the history of the case confirmed the diagnosis of aneurysm of the aorta.

Bergonie [1] has used the radioscope for the diagnosis of intrathoracic lesions and found that the coincidence between the shadow-changes and the lesions was always perfect. Dulness was represented by opacity and it was also possible to recognize exactly the limits of a hydatid cyst by this method.

Bouchard [2] has employed the Röntgen rays in the diagnosis of pulmonary diseases. He finds that pleural effusion produces darkness on the side in which it exists. Pulmonary infiltration or consolidation also causes the appearance of a shadow, the difference between the two being that one usually occurs at the apex and the other at the base of the heart. Cavities are indicated by lighter areas or clear spaces in the midst of the shadows. He reports several cases in which the diagnosis was doubtful until the fluoroscope had been employed.

Wasserman [3] reports 2 cases in which the diagnosis was finally confirmed by means of the Röntgen rays. In the first there were symptoms of pulmonary infiltration, but it was only when the thorax was examined with the fluoroscope that attention was attracted to the lower part of the field, which was much darker than the upper part, to a very bright spot about 2 cm. to the right of the shadow of the sternum, and just above the shadow of the liver. Upon careful examination of the thorax anteriorly in the corresponding place it was possible to find signs of a cavity, but absolutely impossible posteriorly. The author concludes that in case of a central cavity not giving rise to signs, either anteriorly or posteriorly, it would be impossible to diagnose it except by this method. As the tubercle-bacilli had never been found in the sputum, the discovery of this cavity confirmed the otherwise doubtful diagnosis. In the 2d case there was some dulness in the first intercostal space to the right of the sternum, but no pulsation. When, however, the thorax was examined with the fluoroscope a large pulsating tumor was found in this situation that also reached considerably further to the left than percussion had indicated, and extended quite a distance downward along the descending aorta, rendering it very easy to make a plastic representation of the diseased artery. It is possible by this method to detect an aneurysm too small to give rise to symptoms, and also to make a differential diagnosis between aneurysm and tumor.

Von Basch [4] has been able to recognize the condition of pulmonary swelling and inelasticity, that he has previously described, by means of the Röntgen rays.

Satterthwaite [5] suggests the use of the fluoroscope in connection with percussion. He marks upon the chest-wall the outline as obtained by percussion, then places the Crookes tube at a point directly back of this in order that the rays casting the shadows shall pass perpendicularly through the chest. The important angles are all confirmed by this method and the result is then sketched.

Levy-Dorn [6] records an observation of the intrathoracic conditions **during an attack of asthma** made with the aid of the **fluoroscope.** Before the attack nothing specially interesting was observed excepting the right-sided enlargement of the heart. During the attack he observed the following changes: the left half of the diaphragm sank repeatedly and then rose in a labored fashion, and again descended rapidly, and this continued, expiration

[1] Trib. Med. Jour., Feb. 3, 1897.
[2] Rev. de la Tuberculose, Dec., 1896 ; Gaz. des Hôp., Dec. 22, 1896 ; Ibid , Jan. 5, 1897.
[3] Wien. klin. Woch., Jan. 28, 1897.   [4] Wien. med. Woch., Jan. 30, 1897.
[5] Med. Rec., Apr. 10, 1897.   [6] Berlin. klin. Woch., Nov. 23, 1896.

being difficult and slow and inspiration sudden and complete. At the same time the right half of the diaphragm behaved in an entirely different manner, remaining stationary in both expiration and inspiration. When the patient was directed to take a deep breath the left side made somewhat greater excursions, but the right side still remained fixed. This continued some months, when a severe attack of coughing occurred and the paroxysm was ended. The author concludes from his observation that the position of the left side of the diaphragm was due to marked distention of the left lung, and holds that it furnishes disproof of the theory that bronchial asthma is dependent upon diaphragmatic cramp and confirmation of the view that asthmatic dyspnea may be dependent upon disturbances in the bronchi of one side only.

ANIMAL PARASITES.

Protozoa.—Mathieu and Soupault[1] discuss the pathogenic importance of **amebæ** in the intestines. They note that amebæ are found in large numbers in the liquid stools of healthy persons after salines; they are met with in large numbers in cases of dysentery, but are not always to be found in dysenteric stools, having been absent in certain epidemics with grave manifestations. They have frequently been found when patients presented diarrhea, but no dysenteric manifestations; in the last-named cases they are usually more numerous than in healthy persons, and disappear when the condition is relieved, although occasionally their disappearance bears no relation to the attack. They hold that no certain relation between the form of amebæ found and the clinical variety of diarrhea has been established, and they cast doubt upon the pathogenic significance of the organisms. Finally, as to the existence of certain pathogenic or virulent forms, and certain non-pathogenic forms, they hold that it is premature either to accept or reject this suggestion. Their own inclination is to believe that the amebæ in large number and with increased virulence may occasion grave diarrhea or certain dysenteric affections of the intestines, though they admit that this view is not established.

Wijnhoff[2] has reported the case of a woman of 30 years who suffered with attacks resembling renal colic, followed by bloody and purulent urine. Numerous colorless bodies, identical with the amebæ coli, appeared in the urine after each attack; but in the intervals only encysted bodies and ring-forms were present. In 3 other cases **ameburia** occurred during attacks of strangury and vesical or renal colic; the urine was cloudy, and contained numerous pus-corpuscles, and the formation of daughter-cells out of the large amebæ could be observed. The author believes that the organisms bear an etiologic relation to the attacks. Zechuisen, in abstracting the above report, mentions the case of a medical student who had an almost painless attack of hematuria with blood-casts in the urine and numerous amebæ; after the attack the ring-shaped amebæ were still present.

Leyden and Schaudinn[3] have described a form of amebæ occurring in the liquid removed from patients suffering with ascites. This organism was first found by Leyden in a patient suffering with chronic heart-disease and ascites. Repeated tapping was practised, and the ameba was always present. The organisms were gelatinous cells, often aggregated and presenting active ameboid movements. Small nodes formed upon the processes at times, separated, and developed into new cells. The patient presented nodular masses in the abdomen (found after tapping), and it was believed that she had cancer. Similar

---

[1] Gaz. des Hôpitaux, Oct. 17, 1896.   [2] Centralbl. f. innere Med., No. 52, 1896.
[3] Sitzungsbericht d. Kgl. Pr. Akad. d. Wiss., Berlin, July 30, 1896.

bodies were found in the fluid removed from a case of carcinoma of the stomach with ascites in a man of 63. Dr. Schaudinn made studies of the organisms, and declares them undoubtedly amebæ. [The opinion of the latter is of particular value, as he has been working upon the subject of protozoa for years.]

Janowski [1] has observed **flagellate protozoa** in the feces of 6 cases. In 2 the patients suffered from chronic dysentery; in 1 from typhoid fever; in the other 3 from indifferent diseases. He holds that the trichomonads are of no particular significance, but that they may occasionally give rise to diarrhea. He recommends for treatment calomel and quinin, the latter being also useful when given as a clyster.

Gurwitsch [2] reports 7 cases of **balantidium coli** that he has observed in human beings. The chief symptom of the disease is diarrhea, the stools containing mucus, undigested food, and occasionally blood. The subjective symptoms are those of colitis. In addition to the ordinary encysted ovoid form, he describes another two or three times as large as this which shows distinct traces of segmentation. He holds that this is probably a persistent form, brought about by an attempt to expel the parasite. From the fact that the number of parasites existing was usually proportionate to the severity of the symptoms, he concludes that they had a direct pathogenic action. One patient died of hemorrhage; 5 others harbored other parasites.

Vermes.—Thorpe [3] has made some studies of the occurrence of **filariæ** in the blood of natives of the Fiji or Friendly Islands. In 24 cases seen in the hospital at Suva, Fiji, he found filariæ in 4 of 16 men having no form of elephantoid disease, and in 1 of 4 men having elephantiasis. The remaining 4 cases were women without elephantiasis, and of these 1 had filariæ. These results show that 25% of the Fiji natives have filariæ. Subsequently slides of blood from 100 cases came into his hands, and he found filariæ in 24, or about the same proportion as in his cases. He next studied the subject in the Friendly Islands. In examining the blood of the native Tangans he was struck by the fact that the parasites were quite as common in the daytime as at night. Ninety-six natives were examined both day and night, and in only 2 were the filariæ absent at one time and present at another. In 1 of these they were found during the day alone; in another during the night only. The filaria of the Tangans is in other respects like the Filaria nocturna, but is a little smaller than that found elsewhere. The author believes that the habit of waking frequently during the night to talk or eat is the cause of the loss of periodicity. Statistically he found on the 4 large islands of the group: among males: examined day and night 55, 27 affected; examined only during day 8, 1 affected; only at night 60, 23 affected; among females: examined day and night 41, 13 affected; during day 9, none affected; during night 41, 5 affected. The total was 214 cases examined, and 69 affected, or a proportion of 32.24%.

Manson [4] refers to the frequency of filariasis in Samoa. Dr. Davies sent him blood-films of 56 adult Samoans, each of whom had some form of elephantoid disease, of which 27 contained filaria. In some cases the parasites were enormously abundant. The author states that the slides were in the majority of cases obtained from that part of the population least likely to show filaria in the blood—that is, from subjects of elephantiasis, in whom the filariæ are presumably blocked in the lymphatics. He believes, therefore, that

[1] Zeit. f. klin. Med., vol. xxxi., p. 442.
[2] Russ. Arch. f. Path., kl. Med. u. Bact., Sept., 1896.
[3] Brit. Med. Jour., Oct. 3, 1896.
[4] Ibid., Nov. 7, 1896.

examination might show that practically all adult Samoans harbor the Filaria nocturna.

Sellei[1] reports 19 cases of **Filaria medinensis,** all of which were found in a negro colony that was on exhibition at Budapest. The disease commenced as a small fluctuating tumor, usually on the foot, which in the 3d or 4th week suppurated and opened, leaving a small abscess in which the head of the parasite was found. The longest that he obtained measured 52 cm.

Blanchard[2] reports a case in which a live, thread-like worm, 30 cm. long, which proved to be the **Gordius tricuspidatis,** was vomited by a young man, who had apparently swallowed it in drinking-water about 2 weeks previously. The symptoms during that time had been simply slight discomfort in the hypogastric region.

Brown[3] reports the results of a study of several cases of **trichinosis.** There was considerable leukocytosis, with increase in the number of eosinophile cells, reaching $62\frac{1}{2}\%$ of the leukocytes, and diminution of the polynuclear cells to 6.6%. There was no increase in the excretion of uric acid nor in the elimination of any of the nitrogenous constituents of the urine. The muscles showed great proliferation of the nuclei, the presence of parasites with disintegration of the fibers they inhabited, and extravascular eosinophile cells.

Brooks[4] reports a case of **Distoma hæmatobium.** The patient, who had spent a year in South Africa, did not notice the symptoms until his return to the United States. Toward the end of micturition the urine became bloody and upon examination was found to contain minute coagula imbedded in pus. Within these, or else free in the urine, were a large number of ovoid bodies, with one end drawn out into a sharp spine, which developed rapidly into embryos when placed in fresh water.

Sonderm[5] reports a very similar case. The patient had lived in South Africa, and also observed a small quantity of blood at the end of each micturition; examination of the urine showed, in addition to pus, the presence of the characteristic eggs. Gallic acid improved the symptoms without materially reducing the number of the ova.

Zinn and Jacoby[6] have studied **the fauna of the intestinal tract** in negroes, and have found in 23 native Africans representing various parts of Africa, east and west, Anchylostomum duodenale 21 times, Trichocephalus dispar 8 times, ascaris 8 times, tæniæ 4 times, Anguillula stercoralis 4 times, and amebæ twice. None of the cases showed any sign of anemia. In some of the cases of anchylostomiasis the number of parasites was very great, and the authors ascribe the lack of symptoms to racial peculiarity.

Galgey[7] has recently begun the investigation of the progressive pernicious anemia so common in the natives and especially the coolies of the island of St. Lucia, West Indies. The number of cases admitted to the Victoria Hospital was 209 in 1892, 277 in 1893, and 272 in 1894. Most of the cases were coolies, but the natives are also liable. The patient is weak and dejected, the skin is waxy and pale, and the breathing difficult. Finally, extreme weakness prevents his continuing at work. The author's attention having been called to the frequency of **anchylostomiasis,** he studied one of the fatal cases postmortem and discovered numbers of the worms in the intestine. He then adopted the thymol treatment, giving 40 gr. in 2 doses, and the fol-

[1] Pester med.-chir. Presse, No. 48, 1896.   [2] Bull. de l'Acad. de Méd., May, 1897.
[3] Bull. Johns Hopkins Hosp., Apr., 1897.   [4] Med. Rec., Apr. 3, 1897.
[5] Med. News, May 1, 1897.   [6] Berlin. klin. Woch., No. 36, 1896.
[7] Brit. Med. Jour., Jan. 23, 1897.

lowing day a light diet and brisk purgation. The proof of the nature of the disease is determined by the examination of the evacuations. He appends the histories of 23 cases, all of which were improved under the treatment. Since then fully 60 other cases have undergone the same treatment with the most successful results. Geophragia or earth-eating is very prevalent among the coolies, both children and adults.

Mohlau[1] reports 5 cases of Anchylostomum duodenale ; 2 were apparently imported from Italy and the other 3 seemed to have originated in America. The symptoms of the disease, as he observed them, are the marked anemia, the bronzing of the skin, and a peculiar sensation of warmth in the region of the intestines, which he ascribes to hemorrhage and which he finds always precedes the appearance of blood in the feces. Besides these, there is a peculiar pain, commencing very mildly and increasing in severity, irregular diarrhea, and sometimes a swelling nearly over the pancreas. The diagnosis is, of course, to be made by the discovery of eggs in the feces, and it is usually desirable to administer a cathartic before the examination. [The discovery of anchylostomiasis originating in North America is of considerable interest. We know of no previous case.] Moeller[2] also reports 2 cases occurring in slate-workers in the southern portion of Saxony. In both the diagnosis was made by the discovery of the eggs in the feces. Combination of hydrotherapy—that is, high rectal injections of salt water—and cold applications, and cascara sagrada, produced permanent cure.

Sommer[3] contributes a further paper on the occurrence of **Tænia echinococcus** in the United States. In his first paper[4] he summarized 67 cases. He now adds 33 additional instances, making the whole number 100. Of these latter cases 1 occurred between the ages of 11 and 20, 5 between 21 and 30, 4 between 31 and 40, 6 between 41 and 50, 4 between 51 and 60, 2 between 61 and 70, and 3 between 71 and 80. There were males, 21 ; females, 11 ; not stated, 1. As to the organs affected, he finds in his present series : liver, 22 cases ; lungs, 2 ; bladder, 2 ; pleura, 1 ; peritoneum and omentum, 1 ; mesentery and omentum, 1 ; abdomen, 2 ; omentum, 1 ; brain, 1 ; ventricles, 1. In 1 case the parasites were found in the vomita.

Hagelstam[5] reports 2 cases of anemia caused by the **Bothriocephalus latus.** Both patients were Finns that had emigrated to the United States. He describes the symptoms of the disease as those of profound anemia with slight icterus, the blood showing poikilocytosis and leukocytosis. The diagnosis is made by microscopic examination of the feces.

Daniels[6] states that 2 specimens of a tapeworm allied to the **Tænia Madagascariensis** were found in an adult male, aboriginal Indian at George Town, British Guiana. They were in the jejunum ; both were dead and the heads were not found. One of the specimens was cut and the other uncut. The latter measured 9 in. (23 cm.) in length, and the segments increased in size and length from above downward. The first segment was 0.37 mm. in breadth and 0.07 mm. in length; whilst the 50th was 0.8 mm. in breadth and 0.2 mm. in length ; at the 150th segment the breadth was 1.2 mm. and the length 0.4 mm. ; but at the 250th segment the breadth and length were about the same, 1.7 mm. In the remaining segments the increase was almost entirely in length, the terminal segments (about the 320th) being slightly over 3 mm. in length and little more than half this in width. The most peculiar feature and the one in which it resembled the Tænia Madagascariensis is the

[1] Buffalo Med. Jour., Mar., 1897.
[2] Koresp. bl. d. ärz. ver. v. thuringen.
[3] N. Y. Med. Jour., Aug. 22, 1896.
[4] Ibid., Nov., 1895.
[5] Ibid., Aug. 29, 1896.
[6] Lancet, Nov. 21, 1896.

arrangement in the ripe segment of the eggs in masses or balls visible to the naked eye. The genital pores barely projected and were invariably found on the same side of the segments. The illustrations represent segments enlarged about 9 times, Fig. *d* being even more highly magnified.

Overton[1] reports 2 cases suffering from **tapeworm.** The first patient was given a powerful vermifuge and had passed some of the worm by the rectum, when a violent attack of vomiting came on, during which the rest of the

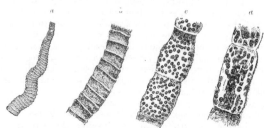

FIG. 4 —*a*, portion of worm just below the head; *b*, portion of worm at about 150th segment, showing genital pores; *c*, *d*, portions of worm between segments 300-320, showing egg masses (Lancet, Nov. 21, 1896).

worm was expelled by the mouth. He also reports another case, in which the patient, after a vermifuge, passed 2 tapeworms, in 1 of which the head was lacking. At intervals of 6 weeks the symptoms would recur, followed in each case by the expulsion of a headless tapeworm ; after the 3d treatment, however, cure apparently took place.

Tretrop and Lambotte[2] found living parasites in the liver and mesentery glands of a native of the Congo, which were from 15 to 18 mm. in length and were recognized as **Pentastomum constrictum.**

Arthropoda.—Henschen[3] reports a case in which the intestinal tract was infested with **maggots.** These had persisted for 7 years and gave rise to a chronic pseudomembranous enteritis. Treatment with filix mas would expel large numbers, but they invariably reappeared.

[1] Med. Rec., Oct. 31, 1896.   [2] Ann. Bull. de la Soc méd. D'Anvers, Nov. 18, 1896.
[3] Rundschau, No. 33, 1896.

GENERAL SURGERY.

BY W. W. KEEN, M. D., AND J. CHALMERS DaCOSTA, M. D.,

OF PHILADELPHIA.

General Review of the Year's Work.—The general trend of surgery during the past year has been in the direction of an enlightened conservatism. Destructive radicalism, recently so popular, is obviously waning. Startling novelties are not common, but laborious studies, careful investigations, and thorough reinvestigations of important subjects constitute the great bulk of the work of surgeons for the past twelve months. Among a host of important matters which have been discussed we may mention the following as of particular note: the real position of iodoform in surgery; formaldehyd as a disinfectant; the use of antistreptococcic serum and the doubts as to its genuine utility; the treatment of inoperable malignant tumors by the mixed toxins of the streptococcus of erysipelas and the micrococcus prodigiosus; orrhotherapy for malignant tumors; the possibility of retarding the growth of or of curing cancer of the female breast by the performance of oöphorectomy; the value of eucain as a local anesthetic and the method of employing it; the treatment of certain forms of neuralgia by intradural section of the spinal nerves; the lack of permanency in the operative cure of epilepsy; forcible correction of the deformity of Pott's disease of the spine; hypertrophy of the prostate gland and the various methods employed in treating it; partial nephrectomy as a substitute in certain cases for complete nephrectomy; the value of the cystoscope in diagnosing renal and vesical disease; treatment of albuminuria by incision or puncture of the kidney; the very important recent studies upon the immediate suture of divided blood-vessels; methods of draining and cleansing an infected abdominal cavity; the technic of appendicitis operations; the value of the intravenous injection of hot saline fluid in the treatment of shock and the collapse of hemorrhage; the ambulatory treatment of fractures; the treatment of certain fractures and dislocations by incision, and the employment of the Röntgen rays in surgical diagnosis.

ASEPSIS AND ANTISEPSIS.

N. Senn[1] discusses ideal **catgut sterilization.** He states that no other surgical procedure has ever enjoyed the confidence of the entire profession as thoroughly as has the catgut ligature. Nussbaum has appropriately said that catgut is without doubt Lister's greatest discovery. Lister's original method of rendering catgut aseptic has been variously modified during the last 25 years. The fact that so many methods have been used is proof positive that no one of them has proved absolutely perfect. Kocher abandoned juniper gut as unsafe after giving it a prolonged trial. Carbolized catgut, sublimated gut, and chromicized gut have been used extensively, but not

[1] Jour. Am. Med. Assoc., Dec. 12, 1896.

infrequently wound-infection could be traced to imperfect sterilization of the material. Dry sterilization has been largely used, but it cannot be relied upon. Catgut should be sterile, should be mildly antiseptic, and of unimpaired tensile strength. Senn says we have all been seeking for a method which would enable us to boil catgut without diminishing its strength, and such a method has recently been found. It has been shown that after catgut is immersed for 48 hours in a 2% solution of formalin it undergoes an unknown chemical change which alters its texture. It can now be boiled with impunity, and boiling actually increases its tensile strength. Hofmeister's method of preparation is as follows : the catgut is wound on a glass plate with projecting edges and the ends of the gut are fastened through holes in the plate. It is immersed in a 2 to 4% aqueous solution of formalin for from 12 to 48 hours. It is then immersed in flowing water at least 12 hours to free the gut from the formalin. It is boiled in water for from 10 to 30 minutes. It is preserved in absolute alcohol containing 5% of glycerin and $\frac{1}{10}$ of 1% of corrosive sublimate. In this method of preparation the gut must be wound tightly around the glass plate and cylinder. Formalin-catgut is absorbable in the tissues, but not so readily as catgut prepared by other methods. Inoculation-experiments prove the formalin-gut to be sterile. It is very strong, the knot is secure, and the material can be boiled and even reboiled any number of times without injuring its texture. Simple sterile catgut is not a safe material because as it lies in the tissues it can act as a culture-medium for microorganisms. Hence every catgut ligature should contain some antiseptic. Hofmeister, as noted above, keeps the gut in an alcoholic solution of corrosive sublimate ; some surgeons immerse it in a carbolic solution; both these antiseptics are irritants, increase primary wound secretion, and thus interfere to some extent with healing by first intention.

Lauenstein has recently proved that it is impossible to render the field of operation absolutely aseptic by any known method of disinfection. Nearly every wound inflicted by the surgeon must contain some pathogenic microbes. Ewald has proved that sterile catgut often contains a toxic substance of unknown composition. This substance when present in sufficient amount has a destructive action upon the cells carrying on repair, transforms them into pus-corpuscles, and produces a limited aseptic suppuration and the formation of sterile pus. Many stitch-abscesses originate from this cause. Senn has come to the conclusion that catgut should not only be sterile, but should be made sufficiently antiseptic to inhibit the growth of pyogenic organisms which enter the wound at the time of operation or which are carried to it by the circulation. He has modified Hofmeister's plan by substituting iodoform for corrosive sublimate. Senn advises hospital authorities and surgeons to prepare their own catgut, and not depend upon the material put up by the manufacturers. Senn's method is as follows : the catgut is formalinized by the method of Hofmeister, being wound, however, upon glass test-tubes or glass drainage-tubes instead of plates. It is boiled for from 12 to 15 minutes, is cut into pieces and tied in bundles, when it is immersed and kept ready for use in the following mixture : 950 parts of absolute alcohol, 50 parts of glycerin, 100 parts of finely pulverized iodoform. The bottle is closed with a well-fitting glass stopper and should be shaken every few days. One of the valuable properties of the iodoform in a recent wound is that it diminishes the amount of primary wound secretion. It does not destroy pus-microbes, but it does inhibit their growth. [The opinion of Prof. Senn that hospitals should prepare their own catgut, is worthy of respectful attention. The formalin-iodoform catgut seems to be a satisfactory material. We have never employed Senn's catgut, but have tried ordinary formalin-gut, and were not satisfied with it. At present we use with great satisfaction the palladium catgut of Johnston, the formula for which will be found in the *Year-Book* for 1896.]

Henry Jellett[1] presents a **modification of Fowler's method of sterilizing catgut.** The method of Fowler, as is well known, consists of sealing up strands of gut in a U-shaped glass tube containing alcohol, raising the temperature of the tube by placing it in a dry sterilizer, and immersing it in boiling water. Jellett calls attention to the fact that raw catgut must be septic because of its origin and its method of preparation. It is made by twisting into cords the prepared submucous tissue of the small intestine of the sheep. The process of twisting brings bacteria which were originally on the outside of the intestine into the centre of the threads. The fat present glues the strands firmly together and encases the bacteria in a sheath which forms an impassable barrier to ordinary means of sterilization. When catgut is introduced into the body the process of absorption serves to bring every particle of it, layer by layer, into contact with the surrounding tissue. Bacteria contained in silk or silkworm-gut may never come in contact with the tissue, but every bacterium present in catgut necessarily does so, and it is this property of being absorbed which makes the absolute asepsis of catgut imperative. In endeavoring to kill bacteria in gut chemical methods are very uncertain because the bacteria are surrounded by fat. The fat must be first removed by ether, but chemical disinfectants require frequent changes of liquid, are troublesome, expensive, and uncertain. Heat is the best antiseptic, but boiling water or steam causes catgut to swell into a shapeless mass and dry heat is likely to make it brittle. Alcohol is a medium in which catgut can be heated without diminution of the tensile strength of the gut. Alcohol boils at 173° F. This is not a great enough heat to sterilize the material, hence the alcohol must be superheated. The author's modification of Fowler's method enables anybody to quickly sterilize catgut. He tells us to roll gut on glass plates and place it in a brass box three-fourths full of alcohol. The box has a screw top provided with an India-rubber washer. This box is immersed in boiling water. It must be able to stand a pressure of 4 pounds to the square inch. Before placing the gut in the box it should be dehydrated by keeping it in absolute alcohol for 3 or 4 days. It must not be rolled tightly on the plate. A coil 90 in. long will lose from $\frac{1}{2}$ to 1 in. in length in preparation, so if rolled too tightly at first it will be greatly weakened after the process is completed. The brass box is placed in a saucepan of cold water, the water is raised to boiling and is boiled for 15 minutes. Do not place the box directly in boiling water. If this is done, it will take some time to heat the box and its contents and the material might be removed before sterilization was complete. The plates of catgut are kept in a mixture of alcohol and glycerin—from 5 to 20% glycerin.

Edebohls'[2] **method of sterilizing catgut** is as follows: he buys the raw material from an importer of jeweler's supplies, raw gut 0 and 100, in coils 5 meters long. He tells us not to buy the smooth white gut; this has been made smooth and white by the use of sandpaper, and it is weak and unreliable. Take away from each coil the fine strand used to fasten it, place the coils in ether to remove fat, and chromicize by placing for 30 hours in the following solution: $1\frac{1}{2}$ gm. of potassium bichromate, 10 gm. of carbolic acid, 10 gm. of glycerin, 480 gm. of water. Dissolve the potassium bichromate in the water, then add the carbolic acid and glycerin. After 30 hours remove the

---

[1] Lancet, Aug. 8, 1896.   [2] Boston M. and S. Jour., Sept. 24, 1896.

catgut with and upon the core and wind it upon frames in lengths of 1 meter. This prevents kinking. The catgut is dried for several days at a temperature not exceeding 40° to 50° C. Higher temperatures might make the moist gut gelatinous, and hence brittle and useless. The drying must be perfect, because if any moisture remains in the gut when high temperatures are applied it will become gelatinous and brittle. After the gut is absolutely dry cut it into pieces 1 meter long, roll the pieces into small coils, pack into 1-ounce glycerin-jelly jars, 20 coils to a jar, pour absolute alcohol into each jar until it is full, and screw down the metal cap. Place the glycerin-jelly jars into a large anatomic jar which contains from 2 to 4 ounces of absolute alcohol; screw down the cover of the anatomic jar, place the whole in an Arnold sterilizer, boil for 5 hours, and then allow it to cool. The firm closure of the jar secures boiling under pressure. This gut is not changed by alcohol. Gut thus chromicized and sterilized remains strong, sterile, and unimpaired in quality for years.

The question of **a cheap and efficient surgical suture-material** is discussed by A. V. Gubaroff.[1] He maintains that hemp and linen thread are worthy of more attention as suture-materials than is usually assigned them. The objection commonly made is that they are difficult to thread and liable to roll up and tangle. He suggests a method of preparation which prevents these difficulties—namely, take linen thread, boil it in soda solution to remove fat, wash it in water and dry; sterilize it in steam and keep it in alcohol for several days. Dip it into 5% solution of celloidin, in alcohol and ether, and dry by stretching upon frames. The threads shrink, become smooth, are threaded with great ease, and do not become tangled when placed in aqueous solutions. They can be sterilized by boiling or by putting them in a steam apparatus, but should not be placed in alcoholic solutions. They keep best dry. We can add 1 : 1000 of corrosive sublimate to the celloidin solution; but if we do so, the thread must be subsequently boiled to remove the superfluous sublimate.

Carl S. Haegeler[2] discusses **airol and other substitutes for iodoform.** He tells us that the three chief objections to the employment of iodoform are its occasional poisonous action, its irritant effects, and its offensive odor. The exact action of iodoform is not known. We are not sure whether it is or is not an antiseptic, and we are not certain that wounds can be infected by the use of unsterilized iodoform. Unquestionably, it produces decomposition-products on which its activity largely depends, the chief one of these being iodin. It is disputed whether it acts upon the organisms, the toxins, or the tissues. In an area of putrefaction the iodoform is decomposed with great rapidity. There can be no question that it has strong antitubercular power. A substitute for iodoform should not be toxic, should not be irritant, should not have a disagreeable odor, and should contain an effective antiseptic material. He tells us that neither iodol nor aristol can be esteemed as substitutes, and dermatol has a very weak antiseptic action. The combination of gallic acid and bismuth with iodin has been recommended by Lüdy. This agent gives off iodin early when introduced into wounds and is called airol. It is not toxic, it acts upon microorganisms like iodoform, it is a valuable drying-powder, it is not at all irritant, and has no disagreeable odor. Haegeler says that it is of no value in erysipelas, because iodin is not set free with sufficient rapidity to keep up with the movement of microorganisms in the lymph-vessels. He thinks it of great value in phlegmonous staphylococcal inflam-

[1] Centralbl. f. Chir., p. 1025, 1896.
[2] Beiträge z. klin. Chir., Bd. 15, H. 1, p. 266, 1896; Ann. of Surg., Mar., 1897.

mations, and likes it very much in recent wounds. It is an efficient stimulant to granulation. We can inject tubercular joints with a 10% emulsion.

P. F. Lomry[1] discusses the **antiseptic value of iodoform.** He considers that wounds which have been infected with staphylococci or streptococci heal better when treated with iodoform than when not so treated. He tells us that laboratory reports on the absence of antiseptic value in iodoform are not to be trusted because the observers have used nutrient material which does not dissolve iodoform. When we place iodoform in living tissues it is found to have a powerful action upon microorganisms. It greatly weakens the power of staphylococci and streptococci pyogenes. It neutralizes the products of many microorganisms; it does not interfere in any degree with the phagocytic power of the white blood-cells—in fact, it actually seems to increase it. In view of the fact that iodoform is probably not germicidal, the sterilized drug should be employed and the dressings changed every day.

E. Huess[2] recommends **tribromophenol bismuth** as a valuable antiseptic. It has very slight poisonous power. It antagonizes suppuration, lessens pain in the wound, and stimulates healing. It greatly quiets pain in burns, decomposes very slowly in the wound, and keeps up a constant action, the tribromophenol attacking the microorganisms, the bismuth serving to dry the parts and to prevent fermentation. This remedy does not promote granulation as strongly as iodoform. It does decidedly promote epithelial growth, is unaltered by light, and possesses some advantages over iodoform.

C. Longard[3] discusses the value of **amyloform,** which is a white powder produced by the chemical combination of starch with formaldehyd. This powder is odorless and non-poisonous, entirely insoluble, and not decomposed even by great heat. Gauze impregnated with amyloform can be subjected to steam without producing any change in the drug. It is a powerful antiseptic, deodorizer, and absorbent. It is unirritant and extremely cheap.

Von Leignek[4] calls attention to the interesting fact that when **catgut ligatures are kept in solutions of corrosive sublimate** the corrosive sublimate is precipitated after a time and the supposed antiseptic solution will not contain a single trace of mercury, it having changed to calomel and been thrown down to the bottom of the vessel. A rubber drainage-tube has the same effect on a corrosive sublimate solution after a time.

Hofmeister[5] recommends formalin for the **sterilization of syringes.** His experiments to determine the effect of formalin upon catgut led him to investigate its action upon leather. He found that ordinary leather after it had been placed for 24 hours in a 2 to 4% solution of formalin could be boiled in water without damaging it to any degree, but if it is boiled without such previous treatment it becomes after boiling a hardened mass which can be easily ground up. He tells us that syringes which consist of glass, metal, and leather are the only ones to which his method of sterilization can be applied. The syringe must be fastened by screws and not by cement. He takes out the piston and places it in ether to remove the fat. He then places it for 24 to 48 hours in a 2 to 4% solution of formalin; after the formalin is washed out the piston is put back, the air is removed, the barrel is filled with water, and the instrument is placed in cold water, the temperature of which is gradually raised to boiling. From time to time this method of treatment must be repeated. The principle of Hofmeister's method is that leather can be boiled in plain water without detriment if previously treated with formalin.

---

[1] Arch. f. klin. Chir., vol. liii., p. 787, 1896.   [2] Therap. Monatsh., H. 4, S. 214, 1896.
[3] Ibid., H. 10, S. 557, 1896.   [4] Wien. klin. Woch., ix., No. 39, 1896.
[5] Centralbl. f. Chir., p. 641, 1896.

H. C. Wood[1] writes upon **formaldehyd,** telling us that the article known commercially as formalin is a 40 % aqueous solution of formaldehyd. The germicidal powers of formaldehyd were discovered by Trillot, in 1888. Not only is it a germicide, but it renders innocuous the toxins of tetanus, diphtheria, and many other organisms. It is of great value for disinfection of rooms. A 1 % solution deodorizes feces (Walter). It is a far safer agent than corrosive sublimate, because it is not actively poisonous, and if a person started to swallow it by mistake it would be at once detected because of its taste and irritant properties. It will satisfactorily disinfect the hands, will disinfect instruments without dulling them, and is a valuable agent in the sterilization of catgut. Wood thinks its use may do away with many of " the tedious procedures at present connected " with the preparation of dressings. He says we should place the dressings in a receptacle of copper or tin, and attach the nozzle of a formaldehyd-forming lamp to the vessel so that the vapor will pass freely through. To wash wounds use a 2 % solution; to irrigate use a ¼ % solution (Willard). Such strengths are not irritant. Strong solutions are irritant even to sound tissues, and are used when we wish a caustic effect, as in chancroids or poisoned wounds. Vaginal gonorrhea is benefited by irrigation with a solution of a strength of 1 : 1000, and the cervix can be painted with a 4 % solution (Von Winckel). Wood suggests to surgeons to try the immediate disinfection of wounds by the vapor of formaldehyd on the ground that this vapor will more thoroughly disinfect recesses and pouches than will any fluid. He further advises the introduction of the vapor into the abdomen after incision in cases of peritonitis.

[The chief use of this agent until lately was as a fixing-material for the laboratory. Mosso and Parletti[2] made a careful study of the properties of formalin, and determined that it almost equals corrosive sublimate as a germicide, but is far less toxic. Laboratory experiments show that a 3 % solution kills the organisms of anthrax in 15 minutes and all other pathogenic organisms in 1 minute. A strong solution is very irritant and produces sloughing of tissue. In the Jefferson Medical College Hospital formalin has been used extensively for irrigation of foul ulcers, abscess-cavities, and sinuses, and for washing infected wounds, and has given much satisfaction. A 2 % solution is the best strength for wounds. Irrigate sinuses or abscess-cavities with a solution of a strength of ¼ to ½ %. Formalin vapor is used for the purpose of sterilizing catheters by R. W. Frank and others. A study of the antiseptic value of formaldehyd has been made by F. C. J. Bird.[3]]

Fürbringer and Freyhan[4] discuss the question of **how to disinfect the hands.** They maintain that it has been demonstrated with certainty that the hands cannot be completely sterilized by the use of soap and water even when associated with the use of antiseptics. Alcohol must be used, and the more alcohol employed the greater the cleanliness. They advise surgeons to place the hands in warm water and scrub them with a brush and soap for at least 5 minutes, rinse them off in sterile water, wash in alcohol for 5 minutes, and, finally, wash in sterile water. They hold that the alcohol is germicidal ; that it helps to remove grease and fat and so opens up the way for the action of a germicide, and that it removes the epiderm itself, which structure always contains bacteria.

Robt. F. Weir,[5] as regards the disinfection of the hands, thinks the weak

[1] Univ. Med. Mag., June, 1897.
[2] Arch. Ital. de Biol., xxiv., 3 ; Brit. Med. Jour., Feb. 8, 1896.
[3] Pharmacy J., Aug. 1 and Sept. 26, 1896.   [4] Deutsch. med. Woch., Feb. 4, 1897.
[5] Med. Rec., Apr. 3, 1897.

spot in aseptic surgery has been in obtaining sterilization of the hands of the surgeon and the skin of the patient. Geppert proved a number of years ago that the hands could not be thoroughly disinfected by corrosive sublimate solutions, and Abbott in 1891 confirmed the views of Geppert. Kocher proved over 15 years ago that carbolic acid was unreliable. Fürbringer advised the employment of alcohol in addition to the mercurial solution. Weir has found that even this plan does not invariably sterilize. He agrees with Reinecke that Kelley's method is not always reliable (washing in a saturated solution of potassium permanganate, then in a saturated solution of oxalic acid, then in sterile water). Weir now employs with great satisfaction chlorin, obtained by a plan which was suggested to him by Wm. Rauschenberger, apothecary of the New York Hospital—that is, mixing in the hands chlorinated lime and washing-soda and adding a little water. Chlorin is evolved when this mixture is rubbed over the hands. It helps to remove a portion of the epiderm and also saponifies fat.

The plan in full is as follows: thoroughly scrub the hands in running hot water with a brush and green soap, cleansing under and around the nails with a piece of soft wool. Something less than a tablespoonful of the lime material is passed into the palm, a piece of washing-soda is placed upon the chlorinated lime, enough water is added to make a cream-like mixture, and this material is rubbed into the hands and arms until the rough granules of soda can be no longer detected and until the material forms a thick paste (will need from 3 to 5 minutes). The next step is to rub the paste under the nails and around their edges by means of a piece of sterile cotton. The hands are now cleaned in sterile water. [We have used this method with entire satisfaction in numerous cases, and we are persuaded of its value. It leaves the hands smooth and soft, and beyond a temporary sensation of heat occasionally felt during its application produces no trouble or annoyance which is at all persistent. We have used it in a clinic 3 times within 2 hours without causing dermatitis.

L. A. Stimson writes to the *Medical Record* (Apr. 10, 1897) in criticism of R. Weir's statement about the introduction of the method into the New York Hospital. Stimson says that Mr. Rauschenberger suggested the method to him and that he used it as long ago as 1893. Its use by Stimson and Hartley in the Hudson Street Hospital was alluded to in the *Ann. of Surg.* for May, 1896.]

The value of **nosophen** and its salts has been a subject of some discussion during the year. Nosophen is obtained by adding iodin to a solution of phenolphtalein. It is a powder, light yellow in color, and free from odor, insoluble in water but freely soluble in an alkaline solution. The technical name of this drug is tetra-iodo-phenol-phtalein. Antinosin is the sodium salt of nosophen and eudoxin is the bismuth salt. A. L. Rix[1] has reported a cure of lupus brought about by nosophen. H. H. Duke[2] looks upon it as a true substitute for iodoform. Howard Lillianthal[3] has reported a case of tuberculous skin disease cured by this drug. Among other interesting articles upon this drug we would mention those of Müller,[4] Sprecher,[5] and Robin.[6] [We have tried this agent extensively and find it very useful. It is free from the odor of iodoform, is not toxic, is not irritant, and does not form cakes like aristol. We agree with Sands that it does not cause dermatitis around the wound. It prevents putrefaction, favors granulation, tends to arrest bleeding,

[1] Med. and Surg. Reporter, Feb. 27, 1897.   [2] Louisville Med. Month., Mar., 1897.
[3] Med. Rec., Oct. 31, 1896.   [4] Aerzte Rdsch., Jan. 2, 1897.
[5] Gaz. med. di Torino, Aug. 27, 1896.   [6] Le Scalpel, Dec. 27, 1896.

and has analgesic properties. Nosophen is not efficient when applied to a sloughing or suppurating wound unless the dead materials are first washed away; to be efficient it must come into contact with living tissue. In the treatment of chancroids it has not proved as satisfactory as iodoform. We have never used nosophen-gauze and have had no experience with antinosin and eudoxin.]

For a consideration of Schleich's formalin-gelatin in wound-treatment, see Wounds, p. 441.

SUPPURATION, GANGRENE, ETC.

Hentschel[1] contributes a study of **pyemia and sepsis.** He classifies the various conditions under the heads of pyemia, septicemia, sapremia, and sepsis. He says that pyemia is exclusively produced by the microorganisms of suppuration. Septicemia is an extremely rare condition in man, and in it the organisms multiply in the blood. Sepsis and sapremia are conditions of intoxication due to the absorption of toxins from local areas of infection. He quotes one case of pyemia in which the diplococcus lanceolatus was found and another case due to the staphylococcus citreus. He quotes as a typical case of sepsis an instance in which toxic absorption took place from a gangrenous focus. In a case of compound fracture of the leg followed by sepsis the blood was found absolutely free from microorganisms. In another case due to another cause the sepsis was produced by a focus of ischiorectal suppuration. There were no bacteria found in the blood.

E. Blondel[2] considers the question of **stitch-abscesses** and how to prevent them. He has returned to the ancient idea which commended the use of alcohol in wounds. He uses as few stitches as possible, and just before tying them wets them and also the wound-edges with alcohol of the strength of 90% and sponges out the wound itself with alcohol. After the suturing is complete the line of suture is covered with iodoform. He says that alcohol causes dryness, removes the grease, coagulates the serum, and promotes cicatrization. [It will be remembered that Le Dran occasionally washed wounds with brandy and that Baron Larrey believed that alcohol improved the condition of a wound. The practice is old and comes up anew from time to time, and we believe has much to commend it.]

The *Indian Med. Rec.* for Mar., 1897, quotes from the *Brit. Med. Jour.* on the proper treatment of inflammation from vaccination when running to excess. If it is found on the 12th or 14th day that the vaccination pustules are becoming confluent and are surrounded by a spreading inflammatory zone, with involvement of the axillary glands and probably with edema of the arm, the area of trouble should be dusted with iodoform and dressed with a dry pad of sterile gauze. The advance of the process will be completely arrested in 24 hours. The fistulæ will dry, the redness pass away, the glands diminish in size, and the edema disappear. This method is greatly to be preferred to the use of hot fomentations or moist antiseptic appliances, which are difficult to use upon an infant and involve the healing of an open wound.

Hugenschmidt[3] considers the **antiseptic properties of saliva.** He undertook the investigation in order to determine why mouth-operations are rarely followed by infection. He found that ordinary microorganisms grow rapidly in the saliva, but that nevertheless this fluid does have a tendency to

---

[1] Centralbl. f. Chir., No. 40, 1896.
[2] Jour. de Méd.; Jour. Am. Med. Assoc., Jan. 30, 1897.
[3] Ann. d. l'Inst. Pasteur, Oct., 1896.

keep down infection. It is alkaline and thus prevents fermentation. It washes away considerable portions of food which tend to lodge on the mucous membrane and dilutes that which remains. Hugenschmidt maintains that saliva stimulates the diapedesis of the white blood-corpuscles in the lymphatics. Even normal saliva contains microbic products, and, therefore, because of its attractive power toward microbes favors phagocytic action, the phagocytosis being due to rapid migration of the leukocytes.

Trenite[1] advises the use of **methylen-blue in the treatment of boils and anthrax.** The methylen is injected into the boil. A solution of the strength of 2 : 1000 is made and about 15 minims of this are injected. He maintains that by this method a boil can be cured in 48 hours. This same treatment is advised in anthrax. In true carbuncle Trenite incises the area of necrosis and removes sloughing material and after this makes the injection. When an injection has been given the wound is packed with iodoform-gauze which has been soaked in a hot solution of common salt.

W. W. Russell[2] calls attention to the possibility of a mistake being made in the diagnosis between **malarial and surgical fever.** In view of the fact that the diagnosis of malaria can be certainly made by the discovery of the hematozoa, in every doubtful case the blood should be examined. He cites a case in which through neglect of this precaution the patient was subjected to an oöphorectomy when nothing was wrong but malaria. The author cites several other cases of mistake to prove his contention. [More often sepsis is mistaken for malaria than malaria for sepsis.]

Jurinky[3] presents a report of 3 cases from Wölfler's clinic in Prague, which exhibit the curative effect of **potassium iodid in actinomycosis.** In 2 cases the head and neck were the seat of disease. Abscesses were incised and from 15 to 30 gr. doses given. Both were cured. In a case of actinomycosis of the appendix the abscess was incised and the iodid was given for several months. The case was cured, but subsequently a small abscess appeared in the scar. It is not known how the drug acts, but it very rapidly stops the pain, and its administration should be continued for some time after all fistulæ have closed. Colvin B. M. Smith[4] records a case of actinomycosis of the cheek which was cured in 2 months by the administration of potassium iodid. Smith recalls the fact that 3 cases were recently successfully treated in the Bristol Royal Infirmary by the same method. He says that in his cases the cure was either spontaneous or resulted from the exhibition of the iodid. It is very improbable that the cure was spontaneous, because it took place coincidently with the exhibition of the iodid after months of no improvement. The patient refused to permit surgical treatment. Herbert B. McIntire,[5] of Cambridge, Mass., records a case of actinomycosis of the chest-wall and lung in which infection was by the bronchial tubes and in which the iodid failed to cure. Parker Syms,[6] of New York, records a case of intraabdominal actinomycosis in which there were discharging fistulæ surrounded by indurated masses. A large swelling over the groin was opened and scraped out, but the woman refused any thorough operative treatment. She was placed under the charge of Dr. Van Arsdale, who administered potassium iodid, and has somewhat improved, but the writer does not think that this case tends to show that iodid has any curative effect.

[1] Jour. de Prat., quoted in Therap. Gaz., Sept. 15, 1896.
[2] Bull. Johns Hopkins Hosp., Nov. and Dec., 1896.
[3] Centralbl. f. Chir., No. 36, 1896.
[5] Boston M. and S. Jour., Jan. 28, 1897.
[4] Lancet, Mar. 13, 1897.
[6] Ann. of Surg., Feb., 1897.

H. Vincent[1] has made a study of the etiology and lesions of **hospital gangrene.** He describes a bacillus which he has found on the false membrane of the surface of the ulcers. He has found this bacillus in every case, and considers it to be the cause of the disease. In some cases it is the only bacillus found, but it is present in greater numbers even when pus cocci and spirilli also exist. He gives a careful description of this bacillus and its properties. An examination of tissue which is attacked by the gangrene exhibits two zones : the superficial, consisting of a false membrane, and a deeper zone, formed of necrotic tissue infiltrated with blood and altered by the action of the organisms. In the neighborhood of the abiding-place of the microbes embryonic tissue exists as a barrier against systemic invasion. The organism is not met with in the blood, and the writer has failed in his attempts to cultivate it on artificial media. From the fact that inoculations in the lower animals have not produced the disease he is inclined to think that the gangrene is limited to the human species. He inoculated several healthy rabbits without any result, and this leads him to infer that many factors are necessary to permit the bacilli to live and multiply. When animals which were the victims of tuberculosis were inoculated with the false membrane they developed typical cases of the disease. [The failure to inoculate animals may mean, as the author suggests, that these animals are not subject to the disease, and may also mean that his bacillus is not really the cause of hospital gangrene.]

Ernest A. T. Steele[2] records a case of acute **spreading gangrene treated with antistreptococcic serum.** The patient was a child 1½ years of age ; 3 weeks before admission to the hospital she had been burned on the calf of the left leg with a red-hot poker. The wound did not heal ; 16 days after this injury she was sick and fretful, and the mother discovered a red spot on the center of the forehead and a small abscess on the lower lip. By the next day the spot had increased to the size of a shilling and had become black in the center. The child was feverish, and there was offensive discharge from the left nostril. She was admitted to the hospital 20 days after the accident to the leg and 4 days after the appearance of the red spot on the forehead. On admission there was a gangrenous spot on the forehead the size of a five-shilling piece ; around the edges of this area the skin was inflamed and undermined. The tissues crepitated from the presence of gas ; the general condition was excessively bad. The pulse was 120, the temperature 101.8°, and she had had a shivering attack before admission. Furthermore, she was drowsy and irritable. The edge of the left lower eyelid was covered with sloughing granulations and there was an offensive seropurulent discharge from both nostrils. On the left leg was an ulcer 1½ in. long and 1 in. broad, which was covered with gray sloughs and showed here and there depressions where the ulcerations had passed into the deeper structures. The child was anesthetized, the edges of the gangrenous area on the forehead were clipped away, and all unhealthy tissue was removed. The part was mopped with nitric acid and the ulcers on the lip and leg were scraped with Volkmann's spoon and cauterized with the acid. The child became temporarily better, but six days afterward it was again necessary to repeat this scraping process. The child was extremely ill and in grave danger. It was decided to administer the antistreptococcic serum. An injection of 5 c.c. was given, and brandy and strychnin were administered internally ; no other local treatment was admitted. The next day the morning temperature was 100.8°. There was a marked change in the appearance of the wounds and ulcers. The gangrene had ceased to spread and the phage-

[1] Ann. de l'Inst. Pasteur, Sept. 25, 1896.   [2] Brit. Med. Jour., Dec. 19, 1896.

denic process in the ulcers had stopped. In the evening the temperature rose to 103.2°, and another injection of 5 c.c. was given. From this date the child steadily improved, although 5 days later suppuration took place in the right elbow-joint which required incision and drainage. Complete recovery ensued.

Obalinski[1] discusses the operative treatment of **suppuration of the posterior mediastinum,** and reports 5 cases. He practises rib-resection near the articulation with the spine. He separates the costal pleura from the ribs and from the thoracic vertebra, thus permitting him to gain ready access to the posterior mediastinum. In 2 cases the pleura was torn, and traumatic pneumothorax arose. The wound was at once packed with gauze ; no infection took place, and the pneumothorax passed away in 2 days. The author advocates this method of procedure when a cervical abscess passes down into the mediastinum, when an abscess takes origin near the spine, when it has caused a fistula in the thoracic region, or when it has followed perforation of the wall of the esophagus.

Samuel Broke[2] reports a case of **blood-poisoning treated by anti- streptococcic serum.** The patient had a whitlow of the thumb which resulted in widespread suppurative cellulitis of the forearm. Free incisions were made. Several days after the incision antistreptococcic serum was ad- ministered. Up to the time the serum was used the swelling was rapidly ex- tending, but a notable decrease took place in the swelling as soon as the serum was employed. The author says it is " difficult to decide " if this improvement was produced by the serum or the incisions. It became necessary in this case to amputate the arm because of threatened gangrene. The patient died 10 days after operation. A. H. Cook and A. R. Cook[3] report 2 cases of blood- poisoning in which antistreptococcic serum was used. One patient suffered from suppurative cellulitis of leg following upon a lacerated wound, the other patient had infection following a punctured wound of the thumb. In case 1 the injections seemed to be followed by great benefit. In case 2 the value of the serum was doubtful.

T. J. Bokenham[4] writes upon the orrhotherapy of blood-poisoning, and makes a plea for exactitude in the use of antistreptococcic serum. He reports a case of erysipelas of head, which was treated by Alfred R. Friel, and which rapidly recovered under serum-treatment. Serum from one of the bullæ showed a pure culture of streptococci. Then follows a report of 2 cases treated by Mr. Stephen Paget. The first case was lymphangitis due to inoculation from a case of septic peritonitis. This case was promptly cured by the use of the serum, which agent prevented the headache and great depression which we expect to accompany septic infection. The second case labored under lymphangitis from mixed infection, and the patient died in spite of the use of serum. Blood examination made during life proved that mixed infection ex- isted, and the prognosis in mixed infection is always worse than in pure strep- tococcus infection. The author concludes that this death from mixed infection does not indicate that the serum is useless.

In a case of infection by staphylococci serum injections had been given without result. Bokenham examined the exudate, found that staphylococci only were present, and advised the surgeons in charge that serum-treatment would probably prove useless.

The author holds that the serum is harmless, that laboratory experiments offer much presumptive evidence that the material is valuable, and that its

[1] Wien. klin. Woch., Dec. 10, 1896.   [2] Brit. Med. Jour., Feb. 27, 1897.
[3] Ibid., Oct. 31, 1896.   [4] Ibid., May 22, 1897.

use does not debar us from employing at the same time other methods of treatment. The serum is obtained from horses, which are immune or very resistant to streptococci, the animals having been rendered resistant by repeated injections of streptococci, or of the germ-free filtered culture-medium in which streptococci have grown, or by a combination of these materials. Bacterial examination should be made to confirm a clinical diagnosis of septic infection.

[The value of antistreptococcic serum is still in doubt. It is an agent which does not appear to act by simply antagonizing toxins, but acts by killing streptococci, and dead streptococci may be virulently poisonous. As Primrose, of Canada, puts it, "We know that there are bacteria which, when killed off, are capable of producing more virulent toxins in their death than during their life." It does not seem proper to say that this agent is absolutely harmless. It may kill large numbers of cocci, and by liberating large amounts of poison may do great harm.]

CYSTS AND TUMORS.

W. Joseph Hearn [1] reports a case of **congenital multilocular cyst of the omentum** in the male. Hearn reviews the literature and tells us that these cases are extremely rare. The patient was 8 years of age. The family physician observed the distended abdomen when the child was born. At the age of 6 weeks the distention had decidedly lessened and remained stationary for the next 6 years. When 6 years of age the abdomen began to increase in size. Aspiration was twice employed, a small amount of brown fluid being drawn off each time. On admission to hospital the abdomen was found greatly distended : greatest circumference was 44 in. The distance between the sternal notch and the pubes was 25 in. Weight was $93\frac{1}{2}$ pounds. There were practically no symptoms except a frequency of micturition and a sense of weight. The abdomen was opened, the cyst incised, and the several compartments drawn out of the wound as they were emptied. The entire cyst was finally delivered, and the point of origin was found to be in the folds of the great omentum, below the margin of the transverse colon. The patient made an excellent recovery, and two weeks after the operation weighed 49 pounds. The weight of the cyst with its contents must have been almost 50 pounds.

Dr. Jacob Frank [2] writes upon **hydatids of the liver.** After considering the etiology and pathology, he discusses the diagnosis and reports 2 cases. The first was that of a woman of 32, born in Russia. The diagnosis made in her case was cyst of the gall-bladder due to obstruction of the common duct. Operation disclosed a hydatid cyst of the liver. The cyst was incised, and as the wall became relaxed it was pulled out and emptied. The peritoneum was sewed about the cyst-wall by a continuous suture, 2 in. of sac were removed, and a drainage-tube and packing were introduced. The patient made a good recovery. The second patient was a man of 28, born in Germany. The diagnosis was biliary calculus. Operation disclosed a hydatid cyst. The peritoneum was stitched around the border of the mass, thus forming a circular surface about the size of a silver dollar closed off from the abdominal cavity ; the aspirator drew off the typical fluid. Gauze was packed over the puncture, the wound dressed, and 4 days later the cyst was incised. The cavity was irrigated with sterile water, the inner surface was curetted, a drainage-tube was introduced, and the wound was dressed. This patient also made a good recovery.

[1] Ann. of Surg., June, 1897.　　　　　[2] Am. Jour. Med. Sci., Oct., 1896.

Dr. Frank offers the following conclusions in regard to the treatment of hydatids of the liver : an incision over the most prominent part of the mass should be made, if a mass can be detected ; but if no tumor is obvious, the guide to incision is the area of hardening and of dulness on percussion. The surgeon should always examine for adhesions, and, if adhesions do not exist, he should produce them by suturing the peritoneum around the mass, thus shutting off the abdominal cavity. The aspirator is used to prove the diagnosis, always bearing in mind the possibility that typical fluid will not appear, as it may be too thick to enter the needle. When it has been found necessary to produce adhesions artificially the surgeon waits for several days before opening the cyst. The opening made in the cyst-wall should be of sufficient size to admit a large-sized drainage-tube. The dressing must be conducted with the strictest antiseptic care. For the first week after operation the cyst-cavity should be washed out with sterile water, after this with carbolic solution, iodin solution, or any of the antiseptic solutions. Frank says in cases in which no adhesions exist it is possible to perform an operation with success in one sitting if great care be employed ; but it is wiser to sew the peritoneum to produce adhesions, and when the adhesions become firm to open the cyst. [It will be observed in a later article that all surgeons do not agree with Frank as to the advisability of suturing the peritoneum to the cyst-wall, at least before the cyst is partially emptied. John O'Conor,[1] of Buenos Ayres, speaks of such a proceeding as " dangerous and useless," and says that the cyst-wall is so thin and tense that sutures will enter the cyst-cavity unless the cyst is previously partially emptied. If needles do enter the cyst-cavity, hydatid fluid will squirt from the punctures and may enter the peritoneal cavity and thus cause the formation of new cysts or the onset of hydatid toxemia. O'Conor surrounds the cyst with sponges, empties the cyst through a cannula, and when the tension is lessened seizes the cyst and draws it to the surface, enlarges the opening in the cyst-wall, removes the sponges, and then sutures the cyst to the parietal wound, suturing to the peritoneum only at the upper and lower angles of the wound.]

E. S. Jackson,[2] of Queensland, furnishes the notes of a case of hydatid cyst of the liver presenting several unusual features. One peculiarity about this cyst was that no endocyst was discovered at the operation or subsequent to the operation. The small cysts numbered many hundreds. No hooklets were discovered in the fluid and there were no daughter-cysts. Since the operation it has been necessary many times to tap cysts which have become prominent ; none of the cysts tapped have been larger than a hen's egg. The case is published in the hope that someone may have seen something similar, and almost with the suspicion that the diagnosis was incorrect. It is possible that it was a form of hydatid or some hitherto undescribed parasite.

John O'Conor,[3] of Buenos Ayres, furnishes a valuable clinical contribution to the surgery of the liver, and in this paper reports 9 interesting cases of hydatid cyst. One case was a hydatid of the liver in a schoolboy of 10. This case recovered. O'Conor, in commenting upon this case, calls attention to what he designates the dangerous and useless practice of introducing sutures through parietes and cyst-wall before the cyst is at least partially emptied. The cyst-walls are so tense and thin that it is impossible to pass sutures without invading the cyst-cavity. He tried to do it in this case, but from each needle-puncture there was a flow of fluid. Some of this fluid entered the peritoneal cavity, but fortunately no ill result followed. In cases in which

[1] Ann. of Surg., May, 1897.   [2] Intercol. Med. Jour. Austral., Sept. 20, 1896.
[3] Ann. of Surg., May, 1897.

hydatid toxemia follows the operation the condition is due to the escape of hydatid fluid into the peritoneal cavity, from which point the poison enters into the system. Such cysts should always be emptied through a medium-sized trocar and cannula, the peritoneal cavity being walled off with sponges. The tension is thus relieved, and the cyst can be grasped with hooks and drawn to the abdominal incision. The trocar-opening is then enlarged, the sponges removed, and the cyst sutured to the abdominal wound. In this last step the peritoneum at the upper and lower ends of the wound is sutured to the cyst, but throughout the rest of the wound the cyst is sutured to the fibrous surface of the incision. The next case was a hydatid tumor of the liver in a patient of 25, in which a transthoracic operation was performed and the patient recovered. An aspirator-needle was introduced into the 4th intercostal space anterior to the axillary line and a few drops of clear liquid were drawn off. A portion of the 4th rib was resected, the costal pleura was opened, and a large cyst was felt beneath the diaphragm. An incision was made through the diaphragm and diaphragmatic pleura, a trocar was inserted into the cyst, and after the cyst had relaxed a portion of it was pulled through the diaphragm and sewed to the wound in the chest-wall. There was no endocyst that appeared. The cavity was irrigated with Condy's fluid, and a large drainage-tube was inserted. Seven weeks after operation during irrigation the endocyst appeared and was removed with forceps. The patient made a good recovery. O'Conor comments on this case, and says that it taught him the valuable fact that if an endocyst is not removed at the time of operation profuse and prolonged suppuration will inevitably occur. Now he always continues the primary irrigation until the endocyst is evacuated. The next case was a hydatid tumor of the liver operated upon by abdominal section. This patient recovered after profuse suppuration and prolonged urticaria from hydatid toxic poisoning. He performed Bond's operation upon this case. That is, after opening the cyst the hand was introduced, the endocyst was removed, the cavity was irrigated with corrosive sublimate solution, the interior of the cyst was dried with sponges and dusted with iodoform-gauze, the opening in the cyst was closed with a continuous silk suture, the mass was returned within the peritoneal cavity, and the external wound was closed. He says that he will never repeat Bond's operation. He considers marsupialization a thoroughly safe procedure, but does not think Bond's operation is safe. He believes that in the ordinary operation very large abdominal incisions should be made, in order to expose the cyst thoroughly and permit of removal of a large portion of the cyst-wall and suture of the remainder of the cyst in folds to the wound. The next case was a hydatid tumor of the liver occurring in a woman of 51 years. The abdomen was opened, the peritoneal cavity was blocked off with sponges, the trocar and cannula were inserted into the liver, and the cyst was struck at a depth of 1 in. Some clear fluid escaped. The trocar was at once reinserted in the cannula in order to prevent collapse of the cyst-wall. A blunt bistoury was passed along the trocar, and an incision $\frac{1}{2}$ in. long was made through the liver-tissue. Violent hemorrhage occurred which was arrested by pressure. A pair of forceps were inserted and opened, when a furious hemorrhage took place. Pressure failed to arrest it, and it was found necessary to insert sutures deep in the liver-substance and apply pressure in association with it. Unfortunately the sutures cut out, and the only hope was to remove the cyst-wall at once. The cyst was at once opened. O'Conor grasped the edges with forceps, and forward traction controlled the hemorrhage. He introduced silk sutures through the parietal wall and no more bleeding occurred. The patient died the next day but one after the operation. He considers that in this case he made some vital mistakes. The first was the introduction of a knife to cut through the healthy liver-substance. Even after he had done this he might have saved the patient had he emptied the cyst through a cannula and closed the external wound. The most lamentable error was the attempt to make an opening into the liver by the use of the forceps. This was a procedure which rendered it impossible for him to retrace his steps, and as the hemorrhage had to be arrested his finger was the only instrument left him with which to reach the cyst. He states that he read [1] with interest a case of **transthoracic hepatotomy,** in which the surgeons strongly advised what they called the *simple method* of pushing a knife into the cyst alongside the trocar, and following this up with a dressing-forceps to dilate the opening. After his experience he is not certain whether to envy or pity the surgeon who has the courage to advance such an opinion. O'Conor says that if in future he should encounter an inch of healthy liver over the hydatid cyst he will do the operation in two, stages. In order that sponge-pressure may be successful in arresting hemorrhage it is necessary to have a firm basis of support; but a torn liver recedes and affords no basis of support, and sutures are unreliable for they tear out. If firm pressure is to be made, the only hope is to have firm adhesion with the parietal wound, and then if hemorrhage does occur we have something solid to press against. The first stage of the operation is to obtain adhesion between the parietal and visceral peritoneum. In the second stage the trocar should be introduced as a guide, but the cautery should be employed to open the cyst.

He reports another case in which suppuration occurred in a hydatid cyst of the liver, and abdominal section was performed by the usual method. The patient made a good recovery. This is the only case of primary suppurating hydatid cyst that he has ever met with, and it is an interesting fact that although the endocyst was gangrenous no constitutional symptoms accompanied the suppuration.

He reports another case of collapsed hydatid cyst of the liver in which abdominal section was performed. This patient had a series of symptoms which suggested congestion of the liver. The physicians had inserted an aspirating-needle a month previously because they suspected hydatids. O'Conor's diagnosis was suppuration in a hydatid following puncture. On opening the abdomen a collapsed cyst was found. It was drawn to the surface, and the collapsed endocyst and a bucketful of fluid were removed. There was no suppuration and no peritonitis. The patient recovered in 67 days. The fever which had followed the tapping a month before was due to hydatid toxic poisoning. He reports another case in which there was a hydatid tumor of the liver treated by transthoracic hepatotomy. The patient recovered. In another case a patient with a hydatid of the liver recovered after a celiotomy. O'Conor states that never in his experience has he been able to detect hydatid fremitus.

J. Bland Sutton [2] writes on **myelomata or myeloid sarcomata.** He has come to the conclusion that it is an error to include myeloid tumors in the genus sarcoma. He holds they should rank as a separate genus under the term myelomata, because red marrow is as distinct a tissue as fat, myomatous, or fibrous tissue. Myelomata arise in the red marrow in the cancellous portions of bones, and the tissue composing them is histologically identical with the red marrow of young bone. When a tumor is cut fresh its surface looks like a piece of fresh liver. The microscope shows us that such growths abound in giant cells imbedded among round and spindle cells, the greater

[1] Lancet, Sept. 12, 1896.   [2] Edinb. Med. Jour., Feb., 1897.

mass of the tumor being composed of giant cells. Such tumors are especially apt to appear in certain bones, notably the tibia and the radius. They are most common in the upper part of the tibia and in the lower end of the radius. Myelomata prefer the head of the fibula rather than the part below, and the lower end of the ulna rather than the part above. Some cases have been reported as occurring in the clavicle, the sternal end being the favorite seat. In the humerus the head of the bone is the usual site, but in the femur the condyloid end is the area most prone to invasion. The patella is a very rare situation for myeloid tumors. As regards the bones of the head, myelomata are peculiar to the jaws. The clinical features are tolerably characteristic. The patients are rarely over 25. The tumor grows slowly and expands the bone equally. As the bony tissue expands it thins until the shell becomes so attenuated that it crepitates under pressure. Here and there the tissue perforates the bony shell, and at the points of perforation there is marked pulsation. Myelomata do not disseminate and do not infect the lymph-glands. If a patient comes under the surgeon's care before the osseous capsule has been perforated, the growth may be extirpated without fear of return. The manner of extirpation varies with the situation of the tumor. Enucleation should not be attempted in the tibia, and in the femur amputation should be performed at some distance above the growth. In the upper limb the lower end of the radius and of the ulna and the upper end of the radius have been excised, with the result that cure has been obtained with the retention of a useful hand. Excision has been practised upon the head of the humerus, the sternal end of the clavicle, and the acromial end of the clavicle, with cure as the result. In the upper jaw the premaxillæ have been removed, this operation sparing the removal of both maxillæ. If the patient does not consult the surgeon until a tumor of the maxilla has fungated, the soft parts will be so invaded that even complete extirpation offers a very slender chance of permanent cure. These tumors are rare, and differ histologically, pathologically, and clinically from the sarcomata.

Dr. Denissenko [1] discovered the fact that **warts** could be **cured by application of the juice of chelidonium majus.** He was led to employ this remedy in the treatment of epithelioma, and he claims that it is of extreme value. He uses it externally and gives it internally to the amount of even 75 gr. a day in an aqueous solution. Locally it is used by hypodermic injection into and about the tumor. The solution employed consists of the extract of chelidonium, glycerin, and distilled water. Denissenko claims that the cancerous cachexia rapidly abates under the influence of this agent and that the tumor greatly diminishes and tends to separate from the sound tissues.

Herbert Snow [2] speaks anew of the value of **opium and cocain in the treatment of cancer.** He tells us that these two drugs possess in a notable degree the power of inhibiting tissue-metabolism—that is to say, that they powerfully sustain the bodily powers. He has long been in the habit of giving opium in cancer with the most beneficial results. Cancer of the female breast produces sooner or later and in every case deposit in the bone-marrow, and this deposit eventually infects the blood-stream. When operations are done, and even when bone-marrow infection exists, we may, by the use of opium, retard recurrence for a long period of time, the patient being apparently in perfect health. For the past three years Snow has been in the habit of combining cocain with the opium. Cocain is of value in sustaining vitality, and its anesthetic powers contribute greatly to the comfort of the indi-

---

[1] Deutsch. med. Zeit., Sept. 24, 1896.　　　[2] Brit. Med. Jour., Sept. 19, 1896.

vidual, especially of one who labors under cancer of the tongue or mouth. In gastric and intestinal cancer this drug is of great value because of its property of preventing vomiting. When Snow has operated on a case in which he anticipates recurrence he places the patient on an opium regimen as soon as convalescence is attained. In this article he reports a number of typical cases to exhibit the great value of these drugs. He tells us that under the opium treatment alone a woman who had been operated on in June, 1877, for advanced mammary cancer with marrow-deposit had no recurrence until December, 1893. One patient remained entirely free from January, 1881, to February, 1885, and 3 from July, 1886, to June, 1893; 3 cases of breast scirrhus operated on in 1891, 2 in 1892, and 2 in 1893, with well-marked marrow-infection, as yet show no evidence of recurrence. A man was admitted in April with a tumor in the abdomen, enlarged liver, extreme emaciation, and a history of persistent vomiting for six months. He evidently labored under cancer of the pylorus. He was placed under cocain and opium, and since beginning this *régime* has not vomited at all and has gained much in strength and comfort. Other cases equally striking are cited by this author.

J. Collins Warren,[1] of Harvard, presents the results of **operations for the cure of cancer of the breast.** He tells us that the old idea was that this condition was incurable, and this idea was true under the circumstances then existing, and the fact that the condition was incurable was due to inadequate operation. Sir James Paget stated that he was not aware of a single instance of recovery. This opinion, however, has been entirely overthrown, although a number of surgeons are still unconvinced. About 15 years ago Volkmann called attention to the necessity of clearing out the axilla. Heidenhain also asserted that it was necessary to remove the fascia of the great pectoral muscle. Mitchell Banks and the younger Gross were among the pioneers in advocating a more radical breast-operation. Halsted's recent work gives convincing evidence of the advantage of removing the pectoral muscles and clearing out the infraclavicular and supraclavicular regions. A frequent source of recurrence is the flaps of skin which are left, and a wide sweep should always be made around this organ in order to remove any infected area. The point to aim at is, not to obtain union by first intention, but rather to remove all of the disease. A clean dissection of the axilla is entirely effectual against a return of the disease in that locality. Warren then discusses certain important points about the anatomy of this region which bear upon the operation necessary to be performed. The operation which he performs now has been developed from the so-called completed operation. By the term completed operation was meant the removal of the mammary gland with a considerable amount of integument and the free dissection of the axilla, the gland and paramammary tissue and integument being removed sufficiently extensively to include the superficial lymphatic vessels which spring from the various breast quadrants and run toward the margin of the pectoralis major muscle. The operation comprises in all cases the removal of the sternal portion of the pectoralis major muscle, division of the pectoralis minor muscle, and occasionally removal of this muscle; dissection of the axilla and the infraclavicular space, and exploration in many cases of the supraclavicular region.

Warren then describes his operation in detail. In 92 consecutive cases in which this operation was performed there were but 2 deaths, 1 from erysipelas and 1 from Bright's disease. The death from erysipelas occurred many years ago. This shows a mortality of but little over 2%. The com-

[1] Boston M. and S. Jour., Nov. 2, 1896.

pleted operation is absolutely essential, as proved by the fact that in only 3 of these cases was it shown by the microscope that the lymphatic glands were not infected. The tables Warren publishes include only the cases in which it was possible to obtain a subsequent history. Taking 3 years as the period which it is considered generally necessary to elapse to pronounce the case as cured, and with 42 cases whose subsequent history he knows, 11 of them are living and well, or 26%. These 42 cases include the 2 fatal cases. If we do not calculate with them included, we have 40 cases with 11 cures, or 27%. There are 15 without recurrence at the end of 2 years. In a series of 28 consecutive cases in his practice there are 14 alive at the present time. Billroth asserts that a patient who has lived one year after operation and shows no sign of recurrence when examined by a competent surgeon may be pronounced cured. In very many cases in which recurrence is said to have occurred at a later date the truth of the matter is that the nodule existed at the time of operation but was not removed. In 33 cases in which the date of recurrence was noted it was found that the disease appeared on an average in 14 months after the operation. The average duration of life in 28 cases in which death was due to recurrence was 32 months. In only 2 of these cases did the disease arise from a benign tumor. There were 2 cases of cancer of the axillary border, a term which Warren has applied to a growth which begins as a nodule of the skin at the point mentioned, and remains localized for a considerable time, but eventually involves all the axilla and breast. Warren then presents his case-records in detail. [Warren insists that, as renewed growth is often encountered in the flaps of skin which are allowed to remain, a large area of skin should be removed. Halsted believes this and removes a very large piece of skin and closes the gap with Thiersch grafts. The younger Gross invariably removed all of the skin over the breast, leaving a considerable gap to heal by granulation. Tausini has recently written upon the necessity of removing considerable skin, and he advises the removal of all the skin covering the breast and also a strip of skin about 4 in. wide from the breast into the axilla, and the partial closure of the gap by dissecting a flap from the back and sliding it forward into the wound. It seems to us that the skin is a dangerous tissue to leave, but that the subcutaneous tissues are much more dangerous. It is necessary to remove a large area of subcutaneous tissue, and with this the skin can be taken, or only a portion of the skin is removed.]

Herbert Snow[1] discusses the insidious **marrow-infection of mammary carcinoma.** He tells us that secondary deposit in the bone-marrow was definitely present in considerable amounts in 80% of the cases of mammary cancer which died. It is very doubtful if the remaining 20% were free from infection of marrow to the end. Out of 150 patients seen in the Out-Patient Service who had cancer of the breast averaging in duration from 10 to 12 months, 90 on their first visit showed well-marked evidences of this condition, 22 showed slighter evidences, and 8 developed them subsequently; total, 120 or 80%. As a rule, when a scirrhous cancer exists in the breast of a woman the lymph-glands of the corresponding axilla are infected in from 6 to 12 weeks. The cancer-cells block up the lymph-channel and the lymph-current regurgitates and passes in abnormal directions. The axillary glands receive lymph from the area of the tumors and from the head of the humerus. When these glands become cancerous the lymph containing cancer-cells regurgitates into the marrow of the humerus. The humerus is, as a rule, the first bone infected. From the edge of the mammary gland some lymphatics pene-

---

[1] Lancet, Jan. 9, 1897.

trate the thoracic wall and carry the lymph to the mediastinal lymph-glands and the thymus gland. The cells which enter into the thymus gland proliferate and directly invade the sternum. After bone-invasion has existed for a considerable length of time fragments of cell-protoplasm pass from the marrow into the circulation, and thus enter into the opposite breast, other bones, or the viscera. The physical signs of marrow-infection are often not positively evident until the disease has existed 18 months, and they may even be delayed until a much later period. The upper $\frac{1}{3}$ of the humerus becomes tender on pressure and the bone feels thicker than its companion of the opposite side. The sternum gradually bulges forward at the junction of the upper and middle portions and the lump is painless. There are very frequently pains in the loins and the scapula which are mistaken for rheumatism. These pains are on the same side as the lesion. Unlike rheumatism they do not affect the articulations. The sternal prominence might be simulated by a natural conformation of the part. It is only when sternal prominence is associated with the gnawing lumbar and scapular pains, and especially when a gradual development has taken place under observation, that entire reliance can be placed upon it as absolute evidence of infection. When infection of the bone-marrow occurs white marrow is formed—a firm material as white as note-paper. When in making a postmortem we find this firm white marrow we can be assured there is cancerous infection even if a microscopic examination is not made.

Snow then records 5 typical cases to illustrate his views, and states that only 5 or 6 times has he seen the sternal protrusion advance to actual tumor-formation with subsequent ulceration. He tells us in conclusion that deposits in the bone-marrow are peculiarly chronic and latent. They may grow unnoticed for 4 or 5 years or even more. They cause hardly any appreciable impairment of health until general blood-diffusion takes place. The marrow is rarely examined at an autopsy unless some palpable bone-lesion exists, and these investigations invite closer attention to it. Many cases which are regarded as osteomyelitis and osteitis deformans have been reported as associated with malignant growths somewhere in the osseous system, and it seems likely that more will eventually pass into the same classification. As a routine symptom marrow-infection for mechanic and anatomic reasons is shown only by cancer of the female breast, but it may follow any form of malignant growth which directly implicates the marrow, as in primary sarcoma of bone or in rectal cylindroma adherent to the sacrum, but under none of these conditions is it insidious. In view of these observations it is impossible to pronounce a patient cured 3 years after the removal of the breast cancer, even when there has been no recurrence, unless we can confidently pronounce that marrow-deposits are absent.

Herbert Snow[1] reports 300 cases of **breast-excision for malignant disease.** He considers these cases carefully and comes to certain definite conclusions. He concludes that infection of bone-marrow is a great obstacle to radical cure. This, as a general rule, occurs within six months of the beginning of the disease and frequently earlier, although the symptoms of it are rarely detected until the second year. In atrophic scirrhus the condition may be delayed for years. Immunity from recurrence for 3 years affords no basis on which to pronounce the disease cured unless insidious marrow-symptoms are absent or unless we have reason to believe that the disease was extirpated before marrow-infection occurred. The most important point in the excision of the female breast is extensive dissection of the subcutaneous connective tissue around the mammary gland from the sternum to the axilla

[1] Brit. Med. Jour., Oct. 17, 1896.

and from the subclavian fossa to the cartilage of the 7th rib. This tissue is the most dangerous tract in which recurrence is apt to appear. It can always be satisfactorily removed by dissecting off a flap of healthy skin, and after its removal we can bring the edges of the skin together and obtain immediate union. Snow asserts that there is absolutely no advantage in destroying an extensive area of skin, and in every single case that he has operated on he has been persuaded that the utmost benefit that surgery could offer was compatible with union of the greater part of the wound by first intention. If the skin is infiltrated, we may be sure that the bone-marrow is infected, and no amount of skin removal will save the patient. He tells us that a startling novelty, which is to be mentioned with incredulous surprise, is amputation at the shoulder-joint in order to secure a covering-flap from the deltoid. If we encounter instances of scirrhus, or even encephaloid, of but 2 or 3 months' duration, the surgeon should endeavor to eradicate the disease permanently by

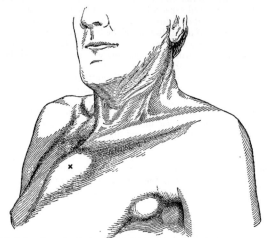

FIG. 5.—The "sternal symptom" of marrow-infection : the characteristic prominence marked **X**
(from photograph by Dr. Johnston English).

removing the mammary gland and a wide area of subcutaneous tissue from around this gland and also the contents of the axilla; but in advanced cases it is futile to risk life by prolonged and heroic measures when we know that there is a deep-seated nidus which we cannot touch. The utmost that we can do in these latter cases is to remove the gross lesions, obtain prompt union of the wound, and by after-treatment with opium and cocain retard the progress of the disease or possibly cause it to remain stationary for years. Partial amputation of the breast for cancer is of course undesirable, excepting for mere purposes of palliation; for even the smallest scirrhus extirpation should be performed. There are 3 exceptions Snow notes to the very just rule that the axillary contents should always be removed. They should not be removed in intracystic cancer-growths, in fairly recent atrophic cases, and in scirrhus appearing close to the sternum, whence the axilla is much more slowly infected than are other regions of the organ, the lymph-current flowing to the thymus and the mediastinal lymph-glands.

George Thomas Beatson,[1] of Glasgow, presents a very remarkable article on **the treatment of inoperable cases of carcinoma of the mamma** and suggests **a new method of treatment,** with illustrative cases. The author says that he has seen a considerable number of cases in which it was obvious that ordinary surgical methods could not be applied with any hope of benefit. In considering these cases he has worked out a plan of treatment which he thinks has not as yet been tried by others. This plan is founded on a conception of the etiology and nature of carcinoma which is radically opposed to the local parasitic theory of the disease. Inoperable cases of cancer may be placed into 2 groups: those which have recurred after an operation has been done, and those in which, although no operation has been done, the disease has advanced too far to permit of thorough removal. He reports 3 cases, one of which illustrates the first group and the other 2 the second. The first case was a woman of 33; the left breast had been removed and the axilla cleared out for cancer, but the growth quickly recurred. It was very evident that the case should be classified as inoperable according to our ordinary conceptions of the limits of operation, and the question had to be decided whether anything at all could be done. Beatson asked himself the question: Can the disease be attacked in any other way than by local removal? He tells us that some 20 years ago he made a study of lactation and gathered a considerable amount of practical information from farmers and shepherds. Certain points struck him as of great interest. He discovered that the secretion of milk, though affected by the general nervous system, had no special nervous supply of its own to control it. Division of the sympathetic and of other nerves produced no result whatever on the secretion of milk. It was clear that the changes that occur in the mammary gland during lactation are almost identical up to a certain point with what occurs in the cancerous breast. In both of these conditions the epithelial cells proliferate, occlude the ducts, and fill the acini of the gland; but in lactation these cells become vacuolated, undergo fatty degeneration, and form milk, while in carcinoma they stop short of that process, penetrate the walls of the ducts and acini, and invade the surrounding tissue. He discovered the remarkable fact that in some countries it is the custom to splay the cow after calving if it is the wish to keep up the supply of milk, for when this is done the cow will go on giving milk indefinitely. This fact seemed to point to one organ holding the control over the secretion of another and separate organ. The fact that struck Beatson most strongly was the local proliferation of epithelium in lactation, the very thing most characteristic of cancer of the breast and of cancer everywhere, differing from it only in the fact that it was held in control by another organ and could either be arrested by that organ or be continued to a further stage where the cells became fatty and passed out of the system as milk. After these observations the author frequently asked himself, Is cancer of the breast due to ovarian irritation, as from some defective step in the cycle of ovarian changes? and if it is due to ovarian irritation, Can proliferation be arrested, or can the cells be forced to go on to fatty degeneration by removal of the ovaries? After trying some experiments upon rabbits and considering much upon these points, he felt that the position of matters was that our present state of knowledge has nothing better to offer than the surgeon's knife when the tumor is limited and can be thoroughly removed, but in the inoperable cases it might be that the administration of thyroid extract would improve the case or work a cure. If this failed, the surgeon should endeavor to arrest the progress of the growth by performing oöphorectomy. He placed the

[1] Lancet, July 11, 1896.

patient upon thyroid tablets pushed until physiologic action was manifest, but at the end of a month there was no obvious change in the growth. He then removed the tubes and ovaries. The right ovary was healthy, the left one a little cystic. The patient made a good recovery; no local application was used on the cancer itself. Two weeks after the operation the administration of thyroid tablets was resumed, the idea being that thyroid extract would be useful as a lymphatic stimulant. Five weeks after operation examination of the diseased area showed a marked change for the better. The large mass of tissue was far less vascular; it was smaller, flatter, and less prominent. Seven weeks after the operation the improvement was still more notable, and 4 months after the operation it was more manifest, while 8 months after operation all traces of cancerous disease had disappeared. Beatson showed the patient to the Society, and it was seen that there were a sound cicatrix and healthy tissues. The patient was apparently in excellent health. It should be stated that microscopic examination by a most competent pathologist proved this growth to have been carcinoma.

The next case Beatson records was a woman of 42 who had had a large tumor of the right breast for 5½ years which had not as yet been operated on. It was evident that the case was inoperable. He placed her in the hospital and watched the progress of the case for a month. In this time the patient grew distinctly worse. Beatson decided to remove the tubes and ovaries. Within 10 days after their removal the pain, which had been very severe, had almost entirely disappeared; the neck which had been stiff and painful moved more freely, and the skin became decidedly less vascular. It may be stated that the uterine adnexa were thick, adherent, and altered in both size and situation. After the operation the patient was placed upon thyroid as was the previous case. She left the hospital, but subsequently became worse because she did not take care of her health, and possibly also because she did not take the thyroid tablets. She returned within 2 months of leaving the hospital, was kept in bed and given her medicine regularly. Under these measures improvement again set in. He exhibited this patient not as a case of cure, but as illustrating the fact that definite changes for the better had taken place in the tumor.

The third case was a woman of 49; she had a large sore on the left breast and the mammary gland was almost entirely destroyed, as if it had been removed by operation. The disease had existed for about 7 years. There were no evidences of any secondary deposits. Examination by a pathologist proved that this ulcer was typically cancerous and not tuberculous. He placed the patient on thyroid tablets, pushing them to their full physiologic effect. During the 3 months they have been taken he has not observed any marked effect on the sore. By itself thyroid extract seems to have little effect on cancerous processes. The question in this case is whether, in the light of what has been observed in the other 2 cases, the removal of the tubes and ovaries would be of any service. The benefit would be very problematical in view of the fact that the woman has passed the menopause, but he is not sure that it would not be right, even though the menopause has set in, to try the effect of removing all the uterine appendages.

The conclusion Beatson draws from the 2 cases he has brought under notice is that we must look in the female to the ovaries as the seat of the exciting cause of carcinoma, certainly of carcinoma of the mamma, in all probability of cancer of the female generative organs generally, and possibly the rest of the body. He has long felt that the parasitic theory is unsatisfactory, and that in concentrating all our energies upon it we are simply losing time. He is satisfied that in the ovary of the female and the testicle of the male we have organs that send out influences more subtle and mysterious than those which come from the nervous system. It may be said that in many cases of cancerous disease there is no change manifest in the ovaries. This statement may arise in the fact that changes have not been looked for, or because the changes are of a delicate nature and require special methods of investigation to detect them, or because the changes are so subtle as to elude detection.

Prof. A. Simpson stated some years ago that removal of both ovaries predisposed to cancer. If this is so, then the theory of the ovarian origin of cancer falls to the ground; but the point that Simpson has overlooked is this: in the cases he refers to the ovaries were removed because they were diseased, and thus these very cases really support the view that cancer in the female is probably due to altered condition of the ovary. If cases can be shown that have had both healthy ovaries removed and have subsequently become the victims of cancer, then the entire theory falls. In recapitulation the author urges the following points: 1. There seems evidence of the ovary and testicle having the control in the human body over local proliferations of epithelium; 2. The removal of the tubes and ovaries has effect on the local proliferation of epithelium which is found in cancer of the breast and aids the tendency which carcinoma naturally possesses to pass into fatty degeneration; 3. This effect is best seen in cases of cancer in young people—the class of cases where removal of the disease by the knife is often very unsatisfactory. [The cases recorded by Beatson are very striking and important. In spite of the fact that Sir Spencer Wells states that he has seen many victims of cancer from which the tubes and ovaries had been previously removed, it seems to be the duty of surgeons to give this novel theory a thorough test. Stanley Boyd, in a recent number of the *Brit. Med. Jour.* (Oct. 2, 1897), reports some cases which seem to confirm the theory that oöphorectomy can cause atrophy of mammary cancer. Boyd suggests that the ovaries may furnish a secretion which in some cases favors the growth of cancer, and that removal of the ovaries in such cases permits the tissues to combat successfully parasitic cells. If a dozen leading surgeons make careful collective investigation, the truth of the matter will be certainly determined.]

Peterson[1] makes a study of the literature of **bacterial treatment of malignant diseases** and of the cases studied in Czerny's clinic, and comes to the conclusion that the treatment is not of the slightest use in cancer; that in very exceptional cases sarcoma disappears under its influence; and that the treatment itself possesses many elements of danger.

Hughes Reid Davies[2] reports a case of a woman aged 53, who had a hard, clearly defined, and movable mass at the axillary border of the right mammary gland distinct from the gland-tissue. There was an adherent, infiltrated mass in the axilla extending into the muscles. Davies advised operation, but the patient's family refused to permit it. As a consequence of this he decided to employ subcutaneous **injections of Coley's fluid.** The patient presented distinct reactions after these injections, but after they had been continued for about a month she became unconscious and died. The usual Jewish objections were interposed in regard to making a postmortem, but external examination showed there was extreme enlargement of the liver. The result of treatment in this case was manifestly *nil.* In the early stage Davies fancied that the rate of growth was checked and the fetor lessened, but the reactions were terribly alarming and induced him to suspend the injections after a few had been given.

[1] Therap. Monatsh., Jan., 1897.   [2] Lancet, Feb. 13, 1897.

George B. Beale[1] reports a case of a woman, aged 67, who had had the left breast removed for cancer and who presented herself with a scirrhous carcinoma of the right breast. Some glands in the left side of the neck were enlarged and painful. The arm was edematous. He tried the treatment of Coley. He gave injections on alternate days from March 22d to May 1st. She gained flesh, had a return of appetite, and became able to sleep well. The glands in the neck shrunk to one-quarter their former size, the tumor in the breast disappeared, the pain disappeared, and the edema almost passed away. It was now considered that the case could be operated upon; the glands of the neck were removed, but did not present any evidence of cancer.

Marmaduke Sheild[2] makes some remarks on a case of recurrent sarcoma of the mammary gland treated by Coley's fluid, with a fatal result. The patient was 44 years of age. Mr. Pick had previously removed the left breast for a myeloid sarcoma; the axilla was at that time apparently free. Within six weeks of the operation, the wound having healed, the disease appeared in the scar, in the axilla, and beneath the clavicle. When Mr. Sheild saw her there were two masses of disease in the centre of the scar. One was the size of a walnut, was of a livid hue, and was crossed by large veins; the other was of smaller size, but was on the point of evacuating through a large mass of disease into the pectoral muscle. The general health was good and there were no evidences of metastasis. The patient was treated with injections of Coley's fluid. There seemed to be no question that the masses were influenced most favorably by the injections. The injections were commenced on the 3d of April. On the 22d a rigor occurred and the temperature rose to 103°. The next two days the symptoms became worse. On the 23d the temperature was 105°, pustules appeared on the legs, with petechial spots on the abdomen, the patient became comatose and drowsy, and died on the 24th.

Sheild sums up the symptoms observed as follows: sharp reaction from the first two injections; after that three injections failed to produce a reaction. After a week's interval severe reaction again followed injection. The effect on the growth was unquestionably very marked and favorable. The injections caused undoubted shrinking and apparent disappearance, this result seeming to be due to inflammatory action rather than any specific effect of the fluid. The postmortem examination showed the evidences of general pyemia. The secondary abscesses contained staphylococcus aureus. This is important, as the original fluid was prepared from streptococci. Sheild has recorded this case because it illustrates both the difficulty and danger that attend methods of treatment the effects of which may easily spread beyond control. In this case the grave nature of the malady justified a perilous mode of treatment. Life was unquestionably shortened by the treatment, but nevertheless so marked was the effect produced upon the growth that he would advise this treatment in cases of sarcoma which appear hopeless when less risky methods are employed. It is interesting to note that this same fluid in the same dose was used for another patient suffering from cancer, and that little or no reaction resulted. The injections were always made with scrupulous care with an aseptic syringe. The fluid was found to be sterile, hence the fatal organisms probably developed in the necrosing tissues of the growths. The mistake in this case was possibly the imperfect disinfection of the skin. Sheild says that the most conflicting testimony exists in regard to the value of this treatment. Prof. Senn has reported 9 failures and says that the method is of no value.

Coley has reported some truly remarkably successful results. It seems to Sheild undoubted that remarkable results have occasionally been brought about

[1] Brit. Med. Jour., July 4, 1896.   [2] Ibid., Jan. 23, 1897.

in the treatment of sarcoma. He says the method is worthy of more extensive trial; the case he has related shows the great importance of making every attempt to prevent the entrance of dangerous organisms into the inflamed tumor.

William B. Coley [1] considers the **therapeutic value of the mixed toxins** of the streptococcus erysipelas and bacillus prodigiosus in the treatment of inoperable malignant tumors. He tells us that a considerable number of cases have been reported by competent observers in which undoubted malignant growths have been permanently cured by an attack of erysipelas. Czerny has reported 2 most important cases. Fehleisen produced erysipelas by inoculation in 7 cases; nearly all the cases showed improvement and in 1 of them the tumor disappeared. The case that led Coley to take up these investigations was one of small round-celled sarcoma of the neck. It had been operated on 5 times by William T. Bull. At the last operation in 1884 it was found impossible to remove the growth entirely and the case was considered hopeless. A few days after this an attack of erysipelas occurred, quickly followed by a second attack. The tumor entirely disappeared. Coley traced the case and found him alive and free from recurrence in 1891. The author then relates the steps of his investigations and how he was led to make the fluid which he now advises for injection. He tells us that the value of all preparations of the toxins depends largely upon the virulence of the original cultures. In most of the successful cases the cultures were obtained from fatal cases of erysipelas. Much larger quantities can be tolerated when injected subcutaneously than when injected directly into a vascular tumor. We should begin with a very small dose, 1 minim of the filtrate or $\frac{1}{2}$ minim of the unfiltered toxins. This dose should be increased each day until the reaction-temperature reaches 103° or 104°. The temperature should be the guide in estimating the dose, and very little benefit will accrue if no reaction is obtained. Usually the injections are given daily, and he aims to get 2 or 3 well-developed reactions every week. If well borne, the treatment may be continued from 2 to 3 weeks. If there is no decided improvement at the end of that time, it might as well be abandoned. In some of the successful cases it has been kept up for three or four months, occasionally an interval of a few days being taken for a rest. By a careful study of the cases which have been treated by this method we are able to answer three important questions: 1. Have these toxins an antagonistic influence upon malignant tumors? 2. In what variety of tumors is the influence most marked? 3. Is this action permanent in character?

The cases include 94 sarcomata and 63 carcinomata. Besides the cases of malignant tumors 8 other cases have been treated with the toxins—2 cases of tuberculosis, 1 of keloid, 2 goiters, 1 recurrent fibro-angioma, 1 fibroma, and 1 mycosis fungoides. Of the sarcomata 45, or more than half, show some improvement. Spindle-cell sarcoma is most apt to show improvement. Melanotic sarcoma is less apt to show it. Osteosarcoma shows little effect. In 1 case of round-cell sarcoma of the neck of very rapid growth the tumor decreased from the size of an orange to the size of a hen's egg in 1 week after 3 injections. The spindle-cell variety forms a large proportion of the successful cases. The results in carcinoma are far from ideal, but are such as to lead us to believe we are working in the right line. The fact that cases of undoubted carcinoma have been cured by incidental erysipelas gives weight to this view.

In a considerable number of cases of inoperable carcinoma Coley has seen

[1] Am. Jour. Med. Sci., Sept., 1896.

improvement follow the injections. In 2 cases the tumor disappeared and the patients are well, one 1 year and 9 months after treatment and the other a year. In a case of recurrent carcinoma of the breast there was very marked benefit under the influence of the toxins. Coley thinks that the chief value of the toxins in carcinoma will be to lessen the chances of recurrence after the primary operation. Coley turns to a consideration of the question, Is the action of the toxins permanent? One case which would remain well for a considerable time can be considered as answering this question. Four cases, all pronounced inoperable by well-known surgeons, in every one of which the diagnosis was confirmed by microscopic examination, are free from recurrence $2\frac{1}{2}$ to $4\frac{1}{2}$ years after treatment. It is proper to regard these cases as permanently cured. The author then records in full 18 cases in which this treatment was employed, and the result in many of them is extraordinary.

AMPUTATIONS.

The **amputation-statistics** at the London Temperance Hospital are presented by W. J. Collins.[1] The table was prepared by Dr. Leonard Wilde, the registrar of the London Temperance Hospital, and includes all amputations performed since Mr. Pearce Gould's retirement in 1888.

Table showing Amputation-mortality from July 1, 1888, to December 31, 1896.

	For disease.		For accident.	
	Cases.	Deaths.	Cases.	Deaths.
At hip	4	. .	. .	. .
Of thigh	9	1	2	. .
Of leg	7	. .	5	. .
Of foot	6	. .	. .	. .
Of toes	12	. .	. .	. .
Of arm	. .	. .	2	. .
Of forearm	2	. .	. .	. .
Of hand	. .	. .	1	. .
Of fingers	19	. .	6	. .
Total	59	1	16	. .

The total number of cases is 75, with 1 death. In only 2 of the above cases was any alcohol administered: one a case of sarcoma of the thigh, which died, the other a case of embolic gangrene with heart-disease, which recovered. Full details of all cases in which alcohol was used are put forth in the annual report of the hospital in accordance with the rule. [These statistics are remarkably favorable, but no limited series of observations can prove that alcohol should not be used. We have never seen harm result from the therapeutic use of alcohol. We consider this agent a drug of great value when properly used. It is worthy of note that the London Temperance Hospital has an unusual mortality in typhoid fever; Osler says the death-rate is 15–16 %.]

A. Primrose[2] contributes a note upon **amputation at the hip-joint in advanced tuberculous disease.** He tells us that upon the question of the advisability of amputation in advanced tuberculous disease of the hip-

[1] Lancet, Jan. 9, 1897. [2] Canad. Pract., Nov., 1896.

joint there is a great divergence of opinion. The very conditions which some authorities maintain contraindicate operation, other authorities hold render it necessary. The association of profuse suppuration with amyloid changes, albuminuria, tuberculous disease in organs, and the extension of the process into the pelvis, has been mentioned in a recent text-book as calling for its performance in order to save life, and yet most of these conditions have been set forth by writers as precluding the possibility of performing a successful amputation. Primrose says that one cannot narrate a train of symptoms either for or against the operation; that numerous considerations must be carefully weighed in each case, and no two patients will present the same identical association of symptoms. The immediate danger from the operation is not as great as has been formerly imagined; but, unfortunately, the prospect of curing the patient is not the best. Primrose then cites a case of tuberculosis of the hip-joint which was first treated by fixation, and next by excision, without the eradication of the disease, and he thinks in such a case as this the question of amputation should be considered. He tells us that Mr. Knaggs has reported an equally severe case which was cured by amputation, and he then relates a case of his own similar to it in which amputation by Furneaux Jordan's method was performed, with the cure of the case. He thinks that the rate of mortality is usually placed far too high, because we do not separate in our statistical tables cases operated upon for tuberculous disease from cases operated upon for other causes. The usual estimated mortality in text-books after amputation at the hip is 60%. The mortality after amputation for injury is 80 or 90%, and, according to Ashhurst, after amputation for disease is 40.2%. Of recent years, however, the mortality after amputation for disease has been very greatly reduced by improvement in technic. Primrose thinks the mortality is in the neighborhood of 10% in amputation for tuberculosis in children.

The operation that he advocates is that of Furneaux Jordan, and is never performed unless excision has previously been done. A primary amputation is never justifiable in tuberculous disease of the hip-joint. The prevention of hemorrhage is a matter of the greatest possible importance. He disbelieves in the use of Wyeth's method when operating upon children. He thinks the method is admirable when applied to an adult with a healthy hip-joint. The method that Primrose advocates is digital compression of the main artery. The femoral artery can be compressed over the pubis. When this is done the amount of blood lost will be very slight and there will be very little subsequent oozing. Digital compression is always possible in children. He thinks that the method suggested by Mr. Howse of removing the limb by successive segments has much to recommend it. In tuberculous disease of the hip demanding amputation Mr. Howse first amputates at the knee and later at the hip-joint, claiming that this method secures to a greater extent freedom from pain; that in many instances the first amputation improves the hip disease; and that in any case the severity of amputation at the hip is very much lessened by the antecedent operation. It is needless to say that the operation of amputation at the hip-joint should only be performed in cases otherwise hopeless, and should be reserved for cases in which excision has previously been performed. Neither amyloid disease nor perforation of the acetabulum is any contraindication to the operation. [Excision of the hip for tuberculosis is decidedly dangerous. The mortality is from 25 to 48%, which is far higher than the mortality of amputation. In not a few cases excision is followed by dissemination of the tuberculosis. Barker and Wright believe in early excision when caseation occurs. Howard Marsh and many others disbelieve in it. We agree with Primrose that mechanical treatment should be given a thorough trial in hip tuberculosis. If mechanical treatment fails, excision is admissible, recognizing its dangers but believing it is justifiable to incur those dangers in preference to sacrificing a limb at once. We disagree with the assertion that amputation is never to be performed unless excision has been previously practised, and we hold that in more severe cases and in very much debilitated cases amputation should be done at once.]

Charles Greene Cumston [1] writes on **amputation of the foot with a dorsal flap.** He tells us that Baudens was the first to perform this operation, having done it in 1839. The 2 cases of this amputation performed by Poncet, of Lyons, show that the dorsal flap makes an excellent stump. The indications for the performance of this operation are the impossibility of finding enough tissue in good condition on the sole of the foot to make a trustworthy flap. In such conditions as perforating ulcer of the sole of the foot and in various atrophic conditions this amputation is useful. Tumors of the heel may require disarticulation of the dorsal flap. The contraindications are loss of vitality of the skin on the dorsal aspect of the body, advanced age of

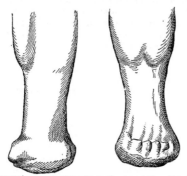

Fig. 6.—Anterior and posterior aspects of the stump after amputation of the foot with a dorsal flap (Charles Greene Cumston, in Ann. of Surg., Dec., 1896).

the patient, and poor general health. In the latter case the question of life is to be more considered than the functional result of the operation. The dorsal flap is composed of the skin, the subcutaneous tissue, the dorsal aponeurosis, the tendons and layer of fibrous tissue, and, lastly, the pediosus muscle with the artery and nerve. This skin, it is true, is thin and elastic, but later it becomes thick and hard because of friction. The cellular tissue contains veins and nerves. The superficial aponeurosis is decidedly dense. The amputation is divided into four steps. In the first the flap is marked out and the soft parts incised. The incision begins in the tendo Achillis below and behind one of the malleoli. The incision is made to follow the dividing-line between the plantar and dorsal aspects. The point of the knife is made to move closely to the bone. It rounds off in the shape of a gaiter over the interdigital groove. The second step is dissecting up the flap. We remember that the flap is to include all the soft parts of the dorsum, and must be particularly careful not to injure the tarsal artery. The dissection is carried up to the tibiotarsal articulation, the surgeon exercising precaution not to lacerate the tissues. The third step is the opening of the tibiotarsal articula-

[1] Ann. of Surg., Dec., 1896.

tion and the disarticulation of the foot. Disarticulation is effected by the ordinary method. The soft parts of the back of the foot are divided if necessary and the insertion of the tendo Achillis is cut off from the os calcis. The fourth step is the sawing of the malleoli and the toilet of the tissues. The malleoli are sawn just above the articulation, care being taken to obtain an even surface. Tendons are trimmed off and nerves are pulled down and cut. The tendo Achillis is sutured to the extensor tendons of the toes. Blood-vessels are sutured, the flap is sutured, and a drainage-tube introduced. Poncet cautions us to mark out the flap as high as possible. Retraction of the skin in this region is very great, and *be sure* to have enough flap. The cicatrix is on the posterior aspect of the heel and is not pressed upon by walking. Three months after operation the patient can use an artificial foot.

Durant, of Lyons, has invented a boot to be worn after this operation.

Charles McBurney[1] advocates **direct intra-abdominal finger-compression** of the common iliac artery during amputation of the hip-joint

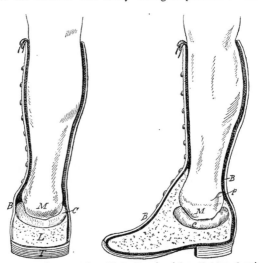

Fig. 7.—Shoe to be worn after amputation of foot with a dorsal flap: *M*, stump; *L*, cork foot; *C*, hair pad; *B*, boot; *T*, heal of boot (Charles Greene Cumston, in Ann. of Surg., Dec., 1896).

as a means of preventing hemorrhage. He has adopted the method in several cases, and he has found it easy and effectual. In the reported cases as much blood as could be safely returned to the body by means of position or the Esmarch bandage was so returned. An incision was then made over the abdominal wall 1½ in. internal to the anterior spine of the ilium, and through this incision an assistant passed his index finger and compressed the common iliac artery. The blood-current beyond the point of compression was arrested and the field of operation was entirely free from a bandage or an appliance of any sort. In his last two cases McBurney made the incision by separating the muscular and aponeurotic fibers according to the plan he devised for the removal of the appendix in interval-cases. [McBurney first described this plan in the *Annals of Surgery*, Aug., 1894. Macewen uses surface abdominal

[1] Ann. of Surg., May, 1897.

pressure, made by the hand of an assistant, to prevent hemorrhage (for details of method see *Annals of Surgery*, vol. i., p. 1, 1894, or Jacobson's *Operations of Surgery*, p. 1134, 3d ed.).]

John A. Wyeth[1] makes a report of 69 cases of **amputation of the hip** done by the author's method; 56 of the patients were males and 13 were females; there were 11 deaths, a mortality-rate of 15.9%. In the 40 cases of sarcoma in which amputation was performed there was a mortality of 10%. In the 22 cases of bone-disease there was a mortality of 13.6%. An analysis

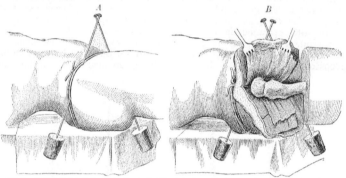

FIG. 8.—Hip-joint amputation : *A*, pins and rubber-tube tourniquet in position, the Esmarch bandage has been removed. *B*, the same, showing the soft parts dissected from the bone and the capsule exposed (John A. Wyeth, Ann. of Surg., Feb., 1897).

of these cases shows that the method of controlling hemorrhage was satisfactory in every case but two. In one case the first incision showed that the constriction was not tight enough. In another case the pins yielded to the pressure, not being sufficiently strong. This operation Wyeth first applied in

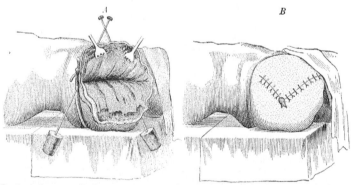

FIG. 9.—*A*, the same, with the disarticulation complete, constrictor still in position *B*, the operation completed (John A. Wyeth, Ann. of Surg., Feb., 1897).

1890. He had used the same method in arresting hemorrhage at the shoulder-joint more than a year before. Wyeth then describes the operation, the

[1] Ann. of Surg., Feb., 1897.

steps of which are well known. He says in his first operation he divided the femur on a line with the incision through the muscles, tied the vessels, removed the bone, and then dissected loose the upper fragment. Finding disarticulation by this method difficult he adopted the suggestion of the late Dr. Murdoch, of Pittsburg, and left the femur intact to facilitate disarticulation.

[We have found the pins and band perfectly satisfactory in controlling hemorrhage. Jacobson thinks it is an objection to the method that it requires a special apparatus which may not be at hand. This distinguished surgeon uses elastic compression by the method of Jordon Lloyd.]

E. T. Elliot[1] reports a case of recurrent myxosarcoma of the scapula in a patient aged 76, who first consulted him when she was 71 years of age. There was a sarcoma of the right scapula. The growth was removed, but recurred in 2 weeks. The growth was again removed by free incisions and the wound was left open and packed with iodoform-gauze. The patient recovered, but the growth again recurred. Since the second operation Elliot has operated 12 times (14 operations in all). He finally removed the entire upper extremity (15th operation). The patient made a good recovery from this serious procedure.

ANESTHESIA AND ANESTHETICS.

Frederic W. Hewitt,[2] the anesthetist of the London Hospital, discusses the **past, present, and future** of anesthesia. He sets forth what anesthesia has done, analyzes the work of Snow and Clover, and shows the value of having a specialist administer the anesthetic. He contrasts the deductions from physiology and the beliefs obtained by practical experience, and thinks that the subject suffers at the hands of certain physicians and physiologists. The giving of an anesthetic is a purely practical matter, and no one is competent to express an opinion upon how it should be given who has not himself had personal experience in the operating-room. Many of the theories that are put forth so freely by physicians would be quickly modified or abandoned were these gentlemen to take a position for a short time as anesthetist in a large hospital. They would realize the important fact that in anesthetizing the human being factors come into play which are not met with in the lower animals. Not long since, Hewitt visited a physiological laboratory where an experiment was being conducted in which the question arose as to whether an animal had ceased to breathe. To his astonishment he saw that respiration was looked upon as existing as long as feeble and occasional muscular contractions about the chest and abdomen persisted, contractions which were without the slightest influence in causing ingress or egress of air. This shows that what the physiologist regards as respiration the anesthetist does not so regard, and that practical experience in giving anesthetics to human beings would greatly assist the physiologist in his investigations. The practice of administering the same anesthetic without regarding the nature of the operation or the type of the subject is a thing of the past. Successful administrators vary their anesthetics and their ways of giving them according to the circumstances of each particular case. Modern surgery requires that all the patients shall be saved, but it may be required that one patient be absolutely immobile, that another be less deeply anesthetized, and that a third be very slightly under the influence of the anesthetic. A very important development in the modern knowledge of the subject is the recognition of the advantage of profound anesthesia over light anesthesia in most instances. It

[1] Lancet, Nov. 7, 1896.   [2] Practitioner, Oct., 1866.

is also a fact learned in comparatively recent times that during the anesthetic state the respiration is apt to be obstructed mechanically, and there is good ground for the belief that this period of obstruction has been the initial factor in most of the cases spoken of as chloroform-syncope. Experience has taught us that within certain limits the state of the patient's heart may be entirely disregarded. It used to be the custom to determine whether or not a patient were fit to take an anesthetic by listening to his heart. The truth of the matter is that patients with strong hearts are more liable to pass into suddenly dangerous condition than those with feebler circulation. A postmortem study of deaths from chloroform will show that in most instances the heart has been perfectly normal. Hewitt does not mean to imply that people with advanced heart-disease or in a condition of extreme asthenia are the best subjects for anesthetics. Another recent addition to our knowledge is the fact that it is a good plan when chloroform-anesthesia is wished for to give the patient first a short course of ether and then continue with chloroform, and this is most readily effected by beginning the administration with gas and ether, or A.-C.-E. mixture and ether, and then after a time giving chloroform. This form of anesthesia is safer than that obtained by giving chloroform from the start. We are now able to obtain anesthesia from nitrous oxid without any of the evidences of asphyxia. It has also been pointed out in giving anesthetics that certain postures are inadvisable and others are of advantage. [There is a world of wisdom in Hewitt's statements that "the responsibilities involved in administering anesthetics are not yet fully realized," and that "the administration is too often placed in the hands of comparatively unskilled men." We have frequently been impressed with the truth of the above assertions. Not a few surgeons pick out the most competent person present to act as personal assistant and let any one at all give the anesthetic, and the "any one" may prove to be unfit for the task. There can be no doubt of the usefulness of one who makes a specialty of giving anesthetics. Every hospital worker realizes the difference between a specialist and an "any body" when he goes away to operate and does not take his assistants. It is absurd to suppose that a person can give ether well by instinct. The post of anesthetist should be regarded as one of trust and responsibility, the duties of which are second in importance only to those of the operator. To ask a person to give an anesthetic should be considered an evidence of confidence, not of disdain.]

Treves[1] publishes an article with the title of "Anesthetics in Operative Surgery." He states his conviction of the great importance and responsibility of the position of anesthetist. A man to most successfully the many demands that are made upon him must have had large opportunities; must be possessed of the power of patient observation, tact, and judgment. The anesthetist is made and not born. This is not the belief of very many. There is a widespread belief that the giving of an anesthetic is a trivial act, and that the power to give it comes with the granting of his diploma. A man cannot give chloroform well unless he has extended practice. He will fail utterly if he follows some method of his own, or if he watches the operation, or attends to anything else excepting the giving of the chloroform. He tells us there are those who think the giving of chloroform a trivial affair, where there is often a stage of struggling when the patient is forced down upon the table as though he were a piece of mechanism possessed of a hardly controllable power to spring into the air. In this state he shrieks and yells and has occasional outbursts of speech which pain the sense of propriety of the relatives. Then comes pouring on large quantities of chloroform and beginning the operation

---

[1] *Practitioner*, Oct., 1866.

before the patient is unconscious. Then more pouring on of chloroform in a hasty, irritable, and even vindictive manner; then comes suspended animation, artificial respiration, and rushings to and fro, and after these things operation may or may not be completed. It is a true assertion that most patients look upon the anesthetic with far more dread than they do the operation. The patient is but ill prepared for this ordeal by an administrator who solemnly displays an apparatus which he manipulates with the stolid ostentation of an executioner, and he is not to be comforted by the jaunty anesthetist who calls for a handkerchief and after placing it over the patient's face chatters of his summer holiday. The anesthetist must appreciate the patient's condition of mind and must sympathize with it.

Regarding the choice of an anesthetic, other things being equal, more depends upon the one who gives it than upon the one which is given. Equally good results are attained by different administrators with different agents. Those who are especially adept in giving ether may not succeed so well with chloroform, and *vice versâ.* An anesthetist of experience should be allowed to give that agent with which he is most familiar or which he regards as best suited to the case. Mr. Treves is convinced, in general, that ether is to be preferred to chloroform. Certain qualities are demanded of the anesthetic. It should be safe, it should not be very disagreeable to inhale, it should produce muscular relaxation, it should not be succeeded by ill effects, it should not lead to the production of hemorrhage. In regard to the safety of anesthetics, as stated before, Treves is assured that ether is infinitely safer than chloroform. In the hands of a thoroughly experienced man there may be no more danger with chloroform than with ether, but in making our estimates as to risk we judge from the success attained by the average administrators and not by the specialists. Chloroform is certainly not suited for indiscriminate use, nor should it be used by people of small experience. There are certainly some cases in which any anesthetic is dangerous. For instance, in intestinal obstruction with great distention of the abdomen and a weak and failing pulse. In cases of this variety, as soon as the anesthetic abolishes the reflexes there is often a torrent of vomit from the mouth and nose and death may immediately ensue. In some cases the pulse and respiration cease and the thorax becomes rigid, the great distention of the abdomen rendering artificial respiration almost impossible. These results are as common with ether as chloroform. In such cases no anesthetic should be given. The patient's capacity to appreciate pain is blunted, and we can often do a formidable operation with little evidence of suffering. After-sickness is much less common after ether has been given than after chloroform has been given, and this is a matter of great importance in abdominal operations. It occasionally happens that vomiting of a most persistent character arises because of some peculiarity due to the patient and the anesthetic, and the same remark applies to hiccough. Occasionally vomiting after an operation is due to iodoform-poisoning. Ether has another disadvantage which chloroform is free from—it is irritant to the respiratory mucous membrane, this irritant effect being especially pronounced when some inflammation of the air-vessels already exists; hence in operations upon the respiratory passages or the pleura chloroform is used instead of ether, and chloroform is preferable in cases in which tracheal or bronchial catarrh exists. It has been stated that one fault in ether is that it produces extreme venous engorgement and leads to much oozing from the field of operation. Mr. Treves does not think the objection well founded. The question is one of administration. When an anesthetic is given by a skilful man the difference between the vascular condition when the patient is under ether and under

17

chloroform is hardly detectable. It is quite true that some administrators who are not skilful in giving ether may put the patient in a state of asphyxia which may impress the operator. Mr. Treves has never noticed that more points require ligature when ether is employed than when chloroform is used, and he thinks that the after-oozing is greater with chloroform than with ether.

Marmaduke Sheild [1] makes a strong plea for the need of better **instruction in the administration of anesthetics.** He thinks the teaching of anesthetics is greatly neglected in most institutions. It is possible for a man to obtain the right to practise without any practical knowledge of giving anesthetics. In order to show the degree of incapacity which exists in this most responsible duty which falls to the lot of medical men, Sheild mentions an actual experience which he had in a remote district, and he thinks that such experiences are too frequently duplicated in private practice. The patient had been given a full meal and some alcohol. The administration of chloroform was begun without examining the mouth for foreign bodies or false teeth and without undoing the corset. The operator noticed that the administrator had no tongue-forceps and no tracheotomy-tube. We know, as a matter of fact, that by careful watching on the part of the operator and considerable good fortune these cases do well ; but we simply court disaster and may barely rescue the individual from the jaws of death. A piece of vomited matter may be hooked out of the larynx just in time to prevent death, and other exciting adventures are liable to occur which impress an operator who is already too busy. We hear much of deaths from anesthetics, but we do not hear of the narrow escapes. We should always remember that no anesthetic is without risk, and we should endeavor to reduce this risk to infinitesimal proportions by great care in administration and by a theoretical as well as a practical knowledge of the subject. Instruction in anesthetics should be compulsory. There is ample opportunity for instruction in the London hospitals, as the amount of material is very large and the number of operations very great.

Sheild thinks the tendency to examine into difficult and obscure subjects to the neglect of common and ordinary ones is a most serious defect in modern medical education. He would establish examinations in anesthetics. He would not expect every medical man to be a highly skilled administrator, but he should know enough to be able to select an appropriate anesthetic for a certain case, and he should be competent to give the common agents with confidence. He should have a thorough knowledge of the preliminary measures necessary for the safety of the patient and of the remedial measures to be employed in case of sudden danger. In remote districts the general practitioner will be forced to administer anesthetics himself in cases which, if treated in the city, would be anesthetized by a skilled assistant. The administration of an anesthetic in such a condition as empyema, for instance, is extremely perilous. The patient's safety can only be insured by long experience and cautious and skilful administration. We, of course, cannot educate all medical men to such a point of excellence, but we should at least instruct them to the degree where they will be fit to estimate the limit of their own capacities and be able to know when a certain case is difficult and dangerous. [The advice in the above article is eminently sound and timely. We ourselves have seen many narrow escapes and have felt several times that peril would have been avoided if the administrator had possessed a little more knowledge. Sheild's criticism of the tendency of modern medical education is true. Examiners multiply subjects, ask many profound questions, and in quest of the deep

[1] Practitioner, Oct., 1896.

and theoretical lose sight of the obvious and practical. The tendency is most deplorable.]

J. Milne Bramwell[1] revives the subject of **hypnotic anesthesia.** He tells us that Esdaile's first mesmeric operation was performed in 1845, and at the end of that year he had reported 100 successful cases. A committee of medical men investigated Esdaile's work and reported in his favor. In 1851 he reported 261 painless capital operations, and many thousand minor ones, and reduced the mortality in the removal of the great tumors of elephantiasis from 50 to 5 %. The author tells us that when he began hypnotic practice 7 years ago he found he could often produce anesthesia. In view of the fact that we already possess reliable anesthetics he looked upon this chiefly as useful in showing that hypnotic phenomena were genuine. Nevertheless, hypnotic anesthesia is not valueless. He reports several cases operated upon without pain by this means: one of double strabismus, one of ankylosis, one of excision of exostosis of the great toe, and many cases of teeth-extraction. Numerous other operations during hypnotic anesthesia have been reported of late, and Bramwell appends a list of the results of other practitioners. The chief objections to hypnotism are the difficulty and uncertainty in inducing primary hypnosis, because of the widely varying susceptibility of different individuals. 94 % of people can be hypnotized, but many preliminary attempts are often necessary, and sometimes hypnosis never becomes deep enough for operative measures. The nervous and hysterical are the most difficult to hypnotize, the healthiest and well-balanced are the easiest. Hypnosis possesses many advantages. When deep hypnosis with anesthesia has been once induced it can be repeated at any time desirable—it not being necessary to reproduce the hypnotic process, a verbal order to sleep being sufficient. The hypnotizer's presence even is not necessary, as the patient can be put to sleep by a written order or by other means suggested during hypnosis. The patient is not obliged to abstain from food or to make any other preparation. The nervous apprehension can be removed by suggestion. The process is pleasant, is free from danger, can be kept up indefinitely, can be stopped immediately; during it the patient can be placed in any position without risk, and will alter that position as the operator commands; gags and other apparatus are not required; analgesia alone can be suggested with great advantage in throat operations. The influence of the muscles can be increased or diminished by suggestion, which is of value in labor cases. There is no tendency to sickness during or after the operation; pain after the operation or during subsequent dressings can be prevented, and the rapidity of the healing process is frequently very marked. [The author makes the assertion that the nervous and hysterical are the most difficult persons to hypnotize and the healthy and well-balanced are the easiest subjects. This view is in direct antagonism to the teachings of Charcot. Charcot asserted that nervous patients, and particularly those laboring under hysteria, are predisposed to the hypnotic state. The absolute safety of the hypnotic state is doubtful. Binet and Férré specifically state that death may occur during hypnosis. The process can never be generally used, because of the difficulty of inducing the hypnotic condition in many individuals. The fact that after a person has been hypnotized it may be possible to hypnotize him easily on another occasion, *even against his own will*, is an objection, as most persons would be unwilling thus to endanger their own liberty in the future. That perfect anesthesia can be obtained by hypnotism is beyond doubt. The experience of Esdaile proves this fact. Guérineau, of Poitiers, amputated a leg successfully under hypnotic anesthesia, and Cloquet am-

[1] Practitioner, Oct., 1896.

putated the breast of a woman who was hypnotized. Cloquet performed his
operation in 1829, and Esdaile did not operate under hypnotism until 1845.
Binet and Férré,[1] Charcot's pupils, state that the hypnotic sleep cannot be
induced in all subjects; that even susceptible subjects must be subjected to a
series of daily hypnotizations before operation; and that sometimes hyperesthesia is produced instead of anesthesia.]

Fränkel[2] sets forth a method of **preventing the disagreeable after-
effects** of ether-anesthesia and chloroform-anesthesia. Quarter of an hour before giving the anesthetic Fränkel administers 1¼ c.c. hypodermically of the
following solution: morphin hydrochlorate, 0.15 gm.; atropin sulfate, 0.015
gm.; chloral hydrate, 0.25 gm.; distilled water, 15 gm. The patients after
taking this injection are very easily influenced by chloroform, and pass into
unconsciousness after the administration of a small amount of an anesthetic.
This mixture was not given to people who had lesions of the heart. [The
elder Gross was a believer in the administration of morphin before giving the
anesthetic, and for many years was accustomed to give it to patients who were
found to be nervous and very apprehensive. It has been asserted that atropin
given before the administration of ether tends to prevent vomiting in the
stage of reaction, but we have never been persuaded of the truth of the
statement. It will be observed in the next article that Silk opposes the use of
morphin, because he believes that this drug may mask the symptoms of a
fatal narcosis from the anesthetic.]

J. W. Silk,[3] anesthetist of King's College Hospital, presents some notes
upon the **preparatory treatment** of patients who are subjected to anesthesia. He says that nitrous oxid should not be given directly after a meal,
nor should it be given with the head in a position which permits the tongue
to fall back over the glottis, but beyond this no previous preparation is required. In regard to ether and chloroform, attention to preliminaries will
not only give comfort to the patient, the anesthetist, and operator, but will
sometimes save a patient's life. As a general fact, it may be stated that an
anesthetic is taken better if the patient has been subjected to what may be
called hospital *régime*—that is, rest of body and mind, regulation of the
evacuations, the use of a bland and easily digestible diet, and the abandonment
of alcohol. We every now and then hear someone suggest that a particular
drug given before the anesthetic is administered may prevent the dangers and
the troubles which occasionally arise, but there is no drug which has a specific
action in the matter. The gastrointestinal system should always be placed in
good condition before giving an anesthetic. Purgatives should be given the
evening before the operation. The stomach should be empty when the anesthetic is administered. This last direction does not mean to carry starvation
to the verge of weakening the patient. Of course, the power of digestion
will be lessened because of the nervousness of the patient, and yet the operation may be so severe as to prohibit the withholding of food for many hours.
The best plan in most cases is to give a cup of hot broth or beef-tea 3 or 4
hours before the operation. Milk and other foods which digest slowly are
not suitable. In patients who are very weak, or on whom a severe operation
is to be done, it will be found useful to give a nutritive enema half an hour
before operation. The enema that Silk recommends consists of the yolk of
an egg, an ounce of beef-tea, an ounce of milk, and an ounce of brandy, the
food elements being peptonized. As a general rule, it is not wise to give

[1] Animal Magnetism, by Binet and Férré.
[2] Zeit. f. prak. Aerzte, 1896; quoted by Bull. gén. de Thérap., Sept. 26, 1896.
[3] Treatment, Mar. 25, 1897.

brandy before operation, although in some instances it may be necessary when the patient is in danger of syncope from fright. The hypodermic use of morphin before operation is deprecated. It has no real advantages, and is apt to mask the symptoms of dangerous narcosis and hence lead to fatal results. Strychnin is a valuable agent in obviating and lessening shock, and some think the tendency to after-sickness is abated by its employment. The position to anesthetize in is, as a rule, the position the patient assumes himself as most comfortable. Chloroform should never be given to a person in the sitting posture. Everything in the shape of belts and stays, which tend to restrict respiratory movement, must be removed.

Clement Lucas [1] thinks that the occurrence of **pneumonia after the administration of an anesthetic** is too common to be explained by antecedent infection or by the effects of cold. He maintains that pneumonia is invariably a germ-disease, and thinks it quite possible that the germs may come from septic secretions. In this connection he quotes the remarks of James Bell, made over 12 years ago in the *Montreal Med. Jour.* Bell maintained that the Clover inhaler possessed every possible disadvantage; that it could not be cleansed, and that patient after patient respired through the same dirty mask in the same dirty rubber bag, each one adding his quota of mouth-secretions, which are possibly specific, cancerous, or tubercular. Lucas says that it would be a good thing to appoint an instrument destruction committee to have absolute power to destroy all out-of-date instruments and relieve hospital surgeons of being obliged to operate with useless tools and appliances. [Prescott has asserted that out of 40,000 etherizations only 3 persons developed lobar pneumonia. The same observer says that broncho-pneumonia and inhalation-pneumonia are more common (*Year-Book*, 1897). Nevertheless we believe profoundly in the use of a clean inhaler.]

Dudley P. Allen [2] has made a study of the effects of anesthesia upon temperature and blood-pressure. His experiments have been made from the standpoint of the clinician rather than that of the physiologist. His conclusions are that animals lose heat in a marked degree under prolonged anesthesia. This loss of heat may be to a great extent prevented by carefully covering up the animal. When an animal is carefully covered up and surrounded with hot bottles the temperature may be actually increased under anesthesia. That these temperature-changes are due to anesthesia is proved by certain facts: (*a*) that temperature-changes in dogs without anesthesia are very slight; (*b*) that temperature-changes in dogs under anesthesia depend on whether the dog was covered or uncovered and whether he was or was not surrounded by hot bottles. Allen found that the temperature after anesthesia ceased tended to return to normal no matter whether it had been above normal or below normal. This loss of heat is somewhat retarded by the administration of ergot or of atropin. The lower temperature quickly returns to normal after the cessation of the giving of ether ; but if the anesthetic be chloroform or the A.-C.-E. mixture, the temperature continues to fall for some time after the administration has ceased. Loss of blood-pressure corresponds closely with loss of heat. The administration of enemata of alcohol tends to bring back the blood-pressure, but renders the return to the normal temperature slower. In a room having a high temperature (93° to 96°) the administration of an anesthetic causes an increase of temperature to a considerable amount, but at the same time a decrease of blood-pressure. These observations seem to indicate that operations in rooms at a high temperature cause the patient more distress and are more perilous than operations in a room of moderate

[1] Lancet, Apr. 3, 1897.   [2] Am. Jour. Med. Sci., Mar., 1897.

temperature with the patient thoroughly protected. Slow operations with loss of blood produce a much greater fall of blood-pressure than operations of much greater severity performed quickly when care is taken to prevent hemorrhage. Allen maintains that in every prolonged operation the patient should be carefully covered to prevent loss of heat, and if he had already lost heat because of injury or exposure artificial heat should invariably be applied. Every care should be taken to limit the loss of blood. In his studies upon human beings he observed 80 patients. During operation there was a temperature-loss varying from 0.2° to 2°; the average loss was about 0.6°, but in some cases there was no loss whatever. [All practical surgeons have long been in agreement as to the absolute necessity of keeping the patient well covered. The theoretical objections against operating in very hot rooms are sustained by experience. We have seen deaths occur which we believe resulted purely from the exhaustion induced by the excessive heat of the operating-room. A year ago one of the editors (DaCosta) was operating for appendicitis. The temperature outside was 98°. The operating-room contained a steam sterilizer, and what the temperature of the room was is purely conjectural. The patient developed thermic fever during operation. The other editor (Keen) had a patient die of thermic fever a few hours after operation. It was midsummer, the temperature outside was 96°, and the room contained a steam sterilizer.]

A. E. Bridger[1] considers **disorders** which are **favored** or produced **by anesthesia.** He reported a case of acute mania which followed directly on the giving of nitrous oxid gas. He also reported cases in which an aortic aneurysm came on very suddenly after the administration of ether, the patient having struggled with considerable violence. The individual had labored under a specific disease and was a drinker, 53 years of age. He reported a case of pneumonia following the administration of ether and also one in which during the administration of chloroform to a morphin *habitué* it was noticed that the stage of excitement was very greatly prolonged.

Gilbert Geoffrey Cottam[2] advocates the administration of **spartein sulphate** in surgical anesthesia. This is given before the administration of an anesthetic, in doses of $\frac{1}{10}$ gr. hypodermically. During the progress of the operation $\frac{1}{15}$ gr. additional can be administered if necessary. He maintains that it strongly antagonizes the depressing influence of chloroform upon the circulation.

Kirk[3] writes on **auscultation of the heart** during chloroform-narcosis. He has made a study of 200 cases. He decides that the effect produced by chloroform on the heart can be assigned to one or both of two causes—either the susceptibility of the patient or the method employed. The following indications show dangerous idiosyncrasy: 1, a very forcible impulse with accentuation of one or both sounds; 2, irregularity before the administration is begun; 3, tachycardia or irregularity during the administration. Victims of syphilis are especially liable to bad results.

Henry J. Garrigues[4] writes on **anesthesia-paralysis.** He tells us that it has been noted after the administration of an anesthetic that in some cases the extensor muscles of the forearm and hand were paralyzed. This phenomenon was explained by the arm having been permitted to roll out and hang over the table-edge so that pressure was brought to bear upon the musculospiral nerve, the paralysis being exactly analogous to that seen in a man who sleeps with the arm hanging over the back of a chair. But there are other

[1] Proc. Soc. of Anesthetists, Jan. 21, 1897.   [2] Therap. Gaz., Nov. 16, 1896.
[3] Brit. Med. Jour., Dec. 12, 1896.   [4] Am. Jour. Med. Sci., Jan., 1897.

kinds of disturbance in the nervous system which may follow or be associated with the administration of anesthetics and which have received but little attention. Dr. Garrigues reports several interesting cases. One of them, a woman, was found to have paralysis of the right arm after recovery from ether, there having been no kind of pressure of the extremity against the table. In another case a left arm was paralyzed, without pressure. Garrigues quotes the well-known article by Budlinger, an assistant of the late Prof. Billroth, in which 9 cases of this sort are described. He also quotes the reports of Placzek of Berlin, Franke of Elberfeld, and Vautrin of Nancy.

In regard to the etiology of anesthesia-paralysis the cases may be divided into two groups, those which are of central origin and those which are of peripheral origin, the latter being by far the most common. These cases may happen it matters not what anesthetic is employed. Many of the cases have occurred after prolonged operations; others have occurred after short operations. Loss of blood may have some effect in predisposing to the paralysis. Children and emaciated individuals are more apt to suffer from it. The related cause of the peripheral cases is pressure, not of necessity pressure against the table, but pressure which is exercised upon the nerve by some position in which the extremity has been placed. When the arm is elevated alongside of the head or when it is brought out strongly from the body, pressure may take place between the clavicle and the first rib. Braun maintains that in such positions the head of the humerus presses upon the brachial plexus. Kron has shown by studies upon the cadaver that by lifting the arm backward and outward when it is in external rotation the median nerve is stretched across the head of the humerus, and that when the forearm is flexed and supinated the ulnar nerve is stretched. But unquestionably in most cases the pressure takes place between the collar-bone and the first rib. The plexus is especially likely to be injured if the nerves are stretched, which stretching is brought about when the head is drawn to the side opposite to that on which the arm is being elevated or when the head is permitted to fall back. Paralysis of the arm, it will be noted, is the most common; but paralysis has also been observed in the extremities and in the face. When the brachial plexus is pressed upon, the 5th and 6th cervical nerves are more apt to be caught than the 7th and 8th cervical and 1st dorsal are. In such a condition we find the deltoid, brachialis anticus, the biceps, and the supinator longus paralyzed, the other muscles having escaped. In some cases the muscles of the shoulder are implicated. If the lower roots are also compressed, the forearm and hand are involved. In some reported cases there was visual disturbance, the palpebral fissure was lessened in size, and there were contracted pupil, amaurosis, and double vision. These conditions are due to trouble with the communicating branch from the first dorsal nerve. There is more or less disturbance of sensation. There may be numbness, there may be absolute insensibility, there may be pain or tenderness on pressure, and sensitive points may be found over the nerves. It has been noted that even when the muscles supplied by the circumflex nerve, the deltoid, and the teres minor are paralyzed the skin over this region is not anesthetic. In some cases the extremities swell. Anesthesia-paralysis of central origin may be due to apoplexy or embolism. People who violently resist the anesthetic and old people with degenerated arteries are most liable to such a condition. It may also be produced in rare instances by primary softening of the brain, brought on by the direct action of the drug on nerve-tissue. The paralysis of central origin may appear as hemiplegia or hemiparesis. It seems likely that the so-called anesthetic death in some cases is due to apoplexy. The prognosis of the lighter cases of peripheral palsy is good, complete recovery being usually soon brought about. In severe cases of plexus-paralysis it may take months or even years to effect a cure. In a central paralysis the prognosis is extremely grave. In giving an anesthetic we should avoid pressure upon special nerves. We should not permit the arms to be raised above the head, but should have them resting easily pressed upon the chest. When leg-holders are employed the parts which are subjected to special pressure should be carefully padded with cotton. The head should rest on a pillow, and if vomiting occur and it is necessary to raise the arm, the head must be bent toward the arm and not away from it. In regard to the prophylaxis of central paralysis, abstain as far as possible from operating on very old persons and shorten the duration of the anesthesia as much as possible. In treating the peripheral paralysis electricity is of the utmost value. Its application shortly after the operation will be found to be very painful, and it is better to wait a week before applying it. A faradic current is the proper one to use, although Krumm recommends galvanism. Massage and hydrotherapy may be associated with the electricity. Strychnin is given internally, and we may also give iron, quinin, arsenic, extract of red marrow, and a nourishing diet.

George H. Bailey [1] considers the **principles of ether-administration.** He prefers to use Clover's gas and ether apparatus. He thinks, in preparing the patient for anesthetization, that we are often inclined to give too little food to old people and possibly to make the interval too long between taking food and operating. A small amount of stimulant just before the operation is in many cases valuable. His own practice is not to examine the patient before operation. As we know little of the causes of death, and the most healthy people are the ones who give the most anxiety, we had better consider every person as apt to succumb to the anesthetic than to lean upon the reed that would most likely fail to give support. In every reported death the statement is made that the patient was examined and found healthy. The attention of the anesthetizer should be centered upon the pulse, the respiration, and the condition of the pupil. Each will point out some special danger if not performing its function in a rhythmic manner. The golden rule as to the position of the patient is, first, make the patient comfortable and then yourself. As a rule, the best position for the patient at the beginning is recumbent with the head and shoulders slightly raised. Bailey stands on the left side, with his left thumb on the superficial temporal as it passes from the zygomatic process and holds the head. After the patient is anesthetized place him in any position required, even if it is necessary to suspend him by the feet. If mucous secretion gathers, sponge out the throat. If the jaws become fixed, employ a Mason's gag to open the mouth. In 2 cases of Bailey's laryngotomy was necessary. The indications for laryngotomy are perfect blueness with fixation of the chest-walls. Bailey is a strong disbeliever in warming the ether. He thinks ether if warmed is liable to produce dangerous symptoms. The pupils may vary from so trivial a cause as sickness with a tendency to slight syncope or the turning of the head on one side to give free exit to the vomit. If with dilated pupils and failing pulse and respiration there is flaccid eyeball, the case is very alarming. We should at once suddenly compress and as suddenly relax the chest-walls in order to expel the poisonous vapor from the lungs. After doing this two or three times it will usually be found that the patient's condition again becomes satisfactory. Time is lost by pulling out the tongue and by applying the stethoscope. If a rally does not come very quickly, artificial respiration must be used. He thinks there is no distinction in complete anesthetic

[1] Practitioner, Oct., 1896.

effects between ether and chloroform, and that either agent can be used efficiently in operations upon the abdomen, the brain, the chest, or eye. Ether given correctly can be used in the same cases as chloroform. In operations about the mouth chloroform is better than ether because ether cannot be as well kept up. He does not agree with the statement that the very young and the very old should not be etherized. He would just as soon give ether in the extremes of life. He says that certainly the young may die under chloroform and that the stimulation of ether benefits the aged. Neither agent is used in organic disease, but then we do not operate in such conditions. In this, the 50th year of the use of ether, we find it in far greater and increasing favor than some time ago.

The administration of ether is considered by F. Woodhouse Braine.[1] He maintains that ether should rank *facile princeps* amongst anesthetics. If he were limited to the use of one agent out of all the anesthetics that have ever been brought forward, he would choose ether. He totally disbelieves the statement that ether should not be given to patients who are below the age of 5 or above the age of 60. He gives it to infants when a few days old as well as to patients over 80. Infants are readily brought under its influence without any cyanosis. It is often a question with an inexperienced anesthetist as to when an infant has reached a proper degree of anesthesia. The writer's method is as follows: place the index finger in the infant's hand and it will be found that during the early part of the administration the finger is tightly grasped, but as insensibility approaches the infant's fingers gradually relax. As soon as the fingers are entirely lissome the operation may be begun. In the adult our guide is the conjunctival reflex. In the infant our guide is the amount of palmar and digital reflex. This method in an infant is greatly preferable to making the conjunctival test, because the conjunctiva loses its sensitiveness very quickly after being touched but a few times with the finger, hence an infant may seem to be thoroughly insensible by the conjunctival test when in reality it is not so. The writer has never seen bronchitis produced in an infant by the administration of ether, but he is very careful to guard against the breathing of cold air for some hours after operation. He does not allow a window to be open, and when possible keeps the child in the room in which the operation was performed for at least six hours. This care not only prevents bronchitis, but antagonizes vomiting, and these results he attributes to the non-stimulation by cold air of the nerves of the lungs with a consequent reflex action on the stomach. After the age of 3 years it is wise to precede the ether by the administration of nitrous oxid. Nitrous oxid is given until the patient is insensible and then the Ormsby inhaler, into which about 2 ounces of ether have been poured, is quickly applied without permitting a single inspiration of air in the interval of transferrence. With nervous individuals and drinkers the gas should be given until the patient is completely insensible before the change is made to ether. Always bear in mind that we cannot get the patient too quickly under the influence of ether. The pulse may be disregarded, for the circulation will always outlast the respiration. It is the respiration which especially requires the etherizer's attention. When ether is being given a slight duskiness of the face is not of any moment at all in fleshy, thick-necked people, especially with people who breathe through the nostrils with the lips closed lividity is apt to become marked. This can usually be prevented by placing a probe between the teeth. It is the absence of oxygen rather than the presence of ether which causes the lividity. If the wedging of the mouth apart by a probe does not cause the return of the

[1] Practitioner, Oct., 1896.

healthy color to the face, let the patient have a few inspirations of pure air, and if these do not produce the desired effect, it becomes the imperative duty of the administrator to get fresh air into the lungs of his patient by the means he is most accustomed to. The patient's life is in his hands and in his hands only. It occasionally happens during artificial respiration when the tongue is drawn forward and the air-passage freed from any foreign body that pressure on the thorax seems to drive air out of the chest, but none enters in to replace it. The obstruction in such a case depends upon the lax vocal chords being forced together by atmospheric pressure. This condition is overcome by the anesthetist placing his lips within those of the patient, closing the patient's nostrils, and making forcible inspiration. The atmospheric pressure is thus removed, the air left in the patient's lungs expands and forces the glottis open and permits air to enter. The after-effects of ether may be summed up in four words—nausea occasionally, sickness seldom.

J. B. Blake[1] furnishes some notes upon the use of **oxygen after ether.** His conclusions are that oxygen administered after ether abridges the time of returning to consciousness and diminishes unpleasant after-effects. It is a valuable cardiac and respiratory stimulant. It is indicated in threatened collapse and is appropriate in private cases, but in hospital practice its effects are not sufficiently beneficial to justify the expense which its routine use would entail.

Sydney Ringer[2] advocates the use of the tincture of **belladonna** for the prevention and cure of ether-bronchitis.

Newman and Ramsay[3] have made some studies upon the **decomposition of chloroform.** They show that chloroform tends to decompose with the formation of hydrochloric acid and the chlorid of carbonyl, and that the chlorid of carbonyl is an agent that is mainly responsible for the after-sickness. This tendency to decomposition can be prevented by keeping a little slacked lime in the bottle of chloroform.

Alexander MacLennan[4] records some cases of **stoppage of respiration** during chloroform-anesthesia which were treated by **tracheotomy.** This operation was done in 3 cases with a successful result in each. He says that obstruction to breathing may be due to tenacious secretion in the larynx or trachea, spasm of the chords, edema of the larynx, vomited matter in the air-passages, or a combination of some of the above conditions.

Waterhouse and Gibbs[5] record an extremely interesting case of arrest of the heart's action and of respiration during chloroform-anesthesia in which **bleeding from the internal jugular vein** was practised, after which the patient recovered. The operation was for the removal of tuberculous glands of the right side of the neck. Just as the diseased glands had been enucleated the patient made several violent attempts at retehing, and in about 30 seconds became deadly pale, the lips became blue, the pupils dilated widely, the respiration stopped, and the pulse ceased. There is no doubt whatever that the action of the heart ceased some seconds before the respiration failed. The patient's mouth was gagged open, the tongue was drawn forward, the foot of the table was raised, and artificial respiration was performed by compression of the chest. Brandy was injected by the nurse. This proceeding of artificial respiration was kept up for 3 minutes. It had no effect. The ear to the chest could detect no sound from the heart or lungs. Everyone in the room considered the patient to be dead. The jugular vein had been cut

[1] Boston M. and S. Jour., Nov. 12, 1896.   [2] Brit. Med. Jour., Nov. 14, 1896.
[3] Lancet, Jan. 23, 1897.   [4] Brit. Med. Jour., Nov. 21, 1896.
                          [5] Ibid., July 18, 1896.

during the operation and clamped. The forceps were now removed and the opening in the vein was enlarged by tearing its margins. A stream of dark blood poured out. The chest was now forcibly compressed and this produced a great flow of blood. Several ounces of blood escaped and after the internal jugular had been clamped artificial respiration was renewed. In less than half a minute the patient began to breathe. Soon the heart was heard and the patient was out of danger. The question which vein surgeons should open in such conditions depends upon the site of operation, but the vessel selected should be as large and as near the heart as possible. This proceeding relieves the distended right ventricle rapidly and thoroughly.

Mollison [1] furnishes postmortem notes of 11 cases of **death during the administration of chloroform.** In the first case it seems likely that chloroform had little if anything to do with the fatal result. The heart was found dilated and flabby and the muscular substance soft, and the kidneys large and congested. The lower lobe of the right lung was collapsed.

Cases II. and X. represent a class of cases in which it is inadvisable to give an anesthetic because of the increased shock and danger of insufflation of vomited matter. This latter accident happened in Case X. Case II. was a man laboring under cancer of the sigmoid flexure; the body was emaciated and the intestines greatly distended. Both sides of the heart were relaxed and flabby and the coronary arteries were tortuous. The tricuspid orifice admitted six fingers and the mitral orifice four fingers. Both lungs were congested. Case X. had also a cancer of the sigmoid, and when placed on the operating-table had fecal vomiting. The intestines were greatly distended with fluid feces, and the autopsy showed that death was due to asphyxia arising from the entry of vomited matter into the air-passages. Excluding cases I., II., and X., we have 8 persons who died because they were put under the influence of chloroform. In only one of these cases was there any evidence that primary cardiac failure was the mode of death; in all the others the evidences of asphyxia were more or less marked. In all of them the heart was abnormal, being either dilated or fatty. The study of these cases seems to Mollison to bear out the conclusion advanced many years ago by Syme, of Edinburgh, that it is necessary to watch the breathing and not the heart. It is not sufficient to watch a heaving abdomen or chest and fondly imagine that the patient is respiring perfectly. There can be no doubt that cases of sudden cardiac failure do occur, but this is much rarer than death by asphyxia, and when it does occur it is a question whether the chloroform is always to blame, as people with feeble hearts may die of shock and fright when an anesthetic is not given. Information as to the mode of death in the absence of a carefully conducted autopsy is absolutely unreliable. In several of these cases Mollison had been assured that the heart failed first, but the postmortem examination did not bear out this assertion.

Mollison here quotes a sentence from Hewitt, who wrote the article upon anesthetics in Treves' *System of Surgery.* Hewitt says: "Errors have been frequently committed in regarding the circulatory depression as the primary factor, the observers having overlooked the initial respiratory symptoms." Further, Hewitt says that "circulatory failure during anesthesia is in the great majority of cases connected with or dependent upon embarrassed or suspended breathing."

Mollison has further reported [2] upon the postmortem findings in 2 cases of death under chloroform. In 1 case the death was due to cardiac failure, although the slight congestion of the lungs and trachea suggests an element of

---

[1] Intercol. Med. Jour. Austral., Aug. 20, 1896.　　　　[2] Ibid., Feb. 20, 1897.

asphyxia. In the other case death was due to partial asphyxia overcoming cardiac power in a heart dilated and degenerated from a continued fever. This mode of death, Mollison says, been called asyphyxial syncope.

R. Hamilton Russell,[1] of Melbourne, endorses Mollison's views, and advises us to " watch the breathing and let the pulse alone."

Leonard Hill[2] contributes a most important article on the **causation of chloroform-syncope.** This article should be read with care. Space does not permit us to do more than present his conclusions, which are of the highest practical importance to the surgeon. He maintains: 1. That chloroform causes primary failure of the circulation and secondary failure of the respiratory center. The respiratory center fails to act partly because of anemia produced by the great fall in arterial tension. This statement is proved by the fact that the activity of the respiratory center can be restored by raising the arterial tension. The depth of anesthesia depends upon the primary fall of the arterial tension, and so does the paralysis of the respiratory center. 2. Chloroform more than any agent known rapidly abolishes the mechanisms of the vascular system which compensate for the hydrostatic effects of gravity. 3. Chloroform abolishes these mechanisms by paralyzing the splanchnic vasomotor tone and by diminishing the power of the respiratory pump. When these mechanisms are entirely destroyed circulation is impossible if the patient is in the feet-down position. 4. Chloroform produces paralytic dilatation of the heart, acting like nitrite of amyl on the musculature of the entire vascular system. 5. There are two forms of chloroform-syncope—that occurring during primary anesthesia and that occurring during prolonged anesthesia. In the syncope which occurs during primary anesthesia the patient struggles, holds his breath, raises the pressure within the chest, congests the venous system greatly, lowers the arterial tension, and finally makes several deep inspirations and thus charges the lungs with chloroform vapor. In the first stage the left heart becomes impoverished, and in the second stage it suddenly fills with blood. This blood is drawn from the lungs and is saturated with chloroform. The chloroform enters into the coronary arteries and the heart is quickly thrown into paralytic dilatation. Respiration and the pulse cease simultaneously or the pulse ceases before respiration. The syncope which happens during prolonged anesthesia arises from gradually giving chloroform to too great an extent. The arterial pressure diminishes more and more and the respiration ceases secondarily because of anemia of the respiratory center. The heart is not paralyzed by chloroform in these cases because the drug is taken in gradually by the shallow respirations and is distributed slowly by the feeble circulation. 6. A patient can be resuscitated from the second form of syncope by artificial respiration and placing him in a horizontal posture. 7. Artificial respiration carried out while the patient is in a horizontal position is the treatment indicated primarily in the first form of syncope. The heart must be rhythmically compressed by squeezing the chest. If these maneuvers do not quickly cause the pulse to appear, the patient should be placed in a vertical position with the feet down. The dilated right heart is thus completely emptied of blood, artificial respiration is kept up during this change of position, and the patient is brought again into the horizontal posture. By rhythmic compression of the chest circulation is maintained through the coronary arteries. If this maneuver fails in the first trial, it is repeated. 8. Placing the patient in the feet-up position or compressing the abdomen will simply increase paralytic dilatation of the heart. In other words, in syncope

[1] Intercol. Med. Jour. Austral., Nov. 20, 1896.   [2] Brit. Med. Jour., Apr. 17, 1897.

occurring during primary anesthesia both of these methods of treatment do harm rather than good. 9. Shock or fear acts like chloroform in tending to abolish the compensatory mechanism for the hydrostatic effects of gravity, and giving the patient chloroform may be the last straw which completely paralyzes the circulation. 10. Pneumogastric inhibition of the heart is of no importance as an agent in the causation of chloroform-syncope. 11. Ether is a vastly safer agent for anesthesia than chloroform. According to Ringer, it is 50 times less dangerous than chloroform. 12. Hill is in entire agreement with the conclusion of the Hyderabad Commission that the inhaler should be removed when the patient struggles or when the respirations are of irregular depth. Hill, in conclusion, says that the work of physiologists and the tracings of the Hyderabad Commission when carefully studied and rightly interpreted prove that paralysis of the circulatory mechanism, and not of the respiratory center, is what the anesthetist must dread. [The chloroform controversy still continues as it has for many years. Syme always taught that chloroform caused death by inducing respiratory failure. The London school has always taught that chloroform causes death by inducing cardiac failure. The followers of Syme watch the respiration for danger-signals, while the adherents of the London school watch the pulse. Hill succeeds in clearing up some disputed points and shows there are two varieties of chloroform-syncope. Hare maintains that while chloroform is a powerful depressant of the respiratory center and heart when given in excess, when properly given, if it produces death, it does so in the same manner as hemorrhage causes death, failure of the respiratory center occurring because it is deprived of blood, and the pulse-failure being due to vasomotor palsy and the heart having no blood to pump. Hare believes in abdominal compression, inversion, bandaging of limbs, and artificial respiration when chloroform-syncope occurs. Leonard Hill's book upon *The Physiology and Pathology of the Cerebral Circulation* is an important contribution to the chloroform discussion.]

Local Anesthesia.—Prof. Ceci,[1] of Pisa, gives a list of **operations** which he has **performed under** the influence of **cocain** or cocain and morphin. Some of these operations are of considerable magnitude. For instance, the radical cure of hernia, laparotomy, vaginal hysterectomy, and extirpation of goitre. He thinks that the addition of morphin for its general effect is a very valuable expedient. In old people he injects a maximum dose of 2 cgm. quarter of an hour before operating. In young people he injects 1 cgm., but he never uses such an injection when a person is under 20 years of age. The cocain he prefers is Merck's, of the strength of 2% dissolved in boric acid. He has a strong solution of a strength of 1 : 100 and a weak solution of the strength of 1 : 200. He warms these solutions to make them more active. He believes in making deep injections, the fluid being thrown in for some distance along the nerve-trunks. Local anesthesia he holds is indicated in operations where we can accurately determine beforehand what procedure must be carried out and where the field of operation is not too extensive. He does not believe in this method for children or for excitable or intractable individuals. The anesthesia by morphin and cocain lasts from 30 to 50 minutes. This observer has never seen poisoning, but has frequently met with thirst and dryness of the month and in some few cases with excitement and loquacity.

Prof. Karl Stoerk[2] discusses the question of cocain-anesthesia and particularly considers the toxic influence of the drug. He agrees with Wölfler that injections of cocain made about the head are more dangerous than injections

---

[1] Brit. Med. Jour., No. 1877.　　　　　　　[2] Wien. med. Woch., No. 44, 1896.

given into the trunk or in the limbs. The amount of $\frac{1}{3}$ of a gr. should never be exceeded in one injection in the mucous membrane of the mouth. Stoerk applies a 20 % solution to the larynx, and has met with only four cases of poisoning as a result of this procedure. He holds that cocain is absorbed much less readily from the larynx than it is from either the pharynx or the esophagus. He states that nervous people are far more apt to be affected unfavorably with cocain than are others. In the milder cases of poisoning the condition resembles hysteria. In the more severe cases the face becomes deadly pale, the pulse becomes rapid, and the respirations shallow. In the very bad cases there is faintness which passes on to collapse or muscular jactitation, with sudden movements, hallucinations, and a feeling of great apprehension. After the acute symptoms have passed away the patient is prostrated and weak for many hours, and is apt to suffer from violent headache. There is no real antidote to cocain. The patient should be placed in a horizontal position and should be given coffee or ether or camphor or injections of musk or inhalations of nitrite of amyl. This writer quotes Doufournier to the effect that the reason toxic symptoms have so often followed applications of cocain to the throat and nose is because the patient in most of these procedures is placed in a sitting posture. He quotes Baracz to the effect that cocain must be used with extreme care in epileptics. [A great many people show slight evidences of cocain-poisoning after the drug is injected, and severe cases of poisoning are not unusual. In the slighter cases the symptoms are often attributed erroneously to fear. Among the symptoms of these slight cases are pallor, incoordination, dimness of vision, tinnitus aurium, headache, tremor, and subsequent sleeplessness for many hours. Cocain is a dangerous drug, and many persons possess pronounced idiosyncrasy toward it. Nervous persons, the insane, epileptics, and drunkards are particularly apt to develop dangerous symptoms. Idiosyncrasy may run in family lines and may exist in even the most stolid and robust individuals. Cocain is often used with a recklessness which is appalling. When first used in an individual very small amounts should be introduced, and if these produce no signs of trouble larger amounts can be given. The urethral use of cocain not rarely produces toxic symptoms.]

John A. Wyeth,[1] in a paper upon cocain-anesthesia, maintains that it is useless to throw cocain into the subcutaneous areolar tissue or even into the deeper corium, such a procedure failing to produce satisfactory anesthesia and carrying with it a certain amount of danger. Injection into the subcutaneous areolar tissue is especially apt to be followed by rapid absorption and by toxic symptoms. The injections should be made into the Malpighian layer, where there is a network of sensory end-organs that are certain to come in contact with the cocain solution. Injection into the Malpighian layer will produce rapid, certain, and safe anesthesia. Dr. Wyeth says that if we wish to inject portions of the body where it is impossible to impede the circulation by the use of the elastic bandage, we should proceed as follows: the needle is carried obliquely through the epiderm until the point. is in the Malpighian layer. Arriving at this point about half a minim of a 4 % solution is forced out. This causes whitening of the epiderm. With the needle still in position an incision from a quarter to half an inch in length is made as far as the anesthesia has spread. The needle is then withdrawn, is reinserted a quarter of an inch from the first point, and another half minim or minim of the solution is forced out at the same level and the incision is extended. From 2 to 4 minims of the solution will enable us to make an incision 1 inch long through the skin and corium and into the subcutaneous areolar tissue. After

[1] Med. News, Dec. 12, 1896.

opening the subcutaneous tissue, if it becomes necessary to prolong the operation, a weaker solution may now be used with advantage. In operating upon an extremity Wyeth uses a 2% solution for the skin. After the completion of the operation the tourniquet is loosened for three or four seconds and then readjusted for several minutes, and this procedure is repeated two or three times. In this way a small quantity of cocain is admitted into the circulation at one time, and this small quantity distributed over a large area produces no ill results. [We have followed a similar method and can endorse its efficiency and safety.]

The use of **eucain** has attracted much interest and attention during the year. This drug was studied by Prof. Charteris, assisted by Dr. McLennan.[1] These observers proved that eucain is far less toxic than cocain. Further, that eucain is slower in onset and of less intensity, but that it is thoroughly efficient as an anesthetic. Dr. George W. Spencer[2] made a careful study of the use of eucain in 20 cases of surgical operation, and he considers that this agent produces the most complete local anesthesia of any drug so far used. It does not lose its strength when kept in solution, and it does not decompose even when boiled. The fact that we can boil the solution without impairing its utility is of great advantage, for we are thus enabled to render it satisfactorily sterile. The amount of eucain used depends upon the severity of the operation. He has usually employed a 2% solution. In one case a dose of 15 grains was injected. In some cases he has used 2 drams of a 5% solution. In no case have any symptoms of poisoning been noted. The time necessary to obtain complete anesthesia varies. In 11 cases the anesthesia was complete within 5 minutes. In 7 cases it was complete in 3 minutes. In 1 case it was complete in 2 minutes. In 1 case in which the tissues were infiltrated with inflammatory exudate the anesthesia was not complete for 10 minutes. When we wish to remove a toenail we should wait at least 5 minutes for the anesthesia to become complete. The duration of the anesthesia varies between 20 minutes and 1 hour. In some of the cases slight local effect followed the use of this drug. Spencer disagrees with the statement of Arthur L. Fuller that eucain hardens the tissues to such a degree that it is difficult to introduce sutures. He has never seen this condition produced by it. [That eucain not unusually causes sloughing is certain. We have noted this occurrence many times, and it constitutes a serious objection to its extensive use. We first thought sloughing might be due to the preliminary use of ethyl chlorid to produce an anesthetic area through which to insert the needle, but we have seen the same accident since the use of ethyl chlorid was abandoned. It has happened when no carbolic acid was used in the solution or in the tissues, and when the fluid was rendered sterile by boiling. We do not mean to say that it always happens, but it frequently does, producing a dry, semi-elastic, tough, and very adherent slough. Sloughing is most apt to occur after operations in fatty tissue, upon the fingers and toes, the prepuce, bursæ, and tendon-sheaths. In a few cases also it has produced constitutional symptoms of considerable danger.]

Eucain in surgery is the title of an article by Drs. Legueu and Lihou.[3] They hold that in physiological action eucain is analogous to cocain, but it has very slight action upon the heart. Cocain slows the pulse and elevates the arterial pressure. Eucain slows the pulse very slightly and has no effect on the arterial pressure. Arterial pressure can be reduced by eucain only when extremely large doses are given. An animal can be killed by very large doses

[1] Brit. Med. Jour., Mar. 27, 1897.   [2] Univ. Med. Mag., Nov., 1896.
[3] Gaz. des Hôpitaux, Nos. 19 and 20, 1897.

of eucain, death being due to respiratory paralysis and not to cardiac failure. Experiments show that eucain is far less toxic than cocain. These observers have used cocain in a large number of cases, including amputation of the fingers, opening of abscesses, etc. They use a solution of the strength of 1 %, and rarely administer over 1½ grains of the drug. In the examination of the bladder by the cystoscope they use a solution in the strength of ½ of 1 %, employing from 4 to 8 ounces of solution. They have never noticed any toxic symptoms. One patient who had previously been operated upon under cocain and had presented toxic symptoms was not affected at all by the eucain. The anesthetic effects have been as thoroughly good as those obtained with cocain. Hemorrhage is more abundant when eucain is used than when cocain is employed, because of the hyperemia induced by the eucain. This hemorrhage, however, always stops readily. It is a great advantage that eucain can be sterilized readily by boiling. Cocain is decomposed when boiled. The anesthetic effects of eucain are more rapidly obtained than those of cocain. The injection is a little more painful than the injection of cocain. [Eucain is sometimes irritant to the urethra. Görl's advice is sound: "Do not use eucain in the urethra if anesthesia is required oftener than once a day." Eucain causes a hyperemic condition, and should never be introduced into a bladder which tends to bleed.]

Dr. Spencer [1] presents a further investigation of eucain hydrochlorat as an anesthetic, with a report of 24 cases, and these additional studies have served to convince him of the great value of the drug. In this latter list of cases are included 3 tracheotomies, the removal of a large nevus, of a fatty tumor, of a portion of the lower lip, and of a melanotic sarcoma, operation for empyema, fistula in ano, thyroid cyst, traumatic gangrene of the finger, phimosis, hydrocele, needle in the hand, Alibert's disease, and dermoid cyst of the ovary; the operators having been Keen, Hearn, Brinton, Jones, DaCosta, Spencer, and others.

Among other articles upon eucain we would call attention to the papers of the following authors: T. J. Yarrow,[2] Martin H. Williams,[3] W. J. Howe and Macleod Yearsley,[4] Joseph S. Gibb,[5] Gaetano Vinci,[6] and E. Vogt.[7]

THE ESOPHAGUS.

[During the past year it has been found that the location of foreign bodies in the esophagus is made certain and easy by the employment of the x-rays. This application of the x-rays will be discussed in a special article devoted to them.]

William T. Bull and John B. Walker[8] report a case of extreme interest in which a **foreign body** was successfully **removed from the esophagus** by external esophagotomy after a lodgement of 22 months. The patient had a fainting attack, and recovering found that she had swallowed a tooth-plate holding two teeth. The physician who was called in could only pass a probang 6 inches. The next day the patient was able to swallow liquids and at the end of 6 weeks could take solids. She remained in good health for about 18 months, when she began to suffer from dysphagia and hoarseness and loss of flesh became apparent. External esophagotomy was performed on the left side. Even when the esophagus was reached the body could not be felt. The tube was opened just above the sternum upon a bougie; 1 in.

---

[1] Med. and Surg. Reporter, Nov. 28, 1896.
[3] Internat. Jour. Surg., June, 1897.
[5] Phila. Polyclinic, Jan. 23, 1897.
[7] Therapist, Mar. 15, 1897.

[2] Med. Rec., Jan. 9, 1897.
[4] Brit. Med. Jour., Jan. 16, 1897.
[6] Therap. Monatsh., Feb., 1897.
[8] Med. Rec., Mar., 6, 1897.

below the incision and back of the first part of the sternum instruments were arrested. Eventually a whalebone bougie was passed into the stomach along the anterior wall of the gullet. A probe inserted alongside of the whalebone entered a pouch on the posterior esophageal wall and came in contact with the plate. The mucous membrane in front of the plate was nicked with scissors and the plate was removed by means of curved artery-forceps. A rubber catheter was inserted through the wound into the esophagus and was passed 4 in. below the point where the tooth-plate had been lodged. The wound was lightly stuffed with gauze about the cavity. For the first 24 hours the patient was fed purely by rectum, but after this period rectal feeding was supplemented by other methods. At this time fluids were first introduced through the catheter. The tube was withdrawn on the 13th day. In 48 hours after removing the tube the patient was fed by means of a stomach-tube, and a day or two later swallowing was permitted and rectal feeding was discontinued. The patient was out of bed 1 week after the operation and the wound was healed in 7 weeks. The length of time intervening between lodgement of the foreign body and its removal by operation makes this case especially noteworthy.

M. Péan [1] records a case in which a **coin lodged in the esophagus** was **located by means of a skiagraph.** Péan decided to perform external esophagotomy. After exposing the esophagus he concluded to endeavor to move the body upward by manipulation without opening the tube. By this means the coin was pressed upward until it was extracted from the month by means of alligator mouth-forceps. Péan tells us that children can swallow foreign bodies of at least 1 in. in diameter, these bodies lodging at the narrowest point of the esophagus, and the child still continuing to take liquids with ease and not complaining of pain. For this reason it is often thought that the foreign body is not in the tube. Both Broca and the author have reported cases in which death resulted from foreign body lodged in the esophagus, the cause of death not having been suspected until postmortem made it evident. It is a great advantage, if possible, to remove bodies without opening the esophagus, because this operation is dangerous and requires prolonged subsequent treatment which entails much discomfort.

The first case in which the skiagraph was used to detect and locate a foreign body in the esophagus was recorded by J. William White in the *Annals of Surgery* for August, 1896. The patient was a child 2 years and 5 months of age, and was brought to White 13 days after having swallowed a jackstone. The patient was able to swallow liquids but refused to swallow solids. A skiagraph was taken and the jackstone was distinctly recognized as it lay a little to the left of the middle line, somewhat above the bifurcation of the trachea. Attempts to reach the body with esophageal forceps failed and gastrotomy was performed. A slender and flexible esophageal explorer, which had fastened to it a stout silk thread 3 feet in length, was passed downward through the pharynx and into the stomach. One end of the thread was brought out of the wound in the stomach and the explorer was withdrawn, leaving the other end of the thread emerging from the mouth. Pieces of gauze of different shapes and various sizes were tied to this string, which thread was drawn up and down until finally a piece of gauze entangled the foreign body and brought it into the stomach, from which viscus it was easily extracted. The stomach-wound was closed and the child made a rapid and complete recovery. White dwells on the great improvement the Röntgen process of diagnosis is over the old method, in which the sur-

[1] Bull. de l'Acad. de Méd., No. 48, 1896.

18

geon came to a conclusion from a study of the history, the subjective symptoms, and the recognition of the presence of the foreign body by instruments. He shows how the Röntgen process enables us to determine the exact location of the foreign body, and hence to choose a suitable method for its removal. At first, on studying the skiagraph, he thought of performing esophagotomy, but on examining the short, fat neck of the patient he concluded that, if the body were at all fixed, it would be very difficult to dislodge it through the largest wound which could be safely made in the neck. In view of the fact that this foreign body was firmly lodged in the canal and was irregular in shape he thought it better to open the stomach and try to remove it, and thus dispense with attacking an inflamed and possibly ulcerated esophagus. The situation of this foreign body rendered any attempt to push it downward extremely hazardous. Such an effort would probably have resulted in perforation of the aorta or the bronchus. The fact that it was impossible to move the jackstone upward by the means employed in the operation vindicated the choice of the stomach-route. White thought of the possibility of keeping the foreign body in view with the fluoroscope while an endeavor was made to remove it by the use of forceps from above, but he did not employ this procedure because the general condition of the patient demanded haste and because the probable inflammation and ulceration of the esophagus contraindicated prolonged instrumentation. He thinks that in cases seen earlier this method might be employed. [Strange to say, within a short time of the performance by White of the above-reported operation Keen recognized a jackstone in the esophagus by the x-rays and removed it by esophagotomy, and A. C. Wood had a similar case, which he treated according to the method suggested by White.]

H. Beeckman Delatour[1] records a case in which a child 4 years of age swallowed an iron washer $\frac{9}{16}$ in. in diameter; 4 days after the accident the boy was brought to the hospital and the fluoroscope was applied. The foreign body was distinctly visible and a skiagraph was taken. Delatour was greatly impressed with the distinctness of the shadow obtained by looking through the fluoroscope, and he decided to attempt removal of the foreign body with a pair of esophageal forceps while he used the fluoroscope. Two days after admission the patient was cloroformed and the foreign body was successfully extracted with the esophageal forceps. Delatour thinks that this proceeding is especially valuable in children with short and thick necks in which external esophagotomy is extremely difficult. [The removal of the foreign body while looking at it with the fluoroscope was suggested by White in the report of his case (previous article).]

Two cases of a halfpenny in the esophagus are reported by Francis Johnston and C. Thurstan Holland.[2] The first case was a child $2\frac{1}{2}$ years of age, who had swallowed a halfpenny 2 days before admission into the hospital. The skiagraph showed the coin in the gullet, and it was easily removed with a coin-catcher. The second case was a child $2\frac{1}{4}$ years of age with a doubtful history of having swallowed a halfpenny. The child came to the hospital 5 months after the alleged accident, laboring under bronchopneumonia. At this time laryngeal stertor and inspiratory dyspnea were noted. These symptoms became constant and involuntary. It was evident that the pneumogastric or recurrent laryngeal nerve was subjected to pressure, but the laryngoscope threw no light upon the question; 13 months after the swallowing of the penny the Röntgen rays were applied and the coin was found. It was removed by means of a coin-catcher.

[1] Med. Rec., May 1, 1897.   [2] Brit. Med. Jour., Dec. 5, 1896.

THE STOMACH.

Péan [1] discusses **gastrectomy.** He has performed 12 pylorectomies with 8 recoveries, and 3 gastroenterostomies with 2 recoveries. He thinks that pylorectomy is applicable in young people who are still in fair health and in cases in which the tumor is small, movable, and unassociated with lymphatic deposits or disseminations. The only cases in which operations should be done are those in which it is possible to leave a portion of the cardiac end. The cut portion of the duodenum should not be attached to this large gap in the stomach. The stomach-opening is sutured and the duodenum attached by means of a Murphy button to the nearest portion of the stomach. When the lymph-glands are involved or when visceral metastases exist pylorectomy should not be attempted, the preferable operation in such cases being gastro-enterostomy by means of a Murphy button.

Willy Meyer [2] presented a patient to the New York Surgical Society on whom he had done **gastroenterostomy for cancer.** He used a Murphy button. The operation had been performed some 3 months before, and the button had not since appeared in the stools. The patient has gained largely in weight since the operation and is free from pain. In 6 previous cases the button has also remained in the stomach.

Emanuel J. Senn,[3] of Chicago, proposes **a new method of gastrostomy** by the formation of a circular valve. He maintains that a gastrostomy should prevent leakage by making a valve of the stomach-wall itself, instead of utilizing other structures for that purpose ; should minimize shock by putting but little strain upon the stomach ; should leave a fistula which is closed during digestion and can be opened when we desire to administer food. He found a prototype of the ideal mechanism in the valves of the veins. These valves permit the blood to flow in one direction only. The author's operation consists in making an abdominal incision in any situation which is desirable, as no muscular structures are required for sphincter-action. The stomach is seized near the great curvature and an assistant forms a cone of this viscus and holds the apex with his fingers or with forceps. Two puck-

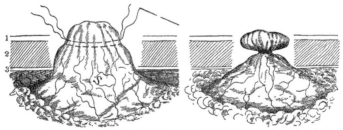

FIG. 10.—Puckering-strings in situ: 1, skin; 2, muscle; 3, peritoneum: S, stomach (E. J. Senn, in Jour. Am. Med. Assoc., Nov. 28, 1896).

FIG. 11.—Puckering-strings tied, forming a constriction (E. J. Senn, in Jour. Amer. Med. Assoc., Nov. 28, 1896).

ering-strings of chromicized catgut are placed parallel to each other $2\frac{1}{2}$ in. below the apex of the cone, the sutures including the serous and muscular coats (Fig. 10). These sutures are drawn tight and thus form a neck (Fig. 11); a portion of the gastrocolic omentum is lifted up, and a cuff is sutured over the

[1] Rev. de Chir., Nov. 10, 1896.　　　　　[2] Ann. of Surg., Mar., 1897.
[3] Jour. Am. Med. Assoc., Nov. 28, 1896.

constriction by means of silk (Fig. 12). The stomach is fastened to the parietal wound with silk sutures, which include the upper portion of the cuff of omentum, the serous and muscular coats of the stomach, and all the abdominal wall except the skin. The skin is closed with silkworm-gut sutures, leaving visible the portion of the stomach which is to form the valve. The stomach can be opened at this time or later, whichever is desired. The opening is made in the center of the portion exposed and should be $1\frac{1}{2}$ in. in

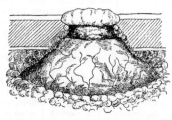

FIG. 12.—Omental cuff covering constriction, and stomach sutured to abdominal-wall (E. J. Senn, in Jour. Am. Med. Assoc., Nov. 28, 1896.

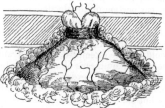

FIG. 13.—Inversion of stomach above constriction, and sutured with Lembert sutures, forming a circular valve (E. J. Senn, in Jour. Am. Med. Assoc., Nov. 28, 1896).

length. A rubber tube is passed into the stomach; the stomach-wall is now inverted, forming a circular valve, and the inversion is maintained by Lembert sutures (Fig. 13). The tube is now withdrawn. The author then records a case in which he performed this operation. The result was most satisfactory. The tube was removed every time after the patient was fed and

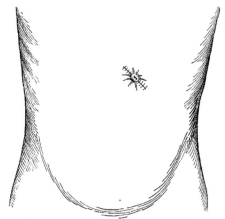

FIG. 14.—Operation completed (E. J. Senn, in Jour. Am. Med. Assoc., Nov. 28, 1896).

there was never the slightest leakage from the fistula. The valve and the constriction were easily passed by the tube, and when the tube was withdrawn the valve would close like a trap-door. Even when the stomach was filled with milk and the patient was told to cough and to move about violently there was not the slightest leakage. [Abbe has performed Senn's operation, and reports that the plan is very satisfactory.]

Fontan[1] describes a **new method of performing gastrostomy.** This method prevents the escape of gastric juice and is very simple in its performance. It is called by Fontan a valve operation. The ordinary abdominal incision is made, the stomach is grasped with forceps and a portion of it pulled outward, and this protruding portion is sutured to the edge of the wound. This hernia is invaginated while the forceps still retain their hold, and the serous surfaces at the ends of the wound are sutured together. The stomach is then incised and a cannula inserted. The author tells us that the cannula lies in a valvular canal, which is shaped like an inverted mitre of a bishop, the gastric surface being formed of the walls of the stomach and the serous surfaces being opposite each other.

Willy Meyer[2] records a case of gastrostomy performed according to **the method of Kader** (first described by Kader in the *Centralbl. f. Chir.*,

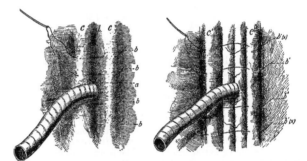

Fig. 15.—Kader's method of gastrostomy (Willy Meyer, in N. Y. Med. Jour., Nov. 7, 1896).

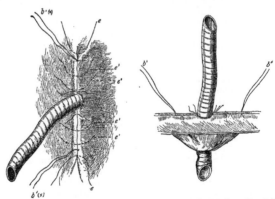

Fig. 16.—Kader's method of gastrostomy (Willy Meyer, in N. Y. Med. Jour., Nov. 7, 1896).

July 11, 1896). Kader stated that he had a case of cicatricial stenosis of the pylorus and esophagus. The abdomen was opened and a long incision was made through the anterior wall of the stomach to perform digital exploration.

[1] Rev. de Chir., Nov. 10, 1896.   [2] N. Y. Med. Jour., Nov. 7, 1896.

The stomach was very small and so slightly movable that it was found impossible to perform any of the ordinary methods of gastrostomy. Kader therefore modified Witzel's method and found the result admirable. His operation, which differs considerably from the Witzel operation, can be performed upon the most difficult cases, and is carried out as follows: an incision 3 or 4 in. long is made parallel with the borders of the ribs and two fingers' breadth distant from them. Kader states, however, that the simple vertical incision can be used, and Meyer thinks it should be used. The rectus muscle is divided by blunt dissection and the posterior sheath of the rectus and the peritoneum are cut. A fold of the stomach is pulled forward in the usual way. If the stomach is movable, the fold is drawn in front of the abdominal wall, the surrounding field being packed with gauze. A small incision is made and a drainage-tube the size of a pencil is introduced into the stomach for a distance of about 2 in. Bleeding is arrested. The drainage-tube is fastened to the stomach by a catgut suture (Fig. 15, *A*). Two Lembert sutures (Fig. 15, *B*) are put on either side of the tube so that they catch and unite a portion of the stomach about ½ in. wide, leaving between a groove ¾ in. wide. These sutures are about ½ in. apart. These sutures catch the serous coat and the muscular coat. By tying them two longitudinal folds are formed (Fig. 15, *C*). The stomach-wall is thus turned inward in the neighborhood of the tube and caused to surround the tube. The drainage-tube is thus surrounded by serous membrane and the canal in which it lies does not pass the stomach-wall obliquely, but enters it perpendicularly. This canal is lengthened by stitching two more folds of the stomach-wall over the first ones (Fig. 16, *C*). These threads are not cut off, but are left long in order to give the surgeon control of the stomach during the rest of the operation. The stomach is now stitched to the peritoneal wound and the posterior sheath of the rectus muscle, the seat of operation thus becoming extraperitoneal. The rectus muscle is sutured with a few stitches, the anterior portion of the sheath is sutured, and the skin closed on either side of the tube. In the case in which the stomach cannot be pulled forward into the wound Kader tells us to apply the deep occlusion-sutures and use them to draw the stomach up against the abdominal wall and thus close off the peritoneal cavity. In the case in which Meyer operated even this procedure could not be carried out, and he was forced to open the stomach within the abdominal cavity. If we wish to establish a permanent fistula, the folds should be made in the perpendicular direction; therefore in cancerous stricture make the folds perpendicular, in cicatricial stricture make them transverse. This operation has been carried out ten times in the clinic of Prof. Mikulicz; three times it was done under the influence of Schleich's infiltration-anesthesia. All ten patients recovered and in all the result was satisfactory.

Meyer then reports his case, in which the operation was performed for cancerous stricture of the esophagus. It gave a most satisfactory result.

Page and Clay[1] report a case of great interest which was seen at the Royal Infirmary, Newcastle-ou-Tyne. There was **obstruction** at the pyloric end of the stomach **due to** kinking produced by the adhesion of a **suppurating gall-bladder.** This condition was confirmed postmortem.

Rutherford Morison,[2] of Newcastle-on-Tyne, publishes his notes on 4 cases of **pyloroplasty.** He says that Loreta's operation is seldom heard of now. It has to be performed in the dark, and is of necessity dangerous. The Heineke-Mikulicz operation has attained a prominent place in surgery. Morison says the diagnosis between cicatricial and malignant stenosis of the pylorus is often one of extreme difficulty, and is in fact frequently impossible.

[1] Brit. Med. Jour., Jan. 23, 1897.   [2] Lancet, Oct. 24, 1896.

In cases in which he has had the pylorus outside of the abdomen he has been unable to say whether an induration were due to malignant disease or inflammatory exudation. The most important element in the diagnosis is probably a long history, as this points strongly against malignant disease. If there is considerable scarring of the stomach-wall and adhesions, the indications are in favor of the non-malignant condition. Morison reports 4 cases in which he performed the Heineke-Mikulicz operation. All of these cases recovered and each of the patients greatly improved in health.

Von Bungner,[1] of Hanan, advises the **combination of gastroenterostomy with enteroanastomosis.** This procedure was originally recommended by Braun. Von Bungner operated upon a case by means of gastroenterostomy, but the operation failed to relieve the pain and vomiting still continued. A week after this operation he performed an enteroanastomosis between the afferent and efferent coils. · The symptoms at once passed away and the patient made a good recovery.

Fricker[2] reports a very remarkable case in which a **large number of foreign bodies** were successfully **removed** from the stomach by **gastrotomy.** The patient, suffering from melancholia, had swallowed with suicidal intent a great number of bodies. The stomach was opened over the most prominent part of the distinct projection ; just beneath the muscles an abscess was entered and was found to contain a crochet-needle $4\frac{1}{2}$ in. in length. The needle lay at the posterior portion of the abscess-cavity and adhered to the parietal peritoneum. No perforation was discovered in the stomach. The stomach was opened above the level of the abscess and Fricker removed from the viscus a door-key, a fork, a couple of teaspoons, two nails, two hairpins, a dozen bits of glass, a steel pen, several needles, a window-fastener, and a number of other materials. The total number of foreign objects was 37. The patient made a good recovery.

William F. Haslam[3] writes on **gastrojejunostomy for pyloric obstruction.** He reports a case in which he performed this operation by means of a Murphy button. The button was passed 140 days after the operation. The patient was very greatly relieved by the operation and gained much in weight and strength. He died 10 months later. The second case was in a woman on whom he performed gastrojejunostomy with a Murphy button. The patient recovered well from the operation and gained in health and strength. A year after the operation the button had not passed. Haslam says that though we divide obstructions of the pylorus pathologically into those due to carcinoma and those due to a fibrous overgrowth, from a clinical point of view they are all worthy of the term malignant, for they tend to cause death, first by obstructing the entry of food into the intestines and secondly by exhaustion produced by repeated attacks of prolonged vomiting ; they differ only in the length of time necessary to kill. A diagnosis before opening the abdomen is very frequently impossible. Even when the abdomen is opened and the growth is handled it may be impossible to tell whether we are dealing with a hard carcinoma or a fibrous stricture. If the patient recovers from the operation, improves rapidly, gains in flesh notably, and is able to return to work, we may hope that cancer was not the cause. There is no great advantage gained by attempting to diagnosticate the exact pathological nature of a growth before operation. If we feel sure there is a growth of the pylorus, we must feel equally sure that the patient will waste and eventually die if the surgeon does not interfere, and it is our duty to interfere. The rapid im-

---

[1] Verhandl. der deutsch. Gesell. f. Chir., XXVth Congress, 1896.
[2] Deutsch. med. Woch., No. 4, 1897.   [3] Birmingham Med. Rev., Apr., 1897.

provement which often follows operation, even when cancer exists, is due to the fact that the growth is of the hard and fibrous type, and as soon as the patient can get a proper supply of food he is able to withstand the slow growth of the tumor. Haslam reminds us that the healthy stomach is always in a state of contraction. If undistended with gas, there is no appreciable cavity; if full, its walls are contracting on the varying amounts of food; but if the walls of the stomach have lost their tonicity and become dilated, as they must do after a pyloric obstruction, they are no longer able to contract and obliterate the cavity of the stomach and are no longer capable of emptying this viscus. As a consequence, after the performance of the operation of gastrojejunostomy vomiting may occur for a time because the contents of the jejunum are being forced into the stomach through the artificial opening. When we examine the abdomen with the flat hand we can often detect a pyloric growth, but not in the normal situation of the pylorus. The growth brings the pylorus down from beneath the liver, and when there are no adhesions the pyloric end of the stomach may even wander about the upper portion of the abdomen. It occasionally happens that we think a growth is freely movable and yet find on opening the abdomen that it had adhesions at the upper part, the growth having spread downward from the pylorus along the anterior wall of the stomach. Haslam believes in opening the abdomen early, and opposes waiting until the patient is worn out by vomiting and starvation and the effects of a distended stomach. An operation to be of real value should be done before the stomach is hopelessly distended and before there is great emaciation. Rapid operation is essential because these patients are weak and emaciated. Regarding the immediate result of operation there is much to be said in favor of **the Murphy button.** It is easy to apply and the operation may be quickly completed, whereas the use of sutures, the favorite type of operation with many, necessitates a prolonged operation. Some object to the Murphy button on the ground that it produces death of tissue, but there is no particular danger in this ring of necrosed tissue, as there are peritoneal adhesions around which effectually shut off the general peritoneal cavity. Another objection is that the opening is too small. This can be obviated by using a large-size button or an oval button. Another objection is that the opening has a tendency to contract; it is probable that some contraction does take place, but even then the opening may be large enough. Another objection is that a foreign body has been left and must be discharged before the patient is out of danger. Haslam says that there is no doubt that the chances seem in favor of the button dropping into the stomach rather than into the intestine. Even if it passes into the intestine it may possibly cause impaction or ulceration or damage of the intestinal wall. Nevertheless a study of the records would not lead us to believe that the chances of serious trouble are very great. If we open the stomach on the posterior wall, the best chance for drainage is afforded, but in order to reach the posterior wall we must perform a difficult and prolonged operation. Those who advocate this route state that the posterior opening facilitates the exit of food, lessens the chances of regurgitation when the patient is supine, and by preventing the accumulation of food in the stomach prevents distention. Haslam says that if the stomach is a mere passive bag, the posterior opening will facilitate the passage of food; but if it has the power of contraction, it will not. The pylorus, it will be remembered, is not situated at the lowest part of the stomach. With the anterior opening and a large and atonic stomach there is risk for a time that the stomach will not get rid of its contents, but when we know that this atonic condition exists we can take particular care not to overload the viscus. It occasionally happens in this operation that there is obstruction in the transverse colon by pressure of a piece of jejunum, or pieces in front of it. This, however, is a very unusual condition, and results when the portion of the jejunum selected was very near the commencement, so that the tension of its mesentery obstructed the colon. We should select a piece of jejunum from its upper end, but not so high up as to have to drag it into position.

[There have been many interesting articles published during the year in relation to gastric ulcer and perforating gastric ulcer. We have selected some of the more striking reports.]

E. Claude Taylor[1] reports a case in which he believes that **perforation of a gastric ulcer** occurred and yet there was recovery without operation. The man had vague symptoms of gastritis for some time. He ate a hearty meal and went to work lifting barrels. He was seized with violent pain and vomited bile-stained material. Five hours afterward he had great pain, collapse, and rigid abdomen. He had passed urine and had had a bowel-movement. He was simply fed by the rectum and got well. Taylor inquires, Should we be in a hurry to operate in such cases, or should we wait as long as the patient is improving? E. A. Seale[2] reports a similar case in which there was recovery after symptoms of perforation. William H. Bennett[3] reports a case of perforating gastric ulcer in which a large opening in the stomach was closed by means of an omental plug. The patient recovered. The procedure was a modification of Senn's original method. The patient was a man who had been seized with the signs of rupture of the stomach 5 hours before admission; a median section was performed and general peritonitis was found to exist. A perforation was discovered 2 in. from the pylorus on the upper aspect. The parts were very adherent. The opening was $\frac{1}{2}$ in. in its longest diameter and was surrounded by a zone of induration 3 in. in diameter. The extent of the induration prevented inversion of the peritoneum by the ordinary method. The trial was made, but the stitches cut out. Bennett turned up a portion of the omentum and pushed as much as was necessary into the perforation, completely closing it just as a cork closes a bottle. This omental plug was fixed in position by a single suture passing through the whole thickness of the plug and of the stomach-walls at the point of perforation and by several other sutures which after transfixing the base of the plug brought the peritoneum on each side into contact with it. These sutures were put in by the Lembert method in order to cause the peritoneum to overlap as much as possible. The abdominal cavity was washed and sponged and the wound was brought together in the usual way. The patient made an excellent recovery.

T. H. Morse[4] reports 3 cases of **perforated gastric ulcer treated by laparotomy;** 2 of these patients recovered and 1 died. The first case was operated on 5 hours after the onset of the symptoms and the second case 4½ hours after the onset of the symptoms, and they both recovered. The third case was operated on 24 hours after the onset of the symptoms, and died of shock. If a case of perforating ulcer is not operated upon, the patient will probably live for about 24 hours. This statement shows how necessary are diagnosis and early operation.

Mr. Arthur E. Barker[5] reported in a clinical lecture 7 cases of perforated gastric ulcer treated by operation, with 3 recoveries. In all of these cases the perforation was on the anterior wall of the stomach. In no instance was there any evidence of a second perforation. In all of the cases excepting one the

[1] Lancet, Dec. 19, 1896.   [2] Ibid., Oct. 10, 1896.
[3] Ibid., Aug. 1, 1896.   [4] Brit. Med. Jour., Feb. 13, 1897.
[5] Lancet, Dec. 5, 1896.

operations were similar. A median incision was made in all. In 3 of them it was necessary to add a transverse cut through the left rectus muscle. In one of them an inguinal incision had been made previously, and this materially facilitated the cleansing of the peritoneal cavity. In all of the cases the peritoneal cavity was cleansed by means of dry sponging rather than irrigation. Great care was taken in 6 of the cases to carry the sponge between the liver and diaphragm, a point in which material is very apt to collect. This procedure was omitted in Case 4 and a subphrenic abscess resulted. Barker has been surprised at the large amount of matter which he has been enabled to dislodge by sponging from between the liver and diaphragm. Great care must be taken to cleanse around and behind the gall-bladder, in the flanks, and in the pelvis. In 2 cases a drainage-tube was inserted through an incision in the flank, but it seemed to be of little benefit. In 4 cases the anterior wound was drained with iodoform-gauze with good results. A portion of gauze was carried down deeply between the liver and diaphragm on each side, another was carried down to the suture-line in the stomach, another was carried behind the gall-bladder. The pieces of gauze were removed on the 5th or 6th day. In no case was the ulcer cut out. The edges were inverted, and the silk stitches were inserted deeply in one or two rows by means of round sewing-needles. In after-treatment Barker advocates feeding by the month. He gives small amounts, frequently repeated, of egg-albumin and water, brandy, beef-tea, and chicken-broth, and begins to give them as soon as the patient recovers from the anesthetic. In addition to this he uses peptonized suppositories in the rectum, alternating every 2 hours with an injection of 5 ounces of hot water. Barker thinks the most important element in success in these cases is early operation. The prognosis is profoundly affected for the worse when it is found that the contents of the stomach have escaped among the intestines. If a solid meal has been taken shortly before perforation and large fragments of food have passed into the peritoneal cavity, profound shock and great distention result. Barker thinks that we should operate early, even in collapse. We had better operate when collapse is present than to take the chance of death involved in waiting for it to pass away. In all of his cases it was necessary to empty the stomach by pressure. This is better done by hand than by washing out. The author does not see how early feeding can injure while the stitches hold firmly. He would feel more anxious as to the consequences of mouth-feeding after 2 or 3 days than at first, because at the later period the stitches might cut out. Great benefit attends early feeding; it rouses the patient from collapse and thus overweighs the risk. Barker says he has been careful in the two patients that recovered to keep them for a long period in bed under strict treatment for the gastric ulcer, as this condition takes a long time to repair thoroughly.

Andrew J. McCosh [1] records a case of perforating gastric ulcer in which recovery followed operation. In this case perforation had occurred gradually and some time before and a limited abscess had formed. When the abdomen was opened it was found that the peritoneum was adherent to the structures beneath. The stomach and liver agglutinated together formed the upper wall of the abscess. At a depth of 2 in. beneath the stomach and liver the abscess-cavity was evacuated. At the bottom of this cavity the finger detected the opening in the stomach. The edges of the stomach-opening were scraped and trimmed and the opening was closed by two rows of sutures. A piece of gauze was brought into contact with the suture-line and was caused to emerge

[1] Med. News, Jan. 16, 1897.

through the abdominal wound ; the rest of the wound was closed with sutures. The patient recovered from the operation and did well.

H. Littlewood,[1] of Leeds, reported 2 cases of perforated gastric ulcer successfully treated by operation. He affirms that the most important factor contributing to a successful result is early diagnosis, so that the operation can be performed within 8 or 10 hours of the period of rupture. In these cases Littlewood excised the ulcer. This was done quickly and easily. He thinks it is an advantage to remove the edges of the ulcer, especially if they are indurated. He believes, however, that there are a number of cases in which excision is not practicable and in which inversion merely should be practised. Littlewood says that the treatment of the peritoneum when there is purulent peritonitis is still an unsettled question. Some wash out, some wipe out. He believes that it is a physical impossibility to cleanse the peritoneum thoroughly by either method. The peritoneum can unquestionably deal successfully with a certain amount of septic material.

J. St. Thomas Clarke,[2] of Leicester, records a case of perforated gastric ulcer in which operation was followed by recovery. After opening the abdomen and inverting the perforation the abdominal opening was covered temporarily with hot sponges, and a second incision was made in the mid-line just above the pubis so as to explore Douglas's pouch. This pouch was found filled with the same turbid fluid which had been noted in the abdomen higher up. The abdominal cavity was irrigated with water at a temperature of 105°, the glass tube being passed between the coils of intestine above the liver, under the liver, and in different regions until the fluid emerged clear. A drainage-tube was inserted into Douglas's pouch and the wound closed, and a drainage-tube passed into the upper opening so as to reach the line of sutures about the ulcer. Dr. Clarke is a firm believer in free irrigation. He does not think that sponging alone can possibly remove all traces of the septic fluid. He believes the second incision a most important factor contributing to the good result.

Herbert P. Hawkins and C. S. Wallace[3] report two cases of operation for perforation of gastric ulcer followed by recovery. In the first case the ulcer was inverted. Another incision was made below the umbilicus and several ounces of turbid fluid were removed from the pelvis. The abdomen was flushed out and each wound was drained. The second case was under the care of Makins and S. G. Toller. The margins of the rupture were freshened by scraping with a Volkmann's spoon and the rupture was inverted. There was no free fluid in the peritoneal cavity and no trace of solid food, and irrigation was not employed. In this second case the perforation had occurred 26 hours previous to operation, but the stomach contained little food at the time of injury. The opening was very small and no solid contents had escaped.

Van Noorden[4] discusses the operative treatment of some **sequelæ of gastric ulcer.** The first case reported was that of a woman who when young had been supposed to have gastric cancer. At the age of 52 she was subjected to operation. A portion of omentum was found adherent to the stomach near the pylorus. The adhesions were cut ; there was a spear-shaped depression on the serous coat of the stomach which was not interfered with. The patient improved very much after operation, but in three months the symptoms returned. They were believed to be due to nervous dyspepsia and disappeared under treatment. In the second case the patient had a gastric ulcer and developed the signs of peritonitis. The abdomen was opened, the

[1] Lancet, Nov. 21, 1896.
[2] Ibid., Mar. 20, 1897.
[3] Brit. Med. Jour., Apr. 10, 1897.
[4] Münch. med. Woch., Sept. 1, 1896.

omentum was found adherent to the stomach, and it was evident that protective adhesions had been formed, but that in spite of them there was perforated peritonitis. An opening was made between the stomach and the transverse colon. Lymph was met with but no pus. The site of perforation was discovered by observing an air-bubble. While preparing to resect a large tear was inflicted upon the stomach and some of the contents of the viscus escaped. The peritoneum was sponged cleaned and the stomach was surrounded with gauze pads. No resection was performed and it was decided to make a fistula. At a later period 4 attempts to close the fistula failed. The patient died some 8 weeks after operation. Postmortem disclosed the fact that there was a small opening on the anterior wall of the stomach near its lower border and passing over to the posterior wall. The stomach was the shape of an hour-glass. [A very able review of the varying views upon the treatment of gastric ulcer will be found in the *Annals of Surgery*, Nov., 1896.]

DISEASES OF THE PERITONEUM AND OF THE INTESTINES.

O'Conor[1] records a **chyle-cyst of the mesentery.** The swelling was distinct in outline, smooth and tense, fluctuating, distinctly movable, and about as large as a cocoanut. Pressure caused a considerable amount of pain. Percussion elicited a dull note. There was no thrill. When the abdomen was opened a greenish-colored cyst was met with. It was covered with large veins and looked much like sarcoma. The adhesions were so dense that removal was found impossible. The tumor was incised and the edges sutured to the abdominal wound, the interior being packed with gauze. The patient made a satisfactory recovery.

Theodore A. Magraw[2] discusses the utility of **omental splints in intestinal surgery.** He presents the records of some cases in which this method was applied with great advantage. He thinks that the omentum should be applied with little disturbance of its blood-vessels. It is a tissue that is well supplied with blood, and it is probable that its power to resist the ill effects produced by feces or pus arises chiefly from its ample blood-supply. It is an error to cut a flap of omentum, because doing so alters profoundly the blood-supply, as some blood-vessels would require to be tied and cut. Omental grafts are valuable purely because of their capacity for rapid adhesion. If this does not take place, their vitality fails. It is not likely that an omental graft, even when it unites quickly to the raw surface, will resist for any great length of time the pressure of feces if the suture gives way. The detachment of the flap from the omentum and its suture to the bowel produce a cord-like band under which strangulation may occur. Magraw is a believer in the application of uncut omentum. He says it should be drawn over the bowels like a sheet, and its extremity must be wrapped about the wounded intestine in order to cover the suture. In this way we can secure admirable support to the bowel, a support which is amply supplied with blood and which does not cause danger of intestinal strangulation. Omental flaps or omental grafts, or the use of neighboring coils of intestine as splints, are to be employed only in cases in which atrophy or disease renders it impossible to draw the omentum down to the wounded surface.

Gilbert Barling[3] furnishes some valuable and practical considerations on **peritonitis due to perforation.** He states that peritonitis from perforation may be due to perforation of the vermiform appendix, bursting of a

---

[1] Brit. Med. Jour., Feb. 13, 1897.   [2] Physician and Surgeon, Oct., 1896.
[3] Birmingham Med. Rev., Dec., 1896.

circumscribed abscess about the appendix, perforation of a gastric ulcer, a duodenal ulcer, or an ulcer of some other part of the intestine, sloughing of a typhoid ulcer, or the rupture of a distended gall-bladder, or a pyosalpinx. The onset is very acute and the progress of inflammation is extremely rapid, and early recognition is of the first importance. The course of perforative peritonitis is for several reasons not always the same : the simple cases are frequently not typical, variations being due partly to the nature of the material which is extravasated and the amount of this material, partly to the position which the damaged part occupies in the abdominal cavity, and partly to the vital resistance possessed by the patient. For instance, rupture of a gall-bladder with extravasation of mucus and bile only is not nearly so dangerous an accident as rupture of a gall-bladder containing pus. If perforation occurs in the stomach, widespread abdominal extravasation is apt to ensue. If perforation occurs in the appendix well behind the cecum, or in the pelvis, the extravasation does not at once spread widely through the abdomen, and the inflammatory process may for a time be limited. The danger of the stomach perforation varies according as to whether the stomach was empty or full and as to whether the person was in a vertical or horizontal position at the time of the accident. Nevertheless, it is usually possible to diagnosticate perforative peritonitis and to determine the seat of primary trouble. The onset is generally marked by very acute pain which may be accompanied by faintness. This symptom is especially prominent in perforation of the stomach. In some cases the pain is widespread at the start ; but, as a rule, it is first local and subsequently becomes general, the locality of the initial pain pointing to the seat of perforation. Local tenderness early in the case corresponds to the seat of perforation ; later in the case it becomes widespread. Soon after perforation the abdomen is not distended ; in fact, it is rather concave from muscular rigidity, and this rigidity may be extreme. In spite of rigid muscles distention eventually becomes prominent. Distention may be due to paralytic distention of the stomach and bowels associated with a large peritoneal effusion. It may sometimes be due to free gas in the belly-cavity which has escaped through the perforation. If there is complete abolition of liver-dulness, it is almost certain that perforation has occurred, from the gas having entered between the front of the liver and the diaphragm. Mere diminution of liver-dulness is not of great diagnostic consequence. If at any part of the abdomen there is a circumscribed area of tympanitic resonance surrounded with comparative dulness and other symptoms indicative of perforation exist, this tympanitic area almost positively points to a collection of free gas which has escaped from the perforation. Vomiting is not very pronounced at the beginning. The patient often vomits once or twice and then the sickness passes away. There may even be no vomiting, only a feeling of nausea existing. As peritonitis finally begins vomiting is very apt to come on, but its frequency and persistence are much influenced by the manner in which the patient is fed. If the patient is fed by the mouth, there will be persistent vomiting; and if the stomach is kept empty, there will be very little vomiting. Obstruction of the bowel is a very common associate of peritonitis whether the peritonitis arises from perforation or not ; but obstruction does not of necessity occur. There may be actual diarrhea or occasional passage of flatus. A case with complete constipation offers a worse prognosis than where there is not complete constipation. The fact that the bowel can act spontaneously or can be emptied by the use of purgatives is an important point in the differential diagnosis between perforative peritonitis and acute intestinal strangulation. The temperature of peritonitis varies extremely and it is very difficult to draw useful conclusions from it, but in perforation a study of the temperature may give the most useful information. Right after the perforation there is either a subnormal temperature, or, if fever has existed before, there is at least a great abatement in the febrile temperature. The worse the shock the more positive is the drop in temperature. After this depression there is apt to be a decided rise, but this rise does not certainly follow. If at the time of perforation there is considerable shock, the pulse will be found to be small, fluttering, and of varying frequency. Whether shock has been pronounced or not some little time after the perforation there will be noted a quickening of the pulse, until in three or four hours it amounts to between 100 and 130. It may become of the hard, wiry character which is supposed to indicate peritonitis, but more often it is the soft pulse met with in septicemia. In making a diagnosis of a case of perforative peritonitis the age and sex should always be considered. In a child the most likely seat of perforation is the vermiform appendix, and in a young, anemic woman it is the stomach ; in the young or middle-aged male we should first suspect the vermiform appendix, and after that the existence of duodenal ulcer.

The history of any previous illness is of great importance. If there is a possibility of typhoid fever, this may clear up the diagnosis. If there is a history of stomach indigestion, perforation of gastric ulcer should be considered. If the patient is a married woman who has been sterile for some time, or has been completely sterile and who presents a history of pelvic inflammation and purulent vaginitis, rupture of pyosalpinx is suspected. The history of previous attacks of hepatic colic would suggest ruptured gall-bladder. In perforation of the vermiform appendix there is often a history of previous attacks of so-called appendicular colic followed by tenderness and possible swelling in the right iliac fossa. In some cases we will obtain additional light by giving an anesthetic and palpating the abdomen to discover any thickening, a procedure, however, which is only undertaken if operative measures are in contemplation. The treatment of perforative peritonitis apart from operation is that of acute peritonitis in general, and does not call for a full description here. Barling, however, dwells upon a few points, especially the question of feeding and the necessity of rest. He restricts what is taken by the mouth to the very smallest quantity, thus keeping vomiting in subjection by having the stomach empty. Vomiting, if allowed to continue, greatly aggravates the distressing thirst. Nourishment is administered by the rectum and thirst is allayed by enemata of plain water. Occasionally fluids, in teaspoonful amounts, are given by the mouth, the amount being gradually increased if vomiting is not excited by their ingestion. If perforation of the stomach is suspected, absolutely nothing should be given by the mouth. If perforation is suspected, absolute rest is imperative because extravasated materials are capable of being localized to one portion of the abdominal cavity, where they may be retained· and shut off by adhesions from the other portion. The slightest movement may serve to widely disseminate extravasation. Great harm is done by moving the patient from place to place.

Barling then discusses the use of opium. He says that one of the chief elements in the production of shock is the severe pain these patients suffer from, and he thinks it is cruel to withhold opium. A sufficient amount should be given to assuage the violent pain and tide the patient over until shock is passed, when the question of operation will be considered. If it is evident that an operation is to be performed, the less opium given the better for the patient, unless the condition is considered almost hopeless, when anything is justifiable which diminishes the patient's suffering. Opium after operation is not desirable. If operation is not resorted to because the indications are not clear, opium should be avoided. It lulls the patient into deceptive calm and misleads the doctor into a sense of fancied security. When perforation is diagnosticated and operation is refused give opium freely. Barling says the influence of aperients in peritonitis has been inculcated in modern times by Mr. Lawson Tait, and our gratitude is due to him for the discovery. The great value of aperients, however, is prophylactic rather than curative. If after an abdominal operation there are any signs of peritonitis, purging does the patient much good ; but when once peritonitis has been thoroughly established purging is commonly difficult to bring about, and although still useful is not nearly so valuable as in the early stage. There is a tendency at present to give aperients freely whenever severe abdominal pain is complained of without special investigation into the cause of the pain. Such a proceeding may do great harm in perforation of the stomach and vermiform appendix. The use of aperients in appendicitis is a remnant of the old idea that fecal impaction exists in the cecum. Now that we know that the appendix itself is the seat of trouble and that it may be perforated or gangrenous, the use of any plan of treatment which disturbs the intestines and omentum about the damaged part can do great injury in the acute stage. If the parts are left at rest, adhesions can form a barrier around the diseased appendix. Although aperients may do harm, opium may do more harm by quieting symptoms of the patient and causing us to misjudge the gravity of his condition.

Barling lays it down as a rule that perforative peritonitis is fatal without surgical interference. It is quite true that cases have been recorded in which perforation of the stomach by round ulcers has been followed by recovery without operation, and occasionally recovery has followed typhoid perforation and perforation of the appendix ; but these recoveries are so few that they may be disregarded. If perforation has been diagnosticated and the condition of the patient and the surrounding circumstances admit of operation, the abdomen should be opened. If the patient is profoundly shocked or if peritonitis has advanced so far as to render the patient moribund, a wise surgeon will not operate. So, too, a surgeon may be without assistants or nurses, and the quarters occupied by the patient may be so miserable as to contraindicate operation. Otherwise invariably operate. If the diagnosis as to the seat of perforation is not certain and an operation is at first exploratory, do median section above the pubis. If it is possible to diagnosticate the site of perforation, the incision should be over that region. Barling says in perforation of the vermiform appendix there is one lesson he has well learned : that is, not to do too much in the very acute condition. The wisest course is to evacuate any extravasation or inflammatory material and introduce drainage. If the appendix is easily found, remove it ; and if it is not easily found, leave it alone and remove it later in the interval if the patient recovers. A lengthened search for the appendix may break down the circumscribed inflammatory products and spread infection. Another reason for caution is that patients in this condition will rarely bear prolonged anesthesia or protracted manipulation. In not a few cases where perforation of the appendix has occurred and where general peritonitis is supposed to exist, in reality the condition is a circumscribed peritonitis occupying the lower half of the abdomen, but not involving the peritoneum above the transverse colon. For this reason Barling hesitates to use irrigation for fear it will tear away limiting adhesions and spread infection to regions that are free from it. In perforation of the stomach and duodenum it is absolutely necessary to close or in some way shut off the perforation from the belly-cavity and to clean the peritoneum by irrigation or sponging. The operation must be done at the earliest possible moment. Every hour which passes adds 5% to the risk of death. The reader will understand, however, that operation is not undertaken during the primary collapse, but is done immediately after this collapse passes away, the period of collapse having been tided over by the use of morphin and stimulants. The abdomen is opened in the mid-line above the umbilicus, in some cases a transverse incision being added to the vertical incision. If on opening the abdomen no evidence of anything wrong is noted, the extravasation is limited, and the surgeon must try to keep it so. Search should be made between the liver and the stomach, where extravasation is most apt to be found. If nothing is detected there, follow along the pylorus and examine the duodenum. When stomach or intestinal contents are found they are carefully sponged away and the perforation is sought for. This is usually on the anterior wall of the stomach or on the lesser curvature; but it may be on the posterior wall, in which case it will be necessary to tear through the lesser omentum or the gastrocolic layer to reach it. It is unnecessary to excise a perforation. It is closed by interrupted Lembert sutures with a wide turning in of the edge. Excision is of no benefit; it consumes time and adds to the risk of the operation. If the perforation cannot be closed, a glass drainage-tube is passed down to it, and gauze is packed about the tube and brought out of the incision. If the stomach-contents have been widely extravasated or if general peritonitis exists, the abdominal cavity should be irrigated with large amounts of hot water or hot normal salt solution. This can only be done throughly when a second opening is made above the pubis; the fluid is introduced in the first incision; the surgeon's hand moves constantly among the intestines, along the colon, between the liver and diaphragm, and in the pelvis, and the fluid is made to emerge from the second incision. If the extravasation is limited and general peritonitis does not exist, irrigation is harmful, as it may break down adhesions and spread infection. In such cases cleansing is effected by sponging the infected area. After cleansing the abdomen drainage should be applied, and if two incisions have been employed drainage is maintained in each. Typhoid perforation is a not very unusual cause of death. The Birmingham general register shows 29 deaths from this cause in the last 20 years; 27 of these perforations were in the small intestine and 2 in the large bowel. In 20 cases in which the exact place of perforation is described in the postmortem notes 17 were within 12 in. and 9 within 6 in. of the ileocecal valve. In these cases there is practically a choice only between operation and certain death, and the mortality from the operation is extremely heavy. Most operators in such cases have opened the abdomen in the middle line, but the postmortem records above quoted suggest the advisability of opening it in the right semilunar line. When the perforation is small and the tissues around are not extensively sloughed invert the edges of the perforation with Lembert sutures. If the conditions are not favorable for this proceeding, Keith's drainage-tube should be passed down to the perforation, gauze-packing should be inserted around the tube, and the incision should be partly closed.

Dieulafoy[1] writes upon **surgical intervention in the peritonitis of typhoid fever.** He says that in typhoid fever it is held that appendicitis can occur, one form due to typhoid, the other form associated with it, and either form can cause perforation. In the first form the lymphatic structure of the appendix becomes the seat of typhoid ulceration and perforation ensues. In the second form true appendicitis complicates typhoid fever. He considers also the other causes of perforative appendicitis, and strongly advocates surgical intervention as the only alternative to death. Dieulafoy

[1] Bull. de l'Acad. de Méd., Oct. 27, 1896.

concludes that in typhoidal appendicitis and appendicular typhoidal peritonitis operation can be performed if the condition of the patient is good. In typhoidal peritonitis operation gives a chance of recovery.

John N. T. Finney [1] discusses the surgical treatment of perforative typhoid ulcer. In this paper we find an elaborate discussion of the history of the surgical treatment of typhoid perforation, the consideration of the conditions under which perforation occurs, an analysis of the symptoms in the reported cases, and a thorough study of all accessible statistics. The author says, if we include all cases that have been reported as operations for perforating typhoid ulcer, together with the six cases which he has collected, we have 52 cases with 17 recoveries, 32.68%. Excluding all doubtful cases we have left 45 cases, of which 11 recovered, a percentage of 26.22. Finney believes that Mikulicz's first case and Dandridge's case should be admitted; this would make a final and, as he thinks, a correct estimate of 47 cases with 13 recoveries, a percentage of 27.65. In 8 of the reported cases a wrong diagnosis was made; 3 were thought to be appendicitis, in 2 a diagnosis of ileus had been made, in 2 the symptoms were supposed to be due to internal obstruction of unknown cause. One was undiagnosticated at the time of operation. The effect upon the mortality of the time of operation is uncertain. Some of the cases operated on earliest died the soonest, and *vice versa.* It would, however, seem reasonable to suppose that the earlier the operation is performed, after the patient has undergone some reaction from the primary shock, the more favorable ought the result to be. The statistics throw but little light upon the disputed question of the respective merits of irrigation and wiping the peritoneum; 8 of the 10 cases in which general peritonitis existed recovered after irrigation. In only 4 cases was wiping practised, and 2 of these recovered. Because all but 2 of the fatal cases were irrigated it would not be fair to say that the irrigation caused death any more than other circumstances. Finney thinks in cases when the inflammatory process has gone beyond circumscribed points, but has not invaded the entire peritoneum, irrigating fluid may possibly disseminate infection. We must of necessity use a fluid so bland as to be practically without antiseptic power. Excision of the ulcer is entirely unnecessary and needlessly prolongs the operation. If the intestinal wall is so damaged that sutures will not hold, it would be unwise to excise the perforation, and it would be far better to pull the damaged loop outside of the abdomen and leave it there for a subsequent resection and anastomosis. Autopsy-records show that the peritoneal surfaces united just as thoroughly in cases when the edges of the ulcer had not been excised as when they had been. The mattress-suture of Halsted possesses great advantages over other sutures and should be used by preference. It is immaterial whether the line of sutures is parallel with the axis of the bowel or at right angles to it. The condition of the bowel-wall and other circumstances determine whether it is necessary to apply more than one row of sutures. The surgeon should always be careful to avoid encroaching upon the lumen of the gut more than necessary. Drainage should invariably be employed. If there is general septic peritonitis, the abdomen is practically an abscess-cavity, and the contents of this abscess-cavity should be thoroughly evacuated and effective drainage should be established. The best drainage is obtained by wicks of bismuth- or iodoform-gauze placed in different parts of the abdominal cavity, the ends being brought out through the abdominal wound, the rest of the wound being sutured. Drainage in the most dependent portion of the abdominal cavity is of great value. The signs which are of most value in recognizing typhoid perforation are sudden, acute abdominal

[1] Ann. of Surg., Mar., 1897.

pain, collapse, and abrupt and decided fall of temperature. Vomiting is often present. The obliteration of liver-dulness, the gurgling sound on respiration, hiccough, etc., are very valuable signs when present. No pathognomonic sign of perforation has yet been put forth. There is one point which promises to be of great aid in doubtful cases; that is, the examination of the blood. Thayer tells us that during typhoid fever there is no increase in the proportion of colorless corpuscles, but there is a tendency toward a diminution in particular at the height of the disease. Finney says in typhoid fever at the beginning the white corpuscles are about normal, the number gradually sinking during the progress of the fever, reaching the lowest point at about the end of the febrile period, at which time they vary from 2000 to 6000 per cubic millimetre. If an inflammatory complication arises, there is immediately a marked increase in the number of leukocytes. We must recall that a slight and temporary leukocytosis has been observed under certain methods of treatment and following a cold bath, but this is too slight and of too short duration to be mistaken for the leukocytosis that follows perforation. Cabot in his recent work on the clinical examination of the blood alludes to the marked leukocytosis which occurs at the time of perforation. So few observations of this sort have been made that systematic study of the blood from the beginning should be made in every case of typhoid fever, as the knowledge of any sudden change may be of great importance if an obscure complication arises. As a rule, perforation is quickly followed by symptoms of peritonitis, the intensity of the symptoms depending largely upon the nature of the infecting agent, the dimensions of the opening, and the area of surface involved. Pyogenic cocci are rarely absent from the intestine. The streptococcus pyogenes is usually found in numbers in the exudate of perforative peritonitis. The autopsy-records of the Johns Hopkins Hospital show 7 deaths from perforating typhoid ulcers. In 6 of these bateriologic examinations were made of the peritoneal exudate. In 4 of the cases there was mixed infection with the streptococcus pyogenes and bacillus coli commune. In 1 there was found the streptococcus alone, in another the colon-bacillus alone. The length of incision should be sufficient to permit the operator to examine the parts thoroughly, to explore completely, and to cleanse satisfactorily. A long incision will heal just as quickly as a short one. When we deal with a case of fully established general peritonitis from perforation of a typhoid ulcer the chances of recovery from operation are somewhat better than 1 in 4. In the treatment of the cases of perforating ulcer 3 things are to be done: 1. Find and close the perforation; 2. Empty and cleanse the peritoneal cavity; 3. Establish and maintain efficient drainage. Finney says that in most cases we should make an oblique incision in the right iliac region, find the cecum, locate the ileum, and draw out coils of ileum through the wound. All the infected intestine is drawn out of the peritoneal cavity—if necessary, the entire small intestine. The peritoneal cavity is carefully wiped out with gauze pads and sponges wrung out of hot salt solution. It is not necessary to irrigate with salt solution; the intestines, which have been covered with hot pads, are next uncovered and irrigated while outside the abdomen with hot salt solution. They are then replaced in the inverse order from that in which they were withdrawn, being wiped dry before replacement. The worst coil is replaced last. The sutured portion is replaced next, and the abdominal wound is packed around with strips of bismuth-gauze, and if necessary a strip of gauze is carried into the pelvis; the abdominal wound is closed tightly, excepting where the gauze drain emerges. If there is much distention, the bowels are moved early by calomel in broken doses, followed by salts and, if necessary, a high enema of turpentine and soap-suds.

Finney sums up his conclusions as follows: 1. Of the so-called diagnostic signs of perforation most reliance is to be placed upon an attack of severe, persistent abdominal pain, associated with nausea and vomiting and marked leukocytosis. 2. The surgical treatment is the only rational one. 3. The only contraindication to surgical operation is a moribund condition of the patient.

Finney then records 3 cases upon which he operated. The first died in 7, the second in 26 hours after operation, and the third recovered. At the end of this useful, thorough, and scientific article is a *résumé* of the cases collected from literature. [Finney is an advocate of operation in these cases, and we think proves his case. The choice is between death and operation. The question whether or not to irrigate is still in debate. It seems possible to cleanse the abdomen thoroughly by wiping if we eviscerate. Irrigation with saline fluid possesses certain merits. The saline fluid is in part absorbed, lessens shock, allays subsequent thirst, aids diuresis, and helps to expel toxins from the blood. The statement that "it is needless to excise an ulcer" voices the opinion of most surgeons. In cases of perforative peritonitis suprapubic and posterior drainage are of value. If a stab is made through the kidney pouch after the plan of Mayo Robson excellent drainage can be established. The increase of leukocytes after perforation seems to offer us a valuable diagnostic point. It is well to remember that leukocytosis occurs after hemorrhage, otherwise the value of the finding of leukocytosis will be overestimated. The blood ought to be regularly studied in every case of typhoid.]

W. G. Spencer[1] reports a remarkable occurrence in the progress of a neglected typhoid fever. This patient was supposed to be suffering from **influenza,** and had had a rupture in the left inguinal region for nine years. When he was admitted into hospital the left half of the scrotum was very much distended, the swelling extending to the inguinal region and the skin being dusky and edematous. The swelling was tympanitic on percussion and opaque to light, fluctuation was present, and the inguinal ring was filled by a firm mass which exhibited succussion on coughing. The temperature was 102.6°. Spencer made a diagnosis of ruptured hernia and made an incision. There was an escape of pus, gas, and flatus, and a mass of sloughing omentum was cut away. There was no bowel found in the sac. The adhesions separating the abdominal cavity were not disturbed. The sloughing hernial sac was treated antiseptically, the sloughs which subsequently formed being removed. For a few days the patient did well, but he soon began to waste with great rapidity, and died 17 days after admission. The postmortem examination disclosed the fact that the **perforation** had been **due to typhoid ulcer.** The oldest perforation was just above the ileocecal valve. There was no question that the patient's illness was due to typhoid fever.

Shattuck[2] reports the case of a Harvard student, 19 years of age, who had typhoid fever with perforation. The perforation occurred within 10 days of the time he took to bed, and was recognized at a consultation which was held 12 hours after the first symptom appeared. The operation was performed by Dr. C. B. Porter. On opening the abdomen there was an escape of turbid serum. No fecal matter was seen, although the odor was somewhat fecal. A coil of intestine bulged from the wound; the intestines were carefully examined, being gradually drawn out and replaced as fast as inspected. The duodenum was reached without finding a perforation. With

---

[1] Lancet, Apr. 10, 1897.　　　　　　[2] Boston M. and S. Jour., Apr. 15, 1897.

the duodenum as a starting-point the entire small intestine was examined. The perforation was found in the cecum. Intestinal sutures were inserted in a diamond-shaped area, the line of sutures being transverse to the bowel-axis; a second row of these inversion sutures was placed over the first. The abdomen was cleansed by wiping and a drainage-wick was placed in each side of the pelvis. The patient died 61 hours after the operation.

E. B. Steel,[1] surgeon-lieutenant of the army medical staff, reports a case of typhoid fever which was complicated by perforation, peritonitis, and relapse, and followed by perityphlitic abscess. This individual had been attacked suddenly with violent abdominal pain; the abdomen was rigid and tender, the temperature was 103.6°, and the pulse was 130. Tenderness was most marked in the right iliac fossa. There was neither a tumor nor dulness on percussion. The previous history suggested walking typhoid fever. For several days the patient showed all the symptoms of acute peritonitis, and on the third day went suddenly into collapse, and it was necessary to administer considerable amounts of opium and morphin. Reaction took place, and for several days the patient presented the usual symptoms of peritonitis. Nine days afterward a crop of well-defined typhoid spots appeared on the abdomen. The condition grew progressively better, the temperature dropping and the symptoms abating, until about 16 days after the case was first seen the temperature began to rise again, and fresh spots appeared indicating relapse; still improvement took place. While the patient was becoming apparently better the pain returned in the right iliac fossa. This pain became very violent, and soon a swelling was detected and a diagnosis was made of suppurating appendicitis. Chloroform was administered and an incision made. Four ounces of pus were evacuated and a drainage-tube inserted. The patient made an excellent recovery.

Armstrong[2] reports the cases in which he operated for typhoid perforation. Three died and 1 recovered. He states that in 23 reported cases in which operation was done and in which the diagnosis was certain only 4 recovered. In spite of the excessive mortality operation is the only thing that offers the slightest chance for life. Even when the patient is in excessively bad condition, overwhelmed with the poison of typhoid fever, operation should still be undertaken, as it is the only chance. If the clinical evidence points to the fact that the perforation has been in the large intestine, or that it is likely to remain local, it is justifiable to wait for abscess-formation; but if the indications are that the perforation has taken place into the general peritoneal cavity, the only chance is laparotomy, inversion of the area, irrigation of the belly with hot saline solution, and free drainage. This operation should, of course, not be performed until reaction from the primary collapse is attained, and it should not be undertaken if the individual be obviously moribund. If a perforation occurs during convalescence, the chances of success from operation are greatly increased. Armstrong uses 2 or 3 rows of inversion sutures and passes them in the long axis of the bowel.

Joseph Price[3] reports 3 cases in which he operated for typhoid perforation, with recovery. The first patient had a typical history of typhoid fever. There were symptoms of perforation, and he could make out an ill-defined tumor on the right side. Two perforating ulcers were discovered in the region of the ileocecal valve. In the second case the character of the ulceration was doubtful, as there was tuberculous trouble in the lungs. In the third case the patient was so far gone that she was unconscious at the time of operation. Dr. Price says that he never attempted to close a filthier peritoneal

[1] Brit. Med. Jour., Jan. 2, 1897. [2] Ibid., Dec. 5, 1896.
[3] Phila. Polyclinic, Nov. 14, 1896.

cavity, and yet recovery followed. He maintains that every case of perforation demands operation, and that operation is the only possible chance that the patient has of life.

L. S. Pilcher [1] presented at a meeting of the New York Surgical Society a specimen of **cancer of the splenic flexure of the colon** which he had removed from a woman 57 years of age. This tumor was as large as a man's fist and yet had produced no symptoms of obstruction. He united the ends of the bowel by the method recently described by Ullmann, which is really a modification of Maunsell's method. The suggestion made by Ullmann was that after the approximation of both the distal and proximal ends a spool of raw vegetable should be inserted and the ends tied about it with an encircling thread of catgut or silk and that then it should be placed within the bowel. Dr. Pilcher used potato ; Ullmann used carrot. The potato placed within the bowel carried with it 2 ends brought into close apposition with a considerable surface. The serous surfaces thus brought together remain held together as long as the core remains in place or until the separation of that portion of the intestine which was strangulated by the cord. Pilcher believes this procedure is a very useful one. This patient died on the 12th day after operation of lockjaw despite the use of antitoxin.

A. J. Bodine [2] presents a new method of performing intestinal anastomosis with special reference to its adaptability to inguinal colostomy and subsequent restoration of the fecal current. He states that intestinal anastomosis when we do not use mechanical aids is an operation of extreme difficulty. Mechanical aids render the operation easier, but they are not absolutely reliable or entirely harmless. The method which he suggests is the outcome of studies made with the idea of improving the spur in inguinal colostomy. It is quite evident that if the spur is level with the skin-surface no fecal matter can enter the lower portion of the colon. The spur, which is formed by suspending the gut over a supporting rod, has neither thickness nor rigidity, and the dragging weight of the intestines pulls its upper border below the level of the skin, and when this happens fecal matter does pass into the lower portion of the intestine. Bodine thought that the mesentery might be folded so that it would stiffen the spur by stitching together both sides of the two limbs of the bend. He tried this on a dog and found it satisfactory. Acute flexion of the gut upon itself forms a septum fully an inch wide, which septum is between 2 rows of sutures. It will at once be seen that simple incision of the center of this spur removes the obstacle to the flow of feces. We therefore have a very simple method of restoring the continuity of the intestine. He has operated upon 5 dogs. He has done enterostomy as advised for intestinal anastomosis, making a temporary anus by excluding the mesentery from between the 2 rows of sutures. He has done colostomy as recommended for permanent anus by folding the mesentery between the 2 limbs of the flexure. The method of anastomosis he now proposes is as follows : the abdomen is opened, a pad is introduced to protect the intestines, and the parietal peritoneum is stitched to the skin with a continuous catgut suture. The lesion which has necessitated operation is sought for and is drawn through the incision until 6 in. of healthy gut protrude on each side of the lesions and beyond the incision. The limbs of this loop are laid side by side, the lesion being the apex. A stitch of fine silk, beginning at the points where exsection is desired, is inserted, uniting the portions of intestine close to the mesenteric border and parallel with it for a distance of 6 in. The sutured loop is then passed into the abdomen until the point where the suturing commenced is on a level with the skin, where it is stitched into the ab-

---

[1] Ann. of Surg., Apr., 1897.   [2] N. Y. Polyclinic, Feb. 15, 1897.

dominal wound with a continuous suture of catgut. This leaves the lesion protruding outside of the abdominal cavity. If it is possible to wait, wait 12 hours, at which time apply cocain and cut off the protruding intestine, including the lesion. This establishes an artificial anus, and we may wait any length of time before attempting to reestablish the continuity of the intestine. When we wish to establish the continuity a finger is passed into the opening of each portion of intestine to define the spur and guide the cutting instrument; the septum is divided with scissors along the median line, the instrument employed being either a pair of scissors or Grant's clamp; the abdominal wound may be closed by any method which the surgeon prefers. Bodine prefers closure by the plan of Szymanowski or Byrd.

Czerny[1] states that he has used **the Murphy button** in 13 cases, with 3 fatalities. In 1 of the cases he used too large a button gangrene occurred and perforation took place. The other 2 cases in which death followed were very unfavorable, the operation being for gangrene of strangulated hernia. Czerny says the button, as a rule, is found in the stools in from 2 to 3 weeks after operation. In a case in which he used the button for gastroenterostomy it had not been found 24 days after operation. Czerny thinks that in the majority of cases the best method for closing intestinal wounds is to double suture. He says that the use of the Murphy button, although it requires practice to become dextrous, can be learned more easily than can the use of the double suture. He remains somewhat anxious for the patient until the button has been discharged. He thinks that this button is a positive advance in the methods of intestinal suture.

Frank,[2] of Chicago, has set forth **a new device for anastomosis.** He uses 2 collars of decalcified bone, with 6 nail-hole perforations at the shoulder of each collar; also a piece of ordinary rubber tube $\frac{7}{8}$ in. in length and $\frac{5}{16}$ in. in diameter. A bone collar is slipped over the rubber tube and is sewed to the tube, the material used to sew with being silk. The other collar is then fitted over the tube and fastened and the instrument is ready for use. The rubber tube over which the collars are fastened being hollow, permits the passage of intestinal contents after it has been placed *in situ.* When the appliance is introduced the intestinal ends are brought over each collar and crowded between the ends of the collar. The 2 collars are forced apart, the rubber tubing is stretched, and the intestinal ends are held in contact by the elasticity of the rubber. This process is sufficient to bring about necrosis of the interposed intestine. The collars after a time dissolve and only a small bit of rubber tube is left in the intestine to pass with the feces.

M. L. Harris[3] has devised a method of **circular enterorrhaphy.** In this method he divides the intestine transversely, being careful to retain the mesentery up to the edge. He now removes the mucous membrane from the distal end of the gut for about $1\frac{1}{2}$ cm. This is readily done with a sharp curette. All of the mucosa ought to be removed. The proximal end is invaginated into the distal end. Three sewing-needles are threaded with fine silk; the first needle transfixes the thickness of the denuded end of the bowel just to one side of the mesentery and at the inner limit of the denudation. It is not pulled all the way through, but the point projects from the caliber of the bowel a little beyond its free edge. A point of this needle picks up a portion of the other end of the bowel transversely just to one side of its mesentery and close to its edge. By drawing the needle back a little it can be used as a lever, and by turning round its point of transfixion in the lower end it will invaginate the upper

---

[1] Centralbl. f. Chir., No. 31, 1896.　　　　　　[2] Medicine, Jan., 1897.
[3] Chicago Med. Rec., Jan., 1897.

end into the lower end, as far as the part is denuded of its mucosa. The same process is repeated with the second needle, at a corresponding point of the bowel on the opposite side of the mesentery, while the third needle is used at the part of the bowel opposite to the mesenteric attachment. The needles are then drawn all the way through and the stitches tied, and thus permanent fixation is secured. By a united or continuous suture the exposed end of the bowel is stitched all round to the invaginated part, the surgeon being careful not to penetrate into the lumen of the gut. If the continuous suture is used, it should be broken at least once, so that when tightened it will not narrow the caliber of the bowel. Two or three stitches are taken on either side of the mesentery. It will be observed when the operation is completed that there are two rows of sutures around the bowel, one at either end, thus keeping the surfaces in accurate apposition regardless of the varying caliber of the bowel. This operation Harris performed on a boy of 8 years, who had a gunshot-wound of the intestine. The boy died in a few hours from shock. Death occurred at too early a period to permit of any conclusions as to the success of any particular method of suture. However, it became evident that the operation could be performed with great facility. The 2d case in which he performed it was a boy of 5 years, who had a large mesenteric tumor. It was found necessary to remove 51 cm. of small intestine. Resection and suture by this method required less than 15 minutes. The boy made a complete recovery and it is now more than 10 months since operation. This operation was tried first upon dogs before being applied to human beings.

Mitchell Banks [1] presented his experiences with the **Murphy button.** He says that in the operation for obstruction rapidity is of the greatest possible importance. The Murphy button is still upon trial; although it has received the approval of a large number of eminent surgeons, some few record serious consequences as the result of its use. Banks records 7 cases in which he used the button. One case of obstruction due to fibrous stricture of the small intestine : excision and death. One case of intussusception of the ileum : excision, end-to-end approximation, and recovery. One case of cancerous stricture of the descending colon : recovery from right lumbar colotomy ; death after subsequent excision. One case of typhlitis followed by suppuration and fecal fistula : end-to-side approximation of the ileum and ascending colon ; death from tubercular disease 11 months afterward. One case of intestinal fistula resulting from strangulated hernia in which a portion of the ileum was removed : the patient recovered from the operation, and died some months after from pelvic abscess. One case of tuberculous matting of the ileum, adhesion having taken place to the bladder and a fistula having formed between the bladder and ileum : end-to-side approximation of ileum to ascending colon was performed ; the patient recovered from the operation and died some months later from tuberculous disease. One case of tuberculous disease of the cecum ; end-to-side insertion of ileum into ascending colon ; the patient recovered, but the operation is of too recent date to be sure of what is going to happen. The patient with intussusception remains fat and well 21 months after operation, showing that the union effected by the button is perfect.

Banks believes that the use of the button will supersede all other methods in intussusception. So far he has not met with any accident from the button, although he knows that others have. Cases have been reported in which buttons were never found again, but the patients have apparently been none the worse. Banks is sure that, if the surgeon and his assistants use the button

---

[1] Brit. Med. Jour., Oct. 24, 1896.

skilfully, they can complete the operation far more quickly than can be done by any other method.

[In endeavoring to estimate the value of various plans of anastomosis we should bear in mind the recent experiments of Ballance and Edmunds.[1] An epitome of these studies will be found in the *Practitioner* (May, 1897). They come to some interesting conclusions—viz., Halsted is right in his statement that intestinal sutures should invariably pass through the tough submucous coat. Lateral anastomosis is, as a rule, easier and less dangerous than end-to-end union. The best method of lateral anastomosis is that of Halsted, and to employ it we do not need mechanical aids. This method gives large openings. End-to-end anastomosis should be performed by suturing. If a mechanical device is used, we should employ one which does not require fastening to the bowel (the button of Murphy). Maunsell's method gives a very perfect union without the formation of an obstructing diaphragm. In using Paul's tubes it is found impossible to invaginate the intestine satisfactorily. The Czerny-Lembert suture obtains solid union, but leads to the formation of a ridge which is practically a diaphragm lessening the calibre of the bowel. The bobbin of Mayo Robson leaves a very small opening. The experiments of Ballance and Edmunds were made upon dogs.]

John Wheelock Elliot[2] furnishes a contribution to the **surgery of the large intestine.** He states that he recently resected a cancer of the ascending colon through the lumbar incision. He found the operation very satisfactory, and believes it to be a new proceeding. The incision was made at the outer border of the quadratus lumborum muscle and curved forward toward the anterior superior iliac spine. The bowel was drawn out and resected with the greatest ease. The divided ends were entirely outside of the body, so that there was absolutely no fear of infecting the peritoneal contents. When the bowel was returned it was in a perfect condition for drainage. This patient recovered. Elliot also records a case of bullet-wound of the colon and a stab-wound of the colon, both of which recovered.

W. A. Garrard[3] reports a case of **carcinoma of the colon** occurring in a child of 12. He states that sarcomatous growths are common in early life, but epithelial carcinoma is excessively rare. In a large number of cases reported by Mr. Cripps in 1890 there was only 1 case of cancer of the colon in an individual under 30. Cancer of the rectum is known to be not very uncommon in young adults, and Garrard is inclined to think that younger people become affected with it more often than was formerly thought to be the case. This patient had labored under constipation for some time, and finally had complete obstruction. The abdomen was opened, the colon was found to be twisted, and the trouble was found to be a stricture in the sigmoid flexure. Colotomy was done, and the bowel was at once opened with a trocar and cannula. The boy recovered without trouble. An examination was then made of the lower end of the colon and rectum when the patient was under an anesthetic. A stricture could be felt under the artificial anus, but not per rectum. Six months after operation he presented himself again, complaining of pain in the artificial anus. There was a hard mass of skin about the colotomy opening, which was ulcerated. The spur was thickened and infiltrated. The naked-eye appearances strongly indicated cancer. During the next few weeks he grew worse and died. Postmortem demonstrated the fact that he labored under colloid columnar-celled carcinoma of the sigmoid flexure. [The above, we believe, is the only case upon record of cancer of the colon at

---

[1] Med.-Chir. Trans., 78th vol.   [2] Ann. of Surg., Mar., 1897.
[3] Quart. Med. Jour., Apr., 1897.

such an early age. Sendler reported a case in a man of 22, and Powell reported a case in a man of 23. Czerny [1] reported a case of only 13 years.]

Archibald Cuff [2] reports an interesting case in which **intestinal obstruction** was **caused by an enterolith.** The patient was a woman 59 years of age. She had the symptoms of obstruction ; the abdomen was opened and a hard mass was felt within the bowel about 3 ft. from the ileocecal valve. The bowel was occluded on each side of the obstruction by the fingers of assistants, an incision was made opposite the mesenteric attachment, and a stone removed. The wound in the bowel and the abdominal incision were then closed. The patient died of exhaustion. The stone is oval, brown in color, and weighs about ½ an ounce—its long diameter is 1½, its short diameter 1 in. Chemically, it is composed of carbonates and phosphates of lime and magnesia. [The collection of such a mass in the ileum so as to cause obstruction is a rare event. Enteroliths are far more common in the large than in the small bowel.]

Francis B. Harrington [3] reports a case of intestinal obstruction due to a large **gall-stone.** When first seen it was supposed that the obstruction was due to malignant disease. The abdomen was opened, a mass was found within the small intestine, the intestine was opened, and a large gall-stone removed. The patient made a good recovery. The stone is cylindrical, has a circumference of 3½ in., a diameter of 1⅛ in., and a length of 1 in. It weighs 170 gr. Robert Wilkinson [4] records a case of acute intestinal obstruction from impacted gall-stone. The patient was not operated upon, and although an unfavorable prognosis had been given gradually improved. Eleven weeks after the onset of the symptoms of obstruction the patient felt a great deal of pain, and examination detected a mass blocking the lower fourth of the rectum. By pressure through the posterior vaginal wall a foreign body was extruded, and found to be a gall-stone the size of a pigeon's egg, faceted, and weighing 5 drams, 41½ gr. The patient became perfectly well. Wilkinson says that this case supports the view of his old teacher, Mr. Mayo Robson, that if we can be reasonably certain that obstruction is due to gall-stone, a palliative line of treatment will probably end in the passage of the foreign body, although many believe that the risk of waiting is greater than is the risk of operative treatment.

F. Kammerer [5] had a patient on whom he had performed unilateral and finally total **exclusion of a part of the intestine for fecal fistula.** The patient was a man who had been operated on three times for appendicitis. After the last operation a fecal fistula developed from which all of the fecal matter passed. After an extensive operation to close the fistula Kammerer implanted the proximal end of the divided ileum into the transverse colon and closed the distal end. Six months later a little fecal matter still escaped from the fistula, and after another attempt at closure by resecting the bowel at the seat of closure he reopened the abdomen and divided the transverse colon immediately before the implantation, thus absolutely excluding from the fecal circulation a portion of the ileum, the weakened colon, and a part of the transverse colon.

Heydenreich [6] states that in the large intestine exclusion with complete closure of the portion excluded produces no ill-effect, but partial exclusion with the formation of a fistula is a better operation. A patient may be relieved of a troublesome fistula by a total exclusion, but it may be necessary at

[1] Münch. med. Woch., No. 11, 1896. [2] Quart. Med. Jour., Apr., 1897.
[3] Boston M. and S. Jour., Aug. 27, 1896. [4] Brit. Med. Jour., Feb. 13, 1897.
[5] Ann. of Surg., Apr., 1897.   [6] Sem. med., Mar., 1897.

any time to operate and make a new fistula. When there is profuse secretion in the portion we contemplate excluding total exclusion must not be brought about. A fistula must be made, and this fistula may close if the secretion becomes slight. The operation of exclusion is really only a palliative procedure, but is very useful in cases in which resection is excessively dangerous. The small intestine is not a suitable field for the operation of exclusion.

F. Kammerer[1] reports 2 cases of fecal fistula treated by total exclusion of a portion of the intestine. He thinks that it is remarkable that unilateral exclusion with implantation into the transverse colon should not be used more frequently for the cure of fecal fistula in the cecum. In malignant tumors of the cecum which are inoperable he does not advise unilateral exclusion, because in such cases there are apt to be ulceration and discharge into the lumen of the bowel. In this article Kammerer reviews extensively the literature dealing with fecal fistula.

D'Arcy Power[2] delivered the Hunterian Lectures for 1897 and discussed the pathology and surgery of **intussusception.** The ileocecal varieties are particularly apt to occur in children. He is a believer in the value of hydrostatic pressure in treatment. The patient should be anesthetized and the large intestine should be gradually filled with hot saline solution, the reservoir being raised not higher than 3 ft. for a child, all the fluid being permitted to remain in the intestines for 10 minutes. As a rule, when this fails the abdomen ought to be opened and an attempt be made to reduce the intussusception by manipulation. When the end of the intussusceptum is gangrenous, when the intussusception is very short, and when it is irreducible because of adhesions of its neck, because of the polypoid tumor or of the bulging of the end of the intussusceptum, the method devised by Barker and Greig Smith should be employed. This method consists in suturing the intestines with the intussusceptum at the neck of the tumor, opening the intestine, removing the portion of the intussusception which lies free, arresting the bleeding, and closing the wound in the intestine. If gangrene exists in the neck of the intussusception or when the intussusception is associated with malignant disease of the gut, it will be necessary to resect the intestine. Mr. Power believes that the Murphy button or the bobbin is most likely to give good results when intestinal resection has been done for intussusception in the small bowel, while Maunsell's operation is indicated for ileocecal and colocolic forms of intussusception.

T. Pickering Pick,[3] after discussing the causation and the symptomatology of acute intussusception in children, takes up the treatment. There are 2 chief plans of treatment: the one seeks to reduce the intussusception by distending the bowel with air or water aided by abdominal manipulation; the other seeks reduction after abdominal section. We should regard an intussusception in the same light as a hernia. No one would think of treating a strangulated hernia with purgatives or enemata, or rest, or opium, or abstinence from food. We ought not to adopt a like plan in intussusception. In a strangulated hernia we apply taxis, and if this fails operate at once, and this is the exact plan which should be employed in intussusception. First, try by introducing air to reduce the invagination. If this fails, promptly open the abdomen and relieve the obstruction. No surgeon would ever think of such a thing as waiting a day or two, or even a few hours, in a case of strangulated hernia before attempting reduction. Yet, strange to say, some surgeons still delay in cases of intussusception. Never delay, but take

---

[1] Med. Rec., Feb. 20, 1897.   [2] Treatment, Mar. 25, 1897.
                    [3] Quart. Med. Jour., Jan., 1897.

active measures at once. Cases of intussusception are on record in which the gut has become gangrenous within 24 hours of the onset of the attack. The plan of distending the bowel with air is safer than distending with water. It is very important to keep the child warm. It should, therefore, be dressed in a woollen jacket and the legs and arms should be covered with woollen bandages. An anesthetic is given and an enema-pipe is introduced into the rectum. This pipe is connected by a piece of rubber tube to a pair of common bellows. The outside of the tube around the anus is carefully packed with wool, which is held in position by an assistant; the child is inverted and held by a nurse, and the bellows are slowly worked. The surgeon has his hand on the child's abdomen so that he can feel the tumor. As the intestine distends the surgeon's hand feels the colon bulge, and he can tell when the colon is distended as far as is safe. If this plan succeeds, the tumor will suddenly disappear from under the hand and the air will become diffused over the entire abdomen, causing a uniform abdominal distention instead of distention of the colon alone. The disappearance of the tumor from under the hand is no proof that the intussusception has been reduced; but the onset of uniform abdominal distention is proof. It happens often on inflating the intestine that the air causes a change in the position of the tumor, so that it slides from beneath the hand, and yet the intussusception is not reduced. Some surgeons have inflated the intestines with carbonic acid gas, generating the gas in the rectum by injecting first citric acid solution and then sodium bicarbonate, the catheter being quickly withdrawn and the nates held together to prevent escape of the gas. This method is not altogether safe; the gas is evolved suddenly and may produce serious symptoms, and we are unable to regulate the amount of the distention.

Senn used inflation with hydrogen gas, but Pick has had no experience with it. It is probable that inflation is useless when the intussusception is beyond the ileocecal valve, but in infants the vast majority of cases are of the ileocecal variety. In introducing fluid into the bowel it will be necessary to proceed with great caution otherwise serious injury may be done.

Forrest has shown that there is little danger of injuring healthy intestines in a young child by injecting water at a pressure of 6 pounds to the inch; but bowel which has been subjected to constriction is not healthy, and is liable to give way under pressure which would inflict no harm on a sound bowel. Fluid should never be injected by means of a syringe, but only by a method of irrigation. The reservoir containing the fluid is placed not more than 3 ft. above the bed. In an infant under 1 year of age 1½ pints of fluid would be used. This amount will completely distend the infantile colon, and the injection of a greater amount will be dangerous. The best fluid to employ is boiled water at a temperature of 100°, containing a dram of salt to the quart. The child is prepared as for inflation. The fluid will be felt to distend the colon gradually. It is allowed to escape after a few minutes. The abdomen is now examined, and if the tumor has disappeared the patient is returned to bed and kept warm. No opiates should be given. If the injection fails, we should not resort to a second attempt. There is a third method of reducing an intussusception, without operation, although it is rarely successful. The method consists in thoroughly anesthetizing the child so that the abdominal muscles are relaxed, seizing the gut between the forefinger and thumb immediately below the tumor, and attempting to push the tumor backward along the course of the colon by a kneading movement. This method can only be applied to the ileocecal or ileocolic varieties.

There is no question that operation in infants is a very severe procedure.

Some surgeons profoundly believe that a section on an infant less than 12 months of age is almost certainly fatal, but this is not so. Many cases are on record in which laparotomy has been successful on very young children. Howard Marsh reported a case of a child under 6 months old. Wiggin has collected 64 cases which have been operated on by laparotomy for intussusception in infants under 1 year of age; 21 of these cases recovered.

Pick says that when the plans of treatment which he has mentioned have been tried and have failed, it is the surgeon's duty to operate. Incision had best be made in the median line, as we are thus enabled to deal readily with all portions of the abdominal cavity. After opening the abdomen care should be taken to prevent the escape of the intestines. If they are permitted to escape, they at once become distended and there is much difficulty in returning them, and the necessary manipulation may burst the intestine and increase the difficulty. The incision in the abdomen should be just large enough to admit 2 fingers. As soon as the peritoneum is opened a flat sponge is introduced to prevent bulging of the intestine. The finger is passed down by the side of the sponge to explore the abdomen. When a tumor is found the finger is carried around it until the lowest limit of it is reached. When this is done the intestine is grasped just below the tumor, and by working along the colon and grasping successive portions of the gut the intussusception is pushed backward and finally reduced. This is all done within the abdomen. If the intussusception has existed for a time and adhesions have formed, or if it is very acute, so that there is much swelling and congestion, the invagination cannot be reduced. In such a case it will be necessary to enlarge the incision and bring the tumor up to the surface of the wound. An attempt is then made to reduce it. On no account should any attempt be made to reduce the invagination by traction on the entering tube. Occasionally it will be found that the invagination is irreducible or the intussusception may be gangrenous. Under these circumstances there are 3 possible methods of procedure : 1. Longitudinal incision into the intussuscipiens, drawing out the intussuscepted part, cutting it off and suturing the intussusceptum to the ends ; 2. Resection of the invaginated gut and end-to-end anastomosis ; 3. The formation of an artificial anus. The first proceeding is best carried out by Maunsell's method. It is seldom necessary to make an artificial anus. In these days, when we can do an end-to-end anastomosis as rapidly as we can make an artificial anus, there seems to be no justification for doing the latter imperfect operation.

Frederick Treves[1] reviews the **surgery of the peritoneum.** He maintains that the Continental operators have indulged in many extravagances in the performance of abdominal operations. Those who come after us will read with interest of operating-rooms built like a diving-tank, of glass tables, " of the ceremonial of washing on the part of the operator, of the rites attending the ostentatious cleansing of the patient, of the surgeon in his robes of white mackintosh and his India-rubber fishing-boots, of the onlookers beyond the pale who are excluded with infinite solicitude from the sacred circle as septic outlaws." Such an exhibition is not a part of surgery, it is rather " a fervent and idolatrous ritual." The people who follow these methods appeal to the infallible test of the bacteriologic laboratory ; but most intelligent surgeons are content to appeal to the test of the patient and to show records of results. What is done in the surgical theatre can be judged by one solitary test, the future of the patient. The results obtained by English surgeons will contrast favorably with those obtained elsewhere in spite of the fact that they do not employ the elaborate ritual above alluded to. These characteristic preparations for operation are

[1] Brit. Med. Jour., Oct. 31, 1896.

unnecessary, and when they are employed no better results are obtained than are gotten from simpler methods. The prolonged exposure and washing of the patient after he is placed on the operating-table are harmful. Treves believes that a simple method, such as the following, is sufficient to secure antiseptic results. The operating-room should be clean and free from dust, the table can be of wood. Some time before the patient enters the operating-room the skin of the abdomen is shaved, is washed with soap and water and then with ether and a solution of corrosive sublimate, and is covered with a compress soaked in a 1 : 20 carbolic solution. This compress should be in position at least five hours before operation. The surgeon is clean, but he does not parade his cleanliness. The macintosh and blankets are clean in a domestic sense ; the towels are sterilized ; the instruments are sterilized by boiling and are kept in a tray containing 1 : 20 carbolic acid solution. Before the operation is begun the solution is largely diluted with boiled water so as to destroy its irritant properties. The sponges are made of Gamgee tissue and are soaked for 24 hours in a 5 % solution of carbolic acid. Before operation the carbolic acid is washed out by sterilized water and each sponge is passed through a clean sponge-washer. Any onlookers can approach the operation just so they neither touch the patient, the sponges, nor the instruments. As to whether these simple precautions are enough, Treves takes as a test the operation of removing the vermiform appendix in the interval. He has performed this 150 times with one death, and he does not think this one case would have been saved if he had adopted the skin-washing and rubber boot ritual. In securing primary union after amputation and after excision of the breast the results obtained cannot be surpassed by any school of the advanced ceremonial. The dressings used are a matter of little moment. The wound is dried, is dusted with iodoform, and is dressed by a pad of wool and a binder. The selection of the dressing used to be a matter of the greatest possible importance. It is now known to be of not the least consequence. A great many wounds do not need any dressing, but are dried, dusted with iodoform, and left exposed to the air under the protection of a cradle. The fact that the iodoform is filled with microorganisms may disturb the bacteriologically minded surgeon, but it disturbs neither the wound nor the patient.

In discussing peritonitis Treves says there can be no doubt that all forms are septic and are due to microorganisms. It is very doubtful if there is such a thing as a rheumatic form of peritonitis. The form due to the pneumococcus has not yet established itself. There is no such thing as idiopathic peritonitis. The constitutional symptoms of peritonitis are the same as those of septicemia, and the patient dies from blood-poisoning and not from inflammation. When peritonitis is developed away from the small intestinal area it is apt to be localized. This is shown by the course of peritonitis in the iliac fossa, in the subphrenic region, and in the pelvis. We have made great advances in the treatment of localized peritonitis, but we have made but little progress in the treatment of diffuse peritonitis. We can open the abdomen, wash it out, and drain it ; but the results are by no means brilliant. The results obtained in the treatment of tuberculous peritonitis have been most admirable. Abdominal section will cure over 60 % of cases, and in 33 % of those who recover the cure is permanent. It is not necessary to indulge in any elaborate preparations for opening an abdomen for tuberculous peritonitis. Simple incision with evacuation is the most successful of all plans of treatment. Treves says that that unfortunate term "toilet of the peritoneum" has wrought infinite harm in abdominal operations. This serous membrane has a wonderful capacity of protecting itself against microorganisms. If the membrane is irritated, this power is diminished and extensive effusion may be brought about by rough manipulation. The surgeon who is infatuated by the term toilet of the peritoneum, who is indifferent to the nature and amount of effusion and seeks to remove it even when it is quite sterile by sponging, rubbing, and flushing, may cause results often disastrous in the extreme. Treves does not counsel us always to leave an extravasation in the abdomen, but he would prefer to leave a few ounces of sterile cyst-fluid than he would to damage the peritoneum beyond hope of recovery by persistent sponging. If the extravasation is both extensive and noxious, it must be removed, and this result is best accomplished by flooding with sterile water with very little handling of the intestines. If drainage of the abdomen is necessary, use the gauze tampon and not the glass drainage-tube. Primary cancer of the peritoneum does not exist. The peritoneum is, however, liable to sarcoma, and this growth is most common from the omentum. The victims of this malady are usually adults of about middle age, although occasionally it is met with in young people. They usually exhibit loss of strength, loss of weight, and loss of color. An omental tumor moves about the front surface, is flat, it may feel hobnailed or quite smooth. The swelling is dull on slight percussion, but may be resonant on deep percussion. After the growth has been pressed down it seems to float up again. There is usually some ascites and more than one lump may be felt. This form of growth is identical pathologically with retroperitoneal sarcoma. Treves has frequently observed diminution in the size of retroperitoneal growths after exploratory laparotomy. In the London Hospital, when a case of ascites needs tapping, puncture is never employed, but a small exploratory incision is used.

In discussing perityphlitis Treves says there is not one bit of evidence that such a condition as appendicular colic exists. The muscular tissue of the appendix is very feeble; the so-called muscular coat, in fact, is composed chiefly of fibrous tissue. In some appendices it is a question whether there is any muscle at all; in any case it is but a thin layer of denuded fibers. Again, the nerve-supply of the appendix is very small. Of course, the great majority of cases of perityphlitis are due to trouble in the appendix, but occasionally the peritonitis is started by trouble in the cecum itself, the appendix itself being sound. He does not allude to cases of cancer or actinomycosis of the cecum, nor even to tuberculous disease of that organ, but to examples of non-malignant, non-parasitic ulceration of the bowel. It is true that when the cecum is found perforated at the bottom of the perityphlitic abscess the perforation has usually come from without and the appendix is the cause. He is aware that an attack of perityphlitis may be brought about by changes in the appendix so slight as to be difficult of recognition. Nevertheless, it occasionally happens that true peritonitis is due to primary ulceration of the cecum. The etiology of perityphlitis is simple. The causal condition is a catarrhal inflammation going on to ulceration, and it is this condition which produces the stricture of the appendix which is so often found. The concretions which may be found in the appendix are formed just as the rhinoliths met with in the nasal passages are formed. Seeds have nothing to do with the production of appendicitis. In very rare cases foreign bodies have been reported found in the appendix, but Treves has never found a genuine foreign body within this structure. It is quite true that the concretions often look like seeds and stones, but a careful examination will show that they are not. The general death-rate in perityphlitis is about 5%. If an abscess form, the mortality may run up to 30 or 40%. If the patient survives an abscess, he is cured of his appendicitis. Treves first proposed interval operation in 1888. The risk of removing the appendix in the period of quiescence is less than 1%. In dealing with cases of appendicitis during an attack operation is rarely necessary before the 5th day. We should condemn in the strongest terms those who operate as soon as the diagnosis is made. There is no sound basis for such a procedure. It is quite true that a fatal attack may commence mildly, but the course of perityphlitis is by no means as erratic as many would have us believe. Very careful observation affords, as a rule, a sound basis for treatment. Violent cases which produce death in 48 hours are exceedingly rare and readily recognized. Of course, in extreme cases an operation cannot be done at too early a period. We are not encouraged to operate by the assurance that simple incision is attended by a death-rate of 18.18%. If there is a strong suspicion of pus, operation should be at once undertaken, and if swelling continues to increase without abatement of the fever, operation should be undertaken. There are few inflammatory conditions in which leeching acts more favorably than in perityphlitis. The application of 5 or 6 leeches in a case where operation seems immediately indicated occasionally appears to arrest the condition. The most active organism in the production of this disease is the bacterium coli commune, and it has pyogenic powers. When an abscess is evident or is suspected the site of incision is determined by mapping out the area of dulness and resistance. If a wound is made too far to the inner side, thus missing the pus and opening the peritoneal cavity, this incision should be sewed up and a fresh one made at the point where the effusion of pus can be reached within the area of adhesion. After incision the abscess-cavity is examined as to its size and shape and diverticula are carefully opened with the finger. No prolonged search is ever made for the appendix. A prolonged search may break down a weak abscess-wall and tear up adhesions which limit the pus from the peritoneal cavity. If any concretion is felt, it should be removed. If the diseased appendix presents itself, it is ligated and taken away. The high mortality accredited to this operation depends upon a blind resolve to excise the vermiform appendix at all hazards. We should evacuate the abscess and remember that the cases in which the least is done do the best. The cavity should not be squeezed out, should not be scraped, should not be sponged, and should not be irrigated. It should be drained by means of iodoform-gauze.

Egbert H. Grandin[1] makes some remarks on **septic peritonitis,** with special reference to the use of the antistreptococcus serum. A few years ago he read a paper upon suppurative peritonitis, and drew the deduction that local suppurative peritonitis will invariably recover after free incision is made and proper drainage inserted, if operation is performed before there has been positive general systemic infection. He also came to the conclusion that general suppurative peritonitis was invariably fatal no matter what treatment was employed. In the present paper he discusses the subject anew on the basis of personal experience. He says that septic peritonitis in the male differs from the same disease in the female only in the absence of certain elements of causation in the first. Of course, in the female there is a useful route for drainage which the male does not possess. His studies have enabled him to be more hopeful in the prognosis of general suppurative peritonitis than was formerly the case. His records for the past 6 years contain 40 cases of local and general suppurative peritonitis. These cases do not include instances of pus deep in the pelvis and accessible by vaginal operation. There were 9 cases of general suppurative peritonitis and 31 cases of local suppurative peritonitis; 31 cases arose from appendicitis, 8 cases from puerperal infection, 1 case from rupture

[1] Med. Rec., Apr. 3, 1897.

of a suppurating ovarian cyst. All of the 31 cases of local suppurative peritonitis recovered after incision and drainage. Out of the 9 cases of general suppurative peritonitis only 1 recovered. In 5 of these cases multiple incisions were made, points of counter-drainage were established, and the peritoneal cavity was freely flushed out. In 3 cases a median incision with flushing of the cavity was the treatment. In the 1 case which recovered multiple incisions were made, copious flushing was practised, drainage was maintained through the incisions, and antistreptococcus serum was injected. This case recovered. The patient was a woman who developed peritonitis, which was apparently secondary to perforative appendicitis. An exploratory incision in the appendix region showed that the appendix was gangrenous and perforated and that the free peritoneal cavity contained foul pus. The appendix was ligated and cut off. Irrigation was practised with hot salt solution and drainage was maintained by strips of gauze. In a few days intense pain developed in the left iliac region; a free incision was made in the left side, opening a cavity containing a pint of pus. This cavity was irrigated and counter-drainage was made into the vagina. The next day an area of dulness was detected in the left side of the abdomen above the level of the umbilicus. A free incision was made here, pus was evacuated, irrigation with saline solution was practised, and gauze was inserted. The patient was given 12½ c.c. of antistreptococcus serum. The next morning the same dose of antistreptococcus serum was administered, and in the afternoon of the same day the two incisions on the left side were joined by another incision. The administration of antistreptococcus serum was kept up and the patient gradually became convalescent and recovered. After the administration of the serum the temperature invariably fell and the pulse-rate became less. The action of the kidneys was powerfully stimulated and the production of pus was greatly limited. The author is not absolutely certain that the serum brought about a cure, but he thinks it so highly probable that in future he will use it, believing that it may do good, and can do no harm.

Bishop[1] discusses **drainage in abdominal surgery.** He thinks that in operations upon the Fallopian tubes drainage is invariably necessary; that it should be employed in any septic operation and in every case where there is any doubt about the asepsis. When the tubes are not involved and when the case is absolutely aseptic drainage does nothing but harm. He then discusses the various materials used for drainage. The fact that a collection of blood exists in the peritoneal cavity is not in itself enough to demand drainage. A small amount of blood will be absorbed and will do no harm. A larger amount will simply serve to block up the drain by clots. Lymph does not require drainage. The only reason for drainage is pus. Drainage of an abscess can be carried out most readily by a gauze drain after the plan of Mikulicz. If we have to drain bile, rubber tubes should be employed. Glass tubes drain bile very well, but the hard inner extremity of the tube produces irritation and the tube is liable to be broken. If we have to drain urine in the region of the kidney, we should use a rubber tube. Tube-drainage should be employed for 48 hours after a lumbar nephrectomy. The action of the diaphragm sucks air into the tissues, and if a tube is not introduced the air is not forced out again. If we drain this region of the body, cover the tube carefully with aseptic cotton-wool or gauze. Drainage-tubes of decalcified bone are not satisfactory and strands of catgut drain very poorly. Horsehair drains should not be used because of the arrangement of the epidermic scales upon the hair, which may cause it to travel into the wound.

[1] Med. Press and Circ., Oct. 28, 1896.

Silkworm-gut is the best material for capillary drainage, but capillary drainage will not remove pus. It will only remove blood-serum or lymph. In the abdomen the best canal of drainage after all is the intestine, which is a natural suction-pump. Action of the bowels at an early period after laparotomy in most instances prevents peritonitis. This is not only because the lower bowel is emptied. The small intestine is practically a long sponge, and when it is in vermicular motion it draws into the lymph-vessels of its walls large amounts of fluid from the peritoneal cavity, forcing this fluid into the blood-current, from which stream it can be excreted. The rhythmic motion of the intestines forces the fecal contents into the rectum and sucks up fluids from the peritoneal cavity, and the removal of these fluids disposes of what might be a culture-medium for bacteria. The bowels should be made to move soon after the operation, because a delay may permit so large an amount of fluid to collect that it cannot be readily disposed of. Bishop believes that we should not wait for signs of peritonitis to give salines, but that we should give them in order to prevent peritonitis. Calomel does very well, but saline purgatives are better. If we place saline fluid in the intestines, that fluid is of a higher sp. gr. than the fluid outside and dialysis takes place. Sodium tartrate produces excellent effects and rarely causes vomiting. It is well to associate the use of salines with the administration of enemata. Some use turpentine enemata, but the most useful enema is soap and water with $\frac{1}{2}$ oz. of castor oil. This is given after two or three doses of the sodium tartrate have been taken.

The **treatment of tuberculous peritonitis** is discussed in the *Jour. des Praticiens*, Sept. 15, 1896. In certain cases a surgical operation is advisable. If ascites exists, operation is of much benefit. In a considerable number of young people the disease can be cured by placing the patient under proper hygienic conditions, by the use of tonics, and by abdominal counterirritation. Some cases are improved by placing iodoform upon the skin of the belly and keeping the drug in place by means of collodion. In some cases puncture of the abdomen does good; in others rectal injections of creasote are of use. Creasote can be given by the rectum mixed with cod-liver oil. In some cases inunctions of ichthyol can be used. [Casassorici and Ligalea apply to the skin of the abdomen tincture of iodin mixed with guaiacol. It is applied in the afternoon during the highest temperature (about 2 gm. of guaiacol to 8 gm. of tincture of iodin). After the material has been applied the abdomen is covered with waterproof and cotton-wool. If the iodin irritates the skin, a mixture of guaiacol and oil can be used.]

G. Lenthal Cheatle[1] writes on a **method of uniting divided intestine.** After a portion of the bowel has been resected, a V-shaped piece of mesentery is removed, and a longitudinal incision is made through all the coats in each end of the divided bowel opposite the mesenteric attachment (Fig. 17, *A*). The length of this incision is equal to the diameter of the bowel at the point of operation. The ends of the intestine are spread out like two fans and the serous surfaces are held against each other (Fig. 17, *B*). The first suture fixes the mesenteric attachments and the two next unite the extremities of the fan-shaped ends. Stitches are now inserted with exactness, all coats being transfixed. When ends are joined it is necessary to suture the longitudinal incision by any method the operator wishes (Fig. 17, *C*).

J. Greig Smith[2] pointed out the proper method of treating a case of **grave abdominal disease before a diagnosis** is made. Suppose a case in which we are in doubt whether a patient has colic (intestinal, biliary, or renal),

---

[1] Lancet, May 22, 1897.
[2] Treatment, Mar. 25, 1897.

20

obstruction, perforation, or effusion of blood. Give an enema of an ounce of brandy or whiskey in 3 ounces of milk. Before giving the enema explore the rectum with the finger for diagnostic purposes. Wrap the patient in hot blankets and surround him with hot bottles. The abdomen is left to be covered separately by a light woollen wrap, which can be easily removed. The surgeon sits by the bedside and watches the patient. The beneficial effects of the alcohol soon become obvious. The surgeon watches the evolution of signs and uses palpation, percussion, and auscultation. The patient's behavior is of much moment. In spasmodic colic the patient makes a tremendous fuss. In visceral perforation the patient makes but little disturbance; he keeps his body rigid, moving his arms and rolling his head. The behavior of the patient in strangulation is between these extremes. Note the condition of the parietes as to tension, distention, spasm, or relaxation, and whether the intestines are moving or quiescent. When peristalsis is active perforation does not exist, because this condition is soon attended with intestinal paresis. In perforation auscultation discovers no sounds in the abdomen except over the seat of trouble, where blowing or rushing sounds are audible. If there is not much distention, abolition of liver-dulness on percussion almost surely means perforation

A   B   C

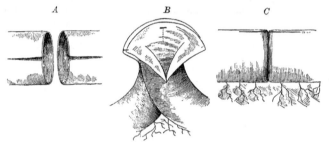

Fig. 17.—A method of uniting divided intestine (G. Lenthal Cheatle, in the Lancet, May 22, 1897).

of a hollow viscus or rupture of an abscess which contains gas. If much distention exists, the sign loses its importance, because it may be due to the bowels having gotten between the liver and abdominal parietes. The phonendoscope is used for auscultation. In colic there are are diffuse sounds; in obstruction accentuated local sounds and rushing noises; in perforation general silence with "rare and remote noises." We can decide whether we are dealing with colic or a dangerous malady. Final diagnosis may be made with the aid of anesthesia. If the patient has simple colic, he "greedily inhales" chloroform, and in a few minutes his condition is seen to be greatly improved. In perforation or strangulation the anesthetic is not taken greedily, the nausea often increases, and the condition is not markedly improved. If we decide that the trouble is only colic, give a full dose of morphin and begin appropriate treatment. At the end of half an hour the diagnosis will have been so far made that the surgeon will have decided whether or not to operate. When operation is decided upon, try to locate the seat of trouble in order to determine the proper place for the incision.

Smith says he places in the front rank these "items of advice": avoid morphin; give nothing by the mouth; give an enema containing alcohol; apply external heat; sit by the patient and watch. As shock passes off the evolution of special signs takes place and we observe these signs.

W. H. Battle[1] describes a case of peritonitis in which **symmetrical edema** of the subcutaneous tissue was noted in both groins. It did not pass into the thighs, being limited by the deep layer of the superficial fascia, but passed outward to the iliac spines and slightly into the flanks. The area of edema was tender and somewhat flushed; the scrotum was edematous. The patient died, and the necrosy showed the existence of acute peritonitis of the pelvic cavity, the cause of which was not discovered.

Robt. Abbe[2] presents a paper upon the prognosis and treatment of **acute general peritonitis,** saying that most infections which originate in the pelvis, in the fossæ about the colon, and in a less degree in the area about the liver and stomach and above to the colon become localized by walls of lymph in the course of a few hours. An infection at a more central point among the coils of the small intestine is rarely limited by lymph. The grave form of acute general peritonitis is almost invariably due to rupture of a hollow viscus (stomach, intestine, appendix, or bladder). Its origin is certainly bacterial, and septicemic infection overwhelms the patient. It is unconfined by any barrier of lymph. The area invaded depends on the stage in which the case is seen. Surgeons who report from 30 to 60 % of cures following operation have included cases which were not true unlimited peritonitis. If infectious material is introduced into the abdominal cavity, the peritoneum endeavors to free itself of this. The most common cause of the disease is appendicitis; next, perforating gastric ulcer; and after this intestinal traumatism, rupture of a pelvic abscess, rupture of urinary bladder, and rupture of gall-bladder. The virulence of the attack varies with the nature of the material introduced. Material from the appendix is more actively poisonous than material from the stomach, or normal urine.

Most perforations of gastric ulcer occur after eating. Weir has collected 97 operations for gastric perforation, with 22 recoveries. Abbe has collected 20 cases, 3 of which are his own. In this series 18 cases labored under general extravasation; 12 of them recovered and 6 died. Abbe believes that future studies will further prove the necessity for operating early after the accident. In gunshot and penetrating wounds of the abdomen operate at the earliest possible minute. It is impossible to be sure that an organ is not injured or that extravasation is not beginning without looking at the "invaded part." If the wound is slight or the shock profound, the wound can be enlarged under cocaine, and if perforation or hemorrhage is discovered the flow is arrested temporarily until the patient recovers from shock, when an appropriate operation is performed. Of 39 cases of gunshot-wound operated on within 12 hours 18 recovered; of 22 cases operated on after 12 hours 5 recovered. If cystitis exists, the chance of grave peritonitis arising is increased. If an inflamed gall-bladder be injured, septic peritonitis will soon arise unless operation is quickly performed, because the bile of an inflamed bladder is filled with bacteria, especially the coli commune. The peritoneum is able to dispose of normal bile fairly well.

Acute general peritonitis from typhoid ulcer differs but little in course and treatment from that due to ulceration of other parts of the alimentary canal.

Finney shows that operation is successful in 26 % of cases. Operation must be performed early. Sharp pain associated with nausea is a signal of perforation. In general peritonitis from appendicitis early operation is of the most urgent importance. In cases which recover albumin and casts are absent from the urine. When the kidneys are choked with bacteria operation is useless. When only the lower segment of the abdomen has been invaded, there

---

[1] Lancet, Mar. 27, 1897.   [2] Med. News, May 29, 1897.

is but one opinion in regard to cleansing the abdominal cavity. The minute septic material appears it is sponged away before it can be diffused. The bowels which present are mopped with sponges, soaked in hot salt solution, and are dried before other coils are drawn up for inspection. When parts are reached which are not much inflamed, a gauze tamponade is pushed among the bowels far from the field of work, a tape is sewed to the tamponade, and a clamp which projects externally is fixed to the tape. One or more tamponades are thrust up and across the abdomen before the pelvis is cleansed. The pelvis is mopped out thoroughly, a packing of iodoform-gauze is placed in the pelvis, the gauze tamponades are withdrawn, and if they are wet from absorbed effusion, pieces of iodoform-gauze are carried in several directions among the coils of bowel. The wound should not be closed.

In the grave cases a long median incision or two lateral cuts are required. A cut for lumbar drainage is only required when the median incision is used. Gauze-packing is far better for drainage than tubes of glass or rubber. When infection is widespread irrigation must be practised. Flush systematically with saline solution as hot as the hand can bear (over 105°). Irrigation with hot saline fluid stimulates the patient and diminishes the power of the endothelium to absorb toxins. If the intestines are distended with gas and fluid, let them emerge from the abdomen, cover them with hot towels, prick them in one or two places with a knife, evacuate gas and fluid feces, and wash away in a stream of hot water. Through one of the openings inject a syringeful of saturated solution of Epsom salt and then close the punctures.

McCosh says that in every bad case we should pass a dose of salts into the bowel through an aspirating-needle and close the puncture with one suture. Salts so introduced cannot be vomited and cause downward peristalsis. If regurgitation exists, lavage of stomach is done before operation, after operation, and whenever regurgitation is renewed. A rectal tube is used to remove gas, and is of great value in promoting downward peristalsis. An ice-coil or light ice-bags upon the abdomen do good and are grateful to the patient. Strychnin is often needed. When the patient is well out of ether and complains of severe pain morphin hypodermically is useful rather than harmful.

George Ryerson Fowler,[1] as to **septic peritonitis from the clinical standpoint,** says that a clinical classification of septic peritonitis is useful to the practitioner. The term diffuse septic peritonitis is preferable to that of general peritonitis, because it is impossible in any case to be sure that every portion of the peritoneum has been attacked. The term perforative peritonitis is useful, and so is the designation circumscribed or local peritonitis. Hematogenous peritonitis is a rare condition. The name is better than cryptogenic septico-pyemia, which some apply to this state. The term puerperal peritonitis is warranted by the frequent occurrence of peritonitis due to this cause, and also to certain clinical peculiarities which belong to this form of the disease. Pelvic peritonitis is used to signify a peritonitis taking origin from the female organs of generation. The term subdiaphragmatic peritonitis should be used instead of subphrenic abscess. Fowler discusses the prognosis of bacterial invasion of the peritoneum. When infection is due to a small number of comparatively nonvirulent germs fatal peritonitis may not arise, but will be favored in its development by prolonged handling. Even a slight injury may be followed by fatal infection if the streptococcus pyogenes gains access to the area of damage. The peritoneum can dispose of a certain quantity of even virulently infectious matter, provided nothing is present to furnish

[1] Med. News, May 15, 1897.

aid and support to bacteria. Bacteria may produce peritonitis even without multiplying, as when they come in contact with the peritoneum, because of conditions which also cause effusion of serum, extravasation of blood, injury to the serous tissue, sloughing of peritoneum, or the entrance at the same time of a substance which serves as nutritive material for the germs; such a material is feces. The route of the invasion affects the prognosis. Peritonitis may arise without the presence of bacteria within the peritoneal cavity, the toxins passing through visceral walls which show no lesion. The serous fluid of the peritoneal cavity is to a certain extent germicidal, but its power is limited. Bacteria in encapsuled abscesses occasionally die (Wieland). The most dangerous method of invasion is perforation of the small bowel; the least dangerous is a wound in the wall of the abdomen. In the first condition there is an escape of great numbers of very virulent bacteria, of toxins formed in the intestine, and of fecal matter, which is an irritant to the serous surface and pabulum for bacteria. The prognosis after intestinal perforation is influenced by the size of the perforation and the rapidity with which bowel-contents escape. In perforation of the small intestine fecal matter is forced out rapidly, and mixed infection of the peritoneum quickly takes place, with the development of diffuse septic peritonitis. When the large intestine is perforated feces may flow out slowly, and limited suppurative peritonitis can occur. Comparatively few bacteria are apt to be introduced through a wound in the belly-wall, and often the peritoneum is able to dispose of them. A wound of the abdominal wall is extremely dangerous if it is associated with contusion of the peritoneal surfaces, the entrance of a foreign body, hemorrhage, or the laceration of a hollow viscus. In degree of danger, midway between rupture of intestine and wound of belly-wall, we may mention invasions due to wounds or perforations of other viscera (kidneys, pancreas, bile-ducts, ureters, etc.), and the rupture of an infectious abscess, entrance of organisms through inflammatory growth of the walls of the intestine or of a hollow viscus, infection by way of the Fallopian tubes, migration of bacteria through an area of nutritive disturbance in the wall of the gut, as in strangulated hernia.

The **treatment** of diffuse peritonitis consists in early free incision and drainage. Fowler thinks that the value of serum-therapy in this disease is as yet uncertain.

Nicholas Senn[1] suggests a **classification of acute peritonitis.** A discussion of the etiology, diagnosis, prognosis, and treatment will mislead unless we employ a comprehensive and definite classification. In order to locate the process or to trace the connection with the organ primarily diseased an anatomic diagnosis is required. Senn makes the following groups for purposes of anatomic diagnosis: Ectoperitonitis—inflammation of the attached side of peritoneum. Endoperitonitis—inflammation of the serous surface of the peritoneum. Parietal peritonitis—inflammation of the serous lining of the peritoneal cavity. Visceral peritonitis—inflammation of the peritoneal coat of any of the abdominal or pelvic organs. Pelvic peritonitis. Diaphragmatic peritonitis.

The following etiologic classification is advocated: Traumatic peritonitis—an injury establishes a communication between the peritoneal cavity and the surface of the body or some of the hollow organs, through which channel pyogenic cocci enter. Idiopathic peritonitis—many doubt if peritonitis can occur without previous injury or suppurative lesion; it is too early to deny absolutely the existence of so-called idiopathic peritonitis, but future bacteriologic study will surely find a microbe in all cases of this sort. Perforative perito-

[1] Med. News, May 8, 1897.

nitis. Metastic peritonitis—arising from infectious processes unconnected with peritoneum; may develop during the existence of an acute infectious disease. Puerperal peritonitis.

The pathologic classification is into: diffuse septic peritonitis; suppurative peritonitis; serous peritonitis; fibrinoplastic peritonitis.

The bacteriologic classification is as follows: streptococcus infection; staphylococcus infection; pneumococcus infection; bacillus coli commune infection; gonococcus infection; tuberculous infection.

Senn's clinical classification is into: ectoperitonitis; diffuse septic peritonitis; perforative peritonitis; circumscribed peritonitis.

APPENDICITIS.

G. F. Shrady,[1] in laying down the **rules for operation in appendicitis,** maintains that increased pulse-rate usually points to the necessity of operating, as it indicates that the case is rapidly progressing. If, in addition to increased pulse-rate, there is a sudden accentuation of pain, delay in ope-

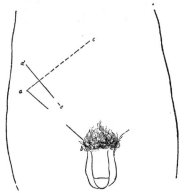

FIG. 18.—*ab*, Poupart's ligament; *a*, anterior superior spine of ilium; *ac*, line joining umbilicus and anterior superior spine; *de*, line of incision recommended by McBurney, parallel with the course of the fibers of the external oblique muscle and its aponeurosis (Van Hook, in Jour. of Am. Med. Assoc., Feb. 20, 1897).

ration will be dangerous. The temperature in appendicitis is not usually high, and it affords no reliable indications for operation. Great prostration confirms the necessity for surgical interference. In some cases immediate surgical intervention is obviously demanded; for instance, when there is a collapsed condition pointing to perforation. As a rule, in appendicitis cases there is, first, a condition marked by very positive symptoms; then these symptoms lessen for a day or two, at which period of time we can make a very careful study of the case. It is wise to refuse to operate during the attack when the pulse-rate lessens, when the pain diminishes, and when the temperature falls. When an abscess forms it is best to wait until firm adhesions have been produced, unless a sudden emergency should happen to arise.

Weller Van Hook[2] has written a very important paper upon the **technic of operations for acute appendicitis,** a paper which is particularly notable for the practical nature of his views. He maintains that the

[1] Treatment, Mar. 25, 1897.   [2] Jour. Am. Med. Assoc., Feb. 20, 1897.

most important part of the operation is the protection of the normal serous coat from infection and the application of a drain of gauze. People who have never operated, or who have operated only occasionally, should be persuaded that the operation for appendicitis is not always an easy and simple affair. It is a matter for surprise, and almost horror, to find that the majority of

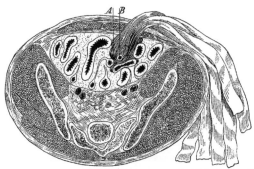

FIG. 19.—To show the application of the gauze when the appendix (*B*) lies in the midst of the small intestine, to the left of the cecum (*A*). This and the preceding drawing were made from photographs of frozen sections made by the writer after having performed the operation described in the text upon the cadaver (Van Hook, in Jour. of Am. Med Assoc , Feb 20, 1897).

writers give an opposite impression, or, like Sonnenburg, boldly assert that the operation is a simple one. It is the positive conviction of Van Hook that 100 cases of acute perforative appendicitis will show a higher percentage of recovery under medical treatment with incision of pointing abscesses than will 100 like cases operated upon by 100 or even 20 surgeons who are gaining

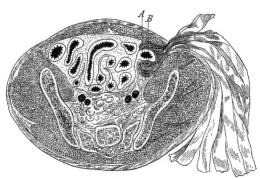

FIG. 20.—To show the relation of gauze strips to the cecum (*A*) and the stump of the appendix (*B*), when the appendix lies between the cecum and the outer abdominal wall (Van Hook, in Jour. of Am. Med. Assoc., Feb. 20, 1897).

their first experience. The loss of life from faulty operations is much greater than is the case with other pelvic and abdominal work. The reason is quite obvious. The operation is an act of violence, and of supreme violence, and is inflicted at the seat of virulent infection. There is no more appalling calamity met with by the surgeon than the passage of pus from the appendicular region to previously uninfected peritoneum. What most marks the man of surgical skill is the ability to prevent this accident during the operation. Every surgeon must make a beginning some time or other ; but, except in cases of urgency, an inexperienced operator must refrain from drawing blood, and experience is to be gained by assisting older surgeons. No one

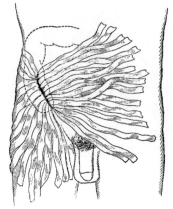

FIG. 21.—To show the appearance of the gauze strips before they are turned over to the right side of the patient's body (Van Hook, in Jour. of Am. Med. Assoc., Feb. 20, 1897).

should begin to operate on such cases without he has both inclination and opportunity to perfect himself in the art, and he will always find that his later cases show better results than his earlier cases. The first goal to be reached by operation is the saving of life, and we must subordinate to this petty con-

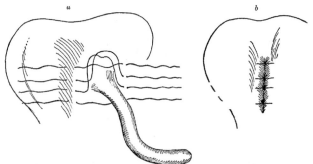

FIG. 22.—*a*, Lembert sutures applied before the appendix is cut off; *b*, Lembert sutures tied after removal of the appendix (Van Hook, in Jour. of Am. Med. Assoc., Feb. 20, 1897).

siderations merely of future comfort and convenience. The secondary objects of operation are the prevention of fistulæ, the prevention of recurrent appendicitis, and the lessening of the chances of hernia. When a surgeon is about to operate outside of a hospital he should first obtain the best nurse accessible. A good assistant is necessary, and should stand opposite the operator and aid in preventing the passage of pus into the sound regions of peritoneum, arrange the sponges and keep them warm, hold retractors, etc. It is well to have an operating-table which permits the placing of the patient in the Trendelenburg position. In an emergency an ordinary kitchen-table or dining-room table will do, and when such a table is used the patient's feet must be fastened to the end so that he cannot slip toward the head of the table, and the end of the table can be raised by placing a box or chair under it. It is not always possible, because of lack of time, to prepare the patient elaborately. Cleansing should never be rough lest it rupture an abscess-wall. Transportation of the patient is very dangerous, as a sudden contraction of the abdominal muscles may force out a great quantity of infectious material from the abscess or from a perforation into the peritoneal cavity itself. The position of the patient depends on circumstances. When pus is discovered at the brim of the pelvis we can prevent the entrance of this fluid into the pelvis by quickly placing the patient in the Trendelenburg position. If the pus flows toward the median line, the patient should be placed upon the right side. These two maneuvers can be carried out simultaneously. The site of the incision depends on the situation of the appendix and the morbid anatomic conditions which exist. The incision should afford direct access to the seat of trouble, excepting where we wish to avoid opening the free peritoneal cavity. The median incision is not used except in those unusual cases in which the cecum and the appendix lie back of the median line. The most useful method of opening the abdomen to reach the appendix in one of its usual positions is that of McArthur or McBurney. It will be remembered that McBurney makes a skin incision 4 inches long, this incision crossing at right angles or nearly at right angles a line drawn from the anterior superior spine of the ilium to the umbilicus. The incision is about 1 in. internal to the spine of the ilium, and the upper third of the incision is above the omphalospinous line. The fasciæ are cut with a knife ; the muscular fibers are separated by blunt dissection. These fibers are held apart by retractors during the operation, and when the operation is completed will come together and almost perfectly close the wound. This method can be used only when good assistants are present and a small incision is required. The principle of this operation should be followed if any incision involve the lateral abdominal region ; that is, the direction of the cut should follow the general course of the fibers of the external oblique muscle ; muscular fibers should be cut as rarely as possible, so as to avoid nerve-trunks. It was with the idea of avoiding injury to the nerves that Kocher recommended that we should make only transverse or oblique incisions unless we happen to be operating in the median line. Van Hook is in entire agreement with Kocher's proposition. He would give up the Langenbuch incision at the side of the rectus muscle, and also longitudinal incisions over the colon. He thinks that the nerves which supply the rectus should not be interfered with, because muscular paralysis weakens the abdominal wall. The oblique incision is useful for another reason. It enables the surgeon to reach freely all ordinary areas of appendix trouble and also makes a wound parallel with the general lines of traction of the abdominal muscles, a wound which does not gape and which is not apt to permit of a subsequent hernia. The length of the incision must be sufficient to permit of necessary manipulation. It should never be so short as to interfere with safe work. There is no special advantage in a very small incision, though, of course, unnecessarily large incisions are not desirable because they increase the liability to hernia. The site of the chief pathologic activity in appendicitis can be in most instances made out, especially when there is swelling or tenderness. In endeavoring to discover swelling or tenderness a rectal or vaginal examination should never be omitted, since it is by no means rare to find that the inflammation is located in or has extended into the pelvis. Pain at the end of micturition is a valuable sign in pointing to inflammation of the vesical peritoneum. A diagnostic localization of the appendix is impossible in gangrenous appendicitis, or in perforative appendicitis in which there is diffuse peritonitis. In these cases there are absence of local swelling and the presence of widely diffused tenderness. It is very important to try to estimate the relation of the focus of inflammation to the ascending colon and to the ileum. The ileum and colon are barriers which limit the spread of infected fluids. An abscess which forms outside of the ascending colon is usually well toward the flank and extends toward the renal and hepatic regions. In such a case we can often make out by percussion the fact that the colon has approached the median line. When the inflammation is located below the mesentery of the ileum it tends to extend into the lesser pelvis, and in this case vaginal or rectal examination is of great importance. When the site of inflammatory activity is internal to the ascending colon and above the mesentery of the ileum the gravest apprehensions arise. We make out this condition by outlining the colon by means of percussion and by determining that the swelling and tenderness are toward the median line. The duration of the inflammation and the area of the swelling are points which will often enable us to have a correct idea of the morbid changes to be encountered. If the suppurative process has existed two or three weeks, there must be much adhesion and multiplication of cells. In an acute and violent condition the process is probably not limited by adhesions. An inflammation which has existed for some time, but which suddenly becomes worse, was probably limited at first, but has extended later into normal serous membrane. Uncertainty in regard to the capacity of the barriers to withstand the spread of the process is greatest between the third day and the end of the first week. Signs of violent inflammation point to local extension of the mischief. When there are mild general symptoms and an area of tumefaction which does not enlarge we are justified in assuming that the process is limited by adhesions. Edema of the skin points to adhesion of the abscess to the wall of the abdomen. Van Hook inquires as to what properties of the peritoneum can we take advantage of in operating. The normal peritoneum possesses an enormous resisting power to infection. One-tenth of the poison which is often thrown into the peritoneal cavity without producing harm would cause fatal infection if placed in the cranial cavity. In operating for appendicitis we can take advantage of this resisting power and venture to inoculate a portion of the serous membrane. Traumatisms, such as mechanical and chemical irritation, drying and cooling, diminish resistance. The chief surgical resource is capillary drainage. In a closed abdomen the serous surfaces are not separated from each other by gas or air, but they lie in contact and are lubricated by serous fluid. If an infecting fluid come between these surfaces, it is disseminated widely and with great rapidity, partly by gravity and partly by capillary action. When about to open an area of infectious matter the usual custom has been to protect the intestines from contact with this matter by means of compresses. When the infected cavity has been evacuated the compresses are removed and pieces of gauze applied in their place to act as drains.

Van Hook strongly urges the application of a preventive capillary drain. Before defilement of the peritoneum has taken place the operator should apply gauze between the parietal serous layer and the region of the infection. Iodoform-gauze is generally the best material, and this gauze rather than the peritoneum beneath it is the surface to be protected by compresses. The ends of the pieces of gauze are inserted in various spaces to prevent the dissemination of poison, not only by establishing capillary action toward the wound, but by occlusion. At the end of the operation the strips are not replaced by fresh gauze for three reasons: first, manipulation favors the entrance of bacteria into the tissues; second, the handling transfers bacteria to clean areas; third, the gauze, if properly applied, will carry away the infectious matter which has escaped arrest by the compresses. The compresses over the gauze can be changed as often as the operator desires.

Gubaroff has asserted that the beneficial action of the gauze extends for $2\frac{1}{2}$ in. on each side of its margin, and Van Hook believes that this statement is true, founding his opinion on a recent autopsy. It is very important for the surgeon to decide before operation whether he has to deal with an inflammatory area which is not mechanically limited, or with a pus-area shut off from sound peritoneum by very thick barriers, or with a genuine abscess-cavity. In a first attack of moderately severe perforative appendicitis there will be no effective adhesions up to the fourth day. Between the fourth and tenth days the new tissue becomes resistant and may be utilized in operative treatment. After the tenth day, if the abscess has not ruptured, it will probably have strong walls.

Van Hook then takes up for discussion the technic of the operation. When adhesions are absent make an incision which gives full command of the region. As soon as the incision has been made a gauze barrier is inserted about the wound so that infectious material may not come in contact with sound peritoneum. For this purpose he uses strips of sterile gauze or iodoform-ganze, each strip being $2\frac{1}{2}$ in. wide, 15 in. long, and 4 layers in thickness. A large retractor is placed under the abdominal wall at the edge of the wound, the parietes are lifted upward and away from the intestines, and the end of a piece of gauze is passed into the abdominal wall between the parietal peritoneum and the intestines at right angles to the incision and carried in for a distance of from 1 to 3 in. The retractor is now moved into another position and another piece of gauze is inserted by the side of the first one, and this process is repeated in every direction until the gauze completely surrounds the region in which the work is to be done. If the focus of trouble is in contact with the lateral parietes, the gauze barrier is applied so as to prevent any possible infection of the pelvis below or the hepatic region above, and for this purpose the incision must be low enough down to enable the surgeon to reach below the appendix. Strips of gauze are carried toward the brim of the pelvis until this avenue is well closed. The temporary use of the Trendelenburg position favors the maneuver. Especial care must be taken to protect the hepatic region from infection, a similar method being used. Strips of packing aid in preventing infection and determine an outward serous discharge. Infectious matter is carried away from the free peritoneal surface and adhesions tend to form. The visible portions of the strips of gauze are covered with compresses wrung out of warm salt solution, and loose coils of bowel are pressed aside by the compresses until the most active seat of disease is reached. The longitudinal muscular band of the colon will lead the surgeon directly to the seat of trouble. When the appendix is reached it will almost invariably be found that feces or purulent matter flow upward. This material must be caught on compresses, which are discarded from time to time and carefully replaced by fresh ones. The cecum must not be lifted up, if doing so increases the danger of infection. Before the appendix is removed a strip of gauze is carried down to the infected region so as to surround the dangerous area. If the cecum can be lifted up without risk of infectious matter gaining entrance to parts of the peritoneal cavity which are not protected by adhesions, a piece of gauze is slipped under it; the appendix is amputated between the temporary ligature on the proximal side and a pair of forceps on the distal side. The projecting mucous membrane is touched with pure carbolic acid and a row of Lembert sutures passed over the stump of the appendix. The temporary ligature is removed, the stump is inverted, and the sutures are tied. The arteries of the meso-appendix are controlled by ligatures or suture-ligatures. If the cecum has not been lifted up, drainage is carried out by additional strips of gauze and also in some cases by a tube. If it is found that infectious material has already passed between the intestines, it is followed up with sponges, is gotten away by gentle pressure, and iodoform-gauze drains are left in contact with the infected peritoneum. It is unwise to lift lengths of intestine from the abdominal cavity to clean them. It is much better to treat them by surrounding with gauze drains. The ends of the strips of gauze should be left very long, so that they hang over the dressings at the side of the patient. The excessive length of the gauze strips favors rapidity of drainage and enables the intra-abdominal portion of the gauze to lift fluid against gravity. The next step in the operation consists in partially closing the wound. Gauze is left to emerge from the portion of the wound which is nearest to the site of inflammation. The wound is closed except at the points of emergence of gauze drains. Stitches are introduced also at the sites of the strands of gauze, and are tied in this region only when the gauze is removed. The question of the technic of the process when adhesions exist is a matter of dispute. All agree that the appendix should be removed if it is near to a focus of inflammation. Others maintain that it should be removed if it can be done without breaking down the wall of the abscess. Some say that it should be removed if it does not constitute a part of the abscess-wall. Some operators say " always remove the appendix," maintaining that operations which leave the appendix are incomplete; that undiscovered abscesses may be left; that convalescence will be prolonged; that fistulæ and sinuses will remain, and that recurrence of trouble will be most probable.

Van Hook reminds us that we operate to save life. The main object to be attained when adhesions have formed is to relieve the tension of the abscess-cavity by outward drainage. To what further extent it is justified to go depends on circumstances. Secondary abscesses do not occur with any frequency, and it is not necessary to remove the appendix to discover and drain a secondary abscess. The extirpation of the appendix in some cases may disseminate the pus widely. The percentage of recurrent attacks after simple drainage is exceedingly small. The operator, especially if inexperienced, should not do too much. Let us remove the appendix if we feel sure that its removal will not disseminate pus or destroy the barrier of adhesions. On opening the abdomen first carefully surround with gauze strips as previously described; next apply gauze about the matted coils of intestines. The surgeon determines by careful palpation what portions of the bowel are nonadherent, requiring isolation from those portions near the appendix by means of packing. The deeper portions of the packing are to be carried back to the posterior layer of the peritoneum. The gauze must be spread out, must touch the neighboring bit of gauze on either side, must be free from knots and kinks, and this is best accomplished by carrying it in on the finger. Every piece of gauze which is used should come to the surface by as direct a route as possible, and the infected area is not to be attacked until the peritoneum is thoroughly protected by gauze. The gauze is to be covered over with pads. When this protection has been secured the infected area is opened and drained. The finger is pushed gently between the coils of intestine until this area is reached. A strip of gauze is then carried into the cavity, and we may, if we wish, have a tubular drain within this gauze. If we decide not to try to remove the appendix, the intestines are retracted with gauze strips and the drains are deeply inserted. Foci of infection which are situated between the ascending colon and the right lateral abdominal wall are usually attacked with ease. The surgeon takes pains to see that the space between the anterior surface of the colon and the abdominal wall, if not obliterated by adhesions, is protected by gauze strips, and that the upper and lower boundaries of the area of infection are protected by gauze-packing. The greatest difficulty in protecting the peritoneum exists when the trouble lies between the colon and the median line and above the mesentery of the ileum. It is often found impossible in these cases to prevent pus passing into the general cavity. If adhesions are absent, the patient must be placed in the Trendelenburg position. The abdomen is opened, the gauze strips are passed as usual around the area of trouble, aseptic compresses are placed so as to catch any infectious materials from the region of the appendix, a drain of gauze is passed down to the appendix, and great care is taken not to disturb even the most delicate adhesions, because if adhesions are disturbed peristaltic action will tend to carry the liberated small intestine in the course of a few hours to a distant part of the abdomen, and this small intestine has infectious material attached to its walls. It has often seemed to surgeons that transperitoneal drainage is more dangerous than direct drainage through the vagina or rectum. When abscesses are situated in the right iliac fossa firm adhesions may exist between the walls of the abscess and the outer abdominal parietes. In such a case the incision should be made to the outside of the focus or even in the loin; the gauze drain should not be removed until between 5 and 8 days, thus allowing time for adhesions to wall off infected areas.

[Van Hook's article is worthy of a careful study and will prove of aid to any one who operates for appendicitis.]

Charles McBurney[1] writes on the **treatment of appendicitis.** He states positively that there is no purely medical measure which is capable of curing the disease. Appendicitis must be placed among surgical diseases. This does not mean that every case requires operation. We are very far from being certain as to the primary cause of appendicitis. McBurney is inclined to the view that the primary cause is probably interference with the drainage of the appendix into the colon. This interference may be brought about by a concretion in the appendix, a stricture, an accumulation of fat causing displacement, or by a kink or twist in the appendix. McBurney has never seen a case of appendicitis in which there was not interference with the drainage. If the appendix is examined before its relations have been disturbed, in many cases the obstruction will be obvious. In a patient not very susceptible to sepsis, a temporary obstruction may cause but slight constitutional symptoms, while in a patient who is very susceptible to sepsis a similar obstruction may cause marked constitutional trouble and may lead to rapid death unless relieved by operation. The preliminary treatment employed is often worse than useless, and the measures that are adopted early in the case are of very great importance as regards the prognosis. It is a grave error to give morphin in the beginning of an attack. It is true that it relieves the patient's pain, but it cloaks the symptoms and prevents an accurate study of the early stage of the condition, and it is upon an accurate study of the early stage of the condition that we found our diagnosis and base our treatment. If a patient is under the influence of morphin, we can-

[1] N. Y. Polyclinic, Jan. 15, 1897.

not detect an increase in the severity of the case or the advent of sepsis. Every patient with acute abdominal pain, whether or not he has nausea, vomiting, prostration, and constipation, should be *suspected* of having appendicitis. Such a patient should be put to bed and subjected to a careful examination. Very little opium or other anodynes should be administered. The patient should be kept at rest and be watched most carefully. If the diagnosis can be made in the first 6 hours, and the patient can be watched for 6 hours longer, the progress of the disease in this time may tell the story. Certainly in 24 hours from the beginning of the attack we are usually able to decide on the diagnosis and the probable course and result of a case. We are thus enabled to make an early choice between operative and palliative procedures. The question of when to operate in an acute attack of appendicitis cannot be answered dogmatically, as no 2 cases are exactly alike. Certain symptoms are watched for and their value considered in each case. McBurney supposes an average case: the patient, let us say, has had one or two attacks of vomiting; the pulse is strong, full, and only moderately frequent; temperature in the neighborhood of 100°; severe abdominal pain, at first diffuse and then settling in the right iliac region. If after 6 hours the patient is no worse, there is no immediate danger. If in 12 hours the severity of the symptoms has not increased, the patient will soon begin to get better; but if the case has steadily become more urgent in 12 hours from the time when the diagnosis was made, an operation will very likely be demanded.

McBurney says that if he can safely permit a patient to get over an acute attack before operating, he prefers to do so; and if in 24 hours from the beginning of an attack the intensity of the symptoms abate, he feels that he can leave the ease to Nature and can postpone operation to an interval. Such an attack ought to subside in 48 to 72 hours. If, however, during the second 24 hours of the attack he is doubtful of the outcome, he always advises an operation. Just as soon as we become sure that the disease is progressing he advises operation.

McBurney feels entirely willing to operate on all cases of appendicitis when the symptoms have practically disappeared. Treves operates when the attacks have been very numerous and when they have been increasing in severity and threatening life. McBurney thinks that when a patient has had two attacks he will as surely have a third as he will have the eleventh after the tenth, and every attack renders an operation more difficult and more risky. Ordinarily in an interval-operation we wait for 2 to 3 weeks after the attack; after this time there is no danger from sepsis and we do not expect a ventral hernia result. The mortality of interval-operations is almost nothing; but in operations done during an acute attack there is decided danger. The period of convalescence will last for at least 6 weeks and the patient may develop a hernia. The question whether it is safe to wait for the attack to pass on and defer operation, requires the best judgment of an experienced man. When we wish to operate in the interval the operation should never be done in less than 2 weeks after the termination of an acute attack, because up to this time a local septic condition may exist. After this period congestion, inflammatory thickening, and danger of sepsis will be absent. McBurney says that he always uses a gauze drain alone, except in cases of general septic peritonitis, in which, in addition to the gauze drain, he passes a glass drainage-tube down to the floor of the pelvis. He uses 10% iodoform-gauze. In the acute eases in which operation is done early it is very rare that the result is fatal. Interval-operations rarely produce a fatal result. When an operation is performed on a patient who has had numerous attacks, and when there are many adhesions and considerable broken-down tissue, there is occasionally a death. The chief cause of death in appendix operations is delay. If a death is due to general septic peritonitis, this rises at a late period of the attack, after the time when the disease should have been recognized, and if there has been no delay, there would have been no septic peritonitis. In cases in which abscesses have formed, each day increases the difficulty and danger of operation. The proper time to operate when the abscess has formed has been very much debated. Treves holds that when pus has been encompassed by barriers the longer we wait the nearer the pus will be to the surface.

McBurney radically differs from Treves, and believes that the pus, instead of approaching the surface, may ascend toward the liver or descend into the pelvis. The sooner abscess-cases are operated on the better. In such cases, if the appendix has not yet softened or broken down, or if only a small amount of peritoneum is involved, the appendix can in most instances be readily removed; but when there is considerable peritonitis, with adhesions and a large amount of pus, the appendix is softened and cannot be recognized, or, if recognized, cannot be removed with safety. A discussion on the removal of the appendix in every case has been carried on in Philadelphia, and some operators maintain that the appendix should always be looked after and removed. As a matter of fact, in some cases it cannot be removed because it cannot be found. It may be buried in the wall of an abscess, and when in this situation it is usually better to abandon the search for fear of making an opening into the intestines. Furthermore, in many cases such a search will occupy a long time and lead to the necessity of greatly enlarging the wound. If the wound is cleansed thoroughly and if free drainage is established, the remnant of the appendix which is left will not be apt to be productive of harm; but if it does cause trouble at a later period, it can be operated upon then. Ill-advised search for the appendix may unquestionably lead to death. McBurney says that, as a rule, the fecal fistulæ which follow the operation for appendicitis close spontaneously; but when they do not close they should be operated upon, the only safe operation being to enter the peritoneal cavity at some other point than through the fistula itself. To enlarge the fistulous opening will lead to wounding of the intestine, but an opening above the fistula can be made easily and with safety. [It is gratifying to find the high authority of McBurney on the side of those who claim that we should not *always* remove the appendix, because in some cases it cannot be found and in others its removal will cause death. McBurney is of the opinion that appendicitis is due to obstruction to drainage of the appendix. This view is forcibly maintained by Dieulafoy, who speaks of the inflamed appendix as a closed vase. Bruns has disputed the view of Dieulafoy, and holds that appendicitis can arise from infection when the appendix is not closed, and septic inflammation does not of necessity arise when the appendix becomes a closed vase. Bruns has seen operations performed for peritonitis of appendicular origin, appendices having been removed which were not closed either partly or completely. Jalaguier maintains that whereas it is frequent to find the outlet from the appendix closed, the closure is the result and not the cause of appendicitis. Pozzi has pointed out that the appendix is a point of least resistance, and may be involved when a general infection exists. Some surgeons believe appendicitis is induced by traumatisms inflicted by the psoas muscle; some that the vestigial nature of the structure makes it especially liable to disease; others that mechanical conditions induce the disease. There is no question that appendices sometimes contain concretions, but their etiologic significance is disputed. There are probably many predisposing causes of appendicitis, and one of these causes is sometimes influenza. What cause is most influential is uncertain.]

Arbuthnot Lane[1] writes on the **milder varieties of appendicitis.** He asserts that the only cause of the inflammation is the presence of fecal matter or some other matter in the appendix, which material the appendix is unable to get rid of. As a rule, it is fecal matter. The fecal matter may be solid or fluid, and fluid feces blocked up in the appendix will produce decided irritation. Some appendices are predisposed to the trouble because of excessive length, manner of attachment, or degree of mobility. When the appendix has been partially or completely occluded at one or more points from cicatrization of an ulcer the accumulation of secretion in the distal portion of the canal is capable of setting up a recurrent attack of inflammation. The difficulty the appendix has in emptying itself is much increased by a loaded condition of the cecum, and people who are habitually constipated are those most liable to appendicular colic. When the appendix becomes anchored it has great difficulty in expelling solid or liquid material from its interior. When the appendix contains material which it cannot expel it inflames. This inflammation may be a temporary condition involving the mucous membrane alone, or it may be so violent that the entire appendix swells and becomes gangrenous. Associated with any degree of inflammation there is a varying amount of peritonitis. In some cases there is just a little plastic lymph thrown out, in others there is a large serous exudate, and in others pus is formed. The character of the peritonitis depends largely upon the number of organisms and their virulence, and intense peritonitis involving the entire abdomen may arise when there is no perforation of the abscess-wall or of the appendix itself. It is by no means always possible to feel a tumor. A tumor, or, to be more accurate, a sense of resistance, can only be felt where matting ensues. When we have serous or purulent inflammation of the peritoneal cavity no mass can be detected, and although the appendix is much enlarged it cannot be palpated because of the rigid abdominal wall and the distension of the intestines with gas. When the appendix contains irritating material which it is unable to expel, the mucous membrane may be ulcerated by the action of organisms and stricture may follow ulceration. In some cases an abscess forms in the wall of the appendix beginning in the lymph-tissue, and these abscesses may burst into the bowel or into the peritoneal cavity. In the majority of cases adhesions form between the appendix and the bowel which is adjacent, and the abscess is thus localized. It is very unfortunate for the patient that the uterine appendages are such near neighbors of the appendix. The majority of females who have appendicitis suffer much from this adjacency, because it is very common to find that a diagnosis has previously been made of disease of the uterus or its appendages. The most common form of appendicitis, and the one most rarely recognized, is that in which the normal appendix makes an effort to force its contents into the cecum. When this process is going on the most variable symptoms may be presented. In most cases the only means of determining that this process exists is recognizing that the appendix is painful on pressure. The so-called McBurney point is of little value because the position of the appendix varies greatly. In a well-marked case of appendicitis there is usually a feeling of gastric discomfort. This is succeeded by pain, which is at first slight and intermittent, but becomes more intense or spreads over the entire abdomen, being most marked in the lower abdomen. There is apt to be vomiting. After a time the severe pain abates, and the whole abdomen is found to be tender to pressure, a spot which corresponds to

[1] Lancet, July 25, 1896.

the situation of the appendix being especially painful. In many cases during the attack it is possible to feel the appendix and to note its location. After the attack passes off there is usually persistent indigestion for a number of weeks. Many cases, however, do not give such a clear history as the above. In some cases vomiting and diarrhea are the only symptoms. In others there may be merely gastric uneasiness. In others there may be frequent micturition, pain being noted in the vesical region when the bladder is distended. Urinary symptoms indicate that the appendix is in relation with the urinary bladder. All symptoms are aggravated during the menstrual period. It is very difficult to distinguish between symptoms due to irritation of a normal appendix and symptoms due to distention of an appendix anchored by inflammation or distention of an appendix the lumen of which is constricted. The symptoms are similar, but, as a rule, are very much more severe when the appendix is damaged. Between the attacks we can usually separate these two conditions by noticing that the normal appendix is not tender and the damaged appendix is. It is important to endeavor to distinguish between these two conditions, because the former requires no operation and can be averted by regulation of the intestinal functions; whereas such treatment is without effect on the latter condition. Operative interference can be safely performed between the attacks, although the surgeon should recognize that it is sometimes wise not to operate. Lane discusses the treatment of appendicitis and lays down the following rule: in mild forms regulation of the intestinal functions will prevent recurrence. If there is great pain in an attack, give morphin, keep the patient quiet, and, if you suspect that the large bowel is loaded, administer an enema. If there are marked pain, vomiting, and general disturbance, give morphin in sufficient dose to keep the patient under its influence. When the intestines are matted about the appendix there is very little cause for anxiety, since in such cases perforation is very unusual; and if an abscess of large size forms, it will spread toward the abdominal wall. The surgeon should not be in a hurry to open these fluid accumulations unless the symptoms are urgent. We know that such conditions not unusually subside, because the colon-bacilli die or lose their virulence. When we open such collections of fluid we should adhere to the strictest antiseptic regulations, in order to prevent the entry of other organisms than those which are present. The colon-bacillus does not appear to exercise any deterrent influence on the healing of wounds, and wounds which contain the colon-bacillus will heal exactly as will sterile wounds. When there is serous or purulent peritonitis the condition is very dangerous. In such conditions, when the surgeon is in doubt, he should interfere and remove the appendix. When an abscess has formed and has not become attached to the abdominal wall, there is great danger that it may burst into the peritoneal cavity. The surgeon may hesitate to expose the patient to the risk of opening an abscess, removing the appendix, and draining through the healthy peritoneum, especially if he has not at command good assistants; but such cases demand operation in many instances immediately. The matted bowel should be wrapped in sterilized iodoform-gauze in order to protect the peritoneal cavity. When the abscess ruptures directly into the peritoneal cavity, or when a perforation of the appendix takes place into the free peritoneal cavity, only prompt interference can possibly do any good. It is far better to wipe the peritoneum thoroughly and then flush it; and if the bowels are not much distended, they should be wrapped in sterile gauze. Lane greatly prefers sterile gauze to gauze containing any irritant germicide. [Lane does not hesitate to give morphin in an attack, but we believe decidedly that it should not be given. Pain will not kill the patient, but by giving the morphin to destroy the pain we may lull the patient and ourselves into a sense of security when beset by the most imminent perils.]

J. W. Elliot[1] describes a **modification of the McBurney incision for appendectomy.** He says that he has done the McBurney operation ten times. When the appendix is normally situated it is easily reached, but when it becomes necessary to enlarge the incision the operation is not altogether satisfactory. If it becomes necessary to retract forcibly the muscles, the tissues are apt to be damaged, so that healing is imperfect. When the wound has to be enlarged the advantage of the McBurney incision is gone, and we have a ragged wound with two layers of muscles which are widely striped, a wound which drains very badly if pus is met with. Elliot advises that the operation should be begun by a horizontal incision through the skin and the aponeurosis of the external oblique. This incision begins half an inch internal to the anterior superior iliac spine and reaches the semilunar line. The fibers of the external oblique are cut across; the fibers of the internal oblique and transversalis are separated as in the McBurney method. The transversalis fascia and peritoneum are opened transversely. If it is necessary to enlarge this incision, we can carry it into the rectus or enlarge it either upward or downward in the semilunar line. He recommends closing the wound by passing two stitches through the entire thickness of the abdominal wall to prevent a dead space, then uniting the edges of the external oblique with a continuous buried suture of silk. He has performed nine of these operations with great satisfaction. As in the operation of McBurney, neither nerves nor vessels are cut, and there is no anesthesia of the skin left as a legacy. When the patient is placed in the Trendelenburg position this incision gives access to the cecal region, and enables the surgeon to dissect the appendix from behind the cecum or from the pelvic ring. This transverse incision passes practically over the base of the appendix and gives more direct ingress than does the incision in the semilunar line.

Floderus[2] considers the **treatment of perforating appendicitis associated with diffuse peritonitis.** He reports a case which was operated upon with success two days after perforation had occurred. The operation was done by Lennander. In suppurating appendicitis the incision should be just above and parallel to Poupart's ligament. Such an incision affords perfect drainage and frequently enables us to open an appendicular abscess back of the peritoneum. The incision parallel to Poupart's ligment is rarely followed by hernia, as it does not cut motor nerves and passes chiefly through tendonous structures. When the surgeon is endeavoring to evacuate an area of appendicular suppuration he must take scrupulous care to protect the general peritoneal cavity from infection. The intestines which are against the abscess-wall should be covered with compresses of sterile gauze saturated with hot normal salt solution, and as soon as pus appears it is mopped up with small compresses. If pus wells up in such great quantities that it cannot be absorbed by the compresses, the patient is placed upon his right side and the assistant makes pressure upon the middle of the abdomen. These maneuvers keep the pus from entering the general peritoneal cavity. When the abscess-cavity is evacuated the surgeon inserts his finger and the cavity is thoroughly cleaned with small compresses. A search is made for the appendix and the diverticulum is removed as near as possible to the cecum. In suppurative cases it is not necessary to ligate the appendix and suture the stump. It is better to clamp it with a pair of hemostats which include the mesentery

---

[1] Boston M. and S. Jour., Oct. 29, 1896.
[2] Arch. f. klin. Chir., Bd. liv., H. 1, 1897.

in the bite and to remove the distal portion of the structure. The forceps are left in place for three or four days. A fecal fistula may form, but this will probably close spontaneously, and in some cases a fecal fistula is actually of value, permitting the escape of gas and favoring the renewal of peristaltic action. After the appendix has been removed the cavity which contains pus is packed with iodoform-gauze, the corners of the wound being approximated by silkworm-gut sutures. It is never wise to irrigate the peritoneal cavity unless pus has escaped into it. If irrigation is necessary, normal salt solution should be employed, and the surgeon keeps on flushing the peritoneum with salt solution until the fluid runs out clear. In some cases the pulse fails during irrigation because of irritation of the splanchnic area, and while this irrigation is being carried out an assistant should carefully watch the pulse. The after-treatment at first consists in stimulants and food to maintain the patient's strength and favor the extrusion of the poison.

Floderns advises that digitalis be given for about three days, and that this drug be succeeded by the use of injections of camphor for one week and the employment of enemata of brandy and grape-sugar. Enemata of brandy and grape-sugar are non-irritant and tend to cause peristaltic movements of the small intestine. Transfusions of salt solution are of benefit by increasing blood-pressure, by increasing the amount of blood, and by preventing a tendency to dryness of tissues. It is always wise to give diuretics. Digitalis and transfusion, of course, tend to produce diuresis. Endeavor to restore peristaltic movements as soon as possible. When the intestines are found much distended at the operation they should be punctured to allow gas to escape. After the operation small doses of calomel frequently repeated followed by a saline cathartic are of value. Repeated enemata are useful in attaining this end, and so is the passage of a rubber tube into the rectum. The patient is not permitted to take food by the mouth until peristaltic power is regained, and is fed by nutritive enemata. The pain which follows operation is due chiefly to distention, and is best treated by enemata and the employment of the tube. Morphin should never be used unless the pain is unbearable, and if it is necessary the dose of $\frac{1}{6}$ gr. should not be exceeded. The great objection to morphin is that it antagonizes peristalsis.

Goulouboff[1] considers the question of whether **appendicitis** can be **an epidemic disease.** He says that in Moscow the disease is very rare, but he has seen it suddenly appear, a great number of people being affected. Appendicitis is due to intestinal microorganisms, and it seems probable that under some favorable conditions the colon-bacilli, streptococci, and staphylococci acquire unusual virulence. Epidemics of appendicitis may be compared to epidemics of tonsillitis, which are not unusual.

Arthur E. Barker[2] furnishes notes on the variety as to time and extent in **the production of inflammatory collections due to appendicitis.** No question is more important than the determination of the time necessary for the formation of a dangerous collection of infectious matter around a damaged appendix. In order to determine this point, Barker has made a study of a large number of cases of appendicitis. These cases may be divided roughly into 3 groups ; (a) those cases in which, because of inflammation and perforation, a serofibrinous peritonitis of greater or less extent has taken place ; (b) those in which an abscess has formed which is incased in plastic matter and is in reality extraperitoneal ; (c) those in which the inflammation is not accompanied by the formation of any fluid outside of the lumen of the appendix. The last group may be left out of consideration for the present. Group (a)

[1] Gaz. méd., Dec. 26, 1896.   [2] Practitioner, Feb., 1897.

includes two classes of cases : (1) those in which there is no evidence of limitation of plastic material, the whole peritoneum being infected ; and (2) those
in which the inflammatory process is widely diffused, but is bounded by plastic matter and is confined to one portion of the abdominal cavity. In group
(*b*) are included (1) cases in which the definitely pointed abscess is within the
peritoneal cavity among the intestines, and (2) those in which the abscess is
behind the cecum, being more or less completely in the areolar tissue of the
pelvis and loin, practically, it will be observed, outside of the general peritoneal cavity. In cases of the variety specified as belonging in class (1) of
group (*a*) ill effects arise with remarkable rapidity. The infection spreads
so quickly because it is virulent and is not limited by plastic material.
This absence of plastic material is due to the effects of the products of the
causative organisms. In such cases acute general septic peritonitis is manifest within a few hours. We note acute pain, fever, vomiting of green
fluid, abdominal distention, and abdominal tenderness, the tenderness, it may
be, being greatest in the right iliac fossa. The prognosis in these cases is
almost hopeless. It is almost impossible to clean thoroughly every portion of
the abdomen. Those rare instances in which a diagnosis of this condition has
been made and which have recovered belong in reality, it seems probable, to
class (2) of group (*a*), cases in which there is infection with less virulent
organisms and in which a certain amount of plastic matter forms and shuts off
a limited portion of the abdomen. Such cases may recover if operated on
early, although their progress is apt to be very rapid. Barker publishes some
very interesting illustrative cases. He states that it is quite clear that wide
differences exist in the speed with which inflammation spreads from the focus
of infection and in the area which may become involved. We have too strong
a tendency to adopt a stereotyped view as to the course of appendicitis. In the
first place, there are anatomic varieties. In the second place, the virulence
of the poison varies very greatly and the power of the body-resistance also
varies. In one case we may have a virulent organism acting on weakened
tissues, no trace of plastic matter being found, and a large serofibrinous effusion filled with septic matter being carried over large areas of peritoneum. In
other instances we have a less intense poison acting on a patient whose tissues
have considerable vital resistance. Here the power of the tissues antagonizes
the poison, and lymph is poured out to wall it in. Between these two extremes occur all sorts of cases. A study of many cases will lead us to be very
cautious in examinations for this disease. We should study each case with
care and endeavor to estimate the type to which it belongs, and should be very
slow to assert dogmatically the time which has passed since the initial disturbance or the extent of the mischief which exists. When we realize the complexity of the process included under the head of appendicitis we will be lenient
in our judgment of all who have found difficulty in the diagnosis and prognosis of such cases.

Robert T. Morris[1] presents **notes on appendicitis.** In 100 cases
which he treated surgically there were 2 deaths. He claims that the death-
rate for the same 100 cases under medical treatment would have been 28 %,
not of necessity in the first attack, but eventually. Appendicitis begins at an
atrium of infection, which is produced in the mucosa or the serosa of the appendix. A common cause of the atrium of infection is traumatism inflicted
by the right psoas muscle. In some cases injury has been inflicted by a concretion, and in rare instances by entozoa. An infective atrium can be produced also by bacterial infection injuring epithelium. An infection-atrium in

[1] Med. Rec., Dec. 26, 1896.

the serosa arises from the extension of inflammation from the serous coat of a neighboring structure. Such an atrium once formed permits the entrance of bacteria or toxins into the appendix tissues. The results resemble those produced by bacterial invasion of the colon, but differ in degree. They differ in degree because of 2 reasons: 1. The outer tube of the appendix prevents rapid swelling of the lymphoid tissue, and as a consequence pressure-anemia occurs in the inner tube, and the compressed tissue becomes a point of least resistance for microorganisms; 2. The chief blood-supply of the appendix comes from one terminal artery, and infective inflammation occludes branches of this artery and bacteria gain the mastery in tissues which are starved of blood. The chief reason why appendicitis is rarer in women than in men has been shown by Robinson. It is because of the fact that in women the appendix is likely to be out of the way of injury by the psoas muscle.

In discussing the diagnosis of appendicitis Morris asserts that the temperature is a matter of no significance whatever in reaching a conclusion. The author positively asserts that the appendix can be palpated. He says that in an acute inflammation the abdomen is boardlike, and palpation is, of course, difficult; but in such a condition it is unnecessary, because we can make the diagnosis without it. In considering the pathology of the disease Morris sets forth his well-known views. In speaking of catarrhal appendicitis he says there is no doubt whatever that catarrh occurs in the beginning of infective appendicitis, and it occurs simultaneously with catarrh of the cecum; but it produces no symptoms which will enable us to make a diagnosis. When symptoms exist sufficiently positive in nature to call for operation the disease has passed beyond the catarrhal stage. Cases of appendicitis can, of course, subside under medical treatment; but patients often die under medical treatment, if not in the first attack, in a later attack, and those who do not die lose a great deal of valuable time by being confined in bed. No one can possibly predict what will become of a patient who is relying on medical treatment.

Morris strongly maintains the value of surgical treatment, because he thinks that each hour of delay permits of more widespread infection, and that each attack renders the ultimately necessary operation more difficult of performance. He believes that a $1\frac{1}{2}$ in. incision is sufficient for many cases—for most cases, in fact, without abscess. This incision greatly reduces the liability to a subsequent hernia. The blunt dissection plan of McBurney is a most excellent procedure. In operating in an abscess-ease adhesions should be broken up and a search made for other abscesses and for the appendix. The free peritoneal cavity can be exposed without any hesitation. Gauze-packing is apt to develop obstruction, and iodoform-ganze may lead to iodoform-poisoning. [We agree with Morris that iodoform-gauze can cause obstruction, and that poisoning is more frequent than is usually supposed and commonly escapes recognition, but nevertheless we do not feel willing to abandon iodoform-ganze. It serves a useful purpose, and we know of no satisfactory substitute. It may be true that the free peritoneal cavity can be exposed without hesitation. We know, in fact, that this is often done. But absence of hesitation on the part of the surgeon may not be equivalent to safety for the patient, and we believe the patient's safety is greater when the free peritoneal cavity is walled off with gauze.]

Byron Robinson [1] writes on the **causes of the pain** in certain cases of chronic appendicitis. He draws his conclusions from many autopsies. In 230 of these autopsies he carefully recorded the conditions in the ceco-appendix region and found that over 70% of adults showed evidence of chronic

[1] Ann. of Surg., Dec., 1896.

peritonitis around the ileo-appendicular apparatus. When the appendix, the cecum, or the lower end of the ileum are in contact with the long range of action of the psoas muscle adhesion is liable to take place, and when this muscle plays upon the bowel, and the bowel contains virulent pathogenic microbes, the injury inflicted by the muscle may be responsible for the migration through the bowel-wall of microbes or toxic products. The same condition of affairs is noticed in the left psoas muscle, to which structure the mesosigmoid can become attached. Of course, the psoas muscle does not cause the peritonitis, but is only a factor leading to the localization of microorganisms. The lower end of the ileum only may be in contact with the muscle. If the appendix ruptures when it is in contact with the psoas, it can become adherent to the muscle, and whenever the psoas muscle acts it will irritate the appendix, induce peristalsis, and cause appendicular colic. All of us have noticed cases of chronic appendicitis in which there were attacks of severe pain unaccompanied by fever, the pain being frequently developed by a long walk or a rough ride. If an appendix is outside of the range of the psoas muscle, exercise does not develop these attacks. Hence we can conclude when a patient with chronic appendicitis suffers considerable pain on muscular exercise, which pain is unaccompanied by elevation of temperature or increased rapidity of the pulse, the trouble is that the appendix is within the range of action of the psoas muscle, and that this muscle is responsible for irritating the diseased appendix into violent peristalsis. [The causative influence of traumatisms inflicted by the psoas muscle, as set forth by Dr. Robinson, is a matter of considerable importance. We believe that the observations above noted are worthy of thoughtful attention. Certain it is that many people who have had appendicitis and who have not been operated upon suffer pain after prolonged or violent exercise.]

J. A. MacDougall[1] calls attention to the fact that in the **treatment of appendicitis** we should consider only acute or inflammatory conditions, for other lesions in this region do not present conditions which are so doubtful or difficult. As the appendix varies in length and in direction, it may give rise to inflammatory phenomena in various situations. Therefore, we should make a rule in any acute inflammation of the abdomen which is not explained otherwise to think of appendicitis as a possible cause. The author considers the predisposing causes of appendicitis to be the situation, the dependent position, the vestigial nature, and the plan of circulation of the appendix. The exciting causes can be divided into catarrhal, ulcerative, and infective. It is probably true that there may be some mechanical causes, as the appendix is liable to become strangulated. Traumatism is not a frequent cause, and this is confirmed by statistics of public schools. The boys in these schools are of the age at which injuries are most frequent, and yet appendicitis is rare among them. It is quite probable that there exists such a condition as catarrhal appendicitis. When this condition exists the mucous membrane becomes congested, the glands overact, the orifice of the appendix is blocked, and as a result the lining membrane of the appendix may be cast off, and when this occurs its regeneration is uncertain. It may be but partially regenerated, a permanent stricture resulting, and at other times granulation-tissue may take the place of the proper lining membrane. The ulcerating form in its relationship with stercoral concretions and foreign bodies has been proved to exist. Concretions act in various ways. Roux, of Lausanne, has proved that a concretion is not in itself dangerous, but becomes a cause of danger because of the changed vital conditions which are apt to occur about it. The presence of a

[1] Brit. Med. Jour., Oct. 10, 1896.

concretion can mechanically produce considerable suffering. The infective form can certainly occur independently of the presence of a concretion, of a foreign body, of ulceration, or catarrh; it may produce gangrene of the appendix, it may cause septic peritonitis without visible perforation, and it is a common cause of general peritonitis. There is no question that the appendix has a strong predisposition to suffer from infection. Ekehorn's experiments have proved that the bacillus coli communis obtained from mild cases of appendicitis is less virulent than that obtained from severe cases, and, therefore, there must be conditions which cause this organism to be at times more virulent or less virulent. Some of these conditions may be found in the degree of tension in the walls of the appendix, in the chemical composition of the contents of the appendix, and in the vital resistance of the individual. Some authors have ascribed the necrotic changes in the appendix to thrombosis and endarteritis, but Hawkins has never been able to find these conditions. The author then discusses the symptoms of appendicitis, the varieties, the diagnosis, the prognosis, and the treatment. When an early operation is decided upon it is usually found to be easy, but may be hard. The abdomen can be opened by either an oblique or a vertical incision. It may be difficult to reach the appendix, or this organ may be found tied down by adhesions, the latter condition being especially common in children. When the appendix is isolated it had better be removed by a circular incision of the peritoneal coat, the retraction of this cuff, the ligation of the mucous canal with fine silk, disinfection of the mucous stump with pure carbolic acid and stitching the peritoneal cuff. When it is found impossible to carry out this proceeding, because of the state of the peritoneum, we can divide the appendix about $\frac{1}{4}$ in. from the cecum after it is ligated and disinfect the stump with pure carbolic acid. In many cases we close the wound without drainage; but if there is even a trace of seropurulent or purulent matter, we must certainly drain. If we do drain, insert a provisional suture to be tied when the drainage is removed, thus obviating the tendency to hernia. When free perforation exists, when there is a rapidly gangrenous process, or when septic or purulent peritonitis has begun, the procedure must be different. If peritonitis exists from some other cause than appendicitis, and if when the patient is anesthetized we discover no evidence of harm in the right iliac fossa, the abdomen should be opened by a median incision. If in doubt as to what is the matter, especially in the adolescent male, suspect the appendix, and first make an exploration of the iliac fossa. When seropurulent or purulent matter is found in the abdomen flush it out with normal salt solution at a temperature of 110°. This fluid can be poured in the cavity out of jugs or can be introduced by means of a large irrigator with a big tube. The appendix should be removed if it can be done easily, but our decision whether to do this or not will be determined by the condition of the patient. If the intestines are found greatly distended, they should be evacuated by incision. Suppose symptoms which call for interference arise after the second day of an appendicitis, a period when it is probable that adhesions are walling in the trouble. In order to reach this diseased appendix we must first open the general peritoneal cavity, and by breaking down adhesions may bring about general peritonitis. McBurney says that although the apparent dangers of causing infection of the noninfected peritoneum are very great, in reality experience shows that the real dangers are not nearly so great. Is the removal of the appendix absolutely necessary? The writer thinks not. If the pus is evacuated, it is justifiable to let the appendix alone. In such a case we should open the abdomen by an oblique incision over the swelling. In some cases it will be found possible to employ Barling's method of stitching the abscess to the parietal peritoneum, and, if we can do this, we will be enabled to protect the general peritoneal cavity. It will be likely, however, that the abscess is in the mass with the coils of intestines, only a thin layer of lymph being on their surface. In such a case iodoform-gauze is packed about the area, the patient is turned on the right side, and the surgeon searches on either edge of the adherent mass to see if pus be presenting there. If pus is not presenting, if pelvic exploration does not discover it, if there is no evidence of its existing behind the cecum, then the finger is directed into the angle between the ileum and the large intestine; it separates adhesions, and when it reaches the focus of trouble is retained there until careful plugging with gauze around the finger walls off the channel which has been made. The finger is withdrawn, pus is sponged up, and a drainage-tube is inserted into the channel which was occupied by the finger. The gauze will be taken out within 48 hours. If it is left in longer, it will be found to be troublesome to remove. There is another way of dealing with the pus-focus, which can occasionally be employed. It may be possible to reach pus behind the cecum by an extraperitoneal incision made 1 inch internal to the anterior superior spine of the ilium. When we operate for distinctly localized abscess about the 8th to the 12th day of the appendicitis, incise freely and make a search for any concretion. The question in such a case is, What shall we do with the appendix? As a rule, it is better to leave the appendix alone. If it is felt lying loose in the pus-cavity or is found projecting from the abscess-wall, it may be removed, and in many cases it is not necessary to ligate. But when the appendix is adherent to the abscess-wall it is a very risky procedure to attempt to remove it, for by so doing we may separate adhesions, and by permitting the escape of septic matter lead to the development of general peritonitis. Or the attempt to remove it may cause intestinal obstruction, the recently separated gut taking on new adhesions and kinking. If from the appendix, which is part of the abscess-wall, fecal matter is escaping into the pus-cavity, no attempt should be made to remove it. Irrigation, the use of gauze-packing, and the employment of frequent enemata will probably be followed by closure of the fistula. If the fistula does not close, it can be closed by operation at a later period. When we come to operate on a fistula of this sort the pus-sac should be thoroughly disinfected, the peritoneal cavity should be protected by gauze, and the gut should be freed by breaking down the adhesions. MacDougall is a believer in the interval-operation when medical means have failed; when the attacks are occurring with increased frequency; when they are so severe as to endanger life, especially if there is an induration, an area of tenderness, or a palpable tumor remaining after the attack; and when there is a constant sense of uneasiness in the iliac fossa. Many surgeons ligate the appendix near its base before its division, but MacDougall prefers the formation of a peritoneal flap after the method of Chiene. Chiene abandoned the ligation of the appendix because he lost a case from intractable vomiting appearing shortly after operation, and apparently due to the tight knot upon the appendix, and he has seen one case in which like symptoms developed, but passed away on the fourth day, at which time, because of softening, tension was relieved. In the debate upon this paper Southam said that it was the custom until quite recently to treat cases of recurrent appendicitis only by medical means. Medical means will relieve the symptoms during an attack, but are powerless to prevent recurrence. He is a believer in the radical cure by the removal of the appendix in the period of quiescence after an attack. He does not believe in removing the appendix after the first attack, because there may never be another attack when this has not been done; but after two well-marked attacks the operation is indicated, especially if the signs persist in a quiescent period. The most important of these signs are tenderness in the appendicular region, swelling, and a sense of resistance. When the appendix is constricted or occluded and bound down with adhesions, particularly if it is distended with fluid which contains a concretion, the patient is always in danger of ulceration and perforation and the formation of pus around the appendix. Southam then reported cases of this sort to illustrate the necessity of surgical operation in recurrent appendicitis. Serious complications are avoided by removing the appendix at an early period.

In the discussion of MacDougall's paper, Rutherford Morison, of Newcastle-on-Tyne, said he also believed in operating where there had been a second attack. He, of course, operates on all cases with abscess and all cases with a very acute beginning. He prefers the oblique incision, because it does not damage the rectus muscle, as an incision in the linea semilunaris is certain to do. Furthermore, the oblique incision, if prolonged into the back, permits of drainage at a dependent situation and allows thorough closure of the anterior portion of the wound, so preventing hernia.

Morison described several kinds of abscess: abscess adherent to the abdominal wall, requiring a simple incision and drainage; cases in which the appendix and the abscess were on the outside of the cecum, in which case the appendix should be removed; cases in which the appendix is behind the cecum with inflammation of the retrocecal tissue, recognized by flexion of the corresponding thigh (in certain of these cases the appendix should be removed); abscess in the pelvis, in which drainage through the vagina in the female and through the rectum in the male is recommended. If an abscess is situated to the inner side of the cecum, the surgeon should practise drainage only, and should not attempt to remove the appendix. The subject was also debated by Charles A. Morton, of Bristol, Jordon Lloyd, of Birmingham, J. Crawford Renton, of Glasgow, T. Jenner Verral, of Brighton, and J. P. Bush, of Bristol.

W. Mitchell Banks said that the statistics of American surgeons filled him with amazement; they seemed to reckon their cases by the score. He has seen a considerable amount of surgical practice in the second city of the British Empire, but any single American surgeon sees more cases in a year than he has seen in all his life. The conclusion he draws is that appendicitis is astonishingly frequent in the United States, or that surgeons operate upon a class of patients which in Liverpool get well without operation. We often find that new operative procedures are employed to too great an extent when first introduced, and later suffer from unmerited condemnation. Operations on the appendix are in the first stage, the stage in which cases are hunted up and triumphs are proclaimed. In many of the cases proper diet, rest, soothing applications, and castor oil would have produced perfectly satisfactory results. Many cases are called appendicitis which have no real cause to be so designated, just as ordinary sore throats are occasionally called diphtheria. Many cases called appendicitis are in reality the old-fashioned typhlitis or colitis, and relapses are almost always due to carelessness in diet, and not to recurrent fits of inherent viciousness upon the part of the appendix. Banks speaks of a case in which the adhesions around the cecum proved that the trouble in reality began in that organ. There seems to be nothing improbable in the old idea that inflammatory products could spread from the interior of the cecum through its unprotected posterior wall and set up trouble in the loose retrocecal connective tissue. Banks says he has opened a great many abscesses which were caused in this manner, and the cases he opened were permanently cured, whereas, if there had been chronic abscess in the appendix, the mischief ought to have returned. He thinks that the case against the appendix has been overstated. It is, however, undoubted that the so-called cases of foudroyant general suppurative peritonitis are caused by intraperitoneal appendicular abscesses which burst. These are the cases where the appendix is in serious trouble and is apt to be found gangrenous. Of course, they should be treated by prompt operation; but Banks denies that these cases are so common as to warrant us in the wholesale operating in which American surgeons would have us indulge. [The ultraconservative view as advocated by Banks is, in our opinion, quite as erroneous and even more dangerous than the ultraradical opinion of those who always operate.]

Mayo Robson [1] reports a series of cases of **appendicitis associated with general peritonitis.** He says the most important points to settle in a case of appendicitis are: Should we operate? and, if so, When? Early operation, performed as soon as the diagnosis is made, will give a much larger rate of recovery than the method of individualizing which most Englishmen still adopt. The removal of the appendix before suppuration or gangrene has taken place, or before firm adhesions form, is a very safe operation. It can be carried out through a small incision with blunt separation of the muscular fibers. If we wait for ulceration to take place, we run the risk of very serious perils and may be forced at any moment to operate under unfavorable circumstances.

Robson then records some striking and interesting cases in proof of his contention. He thinks that cases should be divided into catarrhal, sometimes acute, but generally subacute, and suppurative, which is either acute or subacute. An acute suppurative appendicitis may be followed by perforation or gangrene, and a subacute suppurative appendicitis by a localized abscess. In catarrhal appendicitis operation is not, as a rule, necessary, though it may become necessary because of recurrence of the attack. In suppurative appendicitis operation is always necessary. An acute onset, with a rapid pulse and tenderness over the appendix, without the presence of a tumor, is a condition calling for operation at once. If an attack comes on gradually, if the pulse is not over 100, and if a tumor forms early, we can safely delay. If in the course of any case of appendicitis there is a rigor, with a rise of pulse and temperature, operation should be performed. The pulse is the guide to treatment; the temperature is of but little aid. If opium is given, the general pulse-rate is decreased, and the surgeon may delay too long. When the surgeon is called into a case in which opium has been given it may be necessary for him to reserve his opinion for a few hours, during which period the opium is withheld, and if, during these few hours, the frequency of the pulse increases and the countenance of the patient is seen to be anxious, operation must be performed. If the pain ceases, or is markedly relieved, and this condition is accompanied by pronounced rise in the pulse-rate, gangrene probably exists, and operation must be performed at once. Operation must always be performed if there is abdominal distention with vomiting and rapid pulse. In subacute or catarrhal appendicitis it is well to operate in the quiescent period, as in this period operation is safe. The time to operate is from 2 to 4 weeks after the patient has recovered from the attack. After a second attack it is certain that these seizures are going to recur if the appendix is let alone, and operation should be performed.

In an operation the appendix should almost always be removed. It will occasionally happen that the patient is too ill to bear a protracted search. Sometimes the appendix is not found; Robson had such a case in which

[1] Brit. Med. Jour., Dec. 19, 1896.

pus was evacuated, and in a few weeks the second attack of appendicitis occurred. Sometimes the appendix is so buried in adhesions that it does not seem prudent to separate it, but with very few exceptions the organ should be removed. In the recurrent form it should always be removed, and when there is general peritonitis the perforated or gangrenous appendix ought to be taken away. Doubt arises only where the suppuration is localized and there is fear of opening the general peritoneal cavity in carrying out a search. In such a case the abscess-cavity is evacuated and cleansed. The longitudinal band of the cecum is followed, and this will lead to the appendix. It will be found that the appendix, as a rule, can be removed without greatly disturbing the adhesions ; but even if the peritoneal cavity be opened in our efforts, harm will rarely ensue if the parts are protected with sponges. If a longitudinal band cannot be seen because it is overlapped by inflamed omentum or adherent bowel, it will usually be found possible to feel the hard, rounded appendix when the finger is carried into the abscess-cavity, and when it is felt it can generally be detached. In some cases the appendix actually projects into the abscess and can be removed easily. If none of these conditions exist, a prolonged search is inadvisable. The removal of the appendix is an advantage, because the patient is freed from the danger of subsequent attacks and of the formation of a fecal fistula, and in the search for it we occasionally discover other collections of pus which would be highly dangerous to leave undrained. In operating for general infective peritonitis many patients will die if not operated on early, and in the later stages the percentage of death will be very great. Robson has operated on 6 cases during the year, and has been fortunate enough to save 5 of them. In operating on cases of appendicitis in the quiescent period there is practically no mortality. In operating for acute suppurative cases where the suppuration is limited the mortality is slight. If general peritonitis exists, free irrigation with plain boiled water, or with weak boracic lotion, and very free drainage by several large tubes are desirable. The incision Robson usually employs is 2 to 3 in. in length, somewhat curved, and placed to the inner side of the anterior superior iliac spine, passing over the tender spot known as McBurney's point, which point is usually a guide to the situation of the appendix. When possible, McBurney's method of blunt separation is advisable. In removing the appendix Robson ligates the mesentery with exactitude, makes a circular incision through the peritoneal coat of the appendix and folds this back like a cuff, ligates the mucomuscular portion and amputates it, asepticizes the stump, applies iodoform, turns down the peritoneal cuff and ligates it over the stump. If it is found necessary to ligate the appendix close to the cecum, ligate the stump, invert it into the cecum, and apply Lembert sutures over it. In some cases where the appendix is so much disorganized that it is impossible or undesirable to bring it to the surface apply a catgut ligature around it and cut off the portion beyond the ligature. In closing the abdomen suture peritoneum to peritoneum and muscle to muscle by catgut, and use silkworm-gut for the superficial structures. [Robson's advice always to insist on operating after a second attack is, we believe, sound. A person who has had two attacks is as certain to have a third as a person who has had twelve attacks is certain to have a thirteenth. Many surgeons operate after a first attack, and this procedure is often, though not always, justifiable, though it is not always easy to obtain the consent of the patient. It is not always justifiable to operate after a first attack, because there may never be another. If a first attack was very severe, if it is followed by tenderness or by pain on taking exercise, operation is advisable. That Robson has saved 5 out of 6 cases of general peritonitis is an encouragement to surgeons who are apt to look upon such cases as quite hopeless. Certainly an attempt should be made to save them.]

George R. Fowler [1] presents a study of the **differential diagnosis of lesions of the appendix vermiformis in the adult female.** He tells us that this diagnosis not unusually presents very difficult features, partienlarly in the following respects : 1. The proximity of the appendix to the adnexa may confuse both objective and subjective symptoms ; 2. Acute conditions of one and chronic conditions of the other may coincide ; 3. Acute conditions of both may coexist ; 4. Chronic conditions of both may coexist ; 5. Infectious inflammation of either may cause septic peritonitis, and septic peritonitis may hide the original trouble.

Fowler then reports a case of ruptured right-sided pyosalpinx which had been diagnosticated as appendicitis ; a case of pelvic hematocele which was diagnosticated as appendicitis ; a case of ruptured tubal pregnancy in which a diagnosis of appendicitis was made at first, a proper diagnosis, however, being made before operation ; a case of right-sided hematosalpinx diagnosticated as perforative peritonitis ; a case of ovarian cystoma strangulated from torsion of the pedicle, which was diagnosticated as appendicitis until a vaginal examination discovered the tumor ; a case of perforative peritonitis which resembled ruptured ectopic gestation ; a case of combined acute appendicitis and unruptured tubal gestation combined with suppurative appendicitis ; a case of suppurative appendicitis and pyosalpinx ; a case in which appendicitis had existed 4 years previously, adnexal disease of 3 years' standing, recent impacted gallstone, and dropsy of the gall-bladder ; a case of chronic inflammation of the adnexa, with a neoplasm of the appendix ; a case of left ovarian disease which simulated chronic relapsing appendicitis ; a case of chronic relapsing appendicitis and cystic ovaritis ; a case which gave a history of 3 typical attacks of acute appendicitis, in which operation disclosed an apparently normal appendix and a cystic degeneration of the right ovary ; a case of right pyosalpinx, with adherent and chronically inflamed appendix ; a case of ovarian cystoma and recurrent appendicitis ; a case of chronic appendicitis due to adhesions between the appendix and the stump of a former salpingectomy and oöphorectomy. The main points to be borne in mind in making the diagnosis of appendicitis in the adult female are the following : appendicitis is less frequent in the female than are diseases of the adnexa.   In appendicitis the history is that of a condition coming on acutely ; adnexal disease is apt to show a record of a chronic condition and is usually associated with menstrual disturbances.   In both appendicitis and adnexal diseases there may be acute and radiating pain, or dull and localized pain ; but acute radiating pain is the rule in appendicitis and dull, localized pain in adnexal trouble.   In either condition vomiting may be present, but it is far more frequent in appendicitis.   In adnexal disease we may find tenderness at the site of the appendix, and it may be located elsewhere than in the right iliac fossa in appendicitis.   The reverse, however, is the rule.   The maximum point of tenderness of appendicitis is above the level of the anterior superior spinous process of the ilium.   Vaginal examination which is not forcible rarely discovers tenderness in appendicitis, but readily develops tenderness in disease of the adnexa.   In appendicitis movements of the uterus brought about by the finger rarely produce pain, but are apt to cause pain in tubo-ovarian diseases.   The nearer tenderness is to the bony anterior wall of the pelvis and the median line by external examination or internal examination, the greater is the chance of pelvic inflammation existing, and *vice versa*.   A chill is usually absent in appendicitis, but is fre-

[1] Brooklyn Med. Jour., Apr., 1897.

>b>

quently present in adnexal disease. Fever is apt to be present in appendicitis, but is usually absent in adnexal disease. This rule, of course, is liable to be reversed. Right-sided rigidity of the abdomen is almost invariably present in appendicitis. It is very rarely marked in tubo-ovarian disease, unless the latter condition is complicated with considerable peritonitis.

A tumor in appendicitis is rarely found before the third day; in tubo-ovarian disease it is likely to be found at the first examination. When a tumor exists in appendicitis it is usually located beneath the right rectus muscle opposite the anterior superior iliac spine, or outside of this area. In adnexal trouble it is more easily found by vaginal than by abdominal palpation—in fact, it may be missed entirely by abdominal palpation. An adnexal tumor can be well demonstrated by conjoined touch. It is very rare that an appendical mass can be felt from the vagina. The course of appendicitis is that of an acute trouble, and even in chronic cases there is usually a history of at least one acute attack. In adnexal lesions the course is usually subacute or chronic from the beginning, save when complications intervene. Perforative peritonitis is more common from appendicular trouble than from appendical disease. Perforative peritonitis arising from appendicitis is almost always fatal, because very virulent organisms are set free into the peritoneal cavity. These organisms come from the most dangerous region known—that is, the intestinal canal. The perforative peritonitis of suppurative salpingitis is not nearly so fatal, because the microorganisms are less virulent.

M. Price[1] believes that in all cases in which symptoms closely resembling those of appendicitis appear **free purgation** should be used for the purpose of making the diagnosis clear. If free purgation does not remove the symptoms, it becomes obvious that we are dealing with an inflammation of the appendix or an ulcer of the colon. [Price suggests the use of purgatives for diagnostic purposes. To give purgatives in all cases for diagnosis is not safe. The condition of the patient counts for something. In some cases the administration of powerful purgatives will lessen the chance of recovery when operation is performed.]

William Henry Battle[2] contributes an article upon the **surgical treatment of the diseases of the appendix vermiformis.** He proposes a method of operating for relapsing appendicitis which he thinks has elements of superiority over the methods usually followed. The directions for Battle's operation are as follows: make an incision in the right iliac region with its center corresponding to the point where it is probable that the appendix is attached. The incision is in the direction of the semilunar line and about midway between the iliac spine and the umbilicus. The incision divides the skin and subcutaneous tissue, the external oblique aponeurosis, and the outer portion of the sheath of the right rectus muscle, this part of the incision being an inch from the external margin of the sheath. The rectus muscle is separated from the inner surface of the sheath by means of the surgeon's forefinger and it is retracted toward the middle line. When the edges of the wound are retracted the deep epigastric artery will be visible on the posterior layer of the sheath and can be easily avoided. The posterior layer of the sheath, which is the transversalis fascia, the subperitoneal tissue, and the peritoneum are divided the length of the wound. The small intestines are pushed toward the center of the abdomen, the appendix region is isolated, and the appendix is amputated by the coat-sleeve method, the peritoneum over it being closed by means of Lembert sutures. The abdominal wound is closed by 3 layers of interrupted silk sutures. The deepest sutures bring together the

[1] Med. and Surg. Reporter, Jan. 2, 1897.   [2] Brit. Med. Jour., Apr. 17, 1897.

transversalis fascia and the structures behind the muscle. The rectus muscle is allowed to return to its original position ; the second layer of sutures approximates the external oblique and the anterior portion of the sheath ; the third layer approximates the skin and subcutaneous tissues. In Battle's method the undamaged rectus muscle lies between thoroughly sutured layers which do not accurately correspond, hence the risk of hernia is obviated. The surgeon must be careful not to lose sight of the aponeurosis of the external oblique in suturing. It should always be sutured in order to contribute as much strength as possible. Battle approves of the removal of the appendix after the first attack of appendicitis. Suppurative peritonitis usually takes origin in appendix disease, and early treatment is imperatively necessary. It should be possible to operate some time before vomiting comes on. We should remember, also, that purulent peritonitis is not always associated in its earlier stage with vomiting. [The use of buried silk sutures is liable to lead to trouble in the future. Kangaroo-tendon and chromic gut are better materials. We are not convinced by either McBurney or Battle that muscle is an efficient protection against hernia. The real barriers are the transversalis fascia and the aponeurosis of the external oblique, and the operator who obtains the quickest and soundest union of these structures will be responsible for fewer hernias than other surgeons.]

HERNIA.

Howard A. Lothrop[1] writes upon that obscure condition known as **hernia epigastrica,** and reports 6 cases. These cases are all of interest and worthy of study. In discussing the subject of epigastric hernia he says that we should include under this term all herniæ which are found in the area bounded above by the xiphoid cartilage, below by the umbilicus, and on the sides by the cartilages of the ribs. They so commonly appear in the linea alba in comparison with other sites that they have been termed hernia in the linea alba. The term hernia in the linea alba, however, is unfortunate, as it would also include cases of hernia occurring below the umbilicus and not secondary to the laparotomy. The former term is the preferable one. Such cases were first described in 1743 by Garengeot. He spoke of such a case as a gastrocele, and thought that the stomach was contained in the sac. Something over 100 years ago Richter, in speaking of these cases, stated that the stomach never is in the sac. Maunoir operated successfully in 1882, but until the article by Terrier in 1886 the operation was regarded as too dangerous to be resorted to. This form of hernia is, of course, very rare. In a series of 16,800 cases of all varieties of hernia examined personally by Berger there were 137 cases of epigastric hernia, some of the cases occurring alone, some in combination with other forms of hernia. It is very exceptional to find these cases in individuals less than 18 years of age, and most of the subjects of such a form of hernia are between 25 and 50. Astley Cooper, however, reported 2 congenital cases, and some few cases have been reported as beginning in early childhood. The vast majority of cases are in males of the working-class. As a rule, the onset is insidious. The patient complains for some time of stomach-symptoms before the hernia appears externally or when the hernia is so small as to escape detection without a careful examination. In not a few cases, however, there has been a traumatism followed by very acute local and general symptoms, and the tumor has appeared within a very few hours.

Roth suggests the following classification for such cases : first, cases due

[1] Boston M. and S. Jour., Feb. 25, 1897.

to embryologic defect, the abdominal parietes failing to close in the median line; second, cases due to congenital or acquired thinness of the abdomen; third, Cloquet's theory, which was elaborated by Witzel. This assumes that a slit is formed in the fascia. Into this opening the subperitoneal fat makes its way, subsequently followed by a pouch of peritoneum, which pouch may eventually become occupied by omentum, intestines, or by both. He reports 4 cases due to trauma. This form of hernia may follow almost immediately upon a trauma or some weeks after it. The following causes are set down as productive of a tear in the fascia : a blow in the epigastric region, a fall upon a sharp projection, an injury from a flying missile, sudden and forcible vertical tension upon the muscles of the abdomen, produced, it may be, by coughing or vomiting or by lifting a heavy weight, or by pulling, especially when the arms are lifted and the trunk is extended. Lothrop discusses fully the anatomy of this region and the pathologic anatomy of these herniæ. In discussing the symptoms, he tells us that these cases can be considered clinically under 3 groups : 1. Those in which there are no symptoms of trouble and the tumor is accidentally discovered ; 2. Those which arise insidiously and progress with gradually increasing intensity of symptoms. The symptoms are first referred to the stomach. They are supposed to be due to indigestion, and are made worse by hearty meals and by exercise after eating. Drugs, except morphin, produce no relief. Examination discovers the tumor. The gastric symptoms are probably due to the fact that the omentum pulls on the stomach, the omentum being attached to the hernia. The third group of cases are those in which symptoms follow immediately after the trauma. These cases, as a rule, run a mild course for a great many years, with occasional crises. Adhesions cause the symptoms to become worse. Strangulation is very rare. If the condition is left to run its own course, spontaneous recovery will never take place. Operation, however, is safe and thoroughly curative. Palliative treatment is not to be advised unless there exist some contraindication to operation, such as old age, great prostration, or serious organic disease. The operation is conducted in the same manner as operation for any other hernia. The sac is isolated and opened. If there be a large amount of omentum present, some of it is excised. The contents of the sac are returned to the abdominal cavity and the finger is inserted inside of the ring to see that no adhesions exist at its margin. The sac is excised, the peritoneum is closed with a certain amount of tension, and the abdominal wall is sewed up in layers by buried sutures.

Charles A. Morton [1] records a case of **irreducible hernia.** The patient was a man of 21. When operation was performed it was discovered that irreducibility was due to an omental cyst. Such cysts are extremely rare in any case, but particularly rare in hernial sacs. Mesenteric cysts are occasionally formed by adhesions between the mesenteric folds, fluid which is sometimes chylous collecting in the space thus formed ; but this cyst was of another variety. It resembled the peritoneal sanguineous cysts which have been spoken of by Dr. Fisher.

Stephen Paget [2] writes on the **treatment of cases of strangulated hernia after operation.** He thinks that occasionally the management of these cases is too severe and rigid, and that we often withhold food so long as to actually weaken the patient and interfere with his chances of recovery. Some surgeons have gone so far as to recommend feeding exclusively by the rectum. Under such treatment many cases would die which should recover. There are, of course, two classes of cases of strangulated hernia—what we

[1] Lancet, Dec. 12, 1896. 　　　　　　　　[2] Treatment, Mar. 25, 1897.

might call the sthenic and the asthenic, the asthenic type being met with in people who are aged, ill-nourished, broken down by work, chronic disease, or alcoholism, and especially depressed by pain, vomiting, loss of sleep, and fear of death. Nothing but the most absolute necessity can justify us in keeping these asthenic cases without brandy and food. The reasons given for keeping patients after operation on a rigid plan of treatment are that vomiting must be arrested by keeping the stomach absolutely at rest; that vomiting is very dangerous, as we may rupture a damaged intestine; and that by placing food in the stomach we cause involvement of this injured intestine or damage to it by the passage of feces. Paget questions the validity of these reasons. The vomiting stops of itself. If it lasts beyond a few hours after a successful operation, it is probably due to the anesthetic. When the bowel has been reduced the patient is no more liable to vomit than is a patient on whom any other operation has been done. For the relief of the strangulated hernia small quantities of brandy and milk do not cause vomiting. Therefore, Paget says gives these patients a little brandy just before operation. During the first 12 hours subsequent to operation give small amounts of brandy and water or brandy and iced milk, ½ oz. or 1 oz. every 2 or 3 hours. After the first 12 hours increase the quantity. After the first 24 hours the patient can be allowed to have some tea. Beef-tea is forbidden by some surgeons on the ground that it might cause diarrhea, but a little beef-jelly or beef-tea so strong that it sets to jelly will not cause diarrhea and may often be given with advantage. Opium should not be given; bromid and chloral will produce the good effects of opium without its injurious action. Do not give even a simple enema to move the bowels for at least 7 days. Paget has been speaking of the asthenic cases. All the sthenic cases he says are none the worse for the strict treatment. [That these asthenic patients require stimulation is certain, but that they require it by the stomach in the first 24 hours after operation does not seem so clear. We believe it a sound rule to give nothing by the stomach for the first 24 hours of the post-operative period, giving peptonized milk, brandy, etc., by the rectum.]

Leonard Malloy[1] reports 3 cases of strangulated hernia illustrating the importance of a minor point in the **anatomy of femoral hernia.** Each of these cases was complicated by enlargement of a lymph-gland, so that some doubt was cast on the diagnosis and some complication was encountered in operative treatment. The enlarged gland was the one which Quain tells us is constantly placed in the crural ring, and which Gray states occasionally occupies the interval between the femoral vein and the inner wall of the sheath. Erichsen says that this canal occasionally contains 1 or 2 glands, and Treves has pointed out that an enlarged gland over a hernial sac greatly complicates matters. In the first 2 cases reported by Malloy he thinks that the glandular enlargement was due to the irritation set up by the presence of a hernia in the canal.

Frank P. Williams[2] records a case which he calls masked suppurative peritonitis following violent taxis of strangulated femoral hernia. When the sac was opened it was found to contain the remains of omentum very firmly adherent to it, but no intestine. It was isolated, the internal ring and Poupart's ligament requiring division. A constriction was found at the internal ring. Above the constriction the omentum, being normal, was tied off and amputated, and the stump dropped back. As the sac was about to be ligated before amputation a little pus with a fecal odor was observed coming from the abdominal cavity. Exploration discovered an inverted mass of omentum just

[1] Lancet, Feb. 27, 1897.   [2] Am. Medico.-Surg. Bull., Oct. 31, 1896.

above the ring, from which mass greenish pus welled up in all directions. The incision was enlarged, irrigation with normal salt solution was employed, gauze drains were inserted, a median abdominal incision was made, and gauze drains were packed into Douglas's pouch and on either side of the uterus. No sutures were inserted. The patient died 78 hours after operation, the autopsy exhibiting nothing but indurated omentum and chronic parenchymatous nephritis. [A few months since, a case of strangulated hernia was brought into the Jefferson Medical College Hospital. Forcible taxis had been applied the previous day, and the scrotum was bruised. On operating it was found that the veins of the pampiniform plexus were thrombosed and the perivascular tissue was suppurating. Cultures showed diplococci and colon-bacilli.]

Joseph Ransohoff [1] writes on the **radical cure of umbilical hernia by omphalectomy,** considering in this paper the umbilical hernia of adults only. He considers the various predispositions to recurrence which exist in this form of hernia. In the old operation the remains of the ring were imperfectly approximated, no muscular covering was obtained, interrupted sutures through the whole thickness of the abdominal wall made unequal pressure, and there was a tendency to fat-necrosis and integumentary sloughing. Of late there have been 3 radical improvements made: 1. The umbilical ring is excised; 2. The recti muscles are sutured to each other; 3. The fascia and muscles are sutured by separate layers of buried sutures. Ransohoff then reports three successful cases operated on within two years, a period which he deems is not sufficiently long to justify a positive faith in permanent cure; nevertheless the cure in each case is probably permanent because umbilical hernia when it is going to recur usually does so within a few months of operation. Ransohoff employs a pure metallic suture and thinks it a great aid in permanent cure.

Duplay and Cazin [2] believe that **buried sutures** often cause trouble; that they form points of least resistance and occasionally lead to abscess-formation. They have devised an operation by which they can avoid the use of buried sutures. The sac is drawn well down and tied upon itself, and this knot is kept from slipping by tying a series of knots in the sac or by dividing the sac and tying the two portions together. The external ring and the roof of the canal are sutured by silver wire, which is removed when union has taken place. They report 20 operations, with the most gratifying results.

W. B. Platt [3] writes on the **radical cure of hernia** by implanting a section of sterilized sponge. The patient is kept in bed for 3 weeks. Platt reports 4 cases operated upon by this method.

W. B. De Garmo [4] records **250 Bassini operations** for the cure of inguinal hernia without mortality. These operations were done upon 216 patients, 34 having been operated upon on both sides. Fifty-two of the cases were females and 164 were males. The ages of the patients varied from 5 months to over 80 years. Fifty-five of the operations were on patients under 14, 16 of them were on patients over 60, and 2 were on patients over 80. The cases operated upon in the extremes of life were instances of irreducible or strangulated hernia. Ninety-three of the cases had scrotal hernia, 55 had irreducible hernia, and 16 strangulated hernia. In 55 of the cases it was found necessary to excise some omentum, and this was done by the use of multiple silk ligatures. The largest hernia was 2 ft. in circumference, in a man 53 years of age. The tumor contained omentum, large and small bowel, and a distended bladder. This man stated that

[1] Med. Rec., Jan. 30, 1897. [2] Sem. méd., Nov. 11, 1896.
[3] Bull. Johns Hopkins Hosp., Mar., 1897. [4] Va. Med. Semi-Monthly, June 25, 1897.

22

in urinating he was obliged to press the tumor against the thigh with his hands, but it was only after operation that the exact condition was recognized. Twenty-four hours after operation it was found that he was passing very little urine and the catheter could not be inserted. The next day the bladder was opened through the perineum and free drainage established. There were found in the canal, besides the hernial sac and its contents, the ovary in 3 cases, the testicle in 9, and enlarged veins in a considerable number of cases. It was common to meet with masses of extraperitoneal fat larger than the thumb, in 1 case as large as a good-sized hen's egg. In a number of cases cysts were found which were usually connected with the cord. The time required for the complete healing and discharge of the patient was 14 days in 114 cases; 84 others left the hospital the 21st day. Primary union was obtained in 207 cases. In suppurating cases the infection was invariably immediately beneath the skin, not in the deeper tissue. In 1 case infection was due to a gonorrheal discharge which was not known to exist at the time of operation. Patients whose skin has been abraded by truss-wearing are apt to have suppuration. In only 1 case in which suppuration occurred has recurrence taken place. Double operations were all done at the same time; also some cases of inguinal and umbilical hernia. One man of 52 was operated on the same day for double inguinal and right femoral hernia. In his earlier cases De Garmo used silkworm-gut for suture of the deeper parts, allowing it to remain in. He used it in 12 cases, and in 4 of these much difficulty was experienced later by the sutures coming out. In 8 cases there was no irritation due to the sutures. In 1 case the sutures came out nearly a year after the operation. He therefore abandoned this material and adopted kangaroo-tendon. Kangaroo-tendon gives him perfect satisfaction. The author stated in 1895 that the Bassini operation cured at least 90% of patients. He is now convinced that it will cure at least 95%. Of the 6 recurrences, 3 have been reoperated upon and apparently cured, leaving only 3 lasting recurrences. [De Garmo's paper proves to demonstration that the modern operation for the radical cure of hernia is safe and successful. The fact that suppuration in the operation-wound is apt to arise if the patient has gonorrhea has been encountered in our experience. Before operating on a male for the radical cure of a nonstrangulated hernia it is well to determine if a urethral discharge exists; and if it does exist, operation should be postponed until the urethral disorder is cured. The same trouble De Garmo met with after using silkworm-gut sutures we have seen several times. Kangaroo-tendon, if well prepared, is undoubtedly the best suture-material for hernia operations.]

J. Coplin Stinson [1] writes on the **radical cure of femoral hernia** and the preferable operation. The following operation he considers fulfils the necessary conditions to bring about a cure and obviates the faults of other methods. He makes an incision which begins 1 in. below the spine of the pubis and which is carried upward and outward for about 3 in. parallel with Poupart's ligament. This incision lays bare the sac and the saphenous opening. The superficial fascia is dissected up in order to expose thoroughly Poupart's ligament to the spine of the pubis. The canal and femoral ring are exposed definitely by dissecting up with a blunt dissector the iliac and pubic portions of the fascia lata around the saphenous opening. The sac is free from adhesions to surrounding structures. It is then incised and any internal adhesions are loosened up. If the sac contains omentum, this omentum is removed after ligating the vessels, fixation-ligatures being employed. The neck of the sac is grasped with forceps and pulled down, and the sac with its neck and

[1] Med. Rec., Dec. 5, 1896.

with some of the peritoneum around the neck must be removed, the margins of the cut peritoneum being united by catgut sutures. Fat and glands are then removed from the saphenous opening in the femoral canal. The surgeon retracts the fascia lata, Poupart's ligament, and the deep crural arch, and thus exposes the femoral ring; if it is found that any fat or glands pass into the ring from the subperitoneal connective tissue, such fat or glands are removed. The femoral sheath is grasped with forceps and lifted up, and the inner opening is closed by suturing together the anterior and posterior layers of the sheath, the first stitch being inserted near to the external margin of Gimbernat's ligament, including some of the fibers of this ligament. Several stitches are inserted going toward the femoral vein, the last one being near the septum which separates the ring from the vein, but not close enough to constrict the vein. Poupart's ligament and the deep crural arch are next sutured to the adjacent portions of the fascia lata which covers the pectineus muscle, and to the reflections of the fascia lata which passes behind the femoral sheath, each stitch extending to but not including any muscular fibers of the pectineus. The sutures are passed so as to approach the femoral vein, but near enough to the vein to constrict it. The saphenous opening is closed, the first stitch being inserted close to Poupart's ligament, the needle passing through the pubic portion of the fascia lata on the inner aspect of the saphenous opening and then on the iliac portion of the fascia on the outer side. Suture from above downward, leaving only sufficient room at the lower angle for the full saphenous vein. The skin is closed with catgut or fine silk without drainage. This surgeon prefers a chromicized tendon for the deeper sutures.

Kocher [1] writes on the **radical cure of hernia.** He acknowledges that Bassini's method is useful in certain cases, but he thinks that in subjects who are not in condition to stand a prolonged operation some other method is preferable. Kocher maintains that his own method is safe, even when performed on old subjects, and that whereas suppuration will destroy the result of a Bassini operation, it will not destroy the result of his operation. He discusses 126 cases of inguinal hernia treated by this method. Each one of these cases recovered from the operation. There were 4 relapses. Most of the patients were over 40 years of age. Kocher has modified his operation somewhat from what he originally suggested. He found there was a certain amount of risk of the isolated sac sloughing on account of compression, and he now cuts away the sac. He believes in removing considerable of the protruding peritoneum, and to effect this makes an opening into the peritoneal cavity directly and draws the sac out of this opening, the sac being invaginated so that its serous surface is exposed throughout its whole length. After the sac is removed the peritoneal surface and the other layers of the abdominal wall are sutured.

William B. Coley [2] presents an elaborate article on the **radical cure of hernia,** with a report of 360 cases. He tells us that as late as 1890 Billroth's statistics show a mortality of 6%, with relapses in 32% of cases. Dr. Bull, writing in 1890, reported 3 deaths in 134 cases and 38% of relapses, and came to the conclusion that there is not any prospect of radically curing any form of hernia, most cases relapsing if allowed sufficient time. Sir William MacCormac, in 1893, estimated that the mortality in operations for the radical cure of non-strangulated hernia was 6%. Because of such figures many conservative medical men have been opposed to operations for the radical cure of hernia. That incredulity has given away to a feeling of confidence in the ope-

[1] Centralbl. f. Chir., No. 19, 1897.   [2] Ann. of Surg., Mar., 1897.

ration has been chiefly due to Bassini, of Padua, whose operation has been very generally accepted as the best yet put forth.

Bassini began operating by this method in 1886, and in 1890 published 251 cases, with 1 death and 7 relapses. Robert F. Weir, of New York, was one of the first surgeons in this country to take up Bassini's operation. Bassini's operation is not one of those procedures which give brilliant results only when performed by the inventor. Coley has operated for the radical cure of hernia on 360 cases, with 1 death, a mortality of 0.28 %. This death was due to double pneumonia caused by ether; 326 operations were for inguinal hernia, 25 for femoral hernia, 6 for umbilical hernia, and 3 for ventral hernia. In inguinal hernia 300 cases were sutured with the kangaroo-tendon by Bassini's method, with 2 relapses, 1 with silk suture with 1 relapse; 24 cases of inguinal hernia were treated by sutures of the canal without transplantation of the cord, with 3 relapses. There were 25 cases of femoral hernia without a death and with no relapse; 15 with high ligation of the sac, with purse-string suture of the canal, and 10 with Bassini's method for femoral hernia; 55 operations for inguinal hernia in the female, with no mortality and no relapse. Umbilical and ventral hernia were operated on 9 times, with 4 relapses.

Coley then appends a table of his cases, and it is seen that the total number of Bassini operations is 300, with 1 death and 3 relapses, 280 of these cases having been carefully traced. In 97 % of the cases there was primary union of the wound. The youngest case free from strangulation was 19 months of age, though he operated on 3 cases for strangulation which were all under one year of age. Only 8 cases of nonstrangulated hernia were operated on under four years of age. The oldest patient was 70, the operation being performed for an irreducible omental hernia. Some surgeons have opposed operation for hernia in children, because they think that most cases can be cured by means of trusses, and because they believe the operation in the child is less certain in its results and more dangerous than in the adult. Both of these positions are untrue. In collecting the cases of adult hernia observed in the Hospital for Ruptured and Crippled during the past four years that gave a history of hernia in early life, Coley has already found about 400 such cases. This disproves the idea that all herniæ can be cured by trusses. The operation in children is no more dangerous than in adults. Adding together Broca's, Felizet's, and his own cases, we have 832 cases with 4 deaths, a mortality of less than $\frac{1}{2}$ of 1 %. In fact, the period of childhood and youth is an especially successful period in which to do an operation for the radical cure of hernia. We should not lose sight of the fact that this same period is the most favorable for nature to effect a cure either unaided or aided by a truss. Out of 7000 ruptured children Coley selected 250 to operate on. He does not think that we should operate in children until a truss has been tried for a year or two without benefit. There is an exception to this rule; in femoral hernia operation should be advised at once, for there is almost no chance that a truss will cure. Irreducible hernia, or adherent omentum and hydrocele, suggests the necessity for early operation. In cases where the gut cannot be successfully retained because of lack of care it is generally wise to operate. In the adult operations may be advised in most cases of inguinal and femoral hernia up to the age of 50, unless there be contraindications. Coley advises us not to operate on very large irreducible hernia, especially in stout people. If there are numerous adhesions, it is necessary to remove great masses of omentum, and the operation is thus rendered a formidable procedure; very few of these cases are permanently cured. Inguinal hernia in women yields admirable results when operated on by the Bassini method. The round ligaments should be dissected from the sac and the canal sutured in three layers with kangaroo-tendon. The operation is just the same in the female as in the male, excepting the transplantation of the cord. The round ligament is permitted to drop back beneath the lowermost layer of sutures. In femoral hernia the results are admirable. Six of Coley's cases of femoral hernia were under 10 years of age.

The method of Bassini for the treatment of femoral hernia consists in suture of the canal by two rows of interrupted sutures. He thinks the old method of simply ligating the sac and making no attempt to close the femoral canal should be abandoned.

In discussing rare forms of hernia, cecal and appendical, he states that in 14 cases the cecum and appendix, one or both, were found in the hernial sac. In 6 the appendix alone was found; in but 3 of these was the appendix removed. Three of these cases were of that very rare variety which he has called inguinoperineal. The hernia in these cases is reduced through the inguinal canal, but it passes alongside and beneath the scrotum until it occupies the perineal region. In every case the testis was found in the perineum, at the bottom of the sac; and the maldescent of the testis is undoubtedly responsible for this hernia. In one case it was necessary to remove the testicle; in another this gland was dissected loose and transplanted into the scrotum.

Coley next explains the technic of Bassini's operation, and advises the use of kangaroo-tendon sutures. Sutures should be placed above the cord, the cord passing between the two upper sutures. Many surgeons get an imperfect result in Bassini's operation because they fail to dissect back the aponeurosis of the external oblique sufficiently, especially on the inner side. Coley always uses interrupted sutures for the deeper layer, and unites the aponeurosis with a continuous suture of kangaroo-tendon. The skin is closed with fine catgut. The wound is dressed at the end of a week or ten days after operation. The dressing consists of iodoform-gauze and moist bichlorid gauze. In children the dressing is reinforced by a plaster-of-Paris spica extending from the ribs to the knee. Patients who have been operated on by Bassini's method should be kept in bed for 2 to 2½ weeks, and be permitted to leave the hospital at the end of 2½ to 3 weeks. In but two or three instances has a truss been advised after operation, most patients having been sent out without a support of any kind. Coley believes Bassini's method from a practical and a theoretical standpoint is superior to all other methods. He opposes Packard's contention that the hernial sac does not occupy the inguinal canal at all, but in the large majority of cases of oblique inguinal hernia is really ventral, only making its way out at the external ring, and therefore seeming to pass through the canal. Coley believes that the hernial sac does bear intimate relations to the cord. He has studied the relation of the sac to the cord in 271 cases of inguinal hernia, and in 269 of these cases the sac has been found in intimate contact with the cord. This was true in acquired hernia and in congenital hernia in adults and children. If we dissect with care, we will find the infundibuliform process enclosing both the sac and the cord, the cord itself resting in absolute contact with the sac. The two cases in which this condition did not obtain were both direct hernia, a form of hernia which is much rarer than is generally supposed. In these cases the cord was anterior to the sac and outside of the layer of fascia referred to. A careful study of the evidence will convince us that the cord plays a most important part in the induction of oblique inguinal hernia, and that the operations of Bassini and Halsted have a rational foundation.　Coley then gives a detailed report of his cases. [Coley's study and De Garmo's paper constitute an absolute answer to those who do not believe in the radical operation.　Such a low mortality speaks for itself.　A very important portion of the article is that dealing with the operation in the ease of young children.　The general impression has been that young children are unfavorable subjects.　Coley shows that they are very favorable subjects.　He is, however, judicious and conservative.　He believes that most cases of inguinal hernia in children are capable of cure by a truss, and out of 7000 cases he selected but 250 for operation.　We consider that Coley disproves Packard's hypothesis that in most instances the so-called inguinal hernia is really ventral.]

DISEASES OF THE LIVER, GALL-BLADDER, PANCREAS, AND SPLEEN.

Christopher Martin[1] reports a case of **rupture of the liver** successfully treated by abdominal section.　The symptoms were those of intraperitoneal hemorrhage and peritonitis.　The diagnosis of rupture of the liver was made and operation was performed 30 hours after the accident.　The abdomen was opened in the middle line; an immense quantity of black blood escaped, and the liver was found to be ruptured.　There was a tear between 1 and 2 inches deep on the under surface of the right lobe over the parietal fissure.　The signs of peritonitis were obvious.　The abdomen was cleared of blood by irrigation with hot water and during irrigation a fragment of liver-substance floated up.　The question of how to deal with the rent was somewhat difficult. If it had been on the anterior border or upper surface of the liver, it could have been sutured with catgut or plugged with iodoform-gauze; but as it was on the posterior surface and extended backward and upward suturing and gauze-plugging were both out of the question.　The operator determined to rely on the hemostatic effect of irrigation with hot water, removal of all the effused blood from the peritoneal cavity, and maintenance of drainage.　The abdomen was thoroughly washed out and sponged.　An incision was made above the pubes and a tube was inserted.　A glass drainage-tube was inserted through the epigastric incision and carried down to the rent in the liver.　The abdominal wounds were sewed up with silkworm-gut.　For a number of hours after the operation there was a profuse bloody discharge from the lower drainage-tube and almost nothing from the upper tube.　This patient recovered.

Martin says that the chief causes of death after a rupture of the liver are shock, hemorrhage, and peritonitis.　The injury is excessively fatal, but not absolutely mortal.　There have been some reported instances in which the signs and symptoms all pointed to rupture of the liver, but the patient recovered.　There have been four reported cases where the patient survived the accident many days and died from other causes, in each case a postmortem examination showing that the liver had been ruptured and that spontaneous cure was taking place.　It seems probable, however, that 99 % of such cases die rapidly unless operation is performed.　The operation done on this case saved life because of the free irrigation of the peritoneal cavity with hot water and the thorough drainage.　The irrigation arrested the bleeding from the tear in the liver and removed a great quantity of blood and lymph from the peritoneal cavity.　The drainage-tube is itself a valuable hemostatic.　When the blood is drained away as soon as it is poured out the natural arrest of hemorrhage is promoted.　The progress of peritonitis is checked by the removal of

[1] Birmingham Med. Rev., May, 1897.

the blood, lymph, and bile. The drainage obtained by making the suprapubic opening is a matter of the first importance.

Terrier and Auvray[1] write upon traumatisms of the liver and bile-ducts, and consider 46 cases which are found in literature, of which number 33 recovered and 13 died. The cases which recovered were those operated upon before there had been a great amount of hemorrhage and before marked peritonitis had developed. These surgeons maintain that exploratory laparotomy should be performed as quickly as possible when there is a traumatic injury of the liver. The nature of the lesion is thus definitely recognized and the surgeon is enabled to stop hemorrhage, for the effusion of blood not only produces exhaustion but is liable to infect the peritoneum. When the hemorrhage is arrested or if it has already ceased the wound in the liver is sutured.

Vanverts[2] presents a paper upon the treatment of rupture of the liver. He tells us that after any serious injury of the abdomen the patient passes through a condition of collapse, through a stage when the diagnosis must be uncertain, through a stage when the signs of hemorrhage become apparent, and through a stage of slowly rising complications. The stage of collapse is usually pronounced, but in some cases it is absent. It is treated as any other collapse. During the stage when the diagnosis is uncertain hemorrhage is to be feared and the patient must be kept perfectly quiet and recumbent. An ice-bag is placed over the liver and the patient is watched attentively to determine the first sign of hemorrhage or of peritonitis. The beginning of either hemorrhage or peritonitis calls for immediate laparotomy. The incision should be in the middle line and should be long enough to permit the surgeon to see the liver. The organ must be carefully felt with the finger, especially the upper surface and posterior surface. There are several recognized methods of treating a rupture. We may employ the cautery, we may plug the wound, we may suture it. The best results are obtained by plugging with gauze, one end of the gauze emerging from the abdominal wound. The plug of gauze should be retained at least 48 hours, but should not be left later than the fourth day. If it is removed earlier than 48 hours, hemorrhage may occur. If it is left later than the fourth day, a biliary fistula may result. If it is seen that a large vessel has been lacerated, a ligature should be applied. When there is a laceration extending deeply into the liver-structure the edges of the wound in the liver should be brought together by sutures. When peritonitis begins there is very little chance of saving life, and the only chance is by laparotomy and drainage.

Orville Horwitz[3] publishes a case of rupture of the liver. Five weeks before admission to the hospital this man had a fall in which he struck his right side and testicle. He had been confined to bed for two weeks and had gone about again. Some few days before his admission into hospital a swelling appeared below the margin of the ribs on the right side which was attended with pain. It was soft and the seat of a pseudofluctuation; aspiration brought away 1½ pints of blood. Horwitz found that the abdomen was greatly distended and tender; the swelling was the size of an infant's head at birth. There was a slight diarrhea, the stools being chalky. The left testicle was enormously swollen and there had been an effusion of serum into the tunica vaginalis testis. The temperature was 97°, the pulse 158, and there was some jaundice. An incision was made into the swelling, a large partially organized blood-clot was turned out, and a tear 3½ in. long and 2½ in width was found in the right lobe of the liver. Adhesion had taken place between the peritoneum

---

[1] Rev. de Chir., Oct. 10, 1896. [2] Arch. gén. de Méd., Jan., 1897.
[3] Therap. Gaz., July 15, 1896.

and the liver, limiting a large sac, which contained the blood-clot, and this sac was connected with the peritoneal cavity by an opening $1\frac{1}{2}$ in. in diameter, through which protruded a piece of congested omentum. The abdominal cavity was full of bloody serum. An incision for drainage was made in the left iliac fossa. The cavity was irrigated with saline fluid, a drainage-tube was inserted into the iliac incision, and the wound in the liver was packed with iodoform-gauze. The patient died the next day and no postmortem was permitted. The author states that as far as he has discovered death has invariably resulted from rupture of the liver-substance. [The view that a rupture of the liver is of necessity a fatal accident has gone down before the surgical achievements of recent years. In 1887 Edler published statistics of traumatic injuries of the liver. This table contained 543 cases, the mortality-rate being about 67 %. Incised wounds show a mortality of 64.6 %, gunshot-wounds of 55 %, and ruptures of 85.7 % (Schlatter, in *Beiträge zur klinischen Chirurgie*, Band xv., Heft ii., 1096). The *Annals of Surgery* for April, 1897, reviews Schlatter's work, and herein valuable facts will be found in concise form. Many recoveries have followed direct suture of wounds in the liver.]

F. Winson Ramsay [1] records a case of Glenard's disease in which he practised **fixation of the liver and of both kidneys.** The woman was 39 years of age. She had a tumor in the left hypogastric region, which was found to be a floating left kidney. It was operated on by Vulliet's method—that is, stitched in place by means of the split tendonous structure of the longissimus dorsi muscle. The operation did a great deal of good. In about 6 months a tumor appeared on the right side, which was found to be the right kidney, which organ was anchored by the same method. On sitting up nausea and vomiting returned, and it was discovered that the right lobe of the liver occupied the middle of the abdomen below the umbilicus. The abdomen was opened in the middle line, the left kidney was felt for and was found to be firmly anchored. The right kidney was well fixed, having only slight lateral mobility. The liver moved with great freedom, the suspensory ligament being much elongated. The upper surface of the liver was rubbed with aseptic gauze to promote adhesion. The round ligament was transfixed close to the liver; a silk ligature was passed through it and around it and tied. One end was passed from above downward around the costal cartilage of the 7th rib. The liver was firmly pressed into place and the 2 ends of the ligature were tied. The liver was thus fixed by means of the round ligament and the thoracic wall. As the extreme right lobe of the liver seemed to be mobile, a double suture of kangaroo-tendon was passed through the liver 2 in. from its right border and through the adjacent parietes; when this ligature was tied the liver was fixed in excellent position. The other organs of the abdomen were examined : the spleen was found in normal position ; there was not any lengthening of the mesentery or the mesocolon. The right ovary being cystic it was removed. This patient recovered, with complete relief of all the symptoms.

Tuffier [2] presents a paper upon **neoplasms of the liver** in which he discusses the diagnosis and treatment. He says that it is often impossible to make a diagnosis unless exploratory celiotomy is performed, and in some cases even when exploratory incision has been made we cannot form a diagnosis without puncturing the tumor, and puncture is a dangerous procedure and has proved fatal from hemorrhage in not a few cases. It is always wise to feel the hilum of the liver to determine if enlarged glands exist. Such glands indicate secondary deposit from a malignant growth, and whenever they

[1] Brit. Med. Jour., May 8, 1897.   [2] Gaz. hebdom. de Méd. et de Chir., Jan. 28, 1897.

are found it is unnecessary to make a puncture. Because we do not find them, however, does not prove that a malignant growth is absent. There might be a secondary malignant growth, in which case the glands would not be enlarged, because metastasis would be by way of the venous channels and not by the lymphatic vessels, but a primary cancer of the liver invariably causes enlargement of the glands in the hilum. The question of how to arrest hemorrhage is of vast importance in operating upon the liver. We frequently find the dilated veins surrounded by tissue that crumbles away at a touch, and in such cases the temporary arrest of hemorrhage by compression of the pedicle of the liver by means of the fingers is a valuable procedure. He showed by experiments on animals that he could thus arrest a very severe hemorrhage, and he finds by studies upon the dead body that such pressure can be easily made without producing any damage in the human being. Of course, its exact value can only be determined by clinical experience. He advises that the left index finger be passed through the foramen of Winslow and the structures of the pedicle be compressed with the thumb.

David Drummond and Rutherford Morison[1] report a case of **ascites due to cirrhosis of the liver** cured by operation. The idea of the operation is to remove portal obstruction. Drummond made a series of postmortem studies on cases of cirrhosis of the liver, and in many cases where ascites were absent demonstrated that vascular adhesions existed connecting the parietes to the liver. In one case the cirrhosis had existed for almost 20 years, and yet death resulted from some other cause. In many of these cases free communication was found to exist between the portal and systemic veins. Such a communication seemed to explain the absence of ascites. It seems probable that an enlargement of the channels which normally exist between the portal and systemic circulations is sufficient in some cases to prevent the development of ascites in cirrhosis of the liver, but in most cases an accessory circulation is required. The above facts would lead us to infer that the establishment of a new accessory circulation ought to cure ascites due to liver cirrhosis. Two cases of ascites have been operated on. In the first case the clinical diagnosis was not verified at the operation or by a postmortem examination, and doubts remain as to whether the ascites was really due to liver cirrhosis. The operation in this instance failed to cure. In the second case there was not the slightest doubt of the diagnosis, for the liver was the typical hobnailed liver. In this case the operation proved a brilliant success, and the dying patient was restored to apparently perfect health. The abdomen was opened below the umbilicus; the ascitic fluid was emptied out; the liver was inspected and found to be cirrhotic. The abdomen was dried with sponges and the parietal peritoneum was scrubbed with sponges. The peritoneum covering the liver and the spleen and the portions of the parietal peritoneum opposed to them were specially scrubbed. The omentum was sutured across the anterior abdominal wall. A glass tube was left in Douglas's cul de sac and the abdominal wound was closed by silk sutures. In order to retain the parietal peritoneum in contact with the visceral peritoneum straps were passed circularly over the epigastrium down to the drainage-tube in the hypogastrium. This patient made an absolute recovery.

James F. Gemmel[2] reports a case of hepatic abscess in which he practised aspiration and in which recovery ensued. The diagnosis was rendered certain by introducing a small exploring-needle. About a week after this the swelling was aspirated by means of Allen's surgical pump, about 30 oz. of fluid being withdrawn. The action of the pump was reversed, the cavity was filled with

[1] Brit. Med. Jour., Sept. 19, 1896.　　　　　　　　[2] Lancet, Dec. 19, 1896.

Condy's fluid and was emptied again, and this process was repeated over and over until the fluid ran out clear. The swelling gradually reappeared after this aspiration and then suddenly passed away, the disappearance being followed by a profuse evacuation of pus per anus. [We utterly disbelieve in the treatment of abscess of the liver by aspiration, because pus may get into the peritoneal cavity; because much more damage may be done by a blind puncture than by an open incision; and because aspiration usually fails to cure. Jacobson has pointed out that puncture is useless when multiple abscesses exist.]

John O'Conor[1] publishes a clinical contribution to the **surgery of the liver.** He reports a case of liver-abscess cured by hepatotomy. An incision was made over the swelling; the peritoneum was opened; and the liver was adherent to the parietes; and a director was carried into the liver, where an abscess was found at a depth of a ¼ in. The opening was enlarged by means of forceps, pus was evacuated, a drainage-tube inserted, and the cavity irrigated with Condy's fluid. The patient recovered. In case II. there were abscess of the liver and empyema. The needle of the aspirator was carried into the right pleural cavity and a little pus was removed. An anesthetic was given, a portion of the 6th rib excised near the axillary line, and a great quantity of very foul pus evacuated from the pleural sac. There was found to be a dense and fluctuating swelling pushing up the diaphragm, but there was no opening leading into the pleura. The pleura of the diaphragm and the diaphragm itself were incised. The liver was found to be adherent. A trocar was inserted and 6 pints of pus removed. A drainage-tube was carried into the abscess-cavity and no sutures were introduced into the wound on the chest-wall. This patient improved greatly and got almost well, but later symptoms of septicemia returned and the patient died about 10 weeks after operation. Postmortem examination showed that there was a sinus lined with healthy granulations passing from the upper border to the center of the liver. This was all that remained of the great abscess-cavity. Three inches internal to this sinus a small abscess was found which was superficial in the upper hepatic border, and from this a small sinus passed through the diaphragm into the anterior mediastinum, in which region pus was found, and this mediastinal focus joined the right pleural cavity by a small opening. This case is very instructive, as it shows the fact that even when we have succeeded in reaching a large hepatic abscess a more deadly satellite-abscess may be in existence. Another fact which this case shows is that the aspirating-needle is an unreliable means of looking for small abscesses. The 3d case is one in which abscess of the liver was treated by transthoracic hepatotomy. This patient recovered. It was thought for some little time that the man labored under typhoid fever, and then tuberculosis was suspected; finally, it was determined to explore the liver. There was a tender spot over the liver, and in this region a long hypodermic needle was inserted. Pus was thus discovered. The needle was left in place and a bistoury was carried into the abscess along the needle as a guide. The needle was withdrawn and a pair of forceps was pushed along the blade of the knife; the knife was withdrawn and the blades of the forceps were opened and thus the incision was dilated. A drainage-tube was introduced. This patient recovered. It may be thought that this was a rash manner of opening the abscess, but the patient's condition was so desperate that an anesthetic would probably have proved fatal. He then reports a case of liver-abscess in which hepatotomy was followed by recovery, and another case of liver-abscess in which transthoracic hepatotomy was followed by recovery.

[1] Ann. of Surg., May, 1897.

A. D. Bevan[1] recommends a **new incision in the surgery of the bile-ducts.** He has tried all of the usual incisions and thinks there are objections to each one. These usual incisions do not afford sufficient room for extensive work unless they are made very long, and if they are made very long hernia is apt to ensue. It is impossible for the surgeon to tell before he opens the abdomen for the performance of an operation upon the bile-ducts how extensive an operation may be necessary, and he should make an incision which will be equally suitable for the exploration and simple operation or an operation of great magnitude. Bevan divides his incision into a primary incision and an extended process. The primary incision is used for exploratory purposes or cholecystotomy. It is the shape of an italic letter *ʃ*, along and even through the outer edge of the rectus muscle shown in the heavy line in Fig. 23. The extended parts of the incision are added if required. These

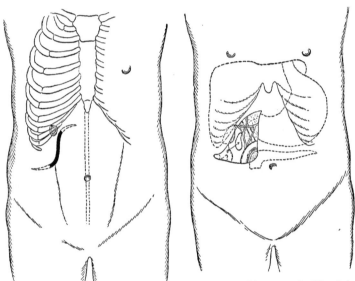

FIG. 23.—A new incision in surgery of the bile-ducts: the heavy line indicates the primary incision; and the light lines, the extended portions of the incision (A. D. Bevan, in Jour. Am. Med. Assoc., June 26, 1897).

FIG. 24.—The abdomen opened and the anterior layer of the lesser omentum removed. The gall-bladder, cystic, hepatic, and common ducts, portal vein, and hepatic artery and branches are in view. Arrow is in the foramen of Winslow (A. D. Bevan, in Jour. Am. Med. Assoc., June 26, 1897).

extended parts are shown in the faint lines in Fig. 23. The extended portions may be an inch in length or 3 in. in length. This incision gives very free access to the gall-bladder and bile-ducts. The edges can be retracted broadly without tension. A very small amount of the abdominal nerve-supply is injured by the incision, even though it is made of considerable length, because the extended parts are practically parallel with the nerve-supply of the abdominal muscles. Partial division of the rectus and of the obliques and transversalis enables us to separate the incision very widely without tension. It is very improbable that a hernia will result, because the incision is close to the costal

[1] Jour. Am. Med. Assoc., June 26, 1897.

348   *GENERAL SURGERY.*

arch. Furthermore, it is well known that a cicatrix in the upper part of the abdomen is not likely to yield and produce a hernia. The structures exposed by this incision are seen in Fig. 24. Bevan closes the incision .by passing silkworm-gut through the entire abdominal wall and then sutures the abdominal muscles and aponeurosis with buried catgut and ties the silkworm-gut sutures.

Carl Beck [1] debates the question, **When shall we operate for cholelithiasis?**—and reports some interesting cases to illustrate his views. His opinions may be summed up as follows : cholecystotomy should be performed as soon as the diagnosis of acute cholecystitis is made, and the same operation should be performed in chronic hydrops of the gall-bladder. It should be performed when acute attacks of biliary colic associated with fever return for a second or third time. It should be performed when jaundice is present for more than 4 weeks. It should be performed in gall-stone ileus. In all obscure cases where signs resembling peritonitis are found in the neighborhood of the gall-bladder exploratory laparotomy should be performed. Beck is a warm advocate of the operation of cholecystotomy, because it does not matter how thoroughly the gall-bladder is exposed small stones are very apt to be retained, and such stones will be discovered only if the opening is left in the gall-bladder for a reasonable time. In the so-called ideal cholecystotomy the gall-bladder is sewed up, and these small stones will not be discovered and will remain.

F. Lange [2] considers the **surgical significance of gall-stones.** He tells us that when retained in the gall-bladder symptoms are very rarely present, but that the symptoms are met with when the stone begins to pass through a cystic duct or the common duct. A large solitary stone may become impacted in a cystic duct, but impaction may be produced by many small stones. If the gall-stone is impacted in the common duct, the symptoms of damming up of the bile are certain to appear, and not unusually inflammation of the gall-bladder or abscess of the liver follows such a condition. It is not uncommon for a large stone to be arrested at the duodenal orifice, and when the stone is arrested in this situation it may form a fistula into the duodenum. The gall-stone may find its way through the wall of the abdomen or into some viscus from any part of the gall system. There is a very serious complication that is liable to be met with in patients with jaundice, and that is a strong tendency to hemorrhage during operations. In operating Lange is a believer in incision parallel to the rib-borders. Small size of the liver constitutes a barrier to the easy performance of the operation, because this organ when it atrophies sinks high up back of the ribs. When the liver is found in this position it is advisable to excise several of the costal cartilages. A very large liver, especially in fat individuals, is a complication. It is better to drain the gall-bladder by means of a long tube. so as to have the benefit of siphonage, and we should remember the liability of this tube to block up with fragments of blood-clot or agglutinated mucus. Irritant solutions should never be injected into the gall-bladder, for they inevitably cause colic, and if they reach the common duct or the hepatic duct will set up inflammation. Normal salt solution or boiled water is the only material proper to inject. Before opening the gall-bladder aspirate away as much of the bile as possible, having first surrounded the gall-bladder with gauze.

F. Lange, in another article,[3] considers the indications for surgical operations on the common bile-duct in cases of gall-stone disease. He tells us that in quite a number of cases in which gall-stones pass the common duct there is

[1] N. Y. Med. Jour., May 8, 1897.   [2] Bull., Johns Hopkins Hosp,. Feb., 1897.
[3] Med. News, May 1, 1897.

not distinct jaundice, and it is very rare that a stone in the common duct produces prolonged and complete obstruction to the flow of bile. Usually more or less bile passes through, and in other cases the stone acts as a ball-valve, as has been shown by Fenger, and allows of a free flow of bile from time to time. The mechanical lesion alone of stone in the common duct is, as a rule, very well tolerated. The degree of obstruction determines whether the stagnating bile will produce sufficient trouble to demand operation. It is quite true that the long persistence of jaundice diminishes the safety of operation because of the great tendency to hemorrhage ; therefore it is wise in cases which require surgical aid to operate before there is persistent jaundice. The group of cases to be noted are those in which complications arise ; complications due to the infectious process, as when we have cholecystitis and cholangitis or ulceration from impaction. It is not unusual for cases to recover in which ulceration occurs by the stone passing into a viscus ; such cases admit of expectant treatment. Suppose that there is a history of a large stone having been passed by the rectum. If attacks of colic are repeated, we may assume the probability that a stone will again pass spontaneously. If the symptoms of absolute obstruction or septic infection become marked, an operation is absolutely demanded. When infection is manifest by acute fever it means acute cholangitis, and surgical operation must be performed. We should first perform cholecystotomy, and the condition of the patient at the time of operation determines whether we shall attack the common duct at that time or not. The majority of cases are chronic or subacute, and may result in dilatation of the duct, atrophy of the glandular structure of the liver, cholangitis, pericholangitis, and abscess of the liver. In view of the danger of these complications the only rational treatment is to perform an operation which relieves the obstruction and promotes a free flow of the bile which is being secreted. [Operations for gall-stone performed early—that is, before the concretion has gotten into the common duct—show almost no mortality. Kehr, of Halberstadt, estimates the mortality of choledochotomy at about 6 %, and of cholecystectomy at 6 %. The same surgeon has reported 127 operations upon the gall-bladder, with 1 death, a remarkable and encouraging showing.]

A. W. Mayo Robson's Hunterian Lectures [1] contain a masterly exposition of the **diseases of the gall-bladder and the bile-ducts,** and are certain to be considered in the future as a most authoritative discussion of the entire subject. After considering congenital malformations, catarrh of the gall-bladder and bile-ducts, and catarrhal cholecystitis Robson takes up suppurative inflammation of the bile-passages, simple empyema, acute cholecystitis, and gangrene of the gall-bladder. In speaking of the treatment of infective and suppurative cholangitis he states that it is useless to apply treatment unless we puncture and drain the infected contents of the bile-passages. Therefore, cholecystotomy must be carried out and drainage must be continued until the bile is sterile or nearly sterile. If the pus is found localized in the liver, the area must be incised and drained. General means of treatment include the following : laxatives, intestinal antiseptics, sedatives for the pain, and the treatment of symptoms as they arise. The first credit of operating for this condition belongs to Terrier.

Robson then presents the subjects of **stricture, ulceration,** and **rupture of the bile-duct** due to injury. In speaking of gunshot-wounds he cites the case reported by Hans Kehr as especially noticeable. In this case there was a gunshot-wound of the gall-bladder ; laparotomy was performed, the wound was sutured, and the patient recovered. Extravasation of healthy

[1] Lancet, May 29, 1897.

bile is by no means as serious as is extravasation of diseased bile, and when a rupture takes place while the gall-bladder is distended or there is disease of the gall-ducts the bile is in an infected condition and causes a diffuse peritonitis which will inevitably end fatally unless an operation is performed at once. Robson speaks of a case in which he opened the abdomen, evacuated several pints of bile and pus, washed out the peritoneal cavity, passed one drainage-tube between the liver and diaphragm, one downward toward the pelvis, and one into the right kidney pouch, and this patient recovered. He alludes to a case reported by Dr. Monier Williams in which typhoid ulceration of the gall-bladder, which perforated, was successfully treated by abdominal section, and refers also to the well-known case of Marmaduke Sheild, in which a patient in the 51st day of typhoid fever was subjected to laparotomy. The gall-bladder was found thick and rigid and congested, with an ulcer the size of a three-penny piece near its neck, and contained 1½ oz. of offensive pus. The abdomen was washed out, the distended intestines were emptied by puncture, and gauze-packing with drainage applied. The patient was cured. When the gall-bladder ruptures from sudden pressure there must be a predisposition to rupture produced by ulceration or by prolonged distention. The danger of such an accident is great in these conditions, and patients with distended gall-bladders should always be operated upon, because otherwise they live in a "fool's paradise." Massage of a distended gall-bladder is futile, and its application is the height of folly. An attempt to force an impacted stone onward by pressure is very likely to rupture the wall of the gall-bladder or bile-ducts or cause perforation through an ulceration. In some cases even when primary perforation takes place an abscess-cavity is formed bounded by lymph, which cavity may again rupture and cause fatal peritonitis. The gall-bladder may perforate into an adjoining organ. It may perforate, for instance, into the liver, producing the signs of abscess of the liver; perforations of the common duct may occur into the pancreas, causing acute pancreatitis. If perforation takes place into the stomach, duodenum, or colon, the course of the perforation is usually encompassed by adhesions and the process takes place quietly. The symptoms of perforation of the bile-passages are those of perforative peritonitis; premonitory symptoms, however, point to the origin of the disease. If a case be not operated upon, death will occur in a few days from toxemia and paralysis of the bowel, although in very exceptional cases the patient may live a week or two. In these cases medical treatment is absolutely useless. If the perforation is even suspected, the abdomen should be opened in the right semilunar line. If pus and bile are discovered, they should be wiped away with gauze; and if the extravasation has extended throughout the abdomen, the entire peritoneal cavity must be flushed with a hot solution of boracic acid. If the patient is in such a condition that prolonged operation is not to be thought of, free drainage may save his life.

Robson calls attention to the fact originally pointed out by Morison that the right kidney pouch is in reality a pocket of the peritoneum; and if a stab-opening from the loin is made into this pouch, a drainage-tube carried through the stab-wound will provide for most efficient drainage. When the whole peritoneal cavity has been soiled a suprapubic incision is made and a tube is introduced for the purpose of drainage. When the patient's condition justifies it the rupture must be sought for, and, when found, in some cases it can be closed by fine sutures of silk or catgut, but, as a rule, it is best to open and drain the gall-bladder at the same time. When there is marked cholecystitis the surgeon considers the question of cholecystectomy, but the operation should not be undertaken when the patient is in a dangerous state. It should be deferred until a later period. The author divides biliary surface fistulæ into pathologic and post-operative. A mucous fistula occasionally follows the operation of cholecystotomy when a cystic obstruction has not been removed. In two such cases Robson brought about a cure by removing the gall-bladder. In another case he followed up the tract and found that the cystic duct was blocked by a calculus, and when this calculus was removed the fistula rapidly healed. A mucous fistula causes but little trouble, as it discharges only about an ounce of fluid daily; but if the opening be permitted to close, accumulation takes place and colic ensues; hence a patient with a mucous fistula must wear a tube or an absorbent pad, or must submit to an operation. The operation of cholecystotomy will not be succeeded by a fistula if the obstruction of the bile-ducts has been removed and if the opening in the gall-bladder be sutured to the aponeurosis and not to the skin. Biliary fistula following operation is a far more serious condition than a mucous fistula. About 30 ounces of bile will flow from the fistula daily. The treatment of such cases consists in removing the cause, but in cases in which this is impossible other means must be considered. When there is no obstruction in the ducts and the fistula is small the application of a Paquelin cautery may effect a cure. In one case Robson opened the abdomen, detached the gall-bladder, and sutured the opening, and cure was brought about. Another method is to dissect the fistula with its peritoneum covering intact over the skin margin, turning in the mucous edges, suturing them, applying one or two layers of buried suture over them, and then closing the skin. When it is impossible to clear the ducts and when the gall-bladder is of sufficient size the operation of cholecystenterostomy should be performed. If the fistula is kept up by gall-stones blocked in the ducts, the ducts may be syringed daily with olive oil or a $\frac{1}{2}\%$ solution of sapo animalis or a solution of turpentine and ether. Biliary intestinal fistulæ are more common than surface fistulæ. This is to be expected because of the adjacency of the duodenum and colon to the gall-bladder. The author then considers intestinal obstruction from gall-stones and states that this is a very unusual condition. It may be produced in several ways. Paralysis of the bowel may follow local peritonitis in the gall-bladder region. The violence of the attack of hepatic colic may lead to volvulus of the small intestine. The obstruction may be due to adhesions left by the local peritonitis of the inflamed region. Finally, obstruction may be mechanically induced by the passage of a very large stone through and into the intestine. There are no symptoms absolutely characteristic of this form of obstruction. A surgeon should not wait beyond the time when the operation may be undertaken with reasonable hope of success. When the abdomen is opened and the stone is felt it may be possible to crush the stone through the intestinal coats; but if this procedure fails, enterotomy should be performed. If the patient's condition is so grave that it is not possible to make a search for the obstruction, temporary relief is afforded by enterotomy or by short-circuiting, and if the obstruction caused is not passed naturally it may be subsequently sought for and removed. The author then makes some remarks on tumors of the gall-bladder and bile-ducts, distention of the gall-bladder, hydrops, and dropsy of the gall-bladder. Hydrops and dropsy mean distention by mucus, and may result from obstruction of the cystic or common ducts, obstruction produced by gall-stones, stricture, tumor of the ducts, or cancer of the head of the pancreas. The mucus results from the secretion of the mucous lining, and the gall-bladder may attain enormous size. When the obstruction is associated with inflammation the fluid may become purulent and empyema of the gall-bladder result. Robson presents the signs of this condition and elaborately discusses the diagnosis, symptoms, and signs of tumor. He says that the treatment of cancer of the gall-bladder may call for cholecystectomy ; but it is very rare that the disease is sufficiently limited to permit of excision. In the 1 case in which he operated he had to associate the cholecystectomy with a partial hepatectomy.

The author presents the subject of **tumor of the bile-ducts** and tells us that the operative treatment for these growths is in its infancy. If possible, the growth should be removed ; but when such a procedure cannot be carried out the gall-bladder or ducts must be opened and drained, or, what is better, drained into the duodenum or jejunum by means of a Murphy button.

Then follows an elaborate consideration of the subject of **cholelithiasis.** The author says that after medical treatment has been fairly tried and has proved unsuccessful a surgical operation should be performed. Cholecystotomy is the operation usually to be aimed at, but very frequently it happens we cannot definitely say what operation is to be done until the abdomen has been opened. The indications for operation are as follows : first, frequently recurring attacks of biliary colic without jaundice, whether the gall-bladder is enlarged or not ; second, enlargement of the gall-bladder without jaundice,. whether or not there is great pain ; third, persistent jaundice which was preceded or accompanied by pain with or without paroxysms resembling ague ; fourth, empyema of the gall-bladder ; fifth, peritonitis of the gall-bladder region ; sixth, abscess around the gall-bladder or bile-ducts (it matters not whether the abscess is over the liver, in the liver, or under the liver) ; seventh, where adhesions are producing pain and sickness ; eighth, fistulæ, mucous, mucopurulent, or biliary ; ninth, persistent jaundice with enlarged gall-bladder due to obstruction in the common duct ; tenth, phlegmonous cholecystitis and gangrene ; eleventh, gunshot-injury or stab-wounds ; twelfth, suspected rupture of the gall-bladder ; thirteenth, some cases of chronic catarrh of the gall-bladder or gall-ducts ; fourteenth, suppurative cholangitis.

Robson says that aspiration of the distended gall-bladder through the unopened abdomen is a dangerous procedure. It is far better to make an exploratory incision than to aspirate. In these operations a narrow and firm sandbag should be placed at the level of the liver on the operating-table under the patient's back. This will bring the common duct several inches nearer the surface, cause the intestines to roll away from the liver, and open the costal angle. The most useful incision is vertical in the right semilunar line. If there be a definite tumor, the incision should be made over the most prominent part of the tumor. If there is an enlarged liver but no tumor, the upper end of the incision will begin at the upper margin of the liver. If there is neither a tumor nor an enlarged liver, the incision will start at the ninth costal cartilage and will pass downward vertically for three inches. If more room is required, it can be obtained by extending the vertical cut or by adding to it a transverse cut either outward or inward from the vertical line. The lumbar incision through which it has been suggested that we can reach the duct without opening the peritoneum is not practicable. In jaundiced patients there is great danger of hemorrhage, and the author thinks that the administration of chlorid of calcium, 30 gr. every 4 hours for a few days before operation, makes the blood more plastic and lessens the danger of excessive bleeding. This procedure was suggested by Dr. A. E. Wright, and the drug may be continued for some time after operation. The operation *par excellence* in the treatment of gall-stones is undoubtedly cholecystotomy or cholecystostomy,

The author then takes up the **technic of the operation,** discusses it most fully, considers the question of fistulæ following cholecystotomy and of calculi in the common duct and the methods applicable to treatment, and in detail the operations of choledocho-duodenostomy, choledochotomy, and cholecystectomy.

The entire article is worthy of the most careful study.

T. C. Railton[1] reports an interesting case of **pancreatic cyst** occurring in a girl 6 months of age. The tumor was aspirated and an operation was performed in which the sac was incised and drained from the infracostal region behind, but the patient died. An interesting fact in this case was that the tumor occupied a lateral position, possibly because of the large size of the liver in the child. This case is the youngest one which is recorded, the youngest previously reported being 17 years of age. There was no history of any injury, and it seems difficult to believe that an injury sustained during birth was responsible for the cyst. G. R. Turner[2] reports a case of pancreatic cyst occurring in a man. The cyst was of very rapid growth. The man was 34 years of age; he had not been injured and was apparently in excellent health, but while at dinner was seized with violent abdominal pain followed by vomiting, constipation, and distention, the symptoms greatly resembling obstruction of the bowels. For a week he improved, and then had a relapse. About a month after the first attack a swelling the size of a hen's egg was detected. This tumor varied in size from time to time and the patient kept on having occasional attacks resembling obstruction. About 9 months after the beginning of his trouble he was admitted into the hospital, and a cystic swelling was detected in the left hypochondriac and upper umbilical regions. There was an interval of resonance between the liver-dulness and the dulness due to the tumor, the superficial veins were not enlarged, and the general health of the patient was excellent. The abdomen was opened; the stomach and great omentum were visible. The cyst could not be seen, but fluctuation could be felt back of the stomach. An exploring-needle was passed through the sac, the cyst was aspirated, and 37 ounces of a thickish fluid of a dark color were withdrawn by the aspirator. The cyst was opened. The opening in the cyst was stitched to the abdominal wound and a drainage-tube was inserted. An examination of the fluid showed that the cyst was pancreatic; the patient made a complete recovery.

Rotter has stated that 75% of pancreatic cysts push forward the posterior wall of the omental cavity so that the stomach and gastrocolic omentum lie in front of them, the transverse colon below them, and the liver above them. If the tumor increases much in size, the stomach is pushed forward and the colon downward, so that the gastrocolic omentum is in front of the cyst. The transverse colon may be pushed downward until it lies back of the symphysis pubis. The case reported belonged to this class, and not to the class in which fluid collects between the layers of the transverse mesocolon. In this latter case the colon lies transversely above the centre of the cyst. In a case in which the fluid collects in the lower layer of the transverse mesocolon the gut lies at the upper border of the tumor. It is quite true that there is a case on record in which a pancreatic cyst in a child was cured by aspiration, but Turner enters a positive protest against this method. Such a procedure is highly dangerous because the stomach, the transverse colon, and the omentum are apt to lie directly in front of the cyst. Exploratory incision should always be made, and after this the cyst can be tapped with safety. An interesting

---

[1] Brit. Med. Jour., Oct 31, 1896.   [2] Lancet, July 4, 1896.

23

case of pancreatic cyst is reported by Charles B. Penrose.[1] There was a lump in the abdomen and the patient suffered from backache, faintness, painful urination, and some loss of flesh. There was no pain in the abdomen; the tumor was smooth and round and obviously cystic, and was without any pelvic attachment. When the abdomen was opened a unilocular pancreatic cyst was discovered containing 2½ gallons of brownish fluid. The anterior wall of the cyst was incised, the margins of the incision were sutured to the upper angle of the abdominal incision, and the remainder of the abdominal incision was closed with sutures. The patient recovered. An examination of the fluid removed from the cyst showed that it was pancreatic. W. W. Keen[2] reported a case of pancreatic cyst in a girl 15 years of age. There was no history of injury or of malaria. The swelling was discovered accidentally some four years before, and was in the upper portion of the left abdomen. There was some dyspepsia because of the large size of the tumor. The tumor was the seat of occasional attacks of severe pain. Four or five months previous to visiting Keen the pain became continuous and the abdominal enlargement rapidly progressed. The patient was not anemic. The left side of the abdomen was filled with a large tumor which was apparently solid. The lower limit of the tumor was 2 in. below the line of the umbilicus and the right side of the tumor extended 4 in. to the right of the umbilicus. The upper border was lost in the hepatic and cardiac dulness. The abdominal wall was very tense. The entire area was dull on percussion, and the colon-resonance separating the kidney from the tumor was found in the left flank. The abdomen did not appear to contain any fluid. The umbilicus was deeply cupped and extremely sensitive. There was no edema of the legs, the heart and lungs were normal, and the uterus and ovaries apparently normal. The patient had never had fatty stools; there was a doubtful sense of fluctuation on percussion. The splenic dulness could not be differentiated from the dulness of the tumor. Examination of the blood showed some diminution of red corpuscles, some increase in white corpuscles, but no alteration in the structure of the white corpuscles; hemoglobin 65%; no plasmodia of malaria. The abdomen was opened, and it became evident that the tumor was a tense cyst, the stomach being spread out in front of it and intimately adherent to it. On attempting to separate the stomach from the cyst-wall the muscular coat of the stomach tore, but the mucous membrane was not injured. The tear was sutured at once. The omentum was in front of the cyst and the descending colon behind it and to the left. It was obvious that the mass was retroperitoneal, probably pancreatic. It became necessary to add a transverse incision to the vertical abdominal incision. The peritoneum below and outside of the stomach was torn through and the cyst-wall was incised. About seven pints of fluid were evacuated. The first fluid that ran out was straw-colored, but the last was chocolate-colored. The fluid was under great pressure and was forced out to a considerable distance from the table. The pancreas could not be recognized with the fingers in the cyst, nor could any stone of the pancreas be detected. The mouth of the cyst was fastened to the abdominal incision and the rest of the incision was closed. The patient recovered. The bacteriologic examination of the fluid first removed showed it to be sterile. The fluid contained 0.4% of urea and a certain amount of serumalbumin and serumglobulin. It was neutral in reaction and of specific gravity 1.017. Bile, mucus, and cholesterin were absent. The iodin-test showed that starch ferment existed, yet this ferment was without effect on food. Prof. Brubaker examined the fluid last removed and reported that starch was rapidly transformed into sugar by it. It was obvious that the

[1] Ann. of Surg., Apr., 1897.   [2] Ibid.

fluid was pancreatic. The cause of the cyst is very obscure. The tension of the cyst was so great that Dr. Keen was at first inclined to think that he was dealing with a solid tumor. He was convinced after the first examination that he was not dealing with the spleen because of the absence of anemia and the absence of a distinctly palpable lower edge. The diagnosis lay between a hydronephrosis, a pancreatic cyst, and a cyst beginning in the gall-bladder or ovary. Ovarian and hepatic disease were ruled out by the results of vaginal examination and by the fact that the tumor was fixed to the left and above. The facts that the urine was normal; that there was an absence of all renal symptoms; that there was no flush-tank symptom, and that the colon was behind the tumor, were against a renal origin. The facts that there was no pronounced loss of weight, no fatty stools, and that the tumor was very much on the left side, made a diagnosis of pancreatic cyst doubtful. The examination of the fluid is particularly interesting when we note that it did not emulsify fats and that it contained a moderate amount of urea. The loss of emulsifying power was probably due to long retention. The fluid which flowed out last did emulsify fats and acted upon starch. Another important fact is that the operation was followed by a slight pancreatic diabetes. Dr. Keen says that if he had depended for a diagnosis on tapping and examining the fluid the presence of urea would possibly have led him to infer that he was dealing with a hydronephrosis. As a matter of fact, urea is sometimes found in old simple cysts; also in ascitic fluid and in pancreatic juice. The percentage of urea was about the same as would have been found in the fluid of a hydronephrosis, but the character of the fluid was markedly different from that of a hydronephrosis. Dr. Keen did not aspirate this tumor because in such cases he looks upon aspiration as a very dangerous performance—far more dangerous than incision and far less likely than incision to give the necessary information. In this case, if an aspirating-needle had been inserted at the most prominent and tense point, it would have passed directly through both walls of the stomach; in addition to this the fluid was in such a high condition of tension that even the small opening of the aspirating-needle would have led to the forcing out of a great quantity of fluid into the peritoneal cavity. The fluid in this case was sterile, but this is not invariably the rule. In dealing with pancreatic cysts only two methods are to be considered: first, incision and drainage; and, second, enucleation. Enucleation is rarely possible, and was impossible in this case. Zweifel says that extirpation has been performed 12 times with 5 deaths. There are 31 reported cases in which incision and drainage have been done, with only 2 deaths. Of the 29 who recovered 10 labored under fistula more or less permanent.

Sendler[1] writes upon **rare tumors of the pancreas.** In one patient a diagnosis was made of malignant disease of the stomach or pancreas. On operation the stomach was found to be very low down, and above it was detected a hard tumor of the pancreas. The lesser omentum was incised longitudinally and a tumor the size of a walnut was removed; the bleeding was free, but was arrested without trouble; the lymph-glands between the pancreas and the duodenum were enlarged and were removed. The patient recovered from the operation. Examination showed that the tumor was tuberculous and that the case was one of primary tuberculosis of the pancreas. In another patient a laparotomy was performed for a supposed cancer of the stomach. The lesser omentum was divided, and it was found that the entire pancreas was enlarged and hard. It was decided that the tumor was an inoperable carcinoma, and no attempt was made to remove it. The patient recovered from

[1] Deutsch. Zeit. f. Chir., vol. xliv.

operation, but the condition gradually grew worse until it was believed that death would soon ensue. Then for no known reason the patient began to improve, and at the end of about a year she was in perfect health. Some three years later the tumor could still be felt, although greatly lessened in size. The condition obviously was not malignant disease of the pancreas, but rather chronic inflammation.

Pereira Guimaraes [1] publishes the report of a case of **hernia of the pancreas** resulting from a bayonet-wound. The tail of the pancreas protruded from the incision; 48 hours after the accident it was restored into the abdomen, the wound was closed, and the patient recovered. The writer states that Quenu has collected 6 cases of pancreatic hernia with one death. In each case the protruded portion had been ligated.

Greiffenhagen [2] writes on the causes of **wandering spleen** and on the methods of operating. He tells us that 5 cases of splenopexy have been placed on record, 4 of which were successful. In Greiffenhagen's case the spleen was found floating during an exploration to determine the condition of a kidney which had previously been sutured. He introduced two sutures through the parietes of the abdomen, through the substance of the spleen, and through the parietes again; a third suture rendered the fixation complete. There was a considerable amount of bleeding from the stitch-holes. The results were most satisfactory. [The opinion generally held by surgeons is that splenectomy is a more certain and not a more dangerous procedure than splenopexy.] J. Bland Sutton [3] tells us that the spleen may travel so wide of its normal seat that it may be brought into contact with any part of the peritoneal cavity from the diaphragm to the pelvic floor. Occasionally it will remain for days in its normal position, and then suddenly slip out and be felt by the patient in the umbilical or iliac region, and then it will pass into the pelvis. Gravity has some influence in causing the spleen to pass into the pelvis, but it is not the only cause. In one case Sutton was able to determine that when the patient lay on the right side the spleen sometimes passed into the right iliac fossa, but sometimes into the left, as if carried on by the intestines like a boat on the water. Wandering spleens are infinitely more common in women than in men, and most of the victims have borne children. A wandering spleen is always liable to engorgement. When we are operating and find a wandering spleen which is engorged, we notice that the engorged organ contracts very greatly after removal or on simple exposure to air before removal. In one case Sutton opened the abdomen and found a spleen reaching from the diaphragm to the uterus. It was withdrawn very gently and supported for a few minutes. Exposure to the air acted as a stimulant, and this enormous spleen shrunk one-third of its original size. A wandering spleen is always liable to axial rotation, and when this happens the organ looks as if it were about to burst. Axial rotation produces the same acute symptoms as ensue on rotation of ovarian cysts and as occur in strangulated hernia. A persistent rotation which completely arrests the splenic circulation permanently occludes the splenic artery and vein and causes atrophy of the spleen. A wandering spleen exercises injurious effects upon adjacent viscera. The spleen is intimately related to the tail of the pancreas, and some disturbance of the pancreas is almost certain to arise when the splenic pedicle is elongated. In some cases the pancreas became incorporated in the pedicle. There is a case on record in which a spleen passed into the pelvis and dragged the tail of the pancreas with it. A wandering spleen pulls upon the stomach, leading to

[1] Progrès méd., Oct. 10, 1896.   [2] Centralbl. f. Chir., Feb. 6, 1897.
[3] Brit. Med. Jour., Jan. 16, 1897.

dilatation of the stomach, accompanied by vomiting and fermentation of food. It happens sometimes that the pulling upon the stomach and duodenum obstructs the common bile-duct and leads to attacks of jaundice. The long pedicle of the wandering spleen is very apt to interfere with the intestines, and such a spleen may become adherent to the small intestine, the colon, the sigmoid flexure, or the appendix. Such adhesions may cause intestinal obstruction, or they may damage the bowel-wall and favor the emigration of microorganisms with all the evil consequences that may ensue. A wandering spleen may cause acute uterine retroflexion and even uterine prolapse. In one published case a wandering spleen dropped into the pelvis and caused prolapse of the uterus, vagina, and bladder. The pressure of the spleen in the pelvis seriously interferes with menstruation. A wandering spleen may endanger life by rupture of the stomach or duodenum, intestinal obstruction, abscess of the spleen, or rupture of the spleen. Wandering spleens may be confounded with various abdominal tumors, such as ovarian cysts, tumors of the kidney, tumors of the omentum, movable kidney, and uterine myomata. It is necessary to bear in mind that ovarian and uterine tumors may simulate wandering spleens. Splenectomy for wandering spleen is a very successful operation, the rate of recovery being fully equal to the rate of recovery after ovariotomy. Sutton has collected the records of 20 cases, with one death. Some surgeons have endeavored to fasten the spleen in the left hypochondriac region, just as we would fasten a movable kidney; but the results demonstrate that such an operation is more dangerous and requires longer confinement than does splenectomy.

Sutton has never seen an evil result from a patient being without a spleen. The spleen is a highly developed lymph-gland of special functions, and there is no more reason to hesitate at removing it than to hesitate to remove enlarged concatenate glands. Many people with wandering spleen are thin and gaunt, and when the spleen is removed they retain this character.

Jonnesco[1] puts on record 2 successful cases of **splenectomy** for ague spleen. Jonuesco says this operation should be performed for malarial spleen after a trial of medical methods, when there is no leukemia, no pronounced cachexia, and no mass of adhesions. In performing this operation tear the adhesions between the spleen and diaphragm, the vessels being cut between two ligatures. The spleen is lifted out of the abdomen, and the vessels of the pedicle are separated and tied individually.

DISEASES OF THE RECTUM AND THE ANUS.

John Campbell[2] considers the value of **the sacral route in operations for diseases of the rectum.** He holds that in rectal cancer this route possesses certain positive advantages. We are able to tell the exact limits of the disease and thus effect a thorough removal, we can easily and completely control hemorrhage, we can reach the tissues which lie between the rectum and sacrum, and are enabled to remove infiltrated lymphatic glands and vessels, and in most instances we do not destroy the sphincter and levator ani muscles. The operation is, of course, a severe one.

Podreze[1] employs the following method of **operation for hemorrhoids:** the patient is anesthetized, the sphincter is dilated, and the rectum is stuffed with cotton-wool above the hemorrhoids. Each group is grasped with forceps and the skin at the base is cut as near as possible to the mucous membrane; a

[1] Progrès méd., No. 12, 1897.   [2] Ibid., Oct. 10, 1896.
[3] Gaz. des Hôpitaux, No. 30, 1896.

needle threaded with silk is introduced into this wound and passed around the base of the pile and out again at the wound. The thread surrounds the base of the pile; it is tied and cut and the hemorrhoid is cut; the skin and mucous membrane are then sutured together. Each pile is treated in the same manner. The rectal plug of wool is removed, a drainage-tube wrapped about with iodoform-gauze is placed in the rectum, and the wound is dressed with gauze.

D. W. S. Samways[1] treats **external piles and anal pruritus** by the application of collodion. This application causes the pile to contract and supports the contracted pile. It acts in the same way as the elastic stocking used in varicose veins of the leg. The collodion is applied on a little cotton-wool each morning after defecation. In pruritus the application of collodion causes smarting for a few minutes, which can be prevented by the previous application of cocain, but there is no itching for 12 to 24 hours after the collodion is applied.

Monin[2] employs the following **ointment in the treatment of hemorrhoids:** 2 oz. of camphor lanolin; 3 drams of castor oil; 1½ drams precipitated chalk; 30 gr. of hydrobromat of cicutin.

Delorme[3] writes upon **Whitehead's method in the treatment of hemorrhoids.** He thinks that this plan should be employed when the hemorrhoids are internal or both internal and external, and when they are very large and form a great, circular mass. In 18 operations performed by Delorme the results were entirely satisfactory and primary union took place in each case. The cicatrix was thoroughly dilatable and there was neither retention nor incontinence of feces. Whitehead's method is a radical cure if the entire pile-bearing area is removed. The surgeon must be careful to preserve the sphincters and must always use strong sutures.

Joseph B. Bacon[4] proposed in 1895 a new method of **treating stricture of the rectum by a plastic operation.** He used the sigmoid flexure to form a new channel around the strictured portion of the canal, and he believes that this method is a certain means of relieving malignant strictures situated above the levator ani muscles. Unfortunately, for strictures above the internal sphincter ani it is not possible to perform any plastic operation which will not be followed by fecal incontinence. Gradual dilatation is unsuccessful in these strictures; the same may be said of forcible divulsion, internal and complete proctotomy, and electrolysis. Complete proctotomy gives temporary relief. For these cases he has recently devised a method which has been successful. The incision of a complete proctotomy has the shape of the letter V when the ends of the stricture retract. If we can prevent this triangle from filling up with fibrous tissue, the severed band of strictured tissue will disappear by absorption. In order to accomplish this a mucous fistula is produced between the stricture and the coccyx, so that the mucous tract will be at the bottom of the wound and prevent the union of the severed stricture-bands. In order to perform this the patient is thoroughly anesthetized, a blunt-pointed aneurysm-needle is threaded with a heavy silk ligature, and just above the internal sphincter and the median line of the posterior rectal wall the gut is punctured; the needle is carried well back into the perirectal tissue and the coccyx and up behind the stricture to above the upper limits of the stenosis. The needle is forced through the rectal wall into the rectum. One end of the ligature is now seized with a blunt hook or dressing-forceps, and one end drawn down through the stricture-opening and the needle withdrawn; the two ends of the

---

[1] Brit. Med. Jour., Nov. 21, 1896.   [2] Méd. mod., Nov. 4, 1896.
[3] Ibid., Oct. 31, 1896.   [4] Quar. Med. Jour., Jan., 1897.

seton are tied and left hanging outside of the anus. It is necessary to leave the seton in place for about three months in order to get a continuous mucous tract. At the end of three months the patient is again anesthetized and the seton withdrawn. A grooved director is passed through the fistulous tract behind the stricture and the intervening stricture-band severed with a Paquelin cautery. In three cases there was partial failure, due to not taking in more tissue above and below the stricture-band, so as to catch all the scar-tissue.

W. J. Chapman [1] reports a case of **prolapse of the rectum** in which he opened the abdomen and practised ventrofixation of the mesorectum, with most satisfactory results.

A. B. Cook [2] writes on the **operative treatment of rectal fistula.** In every case not only should the rectum be examined, but also the lungs, although pulmonary tuberculosis is not of necessity a contraindication to operation. Every sinus must be removed. The sphincter is cut but once, and then at right angles to its fibers. The mucous opening is looked to with care, and pains are taken, especially in females, not to invade the perineum. Antisepsis greatly contributes to favorable results, and the surgeon must himself supervise the after-treatment. If during after-treatment there is an unusual amount of pain or an increase of the discharge, suspect the formation of another abscess. The two chief dangers to be apprehended are hemorrhage and fecal incontinence, but both conditions may be amended by treatment.

Llewellyn Eliot [3] reports 4 cases in which he succeeded in **restoring** a **destroyed sphincter ani,** the muscle having been cut during operation for fistula. Eliot maintains that in cutting for fistula we should dissect out the tract and insert sutures in order to obtain primary union and so preserve the sphincter. In the cases in which he operated for destroyed sphincter he dissected out the scar-tissue and drew the muscular fibers together with silk sutures.

Charles B. Kelsey [4] considers the indications for **celiotomy in diseases of the rectum.** Among these are cancer of the rectum and incurable nonmalignant ulceration. In many cases in which an artificial anus has been formed the surgeon will be obliged later to repair this condition. After the performance of colostomy it occasionally happens that the gut prolapses extensively through the abdominal opening, and a second operation is demanded. In resection of cancer of the rectum by the method of Kraske the peritoneal cavity will be opened. All cases of intussusception marked by bloody discharge and tenesmus, in which the intussusceptions appeared at the anus, are considered by the laity as rectal disease, and many of these cases demand celiotomy. Celiotomy is required for a foreign body in the rectum, for the diagnosis of obscure rectal disease, for extensive rectal prolapse and rupture of the rectum, or, more properly, rupture of the old prolapse, permitting hernia of the small intestine through the anus, and finally for intestinal vesical fistula in the male. There are three well-recognized ways of opening the abdomen in rectal disease—the ventral, the vaginal, and the sacral.

Edward H. Taylor [5] contributes a thorough and lengthy study on the **operative treatment of cancer of the rectum.** He studies anew and with great care the anatomy of this region. He tells us that many surgeons do not regard extensive operations for rectal cancer with much favor, as they believe these operations cannot be carried out as completely as is possible, for instance, in a breast cancer. Nevertheless, we should always remember that in

---

[1] Canadian Pract., Oct., 1896.   [2] Med. News, No. 21, 1896.
[3] Va. Med. Jour., Mar. 12, 1897.   [4] N. Y. Med. Jour., Feb. 27, 1897.
[5] Ann. of Surg., Apr., 1897.

rectal cancer metastases occur late, and this fact gives a more favorable aspect to the situation. Even if we leave behind some glands which are infected, the progress of the disease in these limited areas may be extremely slow. There are numerous examples on record of prolonged life after rectal excision, and many cases have been recorded of non-recurrence for 6, 8, and 10 years. Even if only a very small percentage of radical cures were obtained, it would be much better to operate than to leave sufferers to the miserable end to which this disease dooms them. The mortality of rectum-excision varies from 20 % to 25 %. This means the mortality of the sacral operation. Recently the figures have shown improvement. Czerny's mortality was 5.4 % by the perineal route, 19.4 % by the sacral route; Iversen, 25 %; Albert, 18 %; Ball, 8 %; and Paul, 14 %. There is no question, however, that the high mortality which records have previously shown, will diminish in the future, this diminution being brought about by a more perfect technic, by minute attention to details of operation, and the preparation for operation and careful selection of cases. It is certain that a bad functional result occasionally follows this operation, and the opponents of rectal incision have often made much of this; nevertheless, it has been noted that even in the cases in which the sphincters have been excised there is a fair amount of control, except during attacks of diarrhea. Modern methods of treatment do much in aiding us to preserve the sphincter function of the bowel. When we see a patient with a rectal cancer the first questions are, Should a radical cure be attempted? and, if so, What procedure should be selected? The operation of Kraske has very widely extended the field suitable for operation, and by this method we can remove not only cancers of the upper rectum, but also of the adjacent portions of the colon. The cancers best suited for radical operation are those which are small and movable. We should always try to make out the limits of the growth, observing if it has invaded the perirectal cellular tissue, the glands, the prostate, the bladder, the uterus, the vagina, the saerum, or the seminal vesicles; and in order to determine this several careful examinations should be made. A diagnosis is unfortunately made late rather than early as a rule, because rectal cancer in its beginning often runs an indolent course and seems to be latent. In considering the question of operation we should always take into account the patient's age, his strength, and the condition of the viscera, especially the kidneys. The two main indications in preparatory treatment are to improve the general condition of the patient and to diminish the poisonous nature of the contents of the intestines. There is no known way of making the intestinal tract aseptic. It is impossible to subject it to the action of strong antiseptics. Purgatives used with moderation are of the greatest possible value and cleanse the intestinal tract more efficiently than do all of the recommended antiseptic agents. Resorcin, salicylate of bismuth, and salol, however, can be given with some advantage. The area of ulceration abounds with virulent microorganisms, and in the neighborhood proctitis frequently exists, and for these conditions we should invariably employ frequent rectal irrigation with warm water. Rectal irrigation should be practised every morning and evening for 4 or 5 days before operation, but rectal irrigation and intestinal antiseptics only bring about a moderate amount of disinfection. The most satisfactory way to disinfect the area is by the use of the flushing-curette. The anus is dilated, so that during the flushing free exit is afforded to the stream of water and cancerous debris. This is done immediately before the removal of the growth. Preliminary colotomy was originally employed, because of the numerous unpleasant results which were found after Kraske's operation. Quénu always performs colotomy twelve days before he excises the cancer. This operation enables us to explore satisfactorily the pelvic cavity, determine the condition of the pelvic colon, and examine the lymphatic glands. Furthermore, a preliminary colotomy facilitates disinfection of the rectum by diverting the poison, and enables us to practise thorough irrigation, and thus diminish greatly the chances of infection after operation. Many objections have been urged against it; the first, the necessary lapse of several days between the colotomy and the excision of the growth. In this time the patient's condition may grow worse and the cancer may increase its size. Again, the patient will be subjected to the subsequent closure of the artificial anus, when his condition may not be such as to justify surgical interference. Third, the performance of a preliminary colotomy may make the drawing down of the intestine in Kraske's operation a very difficult matter. This is especially the case where the distention causes the pelvic colon to rise out of the pelvis, it having been fixed in this position when the colotomy was performed. Taylor thinks the procedure has certain advantages, although he has not adopted it in any of his cases. He might be induced to employ it if he were unable to empty the bowel above the cancer by other means, and if he were unable to cleanse satisfactorily the operative field. In endeavoring to select the proper operation to perform, it is well to consider a certain number of types of cancer. First, cancers which begin below the attachment of the levator ani muscles—in reality, anal cancers. Second, those above the levator ani, which are, however, intraperitoneal. Third, those whose lower limit is at the level of the peritoneal cul de sac, the growth extending upward so as to reach to or even involve the pelvic colon. Fourth, cancers which involve the rectum extensively and reach upward for a considerable distance from the anus. If we are dealing with an anal cancer, the surface of the growth is curetted, the rectum is irrigated, and an incision is made in the skin wide of the disease, the external sphincter, of course, being removed. The dissection is carried out with scissors until sound tissue above the growth is reached. The rectum is cut across above the growth and the cut portion of the rectum is sutured to the skin. In suprasphincteric cancer the question to determine is whether the growth does or does not involve the sphincter. In both conditions the perineal operation can be employed. The best method is as follows: make a median posterior incision behind the margin of the anus and extend it deep over the coccyx; starting from the tip of this incision, follow the median raphe forward, thus splitting the posterior portion of the external sphincter and separating the levators ani. The rectum is cleared on its posterior and lateral aspects by the use of the index fingers. A pair of blunt-pointed scissors is now taken; one blade is placed in the wound just behind the anus in the interval between the rectum and the levator ani, and the other blade rests upon the skin. The intervening bridge of tissue is cut and a similar section is made on the opposite side. These lateral incisions are extended in the direction of the middle line in front, cutting the levator muscles all around away from the rectum. When the disease is quite above the sphincter zone this muscle should not be interfered with. The author then discusses elaborately the technic of the sacral and perineal methods for excising cancers above the sphincter zone, and shows why he greatly prefers the sacral method and particularly the osteoplastic resection.

Henry T. Byford[1] presents an article on the **extirpation of the rectum through the vagina,** with utilization of the vagina to replace the lost rectal tissue. He tells us that the sacral method is bloody and severe, and that removal of the rectum by the perineal incision is only applicable when the lower 4 in. mark the area of the disease. He therefore thinks that in some cases

[1] Ann. of Surg., Nov., 1896.

certainly another route is justifiable, and reports a case in which he performed this operation. The vagina was distended by means of retractors. Half an inch below and posterior to the cervix a transverse vaginal incision was made, and the vagina was separated from the underlying connective tissue about the incisions. The tumor and rectum were then separated to and above the level of the brim of the pelvis, large pads of gauze being pushed up to arrest hemorrhage. The rectum below the tumor was separated and the tumor was pulled down to the vulva, which pulling down tore the cul de sac and carried into the vagina two inches of rectum, the front surface of which was covered with peritoneum. The area which included the tumor was excised between two large forceps, and the upper end of the divided rectum was sutured into the vaginal wound, the vagina thus being turned into a rectum. The peritoneal wound was closed and the lower end of the rectum was sewed around with catgut so as to check bleeding, but not to obliterate its caliber; the rest of the vaginal wound was then sutured completely around the rectum.

Byford thinks that this technic in future cases may be improved. It would be well to enlarge the transverse incision by a median incision extending down over the center of the transverse incision—in other words, by making a T-shaped incision. It is well to employ a large amount of packing. The vaginal method has certain advantages. The vagina takes the place of the portion of the rectum which has been removed. We are enabled to remove the rectum as high up as by the sacral route and the mutilation is less, and if the peritoneal cavity is opened the danger is less. An intraperitoneal exploration can be made before the rectum is disturbed. If it is necessary to abandon the operation, we leave a less serious wound than if forced to abandon the large operation, and the patient is left far more comfortable after this operation than after sacral resection.

T. W. Elliott[1] reports a case of **imperforate rectum** in which he performed successfully Kraske's operation. The child was only two days old.

Depage[2] discusses **cancer of the rectum,** the indications for operation, and the technic. In operating on a patient for cancer of the rectum he placed in what he calls the gynecological position, with the pelvis vertical; an incision is made posteriorly, the coccyx is resected, and it may be that one or two of the sacral vertebræ are removed. The rectum is dissected, the surgeon endeavoring to leave as much as possible of the cellular tissue and the peritoneum adherent to it. If possible, the superior hemorrhoidal artery is left intact. The malignant growths of the lymphatics associated with it are removed together in one piece. As soon as the growth has been resected the peritoneal cavity is closed. The upper anal segment should be invaginated into the lower segment; the preservation of the superior hemorrhoidal artery obviates the risk of gangrene. The final step in the operation is the insertion of tampons or applying layers of sutures. Depage very rarely performs a preliminary colostomy. He does so, however, where the condition of the patient is extremely bad and in a case in which the growth is so extensive that removal of the entire rectum is necessary. When we operate on a cancer in the beginning this radical operation should be performed. When we operate on a case which has far advanced we can study out the condition and perform either a radical operation or simply a colostomy, according to the indication.

[1] Med. News, Oct. 17, 1896.   [2] Rev. de Chir., Nov. 10, 1896.

DISEASES OF THE RESPIRATORY SYSTEM.

J. Lacey Firth[1] records **a case of cut-throat treated by immediate suture.** He tells us that Mr. Henry Morris has set forth the advantages of the immediate application of sutures, stating that we can obtain union by first intention ; that natural swallowing can be performed early ; that the distress of feeding by a tube is avoided ; and that we avoid also the painful swallowing attended by escape of food from the wound and troublesome cough, the formation of cicatricial contractions, stricture, and aërial fistula. In a case reported by Firth the wound gaped widely and extended from the left sternomastoid almost to the right one, and passed into the food-passages below the hyoid bone. The wound in the air-passage was oval in shape and about $1\frac{1}{2}$ in. in length transversely. The thyroid cartilage was bare of muscle. The wound was cleansed. It was impossible to suture the wound in the food-passage without penetrating the mucous membrane, because the thyrohyoid membrane and the epiglottis had been cut just below the hyoid bone and there was no tissue below that bone to unite to the upper edge of the lower flap of tissue. The cut edge of the upper portion of the epiglottis was level with the lower border of the hyoid bone and was very closely fixed to it. Sutures of catgut were passed from the hyoid bone and through the epiglottis into the pharynx, and out again below through the flap of tissue consisting of epiglottis and thyrohyoid membrane. Five sutures were employed. The muscles were next sutured. The skin was then sutured, two small tubes being left in the wound for drainage. The head was fixed to the chest in the usual manner and union was obtained by first intention. [In the section on Wounds we have noted a recent article on this same subject by Henry Morris. There is no question that sutures should be inserted and an attempt be made to obtain primary union.]

George Ryerson Fowler[2] writes on the **surgery of intrathoracic tuberculosis.** He tells us that pleural effusions are most frequently tuberculous in origin. Many inflammatory conditions, exclusive of those of traumatic origin, have their origin in a tuberculous process, for few patients who have suffered from pleurisy escape tuberculosis. It used to be maintained that the activity of the pulmonary circulation protected the tissue from tubercular infection, and treatment used to be administered to stimulate the circulation. It is becoming very doubtful if measure directed to this end are beneficial. Laennec long ago maintained that stasis was antagonistic to tubercle, and Bier's observations on the treatment of tubercular joint-disease by the induction of venous congestion appear to confirm the views of Laennec.

It seems likely that Koch's bacilli cause effusion, and that the effused serum inhibits the growth of bacilli. Even when a pleurisy is due to Koch's bacilli the effusion is apt to be sterile, and this suggests the probability that the serum exerts a restraining influence over the development of the organisms, though it unquestionably affords a favorable culture-medium for other organisms. If these views are true, it would be an improper proceeding to evacuate the fluid contents of a pleural cavity at an early stage as long as suppuration does not occur, because the effusion by its pressure and by its antituberculous properties antagonizes the tuberculous process. Among the operative procedures applied in pleuritic effusion we may mention exploratory puncture. The hypodermic syringe is used to the exclusion of almost every other means. The operation must be performed aseptically. The needle must be long enough to penetrate the chest-wall, and the patient must be warned beforehand not to start and not to make any quick inspiration, because a sudden movement may

[1] Brit. Med. Jour., Sept. 12, 1896.   [2] Ann. of Surg., Nov., 1896.

break the needle. When the point of puncture is being selected remember the situation of the heart and the great vessels. In small effusions the fluid may be found at the upper limit of dulness, nothing being found at the lower limit. If puncture extends into the lung-tissue, it should not produce any serious harm. In fact, this measure can be resorted to to differentiate pleurisy with effusion from pneumonia in a doubtful case. Nevertheless, it has been shown that it is possible for such a puncture to be followed by hemorrhage into the pleural cavity. As a matter of fact, it is rarely necessary in exploring for pleural effusion to pass the needle sufficiently deeply to injure the lung. If the fluid is not obtained at one puncture, it may be necessary to puncture in other places to settle the presence of fluid or the character of the fluid. If the patient has been recumbent in one position for a considerable time, fluid obtained from the upper layer may be clear, while fluid obtained from the lower layer may show that suppuration exists. Puncture may enable us to recognize, aided by a microscopic examination, carcinoma and sarcoma. A dry tap may be due to the needle passing into the thick masses or cartilaginous callosities. If the needle fails to fill at the first puncture, the attempt should not be given up until a larger and longer needle has been employed, because the instrument may be blocked up by clots or may have entered an adhesion or thickened pleura. It occasionally happened that after an exploratory puncture in which a small amount of fluid was withdrawn the fluid that was left rapidly disappeared. Thoracentesis in tuberculous pleurisy is indicated when the effused fluid increases the dyspnea greatly or threatens life by displacing the heart and the great vessels. Puncture and evacuation of fluid do not cure the pleurisy itself; they simply remove the effusion. Hippocrates used to advise evacuation of the fluid on the 15th day ; Bowditch said the proper time is 3 weeks. In a case in which there is no fever, or only slight fever, removal of the fluid may not be followed by reaccumulation. Early paracentesis is not safe. The best method of withdrawing the fluid is by means of the aspirator of Dieulafoy or Potain. It is a matter for argument how much of the fluid ought to be withdrawn at a single sitting. The larger the amount present the more may be withdrawn with safety. In a small effusion a comparatively small amount is withdrawn. In a large effusion, particularly one which has existed for some weeks, the entire amount may be evacuated, provided that syncope does not occur. If the evacuation is carried out slowly, syncope and paroxysms of coughing will probably be avoided. It is not necessary to anesthetize to perform thoracentesis. Thoracotomy should be performed if both air and fluid are present in the pleural space, if the effusion is ichorous, or if it is suppurative. In empyema or pneumothorax occurring in a tuberculous individual the advisability of this operation is a matter sometimes difficult to determine. The surgeon must consider the strength of the patient and the history of the progress of the affection. Young individuals with florid phthisis are likely to die soon after the operation. Older people who have kept up a fair degree of strength, although the disease may have existed for several years, do far better after operation. It has been laid down as a rule that suppurative effusions will not disappear without some radical interference; but there are two exceptions to this rule. Rupture may take place into the lungs, drainage of the fluid being obtained through a bronchus. Small collections may be encapsuled and absorbed. As a general thing, however, it is safe to say that when the purulent matter is accessible and the patient's strength permits of it, it is desirable to incise and drain with or without rib-resection. In most cases simple incision will not cure. The author then discusses the relative value and applicability of simple incision, resection of the ribs, trephining of a rib, curettement of the walls of the cavity, and extensive costal resection by the methods of Estlander and Schede. He then considers the direct treatment of tuberculous cavities. The disfavor into which operations upon cavities have fallen is due chiefly to the difficulties and dangers attending methods that have previously been proposed.

Attempts have been made to inject cavities, and enough has been found out to show that systematic treatment of pulmonary cavities is possible. If a circumscribed pulmonary affection exists, and the patient's strength is fairly well maintained, a surgical operation to reach the cavity may be attempted. The only cases suitable for such a proceeding are those in which there exists a slowly progressing and isolated tuberculous focus; but it is not always possible to be sure the disease is stationary or but slowly progressive. To operate, if a case has come to a standstill, will do nothing but harm. The presence or absence of adhesions between the costal and pulmonary pleura is of great importance. These occur in many cases of extensive cavities which are situated superficially; but if they fail to occur, the post-operative progress of the case will be greatly complicated. The exact location of the cavity is of great importance. Only a small area of pulmonary tissue can be reached by the surgeon. The field for operation is bounded above by the clavicle, within by the manubrium, externally by the lesser pectoral muscle, and below by the second rib. It has been maintained that when only one cavity has been operated on adjacent cavities inaccessible to operation have been favorably influenced. It is more difficult still to attack successfully bronchiectatic cavities. It is very difficult to locate them, and they are usually multiple. Mauclaise would limit operation in tuberculous cases to circumscribed cavities that are without peripheral tuberculous infiltration, and to certain cavities of doubtful nature formed at the expense of both lung and pleura, pulmonary abscess consecutive on tuberculous spondylitis, and tuberculous caries of the ribs. Certain cases have been reported as cured by direct incision, and have been called tuberculous abscesses; but these abscesses of the lung are not of necessity tuberculous in origin. When they are tuberculous in origin they arise from a small focus of circumscribed tubercle in which there has been mixed infection with the bacteria of suppuration; but many cases are not tuberculous at all. In reaching a cavity the lung-tissue should be divided with a Paquelin cautery-knife heated to a dull red. If the instrument is inserted slowly, there will be but slight hemorrhage. The pulmonary tissue is not sensitive, and, if the pleura is incised, the anesthetic can be withdrawn. Tuffier proposes to separate the parietal pleura, and thus avoid opening the pleural space; but the proposal has never been generally accepted. Richard expressed the view that the operation in most cases is impracticable. After opening the tuberculous cavity Roux advises that the two layers of the pleura be sutured together. Willard proved by experiment on animals that the pleura can always be made to unite by direct suture, or by drawing the lung into the opening made by the rib-excision and suturing this to the edges of the opening. This should be done before operation; the pleural space is thus excluded and its infection avoided. Resection of the lung would seem to be a rational method of procedure in pulmonary tuberculosis; but when we come to reflect, we remember that the pulmonary structure is more susceptible than any other tissue in the body to infection by the tubercle-bacillus, and its anatomical peculiarities favor extension of the infection and reinfection of parts whose vital resistance has been lowered.

Gluck and Schmidt performed experimental resection on dogs, and these operations led to the hope that the operation could be successfully applied in phthisis, but the experiments on animals have not increased the confidence of surgeons in the possibility of extirpating an entire lung. The latter procedure is not justifiable. Tuffier reports the first successful case of pneumotomy for pulmonary tuberculosis. The disease was limited to the right apex and the diseased area was resected. Two years after the operation there was no return of the disease. Reclus is a disbeliever in resection of diseased portions of the lungs. He says in extensive disease it is useless, and in small foci it is unjustifiable, as the latter frequently disappear under other treatment. Fowler, in conclusion, discusses tuberculous lesions in the mediastinal spaces and tuberculous pericarditis.

J. McFadden Gaston [1] sets forth an improved **method of exploring the thoracic cavity.** He makes a trap-door opening through the wall of the thorax. In performing this operation the arm should be raised above the head. An incision is carried downward through the soft parts and ribs from the 3d to the 8th rib inclusive, in the mid-axillary line, without cutting the pleural lining. A transverse incision is begun over the upper extremity of this cut along the upper border of the 3d or 4th rib, and a single transverse incision over the lower extremity of the first cut along the border of the 7th or 8th rib. These transverse incisions are carried front to the costal cartilage. The pleura in each line is divided by means of scissors, and the detached margin of the flap is elevated; the trap-door opens upon the hinges formed by the costal cartilage and admits of examination of the chest and mediastinum.

J. E. Platt [2] considers treatment of **wounds of the air-passages.** Until a few years ago almost all authorities discountenanced the use of sutures in wounds opening the air-passages. In 1892 Henry Morris recorded a number of cases in which he applied sutures. Pollard advocated the same treatment, reporting 10 cases, of whom 2 died and 7 recovered, with 1 incomplete recovery. Treatment: when the condition permits, chloroform, clean wound, suture the opening. In some cases close the wound entirely; in others put in tracheotomy-tube. If the larynx or trachea is divided near the vocal chords, a tube is best, as edema of the chords may follow. If the epiglottis is injured, do laryngotomy or high tracheotomy before closing the laryngeal wound. Do not use the wound for insertion of the tube, but make a fresh vertical cut. One case in which the tube was used in the wound was followed by stenosis from cicatrization. Silk is the best material for suturing. Feed with liquid food by the month, except when the epiglottis is injured or when the larynx or trachea is divided, or when the pharynx or esophagus is opened—then feed by the rectum. The conclusion reached is that wounds of the throat should be treated by primary sutures when the condition of the patient permits; use antiseptic precautions; use chloroform for the anesthetic; suture the cut muscles; correct the inversion caused by the platysma muscle. Wounds of the air-passage should be closed; make a fresh vertical wound for the tube when one is used; use silk for suturing the larynx or trachea; except in special cases, feed by the mouth. [There can be no doubt that the surgeon's duty is to suture, in the hope of obtaining primary union; and, further, there can be no doubt that primary union can generally be obtained.]

H. Milton [3] gives the description of an operation on the cadaver by which the **mediastinum is exposed** from the thyroid cartilage to the xiphoid. An incision begins at the notch, and by sawing through the sternum the structures beneath are exposed. Another method is to begin at the junction of the xiphoid with the gladiolus and cut up. The author has done this on the living with success. The operation is described on a case of infiltrating

[1] Med. News, Nov. 7, 1896.			[2] Brit. Med. Jour., May 8, 1897.
[3] Lancet, Mar. 27, 1897.

tuberculous disease of sternum with tuberculous mediastinal glands. Remarkably little hemorrhage occurred. The costal respiration ceased, but the diaphragm worked freely. Nearly all the sternum was removed. Little shock followed. The wound was packed with gauze for 48 hours, then closed. Recovery ensued and the respiration was easily carried on.

DISEASES OF THE VASCULAR SYSTEM.

Bose and Vedel[1] publish some experiments on the **effects of intravenous injection** of various solutions. They find that distilled water is very injurious when injected into the veins, but that ordinary water is not harmful or certainly far less harmful than distilled water, and in an emergency it would be quite justifiable to inject common water. Solution of common salt is entirely harmless if the amount of sodium chlorid is not greater than 3 times the amount of sodium chlorid normally present in the blood. The best strength to use is 7 : 1000. Artificial serum is in no sense superior to ordinary saline solution.

Reverdin[2] asserts that **sodium sulfate** administered in small doses is **a valuable styptic agent,** which is particularly useful in hemorrhagic diathesis and epistaxis, capillary hemorrhage, and like conditions. Its great use is in arresting oozing. It will not arrest bleeding from arteries or veins. It increases the rapidity of clotting of the blood, and it can be given intravenously or by the mouth, but hypodermatic injections do not produce styptic results. The dose is $1\frac{1}{2}$ gr. every hour until the bleeding is controlled.

Bienwald[3] reports a case in which he stopped a hemorrhage in a hemophiliac by taking blood from a healthy person and applying it to the oozing wound.

Lewis A. Stimson[4] discusses the use of **intravenous saline injections in shock.** He says that it is well known that these injections are of benefit when administered after a severe operation accompanied by considerable hemorrhage and shock, but it is not so generally known that the same method is of advantage even if shock is not accompanied by hemorrhage. Stimson reports several cases to confirm this statement. He also tells us that in severe septic conditions the use of these injections is of great advantage. He saw them used for this purpose by Prof. Pozzi, of Paris, in a case of puerperal septicemia. Stimson reports a case of his own, and tells us that the good effects of intravenous injections are due to the increase of intraarterial pressure and the freedom with which osmosis is in consequence carried out. It seems also possible to believe that the large additional amount of water favors excretion and metabolism, diminishes the production of harmful compounds, and favors the elimination of those which have been produced. It is not directly curative, but it stimulates the organism and may enable it to recover from shock or to throw off septic attacks, and during this period we can employ other remedial measures. The technic is one of extreme simplicity. A graduated nozzle, which is carefully sterilized, is fitted with a rubber tube 3 ft. long, terminating in a glass nozzle. The solution is prepared by mixing 92 gr. of common salt with a quart of water and sterilizing it by boiling. That amount is secured practically by using a large teaspoonful of salt. The temperature at which it should be injected is 105°. A vein is exposed with a ligature slipped beneath it and the vein opened half across by cutting with scissors. The tube is filled with water, the glass nozzle is passed into the vein, and the ligature is tied so

---

[1] Gaz. des Hôpitaux, p. 398, 1896. [2] Rev. de la Suisse romaine, p. 36, Jan. 20, 1897.
[3] Sem. méd., May 5, 1897. [4] Med. News, Dec. 19, 1896.

as to keep the tube from slipping. The vessel which holds the solution is raised 2 or 3 ft. above the bed and the solution is allowed to run in. Some have maintained that hypodermoclysis is equally beneficial; it is certainly much simpler. [There can be no question that Stimson is right. Again and again have we seen pure shock without hemorrhage successfully combated by saline transfusion, rectal injection of saline fluid, or hypodermoclysis. In grave conditions transfusion is the preferable method. We always use Collin's apparatus. It enables us to measure the amount used and certainly excludes air. We have never used saline transfusion for sepsis, but consider its employment in this condition justifiable. In post-operative anemia the procedure is sometimes of great utility.]

William Horrocks[1] reports an interesting case of **acute aneurysm of the abdominal aorta.** Both iliac arteries were occluded by emboli and the patient was paraplegic. One interesting symptom was the presence of hemoglobin in the urine. The postmortem examination showed that the paraplegia could not have been of spinal origin, because there was no spinal lesion discovered and there was no interference with the circulation in the lumbar arteries.

Charles Watson MacGillivray[2] reports a case of that rare condition, **inguinal aneurysm.** The patient was 64 years of age, and had suffered from an aneurysm for about a year. The artery was tied by Abernethy's method, the incision being somewhat modified to suit the ease. The incision was placed further upward and outward than in the typical Abernethy operation. On the second day there was found to be again slight pulsation in the sac, and this was well marked on the fourth day. This pulsation diminished somewhat, but did not entirely disappear, and 2 months later a bruit again became perceptible. It was evident from a careful study that blood passed into the aneurysm, but chiefly from the distal side. Compression by flexion, tourniquets, weights, and elastic bands below and over the tumor was tried, but it produced only temporary lessening of the signs. Two methods of treatment suggested themselves as worthy of thought : 1. Excision of the aneurysm and tying the branches which entered it ; 2. Cutting down on the distal side and tying all the arteries that entered from below. The first did not seem advisable, as the original size and position of the swelling suggested adhesions to the peritoneum above and to the vein on the inner side. The second method was decided upon. This was carried out and the patient made a complete recovery.

Edmond Souchon[3] reports an interesting case of **high femoral aneurysm** which was cured by the synchronous ligation of the external iliac and superficial femoral arteries below the sac, by excision of the sac, and ligation of the common femoral for hemorrhage. The external iliac was ligated by Sir Astley Cooper's method. The superficial femoral was then ligated below the sac. The intention was to dissect out the sac, but as soon as the integuments were incised it ruptured spontaneously. There was a considerable amount of hemorrhage from the proximal end of the sac. The bleeding orifice was plugged by the finger while a ligature was passed around the artery.

John B. Murphy[4] reports two cases in which after resection of blood-vessels in the human being he practised **end-to-end suture.** In one case the femoral and internal saphenous veins had been injured by a pistol-bullet. An incision was made, the wounds in the saphenous were closed by the use of a continuous silk suture, the profunda branch of the femoral vein was sutured,

[1] Brit. Med. Jour., Jan. 16, 1897.   [2] Lancet, Aug. 29, 1896.
[3] New Orl. M. and S. Jour., Aug., 1896.   [4] N. Y. Med. Rec., Jan. 16, 1897.

and the wounds of the femoral vein were closed by a continuous silk suture. Infection took place from the injury and suppuration occurred. Five weeks later severe hemorrhage began. An incision was made, and it was seen that the hemorrhage was due to a slough an inch in length of the inner side of the femoral artery. The artery was tied above and below the slough and the damaged portion of the vessel removed. The patient recovered without any edema or any signs of circulatory trouble. In the second case the common femoral artery was perforated by a pistol-ball $1\frac{1}{2}$ in. below Poupart's ligament. A considerable portion of the walls of the artery was damaged; the bullet passed downward and backward, and perforated the femoral vein just above the junction of the profunda. The artery was gently clamped and the wounds in the femoral vein secured by continuous silk suture. Half an inch of the continuity of the artery was removed after about 2 in. of the artery had been exposed and the vessel had been isolated. At the proximal end for one-third of an inch the adventitia was turned up, and the proximal end was invaginated into the distal end and held there by 4 double threads. The threads were carried completely through the walls of the artery. A row of sutures was carried around the overlying distal end, passing through the media of the proximal end. The adventitia was then pulled down over the line of junction and sutured, and the clamps were taken away. Pulsation at once returned in the vessel; no edema of the leg ensued, and the circulation of the limb was restored from the moment of operation. As a result of numerous studies by the author, he has reached the conclusion that resection and suturing should only be applied to large-sized vessels, and that the vessels upon which this operation is performed must be handled most delicately, otherwise inflammation will ensue and thrombosis will take place. [The last case was brilliant in the extreme and opens up a new field in the surgery of the arterial system.]

Daniel H. Williams[1] reports a very remarkable case in which there was a **stab-wound of the heart and pericardium.** The pericardium was sutured; the patient recovered, and is alive 3 years afterward. The man was 24 years of age and was stabbed through the 5th costal cartilage. The internal mammary vessels, the pericardium, and the heart were damaged. The wound was 1 in. long, $\frac{3}{4}$ of an in. to the left side of the sternum, and in the long axis of the 5th cartilage. The probe could not be made to enter deeply, but during the night there was a great deal of hemorrhage, cough, pain over the heart, and shock. The following morning a careful examination demonstrated the fact that the knife had passed through the 5th costal cartilage in its long axis deep enough to enter the internal mammary vessels. When the weapon had been withdrawn the cartilage closed behind it and thus prevented the introduction of a probe. It was decided that an operation must be undertaken. The wound was lengthened toward the right side as far as the middle of the sternum, and over the centre of this incision a second incision was made. The second incision was about 6 in. in length and passed over the middle of the cartilage and the 5th rib. The sternum, the cartilage, and about 1 in. of the 5th rib were exposed. The cartilage was separated from its sternal junction and also from its attachment to the rib. Its inner attachments were separated, but its upper ones were left in place. The incised piece was lifted upward, and ready access was given to the internal mammary vessels, which were ligated above and below with catgut. In order to secure more room an incision was made in the 5th intercostal space. A small punctured wound was discovered in the heart. This wound was $\frac{1}{10}$ of an in. in length. The wound in the pericardium was $1\frac{1}{4}$ in. in length. There was no hemorrhage from either the

[1] N. Y. Med. Rec., Mar. 27, 1897.

24

heart or pericardium. The pericardial wound, having been irrigated with normal salt solution at a temperature of 100°, was closed with a continuous catgut suture. The intercostal wound and the subcartilaginous wound were closed with catgut, and the cartilages and the skin with silkworm-gut. The result proved that there was no cardiac, pericardiac, pleural, or wound infection. This patient went on fairly well for about 3 weeks, when evidences appeared of pericarditis with effusion and pleuritis. An incision was made in the 7th intercostal space in order to drain the pleural cavity, and 80 oz. of bloody serum were removed. After the operation adhesive straps were applied to the chest. The patient left the hospital well.

The author tells us that experiments upon the lower animals have been made to determine whether it is feasible to suture the heart and pericardium. Philippov made some of these experiments and Del Vechio made some, and the conclusion was that suture of the heart and pericardium was practicable in the human being. Ferrarresi reports a case in which, as the result of a stab, the left internal mammary artery was cut at the level of the 4th cartilage. He resected from the 3d to the 5th cartilages to reach the internal injury. He decided that the woman's condition did not warrant suturing the heart, so he sterilized the wound, lightly compressing the heart, and arrested bleeding by sterilized tampons. The patient recovered. Turner reports a case of a man who received an incised wound over the left 5th cartilage. The cartilage was split, blood spurted into the air and hissed out at each heart-beat and each respiration, and the pleura filled with blood. The man lived 4½ months. The left pleura became filled with pus, so the 5th rib was resected posteriorly to permit of drainage. The man died finally of what is called cerebral apoplexy. The postmortem showed that the left lung was collapsed, and the pleura adherent to the pericardium; the pericardial and cardiac wounds had healed; the wound in the heart was ¾ in. long, and had penetrated ⅝ in. into the septum between the ventricles, and the left coronary artery had been divided. Dr. Elkton has insisted that it is very difficult to determine the existence of a wound of the pericardium and heart. There is no pathognomonic symptom, and the diagnosis is only reached after a study of all the symptoms. Moullin on one occasion made an attempt to suture a wound of the heart and failed. In most wounds of the heart an antiseptic tampon is used to control hemorrhage and prevent infection. The *Index Catalogue* does not give a single case describing suture of the pericardium or heart in the human subject. [In the Congress of German Surgeons, 1897, Rahn[1] reported a case of stab-wound of the heart. He resected the 5th rib and found a wound of the right ventricle 1½ cm. in length. This wound was closed with 3 silk sutures and the pericardial cavity was packed with gauze. The patient recovered. G. Sandison Bock[2] communicates a case of perforating wound of the pericardium and left ventricle. The wound in the ventricle was sutured by Parrozzani, of Rome. The patient recovered. Durante[3] has reported a case of wound of the left ventricle which was sutured by Fareni. The patient lived several days and died from causes unconnected with the heart-wound. Cappelan[4] reports a case of stab-wound of the left ventricle. He resected the 3d and 4th ribs and sutured the wound in the heart. The patient lived 2½ days.]

E. P. Hershey[5] reports a most interesting case of **sacculated aneurysm of the innominate artery**, which was **treated by the introduction of gold wire and the use of galvanism**; 14-karat gold wire was taken and drawn out to No. 28 gauge, and the jeweler who drew it out conceived

[1] Lancet, vol. i., p. 1306, 1897.   [2] Ibid.   [3] Rev. de Chir., p. 335, 1897.
[4] Norsk Magazin for Loegevidenskaten, Mar., 1896.   [5] Therap. Gaz., Sept. 15, 1896.

the idea of snarling the wire, so that when it passed through the needle it would bunch itself rather than coil. The needle used was a hypodermatic needle with a caliber of about 22, and it was completely insulated by the application of layers of gum-shellac varnish. The current was supplied by a 30-cell galvanic battery, and was passed through a McIntosh milliampèremeter. The patient was prepared antiseptically for the operation. When the insulated needle was passed through the sac blood spurted to a considerable height, but this was arrested the minute the introduction of the wire was begun. The intention was to fill the cavity entirely with wire, it having been supposed that 10 ft. would accomplish this; but after 2½ ft. had been inserted the wire kinked and no more could be introduced. The wire was cut off about 3 in. from the needle; the positive pole of the battery was attached to the wire, and the negative pole was attached to a flat wet sponge covering an iron plate, which plate was placed on the skin of the back directly opposite the aneurysm. As the current passed the patient was at first uneasy and suffered from a certain amount of pain from the negative electrode. The number of cells was gradually increased, the current being kept at 70 ma. The needle as it swung rhythmically was a guide as to what was taking place. During fully three-quarters of an hour the motions of the needle never varied; but when a change took place in the motions of the needle the current was cut down to 60 ma.; as the motion of the needle became less the resistance became greater, until, finally, at the end of one hour and five minutes 40 ma. were used, the motion of the needle being then barely perceptible. At this time, instead of the existence of a soft, pulsating mass characteristic of aneurysm, there was a hard tumor which was very much smaller than the original sac. The needle was hard to remove, coagulated blood cementing it in place. It was gotten out and the wire cut off close to the skin, pressure being made around the point of exit. As soon as the tension was released the wire slipped out of sight, there having been sufficient spring in the mass of wire to pull the single strand into the sac. This man was very greatly improved by the operation. Nine and a half months after operation he is in excellent condition; he still has some pain in the chest, but the symptoms of aneurysm have entirely subsided. This aneurysm was closed by actual clot-formation.

Moore, of London, was the first to practise introduction of wire into the sac. His treatment was not successful. It is not to be wondered at when we reflect that he inserted 25 ft. of wire, and that this was practised before antiseptic details were carried out. Levis tried the introduction of horsehair; Schrotter used Florence silk. Macewen, of Glasgow, has suggested a method of treatment which consists in scratching the inner wall of the aneurysm, thus setting up inflammatory action and thereby strengthening the wall. Considering the fragile character of the sac, this is indeed a hazardous operation.

There have been ten cases reported in which aneurysm has been treated by the combined method of the introduction of wire and the application of electricity. Burresi reported a case in which 17 in. of No. 30 wire were introduced. The current was applied for 25 minutes. A firm clot formed, but the patient died in 100 days.

Barwell passed 10 ft. of steel wire into one division of the sac in a large aneurysm of the ascending and transverse parts of aorta; 10 ma. for one hour and ten minutes. At the end of six hours there were evidences of consolidation. On the fourth day a secondary sac rapidly increased in size. Death occurred on the 7th day. The postmortem showed the first sac contained a considerable amount of fibrin which closely united the sac and the wire. Roosevelt reported a very bad case of aortic aneurysm into which he introduced 225 ft. of fine steel piano-wire, and passed a current of 25 ma. for half an hour. The patient was obviously improved by the operation, but death occurred on the 23d day.

Abbe reported a case in which he introduced 100 ft. of No. 1 aseptic catgut; a portion of the tumor became firmer, but another portion was found to be advancing rapidly. Nine days after this he inserted an aspirating-needle and passed 150 ft. of fine sterilized wire into the sac, and for half an hour employed a current of 50 ma. The anode being applied, followed by 100 ma. for an hour and reversed; cathode the active pole. The tumor-wall was thought to be firmer, but pulsation continued and rupture took place on the second day.

Kerr introduced 6 ft. of silver wire into an aneurysm reaching from the base of the heart to the beginning of the left subclavian artery. He applied a current for 50 minutes. Both pain and pulsation were improved, but death occurred on the 18th day, and postmortem showed that a firm clot had formed about the wire as well as on the sac-wall.

Kerr reported a case of aortic intrapericardial aneurysm in which electrolysis had been tried without success. He then introduced 10 ft. of silver wire and applied a current for half an hour. Six months afterward the patient was in excellent condition, and the case is considered a cure.

Rosenstein reported a case of aneurysm in the ascending portion of the arch. Galvanopuncture was employed twice: first, a single needle was used and 70 ma. were passed for 20 minutes. Thirteen days later this was repeated with two needles. No benefit was observed. Five and a half weeks later something over 2 ft. of wire were passed into the sac. Pulsation disappeared the 7th week and complete recovery followed.

Stewart reported a case of thoracico-abdominal aneurysm into which 2½ ft. of wire were inserted, a current of 70 ma. having been passed for an hour. It ruptured on the ninth day. The postmortem showed that there were firm clots in all parts of the aneurysm, with softened ones of recent origin. Stewart also reported a second case which was greatly benefited by the introduction of fine gold wire, and the application for an hour and a quarter of a current of 80 ma. Taking into consideration these cases that have been reported, we have 30% of cures, 20% benefited, and 50% fatal, and in none of the fatal cases was death due to the operation.

DISEASES OF THE LYMPHATIC SYSTEM.

De Forest Willard[1] writes on **tuberculosis of the superficial lymphatic glands.** He tells us that the seat of invasion is to a great extent influenced by injuries or abrasions. The fact that the legs are but slightly exposed to sources of injury renders tuberculous disease of the lymph-glands of the groin unusual. The hand, though considerably exposed to injury, is protected by hard epithelium; but the face and neck are very liable to scratches, eczema, trivial wounds of the skin and mucous membranes, catarrhal inflammation, etc. A slight area of injury is more apt to give entrance to tubercle-bacilli than are large wounds, probably because in large wounds the tissue-changes are more active. When germs once enter, the vigor of the opposition by the organism depends upon its inherent vital resistance. The first point of arrest of the bacilli is usually in the lymph-nodules, and at this point the organism may be successfully arrested if the tissue-resistance of the individual is at a high level. At times the glands originally infected fail to arrest the

[1] Ann. of Surg., Dec., 1896.

trouble, or a number of bacilli pass the point of infiltration and reach other glands, the route depending upon the direction of the lymph-current. In the neck it may be along through the superficial or the deep glands. Willard commends attention to the diagram prepared by Gerrish, which shows how infection from the brow, eyelids, or outer cheek will be first arrested in the glands of the parotid region, while infection from the frontal, nasal, and deep buccal region will be arrested first in the submaxillary glands, and will then be carried to the superficial cervical. When the infection begins in the deeper tissues of the cheek, or the upper jaw or the cavity of the nose, or the roof or floor of the mouth or the tongue, it will be carried to the internal maxillary glands and thence to the deep cervical. The deep cervical glands may also be infected from the pharynx, the larynx, and the trachea, and the infection may be distributed from them to the superficial mediastinal and the axillary glands. The resisting power of the glands in the groin seems to be lessened by the existence of a syphilitic element, and clinical facts indicate that the bacteria of syphilis and of tuberculosis are not antagonistic.

One method of the arrest of the tuberculous process is the blockage of the lymph-spaces by inflammatory exudate. It is rare for infection to travel into the periglandular connective tissue, and it is still rarer for it to travel in a direction opposite to that of the lymph-stream. In some cases both the superficial and deep glands are affected at the same time. If the lymphatics fail in their power of resistance, the infecting material will be carried into the general circulation and produce distant disease and even miliary tuberculosis. The virulence of a caseous focus is dependent upon the spores rather than the bacilli, and these spores may retain a power of infection for an indefinite period. Willard calls attention to the fact that though he has very frequently seen tuberculosis of different parts of the body ensue on tuberculous disease of the lymph-glands of the neck, he has never seen cervical lymphadenitis result from tuberculosis of the lungs. The author then contrasts certain points of diagnosis. He says that in syphilitic infection we should be able to find the initial lesion or the evidences of the initial lesion, and if the disease be in the second or tertiary stage, we should find obvious evidences of its existence. A simple inflammation or an acute suppurative inflammation is very rapid in progress, and there is either a traumatic cause of the condition, or else the existence of a septic cause, such as scarlatina. In cancerous involvement of glands we can usually find a primary trouble, the enlargement of the glands being secondary to this, as a rule. Primary cancer of lymph-glands is a rare condition. Sarcoma is usually single. It reaches a great size, rarely suppurates, grows rapidly, involves the surrounding tissues, and does not caseate. Secondary lymphosarcoma is a rare condition. Adenomata are single, not multiple. Lipomata are single. Pseudoleukemia shows enlargement of glands in other parts of the body and the affected glands do not caseate. In lymphadenoma there are enlargement of the spleen and increase of the number of white corpuscles in the blood. In tubercular disease it may or may not be possible to find the organism.

Willard is an advocate of early operation, but he does not believe that it is advisable when only 1 or 2 glands are involved to lay open the neck to its entire extent. He would remove the obviously infected glands, but not the non-indurated ones. The operation, when the mass is extensive, is a serious one. The surgeon is often unable to tell before the incision is made whether the deeper glands are implicated or not. He is working among vital parts, and yet the operation must be thorough. A large incision is necessary for safety, and it is sometimes necessary to lay aside the sternomastoid muscle. When the glands have become adherent to the skin this infiltrated tissue should be excised. We should be careful, if possible, not to open the capsule, as the diffusion of tuberculous matter in the wound is a very unfortunate event. Care should be taken not to tear off short branches of the jugular veins. Such an accident is liable to be followed by the entrance of air into veins. If such an opening be made, the fingers should at once close the aperture and then compress the carotid artery against the carotid tubule. The next procedure is to ligate the vein or apply lateral ligature. It has been suggested that in such an accident the wound should be kept full of water to prevent the entrance of air. Willard has not found this nearly so effective as finger-pressure. With pressure on the proximal end of the vein the blood from the distal end will keep the wound clearly filled. Pressure should be continued until the vessel has been secured. Artificial respiration may be practised to prevent immediate collapse, and electricity may be employed if available. Lateral suturing in these cases has proved most satisfactory.

In is rare that the pneumogastric nerve, the descendens noni, or phrenic is injured; but when we lift them from their beds the diaphragm is apt to be interfered with for a time. It has long been observed that dyspnea and congestion of the lungs were more apt to follow neck-operations than operations upon any other part of the body. Injury of the pneumogastric is not necessarily fatal, but is, of course, serious, and will probably be followed by bronchopneumonia, edema, or some other lung-trouble. If we should happen to divide any of these nerves, they should be immediately sutured with fine silk or chromicized gut.

Willard is very fond of using iodin in these conditions, and believes that it markedly inhibits the growth of the microorganisms and stimulates the production of healthy granulation. Iodin injected into sinuses greatly aids in their closure. He has never seen any benefit result from the intraglandular injection of iodoform or chlorid of zinc—in fact, such measures hasten suppuration. If the patient refuses operation, he can gain considerable by the internal use of arsenic, iron, cod-liver oil, potassium iodid, guaiacol, or creasote, by living in good air, and employing proper food. The above means should be employed in both operative and nonoperative cases. Sero-therapy is still in its experimental stage. Antiphthisin gives negative results. He has had no experience with the use of aseptocen and antituberculous serum. Nuclein and protonuclein he has used chiefly locally. These agents favor the production of healthy granulations. A mixture of thymol iodid, or aristol, and protonuclein is of great value in sluggish granulation. [There can be no doubt that in some cases tuberculous glands arise secondarily to enlarged tonsils and adenoids. In such cases R. Sims Woodhead has found bacilli in the tonsils or the adenoids. H. Starck has shown the causative influence of carious teeth. In 113 cases of tuberculous glands 41 were obviously secondary to caries of the teeth, and in 2 cases tubercle-bacilli were found in the teeth-sockets.[1] Nicoll says that in 80% of cases the cause of the glandular enlargement will be found in the nasopharynx, and that many nasopharyngeal catarrhs are tubercular. Dieulafoy has found bacilli in the tonsil and glands of the tongue. It is always to be remembered, however, that numbers of tubercle-bacilli may be found in the mouth of a healthy individual. Another fact of importance to remember is that it is not always possible to make a clinical diagnosis between malignant lymphoma and tuberculous adenitis. It sometimes happens that tuberculous glands attain a large size without softening, and that enlarge-

---

[1] Münch. med. Woch., xliii., 145, 1896.

ments due to malignant lymphoma do soften. In fact, Dietrich has asserted that malignant lymphoma may be combined with glandular tuberculosis.]

J. Crawford Renton,[1] in a discussion of the **treatment of tuberculous glands of the neck**, stated that he recently advocated free excision of the glands, but the result of this procedure is far from satisfactory. In the cervical region it often happens that, after we have removed all of the glands that are enlarged, other glands enlarge and require removal. On account of this repeated enlargement of remaining glands he has recently gone back to the old method of treatment, and now only dissect out glands where softening has commenced and where the smallest possible incision can be made, and where the gland can be removed entire by a small incision after it has been lessened by partial enucleation. [Such a method cannot protect the system from invasion. Thorough extirpation is preferable.]

Harold J. Stiles[2] presented a paper on **tuberculous disease of the cervical glands**. He tells us that the treatment of tuberculous glandular abscess consists in incision, scraping with Volkmann's spoon, the application of pure carbolic acid, and stuffing with iodoformized worsted. The incision should be made parallel to the skin-creases, and, unless the abscess be very small, ought to be large enough to admit the finger. The scraping is kept up until all caseous or purulent matter has been removed from the wall of the cavity. When this has been accomplished the wall of the cavity will feel smooth. The application of pure carbolic acid is an important element in the treatment. Iodoformized worsted is a better agent than iodoform-gauze. It is softer, more elastic, absorbs better, and is a better capillary drain. Another advantage of this iodoform worsted is that it is very convenient for packing sinuses, and it can be prepared freshly with great ease. The carbolic acid does not cause sloughing. It often happens that a deep gland becomes adherent to the cervical fascia, bursts through it, and causes an abscess subcutaneously. In all such subcutaneous collections the surgeon should open the abscess by a moderately large incision and make search for an opening in the deep fascia, and through this opening find the remains of the caseating glands. Caseous and purulent tuberculous adenitis is very difficult to deal with when situated behind the pharynx or in the region in front of the auricle. The most common cause of retropharyngeal abscess in children is tuberculous adenitis. The abscess may be reached by three routes: by the mouth, by Chiene's plan of making an incision at the posterior edge of the sternomastoid, or by Burckhardt's plan of incision in the anterior triangle. The best method is that of Chiene. The great advantage of this over the old method of opening through the mouth is that the abscess can be treated aseptically. Tuberculous adenitis of the preauricular region is under the cervical fascia and close to the parotid gland and the facial nerve, and the tuberculous gland adheres to these structures and also to the skin, and it is seldom proper to attempt to excise it when it is immovable. In fact, a salivary fistula may arise from simply scraping the gland. Scrape it through a very small incision made at its lower part. If the gland is but slightly caseous or is altogether solid, if it has existed for months, and is uninfluenced by general treatment, it should certainly be excised if it is still movable. Excision of a movable gland in this situation is but a trifling operation, and but a slight scar is left. If glands in the neck are adherent to the veins, nerves, and other deep structures, the difficulties are vastly enhanced. In this case we should have large incisions in order to get a clear view of every structure before we cut it, and we should not mistake stretched veins for bands of fascia. A blunt dissector will be a

[1] Brit. Med. Jour., Sept. 12, 1896.   [2] Ibid.

great aid in the operation. If one gland is softened so that it fluctuates, treat this gland by scraping and the use of pure carbolic acid before excising the mass. Do this in order to prevent infection of the wound, and we will then be enabled to suture the wound after completion of the operation. In this operation take care that the patient's hair and the chloroform-mask do not infect the wound. The best apposition is obtained by the use of a continuous suture of horsehair or fine silk, the assistant lifting the edges of the wound and putting them on the stretch while it is being sewed. Stiles says that we must not suppose that he advocates excision in all cases. It should be the rule in adults when the disease is localized to the neck, but there are many instances in young children where it is not advisable. In young children there is generally some local source of infection, the gland-disease is very active, and softening and abscess-formation are almost certain to occur. This makes complete excision a very difficult matter because of the matting together of the structures which ensues. The older the child the more must the question of complete excision be entertained. The operation is not advisable in very young children. It may not be possible to accomplish excision at one operation. It is often wise to do but one side of the neck at a time, and two or even three operations may be necessary in order to eradicate the disease completely. If the patient is approaching adolescence, if he is otherwise in good health, if the disease is of long duration and has resisted all other treatment, and if there be no persistent source of primary infection, excision is to be practised. In case of extensive tuberculous infiltration of both triangles of the neck operate by the plan of Chiene—that is, remove the jugular vein along with the mass of glands. This makes the operation easier and more thorough. In speaking of the points of diagnosis it is commonly stated that when tuberculous glands reach any considerable size they always caseate; but Stiles has seen tuberculous glands as large as pullet's eggs, which exhibited no trace of caseation. Surgeons are apt to speak of such glands as examples of simple lymphomata. The microscope often shows that non-caseous glands are tuberculous.

George Ryerson Fowler [1] reports a case of **elephantiasis of the lower extremity** which was cured by ligation of the external iliac artery. The boy was 16 years of age, and 7 years before he had suffered from double suppurating inguinal adenitis. The mass on the left side was opened, but the right side evacuated itself spontaneously. Shortly after this the lower extromity of the right side began to enlarge, and this increased to a considerable degree. Fowler then submits the measurements of the 2 limbs to show the difference between them. The patient was placed in the Trendelenburg position; a 3-in. vertical incision was made in the right semilunar line and the external iliac artery was ligated by the transperitoneal method. The patient recovered without trouble from the operation and was greatly improved by it; 6 weeks after the operation the legs were practically of the same size. Fowler says that the transperitoneal ligation of the iliac artery is easy, but is no easier than the extraperitoneal method of ligation, and it increases the dangers to the patient because of the possible onset of peritonitis.

Carnochan originally suggested ligation of the femoral below Poupart's ligament in this disease. Hueter suggested ligation of the external iliac artery. Fowler believes this is the first case in which Hueter's suggestion has been carried out.

[1] Brooklyn Med. Jour., Feb., 1897.

DISEASES OF THE THYROID GLAND.

Gayet[1] makes a report on the **treatment of Basedow's disease** by the plan of Jaboulay—that is, by removal of the cervical sympathetic ganglion and division of the nerve below the ganglion. The patient had had an exophthalmic goiter for 5 years; ether was given, and an incision 3 in. in length was made on the left side, beginning about 2 fingers' breadth below the mastoid process and running down close to the posterior edge of the sterno-cleido-mastoid muscle. This muscle was retracted and the structures below exposed. The pneumogastric nerve, the internal jugular vein, and the carotid artery were drawn forward. This maneuver exposed the sympathetic, and the fact that it was the sympathetic which was exposed was made manifest by the dilatation of the pupil when the nerve was irritated. The cervical ganglion was removed with several of its branches, and the trunk of the nerve was cut below the ganglion. On the right side the same operation was performed, differing only in the fact that the trunk of the nerve was sectioned above the ganglion. On the evening of the operation the exophthalmos had absolutely disappeared. Improvement continued during the next day, and on the 8th day the patient left the hospital apparently well. The operation of complete removal of the thyroid gland is not practised in these days because we know it occasions myxedema.

Incomplete removal is the favorite operation. Four-fifths of the patients operated upon recover, but recurrence is common, and often after operation very rapid growth takes place. Sometimes thyroid-intoxication follows operation. The operation of simply exposing an exophthalmic goiter is not often curative, and occasionally the symptoms of systemic intoxication follow its performance. Ligation of the thyroid arteries is an operation of considerable difficulty. The division of the sympathetic nerve is a safe procedure and is easily performed, and the favorable effects seem to be permanent. [Thyroid extract is not useful in true exophthalmic goiter—in fact, it is believed to aggravate the condition. Some hours after the performance of a partial thyroidectomy sudden death may occur, and the cause of such death cannot be determined by autopsy. Delore recently reported such a case. Operation in exophthalmic goiter is often difficult, as the capsule and blood-vessels are very friable and the administration of an anesthetic is fraught with peculiar danger. We disagree entirely with the view of Lemke that exophthalmic goiter is always a surgical disease. It is sometimes a surgical disease. It should pass into the hands of the surgeon if medical treatment fails, or if evidences of grave toxemia are present, and if marked dyspnea exists.]

The *Annals of Surgery* for March, 1897, contains an abstract translation of an article by H. Bergeat, of Tübingen, the abstract having been made by Charles L. Gibson, of New York. Bergeat considers **300 operations for goiter** performed in the Tübingen clinic. He tells us that the proportion of females to males is 2.5 to 1, and that in the male sex goiter is apt to begin between the 14 and 17th years and in the female between the 12th and 16th years. The majority of goiters occur in people who are obliged to perform hard manual labor. The list contains only 2 cases of complete extirpation. The operation of choice has been intraglandular enucleation, but there are a number of examples given of extracapsular extirpation. It is the opinion of the author that we can often combine these 2 methods with advantage. He holds that every nonmalignant goiter which is increasing rapidly in size ought to be operated upon, but we should never operate simply to relieve disfigure-

[1] Lyon méd., No. 30, 1896.

ment. In young people it is well not to be in too much of a hurry to operate, because goiters which begin at the time of puberty may undergo spontaneous cure. Respiratory disturbances are the usual conditions rendering an operation necessary. The majority of these patients had respiratory disturbances; 21 complained of difficulty in swallowing; in 33 the vocal chords of the goiterous side were in a condition of paralysis. There were 89 cases of parenchymatous goiter, 73 of cystic goiter, and 116 of the combined forms. In 53 % the right lobe was the one almost wholly affected, in 22 % the left lobe, in 7 % the middle lobe, and in 18 % the point could not be determined.

The author tells us that the parenchymatous form rarely comes to be operated on until it has lasted for some 14 or 15 years; but the cystic form, as a rule, requires operation within about 4 years. Of the 300 operations, 79 consisted in unilateral extirpation, 176 of enucleation, and 45 of the combined method. In 10 cases the operation was performed without the use of an anesthetic. The author greatly prefers operating without an anesthetic to operating in a state of incomplete anesthesia, because incomplete anesthesia is very unsatisfactory. Besides this, when the patient is not anesthetized the recurrent laryngeal nerve can be recognized if it is grasped. It is very important to arrest hemorrhage. The average length of stay in the hospital after the extirpation of a goiter is 11 days, and after enucleation 9 days. In nearly every case there was some elevation of temperature during the course of the healing of the wound. This was due probably to septic absorption. The ultimate results of 84 of these cases were determined, and two-thirds of them show recurrence in some form.

The conclusion of the author is that one-sided extirpation is favored by the results. Operation for malignant growths of the thyroid is practically useless, and not a case survived operation after a year.

Charles A. Morton[1] discusses the **cause and treatment of sudden dyspnea in goiter,** and also reports a case in which the middle lobe of the thyroid was excised for this condition. He tells us that a person who has a goiter, but who has not suffered from dyspnea at all or who has only suffered moderately, may have a sudden attack which may be fatal. None of the theories that have been advanced to account for this are entirely satisfactory. A very few cases have been caused by hemorrhage into the goiter; but, of course, this condition is excessively rare. The theory of Rose is that the pressure of the enlarged thyroid makes the tracheal rings non-resistant, so that the trachea is apt to be bent and its lumen become obstructed. He thinks that in these cases of sudden dyspnea the trachea becomes kinked from relaxation of the muscles, which maintain the head in such a position as to keep the tube open, and that this is probably brought about either during sleep or anesthesia. But Morton shows that these cases do not occur always during sleep or anesthesia, and that very urgent dyspnea is rarely brought on by the relaxation of the muscles during sleep, for if the position of the neck were the cause of the dyspnea alteration of the position should relieve it, yet this is not the case.

Dr. Hurry thinks that the dyspnea is originated by some unusual exertion; that this unusual exertion, by originating a little dyspnea, leads to the bringing into action of extra muscles of respiration, and when they act the lobes of the thyroid are pressed against the trachea more; but, as a matter of fact, this dyspnea does not always come on because of unusual exertion.

Bristowe believes that the condition is due to inflammatory enlargement of the tissues and edema of the mucous membrane, but we know that this dyspnea is not particularly associated with laryngeal catarrh. Morton inquires if

[1] Bristol Med.-Chir. Jour., Sept., 1896.

pressure on the recurrent laryngeals can be the cause of the dyspnea. Its onset appears to be too sudden to be due to goiter-pressure on the nerves. Moreover, we cannot obtain relief by opening the air-passages above the goiter, and in the case here reported two severe paroxysms of dyspnea came on after the performance of laryngotomy. There is no doubt that a patient who is going about with a very small air-channel may suffer from urgent dyspnea when there is any sudden demand for an unusual quantity of air. This was the cause in Jacobson's case, where fright was responsible for the attack; but all the cases do not show a history of some cause which would make them out of breath. In fact, in some of the reported cases dyspnea came on when the patient was quiet in bed. Morton reports such a case. In this case Morton opened the air-passages above the goiter and passed a tube down the trachea. The dyspnea was relieved and the patient soon was able to breathe as well without the tube as with it. The cause of the paroxysm, therefore, had departed; but after a few whiffs of chloroform were given the extreme dyspnea came on again, and later, while the operation of excision of the isthmus was being performed, dyspnea arose without any apparent exciting cause. We may, of course, assume that the chloroform acted in the same way as the sudden fright; but why, with a cannula in place, did dyspnea come on during operation? In this case Morton performed excision of the isthmus of the thyroid gland, and the result proves that excision of the isthmus alone is not always sufficient to relieve these patients, as in this case it was necessary to retain the tube for weeks after the operation. When we consider the great difficulty of reaching the trachea below the isthmus, the best thing we can do in these urgent cases is to open the air-passages above and pass a long cannula or catheter past the obstruction. If there is room between the isthmus and the cricoid cartilage, that is the best point; but if there is not, laryngotomy must be performed. We cannot expect to get a cannula or catheter down the narrow and devious trachea through the mouth and glottis. The dyspnea is so rapidly fatal that we cannot undertake to excise a lateral lobe, and excision of the isthmus alone is useless. If the goiter is chiefly back of the sternum, we should perform a tracheotomy above the isthmus and attempt to pass a catheter into the right bronchus. After doing this the question will arise as to what form of excision to undertake. The existence of a septic laryngotomy-wound will prevent an aseptic course in the thyroidectomy-wound, and hence the removal of the isthmus alone may be practised with advantage, as excision of the isthmus is nearly always followed by atrophy of the remaining portions of the gland. It has been suggested that division of the fascia in the median line of the neck may give relief, the lateral lobes being thus to a certain extent freed from compression against the trachea; but opening the air-passages above the goiter and passing a catheter beyond the obstruction will be more likely to succeed. We should remember that compression of the trachea by unilateral goiter means compression by a cyst or an adenoma, and not by an ordinary goiter. If a cyst is present, the dyspnea can be relieved by drainage. Dyspnea from an adenoma would require the same treatment as dyspnea from an ordinary goiter.

Riedel[1] reports 2 cases in which there was some **chronic inflammation of the thyroid gland, with the formation of a mass of extreme hardness.** In this condition the tumor is closely adherent to the adjacent tissues, and it is impossible to separate the trachea and large vessels of the neck from the tumor. In the 2 cases reported by the author it was necessary to abandon attempts at removal. In one of these cases thyroid extract was administered without any benefit.

[1] Verhandl. der deutsch. Gesellsch. f. Chir., XXVth Congress, 1896.

DISEASES OF THE MUSCLES AND TENDONS.

Lejars[1] reports a very unusual case of **osteoma of the ligament of the patella,** the tumor having no connection with the patella itself or with the tibia. It was composed of compact bone-tissue and was as large as a walnut. It was necessary to remove it because it interfered with joint-motion. The tumor was removed without seriously injuring the ligament of the patella, and a portion of this ligament which was cut was sutured together. No loss of function followed the operation.

Hartmann[2] makes a study of 22 cases of **wry-neck** operated on in the Rostock clinic. In about one-third of the cases the result was perfect; in two-thirds it was imperfect. The cases were treated by division of the sterno-cleido-mastoid, the division having been sometimes open and sometimes subcutaneous. The author maintains that after division of the sternomastoid the muscle is apt to unite without any shortening, and that the failures in the operation are due to degenerative processes uninfluenced by the operation. Mikulicz recommends the entire removal of the muscle, but Hartmann asserts that this operation has had but a limited range of usefulness. The degenerative processes in the muscle will be arrested spontaneously eventually, and all that will be necessary will be to cut the shortened muscle.

Quervain[3] considers **operations on the spinal accessory nerve for spasmodic torticollis.** He concludes that their chief value as is an abortive. In 61 cases that have been reported there were only 12 cures, although 22 cases were improved. Kocher was so disappointed with operations on the spinal accessory that he devised an operation which consists in completely cutting across all of the muscles which are involved. He treated 12 cases; 7 of them were completely cured. The other 5 are still being treated by manipulations and gymnastics, which Kocher holds must always be employed after this operation. The cross-cutting of the muscles does not cause atrophy, paralysis, nor rigidity of the head.

Andrew J. McCosh[4] records a case of **rupture of the tendon of the quadriceps extensor** treated successfully by suture. This accident is by no means rare, and yet it is very often overlooked. It is very important that these cases should be treated properly soon after the injury. In many of them it is certain that surgical operation is not required, but in the majority of cases when there has been complete rupture either above or below the patella the nonoperative treatment is unsatisfactory. This is especially true of rupture above the patella. Maydl collected 40 such cases, and found that there was complete recovery in only about 60%, and in the 23 cases collected by J. B. Walker there was a complete recovery in 70%. Walker collected 21 cases, with complete recovery in 90% after suture. These operations are not absolutely devoid of risk, and this should be borne in mind. The most favorable time to perform the operation is when the acute stage of joint-hyperemia has passed away—that is, about 5 or 6 days after the accident; but the operation can be performed even when several weeks have passed away. In the first case reported by McCosh there was a delay of 8 weeks, and yet the recovery was perfect, and in the second case there was a similar delay which did not appear to influence the final result. The author reports 3 successful cases. In the first case there was complete separation of the quadriceps extensor tendon from the upper border of the left patella. A 6-in. vertical incision was made, which

[1] Gaz. hebdom. de Méd. et de Chir., Feb. 21, 1897.
[2] Ann. of Surg., Mar., 1897, from Beiträge zur klin. Chir., B. xv., H. iii.
[3] Sem. méd., Oct. 14, 1896.   [4] Ann. of Surg., Mar., 1897.

at once entered the joint and exposed the lower portion of the tendon and the patella. The hardened and irregular end of the tendon and the border of the patella were trimmed off. The operation disclosed the fact that the tendon had been torn directly from its attachment to the bone and had pulled with it some of the periosteum, but the lateral expansions of the tendon were only partially torn off. The joint was irrigated with hot saline solution and 3 drill-holes were made in the upper end of the patella, in which and through the thickness of the tendon silkworm-gut sutures were passed. The synovial membrane and the lacerated portions of the lateral expansions were sutured with catgut. The silkworm-gut sutures were tied and the incision closed by silk sutures without drainage; the limb was hyperextended and put up in a plaster-of-Paris splint, which was worn for 6 weeks. The patient made a complete recovery. [Operation is preferable because it saves months of time and is far more certain in result. It must be done if separation of an inch or more has taken place. If the separation is less than this, it is justifiable, though scarcely desirable, to apply the mechanical treatment if this treatment is found capable of bringing the ends in contact and holding them.]

Janni [1] reports a case of a soldier who during a march was seized with a very violent pain in the middle third of the left leg anteriorly and toward its outer side. This pain passed away after a few days' rest, but returned whenever an attempt was made to walk. This condition kept up for several months. Examination of the painful area showed that there was a small spot where the muscular resistance was less than throughout the rest of the leg. An incision was made and there was found a **rupture in the aponeurosis**. Janni then made some experiments on dogs, and discovered that after there was a small laceration of the fascia without muscle-injury no musele-hernia occurred during either contraction or relaxation. [The author's experiments seem to show that, except under some very extraordinary condition, a muscle is not able to rupture its own sheath, but clinically we know that simple muscular contraction may cause a rupture of the sheath.]

Howard Marsh [2] delivered a clinical lecture on **displacements and injuries of muscles and tendons.** The most familiar examples of displacements of tendons are displacement of the tendon of the peroneus longus to the front of the external malleolus, of the tendon of the tibialis posticus to the front of the internal malleolus, and of the long tendon of the biceps inward or outward from the bicipital groove of the humerus. Displacement of a muscle is a rare condition and but few muscles are liable to it. Muscles which act in a straight line and do not pass over any bony prominence are not liable. The muscles which are liable may be grouped under certain headings: those which have their tendons deflected and which, as they pass around a bony prominence which acts as a pulley, rest in a groove which is bridged over by a ligamentous expansion. We see this in the case of the peroneus longus and the tibialis posticus as they pass behind the malleoli. From a consideration of the deflected course of the extensor digitorum pedis it would seem as if this muscle should be liable to displacement, yet there is no example of this injury on record. The reason of the immunity becomes clear when we consider the structure of the annular ligament. The next group of muscles which are liable are those which pass over bony prominences, and that undergo considerable subjacent movement to one side or the other of the tendon line. This is illustrated by the long head of the biceps cubiti. Those that slip over some bony ridge or projection, as a bundle of the splenius capitis or one of the tendons of the obturator internus. The symptoms of the muscular dislocation

---

[1] Riforma med., Nov., 1896.　　　　　　[2] Brit. Med. Jour., July 25, 1897.

are obvious when the tendons can be seen and felt beneath the skin.   In other cases diagnosis must rest on indirect evidence. In the third group diagnosis may be impossible; the surgeon can only have a suspicion that the injury exists. In this group the history may be of very great assistance in reaching a conclusion. In treating these cases we should place the part in a position so that the muscle is relaxed, and we can then effect reduction by means of manipulation. When reduction has been accomplished, if the muscular sheath is unlacerated, no treatment will be needed; but if the sheath has been lacerated, after-treatment is of the greatest possible importance.   The peroneus longus is an example. As soon as the displacement has been reduced the foot should be placed at right angles with the leg, should be a little bit inverted, and be put up for a month in a splint of leather or plaster-of-Paris.   This will give time for the torn edges of the sheath to grow together.   Gosselin in a case of dislocation of the peroneus endeavored to cause inflammation by permitting the tendon to slip in and out for a few days with a view of securing adhesions, but Marsh doubts very much the advisability of endeavoring to promote inflammation. The question shall we operate always comes up. He has had no experience with operation, and does not know of an instance in which it has been performed.   Published cases show that repair may take place without operation. Whether or not such an operation is advisable cannot be decided until experience has accumulated as to the results of treatment by fixation in an appropriate position.   If we find that the results of this plan are not satisfactory, operation will certainly be indicated. Some would infer that immediate suture might be followed by the formation of adhesions between the tendon and its sheath; but if these should form, they would serve to keep the tendon in place, and at the worst they could only embarrass the action of a single muscle which was already out of gear.   As a matter of fact, though, after an antiseptic operation adhesions are not likely to form.   In speaking of rupture of muscle, Marsh says that he means rupture of single muscles by their own contractions during ordinary movement.   Some examples of such injuries are then submitted.   Marsh discusses **rupture of the ligamentum patellæ,** and reports a case which he sutured.

The treatment consists in the use of a posterior splint, with some means to keep the patella in place, or else suturing.   In many cases the former method has given satisfactory results.   When it is employed the patient should be kept in a horizontal position for two months, and should wear some form of retentive apparatus for from three to six months longer.   Rupture of the quadriceps muscle in the thigh is an injury in regard to which considerable doubt exists.   Some maintain that it will be followed by great impairment of function, and that the patient should not be permitted to walk for months without an apparatus.   The correct view, however, seems to be that in the generality of cases the limb may be safely used for careful walking, without support, within about four months after the accident. A diagnosis of rupture of a muscle depends on a history of muscular effort, a sudden pain, and a sensation as if a part had been struck—possibly a distinct snap and the existence of a gap.   When a tendon is ruptured there may be very little swelling at first, but when a muscle is torn there is usually a great deal of swelling, due to extravasated blood.   In some cases, as when the quadriceps extensor is ruptured, the limb is powerless; but in others, for example, when the tendo-Achillis is torn, the patient may be able to walk with comparatively little difficulty.   Experience shows that when a tendon, for instance the tendo-Achillis, is ruptured, if the limb is placed in a position in which the origin and insertion of the muscles concerned are approximated, and the ends of the tendons are not widely separated, the result is usually good. Whether operative interference is likely to secure a better result is uncertain. Two circumstances justify and may demand interference. First, wide separation of the ruptured ends, which cannot be corrected by other means. Second, a considerable extravasation of blood. If the fleshy parts of the muscle are torn, it is useless to attempt to suture the ends, as the stitches will not hold; but if a large blood-clot is present and near the surface, it will be advisable to expose the swelling by a free aseptic incision and remove the clot. At the same time any available portions of the sheath of the muscle should be sutured.

Perimoff[1] has devised an **operation for the cure of dislocation of the peroneal tendons.** An incision is made, the external malleolus is exposed, and the periosteal bone-flap is lifted up to right angles with the malleolus. This flap has the shape of a trapezoid. The flap-hinge is the posterior border of the external malleolus, and as long as it remains in position the tendon cannot slip forward. The flap is kept upright by driving two nickel nails into the malleolus until bony union has taken place. A plaster-of-Paris bandage is applied and worn for 6 weeks. The nails are removed in the 3d week. [If we are called to a patient who has suffered from this accident for the first time, it is proper to treat him by rest, pads, and bandages. In some 6 weeks the tendon will probably become firmly held. But a patient who has once had this accident is liable to suffer again from a slight cause, and the tendeney to dislocation may become habitual. Operation must then be performed.]

R. Carmichael Worsley[2] reports a case in which he obtained union of the cut tendons of the extensor primi internodii and extensor ossis metacarpi pollicis 5 years after division. The ends were separated by $1\frac{1}{2}$ in. of fibrous tissue, but the result was most satisfactory.

S. E. Milliken[3] publishes an additional paper on his method of **tendon-grafting and muscle-transplantation** as applied to the deformities ensuing upon infantile paralysis. He has operated 14 times on 9 patients. The operations were classified as follows : transplantation of the sartorius muscle into the sheath of the quadriceps extensor of the thigh, transplantation being partial or complete ; grafting the extensor proprius pollicis to the paralyzed tibialis anticus ; attaching the tibialis anticus to the paralyzed extensor longus digitorum ; attaching the extensor proprius pollicis to the paralyzed common extensor ; attaching the gastrocnemius to the paralyzed peroneus longus and brevis ; the extensor longus digitorum was attached to the paralyzed tibialis anticus once ; the extensor proprius pollicis was attached to the paralyzed extensor longus digitorum ; the flexor longus pollicis was transplanted onto the anterior surface of the leg and attached to the tendon of the paralyzed tibialis anticus ; the deltoid was attached to the tendon of the paralyzed triceps of the upper extremity. Milliken tells us we should preserve the sheaths of the tendons and should operate with absolute asepsis. If we follow these rules, we shall be able to obtain primary union and the grafted or transplanted muscle will be most capable of usefulness. In only 1 of his 14 operations did union fail to take place. The functional result of such operations is excellent.

BONE-DISEASES AND FRACTURES.

Cramer,[4] of Cologne, discusses Bardenheuer's method of correcting bone defeets by means of **splitting a metatarsal bone in the long axis** to make

---

[1] Rev. de Chir., Sept., 1896.　　　　　　[2] Brit. Med. Jour., Mar. 20, 1897.
[3] Med. Rec., Nov. 28, 1896.
[4] Verhandl. der deutsch. Gesellsch. f. Chir., XXVth Congress, 1896.

up for the loss of bone in the adjoining metatarsal. In 5 cases he had a most excellent result. In 4 cases he split a metatarsal bone in its long axis and bent the half over to overcome the loss inflicted by removal of the adjacent metatarsal bone. The bone can be very easily divided with a chisel and one of the joint-surfaces is left intact. In not one case did the transferred fragment undergo necrosis.

Delbet [1] writes on the **operative treatment of hallux valgus.** He excises the bursa and resects the projecting portion of the metatarsal bone. The extensor tendon commonly prevents the placing of the toe at once in the correct position; therefore it is well to draw this tendon forward and to anchor it to the metatarsal bone by a sheath made of periosteum. This operation is very satisfactory and corrects the deformity. [Kirmisson maintains that while tendon-contraction does take place, it is secondary and not causative. Regnier, on the contrary, asserts that in young persons the contraction is often primary, and simple tendon-section will cure; whereas in adults the contraction is secondary to arthritis, and cuneiform osteotomy is the proper operation. Our experience is that good results can be obtained in adults by removing with a chisel the projecting portion of the metatarsal bone and leaving the tendon undisturbed. An ordinary osteotomy will often be curative. It is rarely necessary to operate upon children. Dawbarn believes that the operation above advised is insufficient. He makes a half-moon incision on the upper aspect of the joint, the convexity of the cut being outward. The joint is opened and the head of the metatarsal bone removed. The toe is straightened on a sole-splint and the flap sutured. The shortening of the toe causes the contracted and displaced tendon of the extensor proprius to return into place. (See remarks by Weir, Willy Meyer, Dawbarn, L. Pilcher, Wm. T. Bull, A. J. McCosh, in *Annals of Surgery*, April, 1897.)]

Ischwall and Reyer [2] advise the **treatment of bone-cavities by pouring in melted salol,** and say it is an advantage to combine the salol with iodoform, which dissolves in it readily. The cavity to be plugged should be first carefully disinfected.

Ziematzky [3] makes a report on Lannelongue's method of **treating bone-tuberculosis by zinc chlorid injections.** The zinc chlorid is employed in the strength of 10% dissolved in distilled water, and injections are made under the periosteum or ligaments about once a week. A number of punctures are made, 1 minim being injected at each puncture, and about 15 minims being injected at one sitting. The effort is made to surround the tuberculous area with the zinc chlorid. The injection causes considerable pain, and it may be necessary to administer an anesthetic. This drug destroys the bacilli, irritates the tissues, and produces cicatrization. It was used in some 40 cases with most excellent results.

Bayer [4] writes on **Bardenheuer's method for restoring the anterior supports of the foot.** In one case the distal end of the first metatarsal bone had been destroyed, and also the proximal end of the first bone of the toe. The area of necrosis was removed. The lateral ligament of the second metatarso-phalangeal joint was cut; the metatarsal bone was forced inward and against what remained of the proximal phalanx of the great toe. The metatarsal bone was held in place by gauze-packing, which was gradually removed until granulation-tissue prevented the return of the bone to its normal position. A silver-wire suture united the fragment of the phalanx to the distal end of the metatarsal bone. He reports another case in which the fifth metatarsal

[1] Rev. de Chir., p. 329, 1896.
[2] Therap. Gaz., Jan., 1897.
[3] Rev. de Chir., Aug., 1896.
[4] Centralbl. f. Chir., Dec. 27, 1896.

bone was destroyed. The necrosed bone was removed ; the head of the fourth metatarsal was loosened from its ligaments and forced outward to take the place of the fifth metatarsal. In both cases the result was excellent, the 2 anterior points of support of the foot being restored.

Joel E. Goldthwait[1] reports a case of **achillodynia** due to an exostosis of the os caleis associated with an interesting form of bursitis. In this case a skiagraph was taken in which the exostosis was plainly visible. An operation was performed and this projection of bone removed. On drawing aside the tendo-Achillis a bursa of considerable size was opened. The lining membrane of this bursa was in folds because of hypertrophy, and these folds undoubtedly were pinched between the tendon of the bone during exercise, a condition which was responsible for the attacks of severe pain. In such cases we should remove the exostosis and also the bursa.

Kredel[2] reports two cases of **congenital coxa vara.** Both hips were affected and there were other malformations—viz., marked knock-knee and club-feet. The author believes that the deformity arose in utero because of want of room. The deformity is not the same as that met with in rickets, and in these cases of congenital coxa vara there was marked adduction, which is not present in rickets. [Coxa vara was first described by Müller in 1889, and was named by Hofmeister. It is a condition of incurvation of the neck of the femur. The commonly accepted view is that the deformity is rachitic, but Kredel's cases of congenital coxa vara show that the condition may be non-rachitic. Ogston, Czerny, Roth, Hoffer, and others have written upon coxa vara. Ogston's extremely able article was published in the *Practitioner,* April, 1896.]

J. Lynn Thomas[3] reports a case of **double Colles's fracture** in which skiagraphs were taken. He draws attention particularly to the fact that the skiagraphs show fracture of the styloid process of the ulna in each case, and he wonders whether we have not been in error in assuming that fracture of the ulnar styloid is so rarely associated with Colles's fracture.

M. L. Harris describes a **dressing for fracture of the clavicle** which he has used during the past 10 years with gratifying results. Take a piece of roller-bandage 5 or 6 ft. long and lay it over one shoulder like a suspender. Bandage the chest by a bandage 3 or 4 in. in width and about 10 yds. in length. This bandage is applied very firmly. Next take a piece of muslin 3 yds. long and as wide as the length of the arm from the axillary fold to the bend of the elbow ; fold this muslin in the middle, and, beginning at the ends, tear down the centre to within 2 in. of the fold. We thus obtain a four-tail bandage. The arm is passed through the fold so that the untorn portions lie opposite the external surface of the humerus. The tails are passed behind the body and in the same direction, and when these tails are drawn on the arm is pulled backward and inward and the scapula upward and forward, while the tip of the shoulder and with it the outer fragment of the fractured clavicle is carried upward, outward, and backward (Fig. 25).

Tillmanns[4] makes a report on 5 cases of **fracture of the femur** in which the fracture resulted from twisting ; 2 of these patients had locomotor ataxia. The other patients seemed to be well, and the explanation of the occurrence of the fracture was in doubt. Several years afterward Tillmanns followed up the patients who were apparently healthy and found every one of them suffering from locomotor ataxia. Experiments which this surgeon conducted in the dissecting-room tended to prove that a normal healthy femur cannot be broken

---

[1] Boston M. and S. Jour., May 27, 1897. [2] Centralbl. f. Chir., Oct. 17, 1896.
[3] Brit. Med. Jour., Jan. 2, 1897. [4] Berlin. klin. Woch., Aug. 31, 1896.

25

by a moderate twist or strain. In other words, in cases of fractured femur due to slight twists the bone is diseased.

Rudolph Matas[1] makes a report on a **simple method for reduction and fixation of a fracture of the zygomatic arch.** After the aseptic

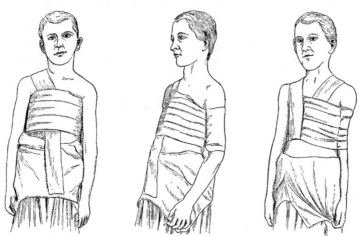

FIG. 25.—Dressing for fracture of the clavicle (Harris, in Chicago Med. Rec., Sept., 1896).

preparation of the skin a large semicircular Hagedorn needle threaded with silk is entered an inch above the middle of the displaced fragments and is carried under the fracture and into the temporal fossa, and emerges again a $\frac{1}{2}$ in. below the inferior border of the fractured arch. A strong piece of silver wire about

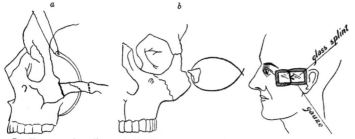

FIG. 26.—*a*, curved needle carrying traction wire under fractured arch; *b*, wire *in situ*, ready for traction to replace displaced fragment; *c*, fracture reduced; apposition maintained by a glass splint (microscopic slide) resting on a layer of iodoform-gauze. The wire is twisted firmly over the glass slide (Matas, in N. Orl. M. and S. Jour , Sept., 1896).

1 ft. in length is attached to the silk and pulled through the needle-track. By twisting the ends of this wire together a loop is formed which permits of traction on the fragments. The fragments are pulled into place by means of traction. An ordinary glass microscope-slide is wrapped in iodoform-gauze and placed over the seat of fracture, and the wire twisted firmly over this. The

[1] New Orl. M. and S. Jour., Sept., 1896.

wire splint and dressings can be removed on the 9th day. This dressing gives an excellent result (Fig. 26).

Robert F. Weir [1] discusses the **replacement of depression in fracture of the malar bone.** The injury is not very common, but when it occurs the resulting deformity is very great. There is trouble in mastication because of pressure on the temporal muscle by the zygomatic end of the fracture; correction of the deformity is very difficult by old methods. Dr. Weir had 2 cases. In these he administered ether, incised the mucous membrane above and external to the canine tooth of the upper jaw, and opened the antrum by the use of a small bone-gouge. He inserted a steel sound through this opening and easily lifted the depressed bone into place, retaining it by packing the antrum with iodoform-gauze. This packing was changed on the 4th day and was dispensed with on the 10th day.

C. J. Edgar [2] reports a case in which the **scapula was fractured by muscular action alone.** Most of the text-books make no allusion to such an occurrence, and some say that fracture of the scapula can only result from direct violence. This man had endeavored to check the progress of a vehicle by catching hold of the spokes of one wheel with both hands.

John B. Roberts [3] makes a thorough study, clinical, pathologic, and experimental, of **fracture of the lower end of the radius** with displacement of the carpal fragment toward the flexor surface of the wrist. He believes that this displacement would be as common as the dorsal displacement if patients fell as frequently on the back of the hand.

A. Herbert Butcher [4] discusses the **treatment of recent transverse**

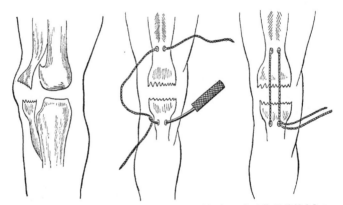

FIG. 27.—A. Herbert Butcher's method of treating recent fractures of patella (Brit. Med. Jour., Sept. 26, 1896).

fracture of the patella. He finds that if we pass a ligature over the anterior portion of the patella, instead of around it, the two ends of the bone can be held together with less traction. In transverse fracture the upper portion of the bone sinks down, the lower edge of the upper fragment is thrown forward, giving a direction forward and downward to the whole upper fragment, instead of directly forward. This is due to the fact that the posterior process

[1] Med. Rec., Mar. 6, 1897.
[3] Am. Jour. Med. Sci., Jan., 1897.
[2] Montreal Med. Jour., Feb., 1897.
[4] Brit. Med. Jour., Sept. 26, 1896.

of the quadriceps tendon ties it down to the femur. Therefore, the fractured edges are more widely separated anteriorly than posteriorly. In order to overcome this condition Mr. Barker, Kocher, and others incise the joint and pass silver wire round the patella. As equally good results can be obtained by keeping out of the joint; Butcher prefers to do so. He takes a handled needle, arms it with a strong carbolized silk ligature which is waxed, and passes this ligature through the quadriceps tendon close to the upper margin of the patella. The needle is withdrawn, leaving the ligature in place. The needle is again threaded with one end of the same ligature, is reentered through the same skin-puncture, and is passed from above downward over the anterior portion of both fragments and brought out below the inferior border of the lower portion of the broken bone. The unthreaded needle is passed over the opposite side, deeply through the ligamentum patellæ, and brought out a little distance from the opposite border through the same skin-puncture which is occupied by one end of the silk ligature, with which it is threaded and withdrawn. The needle, being now unarmed, is threaded with the free end of the silk ligature which was first passed through the quadriceps tendon, and, being inserted through the same skin-puncture, is passed subcutaneously as on the opposite side from above downward and brought out from the ligamentum patellæ at the same puncture already occupied with the opposite end of the ligature. The broken fragments are then rubbed together until crepitus is obtained, the ends of the ligature are tied in a reef-knot, and a posterior splint is worn for a few weeks.

Francis S. Watson [1] sutures a fractured patella by the following method: open the knee-joint by a semicircular incision, the convexity of which is downward, remove clots, bone-fragments, and tissue-shreds, and irrigate the joint with sterilized water. Saw the ends of the fragments off so that they will fit evenly. Each fragment is bored transversely, and the sutures are passed through these openings, the openings being made as far from the fractured edges as possible. This method of drilling the bone is preferable to drilling it vertically, because sutures introduced through transverse holes are far less liable to tear out from the bone than when passed through vertical holes. The suture employed is that suggested by Dr. Lund—three strands of single silkworm-gut braided together. It may be well, in order to insure a good result, that a second suture be passed through the tendons close around the upper and lower ends of the fragments.

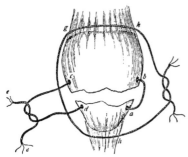

FIG. 28.—Watson's method of suturing fractured patella (Boston M. and S. Jour., Oct. 1, 1896).

George W. Spencer [2] considers the treatment of **fracture of the clavicle** by incision and suture, and reports 2 cases which were operated upon by W. Joseph Hearn. In the 1st case it was found impossible to retain the fracture in position by any of the ordinary dressings. An incision was made; the bone-ends were found to be dentate, and between them lay the lacerated subclavius muscle. The bones were wired together by silver wire and the result

[1] Boston M. and S. Jour., Oct. 1, 1896.   [2] Am. Jour. Med. Sci., Apr., 1978.

was most satisfactory. In the 2d case a small piece of loose bone could be distinctly felt under the skin and over the depression caused by the fall of the outer fragment downward, inward, and forward. The inner end of the outer fragment could not be detected. Hearn, fearing that it might do damage to some important structure, decided to operate. When an incision was made a portion of bone, triangular in outline, was found to have been broken off completely from the inner fragment. This small piece was removed. Another piece of bone was found attached only to the periosteum. This was replaced and held in position by throwing a ligature of kangaroo-tendon around the outer fragment and including the attached piece. In this case, also, the subclavius muscle was between the fragments. The inner end of the outer fragment was long and rigid, and was caught in the remaining fibers of the subclavius muscle, which, fortunately, prevented the sharp ends of the bone from injuring the blood-vessels. The fragments were wired together and the result was most satisfactory.

James Porter Fiske[1] writes on the **ambulatory treatment of fractures.** The splint that he uses is a plaster cast extending from the tips of the toes up to and around the tuberosity of the tibia, so that in walking the body-weight is supported by the upper part of the cast. After reducing the deformity the limb is held in a suitable position and the splint is applied as follows: the limb is bandaged with the ordinary muslin roller from the tips of the toes to the knee-joint; the plaster-of-Paris bandage is applied over this. Cotton-padding is not used because it is desirable that the splint exert equal pressure at each point and so fix firmly. In a great many cases the patient can walk without support as soon as the plaster has become firm; but, as a rule, he is advised to keep his leg in a horizontal position for 24 hours, and if at this time the dressing feels comfortable and there is no swelling of the toes, he is permitted to walk. Fiske has never seen a fracture of the leg but which, at some time during the progress of healing, was suitable for treatment by the ambulatory method. If there is a great deal of swelling due to edema or effusion of blood, equal pressure should be applied, the fragments fixed, the leg raised, and the patient kept recumbent until the swelling disappears, and then the ambulatory dressing can be applied. It is advantageous to apply the ambulatory splint very soon after the accident, the pressure serving to prevent edema. If we are dealing with a compound fracture, the limb should be asepticized, an aseptic dressing applied, and the fragments fixed; if infection does not occur, the ambulatory splint is applied at a later period. If there has been very extensive injury of the soft parts, it is not well to apply the ambulatory splint until the condition of the tissues improves. In most cases solid bony union is not obtained any sooner by this method than by the old method, but the after-treatment is much shortened, as we do not have to contend with the usual stiffness.

The splint is worn from 28 to 35 days. In some cases it has been worn for 6 weeks. After the splint has been removed the hot and cold douche is used upon the leg, and also massage until stiffness has entirely gone. The advantages of the ambulatory method are that the patient is able to be up out of bed and about; that there is but little muscular atrophy or stiffness of the joints; that the duration of after-treatment is much lessened and the general health of the patient is well maintained. The author reports 56 cases of Pott's fracture, in 38 of which the ambulatory splint was applied during the first 24 hours, and in 18 of which the splint was applied from 3 days to 21 days after the receipt of the injury. Besides this he reports 101 cases of fracture of the

[1] Med. News, Feb. 13, 1897.

lower third of the fibula, 7 cases of fracture of the middle third, 2 of the upper third, 9 of the lower third of the tibia, 13 of the middle third of the tibia, 14 of the tibia and fibula, 24 of osteoclasis, and 11 of non-union, treated by this method.

E. H. Bradford,[1] of Boston, writes on the ambulatory treatment of fractures in children. The late Mr. Thomas, of Liverpool, many years ago treated fractures by an ambulatory method, applying the splint which he devised originally for the treatment of tuberculosis of the knee. He treated fractures of the femur, of the patella, and of other bones by this method. Bradford thinks that the ambulatory treatment possesses certain special advantages in dealing with children. He treats cases with a modified Thomas splint, in some cases combined with the use of a plaster-of-Paris bandage. The means that are at our disposal for ambulatory treatment are as follows: plaster-of-Paris with crutches and Thomas's splint, or ring perineal splint and hip traction-splint. In fractures of the leg a splint is used which takes its bearing upon the lower end of the femur. It is not pretended that the ambulatory treatment is to be used in every case; but when it can be used time will be saved, the patient will be more comfortable, and there will be no increase in danger. If dealing with a fracture of the thigh, we can use an ordinary traction-splint with a pelvic band, accompanied by coaptation splints. This can be readily made by fastening a steel rod $\frac{1}{2}$ in. in thickness to a steel bar 1 in. wide and $\frac{1}{4}$ in. thick, bent so as almost to encircle the pelvis and provided with perineal straps. A windlass traction attachment can be added at the bottom, or buckles can be fastened to which the traction-straps are secured. An easily made emergency apparatus was suggested by Dr. Hall, of the Massachusetts Hospital. An ordinary wooden crutch is suspended from the shoulders so that the crutch portion presses in the perineum, the length being such that the crutch projects an inch or two below the sole of the foot; at the bottom of this a bracket of iron is secured, buckles are fastened to it, and the crutch is attached to the leg by straps; when the foot on the sound side is raised by a block the patient can walk about with comparative ease. This form of apparatus is more available in adults than in children. In fractures of the leg in children it is a difficult matter to obtain a bearing on the condyles of the femur or the head of the tibia, because these bones are not completely developed. In such cases the Thomas knee-splint should be used, because it takes its bearings from the perineum. This form of treatment can be applied in all fractures of the lower extremity except where there is great deformity, or where the fracture is in the upper third of the femur. In such cases it will be necessary for the child to remain longer in bed than where the fracture is lower down, because the upper fragment is so extremely short. When the patient becomes convalescent and union is found to be sound the bottom of the splint is removed and the rods are bent to fit in the socket in the sole of the shoe. A bandage is wound around the apparatus and the leg to steady the limb. Thomas's knee-splint, it will be recalled, is made by fastening to an oval ring, made of steel $\frac{1}{4}$ in. in thickness, 2 rods of similar size which are secured at the bottom to an iron bar, which serves as a foot-plate.

W. Bruce,[2] in speaking of **fractures of the lower end of the humerus,** calls attention to the difficulty of keeping the fragments in place and of the ill-results which frequently follow the treatment of such fractures. He thinks such a great mass of callus is thrown out because of bad coaptation and want of proper rest. In this case chloroform should be given before the fracture is set, both for the purpose of diagnosis and to facilitate reduction. In cases where swelling is very great it is well to do nothing for a

[1] Ann. of Surg., Oct., 1896.   [2] Brit. Med. Jour., Oct. 24, 1896.

day or two, but at the earliest opportunity the fracture must be set. The best splint is the trunk of the patient; no arm-splints are required. It is a very great advantage to have no constriction on the limb of the patient. Place the elbow at an acute angle and lay the arm across the chest over a sheet of cotton-wool, apply a bandage including the trunk and the injured limb, and every day open this dressing and examine the fracture. In a little while make gentle passive motions, and later on apply massage. This method of treatment gives the best results of any of which he has knowledge. [The question when to begin passive motion is much disputed. Motion made early moves the joint, but also moves the fragments; movement of the fragments leads to the formation of a large amount of callus, and the large amount of callus forms bone in quantity, which bone blocks the joint. We believe passive motion should not be made for 4 weeks. Dawbarn[1] has recently discussed this question, and our views are in accordance with his.]

George Woolsey,[2] after discussing the use of **massage in the treatment of fractures,** comes to the following conclusions : the treatment of fractures, especially of fractures near joints, by ordinary methods of immobilization or by ambulatory treatment is not entirely satisfactory. By employing massage and passive motion we can shorten the time necessary to obtain bony union by a third or a half and obtain a better functional result. In fractures about or in joints this treatment is especially valuable. If applied very early, it abolishes swelling and relieves pain, hastens the formation of callus, and prevents muscular atrophy and stiffness of the joints and tendons. The patient wears splints, which every day are removed and massage applied for 15 or 20 minutes. This treatment, combined with the ambulatory method, offers the best prospect for a speedy cure. If we are dealing with an oblique fracture of both bones in the leg or arm, or an oblique fracture of the femur or humerus, or a fracture in the middle of the limb with a strong tendency to displacement, we must then immobilize until consolidation takes place.

John B. Roberts[3] warmly advocates the use of **exploratory incision in the treatment of some fractures and dislocations.** He tells us that the employment of the Röntgen rays has often proved that fractures which were thought to be thoroughly reduced really deviate considerably from normal relations. A belief in the value of exploratory incision, which he long ago announced, has been strengthened during recent years. Allis, of Philadelphia, advocates this treatment in fractures of the upper third of the shaft of the femur. Arbuthnot Lane has employed it in fractures of the tibia and fibula near the ankle. McBurney uses it in fractures of the upper end of the humerus complicated with dislocation. Dennis advises it in fracture in which it is difficult to secure thorough coaptation ; but, excepting in fractures of the cranium and patella, most surgeons prefer to obtain imperfect results rather than to advise immediate exposure of the fragments by exploratory incision. Roberts advocates incision in cases in which we are ignorant of the exact lesion or in which we cannot reduce the fragments, or cannot perfectly immobilize, or cannot deal satisfactorily with complications. In these cases the incision is the least of two evils. Fracture of the patella he never treats by incision and suture of the bone, because he has always so far been able to bring the fragments into apposition by a splint, by hooks, or by subcutaneous suture. With aseptic precautions the incision is almost devoid of risk, and many advantages will follow on its performance. We can make out the exact line of separation. We can be certain that we have effected coaptation. Not

[1] N. Y. Polyclinic, July 15, 1897.   [2] Med. News, Mar. 20, 1897.
[3] Ibid., Jan. 16, 1897.

only will the bone-fragments be replaced, but the torn periosteum will be restored, and bands of muscle, fascia, and nerve will be lifted out from between the fragments. We thus lessen the chance of deformity, non-union, neuralgia, atrophy, and ankylosis. When the fragments have been adjusted they can be kept in this position by sutures or pegs, or needles or screws, or ferrules; furthermore, the vessels are ligated and muscles and nerves sutured. Pain is relieved if due to extravasated blood or inflammatory exudate. In some cases where there has been a large amount of interstitial pressure incision averts the danger of gangrene. The pain during the course of treatment is less because the fragments are perfectly immobilized. Fat-embolism is very unlikely to occur, because broken-down fat is permitted to escape. Ankylosis will rarely happen. Repair of the break and restoration of function take place more rapidly than under ordinary methods of treatment. We know that by ordinary methods of treatment it sometimes happens that even a slight change in the axis of the bone will prevent a perfect functional result. We can obviate such a condition by the open incision. In vicious union of fractures open incision with osteotomy is preferable to fracture by the use of the osteoclast. Dislocations which are not easily reduced by manipulation when the anesthetic is administered should also be subjected to open incision. In recent dislocations where manipulation fails and in old dislocations arthrotomy should be performed, a final effort at reduction by manipulation being made just before operation. Open incision and restoration of the dislocation are safer than attempting to drag an old dislocation forcibly into place. After the incision has been made, if restoration is impossible, the head of the bone can be excised.

A. P. Gould[1] has made some remarks on the **treatment of fractures** that are of great practical value. He tells us to take the utmost pains to make an exact diagnosis of the existence, of the position, and of the condition of the fracture, and the number and position of the fragments. Anesthesia is a very great aid in making a diagnosis. It is as much a surgeon's duty to give an anesthetic to aid him in arriving at an exact diagnosis as it is to give an anesthetic for some grave surgical condition. Anesthesia permits diagnosis and greatly facilitates proper treatment. This teaching will be considered by many as rank heresy. The second great aid is the use of the x-rays and the fluorescent screen. After arriving at a diagnosis the surgeon's next duty is to reduce the fractures at once, as the longer we wait the more difficult this reduction will become. Reduction must be complete and not partial. We must not wait in a half-way house, obtaining some improvement to-day in the hope of getting more improvement to-morrow. The surfaces of the fracture are nearly always uneven or jagged, and when these surfaces are accurately put altogether they hold together. Hence a fracture which is once well set rarely slips apart. Recurrence of displacement probably means imperfect reduction. The methods which are suited to secure this perfect adjustment of the fragments vary with different cases. Displacement may be caused by the violence of the traumatism, the action of gravity, or the pull of muscles. The pull of muscles is overcome by relaxation, not by opposing them with extension or counter-extension. The fragments should be thoroughly replaced before a splint or a bandage is applied. We should never trust an apparatus to correct a displacement. All apparatus which are supposed to force a broken collar-bone into position are miserable failures. If we wish to obtain repair of this fracture without deformity, we are obliged to place the patient on his back in bed. We cannot correct the deformity of Colles's fracture by a splint, but we first correct the displacement and then maintain the fragments in their proper

[1] Lancet, June 12, 1897.

position by placing the limb on a splint. Should we or should we not extend to fractures the same development of surgery that we have extended to other injuries and diseases? What can operation do for simple fracture? It can exactly replace fragments, and it can mechanically fix them in place, and in an old ununited fracture it opens up again the medulla and so leads to the formation of a plastic callus. Such an operation, of course, must only be undertaken when we are certain we can maintain an aseptic wound. We must realize that the fitting together of the fragments may be a matter of great difficulty, and that the surgical means of holding the fragments together are not altogether perfect, except in fractures of the patella or uncomplicated oblique fractures of the tibia. These operations are difficult and are not to be undertaken lightly; the cases in which it is necessary to operate are few, but in these few cases the surgeon should put to himself the question whether the difficulties can with reasonable certainty be overcome by operation. If they can be, and he has the necessary means at his command, he ought to operate. Gould would not for a moment advocate a general employment of operations for simple fractures; such a practice would be needless, dangerous, and ill-advised. [The use of an anesthetic for diagnostic purposes is, in our opinion, not only valuable, but often indispensable. In the United States it is taught positively that in examining a case of supposed fracture in which the diagnosis is obscure ether should be administered. In injuries in and about the elbow-joint an examination should be made under ether, unless the x-rays are accessible and clear up the diagnosis.]

DISEASES OF THE JOINTS.

R. W. Lovett[1] writes on the **treatment of sprains.** These injuries may be classified under four headings: contusions, ligamentous injuries, joint-synovitis, and tenosynovitis of the muscles about the injured joint. The use of the word "sprain" is unfortunate, and it is far better to name accurately the special injury which exists. Mild cases of sprains may be most satisfactorily treated by massage daily and the use of a bandage. In severe sprains Lovett has never used immediate massage, because he believes that in a recent severe sprain massage may make the condition more acute. In severe cases he applies the massage only when the heat and sensitiveness disappear. In other words, he applies it at the time it is advisable to stimulate the local circulation. In sprains of the ankle-joint the best results are obtained by immediately applying wet millboard strips over layers of sheet wadding and then applying a tight and even bandage. This dressing is left in place for two or three days, at which time the swelling has largely abated. At this period a severe sprain requires the application of a plaster-of-Paris bandage from the toes to below the knee. This bandage is split, and every two or three days is removed to permit extension of the joint. When the acute symptoms subside massage is begun, and after the application of massage the plaster is reapplied for 24 hours. Gradually the plaster is discontinued, and is replaced by a flannel bandage. The hot and cold douche is valuable in association with massage. It is inadvisable to apply plaster-of-Paris immediately, because in 24 hours there will be a subsidence of the swelling which will leave the plaster loose. If the swelling should happen to increase, constriction will be brought about. Halfway measures are almost useless; cotton bandages and hot water are but makeshifts. Sticking-plaster is better, but lacks precision. We may lay it down

[1] Boston M. and S. Jour., June 17, 1897.

as a rule that a sprain is either slight enough to be treated from the first by massage, or is severe enough to demand efficient fixation for a day or two.

J. O. Mumford,[1] on the **treatment of sprains,** tells us that the old practice of immobilizing sprains is now generally conceded to be impractical. Even in cases in which there is considerable laceration we should use at first the hot and cold douche for about 10 minutes in order to allay pain, then rub and knead the joint for some 15 minutes, and apply a flannel bandage. The part is then rested perfectly for 24 hours. On the 2d day the kneading and stroking are more thoroughly done and a little passive motion is used, and this plan is continued daily. Massage and passive motion are valuable because they keep up the lymphatic circulation and thus aid in carrying off inflammatory exudate, and proper nutrition is maintained by passive motion, which is substituted for the active motions indulged in in health. In a sprained ankle the old treatment of immobilization is objectionable. It leads to the formation of adhesions, functional impairment, and pain, and, if there be tuberculous tendencies, favors the production of a tuberculous joint. The same statement may be made of the wrist, the knee, the shoulder, and other joints. Properly applied, massage will prevent these complications. A very important adjunct to this treatment is the use of a skilfully applied flannel bandage. The surgeon ought to apply this himself. A masseur is seldom acquainted with the general principles of bandaging. The bandage should be broad, cut bias, and cover all the parts as far as the adjacent joint on either side, an extra pad being placed over the injured joint. After the first 24 hours the patient is permitted to go about on crutches, and after the 3d day a little weight is brought upon the foot. Two or 3 weeks are often sufficient time to render a sprained joint actively useful.

Douglas Graham[2] says that in a mild sprain of the foot and ankle, if at the time of the injury the patient is wearing a boot which fits him, let him keep that boot on and walk about with moderation. If the boot is not rendered snug by reason of the swelling, it should be laced more tightly. This is what may be called walking off a sprain. It is the application of automatic massage. Massage properly applied is a plan that is well suited to sprains of all degrees of severity, and it can be used alone or with fixed dressings and bandages. It should not be immediately begun after the reception of the injury. Motion either active or passive should not be encouraged in spite of pain caused by it. Rest and support can usually be obtained in the intervals between the application of massage by the use of a neatly applied bandage ; but if the bandage does not give enough support, then a splint or plaster bandage which can be easily removed should be applied. If the joint is so tender that massage cannot be directly applied, the manipulations should be commenced on healthy tissue some distance above the joint and nearer to the trunk, by gently stroking in the direction of the returning currents of lymph and blood and gradually proceeding downward. The returning currents are by this method pushed along more rapidly and make room for exudations to be carried away. Each hand should make alternate strokes, using the whole palmar surface. After stroking for a few minutes in this manner, deep manipulation, or massage properly so-called, may be brought into play, beginning above the painful joint and gradually approaching the objective point. This maneuver decidedly lessens pain, but does not decrease ordinary sensations. The parts beyond the sprain are treated in the same manner. By this alternate stroking and kneading we will soon be able to apply firm pressure over the joint that was but recently very painful, so that the pressure not only will not hurt, but will be very agreeable, and very soon motion can be added to the

[1] Boston M. and S. Jour., June 17, 1897.   [2] Ibid.

pressure. By these manipulations the effusion and exudation are spread over greater surfaces and brought into more points of contact with veins and lymphatics. Continued bandaging in the treatment of sprains will cause atrophy of the muscles. Rubber bandages should never be used except temporarily—they strangle the tissues ; a cotton-flannel bandage is infinitely more comfortable and renders greater service. Bandages which are cut bias he never uses, because they stretch more at the edges than in the middle, and it is impossible to obtain equable pressure with them.

Graham arrives at the following conclusions: 1. A sprain is a wrench of the joint in which there was partial displacement of the articulating surfaces followed by immediate replacement. 2. The symptoms are pain, swelling, discoloration, and, as a general thing, heat with impaired motion. The swelling may render the diagnosis difficult by hiding a fracture which is underneath. The diagnosis is favored by whatever quickly reduces heat, pain, and swelling, such as massage, bandaging, and elevation. These means are valuable for diagnosis and also for treatment, and recovery under their aid can be brought about in one-third of the time required for recovery under absolute rest and fixed dressings without massage.

Hayward W. Cushing[1] discusses **excision and erasion of the knee-joint.** In the operation as ordinarily performed the knee-joint is laid open by a curved incision in front. The crucial ligaments are divided and the ends of the femur and tibia are resected, great care being taken not to damage the epiphyseal line. The patella may be removed or may be left in place. The ends of the bones are fastened together by nails or by wires, the wound is closed with drainage, and the surgeon hopes for ankylosis. As a rule, sinuses form. This operation, though called excision of the knee, is really excision of the knee-joint. It simply removes the knee-joint, and does not remove the synovial membrane and foci of bone-disease at or beyond the epiphyseal line. It hence becomes perfectly evident that such an operation cannot be considered radical. The operation advised by Cushing is radical. The joint is opened and carefully inspected, and all diseased synovial membrane is removed with scissors and forceps; then the bone is attacked with a chisel, gouge, and curet, rather than a saw. Diseased bone is scooped out; the bones are united by sutures passed through the periosteum ; the wound is closed without drainage and dressed with sterile gauze fixed by plaster-of-Paris. This operation gives primary union in 3 weeks and firm bony union in 8 or 9 months. When the disease is limited this operation is called an erasion ; when the disease is extensive it is called an arthrectomy. If the after-treatment is properly conducted, the leg will be found to be nearly always straight; but we should remember that fixation should be continued as long as there is any tendency to contraction. Do not omit fixation as soon as the operation-wound is healed or as soon as there is apparently bony union, because contraction can occur months afterward. The typical operation of excision should be reserved for the correction of deformity from bony ankylosis.

C. B. Lockwood[2] writes of a new procedure which he calls **osteoplastic excision of the knee.** He has performed this operation on several occasions. It is not done on every case of tuberculous arthritis of the knee, but each case is treated on its merits. Some cases are treated by rest and local applications, some by drainage, some by arthrectomy, some by the ordinary operation of excision, and some by the operation herein described. This operation is used when there is progressive tuberculous arthritis with pulpy synovial membrane and ulcerated cartilage, with but little caries and but little displace-

---

[1] Boston M. and S. Jour., Sept. 17, 1896. [2] Lancet, Mar. 13, 1897.

ment of the ends of the bone. The operation must not be delayed until sinuses form, because it will then be apt to be followed by septic inflammation. The ordinary method of excision has certain great faults; one is that the limb is apt to become flexed and rotated. The skin-incision is of very little importance, just so as it permits the entire disease to be removed. The antero-internal vertical incision of Langenbeck gives better access to the pouches above the patella and saves us from cutting the ligament of the patella, but it does not satisfactorily expose the posterior angles of the joint. The removal of the patella destroys the attachment of the quadriceps extensor femoris muscle, which is one of the chief reasons that flexion of the joint is so apt to follow this operation. In some cases, of course, the patella is in a state of advanced disease and cannot be retained; but even in such cases it is possible to preserve the aponeurosis over it and at its sides. When the patella is sound there is another reason why it should be allowed to remain in place; it may be possible to fasten its sawn surface to the tibia and femur, both of which are sawn to receive it. The ligaments are very important. The crucial ligaments are especially important, as they tend to prevent displacement of the tibia backward and forward. The usual operation of resection of the knee retains the patella, destroys the ligament of the patella, the lateral ligament, the crucial ligaments, and the interlocking articular ends of the bone, and leaves bony surfaces which are unsupported by ligaments and are smooth and flat, and, as a consequence, very easily displaced. In order to meet these objections Lockwood has devised the following operation: a transverse incision is carried across the center of the ligmentum patellæ from one femoral tuberosity to the other; the ligament of the patella is divided and the joint opened. It is not well to open the joint by the vertical incision, nor is it advisable to open it by sawing through the patella transversely. The latter proceeding is objectionable because the patella may be diseased, and, further, because a divided patella is not suitable for fastening to the tibia or femur. When the joint has been opened the knee is bent to a right angle and the joint is carefully inspected. The diseased synovial membrane is thoroughly removed with knife and scissors. It will occasionally be found necessary, in order to reach all of the diseased synovial membrane, to carry the ends of the transverse incision upward. It is convenient to leave untouched the part of the synovial membrane which is behind the femoral condyles until the femur has been sawn. Healthy ligaments ought to be preserved. It remains to be seen whether it is proper to keep both of the crucial ligaments, but it is certainly very difficult to remove all of the synovial membrane without cutting the anterior crucial ligament. The posterior crucial ligament can very often be preserved, but it would be better to destroy both crucial ligaments than to leave any diseased membrane behind. As the internal and external lateral ligaments are outside of the joint, it is very much easier to save them. The articular surface of the patella is now sawn off; and the trochlear surface of the femur is also sawn off so as to leave a flat surface on which the upper portion of the sawn patella will fit. The femur is now raised vertically by an assistant and the greater part of its articular surface taken away by two other cuts which begin at the convexity of the condyles at the edge of the articular cartilage. These saw-cuts are carried obliquely into the intercondylar notch of the femur until they converge, entering the notch at the edges of the articular cartilages and below the notch of the crucial ligaments. These saw-cuts make a groove or hollow in the femur and leave some articular cartilage front and back of the condyles (Fig. 29). The cartilage is to be removed with the sawn bone. The tibia is treated on the same principle as was the femur, two oblique cuts being carried upward from the epiphyseal line to converge at the base of the spine (Fig. 29). The articular cartilages are removed. The advantages of this method of sawing the femur and tibia are as follows: we still preserve the fitting of the tibia into the condyloid notch, and lateral displacement cannot take place. The wedging in of the tibia prevents rotation of that bone, and, further, very large areas of sawn bone are brought into contact and a very small amount of the epiphysis is removed. As the leg is extended the bones become tightly fixed and jam the wedge of the tibia into the notch in the femur, and as long as extension is maintained they remain in this position. The operation is completed by sewing the ligaments of the patella with silk sutures and closing the wound.

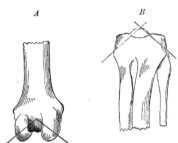

FIG. 29.—*A*, showing section of femur; *B*, showing section of tibia (Lockwood, in Lancet, Mar. 13, 1897).

John Ward Cousins[1] tells us that **excision of the knee-joint** is only to be performed under conditions which are reasonably favorable. There are many contraindications, such as disease in other organs, especially disease of the excretory or nervous system. The very young and the aged are not suitable subjects. Excision should not be practised in acute diseases of the knee-joint; in such conditions amputation is the proper resource. The operation is performed in chronic articular disease in which there are destructive changes within the joint. In some cases it is impossible to arrive at a conclusion as to what should really be done until the joint is opened. The Röntgen rays will undoubtedly prove of great aid to us in coming to conclusions in doubtful cases. Extensive disease does not of necessity condemn the joint to amputation if other features of the case are not unfavorable for excision. The operation is thought to be unsuited to very young children or elderly people. Under the age of 5 the chances of a good result are small; after the age of 10 the results are better; but when we recall that the lower extremity of the femur is not completely ossified until the age of 20, and that the upper epiphysis of the tibia joins the shaft between the 18th and the 25th year, it will become evident that the best period for this operation is between the 15th and the 30th year, because in this period bony union will be more readily obtained. Excision in children does not interfere with the future growth of the limb. The method that Cousins employs to operate he calls jamming the bones. The joint is opened by an anterior incision with the convexity downward. The ligamentum patellæ is divided and the crucial ligaments are cut sufficiently to allow flexion of the joint. The bones are divided beyond their epiphyseal lines and as little bone as possible is removed; necrotic areas are cut out, and the cut bony surfaces are forcibly jammed together. This secures immobility and favors rapid union. The diseased synovial membrane is all dissected away; it is not necessary to employ any peg to hold the bones in position. After jamming has been practised strong catgut sutures can be introduced between the periosteal surfaces and between the cut ends of the ligamentum patellæ. No more of the patella than absolutely necessary should be removed. If there be only slight caries of this bone, the foci of disease can be cleaned out with a sharp spoon. In some cases it will be necessary to remove completely the

[1] Brit. Med. Jour., July 25, 1896.

articular surface and also the concave surface of the femur upon which the patella moves.

Nichans [1] describes a **new method of incising the knee-joint.** He begins the incision 4 in. above the patella, carries it downward along the inner border of the rectus tendon, and then takes it by the side of the patella to the tubercle of the tibia. At its lower extremity he makes a short transverse cut. The tubercle of the tibia is chiselled off and the wound is carried into the joint. When the limb is flexed the patella and the flexor tendons can be pushed aside, when the anterior half of the joint is readily accessible. If exposure of the entire joint is necessary, the lateral and crucial ligaments must be divided. The author believes this operation is of value because it does not injure the extensor tendons of the leg and thoroughly exposes the synovial pouch, which runs up above the patella.

V. P. Gibney [2] writes on the **treatment of stiff and painful joints by superheated dry air.** Gibney uses Tallerman's apparatus. He has reported 8 cases in which the improvement brought about by the superheated dry air was very great.

R. F. Tobin [3] makes a report on **osteotomy of the femur as a treatment for the early stages of tuberculous disease of the hip,** saying that we may take it as granted that in the early stages of morbus coxæ the operative removal of the affected parts gives very unfavorable results, and that we must seek cure by giving rest to the joint, combined with constitutional treatment. There is one unfortunate fact, and that is, that the position of greatest ease for the joint is one which is a position of great awkwardness for the limb, which is flexed, abducted, and everted, and any attempt to straighten the limb will increase the tension of the joint. Extension by weight and pulley, if the weight is heavy enough to keep the leg straight, drags the spine into lordosis; if it is less heavy, the leg becomes less straight and there is less lordosis. Dr. Thomas's splint is an excellent contrivance, of course, to support the limb, but does not overcome during both night and day all the drawbacks of the position. Being satisfied that the awkward position the thigh assumes in cases of morbus coxæ is a great obstacle to obtaining satisfactory results from treatment by rest, Tobin has endeavored to meet the difficulty in the following manner: in the early stages of the disease he performs osteotomy of the femur on a level with the lesser trochanter and places the limb in a straight position as regards the body, allowing the upper fragment to maintain its position of ease.

Alexandroff [4] asserts that atrophy and degeneration of the bones and muscles and **hypertrophy of the subcutaneous layer** beneath the skin go hand in hand **in early coxalgia.** Hypertrophy of the subcutaneous cellular layer of fat increases as the case gets worse, and eventually involves the entire limb. The effacement of the fold between the buttock and the thigh is due to this hypertrophy. The author has devised an instrument to measure the difference of thickness in the layer as contrasted with the thickness of the same tissue on the opposite extremity. Atrophy of the limb associated with hypertrophy of this layer is the most important sign to diagnosticate tuberculous osteoarthritis, and it will be found before other symptoms are manifest. If the above-named conditions are absent, there is no tuberculous lesion of the hip-joint, even if other symptoms would indicate its existence.

A. G. Miller [5] maintains that the **muscular atrophy** which accompanies

[1] Centralbl. f. Chir., No. 16, 1897.   [2] Internat. Med Mag., Apr., 1897.
[3] Brit. Med. Jour., Apr. 24. 1897.   [4] Presse méd , Dec. 9, 1896.
          [5] Edinb. Med. Jour., Sept., 1896.

tuberculosis of the joint results **from a diminished blood-supply** caused by contraction of the main blood-vessels of the limb.

DISLOCATIONS.

Edward Sutcliff[1] records a case of **complete lateral dislocation of the forearm,** resulting from a fall on the right elbow. The forearm was flexed, semipronated, and widened over the elbow-joint. The inner condyle was extremely prominent and the trochlear surface of the humerus could be distinctly made out. The forearm could be readily rotated and the head of the radius could be felt revolving. The patient was anesthetized, and reduction was readily effected by extension around the knee and manipulation of the joint. A perfectly useful joint followed the injury.

W. J. Welsh[2] writes on the treatment of **old dislocations of the elbow.** He says that much force is very dangerous in old dislocations and may do irreparable damage. The olecranon prevents reduction. The proper plan is to cut into the joint, divide the triceps tendon, remove the olecranon, and bring the radius and ulna into place, retaining them there with the hope of establishing ankylosis. He reports a case in which he carried out this procedure with gratifying results.

The treatment of **old dislocations of the shoulder** is considered by F. B. Lund.[3] The obstacles to reduction may be the adhesion of the capsule to the glenoid cavity, the healing of the rent in the capsule behind the head of the bone, thickening or calcification of the capsule, pulling off of the great tuberosity, or filling up of the glenoid cavity. An old dislocation presents a different picture from a recent dislocation. The bony points stand out distinctly because of the atrophy of the deltoid and the scapular muscles. The elbow is not away from the side, because the stretching of the deltoid allows it to fall in. Rotation of the head of the humerus is nearly or quite absent. The arm can be very rarely abducted to a right angle, but abduction is only possible by elevation of the scapula. Backward elevation is not possible. Forward elevation can be carried to a right angle. The author reports from the records of the Boston City Hospital 24 cases, of which 22 were treated by manipulation. The cases reduced by manipulation were of 6 weeks' duration, with the exception of Dr. Burrell's case, which was 8 months. Fourteen of the cases were successful, 13 of them under 6 weeks. There was 1 failure at 6 weeks. In only 1 case of over 6 weeks was the reduction effected by manipulation; there were thus 10 cases in which manipulation failed, and only 1 of these was of less than 7 weeks' duration. In one of these failures resection of the head of the humerus gave an excellent result, and in 1 recurrent case excision of the capsule succeeded. In 2 of the unsuccessful cases the surgical neck was fractured during attempts at reduction. These cases show that when 6 weeks have elapsed after an injury it is improbable that manipulation will succeed in effecting restoration, and its employment may lead to fracture of the humerus or rupture of the axillary artery. If at this late period reduction is to be effected, it must be brought about by arthrotomy with or without resection of the head of the humerus. The results of arthrotomy during the last 6 years are distinctly more encouraging than were the earlier results.

A. H. Tubby,[4] as to the present aspect of the **treatment of congenital displacement of the hip,** says there are 3 methods of treatment: exten-

[1] Lancet, Feb. 27, 1897.
[3] Boston M. and S. Jour., Apr 29, 1897.

[2] Med. Rec., Sept. 19, 1896.
[4] Lancet, May 1, 1897.

sion in recumbency or by apparatus, operation, and forcible reduction. He has tried extension in recumbency in 2 cases, with considerable promise of success. If it is not possible to subject the patients to prolonged recumbency, weight-extension can be put on at night and the extension instrument can be worn during the day, the patient being allowed to walk about. This plan can be used in children under 4, but not in older subjects. Hoffa's operation is an extremely severe procedure and is very frequently followed by unsatisfactory results. The operation of Lorenz has been advocated by a number of surgeons, but Lorenz himself has recently modified his opinion of the value of the operation, and in his recent cases has carried out bloodless reduction with success. Prof. Schede, who has tried operative plans extensively, has come back to treatment by rest combined with extension and abduction. Forcible reduction can be carried out by the maneuvers of Paci as follows : the patient is recumbent; the surgeon flexes the patient's leg on the thigh and the thigh on the pelvis. The movement of the head of the femur downward is assisted by direct pressure. The thigh is now slightly abducted, and is then strongly rotated outward and extended. The movement throws the head of the femur into or on the acetabulum. Paci has reported 15 cases in which the results were admirable. Lannelongue endeavors to fix the head of the femur in its new position by injecting at intervals of 3 or 4 weeks a few drops of a 10% solution of zinc chlorid. Lorenz has modified Paci's method. He lowers the head of the femur by traction, depresses it by forcible flexion, followed by forcible abduction, and fixes the femur by a plaster-of-Paris bandage, to be worn for several months. After the reduction Mikulicz employs an apparatus to make extension with considerable abduction. Tubby himself does not think that it is possible to deepen a shallow acetabulum in such a way that the femur can be retained. In the cases of Lorenz's operation which he has seen the results have not been satisfactory. Hoffa's or Lorenz's method is very rarely necessary, and is only justifiable as a last resource. The best method of treatment will be found to be forcible reduction as practised by Lorenz.

Noble Smith,[1] in an article on **congenital dislocation of the hip,** says that dissections have proved conclusively that malformation of the part is very frequent. The head of the femur may be unnaturally small, the acetabulum may be very shallow. Some observers, however, have maintained that the bony parts of the joint are practically of natural form. Mikulicz believes that the joint is normal at the time of birth. Smith says that these diverse views lead us to infer that in different cases different conditions exist, and it is very important to differentiate between cases in which the bony parts are normal and those in which they are abnormal. The Röntgen rays are very useful in arriving at this conclusion. Smith reports a case in which the rays were used to great advantage. This child when 2 years of age was examined, and was found to have dislocation of both hip-joints. The new joints admitted of free motion, but when the attempt was made to draw the heads of the bone down into position they were arrested by coming in contact with a hard substance which was thought to be the ridges of the acetabula. Smith arrived at the view that this was probably not a congenital dislocation, but a dislocation received during birth. He recommended an attempted reduction under chloroform, but the parents refused to subject the child to this treatment. Two years later the patient was seen again, and was found to have a very awkward gait and increasing lordosis. The case was benefited by applying an apparatus to support the abdomen in a more natural position. Lately a skiagraph of both hips was taken by Mr. Sidney Rowland. The picture shows

[1] Brit. Med. Jour., Dec. 12, 1896.

that the acetabula are well formed, demonstrating that if the heads of the bone had been reduced in the first instance they would have remained *in situ.* The heads of the bones seem to be normal in shape. This picture would go to confirm the clinical judgment that the case was really one of dislocation at birth rather than of congenital dislocation.

VENEREAL DISEASE.

A. Gutheil [1] makes a report upon the use of **argonin in the treatment of gonorrhea.** He claims that, as a rule, injections cause gonococci to disappear from the discharge in about 9 days, the drug producing no irritation. After the disappearance of the gonococci the use of argonin is abandoned and ichthyol is employed for about 3 weeks. The author tells us that a remedy for gonorrhea should kill gonococci, should not add to inflammation, and should not damage the mucous membrane. Solutions of lead and zinc and tannin are not germicidal; corrosive sublimate and potassium permanganate are germicidal, but are very irritating. Argentamin is germicidal, but irritant. Argonin is a white powder, and is a combination of albumin, silver, and an alkali. The strength of solution used is $\frac{1}{2}\%$. [This agent was introduced by Röhmann and Liebrecht as an improvement on Schäffer's argentamin. J. W. Daniel, in a paper in the *Am. Therapist,* states that argonin is not irritant, is not precipitated by chlorids, and is not decomposed by albuminous matter; its use quickly allays ardor urinæ and inflammation. In uncomplicated cases he uses a solution of a strength of 5%, introducing it for the first few days of the attack 6 or 8 times daily by means of a urethral syringe. Later in the case, besides injections by an ordinary syringe, he gives 2 injections a day with a long-nozzle syringe. Jadasohn published a report in *Arch. f. Dermat. u. Syph.* He uses argonin in solution of a strength of 1.5–2%, and maintains that this agent does not coagulate albumin and rapidly kills gonococci; it is not irritant and is very valuable in the treatment of gonorrhea. The fact that argonin is not astringent renders it useless in nonspecific urethritis.]

Geo. Knowles Swinburne has made a favorable report on argonin.[2] He holds that the drug causes rapid disappearance of gonococci and allays inflammation, though *relapses* may occur. D. T. Kreissl [3] thinks highly of argonin. If the duration of the case is less than 5 days, he finds 12 daily injections of 8% solution are usually enough. In cases over 5 to 10 days old injection for 18 days is usually enough. When the gonococci are not found in 3 consecutive examinations, stop the use of argonin and employ for a few days a mild solution of potassium permanganate. Argonin is of little value in chronic cases.

O. Werler [4] claims that **citrate of silver** (itrol) does not irritate the urethra, and kills gonococci passing deeply under the mucous membrane. He uses it in solution of a strength of 1 : 8000, gradually increased up to 1 : 4000.

A. S. Hotaling [5] reports 50 cases of gonorrhea treated with **permanganate of zinc** injections of a strength of gr. ss–ʒj of aqua, gradually increasing to 1½ gr. Alkaline diuretics are given internally. The average period of cessation of discharge was 9 days after beginning treatment.

H. M. Christian,[6] writing on the **duration of acute gonorrhea**

[1] Deutsch. med. Woch., No. 35, 1896.
[2] Jour. Cutan. and Genito-Urin. Dis., Aug., 1896.
[3] Chicago Med. Rec., Jan., 1897.   [4] Berlin. klin. Woch., No. 37, 1896.
[5] Med. News, Nov. 7, 1896.   [6] Therap. Gaz., Jan. 15, 1897.

under treatment, states that the general idea among both the laity and a large number of practitioners is that gonorrhea is a disease that may be cured in 3 weeks. He presents a series of cases from the University of Pennsylvania, Genito-Urinary Department, showing: 1. Gonorrhea is much more serious than usually supposed ; 2. Two-thirds of uncomplicated cases require from 6 to 10 weeks for cure ; 3. Four weeks is necessary in anterior urethra cases ; 4. The importance of urinary examination before declaring a cure is very great. [Christian states several most important facts. We concur entirely with his views on this subject.]

J. Janet,[1] discussing the **abortive treatment of gonorrhea,** claims that in every case in which he used the potassium permanganate before the acute symptoms showed themselves he has been able to suppress the gonorrheal process without complication. The treatment lasts from 8 to 12 days. Janet believes the treatment has its limitations, because few patients can spare the time or expense, and only the specialist can conform to the severe regularity. Vigueron, of Marseilles, has used Janet's method for 5 years, and found it strikingly successful in the first 36 hours of the disease. Guiard, of Paris, believes in weak solutions from 1 : 6000 to 1 : 10,000. Janet agrees with Guiard as to weak solutions, and regards the irrigation of the entire urethra as important, though it may be omitted for the first day or so. An abstract of this debate in the French Assoc. of Genito-Urinary Surgeons will be found in the *Jour. of Cutaneous and Genito-Urin. Dis.,* Feb., 1897.

James Moore[2] considers the internal use of **methylen-blue in gonorrhea.** He gives 3 gr. of methylen-blue three times a day and 15 gr. of potassium citrate three times a day. After the subsidence of acute symptoms he also employs injections of alum solution (gr. 3 to oz. 1 of hot water). It is useful in first attacks, cuts short the acute stage, and lessens the suffering of the patient. The drug is borne to the seat of disease by both the blood and urine, and acts by staining the organisms and the soil in which they grow. [Personally we have not been greatly impressed with the value of this drug in gonorrhea. In first attacks it does seem to shorten somewhat the acute stage, but occasionally it produces strangury.]

König[3] discusses **gonorrheal arthritis,** and advises us invariably to examine the urethra if acute joint-inflammation exists. He says that gonorrheal arthritis is the most usual form of joint-inflammation, many supposed cases of puerperal arthritis and chronic articular rheumatism in females being gonorrheal. The joint most likely to suffer in woman is the wrist, in man the knee. Careful observers have found gonococci in joints, but other organisms may be found. Ankylosis is likely to follow gonorrheal arthritis. If the case is one of simple effusion, the joint should be punctured and injected with carbolic acid. If para-articular infection also exists, the joint must be opened and washed out. Movements are employed if ankylosis threatens. Pain can be relieved by the application of a plaster splint ; but as this favors ankylosis, do not employ it unless driven to it, and try first the administration of potassium iodid (45 gr. a day) and the injection of iodoform emulsion. [The common impression that a joint-inflammation occurring in a person who has a urethral discharge is of necessity gonorrheal rheumatism, is erroneous. Gonorrhea gives a man no immunity from ordinary arthritic inflammation. The diagnosis of gonorrheal rheumatism is not unusually an inference or a guess. Gonorrheal rheumatism begins more gradually than acute rheumatism, and

---

[1] Ann. d. Mal. d. Org. gen.-urin., p. 1013, 1896.   [2] Brit. Med. Jour., Jan. 16, 1897.
[3] Centralbl. f. Chir., No. 48, 1896, abstracted in Ann. of Surg., May, 1897, by Daniel N. Eisendrath.

not only attacks the synovial membrane, but in many instances also the capsule and the tendons about the joint. The case is apt to be prolonged, and ankylosis is common. Suppuration is unusual. The disease attacks one or several joints, but is asymmetrical as a rule.]

An editorial[1] on the **diagnosis and prognosis of chronic gonorrhea,** quoting Kopp,[2] shows how little reliance can be placed on microscopic examination of urethral threads. Von Schlen,[3] of Hanover, added the third glass test. Pezzoli[4] examined the urine and washings from different parts of the urethra, and concluded that the urethral glands and pockets in the acute stages of a gonorrhea are almost always affected; and in cases of chronic anterior urethritis the gonococci will be found oftener in the glands of Littré and pockets of Morgagni than in the anterior urethra itself. In chronic posterior urethritis the prostatic follicles are also involved almost without exception.

Finally, irritant injections must not be overlooked as a means of cure, but can only be of value in the anterior urethra.

Ferd. C. Valentine[5] gives a detailed description of apparatus and technic for irrigation of the urethra and bladder, in both male and female. The solutions used are potassium permanganate, corrosive sublimate, silver nitrate, and cupric sulfate. The apparatus is simple in construction and easy to keep aseptic.

Reginald Harrison[6] considers the **cause of suppurations in male and female generative organs,** occurring in gonorrheal affections. Many forms of gleet, he says, are re-infections from the bladder, though in most instances the prostate is the only part showing indication of contact with septic products, the mucous membrane of the bladder being insensitive to gonococcal influences. He advises examination of the vesical urine obtained by catheter for the gonococci. He employs vesical irrigation with antiseptics, using Condy's fluid, boric acid, and silver nitrate. Borocitrate of magnesium given internally he has found valuable in sterilizing purulent urine; give ʒj t. d. in water; this does not disagree with the stomach. Salicylate and benzoate of sodium together he has also found of use, giving 15 gr. of each t. d. in chloroform-water. He also finds good results in irrigating sinuses, by filling the bladder with the solution and allowing the patient to void it, part escaping by the urethra and part by the sinus.

Chas. C. Godding,[7] writing on **non-venereal bubo,** states that the affection is quite common in the British navy, both in the home and foreign departments. The inguinal glands alone are attacked, the existing cause being a sprain, or an abrasion on the penis or toe, but there may be no appreciable cause. The glands may or may not suppurate. The constitutional condition is usually low before the onset, and progressive debility and anemia follow. In 7 years the yearly average was 733 cases among 56,000 persons, or about 13 per 1000. Three cases are reported with detailed symptoms. He believes the condition to be one of lymphadenitis, and the best treatment increasing doses of arsenic.

J. Clifford Perry,[8] writing on **venereal buboes,** states that the percentage of gonorrheal buboes in the U. S. Marine-Hospital Service is 2½%.

Ducrey states that he has found the **germ of soft chancre,** but the germ fails to fulfil Koeh's law. Taylor claims the soft chancre is not due to a specific germ. The evidence is that a chancroidal bubo is caused by the absorp-

[1] Jour. Cutan. and Genito-Urin. Affections, Mar., 1897.
[2] Internat. Jour. Surg., p. 307, 1893.   [3] Centralbl. f. Krankh. d. Harn. u. Sex. Org., 1893.
[4] Arch. f. Dermat. u. Syph., 1896.   [5] Med. Rec., June 5, 1897.
[6] Lancet, June 26, 1897.   [7] Brit. Med. Jour., Sept. 26, 1896.
[8] Am. Jour. Med. Sci., Nov., 1896.

tion of toxins or ptomaïns resulting from the action of the germs in the chancroid lesion. The author's treatment consists in the injection of 20–30 ℳ of the **benzoate of mercury** in non-suppurating buboes at several points. In a report of 22 cases treated by this method the greatest number of injections was 4, and the time of healing was from 5–26 days, or an average of 13.9 days, as compared with 33.76 days average by the excision method. For suppurating buboes he uses Hayden's method of a skin puncture at the most fluctuating point, evacuation, irrigation with peroxid of hydrogen, then with corrosive sublimate 1 : 1000, then filling with warm 10 % emulsion of iodoform in vaselin and applying cold bichlorid dressing.

R. Percy Crandell,[1] on **venereal disease in the navy and its prevention,** states that the loss to the service from this cause is equal to 122 men for 6 months, or 721 cases out of 10,625 men. His conclusions are : 1. Circumcision is advisable before or immediately after enlistment ; 2. Applicants should be placed on probation before final enlistment ; 3. Periodical examination of crew should be insisted upon ; 4. Examining parties going ashore, before going and after returning ; 5. Using individual washing materials should be a rule ; 6. Registration and inspection of prostitutes would prove an aid.

R. A. Stirling[2] calls attention to **gleet of syphilitic origin** appearing about 2 months after the primary lesion. He believes this to be a very early secondary manifestation and antecedent to the symmetrical redness on the faucial pillars. This gleet is contagious, and is rebellious to antisyphilitic treatment, responding to injection of zinc chlorid gr. ss, ℨj of aqua, gradually increased in strength. This discharge is not due to ulceration or mucous patches. It is an infectious syphilitic discharge. Its continuance is the probable cause of the stenosis which is not unusual in syphilitics.

Chas. G. Cumston,[3] writing on **epididymitis of tertiary syphilitic origin,** states that this symptom may appear from 2 to 20 years after the chancre, attacking preferably those from 35 to 45 years of age, venereal excess being the usual exciting cause. He reports a case which was supposed to be tuberculosis of testicle, but after a course of mixed treatment recovery took place. The affection begins in a subacute form, with or without pain. In syphiloma of the epididymis the caput or the whole organ may be involved, is firm and resistant, irregular, with indurated spots, and lacks the adhesions found in gonorrheal epididymo-orchitis, and is unilateral. There is also a tendency to selerosis or gumma. Tertiary syphilitic epididymitis may be mistaken for gonorrheal, tuberculous, or malignant tumor, or cyst.

An editorial[4] on **syphilis of the kidneys and its treatment** states that it is established that syphilis may attack the kidneys both in the secondary and tertiary stages ; its frequency is not settled, writers varying widely. The symptoms in early secondary attacks develop about 2 or 3 months after a chancre. There is edema or frequency of urination, headache, and digestive trouble. The urine shows blood and casts. Late nephritic lesions are like ordinary chronic nephritis.

Welander[5] concludes that mercury must be given cautiously, and that nephritis due to secondary syphilis is rarer than that caused by full doses of mercury. It is important therefore, in treating syphilis, to examine the urine frequently, and when albuminuria and cylindruria are seen to be cautious in the administration of mercury.

Arthur H. Ward,[6] writing on **the primary lesion of syphilis,** advo-

[1] Med. News, June 12, 1897.   [2] Intercol. Med. Jour. of Australasia, Nov. 20, 1896.
[3] Ann. of Surg., Mar., 1897.   [4] Therap. Gaz., Feb. 15, 1897.
[5] Arch. f. Dermat. u. Syph., Bd. xxxvii., H. 3.   [6] Brit. Med. Jour., Oct. 24, 1896.

cates the microbic theory of syphilis, holding that the lesions are caused by the toxins, and the induration is due to chemotaxic action causing migration of leukocytes. He enters quite fully into the pathology of the disease.

Lane[1] discusses the **treatment of syphilis** by the intravenous use of mercury. He uses a solution of cyanid of mercury of a strength of 1%, and in the average case injects $1\frac{1}{4}$ gr. (20$\mathfrak{m}$). In a severe case for the first few injections he uses double this quantity. Injections are used at first every other day, but are soon given every day. The skin over the elbow is rendered sterile, a fillet is tied around the arm, the needle is introduced into a prominent vein in front of the elbow, the fillet is loosened, the mercury is injected, and the needle is withdrawn. The author maintains that the method is entirely safe, causes rapid improvement, is painless, does not disturb the intestinal tract, and can be easily regulated according to the susceptibility of patients. He strongly commends this mode of using mercury in cerebral syphilis. It occasionally happens that the method cannot be used because of the impossibility in some individuals of making the veins prominent.

DISEASES OF THE BRAIN AND OF THE NERVES.

J. Leonard Corning[2] recommends the use of **congealed oils to prevent the reunion of nerves** after subcutaneous division. He introduces an oil in the wound after the nerve-trunk has been divided, and applies cold to congeal the oil. The melting-point of the oil should be at least 3° above the normal blood-temperature. A good non-irritant oil may be obtained by melting oil of theobroma over a water-bath and adding paraffin until the melting-point of the mixture is over 105°.

Robert Abbe[3] writes on the **intradural section of the spinal nerves for neuralgia**, and reports 3 cases in which he divided portions of the posterior roots of the brachial plexus or resected them at their origin from the cord. The field of this operation, though necessarily small, will probably prove to be important, especially in cases of acute neuritis starting in the peripheral nerve and ascending.

Mayo Robson[4] reports a case in which the **spinal cord of a rabbit** was successfully **used as a graft** in the median nerve of a man of 29 ; 7 months before, he had fallen on a scythe, which had produced a deep cut on the inferior and inner aspect of the arm, dividing the brachial artery. At the time of injury a surgeon had tied the artery and sutured a divided nerve. It was evident that there had been a complete division of the median, ulnar, and internal cutaneous nerves, and it was decided to operate. An incision was made along the line of cicatrix and a transverse incision was added to this 1 in. above the elbow. The ulnar nerve was firmly anchored in fibrous tissue and the lower end of the proximal portion was bulbous and connected by fibrous tissue to the upper end of the distal portion. The severed internal cutaneous nerve was discovered and sutured. About the middle of the upper arm the bulbous end of the upper segment of the median nerve was discovered. The upper end of the lower segment was found just above the elbow. The fibrous tissue between the ends of the ulnar nerve was excised and the two portions of nerve united by grafting strands of the sciatic nerve of the rabbit, so as to fill up the gap and produce continuity. The ends of the median nerve could not be brought nearer together than $2\frac{1}{2}$ in. The spinal cord was dissected from a recently killed rabbit, and this was used as a graft to join the ends of the

[1] Brit. Med. Jour., Dec. 12, 1896. [2] Med. Rec., Dec. 5, 1896.
[3] Boston M. and S. Jour., Oct. 18, 1896. [4] Brit. Med. Jour., Oct. 31, 1896.

median nerve. Fine catgut was the suture-material employed. The edges of the wound were approximated and the arm placed on a right-angled splint. Healing took place by first intention, and 10 days after the operation sensation was obviously returning, and in another week it returned more markedly. After about 4 months the nutrition of the hand was very greatly improved. It felt warmer and the man was able to pick up small objects. The power of flexion of the wrist and abduction of the thumb was increased, but there was no sensation over the ulnar distribution. Six years after the operation the right forearm is only $\frac{1}{8}$ in. less in circumference than the left forearm. All the muscles except the abductor of the thumb are as well developed on the right side as on the left, this being true even of the interossei. The movements of the arm are completely restored, and are almost as perfect as those of the left arm. Flexion of the fingers and the grasp have completely returned, sensation is entirely restored, and the electrical reactions, except those exhibited by the abductor of the thumb, are normal. In this case, although recovery has been slow it is complete, except in regard to the abductor pollicis. This case demonstrates absolutely that we can restore nerve-continuity by grafting. We do not know whether the rabbit's cord assumed the function of the nerve, or whether it simply acted as a basis on which nerve-tissue was constructed. Why it is that the restoration of function in the ulnar area required a longer time than in the median distribution it is impossible to say. [A great variety of plans have been employed in endeavoring to restore nerve-function after a loss of nerve-substance. A plan which suits one case may not suit another. Von Bergmann has proposed in some cases to shorten the limb by bone-resection, so as to permit the approximation of the separated ends of the nerve. Létiévant has suggested the attachment of the proximal end of the peripheral portion of a cut nerve-trunk to a near-by uncut nerve-trunk. A flap may be formed on the central stump, or flaps can be made upon both the central stump and the peripheral stump. The suture *à distance* may be employed, catgut passing from cut end to cut end (Assaky). Vanlair employs a tubular suture. Schüller stretches the nerve. Other surgeons have implanted a piece of nerve from one of the lower animals or from a recently amputated human limb. When two nerves which run in the same direction and near each other are cut obliquely Tillmanns sutures the long central stump to the short peripheral stump, and *vice versa*. Huber, of Ann Arbor, recently reviewed this subject most ably and reported some striking experiments of his own. He tells us that nerve-implantation has been performed 14 times, success being obtained in but 3 cases, and he asserts that the implanted portion always degenerates and serves only as a support for growing axis-cylinders. Robson's case is a brilliant success and is unique.]

A. E. Morison[1] describes a **method for locating the fissure of Rolando:** "The measurements may be made with a piece of sterilized silk marked off by knots to form the triangle, or by defining the sides of the triangle by means of the surgeon's finger, whose length is already known. A point is taken half-way between the glabella and the external occipital protuberance, and the breadth of the little finger behind it (about $\frac{1}{2}$ in.) indicates the apex of the triangle. An isosceles triangle is then mapped out on the scalp; its sides are $3\frac{3}{4}$ in. long. One lies in the middle line forward from the point mentioned above. The base measures $4\frac{1}{2}$ in., and is anterior. The posterior side of the triangle is over the fissure of Rolando. Trigonometrically the apical angle of this triangle is 67° 27′ 52″, and this is practically identical with the angle formed by the fissure and the middle line of the skull worked

---

[1] Brit. Med. Jour., No. 1868, 1896.

out by other methods, and, from an examination of a large number of skulls of various sizes, is constant and correct."

R. Abbe[1] reports a case in which he **implanted some rubber tissue under the dura mater.** A year has passed since the operation and no ill effects whatever have become manifest. The patient suffered from Jacksonian epilepsy. Adhesions between the dura and the brain were found over the arm-center. These adhesions were broken up and a bit of rubber tissue was placed between the brain and the dura and the dura sutured over it.

Payr[2] describes some instruments he has devised with the object of **exploring the cranial cavity by means of small perforations** made in the bones. He uses a fine drill and syringe, straight and curved needles, capillary glass tubes, a glass rod (one end of which is right-angled and drawn into a thread), and also harpoons. The author has made many experiments on animals in order to discover whether it were possible by the use of small perforations in the cranium to determine the existence of a fluid collection in the brain or under the meninges, and the nature of the fluid removed, to secure minute portions of brain-substance for histologic examination, and to prove the existence or absence of pulsatile movements of the dura. Pulsation of this membrane can be shown by the mounting of the fluid in the capillary glass tube which is passed into the cranial cavity through the drill-hole, and it can also be shown by movements of the glass rod when that is inserted. He tells us that we may determine if the collection of fluid is pus, hydatid material, or blood by the use of an exploring-syringe. The situation of the growth and its nature can be ascertained if we remove a small portion by the harpoon. Through one of these drill-holes we can penetrate the lateral ventricle, and it is even possible that by a ligature passed through 2 drill-holes we could arrest hemorrhage from the middle meningeal or a venous sinus. [The above procedures appear to us fanciful, dangerous, unsurgical, and unsatisfactory. It is certainly safer to trephine and explore than to plunge instruments into the brain on the trust to Providence principle.]

Gilbert Barling[3] reports 3 cases of **otitis media with brain-abscesses.** In the 1st case otitis media was followed by extradural suppuration and abscess of the cerebellum. Operation was followed by recovery. In the 2d case otitis media was followed by abscess of the cerebellum, and trephining was followed by death. Necropsy showed the existence of a second abscess. In the 3d case cerebral abscess followed otitis media, and recovery ensued upon operation.

Marchant and Herbet[4] write on **resection of the Gasserian ganglion.** They come to the conclusion that some forms of facial neuralgia are due to lesion of the ganglion. This lesion is inflammatory in nature, and the proper treatment is destruction of the ganglion. In some cases in which there has been no ganglionic lesion and yet the neuralgia has ceased after the ganglion has been extirpated, we must assume that the cure has been brought about by destruction of this nerve-center. The best route to reach the ganglion is the entrance through the temporosphenoidal region, because by this route we are readily led to the ganglion by finding the inferior maxillary division in the foramen ovale. Complete extirpation is certainly possible, but in the majority of the cases which have been recorded incomplete destruction was practised by means of cureting or crushing. Some surgeons only resect the branches of the ganglion. The accidents which most commonly result from the operation are hemorrhage from the middle meningeal or the dural vessels and cerebral

[1] Ann. of Surg., Jan., 1897.
[3] Brit. Med. Jour., June 12, 1897.
[2] Centralbl. f. Chir., No. 31, 1896.
[4] Rev. de Chir., Apr., 1897.

compression. Septic infection may take place, and secondary hemorrhage may occur, as may iodoform-poisoning and eye-trouble. Immediately after the operation anesthesia is noted in the area supplied by the three chief branches of the ganglion, but this anesthesia is not persistent. Relapse is less common after destruction of the ganglion than after removal of its main branches. An examination of the statistics would not indicate that complete removal of the ganglion gives a better result than simple destruction of it. Out of 95 recorded cases there were 17 deaths. By the temporal route the death-rate is $12\frac{1}{2}\%$. In Rose's method the death-rate is $20\frac{1}{2}\%$. The mortality is the same for complete extirpation of the ganglion as for incomplete removal of it.

Louis McLane Tiffany[1] makes an elaborate study of **intracranial operations for the cure of facial neuralgia.** He says that a consideration of operative measures resolves itself at the present time into a consideration of intracranial operations for the removal of the Gasserian ganglion and nerves, or either of these structures. The history of operative measures for the relief of neuralgia shows that the first operations were done on peripheral nerves, and that surgeons gradually advanced in the central direction. With each advance toward the center fresh hopes of cure were raised. The removal of Meckel's ganglion and the superior maxillary nerve excited confident hopes. Peripheral operations will cure many cases, but not all of them. In some cases the trouble returns, and the question to be considered is whether or not the ganglion of Gasser when removed absolutely cuts off the pain-route in nearly all cases. Tiffany is careful to state " in nearly all cases," because it is beyond question that some cases of neuralgia are expressive of a central lesion. The credit of first removing this ganglion is accorded to Rose. Andrews, of Chicago, had thought out a similar method, but Rose operated before him. The Hartley-Krause operation has been more frequently done than any other procedure. Doyen has devised a method of reaching the ganglion by the temporal route. Tiffany then describes Doyen's operation. The total number of Gasserian-ganglion operations collected is 108; nearly $\frac{2}{3}$ of these were operated upon by the Hartley-Krause method, $\frac{1}{4}$ by Rose's method, 7 by Horsley's method, 4 by Doyen's method, 4 by a method of Quenu, 1 by Navarro's plan. There were 47 operators. The patients varied in age from 20 years to 79, and there were more men than women. The right side was twice as often affected as the left side. In 22 cases all of the divisions were affected; in 10 cases only the 3d division; in 6 cases only the 2d division. In the remaining cases the 2d and 3d divisions were affected. There was no instance in which the 1st alone was the seat of pain; the 2d and 3d were always affected with it. In fact, it is a question whether, when the 1st division is affected, it is not affected reflexly. There seems to be nothing that we can with justice claim as the cause of facial neuralgia. In some cases spasm of the facial muscles accompanied the pain, but there was no case in which the musele-spasm sometimes accompanied the pain and sometimes did not. In some cases, when the patient made an effort to keep the face-muscles quiet during the pain, trembling of the corresponding side of the face occurred. The areas of distribution of the pain correspond to the divisions of the fifth nerve above. Paroxysms can be induced by moving or handling the involved area. There are very generally extremely hyperesthetic points which when touched cause a pain-paroxysm. There may be a scarlet flush over the pain-area during a paroxysm. Heat and cold may also serve to develop pain-paroxysms. A central operation is rarely seriously considered by the patient until the materia medica has been exhausted and peripheral operations have been performed

[1] Ann. of Surg., Nov., 1896.

without avail. Many of these patients become addicted to morphin. The one persistent condition which is found present in the victims of facial neuralgia is arterial sclerosis, and it exists in the ganglion as well as in the branches. It is not certain, however, that a sclerosis is more positive in the Gasserian ganglion and branches the subject of pain than in the Gasserian ganglion and branches not the subject of pain on the opposite side of the same individual. The best operation is the Hartley-Krause method. This gives excellent access to the ganglion, which can be seen well together with its branches. If we decide that removal of the sensory route near to the ganglion is expedient, it can readily be performed; and again, motion of the lower jaw cannot be impaired, as it may be by the Rose operation. The osseous flap can be cut with a chisel, circular saw, etc., but it must be large enough to admit of safe work. The opening must be as low down as the zygoma. Preliminary ligation of a carotid artery may predispose to necrosis of the flap, soft and osseous. If ligation is decided upon as advisable, it is a question whether it should not be done very shortly before the Hartley-Krause operation. There seems to be no special advantage in replacing the bone-flap, as the temporal fascia makes a very firm scar. The advantage of not replacing the flap is that we leave a permanent route by which the interior of the head can be reached at any time without trouble. The dura can be separated from the base very easily by a piece of cotton held in forceps, the cotton pressure serving to diminish the bleeding. If there is excessive bleeding, gauze-packing applied for a short time will arrest the flow of blood and permit the continuation of the operation. The bleeding is venous and comes from vessels which pass between the bone and the dura. The middle meningeal artery may, of course, be wounded. The 2d branch is the first one which comes into view, then the 3d is found and the ganglion is exposed. The lifting of the brain from the floor of the skull is rendered much easier by making an incision in the dura and evacuating some of the cerebrospinal fluid. There is no doubt that the ganglion and branches can be removed after they have been thoroughly exposed, but the advisability of so removing them is questionable. The first branch is never affected alone, although it may be involved reflexly, and when the first division is removed there is apt to be trouble of one sort or another. The eye-involvement manifests itself by corneal anesthesia and panophthalmitis. The above are the two chief reasons why it is not advisable to take away the upper portion of the ganglion and the 1st branch, but rather to remove the 2d and 3d branches with the corresponding portions of the ganglion. The ganglion should always be uncovered, and the portion indicated excised. We should consider the expediency of trying to save the motor fibers which accompany the 3d branch. Tiffany says that, as a rule, he has not taken the pains to do this, yet he has thought that he recognized them, being able in one case to make the muscles of mastication contract by passing a tenaculum into the 3d branch close to the bone. Another reason why it is desirable to leave the motor route is that it might become necessary at a future time to operate on the other Gasserian ganglion, and, if we did the ordinary operation, there would be bilateral paralysis of the muscles of mastication. The motor root should be spared, as it often can be. The operation should be finished at one sitting, if this is possible, and the wound should be drained. Entire closure of the wound without drainage will be likely to make trouble. Of the 108 reported cases, 24 died. Tiffany then analyzes the causes of death. The study of the cases proves conclusively that intracranial excision of the 5th nerve relieves pain, certainly for a time, and possibly permanently; but pain may recur again, possibly in the territory which was presided over by the excised branch, possibly in other branches. If the Gasserian ganglion is removed, there is never recurrence of pain ; that is, after known removal pain does not recur, but in cases in which the ganglion has been picked or curetted away we do not know that it has been entirely removed, and in some of these cases pain has recurred. In cases in which pain has recurred after operations on the ganglion the operation has been attempted removal rather than known removal.

Conjunctivitis, anesthesia of the cornea, and ulcer of the cornea have been frequently observed on the side of operation, but when the eye is protected from injury it recovers as a rule. Ross, Krönlein, Keen, and Tiffany have been obliged to enucleate an eye after operation. Sewing the lids together avoids irritation from the presence of foreign bodies. Such results show the importance of leaving the first branch, and thus avoiding eye-injury. If eye-irritation occur, the organ should be covered with a watch-glass. Ordinary sensation in the nerve-trajectory is abolished over a small area and is irregularly present over a larger area. We often find ordinary sensation where pain-sensation is abolished. The secretion of saliva is unaffected. It is not always possible to say what cases require the central operation, but the following suggestions may be of assistance to the surgeon : intracranial operation is to be considered if more than one branch of the nerve is affected ; if the painful area receives filaments from the branches near the exit from the head, the tongue, the temporal region, etc. If the pain is not due to constitutional disease; if there is any cause central to the ganglion ; if other measures have failed ; the operation which Tiffany advises is the removal of the lower $\frac{2}{3}$ of the ganglion with the 2d and 3d branches as far as their points of exit from the skull all in one piece, the upper 3d of the ganglion and 1st branch not being excised. Tiffany then presents an epitome of all the published cases.

H. M. Thomas and W. W. Keen[1] report a successful case of **removal of a large tumor** from the left frontal region in which the lateral ventricle was opened and packed with iodoform-gauze. The tumor weighed 2½ oz., and its dimensions were 3½ by 2⅛ by 1₁₆⁹ in. After the tumor had been removed a clot was seen at the bottom of the cavity. Keen removed this by lifting it out. He then discovered that he had opened directly into the ventricle at a point where the anterior cornua joins the main cavity. A piece of iodoform-gauze was carried into the cavity occupied by the tumor, the end of the gauze filling the anterior portion of the lateral ventricle. This patient was greatly improved. Five months after operation he had no head-symptoms, was perfectly free from headache, and was in excellent health and spirits. Exophthalmos of the left eye, which was marked, had disappeared, and the muscles of the face on the two sides acted equally. The vision of the left eye had improved somewhat, but he still was unable to see well enough to walk alone.

B. Sachs and A. G. Gerster[2] write on the **surgical treatment of focal epilepsy,** and consider 19 cases upon which they operated. They report 3 of these cases cured, 5 improved, and 11 unimproved ; 3 of the 11 died as a result of the operation. The authors have come to the conclusion that, if a long time has elapsed since the injury, operation will fail, and that in most cases operation is not of benefit. They advise operation in cases of essential epilepsy in which the onset of the disease or the traumatism was but 1 or 2 years previously. If there is obvious skull-injury, surgical operation is advisable, even if years have passed. In many cases ordinary simple trephining is enough, and this is particularly true in cases in which the epilepsy is due to a cystic condition of the brain or in which there was an injury of the skull. If the epilepsy has lasted a very short time, and if the evidence indicates the

[1] Am. Jour. Med. Sci., Nov., 1896.   [2] Ann. of Surg., Feb., 1897.

existence of a very limited area of disease, a portion of the cortex should be excised. Remember that cortical lesions are frequently microscopic, and the mere fact that the tissue appears normal does not contraindicate excision of the area. It is justifiable to attempt surgical treatment in epilepsy associated with infantile palsies of cerebral origin, if the palsy is not too old. In long-standing cases of epilepsy no surgical procedure is of any use.

Charles B. Nancrede[1] writes on the **operative treatment of Jacksonian epilepsy,** and comes to the following conclusions: Removal of a discharging lesion in cortical and Jacksonian epilepsy is palliative only, the operative scar infallibly becoming a new source of irritation. The sooner the operation is done after the establishment of the disease the more prolonged will be the immunity. It is possible that trephining performed very early may cure, especially if we find any really reliable method to lessen the area of the scar and to prevent adhesions between the brain and the membranes. In competent hands the operation is not so dangerous as to forbid our urging trephining in this class of epilepsies, especially when done early, because the chance of a prolonged immunity is greater and the fits are likely to be lighter and to recur at greater intervals after the relapse than before the trephining. When the intervals between the fits are so short that the paroxysms are practically continuous the removal of the discharging-center is a life-saving measure. It is a great mistake to permit the patient to resume work early, particularly manual work, after one of these operations, because muscular effort may lead to congestion of the encephalon and the reestablishment of the convulsions. Operation removes but one of the factors causative of epilepsy, but the too ready response to stimuli still remains and can only disappear, if it ever disappears, after a prolonged period. The individual must avoid everything which may excite acute cerebral congestion or constant congestion. He, therefore, must avoid excitement of mind and body and mental strain for a prolonged period or possibly for the remainder of his life. [There can be no doubt that the high anticipations which were once entertained as to the curability of epilepsy by operation have not been realized. Von Bergmann does not think that permanent cure can be obtained. Occasionally a case is really cured; sometimes operation renders a patient more amenable to medical treatment and leads to prolonged improvement. As a rule, the most we can expect is improvement, which may be very temporary, but which not infrequently lasts for a year or more. We believe, with Dana, that freedom from fits for a year or more is worth the suffering and slight risk incurred by operation. Early operations upon cases of traumatic origin offer the best prospects of gain.]

William N. Bullard[2] makes a statistical study to determine the **permanent or later results of fractures of the skull.** His conclusions are as follows: Out of 70 persons who had had fracture of the skull, 37 presented no symptoms when examined some time later; only 7 presented serious symptoms, and in 4 of these it is very doubtful if the symptoms were due to the injury. The most frequent consequences were headache, deafness, dizziness, and inability to resist the action of alcohol. Out of 15 cases in which operation (trephining, etc.) had been performed, 12 had no symptoms. In one it was doubtful whether the symptoms were due to the injury; in another the symptoms were very slight. The other was deaf, but had no other trouble. We are, therefore, justified in concluding that those cases in which trephining was performed have shown much better results than those in which no operation was performed.

[1] Ann. of Surg., Aug., 1896.   [2] Boston M. and S. Jour., Apr. 29, 1897.

DISEASES OF THE SPINAL COLUMN AND SPINAL CORD.

Enderlen [1] maintains that in **fracture of the lumbar region of the spinal column** operation is not justifiable unless the fracture involves the arch of the vertebra and is comminuted or complicated, or unless bone-fragments have damaged the cord. If such complications do not exist, it is a difficult or impossible matter to diagnosticate fracture from concussion and bruising of the cord, and an early operation is never to be thought of in either one of these conditions. The author is also opposed to operating for the removal of a blood-clot, because the clot may undergo absorption by process of nature after the lapse of, it may be, months, or even, as in one instance on record, after the period of 2½ years. Cases have been reported in which it is claimed that the operation proved of great benefit; but it is uncertain whether the benefit was due to nature or the operation. Even when the cord is subjected to pressure it is not well to operate early, and we should allow some three weeks to pass before we operate. In 95% of all cases the vertebral body is the seat of the injury. The reports of cases operated on would indicate that fracture of the arches has been almost as common as fracture of the body. In view of the fact that postmortem observations show that 95% of the fractures met with are fractures of the body, we would of necessity conclude that fractures of the body are far graver in their consequences than fractures of the arch, and fractures of the arch are more readily reached for surgical treatment. The author reports a case in which there was fracture of the 6th dorsal and 1st lumbar vertebræ, followed by anesthesia and sphincter-paralysis. Some 6 months later the patient died of phthisis. The postmortem examination showed that there had been a slight injury of the 5th and 6th dorsal vertebræ and a fracture of the body of the first lumbar vertebra, fragments of which had been driven into the spinal cord. There was an almost complete transverse cord-injury.

De Forest Willard [2] writes on **laminectomy in spinal caries paraplegia.** He concludes that the prognosis in the paraplegia of Pott's disease is hopeful, except in those cases in which the cord has been actually destroyed. Laminectomy should not be undertaken until the patient has been treated for at least a year by rest, fixation, extension, and the administration of alteratives. The operation is extremely dangerous : 24% die from immediate shock, 36% die within 1 month, 46% die within 1 year, and 65% are not improved by the operation. The dangers are from hemorrhage, shock, and reflex disturbances from manipulation of the cord. Nevertheless, the operation is called for in selected cases when careful and persistent treatment has failed. [Willard's conclusions are eminently wise. Laminectomy is only to be thought of in a few selected cases.]

Chipault [3] discusses **acute osteomyelitis of the vertebræ** and reports 3 cases, with a notice of 28 cases seen by others. His conclusions are that the vertebræ may be alone the seat of trouble, or other bones may also be affected, and there may be various visceral lesions. In only a few cases have the causative germs been sought for. In 4 cases staphylococcus pyogenes aureus was discovered, and in another case staphylococcus pyogenes was found ; 19 cases out of 23 were males, and all the cases but 4 were less than 20 years of age. In some cases the exciting cause has been traumatism, in others fatigue and chilling of the surface of the body. The changes induced are identical with those of osteomyelitis anywhere. The lumbar region is the most commonly affected. The arches are affected more frequently than the bodies, and the bodies more

[1] Deutsch. Zeit. f. Chir., Bd. xliii., p. 329.   [2] Jour. Nerv. and Ment. Dis., Apr., 1897.
[3] Gaz. des Hôpitaux, Dec. 12, 1896.

commonly than the lateral portions of the vertebræ, but in some cases several portions of the vertebræ are attacked. In only 2 cases in which the vertebral bodies were involved was there spinal curvature. The absence of this spinal curvature, Chipault tells us, is due to the dorsal decubitus and the hyperostosis which quickly ensues. The vertebral joints may become involved, or pus may collect. The situation of the collection of pus varies with the situation of disease. If the bodies are diseased, the pus will pass forward, forming a retropharyngeal abscess, a mediastinal abscess, a psoas abscess, or a pelvic abscess. If the posterior parts of the vertebræ are diseased, a dorsal abscess is formed. Inflammation of the cellular tissue about the membranes of the cord, of the membranes themselves, or of the cord, may occur. The general symptoms of vertebral osteomyelitis are high fever, weak and rapid pulse, delirium, diarrhea, and the passage of small amounts of albuminous urine. The local symptoms are influenced by the seat of trouble. When the posterior portion of the vertebræ is the seat of disease brawny swelling can be made out, the swelling being in the middle line, in the neck, on one side, or in the middle line in the dorsal and lumbar regions, but always on one side in the sacral region. Fluctuation is very rarely detected. When the bodies of the vertebræ are attacked spinal rigidity and acute sensibility are noted, with other symptoms which depend on the region attacked. In some cases meningomyelitis may be present. The treatment consists in incision, removal of the pus and any sequestra, disinfection, and drainage. [The pressure-symptoms of acute osteomyelitis come on very suddenly. This is in contrast with tuberculous disease, in which there is a gradual onset of pressure-symptoms after a prolonged period dominated by evidences of irritation. The sudden onset of pressure-symptoms has led Müller to attribute them to edema of the cord. Makins and Abbott discussed this subject most carefully last year. See *Year-Book* for 1897.]

Thelwall Thomas [1] reports two interesting cases in which he succeeded in curing sacral meningoceles by excision.

F. Calot [2] writes on the **treatment of the deformity of Pott's disease.** His method is as follows: the patient is anesthetized and laid upon his face. One assistant takes hold of the hands and another assistant grasps the feet, and strong traction is made. An assistant supports the pelvis and lower abdomen, another the upper abdomen and chest. It is often necessary to resect the spines of the projecting vertebræ and remove the thickened skin above these spines. After this operation has been performed the surgeon is able to apply pressure where it is needed. In some cases when the deformity is maintained by bone-deposit the author resects the spines and laminæ and performs cuneiform osteotomy of the ankylosed bodies of the vertebræ. Whatever means are taken to correct this deformity should be followed by the application of a plaster-jacket for the head, neck, trunk, and pelvis. This jacket is worn for 3 months, when a fresh one is applied, which is also worn for 3 months. The patient then has placed upon him a poroplastic jacket and is allowed to walk about. Calot has operated on 37 patients without a death; 5 of the patients were straightened forcibly. In 30 resection of the vertebral spines, and in 2 cuneiform osteotomy was performed. Several of the patients had been deformed as long as eight years. Some of the operations were performed when the disease was active, some when it was passive. The results in some of the cases were very remarkable. Calot tells us that in the early stages of Pott's disease we should apply pressure over the diseased

[1] Liverpool Med.-Chir. Jour., Jan., 1897.   [2] Arch. Prov. de Chir., Feb., 1897.

area and use extension in order to prevent deformity. [Calot was preceded by Chipault in treating the deformity of Pott's disease by forcible correction.]

DISEASES OF THE PENIS, THE URETHRA, AND THE TESTICLE.

Arthur H. Ward[1] reports a case of **persistent priapism.** The patient was unmarried and 32 years of age, and came to the hospital with the statement that his penis had been continuously erect for 5 days. There had been no illness or accident, the patient was temperate, and there was no evidence of malaria; 8 days before admission he had had sexual intercourse; 5 days before admission he arose at night to make water, and on returning to bed erection occurred and continued. There was no emission and no sexual desire, and turning in bed caused much pain in the body of the penis. The erection was limited to the corpora cavernosa, the glans and corpus spongiosum being flaccid. Pulse and temperature were normal. There were no signs of local hemorrhage. Micturition was accompanied by pain and straining, and a soft catheter was used. The spleen was enlarged. The penis was treated with lead water and laudanum and the patient given cathartics, diuretics, and anodynes. Later potassium iodid was administered internally. Gradually the penis became less rigid, and on the 7th day fluctuation was detected over the corpora cavernosa and the spleen was found to have increased in size. Arsenic was added to the treatment. Examination of the blood showed that leukocythemia existed. By the end of the 8th week the penis was normal and the patient was able to have normal erections without pain. The author believes that the priapism was due to spontaneous thrombosis of the corpora cavernosa, caused by erection when the blood was leukocythemic. It would have been possible to squeeze out blood-clots through incisions, but incisions in such a case might be followed by disastrous infection, and might leave as a legacy distortion from trabecular adhesions. Incisions are only justifiable if suppuration occurs. The fact that the corpus spongiosum was not involved proves that the condition was not due to reflex irritation or cerebral excitement, and the same fact is proved by the persistence of the priapism for weeks. The author publishes a table containing the records of 12 cases of priapism.

J. N. Bartholomew[2] writes upon the **radical cure of hydrocele** by a new ambulatory method. An incision $\frac{1}{4}$ in. in length is made at the most dependent portion, the incision reaching to but not passing into the tunica vaginalis. The sac is dissected loose from the infundibuliform fascia and is loosened up to the epididymis. The sac is now opened, and the wall of the empty sac is pulled through the small incision and cut off close to the epididymis. The testicle is examined, and any granulations or cartilaginous bodies are removed. The incision contracts to $\frac{1}{2}$ of its original length, requires no stitches, and serves to drain the parts. After the completion of the operation the testicle is strapped as in a case of epididymitis, and the patient is permitted to walk about.

E. A. Southam[3] discusses the radical cure of hydrocele by excision of the sac and furnishes notes of 22 cases. Southam does not employ drainage, but after the operation elevates the scrotum and applies pressure by means of wood-wool pads. This radical operation should be performed in the following conditions: if the patient wishes a radical cure, but does not care to take the risk of a failure of the method of injection; if the hydrocele is old, with thick and rigid walls; when injection has failed; when a sac suppurates after tapping;

---

[1] Lancet, Apr. 24, 1897.   [2] Jour. Am. Med. Assoc., Apr. 24, 1897.
[3] Lancet, Mar. 20, 1897.

when a hematocele forms after tapping; when an inguinal hernia exists with hydrocele and we desire to cure the hernia radically; when, as a consequence of previous tapping, the testicle adheres to the scrotum; if the hydrocele is multilocular; if the hydrocele is encysted.

Weissblatt [1] reports a case of **fracture of the penis.** The patient when drunk had bent the penis violently. The next morning the organ was enormously swollen and discolored. On one side there was distinct thickening, due to laceration of a corpus cavernosum. The patient was placed in bed and treated by the local use of lead-water and laudanum and cold, and recovered in 2 weeks, although the spot of thickening remained. In 6 weeks the patient was able to indulge in sexual intercourse, although there was an area of thickening still existing the size of a pea.

Gwilym G. Davis [2] advises the following **method of amputating the penis :** bleeding is controlled by a rubber tube caught around the base of the penis; a circular incision is made through the skin to the tunica albuginea; an incision is made through the spongy body, the urethra is dissected up for half an inch, and the cavernous bodies are cut transversely at this point. Vessels are ligated with fine gut; the catgut sutures are passed through the outer edge and substance of the cavernous bodies on each side. When these are tied the cut surface is folded in the middle and forms a straight union upward from the projecting urethra. The urethra is slit in 3 places so as to form 3 flaps reaching back to the cavernous bodies. The corners of the flaps are cut off, leaving 3 triangular flaps which, when opened out, make one large triangle, the apex of which is above and the base below. The skin is sutured to these flaps by catgut.

W. G. Handley [3] advocates the performance of **inguinal instead of scrotal orchidectomy.** An incision is made in the line of the cord and over the external abdominal ring. This incision is slightly curved, its convexity being downward and outward, and is about 1½ in. long. The cord is isolated and pulled upward. Traction is kept up upon the cord, and the tissues are freed from the advancing cord and testicle by means of a blunt dissector. The testicle is taken out of the incision and removed, and the cord treated as usual. The scrotum should be invaginated through the wound in order to find and tie bleeding points. The incision is closed by a continuous horsehair suture. This wound, unlike a wound in the scrotum, can be approximated with accuracy, and infection is far rarer after inguinal than after scrotal orchidectomy. In the new operation there is no risk of hemorrhage in the tissues after castration, and the wound can be dressed and thoroughly protected with ease.

Ramon Guitéras,[4] in an article upon the treatment of stricture of the male urethra, describes the **treatment of stricture** by means of Fort's linear electrolyzer. The author states that the instrument resembles in outline the Maisonneuve urethrotome, although the blade is dull and is made of platinum. The blade of the instrument is connected with the negative pole of a galvanic battery. The chamois-covered positive pole is placed over the pubis or thigh, and the guide is carried into the urethra until the blade comes in contact with the stricture, when the current is turned on and the blade passes through the stricture. The current is turned off, and, if there be another stricture, the instrument is passed on until the next constriction is encountered, when the instrument is passed through it in the same way. The blade does not become heated and the operation causes very little pain. The current-strength is from 10–20 ma. It requires from 30 sec. to 4 min. to pass through a stricture.

[1] Deutsch. med. Zeit., Dec. 24, 1896.
[2] Univ. Med. Mag., Jan., 1897.
[3] Lancet, Dec. 12, 1896.
[4] Med. Rec., Nov. 14, 1896.

The operation brings the urethra up to the size of a No. 18 F. sound. After the use of Fort's instrument the urethra can be enlarged still more by the passage of larger bougies, or, if the stricture is anterior, by the performance of internal urethrotomy. This operation does not lacerate as much as does the operation of Maisonneuve, is not so painful, is not attended with hemorrhage nor followed by infection, and micturition afterward is but slightly painful.

Guitéras's conclusions on the treatment of stricture are as follows : Whatever treatment is employed urinary antiseptics must be given. If the meatus is small, the beginning of treatment is meatotomy. If possible, dilatation should be employed rather than cutting. In very small strictures continuous dilatation gives excellent results. It should always be used to enlarge the urethra for gradual dilatation or for the introduction of a guide if cutting is necessary. Oberlander's dilator is the best instrument for gradual dilatation. If dilatation fails to cure, urethrotomy must be performed. If a filiform bougie is passed only with great trouble, do not carry a tunnelled catheter over it unless it is proposed to operate at once, because to do so lacerates the urethra. If an operation becomes necessary to cure a small anterior stricture, most surgeons advocate internal urethrotomy by the plan of Maisonneuve ; but Fort's operation is safer. If it is necessary to cut an anterior stricture the caliber of which is over 18 F., use Otis's urethrotome. If a perineal operation is necessary, avoid Cook's operation if possible. In a perineal operation it is well to use the tunnelled catheter threaded over a filiform as a guide. No special method of section is applicable to all cases. Never do perineal section without a guide unless obliged to ; and if we can use a guide, use the largest one which can be inserted. There is no operation which will permanently cure a small and densely fibrous stricture of long standing. After operation such cases must be watched as long as the man lives.

Fort, in a letter to the *Medical Record*, Jan. 9, 1897, corrects some statements made by Guitéras about the operation of linear electrolysis. He says his instrument in nowise resembles the urethrotome of Maisonneuve, as it is composed of but one piece, and is like a whip which has a platinum blade projecting near the center. The operation lasts generally from 20 to 30 sec., and should never last longer than 1 min. After operation pass, not an 18 F. sound, but a No. 22-24 F. After operation it is never necessary to perform internal urethrotomy. [There can be no question that Fort's method is a great improvement upon the older plan of electrolysis. The older operation has been completely abandoned, because results were often bad and never permanent, healthy tissue as well as diseased tissue being acted on by the current. Fort's instrument enables us to act purely upon diseased tissue. This operation causes so slight an amount of pain that it is not necessary to cocainize the urethra, and the patient is not confined to bed. It is claimed by some that the cure is permanent, but this point is doubtful. The method of Fort has been practised and praised by Chas. Chassaignac, Bruce Clarke, Stevenson, Charles, Beni Madhab Baso, and others.]

A. J. Jonas[1] discusses **retrograde catheterization in impermeable deep urethral strictures,** and reports 4 cases. He says we may completely loose the proximal end of the urethra when performing a perineal operation for impermeable stricture. If this happens, attempt to discover the lost tube by making pressure above the pubes and in the rectum, in the hope that a stream of water will flow from the proximal end of the divided urethra and so disclose the situation of the canal. If we cannot discover the lost urethra by this means, perform suprapubic cystotomy and follow this by retrograde cath-

[1] Med. Rec., Feb. 6, 1897.

eterization. The passage of a catheter from behind forward furnishes a guide to enter and enables us to complete the formation of a channel. Jonas uses a large elastic tube for retrograde sounding, thinking it safer than a metal instrument. . This tube is kept in place for a time to secure perineal drainage. In impermeable stricture the cicatricial structure should be extirpated. No instrument is passed through the anterior urethra until the perineal drainage-tube has been permanently removed (when urine has become clear and nearly free from epithelium, triple phosphate, etc.). When the perineal tube is removed a sound is introduced from the meatus every day, the size of the instrument being progressively increased until a full-sized one can be used. [The practicability of safely excising large areas of diseased urethra has been proved by Eugene Fuller,[1] who in 1 case excised the entire bulb, 1 in. of penile urethra in front of the bulb, and the anterior $\frac{1}{2}$ in. of the membranous urethra. In another case he took away $1\frac{3}{4}$ in. of urethra. The results were excellent. Fuller doubts the value of grafts in these cases. His custom is, after completing the resection, to make a low cut dividing "the deepest portion of the membranous urethra, the lowest portion of the perineal structures, and some of the circular fibers of the sphincter ani." By this route a rubber drainage-tube is carried into the bladder. A rubber catheter is passed from the meatus to the perineal tube. The perineal structures about the catheter are sutured. The urethral tube is retained for a week or 10 days.]

L. Bolton Bangs[2] considers **stricture of the urethra in male children.** Most cases reported have been congenital malformations; some have been due to traumatism. Acquired stricture from non-traumatic post-natal causes has received but scant attention. Cases are upon record of children of 2 years of age or more who have received blows upon the perineum or who suffered from injury of the urethra by calculus, and who later in life presented symptoms of extreme gravity. Such cases should be treated at an early period after the accident, and the tissues of the urethra should be saved by the performance of perineal section and the securing of drainage. In a child who has been subjected to a perineal bruise and has been improperly treated stricture will develop very rapidly. The etiology of acquired stricture is often uncertain. In some there is positive history of gonorrhea, in some there is an uncertain history of an inflammation; in many there is no evidence of a preceding inflammatory condition. Many of these obscure cases of stricture in young adults arise from an extension into the urethra of balanoposthitis. Bangs reviews the literature of the subject and reports 2 cases: 1 a boy 3 years and 5 months old, and 1 a boy of 15, in which it seemed probable that the strictures arose from the urethral extension of a balanoposthitis.

DISEASES OF THE BLADDER AND PROSTATE.

L. Conitzer[3] writes on the **diagnosis and treatment of tuberculosis of the prostate.** He tells us that this disease is more common than is usually supposed. It is frequently impossible to tell at the postmortem which portion of the tract was the original seat of disease; but in the studies by Kzrywicki it is seen that out of 15 cases of tuberculosis of the genito-urinary tract 14 had tuberculosis of the prostate, and that the process had its beginning in the prostate, as the most ancient deposits were found in this organ and spread from it as a central focus. There are multiple foci which undergo cascation and increase in area, and occasionally, though rarely, run together. These

[1] Med. News, July 25, 1896.   [2] Med. Rec., Apr. 10, 1897.
[2] Centralbl. f. d. Krankh. d. Harn, u. Sex.-Org., p. 14, 1897.

deposits, as a rule, break into the bladder, the rectum, the urethra, or the perineum, and where they break they leave a fistula. The bladder is very likely to be attacked, and the process may advance up the ureter to the kidney, and may lead even to general tuberculosis. In some cases the disease reaches the seminal vesicles and the epididymis. It seems in some cases as if infection by gonococci had prepared the soil for the tuberculous process. The author then reports a case in which the diagnosis was made by observing abscesses. There was difficulty in urination associated with rectal tenesmus, and pain which passed into the perineum and was greatly increased by walking. The patient was weak and lost a great deal of flesh ; but there was no mucopurulent urethral discharge and no hematuria. In these cases catheterization is painful, due in early conditions to prostatic swelling, in later conditions to ulceration. Rectal examination shows that one lobe is probably larger than the other, and that the gland is sensitive on pressure. An area of softening may in some cases be detected by the finger. The condition of the urine depends upon the condition of the bladder ; if it is tuberculous, the urine will be cloudy and purulent and almost invariably acid. We may find bacilli in the urinary sediment or may not, and the fact that we do not find them does not forbid the diagnosis of tuberculosis. The cystoscopic examination is of very great importance, as we can determine by it whether or not the bladder is affected. In early stages of the disease miliary tuberculosis may be present; in later stages, ulceration. If · the bladder is not affected, the diagnosis of the disease may be made by pressing out the prostatic secretion and making a bacteriologic examination. The prognosis is, of course, unfavorable, although cure occurs in some few instances. It is always necessary to examine into the condition of the seminal vesicles, as they are very frequently involved. The proper treatment depends on making an early diagnosis. Mansedel wrote in 1892 that the opportunity for operation comes with the formation of abscesses. The author refers to three of Czerny's cases, in one of which the entire gland was converted into a caseous mass. He approves strongly of the saying of Guyon that it is as necessary in the patient with urinary trouble to examine the prostate frequently, as in the patient with rheumatism to examine the heart frequently. [N. Senn, in his address before the American Surgical Association in May, 1896, discusses thoroughly the subject of tuberculosis of the prostate. He says it is a proved fact that the prostate can be the seat of primary tuberculosis, and that it usually occurs in young adults. This distinguished observer states that the symptoms resemble those of chronic prostatitis ; hectic fever and wasting are only observed if other organs are also involved. During the early stage of the disease parenchymatous injections of iodoform-glycerin emulsion are indicated.]

The British Medical Association, at the Carlisle meeting in July, 1896, discussed **the surgical treatment of prostatic hypertrophy.** David MacEwan[1] opened the discussion. His views are as follows: Mercier devised the operation of urethral prostatectomy in 1856, but the proceeding was generally looked upon as a surgical freak. The first positive step in the road of progress was when Sir Henry Thompson and Mr. Harrison proposed bladder-drainage as a treatment for prostatic cystitis. It was discovered that the operation of lithotomy when accompanied by removal of a portion of the gland, was occasionally followed by very great improvement in the symptoms of prostatic trouble, and this led to the operation of perineal prostatectomy. McGill, in 1889, called attention to the value of the suprapubic route and introduced the operation of suprapubic prostatectomy. Further advance has been made by the introduction of combined operations, as in the methods of Bellfield, Nicoll,

[1] Brit. Med. Jour., Oct. 10, 1896.

and Alexander. In 1893 J. William White brought to the attention of the profession the operation of **double orchotomy.** [The term orchotomy is used by some and orchectomy by others. We believe neither is correct. To signify the removal of the testicle the proper word is orchiectomy or orchideetomy.] To obtain a knowledge of the results of double orchotomy we turn to White's table of 111 cases. White's conclusions are that in 82% of the cases rapid prostatic atrophy follows operation. In 52% cystitis disappears or greatly lessens. In 66% more or less vesical contractility returns. In 83% the troublesome symptoms are ameliorated, and in 46.4% the local conditions become practically normal. The mortality is 18%; but if we exclude unsuitable cases, it is 7.1%. MacEwan says that one cannot examine this table closely without noting that the details of many of the cases are too insufficient and vague to admit of a just judgment as to the amount of success which followed the operation. The previous histories are very meager in many cases, especially as to the employment of the catheter, and many are reported too soon after operation to permit of the formation of an estimate as to the permanency of the result. In many cases other methods of treatment were also employed at the same time, and this makes it difficult to say how much of the relief was due to the orchotomy and how much to the auxiliary measures. Nevertheless, this table shows that in a large number of cases the operation has caused a diminution of the obstruction and an amelioration of the concomitant evils. The author has collected a number of reports of cases published since White's paper. The number of operations has been 52; 42 of these were successful, 4 were not improved, and 6 died; 38 of these cases were reported with fulness, and the prostate diminished in size in 17 of the 38; in 6 no diminution occurred; in the remaining cases the symptoms were relieved, but the size of the prostate is not given. The best method of performing the operation is to make a 2-in. incision through the lower portion of the raphe, both glands being delivered through the one opening. When the cord is divided the vessels should be tied separately. Ligation *en masse* increases the risk of suppuration. The author then reports 3 cases of his own, all of which were improved.

He next discusses the rationale of the shrinkage of the prostate. In considering the amelioration of the functional symptoms he says that the lessening of the congestion accounts for the relief of pain and tenèsmus. The cystitis is relieved, because the mucous membrane is brought to a healthier state by better circulation and partly because the bladder obtains some physiologic rest when the obstruction is lessened. If the walls of the bladder are thick and sacculated, the most that the operation can do is to effect a small amount of improvement, and no benefit at all can be obtained if the pyogenic infection has extended up the urinary tract and pyelonephritis has developed. The return of the functional power of the bladder is chiefly due to the removal of the obstruction. It has been noticed that the operation is occasionally followed by mental disturbance, but the majority of these cases have not resulted directly from the operation, but are due to septic absorption or uremia. Orchotomy performed for disease of the testicles is never followed by mental disturbance, and it is therefore a just inference that maniacal states which arise after the operation has been performed for enlarged prostate result because of associated morbid conditions. In regard to unilateral orchotomy the evidence does not show that atrophy of half of the prostate is an ordinary consequence of removal of the corresponding testicle in cases of disease. A few cases of unilateral orchidectomy have been reported, but a correct decision can only be reached after further experience.

Mr. Harrison proposed as a substitute-operation resection of the vas deferens. If it can be shown that this operation is capable of producing as good results, it should receive the preference. It is safe, it is easy of performance, and would be more acceptable to the patient. White found on experiments in dogs that the operation produced loss of weight in the gland in every dog that died after 8 days. Guyon thinks that the operation produced some effect, although not nearly as great as that produced by bilateral orchotomy. Pavone thinks that bilateral resection brings about the same atrophy as White's operation. We may conclude that division of the vas occasionally induces atrophy of the prostate, but that the bulk of evidence seems to show that but little change occurs in the testicles; 37 cases of this operation have been reported, and 26 of these are said to have been successful. In 3 there was some improvement; 4 were failures, and 4 died from causes not connected with the operation. In a few of the cases it is mentioned that distinct shrinkage occurred in the prostrate; but this diminution is not so positive as we find recorded as following orchotomy. Guyon records a case in which the operation brought relief, but the diminution in the size of the prostate was scarcely appreciable. In Helferich's 10 cases, 8 of which were successful, there was a diminution of the size of the prostate in only a minority. Atrophic changes are said to take place more slowly than after orchotomy, and it is possible that these cases may have been published too early. More positive statements are made in regard to the effect upon the functional symptoms. Definite amelioration has occurred in 26 of the cases. There is no mention of specific mental disturbance except in one case by Dunstrey, of Leipsic, in which there was a diminution of bodily and mental vigor lasting 14 days, the patient's former briskness never being quite restored. The operation can be performed without an anesthetic. The vas is separated from the other structures of the cord, is caught between the finger and thumb a little below the external ring, an incision is made through the skin, an aneurysm-needle passed beneath the vas, and this structure isolated a short distance above and below. The needle is armed with a double catgut ligature and withdrawn. The vas is tied in two places and the intervening portion is cut away; the wound requires no sutures. Mr. Harrison says that we should attack only one vas at a time, and if the object is not sufficiently attained we may then attack the other. It is probably wiser, however, to deal with both sides simultaneously.

The author of this paper concludes that in a considerable proportion of cases castration brings about more or less atrophy of the enlarged prostate. The atrophy occurs most easily in the soft and elastic forms of hypertrophy, but it may also take place in the hard even when associated with general arteriosclerosis. The best effect is obtained when the enlargement of the gland is general. Sessile enlargement of the median portion may yield to castration, but intravesicular outgrowths are better treated by prostatectomy. Cystitis when not far advanced may be relieved or even cured. If the cystitis is associated with septic infection of the kidneys and with distressing bladder-symptoms, drainage of the bladder will be of more value. Vesical contractility may be restored even after years of catheter-life. Even if voluntary power does not return, the operation may bring relief to the patient if catheterism has been difficult, painful, and frequently necessary. With the exception mentioned double orchotomy will give as good results as prostatectomy, with a smaller death-rate. Resection of the vas acts more slowly in reducing hypertrophy of the prostate. It is a simpler operation, will be looked upon by the patient as more acceptable, and can therefore be recommended earlier.

Reginald Harrison, in discussing the paper of MacEwan, said that there can be no doubt that the removal of the testes or their atrophy, however obtained, is liable to be followed by shrinkage in the size of the normal prostate. The facts which have been gathered are sufficient to warrant a trial of vasectomy either on one or both sides. The cases in which Harrison has practised vasectomy may be divided into 2 groups: first, those in which only 1 vas has been divided; second, those in which both vasa have been resected either simultaneously or at intervals of some days. This surgeon has performed single vasectomy 12 times and double vasectomy 10 times. Of the 12 cases of single vasectomy, 7 derived permanent benefit from the operation. In the remaining cases there was either no benefit or the patient could not be traced. If both vasa are divided, it is well to have an interval of a month or so between the operations. The risk is less, and it might happen that the operation on the single vas relieved the too frequent micturition. Out of the 10 cases of double vasectomy there was very great benefit in 5, benefit which Harrison believes to be lasting. Of the remaining 5, 2 have not derived much advantage from it, 2 cannot be traced, while the 5th case is a recent one. That many of the troubles connected with enlargement of the prostate may be combated by castration or vasectomy is undoubted, but there are some pathologic conditions of the prostate which are not influenced by either procedure. Harrison does not oppose the operation of castration, but he calls attention to the fact that besides the mortality which attends it certain distressing mental disturbances are liable to follow it.

C. W. Mansell Moullin said that there is no single method of treatment for cases of enlargement of the prostate, and that statistics on such a subject drawn from all sorts of cases by different surgeons of different nationalities are worthless. There are undoubtedly many cases in which treatment by the catheter can be practised, and also many in which the prostate should be removed by the suprapubic or the perineal route. It is true that the mortality of suprapubic cystotomy is estimated at as high a figure as 20%, but the estimate is scarcely fair, because in 75% of the cases cystitis and pyelonephritis were present. Suprapubic prostatectomy performed when the urine is aseptic and the kidneys are sound has a very different result.

Mayo Robson published a series of 11 cases, with only 1 fatality. Moullin performed the operation 5 times without a death. He performed orchotomy 11 times, with an excellent result in 6 cases and relief in 2; 3 died, from heart-failure, apoplexy, and uremia respectively. He has always performed the bilateral operation, and does not think the unilateral operation is likely to be useful when there is marked inequality of the lobes. He has performed vasectomy 3 times, twice with conspicuous benefit, although the prostate did not diminish much in size.

[J. William White[1] believes that a patient with moderate prostatic enlargement, little or no pain, and 3 or 4 oz. of clear residual urine, and especially if he is not very old, retains sexual capacity, has healthy kidneys, and is in good general condition, should not be subjected to castration, and should be instructed in the use of a catheter. If such a patient develops severe pain which is not controllable by remedies, or if the amount of residual urine rises to 12 oz. or more, vasectomy is indicated. If a patient has decided enlargement, with 8–10 oz. of fetid or mucopurulent residual urine, with pain and difficulty in passing a catheter, an operation must be performed. If a patient is becoming old and the sexual power is weak, vasectomy is performed. If a patient is younger and sexual power is good, prostatectomy is indicated. Vasectomy is employed if there is renal disease and failure of the general health in a man well

[1] Univ. Med. Mag., Apr., 1897.

advanced in years. Castration is employed in a very old man with good general condition and healthy kidneys. In very serious cases of enlargement in which there is cystitis, with retention of urine, and in which the use of the catheter is difficult and painful, castration is indicated, though vasectomy may be first tried.]

A. T. Cabot[1] considers the question of **castration for enlarged prostate.** He says it was a great surprise to find that the mortality of this operation was high. Experience has shown that this mortality was not an accident, happening in the first 100 cases. Many patients who submit to castration are already suffering from disease of the bladder and kidneys that is tending to a fatal issue, and many of them die from this disease rather than from operation. White recognized this fact, and in his first series eliminated 13 of the 20 fatal cases, bringing the collected death-rate down from 18% to 7%. Such a revision of statistics in proper if we are comparing this with other operations performed upon persons in good health, but it is improper when we are making a comparison with other operations carried out upon the same variety of patients. It is this latter comparison which Cabot proposes to make. It is evidently improper to rule out cases in which death from pyelonephritis followed operation unless similar cases are excluded from the statistics of the other operations. It would seem better to take all cases as they come, trusting that they will distribute themselves with reasonable fairness through the different sets of statistics. He has excluded from this table cases in which other serious conditions existed to complicate the prostatic hypertrophy, conditions such as vesical stone and tuberculosis. When White's table is revised on the same lines we reduce his cases to 104, with 19 deaths, a mortality of 18%. Cabot has obtained reports of 99 other cases, of which 20 died. When these are added to White's cases we have a total of 203 cases with 39 deaths, the mortality for the entire series being 19.4%. So high a death-rate from so slight an operation is surprising. We should remember that an operation performed for the relief of a serious pathologic state has its danger much increased if it does not completely and at once relieve the condition. When an operation is performed for enlarged prostate the obstruction is slowly removed by shrinkage, but the shrinkage is slow and is of slight immediate use in stopping the back-pressure on the kidneys. This is a source of great danger and goes a long distance toward explaining why there is such a trivial difference in the mortality of castration and prostatectomy. The latter operation is far more severe, but it provides for ample drainage. Prostatectomy is an operation in which skill and a correct technic make the greatest difference in the fatality. As a consequence, the statistics show a constant improvement in the rate of mortality. White found, when his paper was written in 1893, that the more modern statistics of prostatectomy show a mortality of 14.9%. Cabot advances the belief that the correct death-rate of prostatectomy is under 20%, hence the operation stands upon the same footing as castration in its fatality when applied to all cases of advanced hypertrophy. Among all the reported cases of castration performed in middle life or advanced age there is not one in which there has been any **loss of masculine characteristics.** It is too early to state whether these patients will show diminished vigor as age advances, although there are some facts which should lead us to be watchful for evidence upon this point. We know that some neurologists believe that these glands exert an influence upon the nervous system even in old age, and Brown-Séquard's experiments in the use of animal extracts led him to believe that they have a distinct power of improving nutrition and increasing the force of the

[1] Ann. of Surg., Sept., 1896.

nerve-centres. In 99 cases of orchotomy mental disturbance followed 11 times immediately upon the operation. In 6 cases the condition was maniacal, in 5 there was loss of mental balance, and in several a melancholic tendency arose. Of the 6 maniacal patients 1 had previously shown symptoms of mania. Cabot reports a case of his own in which mental disturbance followed the operation and in which testiculin was administered with the greatest benefit. In some cases the operation has a decidedly depressing effect upon the strength, leading to severe shock. In other cases the patients have reacted well from the operation and the wounds have healed, but at the end of a short time they failed without any marked change in the symptoms and died. When a postmortem is performed on such a case it is usually found that pyelonephritis existed, but nevertheless it is important to note that those patients who carry successfully partially disabled kidneys for a considerable time succumb after a slight operation without any symptoms pointing to an increase of the renal condition, seeming to show that by the removal of the glands the vital force of the individual was diminished. It has been noticed after this operation that patients frequently suffer from flushes of heat similar to those experienced by women at the menopause, and even distinctly hysterical phenomena have been noted. Nevertheless, it is proper to state that in some cases nervous excitability which existed before has been relieved by the operation. In order to determine the real result it is necessary that the patient be under observation for a considerable length of time, for it often happens that while the patient is in the hospital he seems to have obtained very decided relief, but after he resumes his less regular habits of life this relief is found to be transitory. Indeed, the time which has passed since the operation first began to be practised is too short to determine the permanency of results, but we know definitely that in a few cases relapses have occurred and irritability and obstruction have returned.

Cabot's tables show that 79 cases survived operation; in 18 of these cases the reports were meager, and we are left with 61 cases to study; 5 of these were not improved; 1 improved for a time but later suffered a relapse. In 4 cases the catheter was still used, but entered with greater ease. In 27 cases retention, which had existed at the time of operation, disappeared. In 2 cases catheter-life, of 11 years, in 1 of 18 years, was cured by the operation. In the remaining 24 the power of urination was not entirely lost, but had been greatly impaired. In all these there was decided improvement. These facts show that in 9.8 % of cases there was failure, in 6.6 % moderate improvement, and in 83.6 % very great improvement. If further experience justifies these statements, we shall be able to say to the patient he has 8 chances in 10 of getting through the operation all right, and if he gets through it all right he has a little more than 8 chances in 10 of obtaining positive relief.

In comparing these results with those of suprapubic prostatectomy we may take the cases in Moullin's table which occurred after 1889—42 cases; 6 of these cases are too vague for consideration, which leaves us 36 cases; 8.3 % were not improved, 8.3 % were somewhat improved, in 83.8 % the power of urination was restored. We thus see that the two operations were remarkably parallel in their results both as to mortality and restoration of function. The author then considers the changes in the prostate which follow castration and lead to a diminution in its volume. It seems to be certain that myomatous tissue of the prostate is not affected by castration, and it is very difficult to determine whether the conditions in the prostate found after death are due to changes following castration or are degenerative changes already present in a pathologic organ before the operation was performed.

The second theory accounts for the reduction in size by supposing it to arise from changes in vascularity. This theory best explains the quick relief which immediately follows operation. The fact that retention may be relieved and yet subsequently recur opposes any belief in early anatomic changes. The phenomena are better explained by the vascular theory. It is probable that the alteration in the blood-supply plays a considerable part in the changes observed in the prostate, while the atrophy and disappearance of portions of the gland may bring about a final, permanent reduction in the size of the organ. Observations made during the past year have not borne out the suggestion that the third lobe is especially likely to shrink after castration. Whereas there is uncertainty as to the means by which shrinkage of the prostate is brought about, there is no doubt whatever that in the greater number of the patients operated on there is a considerable diminution in size.

The author then considers the **choice of operation.** A large and succulent prostate gives the best chance of improvement by castration, and if the obstruction is due to close apposition of the lateral lobes, relief after castration may be confidently expected. This is especially true if the bladder is free from bacterial infection. Such cases are not especially favorable for prostatectomy, because they require the removal of large portions of the gland, and such an operation is decidedly serious. If the obstruction is due to a valvular third lobe or to masses which pass into the bladder and encroach on the urethral orifice, castration is not particularly efficient, and this condition is well treated by prostatectomy. Between these two conditions we have every degree of combination of obstruction by pressure and by valve, and these cases constitute debatable ground; but there is one thing which is undoubted, and that is, when the urine is still aseptic we may venture to do an orchotomy, but if the urine contain pus, we should prefer the suprapubic operation. In cases in which there is great dilatation of the bladder after long, chronic retention we know that hemorrhagic cystitis or pyelonephritis may follow an attempt to establish catheter-life. In such a case it seems possible that orchotomy may permit the distended viscus to relieve itself gradually without any danger of infection. Myomatous and fibrous prostates are not especially affected by orchotomy. In considering ligature and division of the vas deferens, Cabot says he has obtained reports of 22 cases, which gave a most unfavorable showing, for 7 of these cases died. Two of these deaths were due to hemiplegia; 1 was a suicide, the man having become maniacal after operation. The other deaths were due to internal conditions, generally of the kidneys. Of the remaining 15, 3 showed no relief; in 5 improvement was marked, but 1 of these afterward relapsed; in 7 there was great improvement. The operation seems to have no advantage over castration in point of mortality, while it is less satisfactory in obtaining relief. The records of unilateral castration are not of positive value. In some cases there was a decided diminution of the corresponding lobe of the prostate, while in others no change could be detected in the gland.

The author's conclusions are as follows: prostatectomy has a slight advantage in the matter of mortality over castration, and later improvements in technic will probably render this advantage more marked. Prostatectomy permits of a thorough examination of the bladder and the discovery and correction of other conditions which we know of or suspect, stones being frequently removed in this way without increasing the gravity of the operation. Prostatectomy confines the patient for a longer period and is occasionally followed by a fistula. It is not yet certain whether any permanent loss of vigor follows castration when performed on old men. The nervous defects which sometimes immediately follow the operation suggest the suspicion that with the loss of the testes the system may lose some tonic effect exerted by these organs. The functional results of the two operations seem nearly equal, and the tendency to relapse is about the same after either. The reduction in size of the prostate is largely due to diminution of congestion, but later a degeneration and absorption of considerable portions of the gland may occur. The glandular elements are especially affected by this atrophy. Castration is particularly efficient in large, tense prostates when the obstruction is due to pressure of the lateral lobes upon the urethra. The special field of prostatectomy is in the relief of obstructive projections which act as urethral valves, but a skilful operator may correct any form of enlargement by prostatectomy. Prostatectomy is applicable to more cases than castration, and is the operation to be selected when an inflamed condition of the bladder makes drainage desirable. [White combats many of the statements of Cabot in the same number of the *Annals of Surg.* in which the paper of the Boston surgeon appears (Sept., 1896), and Cabot analyzes White's statements in the *Annals of Surg.* for Jan., 1897. The real status of the question may be obtained by reading these articles.]

Samuel Alexander [1] writes on the **radical treatment of prostatic enlargement by prostatectomy.** He says that we can choose between three plans of proceeding: 1. Having the patient use a catheter for the rest of his life; 2. Removing the obstruction; 3. Establishing and maintaining an artificial channel. We cannot estimate too highly the usefulness of careful catheterism. A great many people who have even decided prostatic enlargement may live comfortably for many years if a catheter is regularly and properly used; but there are certain patients who are unable to use a catheter or who refuse to use it, and there are other patients to whom the proceeding does not give relief. In such conditions we must choose another method. As soon as it is recognized that palliative treatment is failing in its design we should employ some radical method of procedure. The conditions which call for operation are as follows: Retention of urine due to prostatic growth around the internal orifice of the urethra, or in the prostatic urethra, which makes the patient absolutely dependent upon the catheter. When vesical irritability continues and cannot be entirely relieved by the use of a catheter and bladder-washing; such patients are liable to develop seizures of hematuria and inflammation of the bladder. Again, when in spite of the careful employment of a catheter the amount of residual urine steadily increases and the expulsive force of the bladder steadily diminishes. When the use of a catheter becomes more difficult progressively and when the use of an instrument gives rise to hemorrhage. When the use of a catheter is followed frequently by cystitis. When cystitis continues and cannot be arrested by treatment. When the patient cannot use a catheter or will not use it, or will not take the requisite antiseptic precautions to make the procedure safe. An operation should fulfil three conditions: at once completely remove the obstruction; do but little injury to the mucous membrane; enable us to establish through drainage. The operation which Alexander prefers is an addition to or modification of Nicoll's operation.

Oppler [2] **sterilizes catheters by the use of formalin.** A 2% solution of formalin is placed in an apparatus and the catheters are exposed to the vapor for 6 hours. The catheters lie in a tray above the formalin-solution.

Reginald Harrison [3] reports an interesting case of **extroversion of the**

---

[1] Med. Rec., Dec. 12, 1896. [2] Centralbl. f. Chir., Jan. 9, 1897.
[3] Med. Rec., May 1, 1897.

bladder which he treated successfully by the performance of left nephrectomy and transplantation of the right meter in the loin.

F. Tilden Brown[1] discusses the value of **air-distention of the bladder in suprapubic cystotomy.** Some time since he wrote to a number of surgeons to find their views on the best means of rendering the bladder accessible in the suprapubic operation. He found the views were very diverse : 23 use water rather than air for vesical distention, with or without other aids ; only 3 use air-distention alone of the bladder ; 10 of these surgeons use Petersen's bag ; 12 use the Trendelenburg position, or some modification of it, in addition to other artificial aids ; 4 never use the Trendelenburg position ; 1 uses the Trendelenburg position only. The author thinks that air-distention is of very great value. The bag of Petersen is effective, but it is troublesome and not altogether safe. If air is used, the bag is not required, and we should abandon the use of the bag in favor of air. The use of air was first suggested by Bristow in 1893, and was first put in practice by Keen a month later. Bristow showed that a diseased bladder may be readily ruptured. Water is incompressible ; air is extremely compressible ; hence a diseased bladder is less likely to rupture from air than from water. He further said that, if the bladder could be dilated by anything, it could be best accomplished by the use of air. With the conclusions of Bristow Brown agrees. He quotes Richardson, of Boston, to the effect that by air-distention the prevesical space may be made to reach very high above the pubes. The injection was made by Keen with a Davidson syringe ; but Brown maintains that this syringe will frequently fail when used to pump air. The most useful apparatus to employ is the pocket-bicycle air-pump. This instrument may also be used for making the air-test of a ruptured bladder, as has been alluded to by Keen. Keen's plan in this condition is to insert a catheter and empty the bladder of any urine which is present, and after the urine flows out connect the catheter with a disinfected Davidson syringe over the distal end of which a mass of absorbent cotton is tied. Air is pumped into the bladder, and if there is no rupture we can make out the tympanitic and rounded bladder above the pubes. If there is a rupture, the air will pass into the general peritoneal cavity. In order to distend the bladder with air previous to cystotomy Brown says we should pass a soft-rubber catheter into the bladder and retain it by a bandage. The bladder is washed out, and the Trendelenburg position is not used unless the patient has a pendulous abdomen or it is noticed that light will reach the bladder best when the hips are elevated. The air-apparatus is attached to the catheter and left lying on the towel stretched across the thighs. An incision is made above the pubes until the transversalis fascia is exposed, and the pump is then used to bring the bladder closely against this fascia ; the lumen of the catheter is closed by an artery clamp, the peritoneum, if seen, is lifted upward, and the bladder is opened. Each in-and-out piston-action of this air-pump is about equal to moving 1 oz: of water.

Eugene Fuller[2] writes on **operative interference in aggravated instances of seminal vesiculitis.** He claims that chronic nontuberculous conditions may be treated successfully by extirpating the sac, but that this proceeding should be applied only to extreme cases associated with severe subjective symptoms. Before extirpation is employed stripping should be tried, extirpation being resorted to only when stripping and incision have failed. Kraske's incision is the best method. The sexual functions can be maintained perfectly when but one seminal vesicle is strong and healthy. A sub-

---

[1] Ann. of Surg., Feb., 1897.   [2] Jour. Cutan. and Genito-Urin. Dis., Sept., 1896.

acute epididymitis is to be expected after the performance of the operation, but the corresponding testicle does not atrophy.

Henry Morris[1] advocates the employment of **bimanual examination of the urinary bladder** in diagnosticating vesical hematuria from renal hematuria. He thinks that this procedure is a matter of the very greatest importance. It is useful in the male, and is even more useful in the female. He cites several cases in which he was enabled to make a diagnosis by this method.

D. F. Keegan[2] furnishes some notes upon **stone in the bladder.** He tells us that the majority of vesical calculi we encounter in girls and women should be removed by litholapaxy. There remain two other modes of removing stone from the female bladder—vaginal lithotomy and suprapubic lithotomy, but it is very rarely that either of these operations should be employed. He furnishes a report of 20 cases of stone in females, 18 of which were treated by litholapaxy. He agrees with Mr. Gilbert Barling, that in boys lateral lithotomy and litholapaxy are safer than suprapubic lithotomy. Indian surgeons long ago reached the same conclusions as Mr. Barling. Keegan presents the records of 780 operations performed on boys for vesical stone, and there were only 2 suprapubic lithotomies and 2 median lithotomies in the entire list. The litholapaxies were nearly twice as many as lateral lithotomies. The stay in the hospital was four times as long after lateral lithotomy as after litholapaxy. The death-rate from litholapaxy was less than half that which followed lateral lithotomy. In 509 litholapaxies in boys the percentage of deaths was 2.35. Unquestionably the best operation for a boy 7 or 8 years of age, who has a urethra of normal caliber and suffers from a small and uncomplicated stone, is litholapaxy. A surgeon is not justified in cutting such a boy because he does not have the necessary instruments for litholapaxy, or because he does not know how to use them successfully. The case should be referred to some individual who is able to perform it. In considering the comparative safety of litholapaxy, lateral lithotomy, and suprapubic lithotomy in patients of all ages, the author shows a death-rate of 3.9% for litholapaxy, 11.2% for lateral lithotomy, and 42.17% for suprapubic lithotomy. Suprapubic lithotomy should be very rarely employed. An expert litholapaxist may attack a stone that weighs between 2 and 4 oz. with absolute confidence. If he meet with a stone which cannot be attacked successfully with a No. 16 or 18 lithotrite, lateral lithotomy or perineal lithotrity is preferable to the suprapubic method. It seems certain that in India, in the next decade, peritoneal lithotrity will occupy the place now held by lateral lithotomy in dealing with very large and hard calculi in adult males. Experience proves that suprapubic lithotomy is not more successful than lateral lithotomy in dealing with very large calculi, and perineal lithotrity should be given a fair trial in these extremely difficult cases.

Godfrey Goodman[3] employed the **phonendoscope** attached to a stone-sound in detecting stone in the bladder, after the ordinary method failed to deteet stone. The sound of the contact of the instrument with the stone was very positive.

Reginald Harrison[4] delivered the Bradshaw Lecture for 1896 upon **vesical stone in prostatic disorders.** He considers the various means for relieving prostatic hypertrophy and vesical calculi, agreeing with Dr. Cabot's opinion that castration is especially successful in dealing with large, dense prostates, in which the lateral lobes make pressure upon the urethra, but that the operation is of little value if the prostate is myomatous and fibrous.

[1] Lancet, Oct. 31, 1896.
[2] Ibid., Jan. 9, 1897.
[3] Brit. Med. Jour., Jan. 9, 1897.
[4] Ibid., Dec. 12, 1896.

P. J. Freyer,[1] on the best **methods of removing large calculi from the bladder,** inquires, What are we to regard as a large stone? It is impossible to draw a definite line, but we shall be assisted by considering the advantage of the patient and the operator's experience. A stone of 1½ oz. would be small in an adult but large in a child of 3 or 4 years, as large comparatively as a stone of 3 oz. in an adult. Again, a novice in the operation would regard a stone of ½ oz. as a huge one, whereas an expert would look upon it as a very ordinary affair. We may define a large stone as one weighing 2 oz. and upward. Bigelow's method is undoubtedly the best for calculi of all sizes, provided only that this operation is feasible. Calculi of about 3 oz. in the adult, and of a corresponding weight in the child, should be removed by a perineal lithotomy, and beyond that by suprapubic incision. The author has removed stones of 6 and 8 oz., however, by the Bigelow method, and larger stones have been removed by other operators. The author would lay it down as an absolute rule that in no case in the male or female, adult or child, should a stone, whether small or large, be subjected to a cutting operation until after a trial litholapaxy is found not feasible.

Richard Baker[2] records **200 cases of litholapaxy,** with a mortality-rate of 1%. The largest stone weighed 2 oz. 3 drams 10 gr. There were 195 males and 5 females.

W. S. Forbes[3] reports an interesting **case of litholapaxy,** in which he successfully removed from the bladder of a man 30 years of age a willow twig 7 in. long, heavily encrusted with urinary salts.

DISEASES OF THE KIDNEYS AND THE URETERS.

Maurice Richardson[4] reports 2 cases of **wound of the kidney.** In each of these cases only the liver and kidney were damaged. There was some bleeding into the abdominal cavity from hemorrhage back of the peritoneum. In each case there had been complete perforation of the kidney and some of its secreting structure had been destroyed. In each case it was necessary to make extensive exploration before determining what was to be done. In 1 case the renal vein and the pelvis of the kidney were very badly lacerated. In the other case they were uninjured. In the 1st case nephrectomy was performed and death ensued. In the 2d case drainage was introduced and the patient recovered. It seems that in the case in which nephrectomy was performed death was due to failure of the other kidney to carry on the work of excretion. The surgeon in such a case as this wonders if he might have saved the injured kidney; whether the best proceeding would not have been simply to drain, believing that, even though injured, it might perform a certain amount of excretory function. Of course, the doubt arises whether gangrene would follow with certainty with laceration of the renal vein, although it is possible that the well-recognized anomalies of the kidney-vessels might keep up the organ's vitality. The question whether or not it is better to treat all wounds of the kidney by a conservative plan can only be certainly determined by additional experience.

Albarran[5] reports 66 **operations upon kidneys** with 6 deaths, a mortality of 9%. He performed 7 complete nephrectomies with 1 death, 1 partial nephrectomy which was successful, 24 nephrotomies with 2 deaths, 5 nephrolithotomies with 2 deaths, 1 case of anuria operated on on the 10th day and

[1] Brit. Med. Jour., Nov. 7, 1896.   [2] Lancet, Oct. 10, 1896.
[3] Jour. Am. Med. Assoc., Nov. 28, 1896.   [4] Ann. of Surg., Dec., 1896.
                    [5] Rev. de Chir., Nov. 10, 1896.

followed by death, 23 operations for floating kidney without a death, and 4 exploratory nephrotomies without a death. After a number of these operations very grave reflex phenomena occurred, and they were invariably accompanied by oliguria. The most pronounced symptoms were intractable vomiting and epigastric pain, or pain in the lumbar region. The pupils were contracted, the patient was pallid, the pulse small and very rapid, and the temperature normal. These symptoms rarely last beyond 24 or 36 hours, but in some cases they continue despite the intravenous use of artificial serum. In 1 of the nephrorrhaphy cases the symptoms lasted for 2 days, and in another for 3 days, disappearing in both on the administration of hot alcoholic drinks. [We have witnessed such phenomena upon several occasions.]

E. Hurry Fenwick,[1] writing on the use of the **cystoscope,** maintains that this instrument enables us to lower the mortality of the operation of **nephrectomy.** He cautions us not to examine with the cystoscope any patient who is known to have tuberculosis of the epididymis or prostate or malignant disease of the bladder, but in all other cases the examination should be made, the surgeon being ready to operate at once on completion of the examination. The cystoscope must be used with great care, otherwise it may produce death, causing kidney-trouble secondary to ascending sepsis. Every case of pronounced hematuria should be examined with the cystoscope, a kidney-operation or bladder-operation being carried out if necessary on the termination of the examination. In every case of severe pyelitis unassociated with trouble in the genital or lower urinary tracts the cystoscope will show if both kidneys are present or if one is absent, and will point out the diseased kidney. A better mode of exploration in women is catheterization of the ureters. [The value of the cystoscope is very great if it is used by a trained and skilful man. When used by an untrained man no information of value can be obtained, and great damage may be done. A cystoscope in the hands of an expert is an instrument of surgery; in the hands of a bungler it is a deadly weapon.]

Albarran[2] discusses the **enlargement of the kidney and polyuria** which take place in attacks of **intermittent hydronephrosis.** He thinks that in the early stages of the disease the enlargement is chiefly due to congestion, and not to retention of urine in the pelvis of the kidney. He says that when there is complete retention of urine in the bladder the kidneys increase one-third in volume, and, if this retention is not soon relieved, ecchymoses arise in the parenchyma of the kidneys, and blood-clots may be formed. If the ureter is ligated, the kidney increases greatly in size for the first few hours, and yet very little urine collects in the pelvis. Albarran operated on a patient who suffered from intermittent hydronephrosis, and there was not a sign of dilatation of the pelvis or of the kidney at the operation. In 3 other cases he made the same observation. He has seen 2 cases of intermittent hydronephrosis with movable kidney in which hemorrhage occurred with the attacks of pain, and in which operation showed there was no dilatation whatever resulting from pressure. The polyuria which commonly follows an attack is due to excessive urinary secretion, and not to the flow of urine which has previously been retained in the pelvis of the kidney. Albarran reports a case in which there was extreme polyuria with but very slight increase in the size of the kidney, and in which operation proved that the pelvis of the kidney was not dilated. [This view is radically opposed to accepted teaching, but Albarran's report renders it highly probable that he is right.]

[1] Brit. Med. Jour., Feb. 27, 1897.   [2] Ann. d. Mal. d. Org. gen.-urin., No. 11, Nov., 1896.

Tuffier [1] considers the surgical treatment of **tuberculosis of the kidney.** We now know that primary tuberculosis may occur in the kidney, and that this condition may remain local for a considerable length of time. Operation is only to be performed when medical treatment has failed, and it is employed in the treatment of complications rather than in an attempt to cure the primary tuberculosis. Tuffier has operated on 15 cases. He tells us that the most common indication for operation is infection from renal products which are septic. This infection is manifested by various symptoms. We may have the symptoms of pyelonephritis or of large collections of tuberculous matter without pyuria. The last-named condition is difficult to diagnosticate from tumors of the kidney, liver, or spleen. We are likely to have present hectic fever and emaciation. In cases of this sort Tuffier has operated 9 times. He has performed 5 nephrotomies, with 1 death from operation; 2 secondary nephrectomies after nephrotomy; and 1 complete primary nephrectomy. The operations are too recent to judge of the final result.

J. William White and Alfred C. Wood [2] discuss **surgical affections of the kidneys.** They think the tendency of the profession is to be too conservative in dealing with these conditions, and that a surgeon should by rights have charge of a chronic painful affection of the kidney. One serious obstacle to advancement in this branch of surgery is the trouble in reaching a certain diagnosis. Renal symptoms may follow abscess-formation and spinal caries. A perirenal abscess may be caused by the extension of an appendicular abscess or a subphrenic abscess, and diffuse suppuration about the kidney may be mixed up with hydronephrosis, pyonephrosis, or tumor of the kidney. A smooth stone may be impacted in the parenchyma of the kidney and give rise to no symptoms; but, as a rule, the patient has distinct symptoms—namely, pain in the loin, which is fixed or radiates toward the genital organs or the upper portion of the thigh; irritable bladder; gravel, blood, and pus in the urine; acid urine; and attacks of renal colic. Palpation is only occasionally of use. Morris has pointed out the extreme difficulty of determining the presence of a calculus by direct palpation of the kidney. The use of the Röntgen rays may be of great aid to diagnosis. When there is an abscess of the kidney fever is apt to exist. The most common symptoms of hydronephrosis and pyonephrosis are the dull, heavy, persistent pain in the loin; and after a time the appearance of a distinct tumor, or at least fulness. In pyonephrosis the urine contains pus. Of course, pus may be found in cysts; but when the pus comes from the kidney the urine is usually acid, while in pus from the bladder the urine is usually alkaline and the microscope will probably detect characteristic elements. The writers approve of Tuffier's classification of movable kidneys, namely, into the painful, the dyspeptic, and the neurasthenic. They do not believe that the cause of movable kidney has been certainly made out, but it is probable that several causative influences are at work in the production of this condition; for instance, the absorption of the fatty capsule, pregnancy, pendulous abdomen, the presence of a mesonephron, heredity, etc. The paper then discusses anuria and various operations which are performed upon the kidney. [The surgeon must be very cautious before deciding to perform nephrectomy. A great many patients die some time after this operation because of the failure of the other kidney to undergo compensating hypertrophy. Wagner's dictum that a kidney must not be removed unless the existing disease threatens life, is a good star to steer by. Before doing a nephrectomy the surgeon should ascertain that another kidney exists and that it is competent. The first point can usually be determined by watching the ureteral orifices with a cys-

[1] Brit. Med Jour., Apr. 3, 1897   [2] Ann. of Surg., Jan, 1897.

toscope; the second, by catheterizing the ureters. In some cases partial nephrectomy can be performed instead of complete extirpation. The value of this procedure in some wounds, innocent tumors, imbedded calculi, and localized abscess has been amply demonstrated. The catheterization-test is not absolute, as in horseshoe-kidney there may be two ureters and but one kidney. Exploratory incision is the real, positive test.]

J. Wesley Bovée[1] discusses **uretero-ureteral anastomosis.** The pioneers in this work have been Pawlik, Kelly, Fenger, and Van Hook. The first operation on man was performed by Schopf, in 1886 ; 11 cases have been recorded, and Bovée adds another case in his own experience. There has been much discussion as to the actual length of the ureter, the estimates being from 10 to 16 in. Cabot shows that bands from the fibrous coat of the ureter are connected intimately with the peritoneum, and that in three points the caliber of the ureter is distinctly diminished. Bovée discusses the anatomy of the ureter fully and considers the recorded cases of uretero-ureteral anastomosis. He advocates cutting the ureter obliquely and applying rectangular sutures, alternating with interrupted sutures. He does not use drainage except in pus-cases. He tells us that, next to ureteral anastomosis, bladder-graft is decidedly the best alternative. It has been performed by Penrose, Kelly, and others. Van Hook has suggested sewing a part of the bladder-wall into the form of a canal when it is necessary to meet a short portion of the ureter. Most of the operations have been done within the peritoneal cavity. The only extraperitoneal operation was done by Baumann. Van Hook believes that rectal implantation is very dangerous, and should only be performed when the bladder has become badly diseased. When it is done the vesical opening of the ureter must be removed in order to preserve the natural valve. Nichaus in one case successfully implanted the ureter in the urethra. The author concludes that the operation of uretero-ureteral anastomosis when possible is preferable to any other form of ureteral grafting, to nephrectomy, and to ligation of the ureter. It should be performed either by lateral implantation or oblique end-to-end anastomosis, although we can with safety use the transverse end-to-end or the end-in-end method. He maintains that constriction of the caliber does not usually follow suturing of complete transverse section. Nephrectomy for transverse injury of the ureter alone is an unjustifiable procedure. Simple ligation of the ureter to produce cessation of kidney function is too uncertain to justify its performance. Drainage is not required if the wound is perfectly closed and the tissues are aseptic.

Arpad G. Gerster[2] furnishes a contribution to the **surgery of the kidney and the ureter.** He reports a case of hydronephrosis of traumatic origin in which nephrotomy was performed, the nephrotomy being followed by a plastic operation on the proximal orifice of the ureter. The patient was cured. He reports a successful case of nephrectomy for a hydronephrotic floating kidney ; a case in which closure of the ureter followed nephrectomy, and cure succeeded on extirpation of the ureter; and a case of double pyelitis with intense cystitis, in which nephrectomy of the left side caused temporary improvement. He also records a case of hydatid of the right kidney which was cured by exposure of the tumor, incision, and evacuation. He makes a plea for earlier operations in acute inflammations of the kidney, and gives the history of a case to prove his point. He records cases to illustrate the rapidity with which the kidney may become involved in septic processes. He also discusses tumor of the kidney and some other interesting conditions. He arrives at the following conclusions: that early nephrotomy should be per-

---

[1] Ann. of Surg., Jan., 1897. [2] Am. Jour. Med. Sci., June, 1897.

formed in suppurative processes and infection of the kidney and in acute, non-suppurative forms of nephritis. He reports two cases of tumor in which extirpation was followed by cure.

Jordan Lloyd [1] considers the **impaction of stone in the ureter.** He says that when the ureter is partially obstructed with stone the urine secreted is of low specific gravity, poor in urea, and does not contain albumin. The symptoms vary according to the point at which impaction has occurred. Impaction close to the bladder produces symptoms simulating the classical symptoms of stone in the bladder. Impaction higher up simulates renal stone. There is usually hematuria, and pus as a rule is found. A sharp, stabbing-pain can usually be elicited by forcibly prodding the loin. If the symptoms point to kidney stone, but prodding the loin causes no pain, the probability is that the stone is in the ureter. Exercise increases the pain of renal stone, but does not increase the pain of ureteral stone. He reports three cases of ureteral stone.

Christian Fenger [2] writes upon **operation for valvular stricture of the ureter.** Pelviotomy was performed and four stones removed from the ureter above a valvular stricture, and this stricture was treated by longitudinal ureterotomy over the stricture, excision of the stricture, and a plastic operation on the ureter. The wound in the pelvis was left open after a bougie had been passed into the ureter. The wound healed in six weeks and the patient made a complete recovery. In this case Fenger made the incision between the 12th rib and the rim of the pelvis forward for about 9 in. from the border of the erector spinæ muscle, and after isolation of the pelvis, which he found somewhat dilated, he laid bare the ureter and felt a nodular mass 2 in. below the pelvis. When he incised the pelvis longitudinally about one ounce of urine escaped. On passing the little finger down the ureter for about an inch he could not feel a stone, but on manipulating the ureter with the other hand he succeeded in squeezing four stones up into the pelvis and removed them from the wound. When the sound was passed down from the pelvis into the ureter it was arrested $2\frac{1}{4}$ in. below the pelvis at a point where palpation detected thickening. A longitudinal incision $\frac{3}{8}$ in. long was made into the ureter upon the end of the sound, above, through, and below a transverse valvular stricture. An instrument passed through an opening below the stricture easily entered the bladder. The longitudinal wound was held open, and this part of the urethra was stretched over the index finger while the valvular stricture was cut off from within by scissors, the muscular coat of the ureter being left intact. A plastic operation was now performed on the ureter after the method which Fenger proposed in 1894.

Willy Meyer [3] writes on **catheterism of the ureters** in the male with the help of the ureter cystoscope, and makes a report of 7 cases. He shows that Kelly's method is not suitable to men, because of the limits of dilatability of the urethra and the presence of the prostate gland. He uses Casper's instrument, but the urethra must be sufficiently large to permit the passage of the instruments, the bladder must have a capacity of at least 4 or 5 ounces, and the fluid within the bladder must be kept transparent. He reports 7 cases in which he successfully catheterized the ureter. The bladder should first be washed and cocainized, and should be filled with clear fluid before the instrument is introduced.

Hugo Maas [4] writes on **suppuration of the fatty capsule of the kidney,** a tissue very prone to suppuration because of its vascularity. Pus formed in such a deep-seated situation reaches the surface very slowly, and a large

[1] Brit. Med. Jour., Oct. 24, 1896.   [2] Am. Jour. Med. Sci., Dec., 1896.
[3] Med. Rec., May 1, 1897.   [4] Ann. of Surg., May, 1897.

retroperitoneal abscess forms which endangers important organs because of their proximity. No one causative factor of this suppuration has been elicited. In some cases it follows pyelonephritis, calculous pyelitis, or gonorrheal suppuration in the pelvic fascia, metastasis from carbuncles, from empyema and other foci of suppuration. Israel, it will be remembered, reported a case in which carbuncle was associated with a perinephric abscess. Twenty-two cases of perinephric abscess are reported, with 5 deaths. [These abscesses are often due to traumatism, a very slight bruise, or wrench or twist leading to a trivial hemorrhage and so establishing a point of least resistance. Violent coughing may also be causative. Niebergall [1] has insisted on the causative influence of slight traumatisms in producing these suppurations, and mentions the following : taking a false step, riding in a jolting wagon, riding horseback, digging, stamping violently with the feet, carrying a heavy load, or lifting a great weight.]

Oscar Bloch [2] records a case in which half the **kidney invaded by a morbid growth** was removed. He says that when we have come to the conclusion that an operation is necessary in a kidney-case the question always arises as to the existence or condition of the other kidney. Surgeons have endeavored to clear up this doubt in many ways. Under these circumstances we naturally ask if it be not our duty to save as much as may be of the kidney-structure ; in other words, to perform partial excision instead of total extirpation of the entire organ. If this operation is possible, it is very much better, as when we leave a man with a single kidney he will fare very badly if this becomes the seat of disease. There are but very few cases in literature in which a partial removal has been performed. This is chiefly due to the apprehension of hemorrhage during the operation and partly to the fear that the kidney-wound would not heal, but would leave a fistula as a legacy. Experiments on animals have shown that these fears are unfounded. Bleeding can be controlled and the kidney-wound may heal—in fact, may heal with great rapidity. A case is reported by Bloch of a patient who suffered from pain and hematuria. An incision was made and the growth was found in the kidney. The tumor was in the lower third of the kidney. The portion of the kidney containing the tumor was excised, only one artery bleeding, which was easily seized. The incision, which was transverse, began at the lower part of the pelvis and ended at the convex part of the kidney. A piece the size of half a normal kidney remained. Two bleeding arteries in the hilus were ligated. The surfaces of the wounds in the lower part of the kidney were brought together with 3 sutures of catgut, each suture grasping the wound on the convex part of the kidney and including distinct bridges of tissue ; the bleeding was slight. Only 3 sutures were applied to the convex part of the kidney, for fear of stasis of blood between the surfaces of the wound ; yet gaps were nowhere to be seen between the sutures. The portion of the kidney left was 7 cm. long and 5 to 6 cm. broad. The cavity in which the kidney rested was dried with gauze ; the pedicle was carefully palpated and found to be sound. The interior of the capsule was cleaned and sutured with catgut sutures, so that it covered the stump ; but room was left to permit of free drainage. The stump of the kidney was replaced quite under the diaphragm. The vertical portion of the wound was closed with 3 deep sutures. Five ligatures were applied to the arteries in the muscle-wound and a drainage-tube and a bit of iodoform-gauze were inserted. The muscle-wound was closed with 11 catgut sutures. This patient completely recovered, and 9 months after operation he was perfectly well, and there was no blood in the urine. Examination of the tumor showed that it was an adenoma

---

[1] Deutsch. med. Zeit., Aug., 1896. [2] Brit. Med. Jour., Oct. 17, 1896.

28

undergoing degenerative changes from bleeding in the tissues. At the site of amputation the kidney-tissue was proved by the microscope to be normal. The author then discusses reported cases in which partial nephrectomy has been performed

W. F. Brook [1] reports 2 cases of **nephrolithotomy** to illustrate the value of heavy percussion in the loin in the diagnosis of renal calculus. In one of these cases deep pressure over the kidney caused pain, and heavy percussion below the tip of the last rib caused acute pain in the loin. In the second case the kidney on palpation was not tender, but heavy percussion over the kidney in the back caused stabbing-pain in the loin. The author calls attention to the similarity of the symptoms in both cases. In one case the most acute pain was at McBurney's point; in the other case at a corresponding spot on the left side. In both the classical symptoms of renal calculus were absent. Neither blood nor pus was found. In the absence of the acute, stabbing-pain on percussion in the loin it would have been impossible to diagnosticate the stone in either case. Jordan Lloyd first drew attention to this symptom.

Reginald Harrison,[2] in an address before the Medical Society of London, considered the **treatment of some forms of albuminuria by renipuncture.** Early in the present year Mr. Harrison narrated 3 cases in which albuminuria completely disappeared after digital exploration and puncture or splitting of the kidney-capsule. The operations were undertaken for another purpose, but the result in each case was good. The first case was scarlatinal nephritis, the second was nephritis from exposure, and the third was nephritis from grippe. Newman, of Glasgow, has reported 2 cases of albuminuria which ceased after the performance of nephrorrhaphy, and Hoeber, of Homburg, reports a case in which albuminuria disappeared after an incision. Harrison believes that in these cases the albumin disappeared as the result of the operation. In one class of cases the tension was due to inflammatory hyperemia and in the other to mechanical obstruction of the vessels. Analogues may be found in other portions of the body. Iridectomy is performed in glaucoma; puncture or limited incision may be of great benefit in acute orchitis, relieving tension and preventing damage to secreting structure. The kidney is capable of gradual distention, but cannot distend from sudden force. We might infer that, as the kidney is normally a double organ, both glands must be submitted to the operation, inasmuch as in ordinary nephritis both kidneys are similarly involved. This does not, however, of necessity follow. Strong sympathies exist between two glands, and impressions upon one gland may be reflected to the other, and relief afforded to one kidney usually assists the other. When the excretory power of one side is lessened or arrested the other organ takes up the whole of the work. This operation may be employed in scarlatinal nephritis, in which the albumin does not disappear from the urine rapidly and completely. There are 2 groups of these cases: in the first the kidney-trouble is grave from the very start; in the second group the symptoms do not tend toward recovery even after a considerable time. In these cases the kidney should be exposed by a moderate incision in the loin. The operator should feel the organ both in front and behind, aided by pressure exercised by the hand of an assistant over the front of the abdomen. If, with albumin in the urine, the kidney is found in a state of tension, 3 or 4 punctures may be made through the capsule in various directions, and if the organ is in a high state of tension a limited incision should be made in the cortex. The wound should be packed with gauze or a drainage-tube should be inserted. The fact that tension exists in the kidney can readily be made out when an ex-

---

[1] Brit. Med. Jour., Dec. 19, 1896.   [2] Ibid., Oct. 17, 1896.

amination is made. In some instances it will be so marked that the organ will resemble a bursting plum. [In the case reported by Keen and Stewart the capsule of the kidney was incised and a portion of the organ was removed for microscopic examination.[1]]

Willy Meyer[2] writes on **early diagnosis and early nephrectomy for tuberculosis of the kidney.** He is a profound believer in the value of a cystoscopic examination of the bladder and catheterization of the ureters. He reports a case in which there was a tuberculous kidney, the process passing down the ureter to the bladder, an injected area on the bladder-surface near the mouth of the ureter being seen. An operation showed the kidney to be tuberculous. Tubercle-bacilli were found in the urine in these cases. He tells us that a recent appearance of frequent micturition in a hitherto healthy individual who has not been infected with gonorrhea is very suggestive of tuberculous kidney, especially if this is associated with permanent, or more particularly intermittent, voiding of turbid urine with or without blood. If, in a case with such symptoms, the cystoscopic examination shows a healthy bladder with one ureteral opening clearly inflamed or swollen, we are certainly dealing with primary tuberculosis of the kidney to which the inflamed ureter belongs.

F. Tilden Brown[3] has made an elaborate study of **renal tuberculosis.** He takes up for consideration the methods of infection, the pathology, the symptomatology, and diagnosis. He tells us that the early symptoms will depend somewhat upon the mode of infection—whether it was arterial or ureteral. Invasion by the vessels may be nearly or quite without symptoms until the disease has advanced to a considerable degree. A careful urinary analysis always permits of a comparatively early diagnosis. The following is a summary of the different symptoms and signs of the disease: the existence of a tumor which corresponds to the position of a kidney; this tumor may or may not be painful on palpation. It may be the seat of spontaneous pain which is often intermittent, or it may be a center from which pains radiate to different portions of the abdomen, spine, groin, outer side of the thigh, or the opposite and healthy kidney. It is well to remember, however, that there may be no obvious enlargement of the kidney. The other symptoms to be mentioned are pallor and emaciation, edema of the lower extremities, reaction after the injection of tuberculin, albuminuria, moderate fever, night-sweats, dysuria, pyuria, hematuria with acid urine, turbid urine seen by the cystoscope emerging from the ureter, and the finding of tubercle-bacilli in that urine which we know to come from one or the other kidney as obtained by ureteral catheterism. Emaciation is of little importance, because it is such a common symptom of disease, and many patients do not show emaciation for a considerable time; the same remarks apply to pallor and cachexia. Edema of the extremities results simply from impairment in the quality and alteration of the quantity of the blood. The existence of albuminuria in tuberculous kidney has been a matter of great dispute. The reason of this divergence of view can be readily explained. When the tuberculous lesion is in free communication with the urinary tract serum, leukocytes, and blood-corpuscles mix with the urine in greater or less quantity, and in such a condition boiling and the acid-test show the presence of so-called albumin. In this sense slight albuminuria is a not infrequent symptom of renal tuberculosis. But when the tuberculous focus is still enclosed in the parenchyma these products are not mixed with the urine, and the uriniferous tubules and glomeruli which are undisturbed are functionating normally, and albuminuria is very rare. If albuminuria does appear, it

---

[1] Lancet, Sept. 24, 1897.   [2] Med. News, May 1, 1897.
[3] N. Y. Med. Jour., Mar. 20, 1897.

will be associated with the presence of casts and tuberculous epithelium. Such a condition arises from nephritis due to overaction of the excreting channels brought about by the irritating waste-products of the system at large. Undoubtedly in many cases of renal tuberculosis there is no albumin in the urine, but we can only definitely settle this question when able certainly to distinguish between globulins and true albumins.

The reaction to tuberculin is a very uncertain diagnostic test; at least it is uncertain in human beings. Escherich's report shows that its importance in diagnosis is limited. If, however, we have a patient with a slightly enlarged or tender kidney, with a moderate evening pyrexia and slight polyuria, and if tuberculin in such a case produces a distinct reaction, we should suspect the existence of renal tuberculosis, order the patient a change of climate, and institute restorative treatment. Dysuria cannot be called a symptom of kidney disease unless associated with tuberculous lesions of the lower portion of the urinary tract. In most of the victims of tuberculous kidney there is discomfort arising from frequency of urination rather than from real pain. Enlargement of the kidney is a noticeable symptom in the well-advanced cases of both varieties of the disease. In the ascending variety intermittent hydronephrosis may occur. An enlarged kidney is usually uncomfortable or painful on palpation, and is commonly the seat of attacks of local and radiating pain. In nearly all cases of tuberculosis of the kidney there is a slight afternoon or evening pyrexia, possibly not more than 0.5°. This symptom would tend to exclude calculus, and a septic kidney would be associated with a far greater rise of temperature. In the later stages of tuberculosis of the kidney the afternoon temperature will be frequently as high as 103°, and night-sweats will probably occur. In the early stages of the disease the pulse is not particularly involved, but later in the case it becomes rapid and weak. Polyuria is one of the earliest symptoms which attend the formation of a tuberculous area in the kidney. Pyuria and hematuria ocenr only when the tuberculous focus is in communication with the urinary tract. Pyuria of tuberculous kidney is an acid urine, and when pyuria exists there is nearly always hematuria. The blood may be present in small amounts or in very large amounts, and the bleeding may take place at long intervals—months, it may be even years. Frequency of micturition is the symptom most apparent to the patient, and it is the symptom for which he usually comes to seek relief. If this polyuria is marked at night as well as in the day, the suspicion of the existence of tubercle is increased. At periods during the progress of the disease the frequency of micturition is for a time abated. When the cystoscope shows turbid urine emerging from the ureter which belongs to an enlarged and tender kidney, and when this urine is withdrawn from the bladder by a sterile catheter, or, better still, when it is brought into a centrifugating tube by means of Casper's or Nitze's instrument, and it is found to contain bacilli, or if it is found that injection of this urine into a guinea-pig produces tubercles, the diagnosis is certain. If there are lesions of the bladder, of course the diagnosis is somewhat obscure. The microorganisms which most resemble the bacillus of tubercle are the lepra-bacillus and the smegma-bacillus. All grades of this disease may be classified for the purpose of preliminary treatment under two heads. The rich must be sent to another climate, pay scrupulous attention to hygiene and alimentation, and take invigorating drugs. An attempt may be made in the poor to approximate the treatment outlined for the rich, and if it is possible for the poor man to go away and live in another climate, he should do so. Theoretically it would seem that the treatment of these early cases should be a radical surgical operation, but practically it has been shown that the impairment of the strength which temporarily follows upon nephrectomy does the individual great harm when there is an early tuberculous lesion. It is very probable that there is another lesion in the body somewhere besides the one in the kidney ; even if this lesion is not active, any impairment of the individual's health and strength may cause its rapid progress and dissemination. If this small tubercular focus in the kidney is found at an early period, and the individual is in an excellent state of health, a nephrectomy would probably be the best thing for the patient ; but because a number of these early cases can be cured by other than surgical measures it is thought right to employ them before advising operation. In some cases it occasionally happens that this form of treatment must be delayed until some urgent condition has been relieved surgically. For instance, the sudden appearance of marked pyuria, with fever, in a patient with enlarged and tender kidney, or the sudden onset of severe hematuria with moderate fever, calls for operation. When these symptoms are present in the early stage of the disease nephrectomy is indicated unless there is a tuberculous focus in the other kidney. Nephrectomy should also be performed when the individual has had every advantage of climate and medical treatment and yet the tuberculous focus is advancing. The evidences of this advance are loss of appetite and strength, diminution in weight, increase in the pyuria, the pain, the fever, and the size of the kidney. We would not entertain the idea of radical surgical cure when in addition to an undoubted area of tuberculosis in the kidney the lower urinary tract is positively involved, when it is probable that the other kidney is affected, when in the male the prostate, seminal vesicles, or testes are attacked, and in the female the bladder, peritoneum, Fallopian tubes, or ovaries ; but even in these cases, when the chief trouble is certainly in one kidney and the ureter is unable to afford adequate drainage, operation may be performed as a tentative rather than as a curative measure. It is in this sort of case that surgeons were formerly in the habit of recommending nephrotomy, but Brown believes that nephrectomy is preferable. If in the advanced cases serious renal hemorrhage occurs, nephrectomy is the only proper treatment. The figures of Continental surgeons show a mortality from nephrotomy of 13 %, and from nephrectomy of 30 %. In some statistics Brown has collected in New York, out of 28 nephrectomies there were 2 deaths, a mortality of 7.1 %. These nephrectomies were not all done for tuberculosis, but the operative mortality of nephrectomy performed for tuberculosis is certainly as low as the mortality for nephrectomy performed for any condition requiring operation. The author then discusses the methods of performing nephrectomy.

Bayard Holmes [1] writes on **tuberculosis of the kidney** and records some interesting cases ; his conclusions are as follows : tuberculosis of the kidneys is rather a common disease ; it usually begins in the kidney, passes down the ureter to the bladder, and ascends to the other kidney, and is for a long time a unilateral trouble. It is progressive, and destruction cannot be arrested by medication, and offers a very unfavorable prognosis. Diagnosis is made by the symptoms of cystitis, with the low temperature and rapid pulse and dilated heart, tubercle-bacilli in the urine, tuberculosis of the bladder about the ureteral orifice of the diseased kidney, pyuria or hematuria, with diminution of the normal constituents of the urine from the diseased kidney, normal urine in increased amount from the sound kidney, sometimes pain, tenderness, and enlargement in the situation of the diseased kidney. When one kidney is healthy and the other diseased the indications are absolute for removal of the tuberculous organ together with its ureter ; but if both kidneys

[1] Jour. Am. Med. Assoc., Sept. 5, 1896.

are diseased, no operation should be undertaken. The fact that the other kidney is competent can be proved by repeated catheterization of the ureters before nephrectomy. For some days before the removal of the kidney toxic elements should be eliminated from the blood by the use of a liquid diet, irrigation of the colon, and hydration of the system. The safer operation is extraperitoneal lumbar nephrectomy. In women the ureter should be completely removed through the vagina. Any remaining tuberculosis of the bladder should be treated locally by curetting or excision. Catheterization of the ureter is not dangerous, and can easily be carried out in women by Simon's cystoscope or the cystoscope of Pawlik or Kelly; in men we may use the instrument of Casper.

WOUNDS, BURNS, ULCERS, SHOCK, ETC.

William Turner[1] presents some remarks on **wounds of the heart** and furnishes the notes of a case in which death took place $4\frac{1}{2}$ months subsequent to a heart-wound, cicatrization being shown by the postmortem examination. He tells us that there is a firm belief in the popular mind that the heart is the most vital structure of an animal, and that in order to destroy an animal with the utmost certainty the effort should be made to injure the heart. Hunters act on this idea. The rules of the army direct that when a person is to be executed the firing-party must point their weapons at the heart of the culprit, with the idea that suffering will thus be minimized. It has been supposed that if the substance of the heart be even touched by a foreign body the action of that organ must necessarily cease immediately. The experience of most surgeons, however, positively disproves these notions. Turner saw a child of 2 years with a sewing-needle driven into the heart. The needle had disappeared in the chest, but its head could be felt beneath the skin knocking against the finger with each heart-beat. The needle was cut down upon and extracted, and no harm apparently resulted to the heart or the child. Some years ago the dead body of a man was discovered by the police. There was a series of some 10 or 12 wounds over the region of the heart. A large butcher-knife was buried in one of these wounds, and the right hand, covered with blood, grasped the handle of the knife. There could not be the possibility of a doubt that these wounds were self-inflicted. At the postmortem it was found that three of the wounds had penetrated the cavity of the heart and caused laceration of the heart-walls. It followed, therefore, that after the heart had been at least twice penetrated by a large butcher-knife and very greatly damaged, the individual had retained sufficient physical strength and mental determination to inflict a third wound on the same organ. Most of the records point to the fact that wounds of the heart are seldom, if ever, immediately fatal. Out of 29 collected cases only 2 were fatal within 48 hours. A stag ran 60 yards after being shot through the heart. An examination showed that the left auricle had been practically destroyed and that the left ventricle had been completely torn through. There is a thoroughly authenticated case in which a bullet was found imbedded in the substance of a soldier's heart six years after he had been wounded, he having died from another cause.

Turner then cites some interesting examples of penetrating wounds of the heart which were not immediately fatal. In his own case, which he then proceeds to describe, there was a cicatrized wound over the intraventricular septum. The patient was a Maltese, who was admitted to the hospital collapsed and bleeding from a wound in the left side of the chest over the heart. He had been stabbed in a quarrel. There was a considerable amount of arterial blood

[1] Brit. Med. Jour., Nov. 14, 1896.

issuing from the wound synchronous with cardiac systole, and air was also passing out with hissing noises on each movement of respiration. The heart's sounds were muffled and the pulse at the wrist was scarcely to be detected. The patient seemed to be on the verge of death, but he gradually improved. A month after the injury the discharge was purulent and abundant, and the pleural sac was converted into a large suppurating cavity; the 5th rib was resected posteriorly to permit of drainage. 4½ months after the injury the patient was allowed to sit up, but one morning he had a convulsion and died. The postmortem showed that he died of an apoplectic clot. Examination showed that there was a cicatrix in the pericardium corresponding to the external wound, and immediately subjacent to this was discovered a cicatrix on the anterior surface of the heart itself. This second cicatrix was ¾ in. in extent, and was placed over the intraventricular septum about 1½ in. from the apex. It was found on section to have penetrated ⅝ in. into the muscular substance of the heart, the left coronary artery and vein having been divided. It seemed certain that after infliction of the wound the' pericardium must have filled up with blood, and yet cardiac action was not thereby arrested. [The subject of wounds of the heart is discussed in the section upon the Vascular System, p. 369.]

Charles H. Lemon [1] writes on **gunshot-wounds of the kidney,** and reports 2 cases. These lesions are not common, because the kidneys are deeply placed. Years ago Larrey and Dupuytren recognized the necessity of providing free drainage in kidney-wounds, but during the War of the Rebellion surgeons neglected this advice. The *Surgical History of the War of the Rebellion* contains the reports of 78 cases of gunshot-wounds of the kidneys, and but 26 of these recovered. Every one was treated upon the expectant plan, and no incisions were made for exploration. Accumulated experience has shown that in penetrating wounds of the kidney adjacent viscera are often wounded, but that, unlike incised wounds, there is rarely infiltration of the retroperitoneal tissues. The author commends to the attention of those who are interested in this subject the paper read by Prof. Keen before the American Surgical Association this year. Among those tabulated are all cases of traumatism of the kidney reported since 1878. In this last are 19 cases of gunshot-wound of the kidney. Of these 19 cases 10 recovered. Lemon relates 2 cases which happened in his practice, both of which recovered. In the first case he made an exploratory lumbar incision exposing the left kidney along the track of the bullet. The perinephric tissue was found to contain clotted blood and urine, and the wound was discovered on the inner convex border of the kidney. When a probe was introduced it was demonstrable that the ball had not lodged in the kidney. The direction of the bullet was such that it was evident that the pelvis of the kidney had not been penetrated anteriorly. No further exploration was made. In order to arrest hemorrhage the tear was plugged with iodoform-gauze. The deep structures of the back were sutured with catgut and a gauze drain inserted along the track of the bullet. In the second case an exploratory incision was also made. The incision was made in the right loin parallel to the last rib, to expose the kidney. The kidney was thoroughly exposed, and a wound found in it which easily admitted the index-finger on the posterior surface about its center an inch external to the pelvis. There was little or no extravasation of urine and no clotted blood in the perinephric tissue. The wound was closed after a strip of gauze had been packed into the opening on the posterior surface of the kidney. The author quotes approvingly the words of Prof. Keen : " If the surgeon has reasonable evidence that the

[1] Jour. Am. Med. Assoc., Jan. 9, 1897.

kidney has been probably traversed by a ball (and all the more so if it is certain that it has been so wounded) and the patient is evidently in grave danger, as shown by the general symptoms of internal hemorrhage and by the physical signs of a large lumbar hematoma, or of intraperitoneal bleeding, I take it for granted that all of us would recommend an exploratory operation with a view of determining the extent of the injury to the kidney and the proper treatment."

Assistant Surgeon A. Wells[1] reports 2 cases of **snakebite** treated successfully by the use of **potassium permanganate and strychnin.** In the first case the remedies were administered by means of the stomach; in the second he enlarged the punctures made by the fangs of the snake's teeth and introduced the permanganate crystals, injected strychnin in the arm, and gave the permanganate internally in solution in doses of 5 gr.; both patients were cured.

H. P. Keatinge[2] reports a case of **snakebite treated by antivenene serum.** A child was bitten on the forearm by an Egyptian cobra; she almost instantly became unconscious. The village barber made several small incisions on the arm and forearm. When brought to the hospital she was cold and collapsed, pulseless, with rambling delirium. It was found that the forearm had been coated with Nile mud, which is a favorite native remedy; 3 in. below the bend of the elbow 2 distinct holes were seen passing through the skin and corresponding to the fangs of the serpent. It was noted that the pupillary reflexes were absent; the pupils were moderately dilated. The child became comatose. Twenty c.c. of antivenene serum were injected under the abdominal skin. In 4 hours her condition was distinctly improved. Ten c.c. of the antivenene serum were again injected. She then slept during the night and the next morning was notably better. The serum used was **Calmette's antivenene serum.** Another case of recovery is reported by Surgeon-major S. J. Rennie.[3] L. S. Alexander[4] reports a case of rattlesnake-bite treated by **rattlesnake-bile.** An incision was made in the bitten area and the bile was poured into the wound. No other treatment was employed except the administration internally of ammonium carbonate. There was not a particle of swelling and the man suffered no inconvenience of any description. Surgeon-captain C. W. R. Healey[5] reports a case of snakebite which was treated as follows: the wounds were enlarged, a strong solution of potassium permanganate was applied, a ligature was tied at the base of the injured finger, the hand was placed in hot water, and bleeding was encouraged by pressure from above downward. The man was given aromatic spirits of ammonia, which he vomited, and after that he was given some brandy, which he retained. The patient was subsequently placed in bed and given strychnin hypodermically. In spite of this treatment he died. Ram Dhari Sinha[6] reports a case of snakebite treated successfully with **liquor ammonia.**

Ottinger[7] maintains that **venomous insect-stings** should be treated by the application of **pure ichthyol,** or a mixture of equal parts of ichthyol and lanolin. This remedy mitigates the pain and greatly lessens the inflammatory reaction. If, when the surgeon first calls, swelling already exists, ichthyol is applied, sheet India-rubber is laid over this, and an ice-bag placed on the India-rubber tissue. Ottinger advises the administration internally in such a case of 10-drop doses of a mixture of equal parts of ichthyol and spirit of ether. V. Dinshaw[8] reports the case of a boy who was stung by a scor-

[1] Indian Med. Rec., Apr. 1, 1897.
[3] Ibid., Nov. 21, 1896.
[5] Indian Med. Rec., Jan. 26, 1897.
[7] N. Am. Pract., Feb., 1897.

[2] Brit. Med. Jour., Jan. 2, 1897.
[4] Med. Rec., Sept. 5, 1896.
[6] Ibid., Nov. 1, 1896.
[8] Indian Med. Rec., Jan. 1, 1897.

pion. His relatives administered musk, which produced no improvement. The surgeon ordered arrack, which is a strong spirit, giving half an ounce with an equal quantity of water. Two doses were given within 5 minutes. Next, 10℔ of aromatic spirits of ammonia in an ounce of water were given. Three doses of this were administered, when the patient began to improve. In this case the symptoms were extremely grave, but the patient made a complete recovery. Patients who are stung by scorpions develop all the signs of collapse.

E. M. Foote[1] writes on the effect of **formalin-gelatin in suppurating wounds.** He has made a number of clinical experiments in the use of this agent, and concludes that the formalin possesses a distinct antiseptic action.

SKIAGRAPHY.

[During the year there have been many interesting cases reported of the use of the Röntgen rays, and surgeons have come to a more accurate conclusion as to the value of this new process, the relative value of the fluorescent screen and the skiagraph, of the methods of locating the exact situation of a foreign body by the process, and of the destructive effects and erroneous conclusions which may occasionally follow upon its use.]

J. E. Stubbard[2] has compared 73 cases of pulmonary tuberculosis, examined by **the Röntgen rays,** with 15 normal individuals. His conclusions are as follows: 1. Slight haziness indicates the beginning of tuberculous infiltration, which may or may not be accompanied by dulness on percussion. 2. Decided shadows indicate consolidation, the extent of which is in direct relation to the comparative density of the shadow thrown on the fluoroscope. 3. Circumscribed bright spots surrounded by narrow rings of dark shadow or located in the midst of dark areas indicate cavities. 4. Intense darkness, especially at the lower portion of the lung, indicates old pleuritic thickenings over consolidated lung-tissue.

Surgeon-major Whitehead[3] has published a skiagraph of a **case of fractured femur.** This picture appeared to be a recent fracture of the lower end of the femur, in which there were considerable deformity and overriding of the lower end of the upper fragment, whereas in reality the picture was of a fracture close above the knee-joint which occurred six months ago. The lower end of the upper fragment was jagged and irregular, as if Nature had made an attempt to round it off, and no projection of bone could be felt at the seat of fracture. There was half an inch of shortening and the man walked without pain or trouble. From a surgical point of view the result is as good as could have been expected. It is not probable that the bone is really as sharp as it appears to be in the skiagraph. It is probable that the x-rays traversed the more recent callous material, which really does round off the end, without throwing a shadow on the plate.

Edmund Gwen, in speaking of a similar case of his own, suggests a misuse to which skiagraphy may be put in the future. He inquires what a British jury may think when a skiagraph of a case is being explained by a sharp advocate of a claimant for damages for malpraxis. In Mr. Owen's ease the x-rays showed a deformity which really did not matter, as the result is as good as the surgeon could achieve, and the author remarks that imaginative patients may consider themselves badly treated if they have their broken bones skiagraphed.]

Herbert B. Perry[4] has reported an interesting case in which he was able to

---

[1] Med. News, Nov. 14, 1896.   [2] Med. Rec., May 22, 1897.
[3] Lancet, Mar. 20, 1897.   [4] Med. News, Mar. 20, 1897.

demonstrate by the x-rays the presence of the point of a pair of **scissors in the knee-joint.** He performed an operation and removed the foreign body. He located the foreign body in the joint first by the use of a fluorescent screen. In order to have some landmarks to work by in performing the operation he took a long, flat key, smeared the point with ink, and passed it between the light and the knee and the knee and the screen until it was seen to touch the skin at the location of the foreign body. In this manner the distal and proximal ends of the scissors-point were noticed on the external and internal surfaces of the knee. The mark was afterward made indelible with nitrat of silver.

Leonard Freeman[1] publishes several **interesting skiagraphs.** He records one case in which a diagnosis was made of epiphyseal separation of the wrist. After 14 weeks two skiagraphs were taken, when it was seen that the anterior half of the right epiphyseal line was obscured by a shadow representing a growth of new bone, the border of the epiphysis being tilted downward from the shaft. The bone, therefore, was in an apparently incorrect position, yet the final result was good. He also publishes a picture of a fracture of both bones of the forearm, another through the lower extremities, and a fracture of the styloid processes of the radius and ulna.

F. J. Clendinnen[2] publishes **skiagraphs of the blood-vessels** of the ankle and knee-joint. In order to obtain these he injects the arteries with a solution of red lead. The bone offers less resistance to the rays than the injected vessels, and the arteries can be seen back of the bone as well as in front of it. This method promises to be useful in the study of anatomy and pathology.

Eugene R. Corson[3] records 4 cases, with skiagraphs, of injuries which had been diagnosticated as **Colles's fracture.** He shows that there had been no fracture of the radius, the great deformity being due to arrachement of the ligaments from excessive flexion of the wrist. It is very important to treat this sprain. If there is simply a fracture of the radius without a tear of the ligaments, almost any treatment is successful; but, as shown by Hamilton, a severe·sprain will be followed by marked deformity, and it is in the latter cases that suits for malpractice are apt to be brought.

Schier[4] makes a report upon the value of the Röntgen rays in detecting **bullets in the head.** In a patient who was shot five years previously in the right brow the symptoms indicated that the bullet might be lodged in the ethmoid bone. The skiagraph taken from different directions showed that the bullet was located near the petrous portion of the right temporal bone, in the neighborhood of the Gasserian ganglion.

Willy Meyer[5] makes a report of a man who had attempted suicide by shooting himself in the right temporal region; he had been trephined, but no search for the bullet had been made. The patient recovered from the operation, but motor symptoms developed in the left arm and leg. X-ray photographs faintly revealed **three foreign bodies** in line with each other, two of them evidently the split bullet, the third either a part of the bullet or a splinter of bone. Two of the foreign bodies are on one side of the median line and one is on the other. The case is looked upon as beyond surgical relief. It is interesting to note that exposure to the x-rays brought about an extensive loss of hair over the posterior half of the head. Philip D. Bunce[6] reports a case in which a bullet was located in the motor area of the brain with x-rays. Operation was not advised because it was believed that the destructive changes

[1] Ann. of Surg., Apr., 1897.   [2] Intercol. Med. Jour. Austral., Jan. 20, 1897.
[3] Med. Rec., May 8, 1897.   [4] Wien. med. Presse, No. 33, 1896.
[5] Ann. of Surg., Apr., 1897.   [6] Med. Rec., Apr. 17, 1897.

in the brain were permanent. Brissaus and Londe[1] report a case in which a pistol-bullet imbedded in the brain was successfully skiagraphed. As the ball was situated in the temporal region, it was obvious that the existing hemiplegia was not due to the presence of the bullet, but resulted from injury the bullet had wrought in its passage, hence that no surgical operation was justifiable. L. E. Henschen and K. G. Sennauer[1] have reported an important case in which the x-rays showed a bullet in the brain. Two skiagraphs were taken. The first showed the ball in the occipital region; the second showed it to the right of the median line. An operation was performed, the ball was removed, and the patient recovered.

J. William White, Arthur W. Goodspeed, and Charles L. Leonard[3] report an interesting series of cases in which the x-rays were used, and discuss the subject of **the value of the x-rays.** They tell us that the most obvious and simplest use of the skiagraph is in detecting foreign bodies imbedded in any of the tissues. They then discuss the cases in which foreign bodies have been found in certain organs and viscera, and the detection of foreign bodies within the organism itself, such as renal, vesical, and prostatic calculi.

George R. Fowler[4] reports a case of **lateral dislocation of the elbow-joint** in which the skiagraph failed to make the injury evident. This was due to the fact that the individual who used the apparatus was not aware that there was likely to be a lateral dislocation. Under an anesthetic lateral dislocation was perfectly evident to the examiner's fingers. He also reports a case of **gunshot-wound of the head** in which the bullet was located by means of the Röntgen rays and the telephonic probe and was removed by operation.

A. P. Laurie and John T. Leon[5] report a case in which a **vesical calculus** was successfully skiagraphed after an exposure of 7 min.

Sidney Rowland[6] presents a study of **the x-rays and their application.** In the region of the skull their use is practically confined to the discovery of foreign bodies. The conditions are not very favorable, for the skull forms a more or less opaque screen; but bone is not absolutely opaque, and by prolonged exposure it is possible to locate a bullet in the brain. A tuberculous focus in the cervical spine can be made out. In discussing the use of the x-rays in the thorax he tells us that by the use of the plate a skiagraph of the heart can be obtained; but a skiagraph is only a shadow of the outline of the heart, nothing is shown of the condition of the valves or cavities. For the diagnosis of foreign bodies in the trachea and bronchi, or imbedded in the substance of the lung, the skiagraph will reveal all that can be desired, providing these bodies are opaque to the x-rays. The rays are especially useful in the case of children who have swallowed marbles and small coins. In making a diagnosis of spinal caries the sternum and ribs act as a screen to the rays; but if the rays are directed, by adjusting the tube laterally to the sternum, so as to traverse an intercostal space, the difficulty will be overcome and we shall be enabled to obtain a slight oblique spinal projection. In the abdomen the rays are valuable in detecting foreign bodies, locating a Murphy button, and diagnosticating lumbar caries, fracture, or dislocation. If the surgeon is going to operate for a foreign body, it should be seen just before operation; otherwise the position may be altered by the peristaltic action of the intestines. The question as to the value of the x-rays in the diagnosis of vesical or renal calculus is still open. If the bladder shows no shadow upon it, that is no evi-

[1] Med. Press and Circ., N. S., vol. lxii., No. 2984.
[2] Nordiskt Medicinskt, Arkiv, 1897.   [3] Am. Jour. Med. Sci., Aug., 1896.
[4] Brooklyn Med. Jour., Dec., 1896   [5] Lancet, Jan. 16, 1897.
        [6] Brit. Med. Jour., Oct. 3, 1896.

denee that a stone does not exist in the kidney; but if a decided shadow exists, proof is positive that a foreign body is present. In some cases a positive diagnosis can be given, but in any case the information should be sought for. The limbs prove themselves most adapted to the purposes of the skiagraph. It is in the elbow-joint that the greatest use will probably be found for the skiagraph in surgery. This joint is very easily skiagraphed, and we are able to distinguish between separated epiphysis, epicondylar fractures, and many other intricate combinations of lesions. We can also use the fluorescent screen without elaborate precautions. In the forearm and wrist the application is practically limited to the diagnosis of fractures and the recognition of the position of foreign bodies. It is not a simple matter to diagnosticate a dislocation of the metacarpal bones with the aid of a skiagraph, as here a side view is difficult to obtain, and an anteroposterior view does not give us all the information we desire, and it is in this direction that displacement must occur.

In considering the lower extremity, what we have said about the upper extromity also applies. The hip-joint presents several conditions in which early diagnosis is invaluable, but it is often very difficult to obtain a satisfactory skiagraph. In most cases, however, there is no difficulty in obtaining one. In early tuberculous disease we may be able to make a diagnosis by the skiagraph. In cases of congenital dislocation the process gives us valuable information as to the extent of the acetabular rim. [In a later article Sidney Rowland considers the method of using the Röntgen apparatus, and tells us that the rays occasionally produce some very curious effects upon the skin. In one case there was exfoliation of the skin and nails of the hands.]

Robert G. LeConte[1] reports an interesting case in which a **bullet** deeply imbedded **in the tissues of the neck** was located by a skiagraph.

E. E. King[2] records an interesting case in which **lesions of the skin,** hair, and nails were produced by the action of the x-rays.

Maurice H. Richardson[3] presents a series of **22 cases,** illustrating the importance of the use of the x-rays in the routine office practice of a general practitioner, taken, as he says, by one who knew nothing about photography, nothing about electricity, and very little about physics. He advises the use of the Röntgen rays as an aid to diagnosis, and insists upon their value because of the medico-legal aspect of many of these cases. When it has been employed the surgeon is able to locate the exact situation of the fragments in fractures, which is of the utmost value in routine practice.

W. S. Forbes[4] reports a case in which he obtained a skiagraph showing a **crochet-needle** 3 in. long **in a girl's bladder,** the needle being imbedded in a mass of uric-acid incrustation.

Henry Morris[5] says that, owing to the position of the kidney close to the vertebral column and deep beneath the muscles and ribs, the x-rays have not as yet been of use in diagnosticating **biliary or renal calculi.** Calculi formed of lime salts show a deeper shade than those composed of uric acid and urates. Over-exposure often causes failure in skiagraphing calculi, and Morris suggests as short an exposure as possible, supposing the rays are strong enough to reach the renal region. James Swain[6] objects to Mr. Morris's assertion that the Röntgen rays are not of assistance in diagnosticating renal calculi. He succeeded in skiagraphing an oxalate stone and successfully removed it, and in another case he has skiagraphed a stone which the patient will not have removed. He also knows of another case in which the stone was skiagraphed

[1] Ann. of Surg., Aug., 1896.
[3] Med. News, Dec., 1896.
[5] Lancet, Nov. 14, 1896.
[2] Canad. Pract., Nov., 1896.
[4] Jour. Am. Med. Assoc., June 26, 1897.
[6] Ibid., Dec. 5, 1896.

and removed. Chappins and Channel have shown that calculi in the urinary passages may be demonstrated by the x-rays, and, further, that it is often possible to determine by skiagraphy the character of the stone, the composition, and causation, by differences in the appearance of the skiagraphs.

Francis Johnston and C. Thurston Holland [1] report 2 cases of **halfpenny in the esophagus** recognized by means of the x-rays. In one case the child had swallowed the halfpenny 2 days before, and the skiagraph showed the coin distinctly in the gullet. The second case had a doubtful history of having swallowed a halfpenny 5 months before, and the coin was distinctly visible by means of the x-ray. In Case I. the coin could be seen most distinctly with the fluorescent screen. In Case II. the screen showed the coin faintly apparent behind the upper part of the sternum, but the attempt to obtain a radiagraph was unsuccessful.

H. Beeckman Delatour [2] has reported a case in which he removed a foreign body from the esophagus by esophageal forceps guided by the fluoroscope. The patient had swallowed an iron washer $\frac{9}{16}$ in. in diameter. The object was so distinctly visible when looked at by the fluoroscope that Delatour at once thought of the possibility of passing a pair of forceps guided by the fluoroscope and grasping the washer from above. The fluoroscope was applied to the back and showed the disk. A pair of flexible bullet-forceps were then passed into the esophagus and were visible in the fluoroscope; the forceps were made to grasp the washer, and had withdrawn it about an inch when the child made some efforts at swallowing which dislodged it from the grasp of the forceps and it slipped back to its former position. More chloroform was given and an attempt was made with a pair of alligator-forceps, with the same result. In the third attempt a pair of esophageal forceps were passed until they were seen to be $\frac{1}{2}$ in. below the washer; they were then opened and closed, and seen to grasp the foreign body, which was then successfully withdrawn. [White expressed the view that such a procedure might be successful 9 months before the appearance of Delatour's article.]

W. B. Bannister [3] reports a case of **x-ray traumatism** due to exposure for four hours in two sittings, a slight redness resulting. About a month later the patient was exposed to the x-rays for twelve hours during four days. This was followed by necrosis of the abdominal skin over an area 12 by 15 in., and the patient was confined to bed for a month. The beard on the chin and the thumb-nail were destroyed, and there was agonizing pain of a burning character. The author attributes this effect to action upon the terminal nerve-filaments, probably on the vasomotor nerves.

J. William White [4] records a case in which a jackstone was detected in the esophagus by means of skiagraphy. [This case was reported in the *Year-Book* for 1897. W. W. Keen and A. C. Wood have reported similar cases.]

Péan [5] has written upon the value of skiagraphy in detecting foreign bodies in the esophagus and has reported a recent case. A child had swallowed a coin ten days before. Because the child was still able to swallow liquids the physician had decided that the coin had gone into the stomach, but a skiagraph showed that the coin was lodged, and led Péan to decide upon the performance of an operation. The fact that in many cases after foreign bodies have been lodged the individual can still swallow liquids may lead to the lapse of considerable time before there is a recognition of the real condition. Skiagraphy enables the surgeon to know that a foreign body is present, enables him to

[1] Brit. Med. Jour., Dec. 5, 1896.   [2] Med. Rec., May 1. 1897.
[3] Ibid., Jan. 23, 1897.   [4] Ann. of Surg., Aug., 1896.
[5] Bull. de l'Acad. de Méd., No. 48, 1896.

determine accurately its situation, and also to decide upon the operation which is most suitable.

O. L. Schmidt[1] has published an interesting skiagraph of an **aortic aneurysm.** An exposure of seven minutes was required to take the picture, the plate being placed on the chest and the discharge-tube back of the patient. The picture shows the inner ends of the clavicles, the sternum, the diaphragm, and the upper border of the liver. The heart throws a triangular shadow; the aneurysm is seen as a large round shadow in the centre of the picture. The second picture was taken with the plate posterior and the discharge-tube in front, and this showed that the aneurysm had extended downward on the side of the vertebral column. The patient died some weeks later, and postmortem examination showed that the aneurysm was almost the same size as was indicated in the picture.

Henry C. Drury[2] reports a case in which a man was exposed to the *x*-rays for an hour in an attempt to obtain a skiagraph of the region of the kidney. Three hours later he had an attack of nausea which soon passed away. Six days after this he was again exposed to the rays for 1½ hours. After leaving the laboratory he was again nauseated; next day the abdomen was reddened, and on the third day this redness had become very marked. On the fourth day a crop of vesicles appeared, which increased in size and number and became confluent and then ruptured. 18 days after the second exposure there was a patch on the abdomen like eczema, from which the **epidermis** had **exfoliated.** This patch gave origin to a profuse seropurulent discharge and was 7½ by 8¼ inches in area. In 16 weeks there had been some healing, but there was still a considerable area which was covered by a false membrane.

William S. Hedley[3] tells us that in using the *x*-rays we must be careful not to produce on the plate **artificial deformities;** that is, the shadows must be thrown upon a flat surface, never upon a curved one. It therefore becomes obvious that sensitized paper must not be adapted to the curves of the body, as this would make the skiagraph absolutely misleading.

Samuel Lloyd[4] has recently shown the value of the *x*-rays before and after **osteotomy.** The case was that of a girl whose femora were crossed. Each thigh bone was subjected to osteotomy and was produced in the position for reunion. The fact that the union was perfect was determined by the use of the *x*-ray apparatus. The bones could be seen very readily by placing the Crookes tube under the operating-table and holding the fluoroscope above the thigh bones. The observer has also had most satisfactory results in studying fractures about the knee and elbow and diseases of the bones of the hand.

W. S. Hedley[5] considers the **usefulness of the x-rays in medicine and surgery.** He tells us that in fractures of the extremities the use of this process has become almost routine, not only to recognize the existence of fractures before reduction, but to study them for the application of splints. Foreign bodies in the esophagus have been clearly shown. Luxations of the hip have sometimes been recognized, and renal and vesical calculi have been darkly defined, but no results as practically useful as those obtained by the skiagraph in the surgery of the extremities have yet accrued to medicine. The skeleton of the thorax is readily seen, and organ after organ is beginning dimly to take form. The light space occupied by the lungs can be contrasted with the dark lines of the ribs, the diaphragm is visible to the extent of its movements, and the shadow of the living heart in action can be thrown upon the screen.

[1] Medicine, Apr., 1897.   [2] Brit. Med. Journ., Nov. 7, 1896.
[3] Lancet, Apr. 3, 1897.   [4] Jour. Am. Med. Assoc., Apr. 24, 1897.
[5] Treatment, Mar. 25, 1897.

Bouchard has shown by this means the presence of fluid in the pleura, and he has also demonstrated cardiac hypertrophy and aortic aneurysm. The convex surface of the liver is clearly seen, and a hydatid cyst has been demonstrated there, but the lower surface of the liver has not been defined. The kidney cannot be differentiated. When the stomach is distended with gas it can be made out as a light spot on a dark background, but it is not possible to verify the existence of a large cancer of that organ. The *x*-rays have not yet established any claim to therapeutic usefulness. They are not fatal to the diphtheria-bacillus. It is stated that when they were applied to a cancer of the mouth pain was diminished by prolonged and frequent exposure. Despergnes has reported a case of cancer of the stomach treated in this way, and he claims that the general condition of the patient was improved, the pain disappeared, and there was a diminution in the size of the stomach. In view, however, of what is known of the effects of suggestion in relieving the pain of cancer, even for a long time, these observations must very largely increase in number before they are seriously considered. There can be no doubt that the *x*-rays occasionally produce traumatic effects—severe dermatitis and ulceration. Crocker reported a very striking example of this in the *British Medical Journal* of January 2, 1897. Daniel, of the University of Virginia, it is stated by the *New York Medical Record*, secured a simple depilatory action without any inflammation.

Edmund E. King[1] describes cases in which marked **changes** were produced **in the skin,** hair, and nails of an individual he was operating on by the *x*-ray apparatus.

W. H. Peck[2] considers recent contributions in skiagraphy and discusses reported cases of *x*-ray dermatitis.

[1] Canad. Pract., Nov., 1896.　　　　　　　　　[2] Medicine, Jan., 1897.

OBSTETRICS.

By BARTON COOKE HIRST, M. D., and W. A. NEWMAN DORLAND, M. D.,

OF PHILADELPHIA.

The Chief Features of the Year's Work.—The much-mooted question, Shall we or shall we not favor the higher education of midwives? has agitated obstetric circles in this country and in England. There are two ways in which it may be answered : either we must admit these women to a recognized standing in obstetrics, and then, of course, they must be educated for the safety of the women who entrust their lives and health to their care; or else they should be prohibited from practising their calling, and their places filled by well-educated medical men. In this country we have no place for midwives save in the foreign colonies in the hearts of our great cities, where they are mainly found, and even here they should be supplanted by skilled men, and thereby the continued mortality from puerperal sepsis be greatly diminished. The serum-therapy of puerperal sepsis is following the usual course pursued thus far by the various antitoxins, as of tuberculosis and diphtheria. The cases hitherto reported in which it has been employed clearly demonstrate that at the best it can have but a very limited field of usefulness in puerperal infection. The same may be said for vaginal section for extrauterine gestation, which has been advocated in some parts of the globe. If ever an operation to be desired, it must of necessity be only under the most unusual circumstances. The study of the fetal appendages has been most assiduously pursued, and our knowledge of their methods of growth and development, the pathologic changes to which they are subject, and their effects upon maternal and fetal tissues is daily becoming more rounded and accurate. Notably is this true of the placenta and of that curious and grave condition—malignant deciduoma. The dangers of labor after antefixation of the uterus are now well recognized, and operations are being done mainly after the period of sexual activity is over. Owing to its greater mortality and the increased difficulty in its performance, the operation of symphysiotomy, as was predicted last year, has been largely abandoned in favor of Cesarean section.

PRELIMINARY AND GENERAL CONSIDERATIONS.

The Question of Midwives.—R. R. Rentoul[1] enters an earnest protest against the licensing of midwives in England, rightly claiming that it is a movement not in the best interests of public health and of public safety. He argues that the proposal to supply the poor with midwifery practitioners only partly trained in obstetrics, and wholly untrained in medicine and surgery, is a distinctly retrograde step and conducive to the production of crime, in that it

---

[1] Lancet, Jan. 16, 1897.

will aid in concealing criminal stillbirths and the nefarious business of the abortion-monger. He believes that with the existing arrangements of the poor-law medical service in the United Kingdom, and without establishing any partially educated midwifery practitioners, they have now the means by which all poor pregnant women can be supplied with fully educated medical attendants. In addition, through the workings of the various nursing-associations, suitable nursing can be provided free of cost for such worthy poor. For those women who are willing to pay a part of the medical fee, maternity clubs and provident dispensaries have been provided. [Our views upon this very vital question have already been given here, and our stand remains firm for the higher education of the obstetric student and the unequivocal denunciation of the licensing of midwives.]

Telegony.—[It has long been believed and tacitly acknowledged by many honest observers that the progeny of one sire may be influenced in color, formation, or other outstanding characteristic by a previous sire, by which the mother has produced offspring. Especially is such a belief rife among veterinarians and horse-breeders, and several well-known cases have often been quoted in support of this theory. This is also true of some instances in the history of medicine and obstetrics.] In an able paper A. L. Bell[1] endeavors to disprove such a belief. He states that to account for the influence of a previous sire there are two theories advanced : 1. That the spermatozoa of the first sire pass up the Fallopian tubes to the ovaries and are absorbed by the unripe ova contained therein ; and that these spermatozoa, though of insufficient power to fertilize the unripe ovum, have yet sufficient power to alter the development of that ovum subsequently, when it is fertilized by the spermatozoa of the second sire. 2. That there is an interchange of constituent parts of the fetal and maternal blood-currents, the exact amount of interchange not being defined. It is asserted that some part of the fetal blood enters the maternal circulation— not perhaps as blood, but in one form or other—and the fetal element thus given up to the mother is kept by her and enables her to impress the characteristics of the offspring of a previous sire on subsequent offspring of a different sire ; that is to say, the first sire impresses his own offspring with certain of his own characteristics ; this offspring impresses the mother through the blood-current ; the mother, in turn, transmits the peculiarities of the first sire to her subsequent progeny by means of the blood-element she is said to have received from her first offspring.

In refutation of the first assertion, Bell claims that when a spermatozoon is absorbed into an unripe ovum it must surely die, so far as its individual existence is concerned, by becoming part of the ovum ; and it seems incredible that a dead sperm-cell can exert any influence on the development of an ovum by which it was absorbed months before, unless the ovum possesses some special power of preserving not only *its own latent* power, but the potency of the sperm-cell on which it depends for the special growth intended by Nature. As regards the second theory, Bell supposes for argument that this influence of a previous sire exists in fact ; he is then driven of necessity to the conclusion that the fetus actually gives up to the mother, besides the waste-products, some essential part of its blood, carrying with it the key to hereditary transmission. If so, then the blood of the mother must become more and more mixed with each succeeding pregnancy, and be liable, therefore, to impress on her offspring the peculiarities, not of *one sire* only, but of *every previous sire* to whom she has borne offspring. It is impossible adequately to comprehend where such a theory would lead us, utterly at variance as it is with what we know of the

[1] Indian Med. Rec., Aug. 16, 1896.

definiteness of the physiology of Nature. He further argues that if it be possible for a sire to influence subsequent progeny not his own, it is fair to expect that he will be able to influence subsequent progeny which are his own; so that we should find, at least in a certain number of cases, the children of the same parents consecutively resembling more and more strongly their father; but, so far as he has observed, the first child is just as likely to resemble the father as any of the later children.

THE PHYSIOLOGY OF PREGNANCY.

Obesity as a Cause of Sterility.—J. V. Gaff,[1] in discussing the etiologic importance of obesity in sterility, states that in obese subjects the uterus, tubes, and ovaries will be found firmly packed into the pelvis and surrounded by layers of fat; the fat-cells interspersed between the unstriped muscle-fibers and connective tissue surrounding the follicles are so thick and cause so much pressure that it is impossible for the ovum to escape from the ovary; large masses of fat crowding down upon the cervix bend the canal of the uterus forward, producing an aggravated condition of anteflexion, and thereby effectually preventing the entrance of semen to the uterus. During copulation the uterine round and broad ligaments by their concerted action cause a suction from the vagina toward the ovaries, greatly facilitating the movement of the semen. When they become encumbered with large quantities of fat they are no longer able to perform that function, and the semen is retarded or is lost on its way toward the junction with the ovum in the tube or ovary. Compression of the tubes by masses of fat obstructing the passageway through is another fruitful cause of sterility. [That this relationship between obesity and sterility exists is substantiated by statistics. Kish has enumerated over 200 cases of obesity associated with amenorrhea and sterility, without other appreciable cause. Philbert has described 5 cases wherein pregnancy occurred through adopting a thorough and vigorous system of hydropathic and dietetic treatment. Abortions in obese women are frequent. Stoltz has cited the case of an obese woman who had 5 consecutive abortions which he could attribute to no other cause, and Goubert cites the case of a very fleshy woman who had 8 consecutive abortions from the same cause.] Vedeler[2] has observed 310 cases of primary sterility. All the women had been married more than one year; 72 were married 10 or more years; and of the others, the average duration of marriage was 3 years. In only 50 cases was the husband examined, either directly or indirectly; of this number of men, 38 had certainly had gonorrhea, and probably more. In 34 cases of the wives of these men, 11 suffered from perimetritis, 10 from ovariosalpingitis, 3 from metritis, 2 from cystitis and vulvitis, and 8 from vulvovaginitis. If this proportion existed in the entire number of husbands of the remaining 260 women, 235 would have had gonorrhea, and 210 would have infected their wives. As a matter of fact, in 198 sterile women the same inflammatory processes were found as in those whose husbands had undoubtedly had gonorrhea; 64%, therefore, suffered from this disease. The abnormal conditions which were found to exist in the 310 women were as follows: 1. Inflammatory processes: 66 suffered from perimetritis, 45 from salpingitis, 42 from metritis, 18 from vulvovaginitis, 15 from ureterocystitis, 12 from endometritis; in all, 108 cases. 2. Non-inflammatory conditions: (a) Anatomic abnormalities: atrophy of the uterus, 22 cases; persistent hymen, 7 cases; stenosis of the external os, 6 cases; conical cervix, 3 cases; defective uterus or vagina, 2 cases; unclassified, 27 cases; in

[1] Jour. Am. Med. Assoc., Jan. 23, 1897.　　[2] Am. Medico-Surg. Bull., Mar. 25, 1897.

all, 67 cases. (*b*) Pathologic-anatomic abnormalities: uterine fibroid, 23 cases; ovarian cyst, 5 cases; uterine polypus, 2 cases; vaginismus, 7 cases; hematocele, 4 cases; syphilis, 3 cases; chancre, 1 case; in all, 45 cases. The author believes that the cause of the sterility lay in the men in 70% of cases, and in the women in 30%.

Precocious Puberty.—An interesting case is reported by A. J. Price.[1] The patient, aged 6 years and 7 months, presented a luxurious growth of downy fur on the face, well marked on the upper lip; the body was shapely, the curves graceful, the hips broad, the breasts well developed, and the mons veneris, which was thickly covered with hair, suggested the appearance of a woman past puberty. The sexual organs were normal in formation, with the exception of a slightly hypertrophied clitoris. Her voice was as coarse as that of an adult woman. The hair on the pubis and under the arms was first noticed at the age of 18 months. Early in her 4th year blood-stains were frequently found on her undergarments, which the parents did not attribute to menstruation until a few months later—during the latter half of her 4th year —when that function set in more perceptibly and regularly. The child never showed any disposition to play with other children, but rather sought the company of older persons, and was bright and reasonable beyond her years.

Ovulation, Menstruation, and Conception.—Strassmann[2] reports the results of a series of experiments to determine the causation of menstruation. Eight experiments were performed upon bitches, the abdomen being opened under antiseptic precautions and sterile fluid injected into the ovary. It was found that the increase in the vascular tension of the ovary which followed such injections produced the phenomena of menstruation, including the characteristic changes in the mucous membrane of the uterus. Strassmann finds in the results of his experiments an explanation of the discharge of blood which has been so often observed to follow the removal of one or both ovaries or any operation that interferes with the nervous supply of the genital organs. His experiments and the observations of operators show that menstruation results from an altered condition in the vascular tension of the ovaries produced by a nervous stimulus. The results of his most interesting studies may be summarized in the following description: the ripening of the ovum produces an increase in the vascular tension of the ovary, causing nervous stimulus to be transmitted to the uterus and bringing about the characteristic enlargement and turgescence of that organ and its lining membrane which are observed at menstruation. This increased vascularity of the womb prepares it to nourish the ovum if impregnated. When conception does not occur the ovum escapes, and with it are discharged the surplus blood-supply and epithelial soil which were prepared for it. As has been stated by others, each menstruation is the birth of an unimpregnated ovum. This teaches us that conception most readily occurs, outside the uterus, within the tube, pregnancy usually beginning as an extrauterine or ectopic gestation. Conception most frequently occurs not immediately after menstruation, as has been supposed, but during the 2 weeks immediately preceding a menstrual period. Menstruation itself is a sign that conception has not occurred. In reckoning the date of confinement the last day of the last menstrual period, which has usually been taken, should not be considered as the probable time of conception, but a period preceding by a week or ten days the first menstrual epoch at which menstruation did not occur. Thus, if the last day of the last menstrual period is stated to be the first of a given month, the period of gestation should be counted, not from this date, but from the 20th or possibly the 25th of this

[1] New Orl. M. and S. Jour., Aug., 1896.   [2] Arch. f. Gynäk., Bd. lii., H. 1, 1896.

month. It is believed that a more accurate estimation of the date of confinement can be obtained by reckoning in accordance with these results. [This will be a most desirable result if experience will verify the deductions of the writer.]

Stansbury Sutton and Gordon [1] relate two extraordinary cases for which they do not profess to account. On October 20, 1892, Sutton removed 2 large multilocular ovarian cysts from a woman aged 28. The ligatures lay close to the uterine cornua. On June 10, 1894, the patient gave birth to a male child weighing 10½ pounds. On February 25, 1896, she was again delivered. Gordon in March, 1894, removed both ovaries and tubes from a woman aged 33, the subject of chronic pelvic disease. From a few months after the operation she menstruated regularly till June, 1895, when she became pregnant, and was delivered of a healthy child in March, 1896. The only explanation is that the stump of one tube must have opened, allowing an ovum from a piece of ovarian tissue to pass through into the uterus. In a second case, in which pregnancy followed 3 years after operation, it was not absolutely certain that both ovaries were removed.

Superfetation.—P. Gustin [2] reports a case of a woman convalescing from typhoid fever who expelled a fetus of 3 months and one of 6 weeks. A. L. Bailey [3] records a twin pregnancy in which a 4-months fetus was expelled, followed by the birth of a full-term fetus. The small child was wrinkled and flattened out, and the cord shrivelled up like a string; the placenta was anastomosed with the larger one and showed calcareous degeneration of the whole side whence was given off the small cord. [This was undoubtedly a case of fœtus papyraceus, and not an instance of superfetation.] In addition Bailey records a true instance of superfetation, a full-term child being delivered together with one of 4 or 5 months. H. W. Mills [4] relates the case of a woman, aged 42 years, who, in her first pregnancy, aborted at 3 months. Six months later she miscarried in her second pregnancy, discharging a fetus of about 16 weeks and a fresh, healthy ovum of about 7 weeks.

Placental Tissue, Fresh and Old.—In a paper read before the Obstetric Society of London, Nov. 4, 1896, T. W. Eden stated that the placenta, like other caducous structures, commences to degenerate for an appreciable time before it is cast off, and, in fact, this is the immediate cause of its being shed. The first and most important change is slowly progressing obliteration of a certain number of branches of the allantoid (umbilical) arteries, principally in the marginal cotyledons, the affection being in the nature of endarteritis. The corresponding capillaries and veins remain unaltered until the circulation through them is suspended by the ultimate complete obliteration of the arterial branches supplying them. Then they become thrombosed. This process may be detected as early as the seventh month, and at term the total number of arteries affected is considerable, though few of them become altogether obliterated, except in the marginal cotyledons. The first effect of the diminished blood-supply is atrophy and degeneration of the epithelial covering of the villi, which undergoes hyaline or fibrous degeneration (coagulation-necrosis). Layers of true fibrin are deposited over the degenerated areas from the maternal blood. In this way the villi become enclosed in thick layers of fibrinous material, and neighboring villi become welded together. Scattered areas of consolidation are thus formed in the spongy placental tissue, to which the name of "white infarct" has been applied. Some of these may attain the size of a pea or a filbert, and even an entire cotyledon may be consolidated.

[1] Am. Gyn. and Obst. Jour., July, 1896. [2] Arch. de Gynéc. et de Tocol., July, 1896.
[3] Med. Age, Aug. 10, 1896. [4] Lancet, Mar. 13, 1897.

The structures involved in the areas of degeneration become atrophied, and in the larger infarcts are seen evidences of fatty and calcareous degeneration. Another form of consolidation, known as the "non-fibrinous infarct," sometimes occurs in the ripe placenta. This form is probably due to blocking of the maternal arteries, and not to fetal endarteritis. It is clear that a process similar to that of fibrinous infarction occurs in the extraplacental chorion, causing atrophy and disappearance of its villi. Infarction represents the extension to the placental chorion, during the later months of gestation, of changes that occur with regularity in the extraplacental chorion during the earlier months. It is not a pathologic change, but is the natural outcome of the processes of evolution and decline. Thrombosis of the subplacental sinuses has been stated by Friedländer and Minot to occur as early as the seventh month; but as the number of sinuses affected is not great, and as there is free anastomosis, the intervillous circulation is probably not materially hindered. The superficial layer of the serotina is the seat of a degenerative process akin to that affecting the chorionic epithelium. The change begins in the intercellular substance, which is converted into a deeply staining fibrillated material allied to fibrin. The protoplasm of the decidual cells is involved and ultimately their nuclei break up and disappear. The change begins at the surface, but often extends irregularly into the deeper layers. Fibrin from the maternal blood is deposited on the degenerated surface. At term coiling serotinal arteries may sometimes be found thrombosed for a considerable distance, and veins are often more or less completely blocked by deposits of fibrin.

Occasionally this process of separation fails to take place, and then there results the condition known as retained placenta. By *retained placenta* is meant one which has been retained in utero after the death of the fetus, irrespective of the period of gestation to which it belongs or of the length of time that has elapsed between the death of the fetus and the evacuation of the uterus. There are two factors to be borne in mind : 1. The morbid condition leading to the death of the fetus, which may have directly affected the placenta; and, 2. The arrest of the fetal circulation—*i. e.*, the death of the villi. Changes due to the first factor may be called primary, and those due to the second factor secondary. When the changes are far advanced the difficulty of distinguishing primary from secondary changes is very great.

For practical purposes it is necessary to distinguish two groups : (*a*) cases in which the placenta has been retained for only a short time after the death of the fetus, which is born in a nonmacerated or but slightly macerated condition ; and (*b*) cases in which the placenta has been retained a considerable time and the fetus is more or less markedly macerated. In the second group the primary changes are obscured by the superimposed secondary changes, so that the best chance of studying the primary changes occurs in the first group. The secondary changes, on the other hand, are more pronounced in the second group, though their beginnings may be found in the first. In the past no serious attempt has been made to distinguish between primary and secondary changes, and much careful work has therefore been invalidated.

When the fetus perishes the placenta may remain attached to the uterine wall and the maternal circulation through the intervenous spaces continue, although the fetal circulation through the villi has ceased. Although technically dead, therefore, the villi remain in contact with the maternal blood, and are thus preserved from decay ; so much so that, after retention for several weeks, areas of villi may be found that can scarcely be distinguished from those of a living placenta. At the same time the villi never appear to show the least trace of growth or multiplication, and in retained placenta signs of recent activity are altogether wanting. The condition of the extraplacental tissue is in marked contrast to that of the placenta proper. The membranes, the cord, and the tissues of the fetus itself necrose with rapidity, because there is nothing to preserve them from the fate of dead organic matter. When the maternal circulation through the intervillous spaces is maintained no marked change occurs in the placental villi, but gradually that circulation is arrested and, as the villi become cut off from the maternal blood, they perish. We have thus to trace: 1, the arrest of the maternal circulation; 2, the changes that result to the villi; and, 3, the changes in the extraplacental tissues. The arrest of the maternal circulation occurs by a process similar to that already described, in connection with the formation of white infarcts in the living placenta. The obliteration of the intervillous spaces in the retained placenta appears to be due rather to progressive failure of the maternal circulation from shrinking of the uterus and loss of the stimulus of the growing ovum than to fetal arterial changes. The maternal blood consequently clots more readily and deposits fibrin more freely than in the living placenta. The intervillous spaces are first obliterated around infarcts and upon the fetal and maternal surfaces of the placenta. In this manner the retained placenta becomes extensively consolidated, and its tissues present microscopic characters closely allied to those of infarcts, and differing widely from those of spongy, placental tissue.

The changes in the villi are practically the same as in the middle and inner zones of large infarcts in the living placenta. They undergo atrophy and necrosis, lose their epithelial covering, then their connective tissue, stroma, and blood-vessels, and, finally, their nuclei. In addition, large areas of placenta may become consolidated by the process of noufibrinous infarction. Extensive fatty degeneration usually occurs in all the consolidated areas, and calcareous deposits are also abundant.

The most frequent cause of the death of the fetus in the earlier months of gestation appears to be some pathologic condition of the decidua, and we must be careful to distinguish between the primary and secondary changes. In a retained placenta of the 5th month or later the compact layer is generally fused with a superjacent stratum, consisting of several rows of villi imbedded in fibrin and blood-clot. Its structure is barely recognizable. The spongy layer, as a rule, is much less altered, but is generally thinned and atrophied, though the characteristic decidual cells are distinct and the vessels often full of blood. The process of fibrinous degeneration never affects this layer except to a very slight degree—a point of importance when we consider that any process tending to consolidate this stratum would inevitably render separation of the placenta difficult.

The amnion always necroses after the death of the fetus, though the changes proceed less rapidly over the placenta than over the extraplacental chorion. The extraplacental chorion and decidua vera also necrose in all cases, but not so rapidly as the amnion, being longest preserved in the neighborhood of the placental margin, perishing soonest in parts most distant from it.

The changes in a retained ovum that follow death may be summed up as follows: 1. Necrosis, commencing at once, of, *a*, the body of the fetus; *b*, the umbilical cord; *c*, the amnion; *d*, the extraplacental chorion and decidua vera. 2. Gradual arrest of the maternal circulation through the placenta by thrombosis of the intervillous spaces. 3. Necrosis of the various divisions of the placental chorion, as they become shut off from the maternal blood. 4. Fatty and calcareous degeneration of the necrosing tissues.

[The foregoing is a valuable addition to the paper contributed by Eden last year on the development of the placenta, which was reported in the last volume of the *Year-Book.*]

W. E. Fothergill[1] denies that in "placental polypus" and "sarcous" or "fleshy" mole placental tissue can remain fresh and comparatively unaltered for many months after the death of the fetus. He believes that after the fetal circulation has ceased no constructive process continues in the fetal elements of the placenta, and he finds no trace of division in either epiblastic or mesoblastic fetal cells of a placenta whose embryo has been dead any length of time. The fetal tissues may increase in size, but only through the swelling of degenerative processes. The placenta has been supposed to grow after the death of the fetus in ectopic gestation, but recent investigation has shown that all progressive changes that occur are in the blood-clot, and that none but degenerative processes occur in the villi.

Diagnosis of the Location of the Placental Attachment by External Palpation.—Tribondani[2] has been studying this subject at the Clinica Ostetrica of Pavia, examining the uterus of the patients immediately after the expulsion of the fetus to confirm his diagnosis made from external palpation beforehand. He announces as the result of his experience that the location of the placental attachment can be accurately determined by the following indications: 1. It is attached to the posterior wall if the tube and round ligaments are found on the anterior surface of the uterus, converging toward the top ; if the anterior surface is rather flat, and if the beat of the fetal heart, the parts of the fetus, and its movements can be clearly distinguished from the front. 2. It is attached to the front wall if the tubes and the round ligaments are found on the sides of the uterus parallel to its vertical axis, if the anterior wall is very convex, and the fetal heart and movements, and the fetus itself, are not easily distinguished from the front. 3. When the placenta is attached to the fundus the latter is remarkably convex, almost hemispheric, and the points of attachment of the tubes and ligaments are much below its edge. 4. When the placenta is attached to the side wall the uterus is very prominent on that side, and the attachments of the uterine adnexa are found much higher on that side.

Placental Transmission of Disease.—E. H. Grandin[3] asserts that there is but one acute disease which a woman is not able to transmit to her child in utero, and that is anthrax. There is, however, but one undoubted case on record of transmission of tuberculosis. This is not unexpected when we remember that markedly tuberculous women are not prone to conceive. As to how the transference of disease from mother to child is effected, the theory that fits known facts, and which we must at the present day accept, is that which credits the leukocytes with the process. Let a healthy woman become diseased, and at once the leukocytes in her blood-system carry the infection to the intervillous spaces. Here they are met by the barrier against disease established by the healthy placenta which contains healthy leukocytes with the property of resisting the entrance of disease-germs. The phagocytic action of these healthy leukocytes comes into play, destroys at once the leukocytes bearing disease, and the fetus is protected. Let the woman, however, be diseased at the time of conception, or let her become so very shortly afterward, and we have at the outset a diseased placenta, or one which becomes diseased as it is forming. Such a placenta either contains no healthy leukocytes, or else those with but feeble resisting-powers. Disease may, therefore, be readily transmitted to the fetus.

[1] Brit. Med. Jour., May 9, 1896.   [2] Gaz. degli Osped. e delle Clin., Feb. 7, 1897.
[3] N. Am. Pract., Aug., 1896.

Etienne[1] records the examination of a fetus which had been aborted in the fifth month of pregnancy from an 18-year-old mother on the 29th day after she had been seized with typhoid fever. The spleen and intestines of the child showed no signs of the disease, and the placenta was healthy. A careful culture-examination of the blood from the right side of the heart and from the spleen, liver, and placenta revealed an abundance of typhoid bacilli. The fetus, Etienne believes, had died of typical acute blood-poisoning from a large dose of the bacillus before the occurrence of any local change.

Partus Serotinus.—Reckoning from the cessation of the last menses, the first feeling of life, and the objective signs, Szaszy[2] reports a case in which gestation lasted 330 days. The child was normally developed and 49 cm. long. Ross[3] records a pregnancy lasting 311 days. The condition of the child at delivery coincided with these figures. Wigodsky[4] reports the case of a patient who carried her child 11 months. She was 28 years old and a multipara. The beginning of her last menstruation was Sept. 7; life was felt first toward the end of January; labor occurred on Aug. 13. The pregnancy was normal, but labor was somewhat protracted on account of the large size of the shoulders (18.5 cm.). Forceps were used and an encephalic fetus was delivered alive.

THE DIAGNOSIS OF PREGNANCY.

The diagnosis of pregnancy by the changes in the microscopic appearance of the urinary phosphates is discussed by W. E. Parke.[5] This means of early diagnosis was first suggested by W. B. Gray in 1887, who claimed that he could form an absolute diagnosis within 20 days after conception. Parke has studied about 75 specimens of urine of women known or thought to be pregnant, and he concludes that the change in the urinary phosphates pointed out by Gray occurs in a very large percentage of pregnant women, but that it is not equally pronounced in the urine at the same period of gestation in different women, nor at consecutive examinations of the urine of the same woman. When recognized, however, it forms a strongly presumptive evidence of pregnancy, and is recognizable very early, and is, therefore, of greatest value when other signs are of the least value, or not present at all. Moreover, a diagnosis of probable pregnancy can be made without a physical examination or without exciting the suspicion of the patient. The normal triple phosphate is more or less of a stellate figure, and markedly feathery. Sometimes the stella is segmented, and one leaflet stands alone. Whether we see it in bold relief as a star or dismembered as a solitary leaflet of the same, the feathery character is always to be remarked on both sides of the center fiber of each leaflet. As soon as conception occurs, or within 20 days thereafter, the feathery portions of the stella or segment thereof begin to disintegrate. This process may advance from the apex toward the base of the crystal, or it may declare itself by destroying progressively the feathery continuation of one-half the leaflet, the center fiber of the same determining and defining its boundaries. Past the middle of the seventh month the phosphates begin somewhat to approximate their original form and general character, and at the accouchement can scarcely be differentiated from the normal. If the fetus should perish during the gestation, the phosphates at once recover their normal character in all respects. To prepare the urine for

[1] Gaz. hebdom. de Méd. et de Chir., No. 16, 1896.   [2] Canad. Pract., Dec., 1896.
[3] Austral. Med. Gaz., Apr. 20, 1896.   [4] Centralbl. f. Gynäk., No. 1, 1897.
                    [5] Am. Gyn. and Obst. Jour., Sept., 1896.

examination take about 1¼ in. in a small test-tube and add about ⅓ as much of Tyson's magnesian fluid; this will throw down the triple phosphates in 15 or 20 minutes, and furnish the necessary material for microscopic examination. *Tyson's fluid* is composed of 1 part each of ammonium muriate, aqua ammonia, and magnesium sulfat, and 8 parts of distilled water.

HYGIENE OF PREGNANCY.

Care of Pregnant Women.—Pinard[1] calls attention to the fact that it is very important that women should be kept at rest toward the end of pregnancy. Hard work is an evil both for the mother and for the child. He has made a comparison of cases of women who sought relief at the Lying-in Hospital, usually after the first pains occurred, and those of women carefully nursed in a refuge for the pregnant. The average weight of the Lying-in Hospital children was 3010 gm. That of the children born after the mothers had been at least ten days in a refuge was 3290 gm. A maximum average of 3366 gm. was reached in cases in which the mothers had resided for some time in the wards of the Baudelocque Lying-in Hospital. Pinard remarks, however, that there were more primiparæ in the refuge and more multiparæ in relatively better circumstances in the hospital. Preliminary rest was found to have a particularly good influence on the duration of labor. Out of 1000 women who worked till labor began, 482 only were delivered on the 280th day of gestation. On the other hand, 660 of the women who had rested were delivered at or after the same date.

PATHOLOGY OF THE FETUS AND OF THE FETAL APPENDAGES.

Malignant Deciduoma.—Cases of this rare and interesting condition have been recorded by J. Cock[2] and Lönnberg and Mannheimer,[3] the latter reporting two cases. Cock, suspecting septic infection in her case, employed the antistreptococcic serum, without, however, beneficial results. A comprehensive study of this neoplasm has been made by H. R. Spencer[4] and Newman Dorland.[5] Spencer tabulates 40 cases, while Dorland reports 52 cases, including all authentic reports up to date. Spencer remarks that the disease appears to be almost entirely confined to multiparæ, and in some cases there had been a long interval between the last two pregnancies. He regards deciduoma malignum as a distinct pathologic entity arising from the products of conception. Dorland remarks that the trend of opinion is toward the fetal origin of the disease, the fetal epithelial covering of the placenta—the so-called syncytium—probably first becoming involved in the degenerative process. The growth must be regarded as the most malignant of all forms of malignant tumors, as is demonstrated by its early and exceedingly rapid development, the great tendency to recurrence and to the formation of metastases, and the high mortality-record. In 59.6% the symptoms manifested themselves either at once after labor or within 4 weeks' time. In 78.97% death occurred within 6 months of the appearance of the symptoms. Thirty-eight of the 52 cases died of the primary condition or from a recurrence of the growth, thus giving an absolute mortality for malignant deciduoma of 73%. In only one instance did the tumor occur in a colored woman. Metastases were noted in 70.76%.

[1] Gaz. des Hôpitaux, Nov. 28, 1895. [2] Brit. Med. Jour., Dec. 26, 1896.
[3] Centralbl. f. Gynäk., No. 18, 1896. [4] Quart. Med. Jour., July, 1896.
[5] Univ. Med. Mag., July, 1897.

These secondary deposits were found in the following situations in the order of their frequency: lungs, 78.37 % ; vagina, 54 % ; spleen, kidneys, and ovary, each 13.51 % ; liver, broad ligament, and pelvis, each 10.8 % ; brain, 5.4 % ; and the colon, right iliac fossa, diaphragm, tenth rib, gluteal region, abdominal wall, bladder, peritoneal cavity, mesenteric glands, prevertebral glands, face, stomach, pancreas, left labium, and abdominal lymphatics, each 2.7 %. Only twice did the tumor appear in primiparæ. Once it followed a tubal gestation in a single girl of 17 ; 12 times it occurred after abortions ; 17 times it followed labor at term ; and 20 times it occurred subsequently to the discharge of a hydatidiform mole.

Cervical Pregnancy.—Trotta[1] reports the case of a woman, aged 40, who aborted at 2 months in her first pregnancy. She had a myoma upon the anterior wall of the uterus, which shut off the cavity of the womb from the cervix. The uterus was extirpated because of the tumor, and on examination it was found that the condition present was virtually an extra-uterine pregnancy, the decidua developing above the tumor in the cavity of the uterus, while the ovum had lodged below within the cervix. [The rare condition called " cervical pregnancy " was present in this case.]

Umbilical Cord.—A. C. Wood[2] records a very interesting and rare condition of the cord, namely, the so-called *mesocord*, further complicating an anencephalic birth. The cord, inserted centrally as usual, was adherent from this point to the margin of the placenta ; the blood-vessels radiated from the central point of insertion (see Plate 1).

Lefèvre[3] describes 151 cases which he has collected from literature in which the cord lost itself in the membranes some distance from the edge of the placenta (*velamentous insertion of the cord*). The condition is most frequent in twin pregnancy. It exposes the fetus to dangers during pregnancy as well as in labor. It may involve premature rupture of the membranes during gestation ; no other reason could be found in at least 6 cases. Membranous insertion of the cord may cause premature labor, and Lefèvre believes that this anomaly of the funis explains certain cases of hydramnios and fetal dropsy. In labor Lefèvre finds that some cases of premature rupture of the membranes is due to membranous insertion, but it appears that this is not so frequent an accident in labor as in pregnancy. Membranous insertion is a predisposing cause of prolapse of the funis ; in 2 out of the 151 cases the fetus was killed during labor through this anomaly, but it must be remembered that in both the death was due to pressure on the membranous insertion, and in no instance to tearing off of the cord. It would seem, in fact, that a labor-pain would not cause the fetus to tear off a cord of this kind, though it is easy to understand how it may cause great danger from pressure.

The Amnion.—D. S. Robinson[4] records a case of supplementary amniotic sac which preceded the normal sac and protruded from the vulvar orifice. Examination after the delivery of the placenta showed that the accessory sac had been developed from the amniotic sheath of the cord ; its capacity was about 2 liters.

Maternal Impressions.—Contributions on this interesting subject have been made by G. E. Gilpin,[5] L. Driesbach,[6] W. T. Councilman,[7] J. I. Smith,[8] A. C. Hatfield,[9] J. J. Parker,[10] and W. F. Batman.[11] Councilman claims that

[1] Atti della soc. ital di ost. e gin., vol. ii., 1896.   [2] Univ. Med. Mag., Sept., 1896.
[3] Thèse de Paris, 1896.   [4] Med. Rec., Sept. 5, 1896.
[5] Med. Brief, Apr., 1896.   [6] New Orl. M. and S. Jour., Oct., 1896.
[7] Boston M. and S. Jour., Jan. 14, 1897   [8] Med. Council, Aug., 1896.
[9] Med. Brief, Jan , 1897.   [10] Ibid., Oct., 1896.
[11] Jour. Am. Med. Assoc., Nov. 14, 1896.

PLATE 1

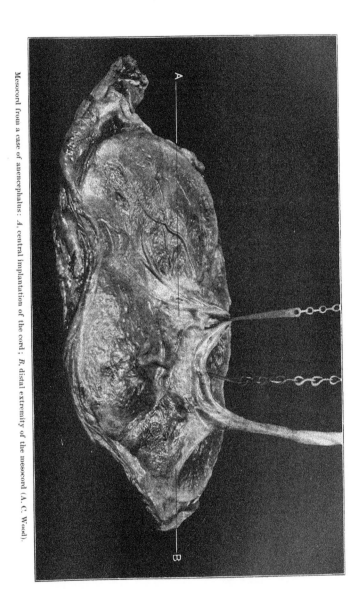

A

B

Mescord from a case of anencephalus: *A*, central implantation of the cord; *B*, distal extremity of the mesocord (A. C. Wood).

there is no scientific foundation for the belief in the so-called maternal impressions, and that no proof exists that they can have any effect on the developing embryo. All malformations seen in man are found in the lower mammalia, on whom the influence of impressions cannot be supposed to be of much importance; and they are also found in birds.

Fetal Monstrosities.—An unusual number of rare and exceedingly interesting specimens of fetal malformation have been recorded during the year. These include the following: Bäcker,[1] a fœtus papyraceus of 2 months' development; H. F. Lewis,[2] a case of iniencephalus; F. H. Allen,[3] a case of cyclopia; C. Douglas,[4] and Brayn and Stuck,[5] each a case of hemicephalus; Newman Dorland,[6] a case of diprosopus; A. Brothers,[7] A. C. Dutt,[8] F. Bolster,[9] and S. Mellor,[10] each a case of anencephalus; Dujon,[11] a case of syncephalus in a sheep; I. Miller,[12] a case of exencephalia with supplemental sac; W. J. C. Coulthard,[13] 1 case, R. H. D. Mahon,[14] 2 cases, and J. L. Kerr,[15] 2 cases of anencephalus; C. N. Ballard,[16] a case of exencephalus; E. H. Root,[17] a case of monomphalic ischiopagus; M. V. Ball,[18] a case of notoencephalus; K. Maydl,[19] a case of inclusio fœtalis abdominalis; Lop and Pujol,[20] a case of iniencephalus or retroflexion of the fetus; Chaillons and Desfosses,[21] a case of hemimelus; A. Stern,[22] a case of perodactylus symmetricus in a female child 6 years of age; E. A. Tucker,[23] 2 cases of intrauterine amputation; M. Günsburg,[24] a case of paracephalus in a quadruplet birth; W. Bradley,[25] an unusual succession of monsters, the patient giving birth first to a 7 months' anencephalic fetus; 18 months later to a full-term anencephalic fetus with a cystic tumor extending from the edges of the bones of the base of the skull; it started from the top of the forehead, forming three folds, and hanging down the back to the middle of the dorsal region; it was covered with fine hair and was soft; 3 years later a third anencephalic fetus was born at the 7th or 8th month; C. G. Grant,[26] a case of ectocardia, the child living for nearly 6 hours; S. K. Church,[27] a case of exomphalos, living for 36 hours; Joachimsthal,[28] a fetal malformation resulting from advanced extrauterine pregnancy; in addition to marked distortion of the extremities there was a large meningocele; L. Wendling,[29] a case of hydrorrachis; and J. H. Raymond,[30] a case of congenital irreducible umbilical hernia occurring in a double uterus. In Ball's case the fetus presented on the posterior portion of the head a huge tumor larger than the head itself, which contained the cerebral hemispheres; the child lived for about 15 minutes after birth. Sangalli's case showed projecting from the mouth of a female fetus a large mass of rudimentary connective and epithelial tissue, containing cells in process of transformation into bone-corpuscles and muscular fibers, both organic and striated;

[1] Centralbl. f. Gynäk., No. 28 1896.
[2] Jour. Am. Med. Assoc., Feb. 27, 1897.
[3] Med. Rec, Aug. 15, 1896.
[4] Brit. Med. Jour., Jan. 30, 1897.
[5] Ibid., Dec. 19, 1896.
[6] Univ. Med. Mag., Nov., 1896.
[7] Arch. of Pediatrics, Aug., 1896.
[8] Brit. Med. Jour., May 1, 1897.
[9] Ibid., May 29, 1897.
[10] Lancet, June 26, 1897.
[11] Jour. de Méd. de Paris, Jan. 24, 1897.
[12] N. Y. Med. Jour., May 1, 1897.
[13] Lancet, Oct. 17, 1896.
[14] Ibid., Sept. 12, 1896.
[15] Ibid., Aug. 8, 1896.
[16] Am. Gyn. and Obst. Jour., Dec., 1896.
[17] Jour. Am. Med. Assoc., Dec. 12, 1896.
[18] Phila. Polyclinic, July 4, 1896.
[19] Wien. klin. Rundschau, x., No. 17, p. 295, 1896.
[20] Rev. Obstét. Internat., No. 52, June 1, 1896.
[21] Bull. de la Soc. anat. de Paris, 5 S., x., p. 308, 1896.
[22] Am. Jour. of Obst., Mar., 1897.
[23] Am. Gyn. and Obst. Jour., Sept., 1896.
[24] Edinb. Med. Jour., Aug., 1896.
[25] Brit. Med. Jour., Jan. 9, 1897.
[26] Ibid., Dec. 5, 1896.
[27] N. Y. Med. Jour., Jan. 16, 1897.
[28] Berlin. klin. Woch., Jan. 25, 1897.
[29] Wien. med. Woch., Nov. 28, 1896.
[70] Med. Rec., Oct. 10, 1896.

g strength t
ging on lal
gauze
vera[1]

th st
d, and
ved the u
en the ta
rer was able
33d week, w
The infant w
ame normal in stre
illustrating the si
and thus confirms
ech gave the drug i
and second doses w
g ceased. With the e
effects were observed. I
m, tincture of iodin, and coc

rdiac Disease.—L. Demel
g 5162 cases of labor in the so
d through 162 pregnancies, in
r symptom attributable to the ha
be attributable to the heart-lesons
or grave), 23 cases; bronchtis,
minuria (cardiac), 12; gastrokpat

, Aug., 1896.   [2] Cenralbl.
ug. 15, 1896.   [4] L'bstét., u

: uterine emorrhages of pregnancy, 9 ; postpartum hemor-

mothers die a mortality of only 3%. This small mortality,
th tha giv by other obstetricians, he attributes to the fact
e. the heart not examined unless serious, often fatal, heart-
st ; and man mild cases of true cardiac disease go through preg-
childbirth unobserved. One of the fatal cases was due to uremic
ie other occurred in a rachitic patient with a fatty degenerated
relates 2 cases which the patients became cyanotic, with much-
d heart and respiratory action, yet recovered. One of these,
ly ill with her fit parturition, passed through a second without a
tom. The total ortality was 15 out of the 162, including 4 abor-
11 deaths of premature infants.

follows : mitral insufficiency, 22 cases ; mitral
aortic, 2 : aortic and mitral, 4 ; myocarditis, 2 ;

n therapeutic deductions: "The mere finding of a
patient motive for intervention. Conception, child-
ble and even perfectly easy among those with car-

2 grand conditions : (1) the anatomic-physi-
; (2) the anatomic-physiologic state of the large

labor, even the interruption of pregnancy,
when menacing accidents appear more or
spontaneous tendency to the expulsion of the
should be followed in turn : (1) medical
e powerful action ought not to be mis-
interruption of pregnancy in the gravest
n the occurrence of a perfectly spon-
women with heart-disease, and they also
n is a localized form of cardiac dropsy.
patient, the subject of chronic heart-dis-
1 miscarriage without distressing cardiac
ney, however, she began to suffer from
Pregnancy is always liable to cause seri-
ary circulation and to throw additional
suffer from mitral lesions, which rapidly
ntly manifest toward the fifth or sixth
dyspnea and hemoptysis. It is yet obvi-
ain point may suffer no inconvenience from
e must not be drawn in advising or with-
wishes and ideas of the patient must be
and injurious effect upon the heart of with-
he lesion and the absence or presence of
noticed, the latter forming a decided bar
treatment upon this condition should deter-
tion and surroundings of the patient and
ed rest, if necessary, should be considered.
—2 or 3 liters should be taken daily from
ney. This is a powerful aid to the circu-

tét. et Gynéc. de Paris, Apr., 1897.

there were also scales of bone and formless tracts of pale and red muscular fibers. The head of Günsburg's ease resembled a fleshy malformed mass, broad in its upper and narrow in its lower part. The occipital bone was absent, and the facial portions of the frontal bones also. The eyes, mouth, and ears were absent; the nose was normal. In the middle part of the face and from prominences corresponding to the zygomatic bones two muscular masses passed downward and ended by converging in the region of the clavicles. Similar muscular masses passed from the posterior part of the head to the back. The sternum was absent, and in its place was a thin membrane, under which one could see the organs of the thoracic cavity. The upper limbs were deformed. The forearm ended in three eminences resembling fingers. The abdomen showed a fissure through which a portion of the intestine was prolapsed. Dorland's case (see Fig. 31) was one of *diprosopus tetrophthalmus*

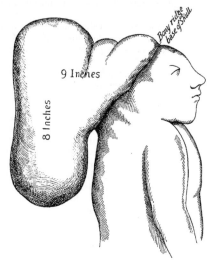

Fig 30.—Bradley's case of cystic anencephalus. From a sketch taken at the time (Brit Med. Jour., Jan. 9, 1897).

with four eyes but only two ears—referred to him by his brother-in-law, Dr. J. B. Thompson, of Siam. The child survived 15 days, dying eventually of inanition induced by inability to retain the nourishment taken, the milk introduced through one mouth being regurgitated through the other, thus proving the existence of a common esophagus opening into the two oral cavities. In Allen's ease the nasal bones were absent, while the orbits were united, thereby forming a large, quadrangular eye, situated near the center of the face; a fleshy teat hung over it. The child survived 30 minutes. Lewis has collected 22 cases of iniencephalus, including his own.

Olano[1] performed an autopsy upon a well-formed woman, aged 39, who had died after 4 days of labor-pains and an unsuccessful attempt to deliver the child by forceps. The fundus of the uterus was just under the liver. It con-

[1] St. Louis M. and S. Jour., Apr., 1897.

tained a well-formed female fetus with the head downward, which measured 68 cm. (27 in.), and weighed 10,000 gm. (26 pounds). The mother had had 3 normal and 2 premature confinements. The woman was said to be much beyond term.

Councilman [1] quotes some interesting observations as to the frequency of malformations. Peusch has found that malformations are more frequent in

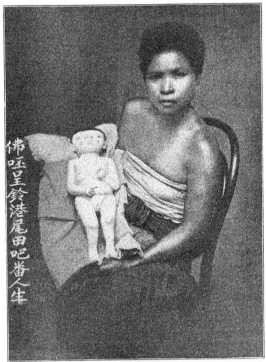

佛哑呈鈴港尾田吧番人生

Fɪɢ. 31.—A diprosopic monstrosity (Dorland, in Univ. Med. Mag., Nov , 1896).

illegitimate than in legitimate children. All malformations are more frequent in females than in males. In 100,000 births Peusch has found 454 simple malformations, 61 single monstrosities, and 2 double monstrosities. There is a considerable difference in the species of animal in the frequency with which malformations are found. They are more common in the hog, cat, and cow than they are in the horse and goat. In general, malformations are due to excess of development, defect of development, or to the persistence of embryonic conditions. They are especially apt to occur in those parts of the body in which there is the greatest complexity in development.

[1] Boston M. and S. Jour., Jan. 14, 1897.

THE PATHOLOGY OF PREGNANCY.

The Pernicious Vomiting of Pregnancy.—J. Fabre [1] notes a case of uncontrollable vomiting in a primipara, 18 years of age, who had previously suffered from anemia and hysteria. The vomiting began at the fifth month of pregnancy, and had continued up to $8\frac{1}{2}$ months, with increasing weakness. The fetal heart was not to be heard, yet the vomiting continued, and medicinal means were of no avail; it was therefore decided to induce premature labor, and Krause's method (introduction of a bougie into the uterus) was employed. On the day before this was done the patient was so weak as to require injections of caffein and ether, and of 200 gm. of artificial serum into the subcutaneous tissue of the abdomen. Twelve hours after the introduction of the bougie into the uterus a dead female fetus was delivered by forceps. The vomiting still continued, and the patient died 12 hours later. The only lesions found at the necropsy were those of recent gastritis. [The case is interesting, for the death of the fetus was not followed by a cessation of the vomiting, a circumstance probably due to the fact that here pregnancy was not the sole factor, but had superadded to it the pathologic state of the stomach.]

Kehrer [2] reports the case of a hysteric woman, aged 21, who not long after marriage aborted at 4 months. During this brief pregnancy she had been greatly troubled with nausea and vomiting, which were not relieved by narcotics. She soon became pregnant again, and at once began to suffer severely from nausea. After various remedies had been tried, including the application of a solution of silver nitrat, an effort was made to end the nausea by partially dilating the cervix with the finger. While very brief improvement followed, no permanent cure resulted. The patient's condition became so serious through weakness, loss of flesh, and failing strength that it was determined to empty the uterus. With a view to bringing on labor-pains, Kehrer tamponed the os and cervix with strips of sterile gauze soaked in glycerin. The nausea immediately stopped, and a period of several days, in which the patient was free entirely, followed the use of the tampon. After a short time the symptoms reappeared, when the tampon was again employed with a similarly successful result. Kehrer was able by this method to carry the patient along in pregnancy until the 33d week, when labor was induced, and she was delivered of a living child. The infant was at first partially asphyxiated, but speedily revived, and became normal in strength and weight.

Reeh [3] reports a case illustrating the successful use of basic orexin in the vomiting of pregnancy, and thus confirms the favorable report of Frommel published in 1893. Reeh gave the drug in doses of $4\frac{1}{2}$ gr. in capsules, 3 times daily. The first and second doses were not retained, but after the third dose the vomiting ceased. With the exception of a burning sensation in the mouth no ill-effects were observed. In the case reported nux vomica, bromids, chloroform, tincture of iodin, and cocain had been employed without success.

Valvular Cardiac Disease.—L. Demelin [4] observed 64 cases of cardiac disease among 5162 cases of labor in the service of Tarnier. These 64 women had passed through 162 pregnancies, in 107 of which there was no serious accident or symptom attributable to the heart, a percentage of 66. The accidents that can be attributable to the heart-lesions are classified as follows: dyspnea (notable or grave), 23 cases; bronchitis, 3; syncope, 7; edema (marked), 7; albuminuria (cardiac), 12; gastrohepatic accidents, 2; epistaxis

[1] Marseille Méd., Aug., 1896.   [2] Centralbl. f. Gynäk., No. 15, 1896.
[4] Ibid., No. 37, Aug. 15, 1896.   [3] L'Obstét., Jan. 15, 1896.

and hemoptysis, 5 ; uterine hemorrhages of pregnancy, 9 ; postpartum hemorrhages, 7.

Two of the mothers died, a mortality of only 3%. This small mortality, as compared with that given by other obstetricians, he attributes to the fact that, as a rule, the heart is not examined unless serious, often fatal, heart-symptoms exist ; and many mild cases of true cardiac disease go through pregnancy and childbirth unobserved. One of the fatal cases was due to uremic accidents ; the other occurred in a rachitic patient with a fatty degenerated heart. He relates 2 cases in which the patients became cyanotic, with much-embarrassed heart and respiratory action, yet recovered. One of these, dangerously ill with her first parturition, passed through a second without a bad symptom. The fetal mortality was 15 out of the 162, including 4 abortions and 11 deaths of premature infants.

The cardiac lesions were as follows : mitral insufficiency, 22 cases ; mitral stenosis, 6 ; double mitral, 3 ; aortic, 2 ; aortic and mitral, 4 ; myocarditis, 2 ; adhesive pericarditis, 1.

He draws the following therapeutic deductions : " The mere finding of a valvular souffle is an insufficient motive for intervention. Conception, childbirth, and nursing are possible and even perfectly easy among those with cardiac disease.

" All essentially depends on 2 grand conditions : (1) the anatomic-physiologic state of the myocardium ; (2) the anatomic-physiologic state of the large emunctories (liver and kidneys).

" The artificial termination of labor, even the interruption of pregnancy, is demanded in grave cases. But when menacing accidents appear more or less far from term, and without a spontaneous tendency to the expulsion of the fetus, the following therapeutic means should be followed in turn : (1) medical and dietetic means ; (2) bleeding, whose powerful action ought not to be misunderstood or neglected ; (3) artificial interruption of pregnancy in the gravest cases." Bornet and Grimodie[1] mention the occurrence of a perfectly spontaneous form of abortion in pregnant women with heart-disease, and they also believe that hydrorrhea during gestation is a localized form of cardiac dropsy.

Jaccoud[2] relates a case in which a patient, the subject of chronic heart-disease, passed through 3 childbirths and 1 miscarriage without distressing cardiac symptoms. After the fourth pregnancy, however, she began to suffer from symptoms of cardiac break-down. [Pregnancy is always liable to cause serious disturbances of the cardiopulmonary circulation and to throw additional work on the heart. Patients who suffer from mitral lesions, which rapidly affect the lesser circulation, frequently manifest toward the fifth or sixth month gravidocardiac symptoms, as dyspnea and hemoptysis. It is yet obvious that a diseased heart up to a certain point may suffer no inconvenience from pregnancy. A too hard-and-fast line must not be drawn in advising or withholding consent to marriage. The wishes and ideas of the patient must be considered, and also the depressing and injurious effect upon the heart of withholding consent. The degree of the lesion and the absence or presence of gravidocardiac symptoms should be noticed, the latter forming a decided bar to marriage, though the effect of treatment upon this condition should determine the final decision. The occupation and surroundings of the patient and the possibility of her taking prolonged rest, if necessary, should be considered. A milk-diet is of great importance,—2 or 3 liters should be taken daily from the second or third month of pregnancy. This is a powerful aid to the circu-

[1] Bull. et Mém. de la Soc. Obstét. et Gynéc. de Paris, Apr., 1897.
[2] Sem. méd., Sept. 11, 1896.

lation by reason of its diuretic action, and not only are the gravidocardiac symptoms warded off, but the appearance of albumin in the urine is prevented.]

Pregnancy and the Thyroid Gland.—Bignami[1] reports the ease of a patient who passed through her first pregnancy without trouble, but a bronchocele developed during the second, and the thyroid gradually returned to its original size after delivery. During the third pregnancy the swelling reappeared, and there were much constitutional disturbance, dyspnea, and dysphagia. The patient died suddenly in the 8th month, and neither tracheotomy nor Cesarean section could be performed. There was no necropsy. [Pregnancy has a bad effect on all bronchoceles, but there is a true or special bronchocele of pregnancy which does not develop until gestation commences, and disappears or diminishes after delivery, to return at the next pregnancy. It is always vascular, and as dangerous symptoms may set in the induction of premature labor is often advisable.]

Albuminuria and Nephritis in Pregnancy.—[The albuminuria of pregnancy holds, with grave valvular lesions, the foremost place in the pathology of pregnancy, as the ever-increasing literature of the subject indicates.] T. C. Allbutt[2] believes that the opinion that the renal complications of pregnancy are due merely to mechanical pressure is erroneous. In the first place, he claims that pressure by the enlarged uterus upon the renal veins is not readily produced; again, complete thrombosis of the renal veins is not followed by renal symptoms which are averted by collateral circulation. Moreover, swelling of the legs and other signs of venous obstruction are more frequent as pregnancies increase in number, whereas albuminuria and eclampsia are evils of the primipara. Again, other large tumors, as fibroids, do not produce serious kidney-disorders, though disturbances of micturition and even pressure on. the ureters, followed by dilatation of these tubes, and even by pyelitis, may occur. In pregnancy there is little evidence of serious pressure on the ureters, and dilatation of these tubes is rarely a complication. The *puerperal kidney* differs from the *cardiac kidney* in that it is not as hard, is often pale, and presents signs of acute degenerative processes penetrating its tissues. It would seem that two poisons at least are concerned in the production of the disease, the one leading to convulsions, the other to coma. In some not infrequent cases the two acting together produce convulsions followed by coma. It is now generally conceded that there is a toxin as yet unseparated in healthy urine. It is not urea, uric acid, kreatinin, nor potassium chlorid. Thudichum thinks that it lies in the coloring-matters of the urine. Allbutt thinks it most probable that the toxin is absorbed from the bowel, for it is less in amount in a fasting animal, in hibernation, and in the urine after sleep. The point of formation of the toxin is also unknown, but it is probable that the liver is at fault, as is suggested by the frequency of liver-disease in pregnant women. Saft[3] believes that the condition is caused by an autointoxication by some product of tissue-change, as is the origin of the molimina graviditatis and of the nervous disturbances of the pregnant state. Eklund[4] states that if the urine be found to contain albumin the patient should be ordered hot baths, flannel underwear, rest in the recumbent posture, mild diuretics and laxatives, beef-tea with parsley, seltzer water with boiling milk, milk-food, boiled fruit, weak coffee, tea, and chocolate, and compound licorice-powder. It is a matter of great importance that the pregnant woman should learn to procure for herself daily evacuations of the bowels, especially toward the end of pregnancy and in beginning labor. For this purpose dietetic means should be employed chiefly,

[1] Wien. med. Bl., Nos. 4 and 5, 1896.   [2] Lancet, Feb. 27, 1897.
[3] Arch. f. Gynäk., Bd. li., No. 7, 1896.   [4] Edinb. Med. Jour., Dec., 1896.

but in case of failure mild aperients should be used, as caseara, senna, frangula, compound licorice-powder, and enemata of salt and water. Of the very greatest importance during pregnancy, and especially during the puerperal state, is the care of the kidneys, the avoidance of all that would tend to increase the functional activity of these organs, the maintenance of equilibrium, and the proper division of labor between the skin, digestive apparatus, and the kidneys. If any organ can bear a greater exercise of function, it is the skin, and next in order of tolerance the intestinal tract ; the lungs are far more sensitive, but the kidneys most of all. If possible, no puerperal woman should be permitted to leave her bed until her urine is free from albumin.

E. H. Grandin [1] especially emphasizes the value of hot saline irrigation of the intestines in case of uremia either complicating labor or some operative procedure. The strength of the solution should be about 1 %, and the temperature of the water in the receiver about 118° F. From 8 to 10 gallons of water should be allowed to flow into the bowel, the gravity syringe being hung at least 6 feet above the head of the patient. This should be supplemented by the use of croton oil and hypodermics of glonoin, $\frac{1}{75}$ gr., repeated $\frac{1}{2}$-hourly until the physiologic effect has been secured. This drug offers the readiest of all means for relaxing the spasm of the renal capillaries.

Mynlieff [2] insists that when a woman with chronic nephritis becomes pregnant the induction of abortion is indicated on account of the immediate peril of the patient (which increases as pregnancy advances), the certain continuance of the morbid process in the kidneys themselves, the great tendency to flooding and abortion, and the small prospect of the development of the fetus to term. Mynlieff dwells on the responsibilities of the physician who is called in when pregnancy is advanced. The induction of premature labor may then be undertaken at a time which seems most favorable for saving the fetus—that is to say, a little delay may be allowed ; but the history of previous pregnancies must be duly considered, and if it is found that the fetus tends to die at a certain date in pregnancy that date must be anticipated. In any case the life of the mother must be considered first ; hence, up to the last, immediate interference is usually the safest course. The same principle is often best for the fetus when viable, as it may die suddenly earlier than in previous pregnancies.

Sevitsky [3] describes a case in which he noted symptoms of uremia in a primipara 1 month before delivery. On the 2d day after labor the patient became semicomatose and perfectly blind. The urine was found to contain casts and was highly albuminous. Notwithstanding this no convulsions occurred, and the patient made a rapid recovery. From this Sevitsky concludes that uremia alone does not cause puerperal convulsions.

Pregnancy and Labor after Nephrectomy.—Cases are reported by Schramm [4] and E. Tridondani.[5] Schramm's patient was a workingwoman, aged 25 years, who had borne 2 children. She requested the removal of a tumor in her right side which was increasing in size and causing suffering. This proved to be a hydronephrotic kidney, which was removed, the patient making a good recovery. Three years after she asked her physician's advice regarding marriage, and, as her general health was good and the remaining kidney performed its function well, a possible pregnancy did not seem necessarily dangerous. This subsequently occurred and was endured safely, the urine being abundant and containing no casts or kidney-epithelium, but albumin only. The patient was delivered in spontaneous labor of a healthy

[1] Am. Medico-Surg. Bull., Sept. 26, 1896.   [2] Der Frauenarzt, Jan. 1, 1896.
[3] Ann. de Gynéc. et d'Obstét., Aug., 1896.   [4] Berlin. klin. Woch., No. 6, 1896.
[5] Ann. di Ost. e Gin., July, 1896.

child, and made a good recovery. But 2 similar cases (Fritsch, Israel) are recorded.

Tridondani's case was of more than usual interest. A patient, aged 29, came into the Maternity at Pavia suffering from symptoms resembling those of intestinal obstruction, accompanied with pain on micturition and scanty urine. She was in the 8th month of pregnancy, and to the left side of the uterus was a fluctuating tumor. Under treatment, the symptoms improved, and the woman was spontaneously delivered of a male infant. Three months later the abdomen was opened and a cystic kidney (the left) was removed. Recovery was complete. Since then the patient has had 3 pregnancies. In none of the 3 were there any abnormal symptoms. There was no edema, and the urine was normal in quantity and quality. The labors were at term and non-instrumental. The placenta and membranes in each case were healthy, and the puerperium was normal. The infants were born alive, were healthy, and had a weight and size above the average. The author concludes, from a study of this and the 3 other reported cases, that pregnancy occurring in a woman with one kidney does not interfere with her health; that the absence of a kidney does not disturb the progress of gestation, labor, and the puerperium, and that the product of conception does not suffer. He does not, therefore, agree with Schramm, who advises that a woman with a single kidney should not marry, or, if married already, should not become pregnant. It is noteworthy that in the above case the liquor amnii was increased in amount; but it is doubtful whether this was a consequence of the absence of one of the mother's kidneys.

Mental Disease in Pregnancy.—Geo. H. Savage[1] classifies the insanity of pregnancy into—(*a*) mental disorders occurring in the early or later months of pregnancy; (*b*) insanity of labor; (*c*) associated with febrile disorder at the establishment of milk-secretion; (*d*) occurring within the first two weeks subsequent to labor; (*e*) between two and six weeks subsequent to labor; (*f*) insanity of lactation and that of weaning.

Savage does not believe that there is a special, definite form of insanity deserving the name of "puerperal mania." The predisposing causes are similar for all the forms of the disorder, heredity being the most important factor. First pregnancies, especially if after the age of 30, are considered more dangerous than earlier pregnancies. Illegitimacy has a doubtful influence. The induction of premature labor as a cure for insanity Savage believes to be far from justifiable in every instance. Within the first two weeks after delivery maniacal symptoms are most common with puerperal insanity; whereas, if developed later, melancholia is more frequent. Savage questions the advisability of the marriage of neurotics, especially if of a pronounced hysteric tendency, because of the danger involved in childbearing by such persons. The term "puerperal insanity" may be ascribed more justly to a group having sepsis as the etiologic factor. The questions involved as to the treatment have reference to the etiology, the use of hypnotic drugs, the removal from home to more favorable surroundings, or the placing of the patient in an asylum.

Chorea Gravidarum.—An interesting case of major chorea gravidarum is reported by W. E. F. Finley.[2] The patient was a primipara, illegitimately pregnant at 5 months. She had had one previous attack of minor chorea, had had rheumatism, and belonged to a neurotic family. Her expression was idiotic, and she emitted peculiar laughing sounds from time to time, owing to the involuntary contraction of the chest-muscles. She was unable to drink, as the greater part of the liquid ran out of her mouth; her tongue was much swollen and very dirty; from the right side of it she had bitten a piece as

[1] Brit. Gyn. Jour., xliv., p. 559, 1896.   [2] Brit. Med. Jour., Oct. 17, 1896.

large as a shilling, and from the other side one the size of a sixpence. The involuntary movements continued day and night, so that she never got sleep. When put into bed her head was dashed about, sometimes with great violence; the violent motions of her legs threw off the bed-clothes, and at times she herself was thrown from the bed. Iron, iodin, arsenic, bromids, and chloral were all ineffectual, as were also opium and hypodermics of morphin. Labor was induced under chloroform, but on the following day the patient suddenly collapsed and died within an hour.

Peripheral Neuritis in Pregnancy.—G. Elder[1] has recently seen two cases of peripheral neuritis, both in multiparæ; both came on about the sixth month. The symptoms began with tingling and shooting paresthesiæ, which gradually increased until the shooting-pains and feelings of pins and needles were very severe and disturbed health. In both they were chiefly in the hands, but in one of the cases also in the feet. Sensation was affected in both cases to some extent, but there was little or no paresis, although, owing to loss of sensation, no fine work requiring careful coordination could be done by the hands. In neither case could any other cause of neuritis be discovered— alcohol, diphtheria, influenza, pneumonia, albuminuria, glycosuria, typhoid, and lead being excluded. Both began to recover immediately after delivery, and recovery was pretty rapid—in one case in three or four weeks, in the other in three to four months. There could be no doubt, he thought, that the gravid state was the exciting cause of the neuritis. The number of cases of peripheral neuritis, evidently due to pregnancy, reported were very few (he could only find eight cases in all); and nearly all of these had been preceded by severe vomiting, and all had been very severe cases. He was inclined to believe that the cases of peripheral neuritis in pregnancy of a mild type must be very much more common than one would expect from the number of cases reported. That vomiting was not necessary to produce the condition his cases showed, and it was just possible that the vomiting might be due to the same cause as the neuritis, and to be only a concomitant symptom. The neuritis was evidently toxemic in origin, though there was no evidence as to what the exact nature of the poison was. Some recent writers were of opinion that some of the cases of peripheral neuritis found during the puerperium had really commenced during pregnancy. If the symptoms got very severe, it would be one's duty to terminate the labor, as after delivery recovery sets in. [Solowjeff and Polk have each reported a fatal ease of peripheral neuritis in pregnancy. Remembering this fact, that the disease may prove fatal, one must be prepared to induce labor before the disease has advanced too far, for as soon as the uterus is emptied there is naturally a tendency to recovery.]

The Influence Exerted by Pulmonary Disease in the Mother upon the Health of the Fetus.—Chambrelent,[2] in discussing this subject, states that in order to explain disease or death of the fetus in cases of maternal pulmonary affections classical authors invoke particularly three causes: the coughing-efforts of the mother, which provoke abortion, asphyxia and its action upon uterine contractility, and hyperthermia and its role in premature labors. Chambrelent has proved, by a series of experiments, that the influence of these three causes is very mediocre, if not entirely absent, and that it is necessary to take into consideration another factor which the older teachers did not recognize—namely, poisoning of the fetus by the bacilli and their toxins. He has demonstrated that if, after having infected the lung, the pneumococci, streptococci, staphylococci, and the bacilli of tuberculosis should penetrate into the circulatory system of the mother and thus produce a generalized infection,

[1] Lancet, July 25, 1896.   [2] Bull. de l'Acad. de Méd., Sept. 22, 1896.

they will traverse the placenta, and thereby reach the fetus, which they in turn will poison. The proof of this is that he has found in the brain, heart, lung, and peritoneal serosa of the fetus the same microbes as were in the lungs and blood of the mother.

Retroversion of the Pregnant Uterus.—This interesting and serious complication of pregnancy has been studied by M. Cameron[1] and Chaleix and G. Fieux.[2] Cameron believes that in the majority of cases the condition is probably due to previous displacement, but that it occasionally arises acutely from a strain or a fall. Overdistention of the bladder is more frequently an effect than a cause, but once retroversion has taken place an overdistended bladder will tend to aggravate the condition and prevent its cure. In fatal cases death has occurred from the manipulations, or from necrosis of the tissues. The symptoms enumerated in those cases that terminated fatally were : (1) retention of urine ; (2) febrile symptoms ; (3) bearing-down pains at the pelvic outlet, with anxiety and great restlessness ; (4) delirium ; (5) intermittent pulse ; (6) coldness of the extremities, moribund sweats, and convulsions ; (7) in a number of cases rupture of the bladder. He reports a case of pregnancy of 4 months, in which the uterus was retroverted, the bladder being enormously distended. Eighty ounces of urine were drawn off. On the next day blood appeared in the urine ; and later a blood-cast of the ureter, some 15 in. in length, was withdrawn. Ten days later abdominal section was done, and the bladder opened and cleared of blood-clots. The bladder then contracted, and it was possible to reach the uterus. By combined pressure from below through the vagina and traction through the abdominal wound from above the incarcerated uterus was pulled out of the pelvis. The patient made a good recovery, blood disappeared from the urine, and she was delivered, at full term, of a large, healthy child.

Chaleix and Fieux report 3 cases of retained dead fetuses in retroflexed uteri. In the first case the embryo, perishing in the third month of gestation, was expelled 8 months later. It was then of a peculiar greenish color. The second patient had the symptoms of missed abortion at about the sixth or seventh week of pregnancy, and 3 months later expelled the small ovum intact. The third patient expelled an embryo in the fourth month of gestation, 1 month after its death. The authors advance the theory that in extreme retroflexion, with a sharp angle of flexion at the cervical junction, geniculation of the uterine arteries occurs ; also that geniculation and compression of the utero-ovarian arteries take place at the sharp border of the broad ligaments, both of which factors lead to the death of the fetus by diminishing blood-supply to the uterus.

Missed Abortion.—In addition to the foregoing cases occurring in and due to retroflexion of the gravid uterus, additional cases of so-called missed abortion have been recorded by P. G. Griffith,[3] F. R. Eccles,[4] Biot[5] (3 cases), and Graefe.[6] Griffith's case was probably one of twin-pregnancy, with death of one embryo at 4 months and its discharge 2 years after the birth of its twin. Graefe states that he has not yet been able to arrive at any certain information as to the etiology of these cases from microscopic examination, although he has personally observed 11 cases and collected 59 reported ones. Retrograde metamorphosis in the ovum is evident after prolonged retention. The mucous tissue becomes converted into more or less rigid connective tissue, but may even be preserved in places or show patches of growth after months of retention. The more the

[1] Brit. Med. Jour., Oct. 31, 1896.   [2] Am. Gyn. and Obst. Jour., Nov., 1896.
[3] Brit. Med. Jour., Sept. 19, 1896.   [4] Canad. Pract., July, 1896.
[5] Lyon méd., Feb. 28, 1897.   [6] Münch. med. Woch., Nov. 4, 1896.

fruit may be developed at the time of its death, the greater the danger for the mother. The uterus should be emptied as soon as the diagnosis has been established. If this be before 5 months, the uterus may be emptied by dilatation under ether and clearing the uterine cavity with the finger. If the diagnosis be made later than 5 months, premature labor should be induced.

Carcinoma of the Cervix in Pregnancy.—[The rarity of this complication is shown by the fact that in 42,000 cases of pregnancy observed in 3 great obstetric clinics only 22 cases of carcinoma were found.] G. H. Noble[1] has collected 166 cases of carcinoma of the pregnant uterus occurring since 1886, and from the data thus afforded an attempt is made to arrive at some conclusions as to the best methods of treatment. In cases of early pregnancy, when the disease has not yet extended beyond the cervix, vaginal hysterectomy should be performed at once; but if pregnancy is too far advanced to permit of extirpation by the vaginal route, he considers that it is better to perform Freund's operation rather than waste time in emptying the uterus and subsequently extirpating the organ, thus reduced in size, through the vagina. He finds, however, that statistics show that vaginal hysterectomy, when performed in the early weeks of the puerperium, does not appear to be attended with any additional risks. At full term Cesarean section followed by total extirpation is the ideal operation if the fetus cannot be born through the natural passages; but if there is any extension of growth into the parametric tissue, the Cesarean section alone should be done. [He gives no information as to the relative frequency of operable and inoperable cases occurring during pregnancy, but it is probable that in the majority of such cases we could not hold out much hope of a permanent cure after a radical operation. Neither of the above-mentioned authors makes clear the line of action to be adopted when the pregnancy has advanced to the sixth or seventh month, and the carcinomatous infiltration has already passed beyond the limits of the cervical tissue.] As J. Sinclair[2] suggests, in cases of advanced carcinoma at full term the fetal and maternal mortality is very high. If operative measures be adopted for the purpose of extracting the child through the vagina, there is great danger of tearing the cervix or uterus, and also of septic infection. Experience appears to point to the following conclusions with regard to cases at term: (1) spontaneous delivery if possible, even though labor be prolonged, gives the best result for the mother, but the fetal mortality is very high; (2) if the disease be so far advanced that delivery cannot take place without operative interference, the Cesarean operation gives the best result for both mother and child. [Generally speaking, when the disease is not too far advanced the operation of total extirpation should be performed without delay, whatever the period of pregnancy may be. Within the first 4 months of pregnancy the uterus may be extirpated by the vaginal route unemptied; but later it is necessary first to induce abortion, and then, 2 or 3 weeks later, to proceed to vaginal hysterectomy. If septic endometritis follows the abortion—which, when the growth is in a sloughing condition, is not uncommon—the uterus should be extirpated forthwith. Beckman has collected 17 cases in which the unemptied pregnant uterus was removed, within the first 4 months of gestation, by the vaginal route, for carcinoma of the cervix, without a single fatality.]

Traumatisms and Operations during Pregnancy.—Villa[3] has amputated a chronically inflamed cervix during pregnancy, with a good result in curing the local disease and without interrupting the gestation. In another case reflex disturbances were so severe that abortion occurred, although the

---

[1] Am. Jour. of Obst., June, 1896.   [2] Med. Chron., May, 1896.
[3] Ann. di Ost. e Gin., No. 4, 1896.

local treatment was limited to glycerin-tampons and lotions. He has also sutured a torn cervix in pregnancy, without abortion. S. Sutton[1] has removed from one patient a large cyst of the broad ligament and from another both ovaries and tubes during pregnancy, without the induction of abortion. The second patient subsequently gave birth to twins. Mouchet[2] performed a double ovariectomy in the third month of gestation without untoward results. J. D. Jones[3] records a case of strangulated ovarian cyst complicating pregnancy. Twenty-six days after the operation she miscarried at the sixth month. A. C. Butler-Smythe[4] delivered a woman at term, the pregnancy being complicated by an ovarian cyst, which spontaneously ruptured 19 days after labor without and ill effects. [The treatment of this complication—ovarian cyst in pregnancy—is preferably by abdominal section. In cases that are allowed to go to term the prognosis is not so good. Litzmann records 24 deaths in 56 labors (43%); Jetter gives the death-rate at about 30%; Heiberg found in 271 cases that 25% of the mothers and 75% of the children died. Ovariectomy gives a very low mortality for the mother—1% or less; while a large proportion of the cases advance to term, and thereby the fetal mortality is lessened.]

F. W. N. Haultain[5] reports 8 patients in whom pregnancy was complicated by uterine fibromyomata, with 2 deaths. He concludes that fibromyomata of the uterus tend to cause sterility by preventing conception and tending toward abortion, should they be so placed or have attained such dimensions as to cause symptoms of their presence in the non-pregnant condition. As regards diagnosis of pregnancy when fibroids also are present, this is often difficult, the tendency being for the pregnancy, on the one hand, by softening these growths, to change the normal " feel," while, on the other, the irregular hemorrhages due to the fibroid tend to mask the ordinary symptoms of pregnancy. Though in a large number of instances the course of pregnancy is in no way influenced by the coexistence of fibroids, their presence considerably increases the risks of pregnancy by complicating labor in preventing ready expulsion of the ovum and predisposing to severe hemorrhage. The prognosis depends on the site and size of the tumor. Thus, when subperitoneal, unless the growth be of sufficient dimensions to cause severe pressure on surrounding organs, or is incarcerated in the true pelvis and thereby obstructs the passages, little or no inconvenience is, as a rule, to be anticipated. Even in these cases, however, retrograde changes in the tumor—that is, suppuration and necrosis—may occasion fatal consequences. With the interstitial and submucous varieties the association of pregnancy must be considered of grave import.

Bossi[6] stated before the Obstetric Society of France that he had observed 14 cases of fibroids complicating pregnancy. In 5 cases premature labor was brought on, and in 4 of these the tumors disappeared entirely. In the remaining 9 cases, in which labor was normal, the tumors all disappeared during or after labor. Budin recalled an instance in which a lawsuit had been brought against G. Thomas, of New York, by a woman whom he had been treating a long time for a fibroid. She became pregnant and the tumor disappeared. She then sued the doctor for malpractice, claiming that she had been treated for a tumor which had never existed. Dorland has met recently two instances of fibroid complicating pregnancy, in both cases the tumors, which were situated in the anterior uterine wall, disappearing during the puerperium. In one case a transverse presentation was produced, and in the other preparations were made for a Cesarean section; the tumor ascended, however,

[1] Med. Rec., Oct. 10, 1896.
[2] Sem. méd., No. 31, 1896.
[3] Med. Rec., Mar. 20, 1896.
[4] Lancet, Sept. 19, 1896.
[5] Practitioner, No. 337, p. 38, July, 1896.
[6] Sem. méd., No. 19, p. 148, 1896.

during the progress of labor, and the delivery was spontaneous. A. Vander-veer[1] reports 2 cases of uterine fibromata complicating pregnancy, both being operated upon and both recovering; and F. L. Burt[2] records another successful case.

Pregnancy in a Cretin.—C. W. Townsend[3] reports the unique case of a cretin, 7 months pregnant. She was born in Eastern Mass., of American parentage, and was 38 years old. She was 43½ in. in height, and weighed with clothes and in her pregnant condition 65½ pounds. Her catamenia began at the age of 22 years. She was an idiot, and her small size and thickened features presented the characteristic appearance of cretinism. She had, of course, a small pelvis. Cesarean section was performed at full term, July 26, 1896, at the Boston Lying-in Hospital by Dr. Edward Reynolds. The mother made a good recovery. The infant was fairly developed, showing no signs of cretinism. It was a male, weighing three pounds and ten ounces. It was very feeble and lived only four hours.

Antepartum Hemorrhage.—J. B. De Lee[4] gives as the most common causes of *obstetric hemorrhage*, named in the order of the usual time of occurrence, the following: abortion; rupture of a vulvar varix; placenta prævia; premature detachment of the placenta; rupture of a fetal blood-vessel with the membranes in cases of velamentous insertion of the cord; postpartum hemorrhage; puerperal hemorrhage. He reports one case of accidental hemorrhage (premature placental detachment) ending in recovery, and one of placenta prævia with a horseshoe placenta.

G. L. Brodhead[5] also reports 4 cases of premature separation, only 1 recovering. Budin[6] relates the history of 2 cases of antepartum hemorrhage in which the blood came from a rupture in the circular sinus of the placenta. In neither case was the placenta situated in the lower uterine segment, nor was there any reason to believe, as the result of careful examination of the surface, that any separation had occurred before the child was expelled. A black clot in each instance was traced directly up to and into the interior of the ruptured circular sinus. [The possibility of antepartum hemorrhage being sometimes due to this accident had formerly been suggested by Jacquemier and Matthews Duncan, but no clinical facts were brought forward to support the hypothesis until quite lately. At the present moment there are 22 cases on record of hemorrhage due to rupture of the circular sinus. It must be remembered that the so-called *circular sinus of the placenta* is situated at the periphery of the placenta, and does not generally form a complete circle, but is interrupted at various points. In caliber it is about equal to the little finger, but in some cases it is imperfectly developed. The walls of the sinus are very thin, which may explain the fact that rupture sometimes occurs. The blood may accumulate in the uterus between the membranes and the uterine wall, or it may escape externally—more often, perhaps, some escapes and some is retained. It is only after the labor is over and the placenta is examined that the cause of the hemorrhage can be definitely ascertained. The prognosis and treatment are much the same as in cases of hemorrhage due to partial detachment of a normally implanted placenta.]

Placenta Prævia.—Cases of interest are recorded as follows: B. Loughrey,[7] placenta prævia centralis, with twin pregnancy, both children surviving for a short time; C. Pierson,[8] partial placenta prævia, delivery by version, with

[1] Med. News, Dec. 12, 1896.
[2] Med. Rec., Oct. 17, 1896.
[3] Arch. of Pediatrics, Jan., 1897.
[4] Chicago Med. Rec., Sept., 1896.
[5] Med. Rec., Feb. 27, 1897.
[6] Presse méd., No. 64, 1896.
[7] Intercol. Med. Jour. Austral., Dec. 20, 1896.
[8] New Orl. M. and S. Jour., July, 1896.

inversion of the uterus, which was the seat of a fibroid tumor; replacement by manipulation; C. A. Thomman,[1] placenta prævia centralis, with masculine pelvis; podalic version was performed with craniotomy of the after-coming head; and T. B. Nariman,[2] 7 cases of placenta prævia in 1100 cases of labor. Füth[3] tabulates the statistics he obtained from midwives in Koblenz with reference to cases of placenta prævia occurring in their practice. The material embraced 50 mothers and 53 children. A physician was present in 44 of these cases. Of the 50 mothers, 19 (38%) died, 2 before delivery, 2 during delivery, and 15 after delivery. Of these last, 4 died from loss of blood, 6 from septic infection, 4 from the effects of previous hemorrhage, and 1 from an unknown cause. Of the 53 children, 32 were born dead and 10 others died in the first 9 days. Only 11 (20.8%) outlived a month. In 12 cases (2 of them fatal) the first hemorrhage appeared just before labor-pains. In 38 cases between the first hemorrhage and labor there was an interval of days, weeks, or even of months, during which time the physician, or sometimes the midwife, tamponed the vagina. Füth believes that many of the mothers might have been saved if the physicians had followed the two cardinal principles that ought to govern these cases: 1. As soon as a diagnosis of placenta prævia is made labor ought to be induced; 2. Only that form of treatment is advisable which stops the hemorrhage and rapidly dilates the cervix, so that the doctor may be by the bedside until the child is delivered. This is especially necessary in the country, where it may take hours to get a physician. These ends are best accomplished by an intrauterine colpeurynter with continued traction upon its tube, followed—as soon as dilatation permits—by podalic version.

ABORTION.

Interesting cases are recorded by C. E. Purslow,[4] J. McCaw,[5] and C. D. Spivak.[6] In Purslow's case the fetus, about 6 in. long, was enclosed in the intact amniotic sac with the liquor amnii; there was no trace of the chorionic or placental tissue on the outer surface of the amnion, and the fetus could be plainly seen through the walls of the sac. Two similar cases have been recorded, one from France and the other by Dorland. Spivak's case was remarkable in that there occurred a delivery at term after 10 previous consecutive abortions. McCaw's patient was septic before the advent of labor, which was presumably due to the septic condition.

Schwab[7] declares that quinin is an undeniable oxytocic, acting directly upon the uterine muscular tissue and making the uterine contractions stronger, longer, and more frequent, but at the same time preserving their physiologic condition—*i. e.* they remain intermittent. It acts rapidly in from 20 to 30 minutes. It is indicated when uterine contractions are insufficient or inertia exists during the dilatation of the cervix, and when the health of mother or child is threatened, especially when the membranes have ruptured and delivery must be hastened.

Daniel[8] reports the case of a 37-year-old 18-para, who has aborted in the last 16 pregnancies at between the 4th and the 7th months. The first child was born in 1880, and the second in April, 1882; both are grown and healthy. In 1882 the husband became a house-painter, and soon after developed lead-colic, followed by paralytic symptoms. Frequently he would give up his

[1] Indian Med. Rec., Nov. 1, 1896.   [2] Indian Med.-chir. Rev., Jan., 1896.
[3] Centralbl. f. Gynäk., No. 36, 1896.   [4] Lancet, Feb. 13, 1897.
[5] Ibid., Oct. 13, 1896.   [6] Am. Gyn. and Obst. Jour., Oct., 1896.
[7] Jour. de Méd. de Paris, Nov. 29, 1896. [8] Jour. d'Accouch., May 17, 1896.

work for months, but would be obliged to resume it for a livelihood. In 1884 the wife aborted, and 15 abortions have followed. Her health seemed to improve during the first one or two months of pregnancy. Suddenly she would be attacked by a nervous rigor, with a sensation of fear. In the morning the breasts would be found flaccid, and within a week the dead fetus would be expelled. The patient would feel well in a few days again. She seemed free from any of the symptoms from which her husband suffered, and had not been subject to either tubercle, syphilis, or alcoholism.

Syphilis as a cause of abortion is discussed by J. A. Ouimet.[1] While abortion among syphilitics is more or less frequent at all periods, it becomes more so as the 7th month approaches, the maximum of frequency being between the 6th and 7th months. Almost all observers attribute the cause of abortion to the fetus itself, which is usually dead and often macerated. The belief to-day is that the influence of the father is far from being as marked as that of the mother. Syphilis in the father, however, certainly has an effect upon pregnancy.

Crosti[2] believes that abortion during the first 8 or 10 weeks is caused by changes in the ovum, and not by any pathologic conditions of the maternal structures. In 3 cases he has observed that when the ovum is thrown off immediately after the death of the embryo the capillary vessels in the chorionic villi are atrophic, while the villi themselves are well preserved, and the epithelium covering them appears perfectly normal, being nourished as before from the decidua. From these observations (atrophy of the capillaries and persistence of the epithelium) the author concludes that abortion is due to the ovum, for if fetal death came through the maternal organism the epithelium of the chorion would be the first structure affected.

Berry Hart,[3] in a short paper on the nature and diagnosis of so-called *fleshy mole,* discusses the symptoms and pathology of this condition. By the term "fleshy mole" is meant "a form of abortion in which part of the aborting ovum, usually at or about the second month, is retained for many months, and is ultimately discharged in a much altered condition." As is well known, the altered appearance depends chiefly on hemorrhages between the chorion and decidua. Hart regards the condition as a rare one. The first factor in the production of a fleshy mole is the death of the fetus, and this is followed by shrinking of the chorionic sac and blood-extravasation among the villi—that is to say, between the chorion and decidua serotina and reflexa. As a result of the hemorrhages, numerous small, rounded protrusions are seen when the interior of the sac is examined. The fetus may entirely disappear, or may be represented by a small, shrunken remnant. In most cases moles of this kind are expelled within 6 months of conception, but in some cases they have been retained until the 11th month; but Hart has never met with any recorded case in which retention has exceeded this period. The diagnosis of cases of this kind is not easy, and in some instances is impossible.

Treatment of Abortion.—[But little progress in the treatment of abortion has been noted during the year.] In the line of prophylaxis, W. F. Metcalf[4] suggests that the rhythm of the body of the uterus is controlled by the hypogastric and ovarian plexuses of the sympathetic, and that pathologic conditions in the rectum, bladder, breasts, or other portions of the body may increase this rhythm, as may also cathartics and other drugs, and mental emotion. The nerve-supply of the cervix is largely cerebrospinal, from the third and fourth sacral; it has no rhythm and guards the opening against the expulsion

---

[1] La Clinique, Dec., 1896.
[3] Brit. Med. Jour., Oct. 24, 1896.
[2] Centralbl. f. Gynäk., No. 9, S. 263, 1896.
[4] Physician and Surgeon, Oct., 1896.

of the uterine contents. Extensive laceration of the cervix may destroy this function, and to guard against a recurrence of abortion such tears should be repaired. He recommends in threatened abortion the administration of fluid extract of viburnum prunifolium, as does also M. Gutierrez.[1] In cases of incomplete abortion A. M. Stuart[2] proposes the following method of treatment: after thorough antisepsis of the vulva and vagina, a Bozeman's intrauterine douche is introduced through the internal os, and a hot creolin solution allowed to flow through; then all loose clots and débris are removed by the dull curet; the cavity is again washed, and the process repeated until nothing remains but the firm decidual tissue which clings to the uterine wall; finally, the uterus is packed from the fundus to the external os with iodoform-gauze, and the patient is given quinin, strychnin, and repeated doses of ergot. The inert uterus is stimulated to contract, and the blood, unable to escape, distends the cavity and flows in between the decidua and uterine wall, dislodging the former. In treating post-abortional retention of the placenta Chaleix-Vivie[3] regards curettage as the only process that will meet all the indications of that condition.

EXTRAUTERINE PREGNANCY.

[An unusual number of interesting cases of ectopic pregnancy have been reported during the year, and a large number of papers of more than ordinary merit have appeared from the pens of leading obstetricians and gynecologists.] Among the cases of **tubal pregnancy** deserving special mention are the following: W. G. Macdonald,[4] 7 cases with 2 deaths; B. Holmes,[5] a right tubal gestation, the operation being followed by a fæcal fistula and ultimate recovery; Thibault,[6] an aborted right tubal gestation; W. B. Chase,[7] a case of secondary right-sided subperitoneal and intraligamentous ectopic gestation, resulting fatally [this is apparently an undoubted instance of intraligamentous gestation, the existence of which has been questioned by many authorities]; J. C. Stinson,[8] 7 cases of tubal gestation, 1 unruptured, with 2 deaths; E. S. Bailey,[9] a tubo-abdominal pregnancy of the right side; A. H. N. Lewers,[10] a left tubal pregnancy, with profuse hemorrhage, cured by intravenous injection of salt-solution after abdominal section; S. E. Wyman,[11] right tubal gestation; W. T. Lusk,[12] right tubal pregnancy, simulating appendicitis; A. S. Warthin,[13] a case of left-sided ectopic gestation associated with tuberculosis of the tubes, placenta, and fetus—the umbilical cord, fetal organs, and placenta showed areas of tuberculous degeneration; T. A. Helme,[14] 4 cases of ruptured tubal pregnancy, all recovering; R. H. Spencer,[15] 1 successful case with operation; A. H. N. Lewers,[16] a ruptured right tubal pregnancy, with a tubal mole (*i. e.*, an ovum situated in the tube degenerated into a mole) which was the direct cause of the rupture and hemorrhage [this is interesting in that it shows that the death of the ovum and its degeneration into a mole are not necessarily followed by a condition of safety to the patient]; E. S. Boland,[17] 5 cases of tubal pregnancy, all recovering; A. Brothers,[18] a ruptured right tubal

[1] Gaceta Medica de Mexico, May, 1896.   [2] N. Y. Med. Jour., Sept. 26, 1896.
[3] Gaz. hebdom. de Méd. et de Chir., Dec. 27, 1896.
[4] Jour. Am. Med. Assoc., July 25, 1896.   [5] N. Am. Pract., Oct., 1896.
[6] Bull. de la. Soc. Belg. de Gynéc. et d'Obstét., No. 3, 1896.
[7] Brooklyn Med. Jour., May, 1896.   [8] Therap. Gaz., Mar. 15, 1897.
[9] La Clinique, Mar. 15, 1897.   [10] Lancet, Mar. 6, 1897.
[11] Boston M. and S. Jour., Feb. 18, 1897.   [12] Med. News, Dec. 26, 1896.
[13] Ibid., Sept. 19, 1896.   [14] Brit. Med. Jour., June 12, 1897.
[15] Physician and Surgeon, June, 1897.   [16] Lancet, July 4, 1896.
[17] Boston M. and S. Jour., Aug. 13, 1896.   [18] N. Y. Med. Jour., Jan. 2, 1897.

pregnancy, developing shortly as an abdominal pregnancy ; E. Collins,[1] a fatal ease of right tubal gestation, in a woman of 25 ; R. H. Fetherston,[2] a fatal case of interstitial pregnancy ; W. Balls-Headley,[3] a case of fimbrioperitoneal ectopic fetation ; M. D. Mann,[4] 2 cases of ruptured tubal pregnancy, resulting fatally after vaginal operation ; W. G. Wylie,[5] 4 tubal gestations, all recovering ; A. J. McCosh,[6] 15 cases of extrauterine gestation, 1 resulting fatally, and 2 being secondary abdominal pregnancies ; F. Henrotin,[7] a case of early rupture of tubal pregnancy, with profuse hemorrhage (80 oz.), with recovery ; J. D. Malcolm,[8] a right-sided tubal pregnancy, with extensive bowel-adhesions ; A. J. Smith,[9] a ruptured right tubal pregnancy ; H. Gage,[10] 7 cases, 1 resulting fatally ; and T. F. Prewitt,[11] 6 cases, 2 resulting fatally.

Cases possessed of more than usual interest are the following : Leopold,[12] a case of uteroabdominal pregnancy at term, the placenta remaining attached in the uterus ; E. A. Ayres,[13] a case of tuboabdominal pregnancy, with delivery of a living fetus at the 7th month, the patient subsequently dying ; Denis,[14] an abdominal pregnancy of 12 years' standing, the fetus not being calcified nor saponified, the child dying at the 10th month ; Menchard,[15] a twin ectopic gestation at 6 months, one fetus in the tube and the other in the abdominal cavity, the tubal fetus being flattened and of about the size of 3 months ; S. C. Gordon,[16] a case of tuboabdominal pregnancy at the 5th month, with a living fetus at the time of operation ; W. J. Means,[17] a case of secondary abdominal pregnancy after term ; P. Tytler,[18] a ruptured interstitial tubal pregnancy treated successfully by suture of the fissure ; T. F. Prewitt,[19] a unique case of extrauterine pregnancy occurring twice in the same Fallopian tube ; R. Ludlam,[20] a case of extrauterine gestation with the placenta in utero, and the fetal sac within the Fallopian tube ; E. Ekstein,[21] a case of advanced extrauterine pregnancy of 6 years' standing, the fetus being between 6 and 7 months old, and partially mummified ; and H. G. Wetherill,[22] a case of extraperitoneal ectopic gestation, advanced to term, the fetus being macerated and the subject of double talipes varus.

J. B. Sutton[23] records a curious case of tubal abortion. On entering the peritoneal cavity he found a clot the size and shape of the dark outline in Fig. 32, lying in the fold of omentum. It was removed. Beneath it lay a second clot of precisely the same shape, but much larger. On removing this a third clot was found in the rectovaginal fossa of twice the dimensions, but of exactly the same shape as the other clots. A rounded, hard body was felt in the left tube. The clots were in shape reniform ; the exterior of each was laminated like the blood in the wall of a sacculated aneurysm or in the sac of an old hematocele of the tunica vaginalis testis, but the central parts consisted of ordinary clot. The hard body in the tube was a "mole," and on microscopic examination yielded many chorionic villi in cross-section. The ostium abdominale was widely patent and the ampullary wall thick, succulent, and entire. The case was one of "incomplete tubal abortion," but peculiar in this respect :

[1] Lancet, Dec. 19, 1896.
[2] Intercol. Med. Jour. Austral., Sept. 20, 1896.
[3] Ibid., Sept. 20, 1896.
[4] Am. Gyn. and Obst. Jour., July, 1896.
[5] Ibid.
[6] Am. Jour. Med. Sci., Aug., 1896.
[7] Ibid., Nov., 1896.
[8] Brit. Med. Jour., Nov. 28, 1896.
[9] Dublin Jour. Med. Sci., Jan., 1897.
[10] Am. Gyn. and Obst. Jour., Nov., 1896.
[11] Jour. Am. Med. Assoc., Jan. 2, 1897.
[12] Arch. f. Gynäk., Bd. lii., H. 2, 1896.
[13] Med. News, Apr. 17, 1897.
[14] Canad. Pract., Sept., 1896.
[15] Am. Jour. of Obst., July, 1896.
[16] Am. Gyn. and Obst. Jour., July, 1896.
[17] Columbus Med. Jour., Jan. 19, 1897.
[18] Brit. Med. Jour., June 12, 1897.
[19] Med. News, June 19, 1897.
[20] La Clinique, Mar. 15, 1897.
[21] Monatsch. f. Geb. u. Gynäk., iii., No. 6.
[22] Colorado Med. Jour., June, 1896.
[23] Lancet, Feb. 13, 1897.

as the blood collected and distended the tubal ampulla it firmly clotted and was then discharged with pain through the tubal ostium into the rectovaginal pouch. The "delivery," so to speak, of each clot coincided with three definite attacks of "pains" which occurred at monthly intervals. [The only record which is in any way parallel is by Noble. In a case of tubal abortion the blood-clots in the pelvis "were coiled up as though they had been ground through a sausage-machine." This was due to the blood clotting in the tube, and the clot was then forced out as a sausage-shaped mass by the continuance of the bleeding. The shape of the clot represented in the illustration is exactly that assumed by the ampullary section of the Fallopian tube when in the condition of hydrosalpinx.]

A case of inguinal hernia containing a pregnant **Fallopian** tube is reported

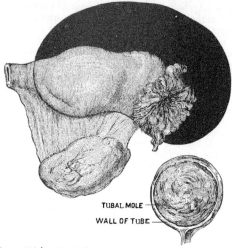

TUBAL MOLE

WALL OF TUBE

FIG. 32 —Figure of a gravid tube. The dark outline represents the shape and size of the smallest clot. It also shows the shape of the ampulla of the tube when distended (Lancet, Feb. 13, 1897).

by Jordan.[1] The woman had undergone several operations for pyosalpinx and vesicovaginal fistula. The pyosalpinx had ruptured into the right broad ligament, the pus finding its way under Poupart's ligament, where it had been evacuated, leaving a scar. The patient had been seized with severe abdominal pain and repeated vomiting, and suspecting pregnancy had visited the clinic for examination. Upon admission she appeared very anemic, with a pinched face and rapid pulse. Above the scar in her right side was a swelling as large as a fist and tympanitic on percussion. Below the scar was another tumor smaller in size, and nonreducible. A third was found to the outer angle of the scar corresponding in position to the internal inguinal ring. This was the size of an apple, soft, irreducible, and painful on palpation. High rectal enemas were administered, and resulted in neither stool nor flatus. Purgatives were not retained. Operation was decided upon 2 days after admission on account of increasing severity of the symptoms of intestinal obstruction. An incision was made parallel to Poupart's ligament, showing a hernial sac containing a large

[1] Münch. med. Woch., No. 1, 1897.

mass of blood-clots, a fetus about 3 months old, the uterine adnexa, and coils of intestine. The wound was cleansed as much as possible and tamponed with gauze. The vomiting continued, and death occurred the following day. It was found at autopsy that the intestinal obstruction was caused by numerous adhesions which were beyond surgical relief.

Ovarian Pregnancy.—[Some authorities deny the possibility of the occurrence of ovarian gestation in the human female, although it occurs as a natural phenomenon in some of the ovo-viviparous osseous fishes, as sharks and rays.] J. Oliver[1] records an interesting case, as follows: the patient was aged 39 years and had been married 12 years; she had had one child, who was born 11 years ago. She began to menstruate at the age of 16 years, and since the birth of the child the discharge, which usually lasted 5 days, had recurred regularly every month until Dec., 1894. In that month and in Jan. and Feb., 1895, there was complete amenorrhea. On March 10, 1895, a substance was passed which appears to have been deciduous membrane. The expulsion of this membrane was effected with but little pain, and was accompanied by a very small quantity of blood-colored discharge. With the exception of this slight discharge of blood on March 10, there was complete amenorrhea in March, April, May, June, and July. On Aug. 26 there was a copious discharge of blood, which persisted for about 12 hours only. Fourteen days later—*i. e.*, about Sept. 9—there was during one day a slight discharge of blood. In October and November there was again complete amenorrhea. On Dec. 25 the menstrual discharge made its appearance and continued to flow for $2\frac{1}{2}$ days, and thereafter it reappeared regularly every 4 weeks until May 14, 1896, when abdominal section was performed. In Jan. and Feb., 1895, she complained a good deal of abdominal pain, but thereafter she experienced but little discomfort and was able to get about as usual, sometimes walking even 3 or 4 miles in one day. The following physical signs were noted on April 18, 1896: the abdomen was prominent and was occupied by a swelling which was located more toward the right than the left side. This swelling, which was almost solid, extended upward from the pubes for $8\frac{1}{2}$ in., and measured transversely at the umbilical level $8\frac{1}{2}$ in. Here and there nodular projections were felt on its right upper half. The girth at the umbilical level was $29\frac{3}{4}$ in. Auscultation detected no sounds over the tumor. Neither breast was full, but colostrum was obtained readily from both. On vaginal examination the cervix was found to be located somewhat toward the right side of the pelvis; it was not soft and the os was not open. The body of the uterus lay behind and was independent of the abdominal tumor. On May 14, 1896, the abdominal cavity was opened. The omentum and small gut were extensively and firmly adherent to the tumor. After freeing these structures the tumor, which originated in the right half of the pelvis, was found to possess a well-defined pedicle. The pedicle was ligated after the manner of dealing with an ordinary ovarian cyst, and the sac containing fetus and placenta was removed intact. The left ovary was apparently healthy. The tumor, which was the right ovary, was found to be a closed sac containing a full-grown fetus with its cord and placenta. The fetus was covered with inspissated sebaceous material, but there was no fluid in the tumor. No breach in the right Fallopian tube could be detected, either at the time of operation or afterward. The patient made an uninterrupted recovery.

Of even greater interest than the foregoing is the case recorded by H. Ludwig.[2] The patient had previously been delivered at term of 5 healthy children, 3 of whom were still living. She became pregnant for the sixth time,

[1] Lancet, July 25, 1896.   [2] Wien. klin. Woch., July 2, 1896.

and on Feb. 20, 1896, labor-pains began. In 6 hours she was delivered of a healthy girl, which presented by the vertex. It was evident that another child remained. Five days later she was admitted into Chrobak's clinic. On examination a living child could be mapped out in the abdomen. The puerperal uterus was about the size of a man's fist, and the appendages on the right side were normal. On the left side a short, thick cord could be felt extending into a tumor which filled the left iliac fossa. By the vagina this tumor was felt pressing down into Douglas's pouch, and the child's head could be made out in the pelvic excavation. The lochia were normal. Abdominal section was performed. The ovum was found attached to the left side of the uterus, from which the placenta appeared to grow. The vascular relations were so intimate that removal of the sac without the uterus was impracticable. The sac was opened and a healthy, well-developed male child extracted, who cried lustily. An elastic ligature was placed on the uterus at the level of the internal os, and uterus and appendages were removed. The cervical canal was cauterized, and the stump treated extraperitoneally. Recovery was delayed by a right-sided pneumonia, but the mother and child left the hospital well at the end of a month. The right tube and ovary were perfectly normal. The left tube could be distinctly traced into a tuboovarian ligament about half an inch wide. The ovarian ligament proper lost itself in the upper part of the sac; from the free end of the tube an ovarian fimbria led into the sac, of which the outer layers appeared to be formed by the remains of the ovary. The sac consisted of 2 parts, one of which, closely attached to the left side of the uterus, was solid, while the other, situated externally, was membranous, and had contained the ovum. The former consisted mainly of a normal placenta, which received from the uterus 2 large vessels—artery and vein; the latter corresponded in its relations to a greatly enlarged ovary, and showed on its surface a number of cystic protrusions—ovarian follicles. Microscopic examination showed the presence of ovarian tissue covering the whole of the membranous portion of the sac; it contained true ovarian tissue, a large number of follicles, and 2 corpora fibrosa. The placental tissue was normal in structure. [The essential points in the diagnosis of ovarian pregnancy have been stated by Veit as complete presence of both tubes and one ovary, the other either being absent or forming part of the sac-wall, while at the same time one ovarian ligament must run into the sac. All these requirements were satisfied in this case, the diagnosis being clinched by the histologic findings.]

Symptoms and Diagnosis of Extrauterine Gestation.—In discussing the present status of ectopic pregnancy, W. G. Macdonald[1] states that *tubal abortion*, or the expulsion of the developing ovum from the fimbriated extremity of the tube into the abdomen, may occur at any time between the second and eighth week of gestation. It is neither a complete discharge into the abdomen nor incomplete, being arrested in the fimbriated extremity, and gives rise to the so-called tuboovarian or tuboabdominal pregnancies. [This is not to be accepted as the inevitable cause of gestation here situated, which may be primary.] Hemorrhage into the membranes of the ovum may occur while it is as yet within the Fallopian tube, and lead to fetal death and the development of a tubal mole. Bleeding more frequently destroys the fetus than the mother in the first four months of gestation. The contention that all ectopic pregnancies continuing until viability are developed between the folds of the broad ligament is not borne out by conditions found on the operating-table or in the laboratory. C. B. Penrose[2] classifies tubal pregnancy as follows: it is *infundibular* when the gestation begins in the infundibulum or in an accessory

---

[1] Jour. Am. Med. Assoc., July 25, 1896.   [2] Univ. Med. Mag., Oct., 1896.

tube-ending. This variety has also been called *tuboovarian*, because in time the gestation-sac may become adherent to the ovary and be bounded by both tube and ovary. The pregnancy is said to be *ampullar* when it begins in the ampulla of the tube; this is the most usual seat of tubal pregnancy. It is called *interstitial* when it begins in the interstitial portion, or in that part of the tube which is in immediate relationship with the uterus. C. S. Bacon[1] remarks that Wyder's proposition to curet the uterus in order to obtain uterine decidua for microscopic examination, which was made a few years ago, and which it was hoped would prove a great addition to our diagnostic resources, has been somewhat disappointing. The failure to find in every case characteristic decidual tissue is probably due to the occurrence of degenerative changes in the uterine decidual membrane which are not yet fully understood. The various descriptions of this membrane do not correspond in all respects. The investigations of Dobbert are among the latest, and his results agree substantially with those of Langhans and others in showing three layers—the superficial compact layer of decidual cells without glands, the middle spongy layer with dilated gland-spaces and little connective tissue, and the deeper layer comprising the bases of the glands and comparatively unchanged connective-tissue cells. After spontaneous expulsion of the decidual membrane only patches of the inner layer are found. The transformation of the uterine membrane into a decidual membrane takes place more rapidly when the fetus is located near the uterus, as in interstitial pregnancy. The change may not be as great in an ampullar pregnancy of 3 months as in an interstitial pregnancy of $1\frac{1}{2}$ months.

According to J. Oliver,[2] a fecundated ovum may develop in some structure in the pelvis outside the uterus, and may even arrive at maturity without exciting any symptom different from that of an ordinary pregnancy, there being throughout this period complete amenorrhea. External hemorrhage is, however, so frequently observed in association with ectopic pregnancy, whether the ovum is enabled to complete its development or dies at a more or less early period of its existence, that it constitutes a common symptom of the disorder. In tubal pregnancy it is probable that the bleeding comes from both the uterus and the tube. When the blood is derived from the Fallopian tube it may make its appearance externally as early as the 20th day after impregnation. During the evolution of an ectopic pregnancy the uterus usually becomes somewhat enlarged, and membranous shreds or pieces are occasionally expelled from this organ, together with more or less free bleeding. As early as the tenth or twelfth week these deciduous membranes may be expelled, but independently of their existence blood may be poured out by the vessels of the uterus as early as the sixth or seventh week.

L. E. Frankenthal[3] has made an extensive study of extrauterine pregnancy occurring twice in the same patient. He is of the firm opinion that in the human female impregnation occurs normally in the tubes for the following reasons: 1. Living spermatozoa have been found in the tubes; 2. The customary site of impregnation in mammals has been proved to be in the tube; 3. The ovum is impermeable after it has graduated the outer third of the tube; 4. The motion of the cilia in the tubes is toward the uterus; 5. That of the muscular fibers is toward the fimbria; and 6. The motion of the uterine cilia is toward the tubes. Impregnation occurring in the tube, any mechanical obstruction or certain pathologic conditions will prevent the advance of the ovum to the uterus. As regards repeated extrauterine pregnancy, he reports 1 case and has collected 12 others.

[1] Ann. of Gyn. and Pediat., Aug., 1896. [2] Lancet, July 11, 1896.
[3] Am. Gyn. and Obst. Jour., Sept., 1896.

Treatment of Extrauterine Gestation.—[But little new has been suggested in the line of treatment.] As C. N. Smith[1] very aptly remarks, in free intraperitoneal hemorrhage, while heart-stimulants, notably strychnin, should be freely employed hypodermically, the greatest stimulus to the heart is the distention of its cavities by blood, or a fluid of similar density. To produce and maintain this stimulation the infusion of normal salt-solution is strongly indicated; this, however, should never be infused into the circulation until the bleeding vessels have been secured. The hemorrhage having been arrested, the salt-solution may be used, and then the removal of the tube and cleansing of the peritoneal cavity can be done. In advanced cases of tubal gestation after extraperitoneal rupture the most satisfactory and clean procedure, and the one especially indicated in an early operation, is the stripping of the placenta and membranes from the sac, ligation of bleeding points, and quilting together of the layers of the broad ligament. If the hemorrhage cannot be controlled by ligation, the sac should be stitched to the edges of the abdominal incision and packed with iodoform-gauze. If the placenta is situated below the pelvis, has an extensive and firm attachment, and its separation promises to be attended with severe hemorrhage, the sac may be stitched to the edges of the incision, the fetus removed, and the placenta left *in situ.* The sac must then be packed with iodoform-gauze, and extreme precautions must be taken to prevent infection of the placenta, which must be removed on the fourth or fifth day, at which time hemorrhage will usually be slight. After the fourth month in these cases operation becomes most formidable. Von Herff[2] concludes from his study of these cases that in removing ectopic gestation-sacs which are complicated by adhesions it is important, whenever possible, to ligate the uterine and ovarian arteries. An attempt should then be made to shell out the sac, beginning at the periphery of the placenta, using clamps and ligatures to control the bleeding. The aperture left should be tamponed with gauze. In rare cases the site of placental attachment must be compressed by a running-stitch; compression of the aorta must be employed, or removal of the uterus with the application of clamps to the bleeding vessels. Gauze-packing is especially valuable when oozing exists or secondary bleeding is feared. W. G. Macdonald[3] has suggested the following method: preliminary ligation of the ovarian and uterine arteries on the side from which the placenta receives its blood-supply; then the placing of a Mickulicz tampon of sterile gauze over the placenta, establishing pressure-atrophy; then preliminary suture of the abdominal walls, the sutures to be tied after the removal of the tampon and placenta; such a tampon may be safely left for three days, and then removed with the placenta and the sutures tied.

F. Henrotin[4] remarks that a question of vital importance is that of operating during profound shock. In these cases the surgeon is called upon to differentiate between temporary fainting from moderate loss of blood and profound shock from excessive hemorrhage. The fainting woman is unconscious during swoons, but rallies from time to time, this being indicated by the variable pulse, slight flushes passing over her face, which shows little anxiety, her body-heat being variable, and the lowering of the head being quickly followed by amelioration. The woman suffering from rapidly progressing, uninterrupted hemorrhage to the point of exsanguination, after the first swoon remains conscious; her pulse steadily becomes weaker until it can no longer be appreciated; her face, which betrays extreme anxiety, is permanently blanched; her body remains constantly cold, and lowering of the head produces but little

---

[1] Ann. of Gyn. and Pediat., Aug., 1896.   [2] Zeit. f. Geburtsh., Bd. vxxiv., H. 1.
[3] Loc. cit.   [4] Am. Jour. Med. Sci., Nov., 1896.

change; she cannot speak above a whisper, and is very still unless she has reached the stage of delirium that immediately precedes death. This differentiation cannot always be absolutely made, as the fainting woman may pass into profound shock from repeated hemorrhages.

Vaginal section for extrauterine pregnancy is discussed by H. Kelly and F. Henrotin.[1] Kelly reports 13 cases so treated, with good results; one patient, comatose when operated upon, died a few days later of nephritis. Cases suitable for this mode of treatment are those that rupture in the early months, including, therefore, the vast majority of all cases. Vaginal puncture and drainage are not a suitable plan of treatment (*a*) in an unruptured extrauterine pregnancy, (*b*) in a recently ruptured one, of (*c*) in advanced extrauterine pregnancy. The most suitable cases are those in which a succession of ruptures has occurred, each time adding to the accumulation of clots in the abdomen. In doing the operation, if the sac is well closed off from the peritoneum, it is a help in bringing away the blood-clots to wash it out at intervals with a normal salt-solution, after which drainage is secured by a strip of plain or washed iodoform-gauze, which is left in for 3 or 4 days. The dangers of the operation are (1) the possibility of a mistaken diagnosis, (2) the risk of opening the peritoneum, (3) the risk of a fatal hemorrhage, and (4) the liability to sepsis through the open vaginal vault. Henrotin prefers this operation for unruptured cases in multiparæ with large vaginæ, in addition to the other indications already given. Especially would he select for this operation patients who are already septic; the dangerous element in the case—hemorrhage—is here to a very great extent eliminated, and by operating through the vagina infection of the peritoneal cavity is prevented. [Vaginal section for whatever cause cannot be recommended for very obvious reasons, notable among which are the danger of sepsis and the inconvenience from lack of room].

CORNUAL PREGNANCY.

H. Briggs[2] reports a case of pelvic hematocele due to rupture of a pregnancy in a rudimentary uterine horn. Operation was followed by cure. He remarks that a cornual pregnancy is liable to any of the diseases or accidents of the normal or ectopic pregnancy. Given a well-developed uterine horn and pregnancy, a natural labor may result; the uterine horn may be styled in all respects a normal horn. Given an ill-developed uterine horn and a pregnancy within it, the obstetric dangers are increased. It is well known that pregnancy in a rudimentary horn has the same tendency to rupture as tubal pregnancy, though the rupture usually has taken place at a later period of gestation in the former than in the latter. His patient had a bifid uterus; the left horn carried a male child till a natural labor at full term closed the pregnancy; the right horn was rudimentary; its pregnancy was, like a tubal pregnancy, abruptly terminated by intraperitoneal rupture. Between these two events there was an interval of 15 months. The uterus, developmentally, was of the type *uterus unicollis cum cornu rudimentaris.* There are 4 known varieties of rudimentary horn: (1) solid throughout; (2) a small tube throughout; (3) solid at both ends and hollow in the middle; (4) patent toward the Fallopian tube, but solid next the other horn. Briggs' case was of the fourth variety. [C. Webster has collected, from Kussmaul, Sänger, and Himmelfarb, 34 cases of pregnancy in a rudimentary uterine horn. In 24 of them rupture occurred and caused maternal death by intraperitoneal hemorrhage.]

[1] Am. Gyn and Obst. Jour. Aug., 1896.   [2] Liverpool Med.-Chir. Jour., July, 1896.

LABOR AND THE PUERPERIUM.

Statistics.—Among the interesting statistics from large institutions mention should be made of the reports of R. C. Norris[1] and H. D. Fry.[2] In the Preston Retreat there were during the year 245 deliveries without a maternal death. Since Norris assumed charge of the institution there have been 745 deliveries with 1 maternal death from chronic nephritis. In 9 cases of the last 245 deliveries a moderate amount of albumin was found. There were 2 cases of grave kidney insufficiency and 1 of eclampsia ; there was 1 case of placenta prævia centralis, 3 of twin pregnancies in primigravidæ, and 8 of minor degrees of pelvic contraction, in only 2 of which was the conjugate diameter below 9 cm. There was 1 complicated labor due to ventrofixation ; and 3 cases of prolapse of the umbilical cord, in all of which the cord was pulseless at the time of examination. In 9.8% the temperature in the puerperium did not rise above 99° F. ; in 81.8% the maximum rise was 100° F. ; in 8.9% the temperature was above 100° F. not longer than 24 hours ; and in 9.3% it remained above 100° F. for varying periods longer than 24 hours. Four of the cases were due to septic absorption. One case of puerperal insanity was noted and cured in 5 weeks' time. There were 6 cases of aspiration-pneumonia in infants, with 2 deaths. There was no case of ophthalmia neonatorum. In 5 female infants a bloody discharge from the genitals was observed. At the Columbia Hospital of Washington there were 252 deliveries during the year, with 2 maternal deaths from uremia, giving a mortality of $\frac{7}{10}$ of 1%. There were 3 twin pregnancies ; 5 cases of uremic poisoning ; 1 of excessive secretion of urine ; 7 of moderate pelvic contraction. Forceps were employed 6 times, or in $2\frac{1}{2}$% of the cases. There was 1 case of placenta prævia partialis ; 1 of subcutaneous emphysema after labor ; 1 of partial premature separation of the placenta ; 34 of malarial complication in the puerperium, the attacks being mild and yielding readily to quinin ; 6 of puerperal sepsis, 1 being treated by the antistreptococcic serum. Of the private statistics, the most interesting are those of W. J. Cree[3] and A. Worcester.[4] Cree reports 330 cases, among which were 165 male children and 186 female children ; 3 twin pregnancies ; 85 primiparæ ; 245 multiparæ ; 1 brow presentation ; 5 breech presentations ; 3 face presentations ; 1 footling and 4 transverse. Forceps were applied 65 times ; 8 times in high position and 57 times in the low. The largest child weighed 14 pounds ; the smallest, 4 pounds. The longest umbilical cord was 42 in. ; the shortest, 8 in. True knots were found in 2 cords. There were 3 cases of placenta prævia and 1 of premature separation of the placenta. Thirty-one perinei were ruptured. There were 1 maternal and 20 infantile deaths ; 1 case each of patulous foramen ovale, bisexual organs, spina bifida, hydrocephalus, and supernumerary little fingers. Worcester records 200 cases, 124 of which were normal as regards labor and the puerperium ; 64 were primiparæ ; 9 cases were premature births, 4 of these being induced. In 37 cases operative assistance was given ; 7 times podalic version was performed ; in 30 cases forceps were used. There were 2 twin pregnancies ; 3 cases of fatal uremia ; and 1 fatal case of pulmonary embolism.

Asepsis in Labor.—[The value of asepsis in obstetrics is recognized the world over, and yet the amount of puerperal sepsis recorded and the large amount unrecorded show a deplorable ignorance or carelessness that is unjustifiable. The subject is one that cannot be too thoroughly ventilated, and the

---

[1] Am. Gyn. and Obst. Jour., Mar., 1897.   [2] Va. Med. Semi-monthly, Feb. 27, 1897.
[3] Physician and Surgeon, Feb., 1897.   [4] Boston M. and S. Jour., Oct. 8, 1896.

papers that are constantly appearing from able hands are ever welcome.] Among those who have contributed articles are G. K. Johnson,[1] R. Braun v. Fernwald,[2] C. E. Skinner,[3] H. L. Williams,[4] C. Godson,[5] E. P. Davis,[6] H. B. Bashore,[7] and C. S. Bacon.[8] Bacon refers to the mortality records of Chicago, which show that puerperal fever kills in that city more women in the prime of life than any other cause except consumption. Godsou reports from the City of London Lying-in Hospital for a period of 10½ years (July 1, 1886–Dec. 31, 1896) 4608 confinements, with 11 deaths, a mortality of 1 in 419, or 2.387 per 1000; in the last 5 years among 2392 deliveries there was no death in which septicemia bore any part. Davis remarks that there are 3 sites after labor at which sepsis may occur—the pelvic floor and perineum, the cervix uteri, and the placental site. After normal labor in a healthy woman the wounds in the cervix and floor are but slight, and are cleansed by the amniotic liquid and blood-serum of the lochia; an occlusion antiseptic dressing is all that is required in such cases. If intrauterine packing is required, iodoform- or bichlorid gauze may be used. Skinner is in favor of vaginal douches of 3% creolin during the puerperal period as a prophylactic measure, using for the purpose a fountain-syringe, well sterilized. He claims that the patients using these douches do not complain of the feeling of soreness in the genitals that is so troublesome to many when they are not resorted to. [We feel that such douching is unnecessary, except when indicated by febrile reaction.] He would also urge early evacuation of the bowels—within 24 hours after labor—to remove the feces and contained microorganisms, and thereby avoid ptomain-absorption. Fernwald remarks that an intrauterine douche should not be given for every elevation of temperature, but ulcers of the vagina or cervix should be looked for and treated if they exist. Iodoform-pencils are of no value for insertion into the uterus after washing it out, and vaginal tampons should never be used. In some cases it is well to swab out the uterine cavity with tincture of iodin.

Anesthesia in Labor.—At the Pirogoff Congress in Cracow Hr. Bukoemski[9] read a paper on the alleviation of pain in normal labor. After careful consideration he concluded that alleviating remedies do not retard labor, they never do harm, and are sometimes of great service. By the tokodynamometer (ether 45 cases and chloroform 8 cases), he determined that when ether is used the pulse and respiration are unchanged. The labor is shortened, albumin is never seen in the urine, the uterine contractions are more powerful, and involution is improved. Ether is a reliable and non-dangerous drug that does not require accurate dosage. Chloroform rather retards labor, but is not injurious to either mother or child. Ether deserves the preference. Both are good and reliable.

Savitsky,[10] as the result of 17 years' experience, recommends antipyrin enemata as an obstetric anesthetic. He administers 1 gm. every 2 to 6 hours, occasionally combining the drug with opium (from 15 to 25 drops of Russian tinctura opii simplex, which contains 1 part of opium to every 10 parts). The pains are always relieved in 15 or 20 minutes after the first dose. Frequently the patient soon falls asleep, which is especially beneficial in cases of spasmodic uterine pains and tetanic contraction of the os; hemorrhage also diminishes. No untoward accessory effects were ever observed by the author.

[1] Chicago Clin. Rev., July, 1896.
[2] Centralbl. f. Gynäk., No. 15, 1896.
[3] N. Y. Med. Jour., Jan. 23, 1897.
[4] Therap. Gaz., Oct. 15, 1896.
[5] Brit. Med. Jour., Jan. 23, 1897.
[6] Therap. Gaz., Mar. 15, 1897.
[7] Med. Rec., Aug. 8, 1896.
[8] Jour. Am. Med. Assoc., Feb. 6, 1897.
[9] Canad. Pract., Jan., 1897.
[10] Vratch, No. 22, 1896.

J. P. Reynolds[1] deplores the unwarranted disuse of ether in the late stage of labor. Instead of conducing to flooding, he claims that the due use of ether saves the mother's courage and strength, and that it preserves uterine contractile power, and thus lessens the risk of hemorrhage. [Anesthesia in labor is of service in a selected class of cases. The routine use of ether or chloroform must be decried as a growing evil; but it would, on the other hand, be dogmatic and inhuman to forbid the anesthetic when there exists some indication for its use, as in dry labor with uterine exhaustion, or in an overwrought nervous individual.]

Posture in Labor.—T. W. Harvey[2] enlarges upon the influence exerted by various positions in the different stages of labor. In the second stage he claims that the posture of general flexion is the most effective. In case there is deflection of the long axis of the fetal ellipse either laterally or in front the woman should be placed on her back in the semi-recumbent position, whereby the uterus is straightened; pressure upon the fundus during the pain will then assist in the expulsion of the child. A change of position will also free an incarcerated lip of the cervix. The knee-chest posture in occipitoposterior cases will often aid in securing rotation if practised early.

Contraction-ring.—Barbour[3] regards *retraction*-ring as a much more accurate and suggestive term than *contraction*-ring. Further, it is wrong to look for this ring in the pregnant uterus; all we find there is a suggestion as to the *place where it will probably develop when retraction has occurred in labor.* The term retraction-ring suggests its nature better than contraction-ring. Contraction is temporary, and will only be found in a frozen section from a patient who has died during a pain. Retraction is permanent, and will always be registered in a frozen section. Further, it is to retraction that its clinical significance belongs. It is to the fact that one portion of the uterine muscle has become permanently shortened and thickened at the expense of the lengthening and thinning of the part below it, and the consequent risk of rupture in the same portion, that this change in labor comes to be of importance, as was first pointed out by Bandl.

Fatty Degeneration of the Uterus during Pregnancy.—L. M. Bossi[4] found the process of fatty degeneration of the muscular fibers of the uterus in active progress in 3 human uteri, 1 removed at the eighth month of pregnancy and the other 2 at term. He inquires whether this is the physiologic condition, and, if so, whether it may not explain the wonderful rapidity with which involution of the uterus after labor normally takes place. It may be asked, further, whether in this fatty degeneration there exists an explanation of some cases of inertia uteri in labor. Bossi has attempted to investigate the subject by the experiments on animals of tying the uterine blood-vessels, but does not regard the results as applicable to the human uterus.

Deflection and Rotation of the Pregnant and Puerperal Uterus.—R. M. Murray[5] remarks that it is a well-known fact that the uterus, growing under the influence of pregnancy, tends to incline more frequently to the right than to the left side of the body. In from 70% to 80% of all cases the uterus inclines to the right side, while in about 20% to 30% it inclines to the left or lies more or less mesially. In addition to this, it undergoes a rotation of more or less degree about its vertical axis, so that one border comes forward and the other recedes. It has, further, generally been believed that in all cases in which the uterus inclines to the right side of the body the rotation is

[1] Boston M. and S. Jour., Oct. 15, 1896. [2] Med. Rec., Nov. 7, 1896.
[3] Edinb. Med. Jour., Nov., 1896 [4] Ann. di Ost. e Gin., Dec., 1896.
[5] Edinb. Med. Jour., Feb., 1897.

such that the left ovary advances, and conversely that in left-sided inclination the right advances. If the uterus expands absolutely symmetrically, it is the only hollow viscus that does ;—the bladder, stomach, intestines, heart, all rotate during distention, and de-rotate when relaxed ; and we may safely assume that the uterus does likewise. Admitting the rotation, we have available an easy explanation of the tendency to deflection or deviation from the middle line which is so universal. For with rotation about the vertical axis there must result a redistribution of the mass of the viscus round that axis. In the unrestrained condition in which the uterus lies in the pelvis this will result in a displacement to one or other side, depending upon the direction of the rotation. Thus, when the uterus rotates so as to bring the left side forward and toward the middle, the uterus will incline toward the right, and when the rotation is in the opposite direction the inclination will be to the left. Murray believes that some relationship exists between left-sided rotation after labor and occipitoposterior position, since in 26 cases of this position the deviation was noted in 18 cases. Schroeder and Schatz give it as their opinion that the side of the uterus which corresponds to the child's back rotates forward, and presumably will deviate accordingly. They would seem to imply that the position of the child was the cause of the deviation, but the grounds on which they do so do not seem quite clear.

Mechanism of the Engagement of the Head in Head-presentations.—[It seems somewhat strange that any room for difference of opinion should still exist as to the common way in which the head presents at the brim. Pinard and Varnier, basing their views on careful clinical and post-mortem research, have seen reason to dissent from the belief that it is the anterior parietal bone that habitually presents, especially in cases of contracted pelvis. Naegele long ago taught that in cases of moderate flattening of the pelvis the head, which lay with its long diameter in the transverse diameter of the brim, became tilted so that the sagittal suture approached more nearly to the promontory of the sacrum, and thus the anterior parietal bone was consequently the presenting part. Pinard and Varnier believe that both in normal and abnormal pelves the fetal head, before it passes through the brim, is not synclitic—that is to say, it is so inclined that the sagittal suture is nearer to the symphysis pubis than it is to the promontory of the sacrum, and that therefore the posterior parietal bone is lower than the anterior. They further hold that the passage of the head through the brim is due to the gradual correction of this lateral inclination, the anterior parietal bone gradually descending until the head is synclitic—that is to say, until the plane of the child's head corresponds with the plane of the pelvic cavity ; but this does not occur until the head has reached the lower part of the pelvic cavity.]

R. de Seigneux [1] gives the results of a series of observations. The position and movements of the head during its passage through the brim were carefully watched in 80 cases. In 43 of the cases the posterior parietal bone presented, the sagittal suture lying nearer to the symphysis than to the promontory of the sacrum. Although this does not fully bear out the wide generalization of Pinard and Varnier, it shows that the presentation of the posterior parietal is infinitely commoner than was generally believed. Among these 53 cases the pelves were all normal except 5, and these only exhibited a moderate amount of contraction. The presentation was found to be synclitic in 19 cases, and during the descent the circumference of the head remained parallel to the plane of the pelvic cavity until the floor of the pelvis was reached. The anterior parietal bone presented only 18 times, although this is

[1] Rev. méd. de la Suisse romaine, May–June, 1896.

the presentation which Naegele and his followers regarded as the usual one both in contracted and normal pelves. At the outlet of the pelvis it should be noticed that in all cases, irrespective of the original mode of presentation, if rotation has not already occurred, the head is inclined so that the anterior parietal bone presents. This fact was long ago pointed out by Matthews Duncan. De Seigneux's observations show that the head may present at the brim in 3 different ways, without leading to any difficulty in its passage through the brim. The nature of the pelvis has no influence on the kind of presentation, but this appears largely to depend on the inclination of the uterus to the plane of the brim. Thus, in primiparæ, in whom the abdominal walls are firm and elastic, the axis of the uterine cavity lies behind the axis of the pelvic brim, and therefore the head presents by its posterior parietal bone; whereas in multiparæ, in whom the laxity of the abdominal walls permits the uterus to fall forward, the anterior parietal bone is the presenting part. The figures further show that when the posterior parietal bone presents this one rides over the anterior, and when the anterior parietal bone presents it rides over the pos-

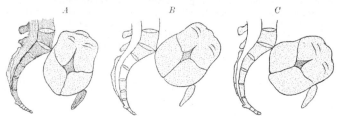

FIG. 33.—*A*, presentation of posterior parietal bone; *B*, synclitic presentation; *C*, presentation of anterior parietal bone (Rev. méd. de la Suisse romaine, May–June, 1896).

terior. When the presentation is synclitic, and there is therefore no inclination of the head in either direction, the parietal bones do not overlap.

Palpation of the Shoulder.—Fabre[1] has studied the relation of the anterior shoulder to the changing positions of the fetus during pregnancy. He says, first, that it can be found with rare exceptions. In 139 patients examined with reference to this point he failed to recognize the shoulder in 5 only, and in these by reason of hydramnios or multiple fetation. One thing that aids in locating the shoulder is the fact that it is found at the level of the fetal heart. By the situation of the anterior shoulder the examiner can determine the degree of engagement, of rotation, and of inclination of the head. Supposing, for example, that the head is normally flexed and is not laterally inclined on the trunk; the distance from the biparietal diameter to the top of the head is 5 cm.; from the biparietal diameter to the bisacromial diameter is (since no lateral inclination of the head is admitted) 8 cm. If it be found by mensuration with the calipers that the height of the shoulders above the symphysis is 13 cm., then the vertex lies at the level of the pelvic brim; and if the shoulder is 8 cm. above the pubic bone, the equator of the head is at the superior strait. Again owing to torsion of the neck of the fetus the anterior shoulder lies on the same side of the mother with the occiput. In a left anterior position the shoulder is at the left of the median line, and conversely. Fabre's observations have shown that at the end of the 8th month the fetus lies in the posterior more frequently than in the anterior position. During the 9th month the occiput gradually glides forward, toward one of the

[1] L'Obstét., May, 1896.

anterior quadrants of the pelvis. Fabre has demonstrated the fact that the head descends synclitically by finding the same distance between the center of the sagittal suture and the anterior shoulder during the labor as after the birth. In contracted pelves, on the other hand, the measurements have shown asynclitism. [These studies bear an interesting and important relation to the results of de Seigneux, as just related.]

Mechanism of Placental Delivery.—According to Ahlfeld,[1] the theory of placental expulsion now credited to Schultze was first taught by Baudelocque. Rigby and Duncan declared that the mechanism of Baudelocque is artificial, resulting from traction on the cord, yet the views of the latter authority are generally accepted in Germany and in France. No demonstration of the Baudelocque-Schultze theory, however, had been offered till the author's investigations in 1881. He then showed that expulsion by the fetal surface was the normal method, and presentation by the margin was an exceptional one, due to irregularity. Fehling and his pupils, Zinsstag and Ziegler, who still adhere to the views of Duncan, refer deliveries by the fetal surface to supposed traction on the placenta developed during the expulsion of the fetus. This assumption is easily disproved by everyday observations. The cord is not drawn tense during labor in normal conditions. Against the contention of Fehling, moreover, are the facts that the placenta could be separated from the uterus by traction on the cord only so far as the passage of air or liquid behind the placenta would permit ; that the insertion of the cord is not always central ; that central inversions of the placenta occur even in marginal and in velamentous insertions.

Duncan teaches that the placental separation begins at the margin, and affirms that the free border is perceptible by the touch at the os uteri, but he does not say how many observations of this kind he has made. Again, the introduction of the hand into the passages disturbs the normal mechanism of placental separation and is not a reliable method of investigation. Ahlfeld made observations in 121 confinements, with the following results : placing a *serre-fine* on the part of the placenta that first presented at the vulva, the *serre-fine* was found at the middle of the fetal surface, after expulsion, in 71 % of cases, at the border in 16 %, on the uterine side near the border in 10.5 %, and on the membranes in 1.9 %. In 85 out of 122 cases (twins occurring once) the membranes covered the uterine surface, in 32 they were on the fetal surface, and in 5 they were between the two situations. Duncan, as an argument for his theory, invokes the assumed fact that hemorrhage does not occur when the placenta descends by its border. But Zinsstag himself has shown that the loss of blood is greatest in these very cases. In 160 confinements he observed hemorrhage exceeding 1000 gm. 34 times. In 24 of the 34 cases the placenta presented according to Duncan. In 50 cases of hemorrhage noted by Ziegler the placenta was expelled 5 times *a la* Schultze, and 45 times by the method of Duncan. Schultze's theory was sustained in 2 cases of Cesarean section observed by Ahlfeld. The placenta bulged at its central portion, the border still remaining adherent. On lifting the edge with the finger blood spurted out from the retroplacental accumulation.

Parturition during Paraplegia.—A. Routh[2] reports a case of labor in a multipara with complete paraplegia below the level of the 6th dorsal vertebra. Labor was painless and required but 12¼ hours for its completion. The only sensation of the patient was a " tight feeling " at the epigastrium during the pains. Involution and lactation were normal. The case proves : 1. That the act of parturition is partly automatic and partly reflex, these actions cor-

1 Zeit. f. Geb. u. Gynäk., Bd. xxxiii., H. 3, 1896.   2 Lancet, June 12, 1897.

responding in the main to the first and second stages of labor respectively ; 2. That direct communication with the brain is not essential to coordinate uterine action, though the brain seems to have a controlling influence upon the pains, helping to make them regular with well-defined intermissions ; 3. That direct communication between the uterus and the lumbar enlargement of the cord, through the medium of the sympathetic ganglia, between the first and third lumbar, is probably essential to the regular and coordinate contraction and retraction of the uterus, as occurs in normal parturition ; 4. It seems also probable that the uterus is able automatically to expel its contents as far as the relaxed part of the genital canal even when deprived absolutely of spinal influence, spinal reflexes being then necessarily absent ; 5. Lactation is not solely due to nervous influence, but partly to chemic changes in the blood.

Nonligation of the Umbilical Cord.—M. B. Kellar[1] enters a plea for this method of treatment of the funis which he has used in more than 2000 cases with good results. He claims that ligation is unnecessary because it is not required at the birth of any other animal, and because there is no danger of hemorrhage without ligation. He asserts that ligation is injurious because it is at times the cause of secondary hemorrhage ; because it interferes with desiccation of the cord, and favors ulceration of the navel, fungoid excrescence, umbilical phlebitis, erysipelas, jaundice, and pyemia, and by preventing a normal escape of blood produces hepatic hyperemia and congestion of the portal circulation.

Involution.—Important studies of the process of involution have been made by McCann[2] and T. B. Stevens and W. S. A. Griffith.[3] McCann's method consisted in measuring with a tape-line from the middle of the fundus uteri to the pubes, taking this at the same hour and with the bladder and the rectum of the patient empty. Septic cases were excluded. Of 37 primiparæ the uterus was found in the true pelvis in 29 before the 13th day. Of 21 multiparæ the womb had entered the pelvis in 13 before the 13th day. Conditions which favored prompt involution were full-term labor, involution being delayed after premature labor, normal or excessive length of the labor, and the parity of the patient, as after repeated labor involution is slower. Contrary to what is commonly held, McCann could not find that lactation furthered involution, but rather predisposed to anemia, which delayed it in many cases. Women who had no secretion of milk whatever often had the most complete involution. Prolonged lactation produced *superinvolution*, a distinctly pathologic condition. He also observed that involution proceeds most rapidly during the first week of the puerperium. After-pains, in these cases, have no effect on involution, but are abnormalities in involution, caused either by retained clots or placental remains, or without known cause, resembling dysmenorrhea.

The measurements of Stevens and Griffith are both vertical and horizontal through the abdominal walls, the vertical being the one to be relied upon, as the transverse are very difficult to obtain. The top of the symphysis pubis is taken as the fixed point from which to measure the height of the fundus uteri. A common "foot" rule is used, the end being pressed against the upper border of the symphysis. The top of the fundus being found, the finger makes a tangent with it and the rule. The distance from the symphysis can then be read on the rule in inches. The bladder and rectum should be empty ; the uterus in the median line and anteverted. The uterus should be in a state of contraction at the time of measurements ; the measurements should be taken at the

---

[1] Pacific Med. Jour., Jan., 1897.   [2] Brit. Med. Jour., No. 1856, 1896.
[3] Tr. Obst. Soc. of London, vol. xxxvii., part iv., 1895.

‾same hour each day. An ordinary temperature-chart can be used to show the curve, by making the 100° line represent the pubes, and each degree above represent one inch. The sources of error are—1, distention of the bladder; 2, distention of the rectum; 3, distention of the small intestine; 4, prolapse of the uterus; 5, retroversion of the uterus; 6, abnormally high uterus; 7, unusual bulk of the uterine muscle; 8, excessive lateral obliquity of the uterus. The pathologic conditions that interfere with the involution of the uterus, and therefore with the descent of the fundus, are—1, retention of portions of placenta and membrane, blood-clots, and lochia; 2, putrid decomposition within the uterus. According to the average chart, the rate of involution is represented by a fall of 2 in. during the first 6 days. After the eighth day the rate of involution is very slow. The average height above the pubes on the first evening is 5¼ in. On the fourteenth day the average height is 2 in., the variation being from 1 to 3 in. It has not been possible to obtain the exact day that the uterus sinks behind the pubes, as most of the cases leave the hospital on the fourteenth day. In one case, on the eighteenth day, it was 1 in. above the pubes. The measurements were taken morning, noon, and evening, and it was found that there were a morning rise and an evening fall, the curve indicating that involution did not progress as rapidly during sleep as during waking hours. The curve in primiparæ was lower in every case by ½ in. than in multiparæ. Age exerted the same influence; the older the woman the higher the curve. In cases of retained products and clots, curetting and intra-uterine washing exerted a marked effect in reducing the curve. With regard to lactation, in those cases in which there was complete absence of lactation the progress of involution was rapid. If lactation was performed, involution was rapid the first few days, diminishing rapidly later. Prematurity of labor delayed involution. Prolonged labor delayed involution for the first few days.

The Excretions of Parturient Women.—Neumann[1] reports the results of his study regarding the excretions of parturient women. His conclusions agree in the main with Winckel's, and show that the excretion of sulfates is lessened during the first 10 days of the puerperal period, being inferior to that usually observed in a healthy adult. The reason for this is found in the fact that such material is voided in the lochia and to some extent by the formation of milk. He also endeavored to estimate the amount of fecal waste which such patients eject during this time. He found that, like the soluble material, less than normal is passed for the first 10 days of the puerperal period. In one instance in which the patient failed to have the bowels thoroughly emptied before labor a very great increase above the normal was noted. He calls attention from this to the practical necessity of having the rectum thoroughly empty before parturition begins.

Effects of Lactation on Menstruation and Impregnation.—L. Remfrey[2] concludes that of nursing-women 57% only have absolute amenorrhea; 43% menstruate more or less, but 20% have absolute regularity. Impregnation does not take place so readily during lactation as at other times; but this is not true to such an extent as has been imagined. If absolute amenorrhea is present during lactation, the chances of impregnation occurring are only 6 out of 100. If menstruation occurs during lactation, the chances are 60 in 100. The more regular a woman is during lactation the more likely is she to become pregnant. During a menstruating lactation the changes in the uterus are presumably similar to those connected with the ordinary monthly periods, and the mucosa forms a nidus for the ovum. In the woman who does

¹ Arch. f. Gynäk., Bd. lii., H. 3, 1896.　　² Tr. Obst. Soc. of London, 1896.

not suckle at all the menses appear, as a rule, sometimes in the first 6 weeks after delivery.

Statistics of Lactation.—[Statistics on this subject are called for, as they throw much light on the health and strength of women in different regions.]

Buchmann[1] observed 126 lying-in women in the obstetric wards of the Halle clinic from February to May, 1895, inclusive. He wished to ascertain the proportion of cases in which the mother was able to suckle her child. Out of the 126 cases, 83 (or 65.9 %) had sufficient milk when discharged between the tenth and twelfth days. The percentages recently reported from Bâsle and Stuttgart are much lower.

Wieden[2] reports from the Freiburg Maternity that out of 525 women in childbed only one-half could suckle thoroughly during the first two weeks, 99 secreted no milk, 49 had imperfect nipples, 46 had fissured nipples, and 44 had insufficient secretion of milk. Only 33 suckled without unfavorable complications. The development of the nipple bore a direct relation to the value of the breast as a secretory organ.

MATERNAL DYSTOCIA.

Pelvic Contraction.—New classifications of deformed pelves are offered by Dohrn[3] and Dorland.[4] Dohrn proposes the following classification, which combines the two systems of classifying by form and by causation: I. *Deformed pelves of normal shape:* 1. Generally contracted pelvis; 2. Abnormally large pelvis. II. *Deformed pelves of abnormal shape:* 1. *Flattened pelves*— (a) Simply flattened pelves: (a) Pelvis plana deventeri, (β) Simple flattened pelves from congenital double dislocation of the hips, (γ) Simple flat rachitic pelvis; (b) Generally contracted flattened pelves. 2. *Deformity from bending of the bones:* (a) Bending of the bones due to osteomalacia; (b) Bending of the bones due to rachitis. 3. *Oblique pelves:* (a) Obliquity due to skoliosis; (b) Obliquity from failure of proper use of one leg; (c) Asymmetry of the sacrum. 4. *Transversely narrow pelves:* (a) Congenital transversely narrow pelves; (b) Kyphotic transversely narrow pelves. 5. *Failure of union at the symphysis.* 6. *Spondylolisthetic pelves.* 7. Deformities due to *exostoses, hypertrophy* of normal bony prominences, early *fractures,* or *neoplasms* of the pelvis.

Dorland's classification is founded on a clinical basis, the pelves being grouped according to the diameter which is most concerned in the contraction. He groups as follows: I. *Anteroposteriorly contracted pelves:* 1. Simple flat pelvis; 2. Spondylolisthesis; 3. Spondylolizema. II. *Obliquely contracted pelves:* 1. The rachitic pelvis; 2. The coxalgic pelvis; 3. The skoliotic pelvis; 4. The osteomalacic pelvis; 5. Naegele's, or the obliquely ovate pelvis; 6. The oblique pelvis due to traumatism (fractures, luxations)—the sitz pelvis. III. *Transversely contracted pelves:* 1. Robert's pelvis; 2. The kyphotic pelvis; 3. The kyphoskoliotic pelvis. IV. *Generally contracted pelves:* 1. The justominor pelvis; 2. The masculine, fetal, funnel-shaped pelvis; 3. The generally contracted and flat pelvis.

[The *relative frequency* of pelvic contractions has been thoroughly studied by a number of observers in this and other countries. No accurate knowledge on this point can be obtained by measuring only cases operated upon, thus omitting the large class of difficult labors often followed by fetal death or maternal injury. Routine examination of women attendant upon clinics or ma-

[1] Centralbl. f. Gynäk., No. 25, 1896.
[2] Medicine, Sept., 1896.
[3] Centralbl. f. Gynäk., No. 16, S. 417, 1896.
[4] Manual of Obstetrics, p. 534.

ternities is essential in arriving at positive conclusions.] J. W. Williams [1] gives the result of his examination of 100 women to determine the pelvic condition present. He designates as contracted only those pelves that presented an oblique conjugate of 11 cm. or less, with an internal conjugate of 9 cm. or less; pelves with shortening of 2 cm. or more. In 2 cases pelves slightly larger than the limit were included in the list, because labor was difficult, 1 case requiring high forceps, the other difficult breech-extraction. In the 100 women 15 had contracted pelves; 4 were rachitic flat pelves; 5 were generally contracted; 1 was coxalgic oblique; 1 was transversely contracted, of the male type. These women were white in 8 cases, and negresses in 7. Eleven of these were born in America. When these cases were reported 13 had been delivered, 7 spontaneously, and 6 by operation. At the recent Congress at Geneva [2] the discussion upon this subject was briefly as follows: Fochier had examined 120 pelves postmortem in the anatomic rooms of the medical faculty of Lyons. He found 27 of these contracted, 1 of them in a remarkable manner, a percentage of contracted pelves of $21\frac{66}{100}$. Among these, 22 were flattened, 10 being simple flat pelves and 12 irregularly flattened. The remainder were rachitic. His clinical observation included 630 pregnant women examined during 1895, among whom were found 120 contracted pelves, $20\frac{16}{100}\%$. Of these, 42 were simple flat pelves, 58 flat rachitic, and 20 generally contracted pelves. All pelves were considered rachitic in which there was a history that the patient had walked later than the average infant. The frequency of transverse presentations in the obstetric clinic at Lyons had led to an effort to find an explanation for this in the peculiar shape of the pelvis among these patients. It was found that in these cases a peculiar flattening of the pelvis was present, which seemed to be an adequate cause for this phenomenon. Rein, of Kiew, Russia, gave the results, gathered from different Russian clinics, of the examination of 54,000 pregnant patients, among whom were found 2005 pelves whose true conjugate was $9\frac{1}{2}$ cm. in flat pelves and 10 cm. in those generally contracted. He could find but 457 cases of markedly contracted pelves. Sufficient deformity to require Cesarean section was exceptional. In the Caucasus rachitis is rare, while in other portions of Russia almost all contracted pelves are rachitic. In the clinic at St. Petersburg but $\frac{6}{10}\%$ of patients examined had contracted pelves. In Russia the most frequent contracted pelvis is the simple flat, and then the generally contracted. Of the 54,000 patients, $1\frac{5}{10}\%$ had simple flat pelves and $1\frac{5}{10}\%$ had generally contracted pelves. But 4 cases of osteomalacia were reported. Kufferath, of Brussels, had recorded pelvic measurements for 10 years in 5000 women, making the same measurements with each. He found 75 contracted pelves, of which 71 were flat, with a true conjugate of less than $9\frac{1}{2}$ cm., while 4 were generally contracted with a true conjugate of not less than 10 cm. As regards treatment, he divided his patients into 4 classes. In the 1st the true conjugate was from 9 to 11 cm.; delivery was effected by the forceps or version, and rarely by symphysiotomy. If the child was dead, the forceps or embryotomy was employed. In the 2d class the true conjugate varied from 9 to 7 cm. Premature labor was induced at $7\frac{1}{2}$ months. If version or forceps failed at term, symphysiotomy was employed. In the 3d class the true conjugate was from 7 to 5 cm. Labor was induced at $7\frac{1}{2}$ months, and symphysiotomy practised if necessary. If the child was at term and the true conjugate from 6 to $5\frac{1}{2}$ cm., Cesarean section was chosen. In the 4th class the true conjugate was less than 5 cm., and abdominal section was employed. Fancourt Barnes, of London, reported the results of the examination of 38,065 pregnant women, among whom were found 150 flat

[1] Bull. Johns Hopkins Hosp., No. 65, 1896.   [2] Am. Jour. Med. Sci., Nov., 1896.

pelves, with a true conjugate less than $9\frac{1}{2}$ cm., and 45 pelves symmetrically contracted, with a true conjugate of less than 10 cm. Treuh, of Amsterdam, gave the results of 22,955 labors. Among these patients 816 contracted pelves were found. Of these, 657 were flattened, with a true conjugate of less than $9\frac{1}{2}$ cm., while 159 pelves were symmetrically contracted, with a true conjugate of less than 10 cm. No cases of osteomalacia were found. In treatment, Treuh had employed the supine posture, or Walcher's position, with success. Pesta-lozza, of Florence, had examined 7962 patients, of whom 2437 had pelves somewhat contracted; 993 of these patients had such slight pelvic contraction that interference was unnecessary. The most frequent forms were rachitic, sym-metrically contracted, and simple flat pelves. In 50 cases an irregular contrac-tion was present. One case of osteomalacia was among the number. Among other operations 3 symphysiotomies and 14 Cesarean operations were performed. The maternal mortality was 8 in 1391 clinic patients, and 95 infants. The most frequent contracted pelves were observed in the south and in the vicinity of Naples. The inhabitants of the north and middle portions of Italy were less often afflicted with disease causing pelvic contraction. Lusk, of New York, reported that in the United States pelvic contraction is exceptional among Americans, rachitis and osteomalacia being practically unknown. Pawlik, of Prague, gave the results of the examination of 29,615 pregnant women in the Austrian Empire: $5\frac{9}{10}\%$ of these patients had flat pelves, $1\frac{9.2}{10}\%$ symmetrically contracted pelves, and $\frac{14}{100}\%$, or 41 patients, had osteomalacia. Morisani, of Naples, among 2769 labors, found deformed pelves in $4\frac{47}{100}\%$. Among these were 50 rachitic pelves and 13 osteomalacic. Most of the rachitic pelves were found in patients from the vicinity of Naples. The osteomalacic cases came from the villages at the foot of Vesuvius, and 3 of these patients had been born in Naples.

Knapp[1] in 4289 cases observed at the University of Prague from 1891 to 1895 found 105 cases of contracted pelvis. Flat and generally contracted pelves, without demonstrable evidences of rachitis, preponderated over the rachitic forms. Osteomalacia was observed in 5 cases. In the 105 cases there was a maternal mortality of 0.95% and a fetal mortality of 31.43%.

The *treatment* of labor in moderate pelvic contraction was discussed at the 64th annual meeting of the British Medical Association at Carlisle.[2] In dis-cussing the relative advantages of forceps and version R. M. Murray stated that the forceps present obvious advantages from the point of view of the safety both of the mother and the child. Thus as to the mother, we have (1) avoidance of risk of uterine rupture, (2) avoidance of intrauterine manipula-tion, and (3) diminished risk of infection; and, as to the fetus, (1) avoidance of traction on the neck, and (2) avoidance of compression of the cord. In justominor pelves the question of turning does not arise, forceps being the only proper operation. In flat pelves version is almost universally recom-mended, while only recently has the accuracy of this view been questioned. Murray had already shown that the diminution in the cranial capacity pro-duced by compression of the forceps is compensated by a vertical expansion, and not by a transverse one. Accordingly, he holds that the explanation of the inefficiency of the ordinary forceps in a flat pelvis is due, not to complica-tions arising from their grasp of the head, but to waste of force arising from error in the line of traction. He therefore urges the use of axis-traction, offer-ing for this purpose the rods devised by himself to be applied to ordinary forceps. He claims these points for axis-traction in flat pelves: (1) the forceps can be applied without difficulty to the anteroposterior diameter of the head

[1] Arch. f. Gynäk., Bd. 51, H. 3, S. 483.   [2] Brit. Med. Jour., p. 1281, Oct. 31, 1896.

and in the transverse or roomy diameter of the pelvis; (2) the grasp of the head, while sufficient to prevent slipping, does not materially compress the head; (3) no amount of practical compression of the head in this direction is capable of causing the least expansion of the biparietal diameter; (4) the mode of grasp favors the development of the Naegele obliquity, and this follows the natural mechanism of delivery in such cases; (5) as compared with version, forceps avoid intrauterine manipulation, traction on the neck of the child, and also the risk of delay during compression of the cord. He has delivered living children in this manner when the brim was not more than 3.25 in., and in one case when it measured 2.75 in. C. E. Buslow agreed with Murray, except that he believes version would sometimes succeed when forceps failed. W. E. Fothergill believed that version in flat pelves had nothing in its favor except its antiquity. He had successfully delivered by axis-traction forceps 6 women in whom the conjugate varied from 3 to $3\frac{1}{2}$ in. A further advantage of forceps besides those mentioned by Murray is that forceps can be applied at any time, however long, after the rupture of the membranes.

R. V. Braun [1] suggests the use of thyroidin in contracted pelvis in order to produce undersize of the fetus.

Puerperal Eclampsia.—The *pathology* of eclampsia has been studied by P. Leusden [2] and J. W. Byers.[3] According to Leusden, there are two forms of puerperal eclampsia. In the one there is found postmortem evidence of acute nephritis added to congenital defects in the kidney, and in the other the so-called nephritis of pregnancy. He regards puerperal eclampsia as the result of a blood-poison from derangement of the function of the kidney. The giant-cell emboli found in the lungs of puerperal subjects appear to have nothing to do with eclampsia; neither have bacteria, nor disease of the placenta, nor necrosis of the liver. Byers especially emphasized the part played by the fetus in the pathology of the disease. He has verified Winckel's observation that when the fetus dies during pregnancy, even in the case of a woman who presents the premonitory symptoms of eclampsia, the danger for the mother is entirely overcome or very much diminished. The extreme view that all cases of eclampsia are the result of renal disease is being abandoned. The following facts are distinctly against the renal theory of causation: 1. Now and then a case is encountered in which no albumin has ever been present, and in some fatal cases the kidneys are quite healthy; 2. All obstetricians have seen women with chronic renal disease become pregnant and never develop convulsions; 3. The certainty of the occurrence of eclampsia is not proportionate to the intensity of the albuminuria; 4. It is very rare for convulsions to occur in acute disease of the kidney apart from pregnancy, except in cases in which the renal affection is associated with some specific disease like scarlatina, when there is *already* a poison circulating in the blood; 5. Sometimes women die comatose in eclampsia, and yet the amount of albumin present has never been more than a trace. The theory of blood-poisoning or toxemia as the cause of eclampsia is supported by the following arguments: 1. It covers all the cases whether albumin is present or not; 2. The clinical history of eclampsia is that of a toxemia; 3. The postmortem appearances. According to Zweifel, multiple thromboses are invariably found in the liver, lungs, and brain in all fatal cases of eclampsia, and certainly indicate the existence in the circulation of some blood-coagulating product of organic change.

Veratrum viride holds its own in the *treatment* of this disease. According to J. C. Edgar,[4] it is second only to chloroform in value, provided the pulse

---

[1] Centralbl. f. Gynäk., No. 27, S. 722, 1896.   [2] Centralbl. f. innere Méd., No. 17, 1896.
[3] Lancet, Jan. 2, 1897.   [4] Med. Rec., Dec. 26, 1896.

be strong as well as rapid; when the pulse is weak morphin hypodermically and chloral per rectum are better. Veratrum viride reduces the pulse-rate and temperature, relaxes the cervical rigidity, and causes prompt diaphoresis and diuresis. C. D. Hurt [1] says that it is suited to the treatment of eclampsia, whether antepartum or postpartum, unless chronic disease or excessive anemia be present. On the other hand, S. Marx [2] questions its true curative and therapeutic worth in cases demanding its use, and W. W. Potter [3] says it is dangerous, uncertain, and deceptive in action. Marx has seen terrible convulsive seizures when the pulse was 60 and alarmingly feeble. [The benefits that generally follow its use are so marked that we are safe in urging its employment in all suitable cases.] Exclusive milk-diet as a prophylactic measure has come into general favor. Potter says it is one of the surest ways to control progressive toxemia. This will also serve to flush the kidneys and thus favor elimination. Marx urges a dietary consisting of milk, buttermilk, kumyss, or matzoon, with the addition of, plenty of water. A. Charpentier [4] remarks that every pregnant woman with albuminuria should be put on an exclusive milk-diet. Ferré [5] regards the milk-treatment to be most efficient from a prophylactic point of view in the treatment of puerperal convulsions, although it does not necessarily cause the other alarming symptoms besides the convulsions to disappear. He has never seen convulsions in a patient subjected for over a week to milk-diet, nor any other trouble of a toxic origin. The alleged disappearance of albuminuria, on the other hand, does not necessarily occur. Ferré speaks with equal decision on this point, declaring that he has never seen so much as an appreciable diminution of albumin even after prolonged milk-diet. The same is the fact with the edema. The above facts are emphasized because he is aware how some obstetricians have very naturally given up milk-diet on account of persistence of albuminuria and edema. Such a step is a mistake, for if the treatment be continued labor will proceed without any convulsions coming on, though the legs remain swollen and the urine albuminous.

There was an important discussion upon eclampsia at the International Congress of Obstetrics and Gynecology [6] in Geneva. Charles, of Lüttich, considered eclampsia a complex disorder. While the reflex element is very pronounced, still the part played by toxins is no less significant. After referring to the autointoxication evident upon examining the various excretory organs, he stated that these retained poisons might result in dyspnea, carcinoma, and paralysis without the development of convulsions, and these cases he would style "imperfect or incomplete eclampsia." While albumin is present in the urine in most cases, it is by no means the inevitable cause of this condition. Among the cases observed by this speaker, the mortality in 151 had been $24\frac{42}{100}\%$ for mothers and $41\frac{83}{100}\%$ for the children. He had observed the usual predominance of primiparæ in this complication. Charpentier urged the most thorough examination of the urine of each pregnant patient. Upon slight indications of albuminuria and diminished excretion he would limit the patient's diet strictly to milk, relying largely upon this for the prevention of eclampsia. In the actual presence of convulsions, if the patient was robust and cyanotic, he would bleed. He would also give chloral with milk through a stomach-tube. The inhalation of chloroform and the subcutaneous injection of normal saline solution are of value. If the patient was not robust and little cyanosis had developed, he would content himself with the use of chloral. In most

[1] Med. Rec., Dec. 26, 1896.
[2] Am. Medico-Surg. Bull., July 18, 1896.
[3] Canad. Pract., Feb., 1897.
[4] N. Am. Pract., July, 1896.
[5] L'Obstét., Nov. 15, 1896.
[6] Centralbl. f. Gynäk., No. 39, 1896.

cases labor came on spontaneously, and delivery followed without assistance. If birth do not end spontaneously, version or forceps are indicated. If the child have perished, craniotomy should be chosen. He did not believe in rapid and forcible dilatation of the birth-canal, but would wait until such could be accomplished without violence. The induction of labor or abortion is rarely indicated in his experience in this condition. Cesarean section could only be performed amid the most favorable surroundings and in rare cases. Halbertsma considered the most important question in the treatment of eclampsia to be whether the obstetrician should wait for the occurrence of labor, or whether he should interfere at once. In serious cases in prolonged labor, when the patient was more than the average age and the pelvis was contracted or multiple pregnancy present, he would actively interfere. He believes that Cesarean section is indicated at the termination of pregnancy in the presence of convulsions. He also urged incision of the cervix in suitable cases. Veit had little confidence in many methods proposed, because he did not think the pathology of the affection sufficiently well established to furnish indications for treatment. He would hasten labor by every safe method, would administer morphin in large doses, and try to obtain profuse perspiration. He did not advise operative treatment in these cases. Byers, of Belfast, had found that morphin tended to lessen the acute catarrhal process in the lungs, which often hastens a fatal issue in eclampsia. He urged the vigorous use of eliminative treatment. When the conditions are favorable he would deliver promptly under chloroform. He urged the importance of rest, milk-diet, purgatives, and warm baths in preventing this complication. In the discussion upon the views previously advanced Tarnier expressed his great confidence in milk-diet as prophylaxis. He would use this not only with patients who had albuminuria, but with those who showed during pregnancy headache, sleeplessness, and other nervous disturbance. In his clinic from the year 1838 to 1887 the maternal mortality was 37 %. From 1889 to 1891 he treated eclampsia with chloroform, chloral, and bleeding, with an increase in the mortality to 38 %. His present treatment consists of bleeding, purgation, the use of chloroform and chloral, with rigid milk-diet, milk being given by a stomach-tube if necessary. Under this treatment the mortality had diminished to 9 %. Since January, 1896, no case of eclampsia had developed in his clinic. Pamard emptied the uterus in these cases as rapidly as possible. He had found that chloroform could be used if necessary for 48 hours to prevent convulsions.

Audebert called attention to the importance of icterus as a prognostic symptom in these cases. In 34 eclamptic patients 4 had icterus, and of these 4, 3 perished.

Queirel, of Marseilles, had but 27 cases of eclampsia in 1200 labors. He ascribed this small number to the employment in his clinic of a milk-diet in all cases in which elimination was deficient.

Morisani, of Naples, drew attention to the fact that the death of the fetus is followed by the cessation of eclamptic fits and also of albuminuria. In the fourth and fifth months of pregnancy he would treat these cases by appropriate medicines. At the eighth month he would hasten labor with every possible means. He would employ incision of the cervix if necessary.

In closing the discussion, Charpentier urged that the effect of drugs be tried in each case before recourse be had to operation. When the conditions are favorable he would promptly use forceps or do version. When dilatation was not sufficient for either of these procedures he would wait and employ medicinal treatment, hoping that the death of the fetus would lessen the convulsions. He believes that the finger and hand should be employed for rapid dilatation.

H. M. Jones[1] urges the value of pilocarpin in eclampsia, and Appleby[2] that of guaiacol locally. J. P. Reynolds[3] prefers prolonged etherization in eclampsia to the use of chloroform. [The depressing influence of ether upon the kidneys would seem to contraindicate its employment in this condition.] J. T. McShane[4] makes a strong plea for the revival of venesection as a specific for puerperal eclampsia. [Venesection cannot be called a specific, but is of immense value in the plethoric type of cases.] Potter[5] claims that if there is high arterial tension—vasomotor spasm—glonoin in full doses is valuable; while Marx[6] also urges the free exhibition of nitroglycerin hypodermically. [In the operative treatment of eclampsia Dührssen's method of cervical incision does not grow rapidly into favor. Halbertsma's method of Cesarean section is only justified when there exists some insuperable mechanical obstruction. Mechanical dilatation of the cervix and the immediate extraction of the fetus appear to be the popular methods of the day, and if properly performed they are safe and efficient.]

Rigidity of the Soft Parts.—Instances of cervical dystocia are recorded by Clivio[7] and Jefferiss.[8] Jefferiss's case was one of total occlusion of the os uteri, relieved by puncture and digital dilatation. Clivio's case was one of cicatricial stenosis, the result of a previous operation for carcinoma. Dilatation was accomplished by incisions and the use of the Tarnier dilator, the fetus being extracted after craniotomy. Clivio discusses operations for the relief of carcinoma, and cites the opinions and experiences of twenty or more different authorities, reaching the conclusion that, in cases of carcinoma of the vaginal portion of the cervix in women who have not reached the menopause, hysterectomy is to be preferred to high amputation of the cervix. When pregnancy complicates carcinoma of the cervix, radical treatment, even if it does endanger the life of the fetus, is to be preferred to a partial operation or to the expectant plan of treatment based on the hope of saving the child.

Perineal Laceration.—G. Coromilas[9] describes the following method by which he has been enabled to shorten labor, diminish pain, and prevent lacerations of the perineum. After proper antiseptic precautions the accoucheur's hands, and the perineum, vagina, and os uteri, are anointed with the following ointment: cocain, 3 gm.; antipyrin, 3 gm.; vaselin, 50 gm. Four fingers of one hand are then passed within the vaginal orifice, and semilunar movements are made, first on one side and then on the other, so as to dilate the perineum. After three or four such powerful movements the fingers of the other hand are introduced and the performance repeated. When the requisite degree of dilatation is achieved, the fingers are passed into the vagina until the index, middle, and ring fingers touch the os uteri, and the same movements made, the perineum being pushed outward with the palmar surface of the hand. A. Milne-Thomson[10] records a central perineal rupture occurring in a young primipara, the tear not involving the sphincter ani nor the fourchet; the child weighed 6½ pounds. Lambertenghi[11] also records a case occurring in a primipara of 17 years. He appends a tabulated report of 91 cases of this abnormality, and various conclusions are drawn from this table. As regards the causation, some writers have sought it in an exaggerated curve of the sacrum, in an abnormal shape of the sacrum, in undue rigidity of the sacroiliac joints, in a very long and high pubes, in retrocession

[1] Brit. Med. Jour., Feb. 6, 1897.   [2] Boston M. and S. Jour., Mar. 18, 1897.
[3] Ibid., Oct. 15, 1896.   [4] Medicine, Aug., 1896.
[5] Ibid.   [6] Ibid.   [7] Ann. di Ost. e Gin., Mar., 1896.
[8] Brit. Med. Jour., Jan. 25, 1897.   [9] Edinb. Med. Jour., Aug., 1896.
[10] New Zealand Med. Jour., July 1, 1896.   [11] Ann. di Ost. e Gin., Jan., 1897.

of the pubic arch, and in abnormal approximation of the ischia. Others have thought that a very long perineum or an abnormally closed condition of the vulva was a potent factor. Some assert that irregular uterine contractions, which destroy the normal dilatation of the birth-canal, are an important factor. As regards the prevention of this accident, insertion of the fingers into the rectum and pressing the head strongly upward have been found efficient by some observers. Others modify the force of uterine contractions by the use of an anesthetic. Episiotomy and the use of forceps have been successful in some hands. In the 91 cases quoted but 1 death occurred, and this was indirectly the result of accident. Under antiseptic precautions and with immediate suture the prognosis for recovery is excellent.

Tumors in Labor.—Sevitsky [1] records a case of labor at term in which the fetal head was arrested by a dermoid tumor of the right ovary. The head was brought to the outlet by forceps, while the tumor, bulging through the anus burst the rectal wall. Its contents were emptied and the fetus then easily extracted, but it was dead. Finally the cyst was drawn down and amputated, the rectal wall being carefully sewn up. There was bad flooding during the third stage of labor, and the patient died in 33 hours of pelvic peritonitis.

Labor after Suspensio Uteri and Vaginofixation.—[The frequency with which backward displacements of the uterus occur, and the increasing use of surgical measures to relieve them, give an especial interest to the report of pregnancies occurring after the various operations for antefixation.]

C. P. Noble,[2] Grusdew,[3] and Dorland [4] have made a thorough study of the effects of these operations upon subsequent gestations and labor. Noble relates two cases of labor occurring in his own practice in which very grave difficulties were encountered, in one case necessitating the performance of a Porro operation. The cause of the obstruction was in both cases the same, and resulted from the fact that the anterior uterine wall and fundus had been fixed by sutures in such a manner that, when the uterus began to enlarge as pregnancy advanced, the fundus and anterior wall were folded on each other so as to form a tumor which occupied the brim of the pelvis. The posterior wall was in both of these instances dangerously thinned as the result of overstretching. The author was led to make a large number of inquiries among American obstetricians; but, curiously enough, could obtain no further evidence that ventrofixation of the uterus led to difficulties during labor. The conclusions he arrived at as the result of his investigations were: (1) that women subjected to this operation are less apt than others to become pregnant; (2) that pregnancy and labor are, as a rule, uncomplicated; (3) that inertia uteri is not infrequently met with; (4) that serious or insuperable obstruction to labor may be produced if the fundus and anterior wall of the uterus are imprisoned below the point of attachment between the uterus and abdominal wall. Noble points out that the operation for ventrofixation of the uterus is performed in different ways by different operators, and that on the method employed depends the presence or absence of difficulties at any subsequent confinement. He believes that the sutures should pass through the upper part of the anterior uterine wall, and that care should be taken that the line of attachment is not too broad or too firm. He alludes to the difficulties in delivery which have been met with after vaginal fixation of the uterus, and considers that from the obstetric standpoint the results have been disastrous. Grusdew reports the results of 123 operations of this character. In 50 of the cases a ventral, vesical, or ventrovesical fixation was performed, in 41, Alexander's operation, and

---

[1] Ann. de Gynéc. et d'Obstét., Aug., 1896.   [2] Am. Gyn. and Obst. Jour., Nov., 1896.
[3] Münch. med. Woch., Nov. 17, 1896.   [4] Univ. Med. Mag., Dec., 1896.

32

in 32, vaginal fixation. In no case of abdominal fixation did relapse occur. Four of these patients became pregnant, one of them after 16 years of sterile matrimony. There was no unusual symptom during the pregnancy, except in one instance. In one case, at operation the uterus was found to be adherent to the inflamed right tube, which was removed. The uterus was then fastened right and left with silkworm-gut to the recti muscles, and with catgut to the vesical peritoneum. Beginning with the second month of pregnancy, there was occasional pain in the right side and straining at micturition. At the end of the fifth month examination by catheter showed the bladder to be situated in the pelvis, underneath the uterus, and extending well to both sides. The urine was perfectly clear. Two of these four cases had normal labors. In the other two pregnancy was not completed at the time of report. Alexander's operation was performed upon 41 women, of whom the subsequent history could be ascertained. It is worth noting that the ligaments were shortened a good deal, in most cases from 3 to 5 inches. There was a recurrence of the posterior displacement in 3 cases, in 1 of them only after labor. Pregnancy occurred in 23 of the patients operated upon, resulting in 5 miscarriages and 18 deliveries at term. One of these was with forceps. Several of the patients complained during pregnancy of more or less pain in the operative scars. Four of the patients treated by vaginal fixation became pregnant. Three of those upon whom Mackenrodt's operation was performed finished the pregnancy normally. In the fourth case the operation recommended by Dührssen, with opening of the peritoneum, had been done. In the second month displacement recurred, and was followed by abortion. In the light of his experience, Grusdew is inclined to reserve the abdominal fixation for those cases in which there are firm adhesions, or in which disease of the adnexa is suspected, preferring for all uncomplicated cases Alexander's operation. The vaginal operations are less advisable, in his opinion, because the strong attachment of the uterus to the vaginal wall is apt to disturb pregnancy, and if that goes on to term relapse is not uncommon. Of course, these objections are most potent in young married women.

Dorland has collected from medical literature every reported case, normal and otherwise, of pregnancy following ventrofixation up to December, 1896, numbering 179 instances. Of this series, in 120 cases, or 62.03%, a normal gestation was noted; in 111 cases, or 62.01%, labor was absolutely normal; in 68 cases, or 37.98%, both gestation and labor were normal; and in 111 cases, or 62.01%, some abnormality was noted, either in gestation, in labor, or in both. Pain more or less severe was experienced in the line of abdominal incision either during gestation or in labor in 16 cases (8.93%); excessive vomiting in 4 cases (2.23%); high position of the cervix at or above the pelvic brim in 10 cases (5.58%); threatened uterine rupture in 9 cases (5.02%); uterine inertia in 5 cases (2.79% of the cases of pregnancy and 22.79% of the cases of dystocia); abortion in 15 cases (8.37%); premature labor in 10 cases (5.58%); gestational disturbances in 15 cases (8.37%); and dystocia in 22 cases (12.29%); abnormal presentation of the fetus in 9 cases (5.02%); ear-presentation once (0.55%); breech-presentation twice (1.11%); transverse presentation 6 times (3.35%), an unusually large percentage of this malposition of the fetus. Version was required 9 times, and forceps 11 times, or in 50% of the cases of dystocia; 3 times Cesarean section was required (1.67% of the pregnancies), and retained placenta was noted in 3 cases. The fetal mortality was 17.87%, and the maternal 1.67%. Lindforst[1] records a case of twin pregnancy after ventrofixation. When 15 years of age the girl, before

[1] N. Am. Pract., Apr., 1897.

she began to menstruate, suffered from prolapsus uteri, the immediate result of lifting a heavy bundle of hay. The prolapse was complete, but she took no means to return the organ for several years. Then she entered a hospital and had what was termed anterior and posterior kolporrhaphy performed. The uterus remained in place but a short time, and 2 years later she came under the observation of the author. The prolapsus was complete, and the mucous membrane was much indurated and hypertrophied. The external os was so small that it could scarcely be detected. The uterus was suspended by the method of Leopold, and a perineorrhaphy by Tait's method. The patient made an uneventful recovery; the uterine sutures, of silkworm-gut, were removed on the 14th day. Eleven months later the patient was again seen and found to be in good condition and pregnant 7 months. The fundus uteri was found 3 finger-breadths above the umbilicus. The cicatrix of the abdominal wound was enlarged in length and breadth and distinctly pigmented. In the middle of the cicatrice the fixed point could be distinctly seen. The bladder was drawn up high, but caused her little inconvenience. Shortly before term she entered a lying-in hospital in labor. The liquor amnii escaped early and the head engaged, but the cervix remained tense and unyielding. The woman's strength began to fail, and it became necessary to deliver. Accordingly, the author made 3 deep incisions in the cervix and delivered with forceps. Another sac then pressed down in the vagina, and it was found to contain another fetus. A profuse hemorrhage occurred from the cervix, and it was necessary to resort to saline injections; but the patient quickly recovered, and passed a normal puerperium. Both children lived, and it was found that the uterus remained in position. The author attributes the difficulty in delivery to the indurated cervix. He does not advise ventrofixation for retroversion.

Successive Pregnancies in a Double Uterus.—Consolas[1] reports a labor in a primipara of 28 years, in which at the time of delivery he found 2 vaginal passages, each leading to a cervix. The left cervix was dilated with the amniotic sac. The right was closed. From the left the delivery occurred without complications, but with the aid of forceps. A second pregnancy occurred, which he also attended. In this he found that the left uterus was empty, the right being the seat of pregnancy. In neither delivery was the septum torn that divided the 2 parts of the vagina.

Delivery in the Moribund.—Decio[2] publishes a table of 18 labors in which women apparently in a dying condition were delivered *per vias naturales:* of these, 6 children, including 1 pair of twins, seem to have lived. Five were born dead. The remainder expired soon after delivery. Turning after various methods was exclusively the means employed in all of the cases. In 6 the mothers were suffering from eclampsia; of these, 5 recovered, including the twin labor case. Three had cerebral apoplexy; of these, 2 recovered. Two with advanced phthisis survived for a few weeks. Four were flooding from placenta prævia; of these, 3 were saved. One with pulmonary congestion recovered. One bleeding from an internal wound was saved, and 1, injured by a fall, died. Decio has also collected 19 cases of Cesarean section performed upon dying women. All were graver cases than those in the table, and all died. In 13 cases the child was alive; 1 labor was of twins, making 14 children saved. In only 2 was the os more or less open.

Rupture of the Uterus.—Fatal cases are recorded by J. Saxl,[3] Cullingworth,[4] J. C. MacEvitt,[5] P. A. Colmer,[6] and Sherwood Dunn.[7] Recoveries after

[1] Am. Medico-Surg. Bull., Jan. 25, 1897.   [2] Ann. di Ost. e Gin., June, 1896.
[3] Med. Rec., Oct. 31, 1896.   [4] Lancet, Sept. 26, 1896.
[5] Med. Rec., Aug. 1, 1896.   [6] Lancet, Mar. 6, 1897.   [7] Pacific Med. Jour., July, 1896.

uterine rupture are recorded by MacEvitt,[1] C. H. Roberts,[2] J. N. Upshur,[3] and Burger.[4] Burger's was a remarkable case of rupture of the uterus in cross-birth. As the patient could not be taken to a hospital and assistance could not be obtained, Burger could do nothing more than make version and extract the fetus. After delivering the placenta the mother's intestines protruded through the rent in the uterus. These were replaced and the hand kept in the uterus until it contracted firmly. The rent in the uterus was tightly closed by its firm contraction, and but little hemorrhage followed. The patient did well until the sixth day, when her husband, while drunk, had intercourse with her violently. She recovered, however, from this and was delivered of a living child 9 months and 6 days after. The placenta was adherent to the site of the former rupture and was delivered manually. A year later the patient died of hemorrhage from adherent placenta before the midwife in attendance could summon a physician.

MacEvitt[5] states that some ruptures are progressive and cannot be recognized until the completion of the disaster. Emphysema at the level of the hypogastric region caused by air in the connective tissue is a symptom not always present; when found it indicates a fatal termination. Roberts states that the child always dies when it escapes into the peritoneal cavity.

Inversion of the Uterus.—Cases of this rare accident are reported by H. S. Kilbourne,[6] J. W. Walker,[7] G. T. Harrison,[8] G. Fowler,[9] W. Lindley,[10] and D. J. Brown.[11] Brown suggests as points of diagnosis between inversio uteri and uterine polypus the following: 1. The circular, not lateral, implantation of the pedicle; 2. The opening of the tubes upon the inferior portion of the tumor; 3. The special sensibility, sometimes accompanied by special contractility, that it offers to pressure and to acupuncture; 4. The half reduction that can always be made in inversions, never in polypi; 5. The absence of the uterus from its ordinary place, ascertained by rectal and vesical examination. As regards prognosis, Crosse says that one-third of the women with puerperal inversion of the uterus die either immediately or within a month.

FETAL DYSTOCIA.

Multiple Pregnancy.—A. Valenta[12] refers again to the extraordinary case of plural pregnancies reported by H. X. Boër in 1808. The patient was aged 40 years, had suffered from epileptic fits, and during a married life of 20 years had given birth to 32 children in 11 pregnancies. Twice she gave birth to quadruplets, 6 times to triplets, and thrice to twins. Twenty-six of the children were boys, 6 were girls. Twenty-eight were born alive and 4 dead. Her first pregnancy was at the age of 14 years and resulted in quadruplets. The mother herself was one of quadruplets, and her mother had a family of 38 children, and died in the puerperium after giving birth to twins. There was a hereditary history of plural births on the father's side, he being himself a twin.

Interesting cases of twin-pregnancy are reported by C. W. Branch,[13] with hydramnios—about 220 oz. of water; Chambrelent and Chemin,[14] with hydramnios, the 1st fetus presenting unilateral fusion of the two kidneys, the 2d

[1] Loc. cit.
[2] Lancet, Dec. 19, 1896.
[3] Va. Med. Semi-monthly, Oct. 23, 1896.
[4] Münch. med. Woch., No. 25, 1896.
[5] Ibid.
[6] Med. Rec., Aug. 15, 1896.
[7] Lancet, Aug. 29, 1896.
[8] Am. Gyn. and Obst. Jour., May, 1897.
[9] Lancet, July 25, 1896.
[10] Med. Rec., Sept. 5, 1896.
[11] Boston M. and S. Jour., Feb. 11, 1897.
[12] Wien. med. Woch., No. 3, 1897.
[13] Brit. Med. Jour., July 11, 1896.
[14] Jour de Méd. de Bordeaux, No. 9, Mar. 1, 1896.

forming an omphalosite peracephalus; J. D. Todee,[1] a living and dead fetus existing together in utero for 1 or 2 months prior to confinement; J. S. Wight,[2] 1 fetus being developed to 7 months and the other to 5 months; the children were both female, there was a single chorion with 2 amnions, both of which were intact, and a common placenta (*uniovial twins*); and C. C. Henry,[3] the mother being in a state of uremic coma for 40 hours, with convulsions and serious brain-disturbance, but ultimately recovering, and the twins being healthy. Kalnikoff[4] reports the case of a woman whom he delivered of a twin 3 days after the spontaneous birth of its brother. He also removed both placentæ. The puerperium was normal and both children lived.

A. L. Bailey[5] records 2 cases of triplets, in one instance the children all being male, and in the other instance all female. Dorland, in Aug., 1896, saw a woman in her 8th month of pregnancy, who 3 weeks later fell into labor while on the street and was admitted to a hospital, where she gave birth to triplets, two boys and a girl.

C. C. Henry[6] and M. Günsburg[7] report instances of quadruplets. Günsburg's case was a peasant woman, 20 years of age, in the 4th month of her 1st pregnancy. Three of the fetuses were normal, the 4th was a monstrosity (see p. 460). Henry's case was a woman 39 years of age, in her 6th pregnancy, who went to term. There were 4 placentas with membranous connection, but no vascular communication; their combined weight was 3 pounds; the aggregate weight of the babies was 16 pounds, as follows: 1st, $3\frac{3}{4}$ pounds; 2d, $4\frac{1}{4}$ pounds; 3d, $3\frac{3}{4}$ pounds; and 4th, $4\frac{1}{4}$ pounds. Two were stillborn, and one eventually survived. [P. Charbonnier[8] gives the proportion of quadruplets to single births as 1 in 400,000; Puech, 1 in 2,074,306; Plenck, 1 in 20,000. The combined tables of Descaner, Spengler-Ploss, Sickel, and Veit, including nearly fifty million births, give the number of quadruplets as about $2\frac{1}{4}$ to the million; in Switzerland, between the years 1881 and 1893 there was one instance in 1,108,092 births. During the last $2\frac{1}{4}$ years a few authentic instances have been recorded, notably one by Bousquet,[9] one by Pergamin,[10] and one by Stahl.[11]

R. A. Hibbs[12] reported a case of quintuplets before the Obstetric Section of the New York Academy of Medicine at its May meeting. The patient had had 6 children previously, and had enjoyed good health up to the time of the present pregnancy. Three months before labor her physician noted that the abdomen was unusually distended. On April 29, at about the 8th month of pregnancy, she was taken in labor. In a few minutes the membranes ruptured and a child presented by the feet and was delivered. In a few minutes more a second child presented by the head and was delivered. Fifteen minutes later the third child presented by the feet and was delivered. The fourth presented by the feet and was delivered. The fifth also presented by the feet and was delivered. All were boys. Three of them lived only a few days, and the remaining two were living in May, when Hibbs saw them. There was only one placenta with the five cords attached.

As regards the management of twin labors, Stephenson[13] concludes that multiple pregnancy is abnormal, and hence more dangerous than usual labor. He believes that different principles should govern these cases from those

[1] Med. Brief, Mar., 1897.
[2] N. Y. Med. Jour., Jan. 16, 1897.
[3] Brooklyn Med. Jour., Oct., 1896.
[4] Monatssch. f. Geb. u. Gynäk., Jan., 1897.
[5] Med. Age, Aug. 10, 1896. [6] Loc. cit. [7] Edinb. Med. Jour., Aug., 1896.
[8] Étude des Grossesses triples et plus que triples, 1895.
[9] Ann. de Gynéc., vol. xlii., p. 55, 1894. [10] St. Petersburg. med. Woch., Suppl. N. 1, 1895.
[11] Tr. Chicago Gynec. Soc., p. 6, 1896. [12] Am. Medico-Surg. Bull., July 18, 1896.
[13] Scottish M. and S. Jour., No. 1, 1897.

which experience has recommended in the treatment of single pregnancies. He would consider the delivery incomplete when the first child was born and the second had not been expelled. With regard to the second twin, the risks are much greater than in single pregnancy for both mother and child, and hence interference must be practised. As regards infant mortality in twin labors, it is on the average $2\frac{1}{4}$ times greater than in single births; inasmuch as twins are usually smaller than the average child and their expulsion more easy, there must be other reasons that bring about the increased mortality. When the element of time is considered, it is found that $\frac{3}{4}$ of the cases end within the first $\frac{1}{2}$ hour without material assistance; 1 in every 4, however, requires artificial aid. The mortality of the second $\frac{1}{2}$ hour after the birth of the first child was 4 times greater than that of the first $\frac{1}{2}$ hour. If the duration of labor be prolonged a $\frac{1}{2}$ hour, the life of the second child is greatly imperilled. It is found that in the first-born of twins, if the head presents, the mortality is greater than in single births; but if the breech or foot presents, the conditions are much more favorable. In the second-born of twins the mortality in head-presentations is almost double. In the cases collected, where the second child was either transverse or in footling presentation, not a single one of these children was lost. To sum up the mortality by presentations, $90\frac{5}{10}\%$ of children lost were in head-presentations; $9\frac{5}{10}\%$ in breech; while there was no mortality in transverse and footling births. The practical conclusion of these studies lies in the fact that so soon as the first child is born the second should be immediately extracted by the feet. In this way the mortality for mothers and children will be rendered as little as possible.

Excessive Size of the Fetus.—A. E. Gallant[1] records a case of dystocia due to disparity between the size of the head of the fetus and the circumference of its shoulders (44 cm.—$17\frac{1}{4}$ in.), the occipitofrontal circumference being 33.5 cm. ($13\frac{1}{8}$ in.). In addition the mother was excessively obese, weighing 220 pounds, the pelvic fat interfering with the distention of the vagina. In 4000 deliveries at the Sloane Maternity the largest child measured 43 cm. around the shoulders.

Fœtus Papyraceus.—Bäcker[2] recently demonstrated at Buda-Pesth a fœtus papyraceus. The mother was a primipara, aged 28, and was delivered at term of a well-developed female child, nearly 19 in. long, weighing 6 lb. 12 oz. On the placenta was the chorion, which bore a second amniotic cavity containing the fœtus papyraceus. This blighted embryo appeared to have reached the 2d month of development. Bäcker preserved the membranes and the placenta as well as the fetus in a 4% solution of formaldehyd: they remained perfect, free from shrinking or opacity.

Goldberger[3] reports a remarkable twin-labor. The waters broke and a fœtus papyraceus, amongst the smallest recorded in literature, escaped. It was $\frac{9}{10}$ in. long, and weighed $5\frac{1}{4}$ gr. The bones showed very well. The other twin, fully developed (delivery being at term) was born apparently without trouble. It had symmetric defects in the skin of the abdomen, about the level of the 12th rib in the anterior axillary line. The right was as big as a thaler-piece, the left was smaller. The edges were irregular, and from them radiated shiny, reddish cicatricial lines. These scars proved that the defects were not due to injury during labor. The base of each "defect"—a fetal ulcer, in fact—was granulating subcutaneous tissue, with scabs at certain points. Both were healed at the end of a fortnight.

Extraordinary Retention in Utero of the Fetal Head.—

[1] Med. Rec., Sept. 5, 1896.   [2] Centralbl. f. Gynäk., No. 28, 1896.
[3] Ibid., No. 30, 1896.

Toth[1] records a case in which the attending physician pulled so vigorously upon the breech of an 8-months' fetus that its neck parted and the head remained in utero, despite all his exertions to remove it. The mother, a young tertipara, recovered with some fever, and enjoyed good health for a year. During this time, irregular hemorrhages and foul-smelling discharge continued, followed by the occasional discharge of bones. At the end of 16 months the cervix was dilated, and the large bones of the skull, which remained, were removed. They were extensively adherent to the uterus, and the free hemorrhage which followed their removal was controlled by tamponade. The patient made a quick recovery.

Dystocia due to Fetal Retention of Urine.—O. Saintu[2] reports the case of a woman upon whom it was decided to induce labor at about the 8th month on account of a contracted pelvis. Saintu delivered the head, shoulders, and thorax with ease, but the rest of the labor was conducted with great difficulty on account of immense distention of the fetal abdomen. The child did not urinate until the next night, when it passed a large quantity of urine, and catheterization removed more. The child died the next evening. At the autopsy the bladder was found to extend to the ensiform cartilage above, and laterally to the sides of the abdomen. The urethra was perfectly patent.

Breech Presentation with Extended Legs.—W. S. A. Griffith and A. W. W. Lea read a paper on this subject before the London Obstetric Society on Jan. 6, 1897. Seventeen cases were briefly described and the following conclusions arrived at : 1. The extension of the legs in incomplete breech presentations may be either primary or secondary. 2. In the primary variety, which occurs before labor has begun, the breech engages readily in the brim, and the diagnosis can be made. 3. In the secondary variety the extension occurs during labor. This form is more frequent than the primary. 4. This complication is more frequent in primiparæ, namely, 70 % of the cases. 5. The prognosis, with regard to the child, is not worse than is that in pelvic presentations in general. 6. Cephalic version is advantageous before labor is advanced. It is not usually possible in the primary, but may be so in the secondary variety. 7. Most cases are delivered naturally. 8. Prophylactic reduction of the leg is required only in exceptional cases. 9. It is probable that flexion of the leg on the thigh is preferable to bringing down the leg into the vagina. 10. If aid is required in the lower part of the pelvis, the soft fillet will usually effect delivery.

OBSTETRIC OPERATIONS.

Induction of Labor.—Kossmann[3] considers that the accidents that have occurred in the induction of labor by the injection of glycerin were caused by the drug being used in large doses for hygroscopic purposes, and not with the more physiologic purpose of stimulating the unstriped muscle. He has used glycerin injections in 2 cases with marked success. He concludes that the injection of 5 c.c. of glycerin into the cervical canal will bring on strong pains without leading to nephritis or any other ill-effect. It is free from the danger of infection which attends injection into the uterine cavity. The introduction of a colpeurynter into the vagina serves to keep up the pains when they have been started, and, therefore, makes further injection of glycerin unnecessary. Kossmann regards this method as being, next to simple vaginal douches, the most harmless method of inducing labor. T. A. Helme[4] does

---

[1] Centralbl. f. Gynäk., No. 24, 1896.
[2] Jour. de Méd. de Paris, July 12, 1896.
[3] Therap. Monatschr., June, 1896.
[4] Lancet, p. 936, Oct. 31, 1896.

the same thing, injecting into the cervix, however, 1½ ounces of pure glycerin.

Stieda[1] contributes an interesting paper upon the employment of elastic bags in inducing labor or abortion. He distinguishes two methods, in one of which the bag is placed within the cervix, while in the other it is carried above the internal os into the lower uterine segment. In connection with this treatment he employed frequent hot douches to soften the parts and promote dilatation. He describes in detail 5 cases in which labor was induced in this manner. In all, a living child was born, while the length of the induced labor varied from 9 to 24 hours, the average being 15 hours. In the case of several of these patients this was a much shorter labor than had occurred previously. In some cases it was necessary to use specula in introducing the bag, but in most this was not found essential. When it was desired to hurry labor traction was made upon the supply-tube through which the bag was filled, and the distended bag was slowly drawn through the cervix; when haste was not desired the bag was allowed to remain until expelled. The precaution was taken to force air out of the bag before its introduction and to fill it with sterile water. In addition to the induced labors, Stieda narrates 3 cases in which he induced abortion by the same method. Here he was equally successful, the abortions being concluded in about 7 hours, the use of the bag being necessary for between 1 and 2 hours. In cases in which traction was made upon the bag the pelvis of the patient was raised so that the traction was exercised downward and backward in the axis of the pelvis. The same method was employed successfully in a case of submucous myoma of the uterus in which the patient declined operation and in which the cervix was dilated; tenaculum-forceps were applied to the tumor, and traction made upon the forceps for 12 hours. At the end of this time it was possible to remove the tumor by enucleation.

Forceps.—A. D. Wilkinson[2] gives the following indications for the use of the forceps: 1. In all pelves in which the diameters are [slightly] below the normal measurements. 2. When the head is in an immovable position, with the chin fixed over the symphysis pubis. 3. When the head is in the superior strait, with the chin to the front. 4. When the head is locked at the pubis, but when flexion is imperfect and fixation of the frontal part of the vertex is the result. 5. When the face is fixed anteriorly, with the chin locked. 6. When the face is fixed laterally. 7. In transverse and oblique positions of the head. 8. When the head is laterally rotated and deeply fixed in the pelvis. 9. In great narrowness and rigidity of the soft parts, when the hand cannot be introduced, or when the fingers soon become exhausted on account of the constriction. 10. In too large heads—as hydrocephalus [this is doubtful]. 11. In placenta prævia and eclampsia. 12. When the extractive methods have been tried and proved insufficient. 13. When the fetus is dead. 14. When the head has been torn from its trunk.

[It is very remarkable how slowly any improvement, although a very real one, makes its way in this country. It is not too much to say that the advantages of axis-traction forceps have been definitely proved by theoretic and practical demonstration, and yet the number of physicians who use these instruments form but a very small proportion of the whole.] S. Milne Murray[3] describes a new modification of his well-known forceps which permits of traction in the pelvic axis being made with still greater scientific accuracy. He points out that the ordinary axis-traction forceps only allow of traction being

---

[1] Monats. f. Geb. u. Gynäk., Bd. v., H. 3, 1897.   [2] West. Med. Rev., Oct. 15, 1896.
[3] Edinb. Med. Jour., Sept., 1896.

made in the pelvic axis when the pelvis is normal, but that when the axis of the inlet is more vertical than usual, as in the justominor pelvis, or more horizontal than usual, as in the flat pelvis, some of the force employed is lost unless provision be made to allow the line of traction to be varied to suit the requirements of the altered canal. Of course, in cases of abnormal pelvis, if ordinary forceps are used, the line of traction is still more faulty than with axis-traction forceps, and in order to do away with this "angle of error" he has devised a pair of forceps which will permit the line of traction to be altered to suit any given case of pelvic deformity. The forceps are identical with those used in the ordinary axis-traction instrument, and the traction-rods are jointed to them in the usual manner. These rods run down the back of the handles, and at a point halfway down they turn backward at a right angle, forming two horizontal bars $4\frac{1}{2}$ in. long, with graduations $\frac{1}{2}$ in. apart. A perforated block with a handle attached by a joint is slid along these horizontal rods and can be fixed at any point by a screw. By means of a sector which moves with the handle that position of the block on the horizontal rods

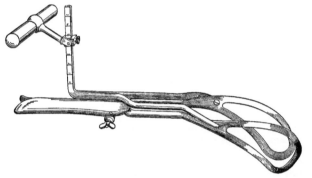

Fig. 34.—Murray's forceps with adjustable axis-traction (Edinb. Med. Jour., Sept., 1896).

can be determined which is necessary in cases in which the pelvic inclination is normal; but if the axis is more vertical than usual, the block is moved forward nearer to the handles, and if the axis is less vertical, it is moved backward away from the handles. By this means we can insure that in all cases the line of traction corresponds with the axis of the pelvis.

Murray[1] also advocates the use of forceps in cases of flattened pelvis in which the head presents transversely in the pelvic brim. He states that the choice of version in these cases has been based upon the belief that the forceps, applied in the anteroposterior diameter of the head, tend to compress it anteroposteriorly, and to cause a bulging of the transverse or biparietal diameter. This would increase the difficulty of extraction, as the biparietal diameter is already brought into relation with the smallest diameter of the pelvic brim. He doubts the truth of this belief, because he has shown by experiment that when the head is grasped over the occiput and forehead that the occipitofrontal diameter may be compressed $1\frac{1}{2}$ in. without increasing the biparietal. A vertical and not a transverse expansion results. The various segments of the cranium slide under each other in a telescopic manner. To

[1] Brit. Med. Jour., No. 1870, 1896.

succeed in delivering the fetal head presenting transversely in the brim of a
flattened pelvis the forceps must not only grasp the head in its anteroposterior
diameter, but must also make traction downward and backward in the axis
of the pelvis. The head naturally passes through the brim, in these cases,
by an exaggeration of Naegele's obliquity, by which the posterior parietal
eminence pivots against the promontory of the sacrum, while the anterior
moulds itself against the pubes. Murray stated that he had delivered living
children when the anteroposterior pelvic diameter was 3¼ in., and even as
little as 2¾ in.

[The value of the Walcher position in pelvic contraction and forceps-
operations is becoming more recognized.] W. E. Fothergill [1] finds that
in about 30 cases measured by him the average increase in the diagonal
conjugate gained by this position was 1 cm., the claim made by Walcher.
He concludes that in high-forceps cases, and after perforation, the position
saves—(1) the strength of the operator, (2) pressure on the head, (3) pressure
on the symphysis, (4) pressure on the perineum by the forceps. In cases of
difficulty at the brim not needing forceps, and in breech cases, the position
saves—(1) exertion to the uterus and abdominal muscles, (2) pressure on the
head, (3) pressure on the pubic symphysis. In all cases, with or without
forceps, in which the perineum is in danger, extension of the legs at the hips
is of advantage in relaxing the integument and subjacent structures at the
vulvar orifice.

Version.—Mensinga [2] performs podalic version with the patient upon
her abdomen. He claims for this method the following advantages : the
outlet of the pelvis is directed above with the patient prone, giving the operator much more room for the insertion of the hand. The operator's hand
and arm are in the position of pronation, giving a better use of the muscles
and tactile sense. This posture also widens and opens the uterus and vagina,
whereby the contraction-ring disappears. There is also less risk of bruising
the soft parts. The patient has a pillow under the chest, her head being
turned to one side, while the operator sits beside her, using either hand for
version. By this posture two dangers are minimized : tearing the uterus from
the vagina and air-embolism. Patients suffer less in this posture. [Version
should always be done under anesthesia, and we cannot see any marked
advantage to be derived from the foregoing procedure.]

Craniotomy.—Hergenhahn [3] tabulates 46 cases of perforation of the
after-coming head. In 25 of these the cranium was opened through the
foramen magnum ; in 2 the opening was through the neck ; in 9 through the
occiput ; in 3 by means of the smaller fontanel ; in 4 through a lateral fontanel ; in 1 through the parietal bone ; and in 2 by means of the base of the
skull. In 29 cases delivery was accomplished by traction on the breech ; in
9 the sharp hook was inserted in the opening of perforation for purposes of
demonstration. In these cases rupture of the uterus occurred once ; the cervix was torn 8 times ; minor lacerations were not infrequent. The mortality
was 5 in the 46 cases ; 1 from eclampsia ; from previous septic infection, 2 ;
from hemorrhage and infection (ruptured hematoma of the vulva) and from
repeated attempts at delivery and mutilation before admission to the hospital,
2. Hergenhahn found that craniotomy should be undertaken in suitable cases
as soon as the fetus has perished. The head should be firmly fixed, after
version, at the pelvic brim and steadied by an assistant. The cranium should
be opened by some form of scissor-perforator through whatever portion is

[1] Brit. Med. Jour., No. 1870, 1896.   [2] Centralbl. f. Gynäk., Nov. 23, 1896.
[3] Arch. f. Gynäk., Bd. li., H. 2, 1896.

most available. The patient is then put in Walcher's position, the finger of the operator is put in the fetal mouth, and by combined traction the brain is expelled and the head moulded and delivered. The prognosis in cases requiring this operation depends on the condition of the patient before operation, many of them having been lacerated and infected by previous attempts at delivery.

Additional cases are recorded by C. E. Purslow[1] and G. F. De Silva,[2] both of whom advocate perforation through the mouth. De Silva gives as the advantages of this method : 1. Safety and the ease with which the object can be accomplished without injury to the maternal parts, which often occurs when perforation is done behind the ear ; 2. So much force is not required as in piercing the mastoid bone ; 3. It easily breaks up the base of the skull. Purslow gives as its disadvantages : 1. The brain-matter will not flow so readily through the opening, but this can be easily overcome by passing the tube of a Higginson's syringe through the hole, and washing out the brain ; 2. The pressure of the perforator on the roof of the mouth tends to cause extension of the head, in which case the mechanism of the delivery of the head may be interfered with, or the perforator may pass through the maxilla and into the orbit, not entering the cranial cavity at all, and even injuring the uterine wall.

Symphysiotomy.—[The wave of reaction has begun, and the operation is limited now to but a very narrow scope, largely because of the difficulty in its performance and because of its higher mortality than that of Cesarean section.] Cases are recorded as follow : Donald,[3] 3 cases ; Swift,[4] the first case performed in Boston or its vicinity ; Heinricus,[5] 1 case, recovery being retarded by a fistula which led to the symphysis, and opened near the mons veneris ; it was accompanied by necrosis of the severed bones ; ultimate recovery occurred with firm union at the pubis ; F. R. McCreery,[6] a case, followed by a fistula and slight separation of the symphysis, with ultimate good recovery ; E. P. Davis[7] and G. M. Boyd,[8] each 1 successful case ; E. A. Ayres,[9] 1 case, the patient dying on the 33d day of pneumonia.

Hansen[10] reports the case of a quartipara whom he delivered 3 years after a delivery by symphysiotomy. The patient had a contracted pelvis, with a conjugate of $3\frac{1}{4}$ in., and was delivered at her first confinement after great difficulty of a dead fetus, which had presented transversely. The second delivery was completed by symphysiotomy, the fetus presenting by the vertex but not engaging at the pelvic brim. Two years later she aborted at the third month, and a year after she presented herself to Hansen in an advanced stage of pregnancy. The general condition was good and locomotion normal, and she continued to perform her daily work. Upon examination it was found that the pubic bones were separated sufficiently to admit the tip of the little finger between them and that there was a marked motion between them in walking. Three weeks later she fell into labor. The fetus presented transversely and soon became impacted in the pelvis, but labor was easily terminated by version. After delivery the pubic bones were found to be separated more than $1\frac{1}{2}$ in. A firm pelvic bandage was applied. Five weeks later the woman was able to walk a quarter of a mile without discomfort. At the time the case was reported the bones were separated about $\frac{1}{2}$ inch.

[1] Brit. Med. Jour., Oct. 31, 1896.
[2] Indian Med. Rec., Dec. 16, 1896.
[3] Edinb. Med. Jour., Dec., 1896.
[4] Boston M. and S. Jour., May 17, 1896.
[5] Monats. f. Geb u. Gynäk., Bd. iii., H. 4, 1896.
[6] Med. Rec., Aug. 15, 1896.
[7] Med. News, Jan. 16, 1897.
[8] Am. Gyn. and Obst. Jour., Sept., 1869.
[9] Med. Rec., Sept. 12, 1896.
[10] Hospitals Tidende, p. 597, June, 1896.

W. Pooth,[1] following the suggestion of Frank, has performed artificial widening in 3 cases of contracted pelvis, inserting a piece of bone between the ends of the pubic bones to keep them separated. The operation is performed through a transverse incision across the symphysis. A piece of each pubic ramus and the anterior part of the symphysis are chiselled off, forming a plate about 3 cm. long and 1½ cm. broad, and including nearly half the thickness of the bones. The posterior part of the symphysis is then separated and the child extracted. The ends of the pubic bones are freshened, and the new plate inserted and fastened by sutures, thus holding the ends of the pubic bones apart about 3 cm. In the 3 cases reported there was complete bony union at the symphysis and no pain or inconvenience of any kind in standing or walking. The diagonal conjugates before and after the operation were, respectively, as follows:

Before, 9½ cm.	After, 11 cm.
" 8¾ cm.	" 10 cm.
" 8¾ cm.	" 10¼ cm.

Cesarean Section.—Cases are recorded as follows: W. R. Wilson,[2] a successful Sänger operation, in a colored girl of 14 years, with an undeveloped nonrachitic pelvis; Strebel,[3] 10 Porro operations from Wyder's clinic at Zurich, with 1 maternal and 1 fetal death; Béchet,[4] 1 successful Sänger operation; Varnier and Delbet,[5] and Pinard and Ségond,[6] each 1 successful Porro operation, the first for complete retroflexion at term, and the second for advanced pelvic contraction; Sinclair,[7] 1 successful Sänger operation; C. N. Van de Poll,[8] 3 successful operations upon the same woman, the last by Porro's method; S. A Bontor,[9] and J. B. De Lee,[10] each 1 successful Sänger operation; A. H. Buckmaster,[11] and G. M. Boyd,[12] each 1 successful Porro operation. Cases of postmortem Cesarean section with delivery of living children are recorded by Erdheim[13] and H. S. Stearns,[14] while Dührssen[15] records a vaginal Cesarean section in a woman who had had vaginal fixation of the uterus. The operation consisted in opening the vault of the vagina and the uterus, performing version and extraction. Mother and child recovered, the puerperal period being but little longer than the usual one. The operation consists in enlarging the vagina, if necessary, by perineal incision, freeing the uterus from the tissues about the cervix, rapid incision of the posterior and anterior lips of the cervix as high as the internal os, followed by version and extraction. After the removal of the placenta the uterus is pulled down, tamponed, and the lines of incision sutured. If indications for removal of the uterus exist, this can be performed with facility.

Hirst,[16] recognizing the fact that Cesarean section may be forced on the general physician in an emergency at any moment, has given a detailed description of its technic for his guidance. If there be time to make arrangements, a period of about 2 weeks before term should be selected. It is unnecessary to excite labor-pains beforehand. The patient should be given a full hot bath 2 days before operation, and should be kept in bed. Admin-

[1] Monats. f. Geb. u. Gynak., Bd. iii , Sept 6, 1896.
[2] Am. Gyn. and Obst. Jour., May, 1897.   [3] Arch. f. Gynäk., Bd. 52, II. 2, 1896.
[4] Progrès méd., No. 46, 1896.   [5] Ann. de Gynéc., Feb., 1897.
[6] Ibid., Feb., 1897.   [7] Med. Chron., vol. v., No. 4, 1896.
[8] Centralbl. f. Gynäk., No. 21, 1896.   [9] Lancet. Mar. 6, 1897.
[10] N. Am. Pract., Jan., 1897.   [11] N. Y. Med. Jour., July 11, 1896.
[12] Am. Gyn. and Obst. Jour., Sept., 1896.   [13] Centralbl. f. Gynäk., No. 14, 1896.
[14] Med. Rec., Aug. 15, 1896.   [15] Thèse. Berlin, 1896.
[16] Am. Jour. Obst., Jan., 1897.

ister the following pill 3 times a day : ℞ Strychnin, gr. $\frac{1}{20}$; digitalis, gr. $\frac{1}{2}$; quinin, gr. 2. M. Secure movements of the bowels daily by 2 drams of Rochelle salt every evening. Examine the heart, lungs, and urine.

Day before Operation.—(1) Diet: gruel for breakfast, soup for dinner, milk-toast for supper. One glass of milk at 10 A. M., 4 P. M., 9 P. M. (2) Medicine : 5 P. M., afternoon before operation, 10 gr. of sulfonal in half a glass of boiling water cooled down to a temperature that permits of its being drunk, if the patient is nervous and has been sleepless ; 9 P. M., half an ounce of Epsom salts in a tumblerful of water. *Evening before Operation.*—(1) Cleanse the abdomen as follows : sterilize for 20 minutes at 240° F. one soft-bristled brush, absorbent cotton, half-dozen towels, gauze, binder, and a long gown. (2) The nurse's and doctor's hands are prepared as for operation : remove rings, scrub with brush, hot water, and tincture of green soap for 10 minutes, clean the nails with a nail-file, scrub the hands and arms with benzene and then with alcohol, immerse the hands and arms in bichlorid solution (1 : 1000) for 2 minutes ; then put on the gown. (3) The abdomen from the ensiform to the symphysis and from flank to flank is scrubbed with a soft-bristled brush, tincture of green soap, and hot water for 10 minutes, paying special attention to the navel and pubis. Wipe the razor with cotton and alcohol, shave the pubis, then scrub thoroughly with alcohol. Cover the abdomen with sterile gauze and apply the binder. *Morning of Operation.*—Give a cup of beef-tea at 7 A. M. The hands of the nurse are cleansed as described ; the articles are resterilized as described. The same cleansing of the abdomen is repeated as described, with the addition that before the alcohol-scrubbing the abdomen is scrubbed with benzene. Wring out a sterile towel in 1 : 1000 bichlorid solution and cover the abdomen with the towel. Put over it a thick layer of sterile cotton. Apply the binder. Catheterize the woman just before anesthesia with a sterile glass catheter in an aseptic manner. Give a vaginal douche of one quart of 1 : 4000 mercuric chlorid solution, followed by a little sterile water. If the bowels have not opened freely, give an anema,—a pint of soapsuds and a dram of turpentine. *The Operation.*—With a large scalpel make a free incision from 2 inches above the umbilicus to just above the symphysis. Enlarge the abdominal opening downward as low as possible with scissors. While an assistant makes the wound gap deliver the womb from the abdominal cavity. The assistant now approximates the edges of the abdominal wound as closely as possible around and above the cervix, at the same time squeezing the latter with outspread hands. Incise the uterine muscle to the extent of an inch with a few rapid but light strokes of the knife, taking care not to wound the membranes. With a rapid movement of the left arm and hand tear the uterine wall down to the internal os. Rupture the membranes, detach the placenta if it be in the way, and push it aside. Seize the child by the most accessible part and deliver. Drop the child with the placenta attached into a sterile sheet spread out over the outstretched arms of an assistant, whose duty it is to revive the child if necessary, and cut the cord. Then follows an easy hysterectomy : ligation of the ovarian arteries and arteries of the round ligaments ; application of clamps ; cutting of the broad ligaments ; preparation of the peritoneal flaps ; amputation of the womb ; ligation of the uterine arteries ; and over-sewing of the stump, which is dropped. The abdominal wall had better be closed by the beginner with close-set interrupted sutures.

PATHOLOGY OF THE PUERPERIUM.

Puerperal Sepsis.—C. J. Cullingworth[1] calls attention to the fact that
there is an undiminished mortality from puerperal sepsis in England and
Wales, and that notwithstanding the general spread of the Listerian method.
In the pathetic statistics given one sees the mortality greater in the decade,
1885–95 than in the previous one, 1875–85, and this worse than 1865–75.
The disease has been almost completely banished from the lying-in hospitals;
hence the trouble must lie in the methods of obstetricians at large. [A more
earnest incentive to prophylaxis in puerperal sepsis cannot be imagined than
this startling fact.] Kortright[2] contributes a paper on the puerperal mortality
in Brooklyn. He finds that during 1895, 224 women died of puerperal causes
in the city of Brooklyn; of these, 76 deaths were due to puerperal sepsis.
The largest number of these cases occurred during the winter months—a fact
often observed by others. Many of these deaths were among persons employing midwives instead of physicians. The writer concludes from his study that
the puerperal death-rate is lower among Americans than among foreigners and
their children. Septic infection is more often fatal where midwives are habitually employed. Kidney-failure is most frequently observed among those who
use alcoholic drinks.

Hirst,[3] in speaking of the etiology of puerperal sepsis, dwells upon the importance of a careful study of the bacteriology of the vaginal secretions. He
remarks that the vagina becomes infected almost immediately after birth. In
a normal condition it contains no pathogenic bacteria, and has strong germicidal powers, which serve to guard a woman against infection. These powers
depend, as far as our present knowledge goes, upon the presence of a special
bacillus and upon the products of its life-processes; upon the leukocytosis due
to chemotactic action; upon phagocytosis; upon the germicidal powers, perhaps, of the anatomic elements of the vagina, of the cervical mucus, and of
the bloody discharge during menstruation and the puerperium. During and
after labor mechanical safeguards of the most effective kind are furnished
against infection. These are the discharge of the liquor amnii, washing out
the vagina; the passage of the child's body; the descent of the placenta and
membranes, and the bloody discharge which follows. Moreover, should the
vagina exceptionally contain pathogenic bacteria, they are likely to be in a
condition of diminished or absent virulence, in which state they will not be
productive of disease unless the tissues with which they come in contact are
reduced in vitality. Bearing these facts in mind, it would seem that the common practice of relying upon vaginal douching for disinfecting the vagina
before labor is faulty, not to say foolish. It has been clearly demonstrated
that the injection of an antiseptic fluid into the vagina will not destroy pathogenic germs there, and will, moreover, rob the woman to a certain extent of
the safeguards against infection that nature provides for her.

E. S. Jackson[4] says that puerperal fevers can only be exactly classified
when we can classify the various bacteria to which they owe their origin.
Among causes, he insists we must admit autoinfection, since the vagina often
contains these bacteria; generally, however, they are introduced from without
from lack of antiseptic precautions. The most rapidly fatal cases are due to
streptococci; staphylococci seem to be less virulent. The gonococcus seems to
produce tubal suppuration and pelvic peritonitis rather than high temperatures
and general peritonitis, and chronic rather than acute cases. Faulty sanitation

[1] Lancet, Mar. 6, 1897.   [2] Brooklyn Med. Jour., No. 2, 1897.
[3] Univ. Med. Mag., Oct., 1896.   [4] Intercol. Med. Jour. Austral., Feb. 20, 1896.

can hardly cause puerperal sepsis, though it may render the system less resistant. Remy[1] speaks of the relationship existing between meconium and sepsis, and insists that the membranes should never be ruptured before complete dilatation of the os without very special reasons. When the waters escape and meconium is mixed with the liquor amnii, the uterine cavity is soiled. If labor be prolonged and antiseptic precautions impracticable, the fluid mixture decomposes rapidly and septic infection becomes certain. Remy distinguished the above conditions in 7 labors under his observation. The mortality was 42%. Antiseptic precautions are, therefore, especially needed in cases of premature rupture of the membranes.

Saft[2] believes that prophylaxis against puerperal infection should consist in diminishing internal examinations as greatly as possible, and in observing absolute antisepsis. G. W. Dobbin[3] reports a fatal case of puerperal sepsis due to infection with the bacillus aërogenes capsulatus.

As to the question of puerperal self-infection, Jewett[4] refers in particular to the relation of pus-producing germs primarily present in the body of the pregnant woman to childbed sepsis, and draws the following conclusions : 1. There is no clinical proof that puerperal infection can occur from normal vaginal secretions. 2. All childbed infection in women previously healthy is by contact. 3. Prophylactic vaginal disinfection as a routine measure is unnecessary, and even in skilled hands is probably injurious. 4. Its general adoption in private practice could scarcely fail to be mischievous. 5. In healthy puerperæ, delivered aseptically, postpartum douching is also contraindicated. 6. A purulent vaginal secretion exposes the woman to puerperal infection. 7. In the presence of such discharges at the beginning of labor the vagina should be rendered as nearly sterile as possible. 8. Concentrated antiseptic solutions should not be used, and the process should be conducted with the least possible mechanical injury to the mucous surfaces. 9. In case of highly infectious secretions the preliminary disinfection should be followed by douching at intervals of 2 or 3 hours during the labor. 10. The safest and most efficient means for correcting vicious secretions is a mild antiseptic douche, repeated once or more daily for several days during the last weeks of pregnancy. 11. Clinically, the amount of discharge, its gross appearance, and that of the mucous and adjacent cutaneous surfaces usually furnish a sufficient guide to its treatment. 12. Probably unclean contact within 24 or 48 hours is an indication for prophylactic disinfection.

Puerperal Purpura Hæmorrhagica.—T. W. Schafer[5] reports the case of a primipara who was delivered by forceps under aseptic conditions. On the fourth day she developed a temperature of 104°, attended with rigors. There was no pain in the abdomen nor tympanites. Examination revealed an exudate near the right broad ligament. Purpura hæmorrhagica appeared suddenly in the lower extremities, below the knees, during the third week following parturition. The attack lasted 2 weeks, the spots alternately appearing and disappearing during final days. Treatment was empirical, in connection with that of the existing pelvic condition.

Puerperal Herpes.—Lutaud[6] describes 5 cases of acute pyrexia occurring between the second and fifth days after confinement or abortion, in each of which the febrile attack terminated by an eruption of facial (usually labial) herpes. In each case the attack was ushered in by rigors, the pyrexia was

[1] Rev. Méd. de l'Est., Mar. 15, 1896. [2] Arch. f. Gynäk., Bd. 52, H. 3, 1896.
[3] Bull. Johns Hopkins Hosp., Feb., 1897.
[4] Am. Gyn. and Obst. Jour., No. 4, p. 417, 1896.
[5] Langsdale's Lancet, No. 4, p. 137, 1896. [6] Jour. de Méd. de Paris, July 12, 1896.

severe, rising to 103° to 104° F., and in each case, after the appearance of the herpes, the patients rapidly recovered. Lutaud calls attention to the disquiet ing nature of these symptoms and their liability to be confounded with those of grave septic infection, and suggests that when strict antiseptic precaution have been taken in the conduct of labor or abortion, and no local condition ca be found to account for the subsequent rigor or pyrexia, it may be well to remember that the explanation of these phenomena may sometimes be found in the occurrence of the herpetic disorder described.

Treatment of Puerperal Sepsis.—[Serumtherapy of puerperal sep sis has commanded a vast amount of attention during the year, and thus far has not given the desired results. In fact, it appears to be a very doubtful metho of procedure.] The most interesting debate was that before the Obstetric Sec tion of the College of Physicians of Philadelphia, on March 18, 1897. Hirs reported 3 cases in which the serum gave no results. He stated that th older plans of treatment will answer in ¾ of the cases, in which, if the serun were used, the results might be attributed to it unjustly. Norris reported case successfully treated with the serum; G. E. Shoemaker a case in which i failed; E. P. Davis, 1 case in which it gave excellent results, and 2 cases in which it failed; and Baldy a case of acute puerperal lymphangitis and phle bitis in which he attributed the death to the use of the serum. J. B. Shobe gave a statistical report of 21 cases, with 4 deaths, a mortality of 19.04%. In the discussion A. C. Abbott remarked that the earlier the period at which the serum is injected the more likely are favorable results to ensue. H thinks that the opinion that Marmorek's serum is specific for all conditions resulting from the invasion of pyogenic streptococci is unwarranted. E. E Montgomery was of the opinion that one should not confine himself alone to the use of antitoxin, but should employ all agents which past experience has demonstrated are beneficial in the condition. In cases in which the poison i not due to the streptococcus the antitoxin is contraindicated and would be prejudicial, since one would be adding another poison which may be sufficient to destroy the patient's life. A bacteriologic examination should be made in every case of sepsis. R. C. Norris remarked that the serum should not be considered as a cure-all any more than should the curet. It probably has but a limited field of usefulness. Dorland, from a study of the literature of the subject, had concluded that the serum-treatment has not met with a flat tering degree of success. The unfavorable results may be attributed to the following three obstacles that must be overcome: 1. The *difficulty in ascertaining in any given case the precise variety of septic infection that may be present.* In cases of mixed infection it is reasonable to believe a favorable result should obtain only upon the administration of a mixed serum. 2. The *intensity of the infection* in any given case must be taken into consideration, and the treat ment by means of the serum regulated thereby. The morbific effects of the infection must increase *pari passu* with the degree of virulence, and upon this factor will depend the amount of blood-alteration present. The general rule is that the earlier the treatment is instituted the better will be the results obtained. The serum, then, should be administered until the desired effects are produced. 3. Another cause of failure must be attributed to the *inability of the blood to regain its proper constitution after grave disorganization has been brought about through the presence in it of the toxins of the germ and of the germ itself.* It stands to reason, therefore, that in all the cases in which the serum-treatment is employed it should from the very first be supple mented by the use of some such remedy as nuclein, which will restore to the blood its nucleinic acid, and thus its defensive properties, whereby it may

successfully resist the further action of the poisonous element. Hirst[1] says that although the antitoxic serum for puerperal sepsis be prepared with the greatest care, there is a possibility that it may contain dangerous toxins, and that the treatment may be more dangerous than the disease. There is a streptococcic infection so virulent that the antitoxin will be of no avail, no matter how strong it may be. There is an undeterminable time in streptococcic infections when the serum will be used too late. The antistreptococcic serum has no antagonistic power over other pathogenic microorganisms. It is not easy to determine during life whether the infection is pure or mixed, though the majority of puerperal infections are due to streptococci. Therefore, the use of the serum must be more or less empirical. Finally, the clinical results of serumtherapy for puerperal infection have not been at all encouraging. Hirst thinks that the plan of treatment for the artificial production of hyperleukocytosis is much more promising. Hofbauer[2] reports the results of, employing Horbaczewski's nuclein in 7 cases of puerperal infection, with favorable results in some cases.

Bar and Tissier[3] have employed the serum in 16 cases, 7 of whom died. In most of the cases this treatment was combined with intrauterine irrigation and curettage. In 1 case the authors attribute the death to the serum; they point out that it is absolutely necessary to make a bacteriologic examination of the uterine discharges before using the serum. In addition to the foregoing, the following cases treated by serum-injections have been recorded during the year: J. D. Williams,[4] 6 cases, 1 resulting fatally; Reddy,[5] 1 successful case, in which the treatment was followed temporarily by hematuria; Gaulard,[6] 2 cases, 1 resulting fatally, the death being attributed to the use of the serum; W. Edmunds,[7] 1 successful case; R. R. Law,[8] 1 successful case; T. H. Moorehead,[9] 1 successful case; P. Coleman and T. G. Wakeling,[10] 1 successful case; J. Adam,[11] 1 successful case; G. H. Mapleton,[12] 1 successful case; C. Coombs,[13] 1 fatal case; C. E. Douglas,[14] 1 case in which the serum had no effect, the patient ultimately recovering under other treatment; Letrain,[15] 1 successful case; A. Veitch,[16] 1 successful case; S. C. Fowler,[17] 1 successful case; A. J. Sharp,[18] 1 successful case; H. L. G. Leask,[19] 1 successful case; McKerron,[20] 3 cases, 1 resulting fatally; Chaleix,[21] 1 fatal case; Ballance and Abbott,[22] 1 successful case. At a discussion on this subject at the Paris Obstetric Society, 39 cases were reported by Charpentier[23] treated by the antistreptococcic serum, with 22 recoveries and 17 deaths. In only 25 cases was the disease confirmed by bacteriologic examination. Of these, in 16 the streptococcus alone was found, and 9 recoveries are recorded; in 8, streptococci in combination with staphylococci or bacterium coli, with 4 recoveries; while in 1 case the Löffler bacillus was noted. Dubrisay related a case of puerperal fever in which the fever developed on the third day, and pure cultures of streptococci were obtained from the cervix. After 4 daily injections of Marmorek's antistreptococcic serum the lochia were found free from streptococci, although the tem-

[1] Univ. Med. Mag., Nov., 1896.
[2] Centralbl. f. Gynäk., No. 17, 1896.
[3] L'Obstét., Mar., 1896.
[4] Brit. Med. Jour., Oct. 31, 1896.
[5] Montréal Med. Jour., Sept., 1896.
[6] L'Obstét., Jan., 1896.
[7] Am. Jour. Med. Sci., Apr., 1897.
[8] Brit. Med. Jour., Jan. 2, 1897.
[9] Ibid., Jan. 23, 1897.
[10] Ibid., Sept. 12, 1896.
[11] Ibid., Dec. 26, 1896.
[12] Ibid., Apr. 24, 1897.
[13] Ibid., Feb. 27, 1897.
[14] Edinb. Med. Jour., Apr., 1897.
[15] Therap. Gaz., Oct. 15, 1896.
[16] Edinb. Med. Jour., Feb., 1897.
[17] Ibid.
[18] Brit. Med. Jour., Feb. 27, 1897.
[19] Canad. Pract., Aug., 1896.
[20] Ibid., Oct. 10, 1896.
[21] Gaz. hebdom. de Méd. et de Chir., Dec. 13, 1896.
[22] Brit. Med. Jour., July 4, 1896.
[23] Centralbl. f. Gynäk., No. 34, 1896.

perature did not fall till 4 days subsequently. Shortly after the last injection the patient had an alarming attack of dyspepsia.

Pozzi [1] suggested another method of serotherapy, consisting in intravenous, followed by hypodermic injections of sterilized water containing sodium chlorid in the proportion of from 7 to 10 in 1000 at a temperature of 104° F.; of this solution from 2 to 5 liters may be injected in the 24 hours. The *rationale* of this treatment is that, in the first place, by raising the intravascular pressure it increases the patient's power of resistance; in the second place, time is given to the blood-making organs to produce new blood-corpuscles for phagocytosis, and to the kidneys to eliminate the toxins.

Kahn [2] reports his results in the treatment of septic puerperal endometritis by the intrauterine injection of steam. The apparatus consists of a kettle heated by an alcohol lamp, to which are attached a thermometer and a hose terminating in an intrauterine applicator having a hollow stem or handle. The thermometer should register 200° C. before the steam is used. He is accustomed to begin with steam at a temperature of 100° C. for 2 minutes, then allowing the temperature to rise to 115° C. for 1 minute. The higher the temperature of the steam the better is the result. Very little complaint of pain is made by patients; in some cases uterine contractions caused after-pains. In cases in which pieces of placenta or membrane have been left within the uterus they must be removed, either by the fingers or curet, before the steam is used. An intrauterine douche is usually employed for 2 or 3 days after the use of the steam. Kalm concludes that the steam increases the sensitiveness of the uterus, stimulates contractions, causes the foul odor of the lochia to disappear, and in no instance have bad after-results been observed. The advantages claimed for this method are its efficiency in destroying bacteria within the uterus, and also its favorable effect upon the general condition of the patient by stimulating the circulation of the blood and lymph.

Baldy [3] records a case of abdominal section for puerperal septicemia. He remarks that in general it may be said that when there is a puerperal salpingitis with resultant pelvic peritonitis, without pus being present, it is permissible to delay operation, keeping the patient under observation. In puerperal cellulitis, that variety in which the infection has found its way from the uterine cavity through the lymph-channels and blood-vessels into the surrounding connective tissue, the problem is a more difficult one. If the tubes and ovaries be distended with pus, abdominal section and removal of the offending organs are indicated; a large proportion of the infiltrated area is thus reached, and drainage of the remainder is favored. Another equally difficult group of cases includes those in which no disease of the pelvic peritoneum, tubes, or connective tissue is demonstrable by examination, and yet absorption of septic material is taking place from the uterus. When intrauterine douches and the application of carbolic acid and gauze-packing fail to relieve the symptoms hysterectomy should be promptly performed. R. R. Kime [4] claims that hysterectomy for puerperal infection has but a limited field of usefulness, as in septic metritis, multiple abscesses in the uterine wall, and thrombophlebitis, if it is possible to be positive in the diagnosis. In doubtful cases he claims that drainage is to be preferred. [The surgery of sepsis puerperalis is a mooted question, and no hard-and-fast rule can be given for all cases. The matter was thoroughly discussed in the last number of the *Year-Book*, and the stand then taken is applicable to-day.]

Gonorrhea in the Puerperium.—A most important contribution on

[1] Sem. méd., July 3, 1896.   [2] Centralbl. f. Gynäk., No. 49, 1896.
[3] N. Am. Pract., Sept., 1896.   [4] Canad. Pract., Aug., 1896.

this subject is made by A. H. Burr,[1] who dwells upon the fact that many cases of sepsis depend upon a previous infection with gonorrheal virus. These cases frequently present symptoms of rheumatoid arthritis during the pyrexia. The majority of males (Ricord estimated 80% for France, and Noeggerath believed the same ratio held good for New York City) have been affected at some period of life with gonorrhea, and Noeggerath held that 90% of males so affected remained uncured, and of every 100 women who had married men formerly affected with gonorrhea hardly 10 remained well. Prince reported that 60% of the blind in Jacksonville, Illinois, were the victims of ophthalmia neonatorum.

Postpartum and Puerperal Hemorrhage.—In speaking of the prevention of postpartum hemorrhage Atthill[2] believes that, to be of any use, ergot should be given for several hours before the termination of labor. He concludes that when ergot and strychnin are given previous to the termination of pregnancy in women having a marked tendency to postpartum bleeding, that this bleeding is prevented; that when so given in ordinary doses no injurious effect on mother or child is observed, but that the commencement of labor seems somewhat delayed. Such practice makes the involution of the uterus more perfect, and hence avoids postpartum disease. Unless the uterus is already acting, this treatment will not bring on premature labor or induce abortion; in cases of threatened abortion ergot and strychnin act as uterine tonics, preventing abortion if the ovum be not blighted; if, however, the ovum be dead, this treatment tends to secure its complete expulsion. [The use of strychnin in this way can be commended; we would hesitate, however, to recommend ergot in any condition prior to or during labor.]

Tarnier[3] stated that the treatment of postpartum hemorrhage was largely diversified and depended upon an accurate diagnosis. All hemorrhages after labor are not of the same origin, but may be classified under two heads : (a) hemorrhages from the cervix or vagina; (b) hemorrhages from the uterus itself. Treatment differs in the two classes of cases. In the former, the diagnosis being made and the vaginal tear recognized, it is seen that the uterus is small, hard, and retracted, and there is no necessity to bring about its contraction. Local compression at the point of injury for a certain period will suffice to arrest the hemorrhage. Sometimes it is not possible, on account of the presence of considerable quantities of blood, to find the bleeding spot in the vaginal fundus, and it is then best to tampon the vagina as carefully as possible.

Schaeffer[4] agrees with those who distrust gauze as a material for uterine tampons in cases of flooding. It often acts, he claims, as a capillary drain, and takes up much blood. He now uses non-absorbent gauze, prepared by impregnating it with gutta-percha. It can be mixed with iodoform or airol. By rolling it up into a ball it can be passed into the uterus, which it distends without absorbing any more blood. As a tampon the gutta-percha gauze retains its elasticity. E. S. Bishop[5] urges the importance of compression of the aorta as a rational and efficient means of checking postpartum hemorrhage. If this is done, the hemorrhage is at once absolutely stopped, and without needless hurry the secondary measures can be employed to empty the uterus of clots in order to bring about firm contraction. The ulnar surface of the closed hand should firmly compress the aorta against the spine, while the other hand is free to compress the uterus. T. Laird,[6] however, remarks that such com-

[1] Jour. Am. Med. Assoc., Aug. 1, 1896.　　　　[2] Brit. Med. Jour., No. 1888, 1897.
[3] Sem. méd., Apr. 11, 1896.　　　　　　　　　　[4] Rev. Obstét. Internat., Dec. 1, 1896.
[5] Lancet, Oct. 31, 1896.　　　　　　　　　　　　[6] Ibid., Dec. 19, 1896.

pression shuts off so many important vessels that it is practically stopping the blood-supply to half of the body, and he would substitute pressure upon the vessels that supply the uterus near the point where they enter that viscus. He does this by introducing the right hand into the womb, while with the left hand he compresses the uterine and ovarian arteries against it on either side, the fingers grasping the left side and the thumb the right. [Herman's method of manual compression is safer and easier of performance.]

Paraplegia after Parturition.—Two cases of this exceedingly rare complication are recorded by J. R. Leeson.[1] Both patients had neurotic tendencies, both labors were precipitate, and both patients had adherent placentæ which had to be artificially removed; in neither case was the bladder or rectum affected. Both cases lasted about the same time, the severer symptoms persisting for about a week, and both recovered slowly and entirely. The paralysis in both cases was probably due to overstimulation and subsequent temporary exhaustion, the shock of the precipitate labor being considerably increased by the prolonged and severe intrauterine irritation necessarily attendant on the removal of the adherent placentæ.

Puerperal Osteomalacia.—J. Ritchie[2] remarks that the pain and muscular weakness which are noticed in the early stages of this disease often lead to a diagnosis of rheumatism or disease of the spinal cord. The fertility of the patient is not diminished—in fact, some have even asserted that it is increased. Ritchie divides the treatment into medical and surgical. Phosphorus and bone-marrow may in some cases lead to a cure. Oöphorectomy cannot be said to produce a definite result, as a relapse may sometimes occur after the operation. The rapid disappearance of the pain after the operation is very noteworthy. If the patient is pregnant, the operation should be postponed until after delivery, unless the disease is progressing very rapidly. There is no evidence that better results follow hysterectomy than oöphorectomy.

Puerperal Thrombosis.—Cases of puerperal pulmonary thrombosis are recorded as follows: T. R. Atkinson,[3] 1 fatal case occurring 2½ months after delivery; Zweifel,[4] 1 fatal case on the 12th day after delivery; Lackie,[5] 1 fatal case on the 12th day of the puerperium; and P. von Tiesenhausen,[6] 3 fatal cases, the only instances met with in 25 years in the St. Petersburg Maternity in 50,000 labors; in all 3 cases the symptoms appeared when the patient first left her bed after labor, in one on the 4th, in another on the 6th, and in the third on the 7th day. Von Tiesenhausen regards whiteness of the lips, followed later by a cyanotic color, as a very characteristic symptom. [Reported cases of this complication show that it occurs most often before the 14th day after birth. It usually follows exertion, and is sometimes not fatal when thrombosis is but partial, in many cases accompanied by peripheral thrombosis also. Beyond immediate stimulation with ammonia and ether nothing can be done for serious pulmonary thrombosis. When a puerperal patient becomes easily faint and breathless she must be kept upon her back, all exertion absolutely avoided, and her nourishment carefully administered. Mental exertion and shock are also potent factors in causing this complication.]

Cases of gangrene of the leg in puerperal women are reported by T. Oliver,[7] 2 cases; and E. R. Rouse,[8] 2 cases, both recovering after amputation. In Oliver's first case right brachioplegia with transitory difficulty of speech

[1] Edinb. Med. Jour., Apr., 1897.
[2] Ibid., May, June, 1896.
[3] Brit. Med. Jour., Jan. 23, 1897.
[4] Centralbl. f. Gynäk., No. 1, 1897.
[5] Edinb. Med. Jour., No. 493, 1896.
[6] St. Petersburg. med. Woch., Oct. 5, 1896.
[7] Lancet, July 4, 1896.
[8] Ibid., p. 1375, Nov. 14, 1896.

occurred 14 days after a normal confinement, and was succeeded by popliteal thrombosis and consequent gangrene of the foot and leg. Amputation above the knee was followed by recovery. In the second case pneumonia appeared 4 days after confinement, and a few days later endocarditis was discovered, followed by embolism of the right popliteal artery. The leg was amputated above the knee, and death occurred 19 days later from pneumonia and exhaustion.

Puerperal Polyneuritis.—Cases are recorded by E. G. Cutler,[1] Köster,[2] G. Elder,[3] W. H. Wells,[4] J. H. W. Rhein,[5] and A. Kennedy.[6] Elder points out that in many instances there is a distinct history of fever during the puerperium; such cases are undoubtedly septic in origin.

Pathology of the Breasts.—A case of true *agalactia* is recorded by J. I. Edgerton,[7] the patient's breasts never showing any engorgement, involution of the uterus and the puerperium being otherwise normal. Her mother and sister had shown the same peculiarity in their pregnancies.

Lactation-atrophy of the uterus is treated of by Vineberg.[8] He states that a true process of atrophy goes on quite independently of even relative debility or anemia. In women who remain feeble after labor or become weak from any cause, external or internal, and in patients who are anemic before pregnancy, the uterus tends to remain large. Subinvolution is, and has long been recognized as, a morbid condition. Vineberg finds that when involution goes on to its full completion the uterus is reduced to a size smaller than that of the non-parous organ. *Postpuerperal superinvolution* is principally seen in nursing-women, and from this circumstance has been termed "lactation-atrophy." It is normal and desirable and is temporary, becoming permanent under rare and unfavorable circumstances. When the lying-in woman cannot suckle, the medical attendant should try to bring about superinvolution. Vineberg believes that this course will save her from the development of a host of maladies due to subinvolution.

PHYSIOLOGY AND PATHOLOGY OF THE NEWBORN.

Variations in Weight in the Newborn Child.—Schaeffer[9] reports his investigations upon this subject in the Heidelberg clinic. His material was 592 healthy infants, observed on the 7th to 14th day after birth, 94 of them being studied daily. It was found that but $14\frac{1}{2}\%$ of these children had made good by the 7th day their initial loss in weight, while 41 % had made good the loss or exceeded it by the 14th day. $44\frac{1}{2}\%$ weighed less 2 weeks after delivery than when born. The lowest weight was seen upon the 3d day, and the greatest gain from the 10th to the 12th. The greatest variation was seen in boys rather than in girls. Young and slender primiparæ gave birth to the lightest children, showing the least tendency to increase in weight. The same was true of mothers who had worked hard during pregnancy, or had been ill. Well-nourished women between the 20th and 29th years of age gave birth to the heaviest children. The character of the mother's recovery from childbirth had little to do with the weight of the child. The development of the father and the peculiarities of race affected the weight of the child considerably. A reason for the loss of weight in the first few days was

[1] Boston M. and S. Jour., Dec. 17, 1896.
[3] Lancet, July 25, 1896.
[5] Univ. Med. Mag., Feb., 1897.
[7] Med. News, Feb. 6, 1897.
[2] Münch. med. Woch., No. 27, 1896.
[4] Phila. Polyclinic, Sept. 12, 1896.
[6] N. Y. Med. Jour., Mar. 27, 1897.
[8] Am. Jour. of Obst., July, 1896.
[9] Arch. f. Gynäk., Bd. 52, H. 2, 1896.

found in the consumption of tissue to maintain the body-warmth. In the first 3 days, when but little fully formed milk is obtained, the excretion of uric acid is greatest. So soon, however, as milk-diet becomes established the quantity of urea increases in the child's urine. Premature children showed greater variations in weight and temperature and in the excretions. The children of tuberculous and syphilitic mothers failed to gain in weight. Icterus resulted from the consumption of tissue to maintain body-warmth. It was furthered by a lack of water in the organism and was often observed in weak, premature, or sick infants. It was also seen in cases in which the meconium was slow in coming away. Artificially fed children increase far less in weight than do those who nurse.

Infantile Syphilis.—An interesting case of post-conceptional syphilitic infection toward the end of pregnancy is recorded by E. Welander.[1] [This is also known as **placental** or **intrauterine** infection, and is the least common method of transmission of the disease.] Cases are also recorded by A. Post.[2] Coutts[3] finds a syphilitic mother much more potent in infecting than a syphilitio father. Marasmus and congenital atrophy of the secretive and absorptive surface of the intestinal tract are considered among the most important symptoms of inherited syphilis. While first symptoms commonly appear in the second month, they may be delayed 12 months. Visceral diseases (eulargement of the spleen and liver) are found in most cases; bone-lesions are less often observed; pain is often absent in syphilitic epiphysitis; suppuration is rare, and is usually seen in the long bones in children old enough to walk. Coutts has found inherited syphilis very feebly contagious, while acquired syphilis is actively so. Jolly[4] reports the case of an infant, 19 days old, who died of purpura hæmorrhagica, in whom autopsy showed intestinal ulceration and lesions characteristic of congenital syphilis. Other possible causes of these phenomena were carefully excluded in making a diagnosis.

Albers-Schönberg[5] gives the results of his studies in the diagnosis of fetal syphilis in the Leipzig clinic. He finds, in common with others, that the mere appearance of sanguinal maceration is not proof that the fetus perished from syphilis. Considerable increase in the weight of the liver and spleen, with increased weight of the placenta, indicates syphilis. On microscopic examination the blood-vessels of the placenta are much encroached upon by an abundant growth of connective-tissue cells. Gradual occlusion of the vessels and anemia and fatty degeneration result.

Melæna Neonatorum.—Swoboda[6] narrates a number of cases of infants dying with passive hemorrhages from the nose, mouth, and intestine. In a number of these postmortem examination revealed the lesions of congenital syphilis. In others septic infection occasioned by the gonococcus was the primary cause of the bleeding. In others a meningitis had developed without the lesions of syphilis. No cause other than a mechanical one from pressure upon the head, or excessive coughing or straining, could be found for the condition. He also reports several cases of bleeding from the nose in infants, in which bacteriologic examination showed the presence of the bacillus of diphtheria as a cause. [His interesting paper serves to illustrate the fact that melena is a symptom only, whose cause must always be sought before the pathology or treatment of a given case becomes evident.]

Icterus Neonatorum.—Knœpfelmacher[7] has studied the icterus of the

---

[1] Nordiskt Medicinskt. Arkiv, Mar., 1896.   [2] Boston M. and S. Jour., July 23, 1896.
[3] Brit. Med. Jour., No. 1843, 1896.   [4] Rev. mens. des Mal. de l'Enfance, Nov., 1896.
[5] Münch. med. Woch., No. 19, 1896.   [6] Wien. klin. Woch., No. 41, 1896.
[7] Ibid., No. 43, 1896.

newborn, and the relation which the condition of the red blood-cells bears to this phenomenon. His conclusions are essentially as follows: in the first weeks of life the number of red blood-cells is not influenced by a condition of icterus. Variations in the number of red corpuscles depend upon changes in the quantity and quality of the blood-plasma. The resisting power of the red corpuscles at birth seems to be fully that possessed by these cells in the adult, and does not seem to be lessened by icterus, however intense. The microscopic examination of the blood of the newborn in these cases shows, during the first days of life, no sign of erythrocytes; but, on the contrary, gives only indications of a vigorous building-up of red blood-cells. [The conclusion of these studies is, in general, that the condition of icterus in the newborn does not influence essentially the red blood-cells.]

Asphyxia Neonatorum.—Schultze [1] draws attention to 2 conditions requiring treatment in asphyxia of the newborn, in which different methods of treatment are indicated and in which it is most important that a differential diagnosis be made. In the first condition the child is blue, its heart is beating, and but a mild stimulation of its skin-reflexes is required to bring about respiration. Sprinkling the chest with cold water is quite sufficient in most of these cases to cause efforts at breathing. In the second class of cases the asphyxia is profound, and the medulla has become so paralyzed that its powers of reflex stimulation are wellnigh exhausted. The most efficient method of rousing this nervous center consists in rhythmic alterations in the vascular tension of the great vessels and the heart. This is best brought about by swinging the child by Schultze's well-known method for 8 or 10 times at intervals of 1 minute, and afterward placing the child in a warm bath. Schultze thinks that the employment of this method produces quite as much result by varying the vascular tension as it does by forcing air into the chest.

G. C. Barker [2] records a shoulder-injury resulting from this method, the infraspinatus and teres minor muscles being ruptured.

Calliano [3] describes a new method of artificial respiration which he has practised with success in cases of asphyxia. The patient is placed in Sylvester's position, and the arms are then drawn up so as fully to expand the thorax, and then fixed above and behind the head by tying the wrists together. In this position respiration is induced by simply pressing with the hands on the thorax some 18 or 20 times a minute. The advantages claimed for this modification of Sylvester's method are: (1) its greater simplicity; (2) the much smaller amount of labor required and lessened fatigue of the operator; (3) the absence of danger from contusion of the shoulder-joints; (4) the ease with which such a method could be taught to and practised by uneducated and untrained people.

Obstetric Paralysis and Injuries to the Child during Labor.— Walton [4] has found, in dissecting the brachial plexus of the newborn infant, that the plexus is in close apposition to the sharp, inner edge of the clavicle. The suprascapular nerve leaves the plexus much higher up, passing outward and backward to the suprascapular notch. Walton believes that this nerve is independently stretched in the separation of the head from the shoulder during birth, the distal point of fixation being the suprascapular notch or the outer edge of the suprascapular spine. It is observed that the muscles supplied below the spines of the scapulæ are most often injured; the rotation of the head, which brings the occiput under the pubes, brings the plexus forward against the clavicle also, shortening the distance from the emerging point of

[1] Centralbl. f. Gynäk., No. 37, 1896. [2] Lancet, May 8, 1897.
[3] Gaz. degli Osped. e delle Clin., Aug. 16, 1896. [4] Boston M. and S. Jour., No. 26, 1896.

the plexus-root from the spine and also the suprascapular notch. [So far as statistics are available they bear out what Walton has stated. The paralysis usually affects the arm upon the side opposite to that to which the occiput was directed during labor, in the first position paralysis of the right arm being most often observed.] As regards prophylaxis, Walton suggests that the second stage of labor be made as short as possible.

Hiebaum[1] refers to a case of labor in a dutipara at the 8th month of pregnancy in which podalic version was resorted to on account of placenta prævia. The child could not be revived, and was found to have suffered a fracture of the occiput and of the vertebral column. On incising the tentorium nothing could be found of the cerebellum but quite a small fragment; the remainder was found suspended in the form of white particles like sand in about 20 c.c. of bloody serum in the left pleural cavity. Schultze[2] notes how in many cases of children suffering from mental or nervous diseases it has been found that at their birth labor was difficult or at least prolonged.

Ritter's Disease.—Dorland[3] reports a case of this curious and exceedingly rare dermic condition of the newborn. The fact that another child in the family had suffered from scarlatina during the later months of gestation, and the well-recognized predisposition of the fetus in utero to acquire the zymotic diseases, are strong reasons for believing that there was in this instance an association between the two diseases. The treatment of the dermatitis should consist in the application of some emollient ointment, as of ichthyol, resorcin, or horic acid, protection of the denuded surface with cotton, and the administration of good milk and tonics, with proper attention to hygiene.

---

[1] Prag. med. Woch., Bd. 21, H. 5, 1896.   [2] Centralbl. f. Gynäk., No. 21, 1896.
[3] Phila. Polyclinic, Sept. 26, 1896.

GYNECOLOGY.

By J. MONTGOMERY BALDY, M. D., and W. A. NEWMAN
DORLAND, M. D.,

OF PHILADELPHIA.

Principal Features of the Year's Work.—The intimate relationship that exists between the nervous system and the sexual apparatus of woman is becoming more clearly appreciated, and the discussion upon this interesting feature of gynecology is probably one of the most important steps that has been taken within recent years in this department of surgery. The baleful influence of gonorrhea in the male is also being brought more prominently before the profession, and the importance of regulating prostitution, not in the woman only, but also in the male, cannot be too highly emphasized. Organotherapy in gynecology cannot as yet be said to hold a very prominent or suggestive place. It is, however, of interest to note the results of experimentation in this line, as in the treatment of uterine fibroids, the phenomena of the menopause, and the various ovarian neuroses. Rectal exploration, as the examination of the urinary tract, is a comparatively new field of study, and will probably develop into just as valuable means of diagnosis as has the latter. The question of bicycling for women is still *in statu quo*, and the arguments for and against constitute most interesting gynecologic reading. Except for the further development and refinement of technic, gynecologic surgery has undergone no radical change. There may be noted a slight inclination of popular favor toward the vaginal route of pelvic exploration, but as yet this has not become pronounced.

PRELIMINARY AND GENERAL CONSIDERATIONS.

Neuroses and Neurasthenia in Women.—A very valuable discussion on the relations of nervous disorders in women to pelvic disease[1] was held at the College of Physicians of Philadelphia Feb. 3, 1897. From the standpoint of the neurologist, S. Weir Mitchell dwelt upon the subjects of epilepsy, insanity, and hysteria. Epileptic attacks are apt to return at the menstrual period with greater frequency than at others, but in no cases seen by him have ablation of the ovaries and termination of menstruation cured an epilepsy. He has never sanctioned such operations when the appendages were sound. Temporary cessation of epileptic attacks is common after operations or changes of environment and habits of life. The insanities of women present a somewhat different case. In women insanity of various types occurs in which the menstrual period is sometimes the originative and sometimes the determinative cause of the mental disease. Because an insane woman is usually worse at her period is no reason why the flow should be stopped by operation any more than that this measure should be resorted to for epilepsy.

---

[1] Univ. Med. Mag., Mar., 1897.

That the climacteric puts an end to these disorders is an old delusion ; in fact, the change of life is quite as likely to make them worse. A great many aggravated cases of hysteria show disease of the pelvic organs, which is so apparent as to make recovery after removal of the ovaries and tubes seem probable. A large percentage of these cases are not made better by operation, but, on the contrary, are often made worse. He is inclined to think that postoperative traumatic insanities are more common after pelvic operations than after others, and this insanity he believes is due to the anesthetic. C. K. Mills remarked that pelvic disease or disturbance is sometimes due to mental or nervous disease. Thus, during the progress of melancholia menstrual disorder or even amenorrhea is not infrequent. A true epilepsy, a true hysteria, or a true melancholia is never absolutely caused by pelvic disease. Neurasthenia, however, in some instances seems to be directly traceable to pelvic disease. Gynecologists should become familiar with certain cases of obsession or monomania, in which pain is referred to perfectly healthy organs. The pains are psychic— in the head, and not in the pelvis. He recalls 3 distinct forms of mental disorders subsequent to pelvic operations : (1) a form of acute mania, (2) delusional insanity, and (3) a form of querulous melancholia. Wharton Sinkler said that operation was not resorted to so often now as formerly in neurotic women. A deplorable number of such operations have been done, with poor success. In Paris, since 1883, 40,000 ovariotomies or hysterectomies have been performed, and during that time about 500,000 were done in all France. Of 300 cases of operation for the relief of neuroses and psychoses collected by Krämer, in 100 the result was doubtful or unfavorable. If pelvic disease exists, it often aggravates all nervous symptoms ; but in many instances the mental disorders and ovarian neuralgic pains seem to be rather the result than the cause of the existing nervous disease. F. X. Dercum believes that pelvic disease is concerned in but a small percentage of the cases of neurasthenia and hysteria in women. Such potent etiologic factors as neuropathic heredity, improper education, overwork, the worries incidental to household duties, the care of children, the daily frictions of life, are too often overlooked. How little local organic disease of itself acts as a factor in the causation of hysteria is shown in the case of uterine carcinoma, in which neurasthenic and hysteric symptoms are notoriously absent. In the male neurasthenic and hysteric conditions cannot be ascribed to pelvic disease. If pelvic disorders are concerned at all in the production of neurasthenia, it must be the spurious or symptomatic form (*neurasthenia symptomatica*). If the pelvic organs really play a rôle in the etiology of neurasthenia and hysteria, it is largely because gynecologists have created that rôle. Among the symptoms presented by hysteric women the one deserving especial attention is the so-called ovarian tenderness or inguinal pain, most marked on the left side when pressure is made. This in reality is situated in the skin and tissues of the abdominal wall, and not within the pelvis, as can be demonstrated by placing one finger on the spot externally and one in the vagina, the finger-tips being approximated. In his opinion operations upon the pelvic organs should be limited to actual diseases, as pyosalpinx and malignant affections. J. H. Lloyd remarked that modern science has almost entirely abolished the idea that hysteria has its seat in the uterus. He does not agree with Mills, however, that hysteria can never be caused by pelvic disease. It is conceivable that it might be started by a diseased ovary, an ovarian tumor, extensive cervical lesion, or lesions of the pelvic floor. It must be recalled, however, that the operation of castration in the female is sometimes followed by grave hysteric troubles, in such a case the very operation designed for relief becoming in turn an exciting cause of still more profound trouble. Another aspect of the case is the fact that some serious nervous condition may arise in cases of real pelvic disease. Thus, a patient may undergo a perfectly proper operation, and may develop insanity as a result of it. This insanity may take the form of melancholia or that of confusional insanity, and there is probably some septic condition that is the primary disturbing cause in these cases to produce the mental condition. B. C. Hirst remarked that a neurasthenic woman, her family, or her physician, will almost surely impute the nervous symptoms of the patient to disease of the sexual organs. A large majority of neurasthenic patients (four-fifths) give an entirely negative result on pelvic examination, except for the ill-development of the sexual organs which is such a constant accompaniment of a feeble nervous system in women. In a small minority of neurasthenic cases the nervous disorders do seem to have had their origin in some pelvic lesion, and slowly disappear when the pelvic disease is cured; but it is usually necessary to unite with the gynecologic treatment a "rest-cure." E. E. Montgomery, while admitting that not infrequently we find patients treated for pelvic lesions in whom the symptoms are thereby aggravated, said that, on the other hand, we find many cases who are subjected to rest-treatment without effective result, for the reason that there is a local lesion which manifests itself as soon as the patient resumes her normal relations. This neglect of consideration of the pelvic lesions seems to be more marked on the part of neurologists. A woman suffering from a mental disease is, at least, entitled to a careful pelvic examination, and any pelvic lesion found should receive appropriate treatment. C. P. Noble remarked that arrested development is the fundamental cause of many cases of nervous diseases simulating diseases of the sexual organs in women. Women with such imperfect development have an unstable nervous system, and are not vigorous or normal women. Many of them have had chlorosis in girlhood. He has seen very marked functional disease of the nervous system caused by operations on the pelvic organs. Remarks prejudicial to operative treatment act by suggestion upon neurasthenic and hysteric patients; neurologists should bear this in mind. G. E. Shoemaker takes it for granted that reputable gynecologists are not given to removing healthy organs for nervous symptoms or for pain only. J. M. Baldy[1] remarked that if it be concluded that in a given case of hysteria pelvic disease does not enter further than as one of many groups of symptoms, the case belongs more properly to the neurologist. He regards cases of hysteria as rare which are dependent exclusively upon abnormalities of the sexual organs, but believes that anatomic changes and abnormal irritation of the sexual organs are conditions especially fitted to cause hysteric manifestations. In true hysteria it is folly to resort to surgical interference. If one symptom in such women is cured, another takes its place; ovarian pains are replaced by painful stumps, backaches continue, and the general nerve-reflexes are increased by the addition of the depressing nerve-storms of the menopause.

Gonorrhea in Women.—According to B. Gordon,[2] gonorrhea in women manifests itself in the following forms: vulvitis, bartholinitis, urethritis, vaginitis, metritis, perimetritis, parametritis, salpingitis, oöphoritis, and peritonitis. Sometimes the disease extends from the urethra, causing gonorrheal cystitis, ureteritis, and nephritis. Also gonorrheal proctitis, arthritis, phlebitis, endocarditis, pleuritis, meningomyelitis, and conjunctivitis are met with. Albuminuria is said to be observed quite frequently in the acute form of the disease. Neisser[3] calls attention to the difficulty of formulating a positive

---

[1] Phila. Polyclinic, July 18, 1896. [2] Med. Rec., Nov. 21, 1896.
[3] Arch. f. Dermat. u. Syph., Bd. 37, H. 1 and 2, 1897.

diagnosis as to the gonorrheal origin of disease of the adnexa, although this is not so in inflammation of the external mucosa, the secretions of which escape externally. He urges the importance of making a rectal examination. The so-called "creeping" gonorrhea of women, caused by gonococci of lessened virulence, has no well-proved existence. Even from the most chronic cases extremely virulent gonococci can be obtained. Sänger,[1] taking up the subject of residual gonorrhea in women, states that after the disappearance of gonococci in the secretions certain manifestations may remain. The period during which gonococci may persist is not known. It is evident from examination of relatively fresh tubal and ovarian abscesses that in these closed spaces the gonococci do not long survive. It is possible they may disappear from the mucosa of the external genitalia, since lesions are often found in whose discharges gonococci are not discoverable. Sänger gives a rather elaborate description of these residua of gonorrhea, including among others a macular vulvitis and sclerotic adenitis, urethritis, periurethritis, kolpitis, endometritis, metroendometritis, and salpingitis. He holds that the greater number of rectal strictures are of gonorrheal origin. Bumm[2] denies that gonococci lose their virulence, and holds that infection from an old case, if planted on healthy mucosa, produces an acute attack. He states that the gonococci may persist and remain virulent in the genital tract for 5 or 10 years. He still believes that the gonococcus is a pure mucous-membrane parasite, remaining in chronic cases quite superficial, and only exceptionally penetrating into other tissues and acting as the ordinary pyogenic microorganisms do.

Schultz,[3] during the year 1895, carefully examined 174 patients from the venereal department of a hospital for the gonococcus. The organism was sought for in the vulva, vagina, urethra, cervix, uterus, duct of Bartholin's gland, and rectum. Microscopic examination was the only method employed. The examination for gonococci was made many times in each case. He concludes that to make a diagnosis the clinical symptoms are not sufficient, but the proof is found in the presence of the gonococcus. Gonococci were found much more numerous in the urethral than in the cervical secretion, and therefore urethral gonorrhea is of greater importance; infection most frequently takes place from the urethra. It results that when there is cervical gonorrhea or adnexal disease gonorrhea of the uterus is not always present. As regards other microorganisms contained in the cervical canal and uterine cavity, he agrees with the investigations of Stroganoff, that the hyaline mucus of the canal and uterine cavity is free from bacteria. In the writer's opinion the treatment should be prophylactic and local.

Of the earlier symptoms of gonorrheal, as well as of nonspecific, salpingitis, E. M. Madden[4] contributes an interesting paper, but advances nothing new.

Macular kolpitis, according to Sänger,[5] is characterized by dark-red spots disseminated over the walls of the vagina and the cervix uteri, more particularly where there are neither folds nor papillæ. In *chronic gonorrheal granular kolpitis* granulations are found in the same regions, at the apex of which the red color is more intense, and which are distinguished from the nodosities of acute granular kolpitis of pregnancy by their being smaller and harder than the latter. These are best treated by applications of a 50% zinc chlorid solution. For gonorrheal vaginitis Schultz[6] advises local treatment. For cervical gonorrhea he employs intrauterine injections, never using more than 8

---

[1] Arch. f. Dermat. u. Syph., Bd. 37, H. 1 and 2, 1897.   [2] Ibid.
[3] Centralbl. f. Gynäk., No. 28, 1896.   [4] Lancet, Aug., 1896.
[5] Ibid.   [6] Ibid.

minims and allowing the excess to escape. The best injection, he says, is a 10 % solution of silver nitrate; with this treatment the secretions soon become hyaline and diminish in quantity, and the gonococci disappear. The treatment is not contraindicated in chronic, but in acute inflammatory disease of the adnexa. Colic results only in those cases in which the external os is stenosed. [This is not a universal experience. Uterine colic is very prone to result from the use of silver nitrate injected intrauterine, stenosis or no stenosis.]

Both Neisser[1] and Gordon[2] especially recommend the salts of silver (argentamin, argonin, argentum nitricum, actol, itrol), hydrargyrum oxycyanatum, and ichthyol, in the local treatment of the disease. The silver salts destroy the gonococcus, and while penetrating deeply into the tissues do no harm to them. Canova[3] believes there is no remedy so promptly curative as ichthyol. He uses injections of 0.5 % in water with the most satisfactory results. De Smet[4] has obtained excellent results from the use of formalin, washing out the vagina with a 2–3 % solution. Piéry[5] recommends the use of nascent carbonic acid in gonorrheal vaginitis.

Rectal Gonorrhea in Women.—Baer,[6] among 191 cases of gonorrhea in women, noted 67 in which the rectum was involved, gonococci being found in the discharge from the bowel. While infection may result directly from unnatural coitus, the writer believes that in the majority of cases it is due to contact of the vaginal discharge with the rectal mucosa, especially in women with deep perineal lacerations. Infection through thermometers or rectal tubes is doubtful. Few of the patients presented any marked local symptoms, unless there was an ulceration at the anal orifice. These complained of burning pain during defecation, with discharge of pus and blood. Condylomata and eczema were rare. On inspection the rectal mucosa was seen to be deeply congested, the folds swollen and glistening, with erosions which bled easily and were covered with pus. A deep ulceration was found only once, and periproctitis in 2 cases. The treatment consisted in irrigation of the rectum twice daily, through a speculum, with a 3 % solution of boric acid, followed by mercuric chlorid 1 : 8000, in order to destroy the gonococci, half a liter of each being used. The erosions were touched with argentamin, 2 % solution. Ichthyol suppositories were also used with good effect.

The Rectum and the Female Reproductive Organs as Related in Disease.—J. P. Tuttle[7] urges the importance of careful examination of the rectum in cases of obscure and intractable pelvic disease; also in diseases of the digestive tract and lower portion of the spinal cord. Certain cases of pyosalpinx and uterine displacement are characterized mainly by rectal symptoms. Tumors of the uterus, especially fibroids of moderate size, frequently make themselves felt at first through rectal symptoms. Prolapse of the ovary often presents marked symptoms of rectal disease, such as dull aching in the back and sacral region, pain at and following defecation, congestion of the rectal mucosa, constipation, and sometimes hemorrhoidal tumors. The effects of pelvic cellulitis upon the rectum are little understood by the profession in general. Cripps has called attention to its influence in causing stricture through the production of spasmodic contractions and consequent shortening of the levator ani muscles. The extension of the acute inflammation into the rectal wall, the deposit of plastic material about the gut, its ligaments, and bloodvessels, the adhesions between the rectum and uterus with its appen-

[1] Lancet, Aug., 1896.   [2] Ibid.
[3] Centralbl. f. Gynäk., No. 41, 1896.   [4] Jour. de Méd. de Paris, Aug. 16, 1896.
[5] Gaz. hebdom. de Méd. et de Chir., July 12, 1896.
[6] Deutsch. med. Woch., No. 8, 1896.   [7] N. Y. Polyclinic, Sept. 15, 1896.

dages, are all influential in restricting the physiologic action of that organ, and in causing both reflex and organic diseases of it. In all obscure diseases of the rectum, immobility of the uterus, or history of pelvic inflammation, with thickening and inelasticity of the vaginal vault, should have a marked influence upon our procedure. The proper treatment of the results of the cellulitis will in the majority of cases relieve all rectal symptoms. Adhesion of the ovary may be responsible for these symptoms. This organ becomes inflamed, the adjacent peritoneum is involved, and attachment between it and the colon or sigmoid takes place (more properly speaking, the adhesion generally occurs at the mesocolon). If the inflammatory condition be checked at this point, no rectal symptoms of importance will ensue. If, however, the process goes on, bands of adhesive elastic material will be thrown out over the intestine to the mural peritoneum of the iliac fossa, and, when this has been reached, forming a bridge or stricture-band across the intestine which will persistently contract and produce all the symptoms of high stricture of the rectum. Malignant disease of the uterus in its beginning frequently presents symptoms of rectal disease. Diseases of the uterus and its appendages not only simulate rectal disease in producing symptoms referred to that organ, but they sometimes produce actual organic diseases in it. Displacement of the uterus or ovaries, especially prolapse and retroversion, or anteversion with enlarged cervix, and deposit of plastic material from inflammation, are not infrequently the exciting causes of rectal congestion, inflammation, fissure, ulceration, and hemorrhoids. They act first by obstructing the venous circulation of the gut, and, secondly, by exciting a more or less constant spasmodic contraction of the circular fibers of the levator ani and sphincter of the rectum. This congestion and spasm soon lead to hypertrophy of the sphincters, and they then act as a stricture of the anus and produce obstinate constipation with all its consequent rectal, intestinal, and digestive symptoms. Ulceration, both rectal and anal, results from these conditions, and fistula or cicatricial stricture may follow the ulceration. The influence of uterine diseases upon the rectum is no less interesting than that of rectal diseases upon the reproductive organs. Internal hemorrhoids, ulceration of the rectum, prolapse of the third degree, fissure in ano, inflammation and ulceration of the crypts of Morgagni, may all simulate disease of the uterus and its appendages. A. B. Walker[1] emphasizes the value of examination of the sigmoid flexure of the colon, especially for fecal impaction.

AFFECTIONS OF THE VULVA AND VAGINA.

Kraurosis Vulvæ.—Peter[2] reviews the literature on kraurosis vulvæ, reports a case, and more thoroughly investigates its pathologic anatomy. He writes that Breisky, in 1885, first described 12 cases of this peculiar disease, and gave it the name kraurosis. Breisky observed an atrophic contraction of the skin of the vestibule, labia minora, the frenum and prepuce of the clitoris, the inner surface of the labia majora and the border of the perineum. Often, however, only part (one side or posteriorly) of these structures was involved. The skin of the vulva appeared stretched and the normal folds were obliterated; the kraurotic tissue was small and glistening, and of a dull-gray color, with the surrounding tissue reddish-brown. In all cases the disease developed slowly and unobserved, and itching was a symptom in only 4 of the cases. The symptoms of which the patients complained were mostly

---

[1] Ann. of Gyn. and Pediat., Dec., 1896.
[2] Monatsch. f. Geb. u. Gynäk. Bd. iii., H. 4, 1896.

due to the vestibular stenosis. They presented themselves for treatment because cohabitation had become impossible, or because of tears and painful fissures. Since this first paper cases have been reported by Fleischmann (8), Janowski (6), Heitzmann, Ohmann-Dumesnil, Hallowel, and Bartels. The cases described by these authors in no way differed from those of Breisky until Orthmann reported 8 cases (1894) seen in Martin's clinic. These patients complained of burning and vulvar tenesmus ; but it was impossible to determine whether these were the result of itching or pain caused by an inflammatory process. The pain was constant and much increased during micturition and defecation.

The disease has been seen at every age after puberty, in nulliparæ as well as multiparæ, and its etiology cannot be concluded either from the history or observation of the progress of the disease. Orthmann found a small round-cell infiltration of the corium, most marked in the deeper portion, extending to the subcutaneous tissue, with a high grade of atrophic change in all parts of the skin. The involution-process was particularly seen in the corium, which was sclerotic. The epidermis, glands, hair-follicles, and blood-vessels were much smaller than normal. The nerve-tissue was unchanged.

The symptoms of which the writer's patient complained differed in no way from those described. Microscopic sections were prepared by hardening in alcohol, sublimate, and Flemming's solutions, and by Benda's method, and suitably stained. From this investigation, which was most complete, the results of each method being described, he concludes that kraurosis vulvæ in its early stage is a chronic inflammatory hyperplasia of the connective tissue, with a disposition to cicatricial contraction, inflammatory edema of the superficial corium and epidermis, and degeneration of the elastic tissue. As a result of this chronic inflammation and new-growth the other elements of the skin are secondarily affected, and because of the degeneration of the elastic tissue the tears and fissures result. He agrees with Orthmann that the nerve-tissue is not involved, but says that it must have been affected in those cases complaining of pain. He believes that kraurosis should be classified with the other diffuse connective-tissue hypertrophies of the skin, to which group, according to Kaposi, scleroderma and elephantiasis arabum belong. All cases reported have been relieved or cured through dilatation, medicinal applications, ointments, and sitz-baths. [As regards the results of treatment, one must bear in mind that it is the almost universal experience that this disease is exceedingly difficult to cure—a cure most frequently falling short of a surgical removal of the parts ; even then the results might be more encouraging than they are. In view of these indisputable facts the above statement as to the cure in all cases must be accepted with reservation.]

Pruritus of the Genitalia.—H. Robb[1] remarks that in treating a case of pruritus the main thing is to discover the cause. Thus, there should be examined (1) the external genitals for skin-eruptions ; in doing this it will be well to obtain scrapings and examine them with the microscope for parasites. (2) There should next be examined the cervix for signs of leukorrhea, and to ascertain the general condition of the uterus and appendages. (3) An examination should be made per rectum. (4) Chemical and microscopic examination of the urine should never be omitted. The presence of enlarged sebaceous glands or any signs of malignant disease should be carefully looked for. Hemorrhoids or fissures of the anus should be treated, and the vulva should be kept free from all irritating discharges. The general health of the patient should never be forgotten. When the vulva is dry, too frequent bathing should be

[1] Therap. Gaz., Sept. 15, 1896.

avoided and the surface should be kept moist, being treated, not with evaporating lotions, but with ointments. Suppositories containing codein or opium and hyoscyamus at night will often give the patient relief. Local applications include silver nitrate (2 % solution), ointments containing 2 to 10 % of salicylic acid, a mixture of chloroform 1 dram to olive oil 1 ounce, solution of carbolic acid (2 %), and a solution of morphin acetate (12 gr. to the oz.). Internally, potassium bromid and belladonna tend to decrease irritation of the peripheral nerves. Ruge[1] adds disinfection of the genital region with mercuric chlorid. According to Cumston,[2] antipyrin is sometimes of service in calming attacks of pruritus. 50 centigrams are given before dinner and the same dose at bedtime. [And yet, after all is said and done, we are forced to admit that in the majority of cases of pruritus vulvæ the cause cannot be definitely settled, and the treatment must of necessity be empirical. And it must be further admitted that not infrequently the cases remain uncured until nature and time see fit to relieve them.]

Vulvitis and Vaginitis.—According to Marfan,[3] the complications of *gonorrheal vulvovaginitis of little girls* may be grouped under three headings: 1. Those by propagation; 2. Those by inoculation; 3. Those by general infection. Under the first group are included bartholinitis, Rocaz observing a case in an infant of 10 months; phlegmonous vulvitis; anorectal gonorrhea, which is very rare, Horand reporting 4 cases; involvement of the urinary passages, being here confined usually to the anterior portion of the urethra, although very rarely a cystitis may result; infantile cystitis is nearly always coli-bacillary, succeeding to an enteritis or rectitis, the diarrheic fecal material soiling the vulva and the bladder becoming infected by way of the urethra; involvement of the internal genital organs, uterus, ovaries, tubes, and peritoneum. Metritis exists in a goodly number of cases; isolated salpingitis and ovaritis are rare. Peritonitis consecutive to infantile vulvovaginitis is very grave; Marfan has observed 2 cases; it may be acute and rapidly fatal; very rarely it may be acute and yet be cured; or it may take the form of subacute or chronic adhesive pelviperitonitis. Complications by inoculation from a distance include purulent ophthalmia, which is quite frequent in vulvovaginitis. Generalized gonorrheal infection (*gonohemia*) includes gonorrheal arthritis, or gonorrheal rheumatism.

A. H. Goelet[4] calls attention to *senile vaginitis* as encountered after the menopause. If the disease has been neglected, contraction of the cicatricial bands may become so marked as almost to prevent access to the cervix. The appearance of the vaginal mucosa is characteristic in these cases. The rugæ are effaced, and the surface is pale and glistening in spots, with nearly normal mucosa intervening, upon which may be seen minute ecchymoses or apparently elevated, intensely reddened papillæ, consisting of exposed capillary vessels, the epithelium being destroyed. Occasionally the entire mucosa is intensely injected and inflamed, and is coated with an acrid, mucopurulent discharge, mainly derived from the uterus, which is the seat of a senile endometritis. Treatment consists of cleansing with a solution of lysol ($\frac{1}{2}$ to 1 %), followed by the application of a bland, non-irritating antiseptic powder, such as markasol (bismuth borophenate).

Trauma of the Vulva.—Three cases of severe hemorrhage following coitus are reported by Chaleix,[5] one occurring in a " bleeder." C. S. Ford[6]

---

[1] Berlin. klin. Woch., No. 18, 1896.   [2] Ann. of Gyn. and Pediat., Aug., 1896.
[3] Gaz. hebdom. deMéd. et. de Chir., No. 27, Apr. 4, 1897.
[4] Med. Rec., Oct. 17, 1896.   [5] Gaz. hebdom. de Méd. et de Chir., No. 45, 1896.
[6] N. Y. Med. Jour., Jan. 9, 1897.

records a case of fatal hemorrhage from a slight wound of the vulva. The wound was situated at the juncture of the clitoris and labium minus on the left side, a flap of mucous membrane about a third of an inch square being turned back. The patient had been delivered six weeks before, and the injury was received by falling astride the back of a theatre-seat. The veins of the vulva were enlarged as the result of subinvolution.

Vaginal Seborrhea.—It is stated in the *Wien. med. Blat.* of December 24, 1896, that a writer in the *Allg. med. Central-Zeit.*, whose name is not mentioned, describes under this title what he considers to be a special form of vaginal catarrh which occurs commonly in corpulent women, old maids, and pregnant women. It consists in an excessive augmentation of the normal secretion of the vagina, and the secretion is made up chiefly of whitish, fatlike lumps containing numerous pavement-epithelia. The secretion soon disappears under the use of injections of warm water containing a little sodium bicarbonate.

Vaginismus.—F. W. A. Godfrey[1] states that vaginismus may be due to several causes well recognized and described, such as urethral caruncle, eczema of the vulva, ulcerations of various kinds, painful fissures of the fourchet, vaginitis, and sometimes probably to a neurosis for which a local cause cannot be discovered. In addition, he refers to that more common form due to a hyperesthetic condition of the hymen or its remains, which may be a cause of intense suffering and distress. Mere removal of the offending papillæ will not suffice for a cure, but the resulting and remaining reflex muscular spasm must be overcome by systematic dilatation.

Vaginal Stenosis and Atresia.—This subject has been thoroughly studied from an embryologic and clinical point of view by E. H. Lee.[2] He states that of the various forms of vaginal atresia imperforate hymen is the malformation most frequently met with; it is usually congenital, rarely if ever acquired. The operative treatment of this condition when retention of the menstrual fluid has occurred is simple, a crucial incision usually being all that is necessary; should there be an excessive amount of membrane, or the hymen be hard and dense, it may be excised. [The crucial incision should be given the preference when applicable, as it is less likely to be followed by contraction. Vidal and Bockel encircled the margins of the wound with a suture after excision; this is rarely necessary.] In operating two dangers have to be contended with—namely, rupture of the tubes and sepsis. The former is only present when hematosalpinx exists; the latter in whatever portion of the genital tract menstrual fluid may be retained. Rupture of the tubes has been repeatedly observed following drainage of a hematokolpos, the time varying from 4 hours to 10 days after operation; all of the cases terminated fatally, either immediately from shock or subsequently from peritonitis. When dilated the walls of the tubes become very thin and friable, adhesions to the surrounding organs taking place. After evacuation of a hematokolpos severe traction is exerted upon the adherent tubes by the contracting vagina and uterus in their effort to assume their normal location. This, with the direct pressure that is transmitted from the uterus into the tube when the ostium uterinum is dilated, and the abdominal pressure, favors the occurrence of rupture. [This dangerous complication has been so much feared that it has been suggested to drain the tubes before further operative procedure. Hegar and Kalberbach recommended puncture and drainage per rectum, but this method should be condemned, the danger of infection being very great. It should also be considered that the tube, usually greatly displaced, is not

---

[1] Quart. Med. Jour., Jan., 1897.   [2] Medicine, July, 1896.

34

always accessible from this point. Hausmann proposed drainage of the tube by abdominal section, and this method has more to recommend it; by establishing adhesions between the tube and the parietal peritoneum, the general peritoneal cavity may be walled off and the blood drained without danger. The proper and safer method is gradual drainage by aspiration of the nuruptured hymen.] Sepsis, the second danger, can, at the present time, be practically excluded, owing to the improved methods of antisepsis.

Imperforate introitus vaginæ and *imperforate vagina* are parallel conditions to imperforate anus and imperforate rcetum, and may frequently be found associated. The first step in the operative treatment of this condition is to establish a canal between the introitus and the os uteri [if possible]. This is accomplished by dissection through the connective or cicatricial tissue, as much blunt force as possible being used. The canal having been established without opening the bladder or bowel, the most important part of the operation follows—that is, the prevention of contraction. Implantation and transplantation of skin and mucous membrane have been attempted by Küstner, Neugebauer, and others with variable results. Rein considers the transplantation of skin better than implantation, as it is less apt to be followed by contraction. The operative treatment of stenosis, providing it is not extensive, is not as unfavorable as that of atresia, extensive lateral incisions with packing often resulting in complete cure. Should the stenosis be annular, it may be excised, and the mucosa above and below be brought together and sutured; this is, however, apt to result in contraction. The results of operations for complete atresia have been so unsatisfactory that the operation should not be undertaken [except in rare cases].

External acquired stenosis may follow trauma, agglutination of the smaller labia, and kraurosis vulvæ· Atresia caused by the small labia, following inflammatory processes, is usually met with in children; it reaches as far as the urethra, rarely occluding it. The adhesions are not firm, and may be easily divided with the finger or a blunt instrument. The greater proportion of acquired atresias and stenoses are due to childbirth, forming in the puerperium, the result of extensive lacerations of the mucous membrane, puerperal necrosis, infective kolpitis, ulceration, and perikolpitis, always followed by cicatricial contraction and adhesions. Stenosis is the usual result, but complete atresia may follow.

Breisky's atresia retrohymenalis, due to adhesions of the mucous folds, is located directly behind the hymen, but is not connected with it. The adhesions are not preceded by any inflammatory or ulcerated condition of the mucosa, and for this reason have been regarded as physiologic by several authors. This form is usually met with in children; it greatly resembles imperforate hymen, having, when pushed forward, the appearance of a fluctuating, bladder-like tumor of soft consistence and bluish color, protruding into the vulva. It usually ruptures spontaneously; if not, the adhesions are easily broken up by the finger or by some blunt instrument.

Vaginitis adhesiva ulcerosa (Hildebrandt) is a vaginitis appearing in old women, rarely forming before the age of 50 and always after the appearance of the menopause. The patients usually give a history of severe lahor or of erosions and lacerations of the cervix. The upper third of the vagina is the seat of the disease in nearly all cases. The mucosa is smooth, not swollen, light-red in color, and has a bruised appearance. The epithelial layer is entirely destroyed. The papillæ are swollen, and if irritated by the finger or speculum are apt to bleed. The secretion is sticky, thin, milky, often mixed with bloody streaks; it contains pus-corpuscles and pavement-epithelium. The diseased portions always show a great tendency to form adhesions with the portio vaginalis; these are usually extensive, covering the portio and obliterating the anterior and posterior vaults. This condition has frequently been observed in postmortem examinations, when the condition during life had not given rise to symptoms. Operative interference is absolutely contraindicated.

Atresia and stenosis may result from constitutional diseases—aoute exanthemata, cholera, typhoid fever, erysipelas, syphilis, and tuberculosis. Trauma is an important factor in their etiology, such as impalement, the introduction of foreign bodies, operation on the external genitals, and the effect of astringent and cauterizing agents.

Meyer[1] has published a very complete monograph on vaginal atresia, with no fewer than 216 cases carefully tabulated. He does not confirm Kussmaul's doctrine that ill-development of the lower part of the genital tract with atresia is due to fetal inflammation. It is in infancy and childhood that these inflammations occur, such as vulvitis and local lesions in general infectious disorders. The vagina closes, the tissues heal and look healthy after a time, and it is not till puberty that the damage becomes manifest. Then it is easy to understand how the disease might be wrongly considered congenital. Unilateral bematosalpinx, with inflammatory closure of the vagina, is very often observed, and Meyer holds that there is closure of the tube at the ostium from the same inflammation, due to some infective agent. As the agent can cause septic changes in the blood in the tube, the ultimate rupture of the hematosalpinx into the peritoneum or into some visceral cavity exposes the patient to great peril. This explains the high mortality of atresia vaginæ with unilateral hematosalpinx.

In treating the acquired form of atresia, A. Mackenrodt[2] suggests the transplanting of flaps, obtained from prolapse-operations on otherwise healthy women, to the granulating sides of the artificial vagina in cases of complete atresia. Of course, an attempt to restore the vagina is warranted only when the atresia is an acquired one, or, if congenital, when the uterus and tubes are sufficiently developed to carry on the generative functions. In attempting to restore the vagina in such eases great difficulty is experienced in keeping the granulating wound open long enough to allow the epithelium to extend up and cover the whole surface.

Labial Hydrocele.—F. Elliott[3] records a case of hydrocele of the labium.

Vulvovaginal Anus.—Interesting cases of cloaca in women are recorded by F. J. Lutz[4] and J. J. Keyes.[5]

Hermaphrodism.—B. Lewis[6] records a case of male pseudohermaphrodism with marked features of femininity, the patient having had an English mother and an American Indian father. "Her" sexual inclinations have been directed toward the feminine contingent, one of whom she eventually married. "She" has menstruated since the age of 18 with a fair degree of regularity; the flow lasts 2 days, and is accompanied with feelings of malaise, and aching in the back, head, and breasts. Intercourse is pleasurable and is accompanied with the oozing from her vagina of a colorless fluid. Her face is smooth and feminine; her figure lacks the outlines of femininity, and there is a total lack of mammary development. The pubic hair grows as in women, with the apex of the pyramid pointing downward and the base upward. The

[1] Am. Pract. and News, Mar. 20, 1897.
[2] Centralbl. f. Gynäk, No. 21, 1896.
[3] Clinical Reporter, Feb., 1897.
[4] Medicine, Aug., 1896.
[5] Med. Rec., Apr. 3, 1897.
[6] Medicine, Oct., 1896.

arms are feminine, the thighs masculine.   The penis in flaccidity is 2½ in.; in the state of erection, 4½ in.; its circumference at the glans is 2½ in.   The separated halves of the scrotum contain testicles of a size larger than that of many men normally constituted.   The vagina is evidently impractical as a vagina; it appears to end as a blind pouch, and no evidence of uterus or cer-·vix is obtained by either digital or ocular examination.   The meatus urinarius opens into the roof of the vagina at a point 1½ in. from its orifice.   S. Pozzi [1] records a case of a supposed woman having on each side a testicle, a cystic epididymis (or tube), and a rudimentary uterine cornu on the left side forming a hernia in the inguinal canal.

Vulvar and Vaginal Tumors.—Holzmann [2] describes an unusually large fibroma molluscum, which grew from the right labium majus of a woman aged 37.   It had existed for at least 9 years, beginning as a swelling of the

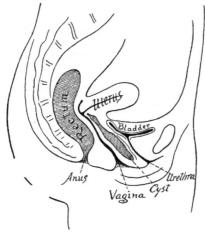

FIG. 35.—Suppurating cyst of the vagina (The Scalpel, Aug., 1896).

labium, which for a time advanced very slowly.   Latterly, as is the case with most new-growths, it advanced rapidly, so that it reached to the knee.   There was little or no pain, and it was successfully removed.   It weighed over 15 pounds.

Turgard [3] reports 3 cases of vaginal cyst.   The first was a nullipara, 36 years old, who thought that she had a prolapsus.   On examination, a tumor the size of a pigeon's egg was found presenting between the labia.   This tumor was so freely movable that it gave the sensation of a hernia, but its true nature was determined by rectal and vaginal exploration.   With cocain the cyst was excised.   The second case occurred in a woman 28 years old, who had had 2 children; during her second confinement her physician discovered the tumor. This was the size of a hazelnut, and was attached to the posterior vaginal wall.   It was excised.   Its contents were thick and of coffee color, probably of hematic origin.   The third case presented a tumor of the vulva.   The labia

[1] Bull. de l'Acad. de Méd., July 28, 1896.   [2] Inaug. Diss., Marburg, 1896.
[3] Sem. gynéc., Apr. 7, 1896.

of the left side were distended with a dull, fluctuating mass. Before marriage the patient had had an abscess of the vulvovaginal gland; during pregnancy the mass appeared as described, but disappeared after confinement. After sitting down suddenly with force the present tumor appeared. It was treated by incision and irrigation, and was considered a vulvovaginal cyst, ruptured by the fall, and producing a hematoma.

Hellier [1] reports an unusual case of suppuration in a vaginal cyst. Fig. 35 shows the site of the abscess-cavity between the vagina and the bladder. The author considered it due to suppuration in a vaginal cyst. The patient, an unmarried girl of 17, first came under notice for leukorrhea, which had troubled her for 2 years. On vulval inspection the physical signs were negative; by the rectum " a soft, elongated swelling was felt in the vagina, reaching from the cervix to the hymen." The vagina was dilated under an anesthetic, and an abscess-cavity was found under the mucous membrane of the vaginal roof and chiefly to the left of the median line. The pus appeared to arise from the os uteri, and was very offensive. Having freely incised the vaginal mucous membrane, the interior of the cavity was scraped and a portion of the cyst-wall excised; the whole surface was then rubbed over with pure phenol and packed with gauze. The patient made a rapid and easy recovery.

To remove papillomata of the vulva Manciere [2] recommends a mixture of flexible collodion 5 parts, and salicylic acid 2 parts, of which a single drop is to be applied to each wart. At one sitting 8 or 10 may be treated in this manner. On the following day the application is made to a number of others, and also to those previously treated. This is kept up daily until all are gone. The collodion does not affect the healthy tissue.

Perineorrhaphy.—Apfelstedt [3] calls attention to the importance of complete approximation of the edges of a recent tear to prevent infection from the lochial discharge. It is important that the stitches should not pass through the rectal wall, as the contents of the bowel might contaminate the wound. A comparatively simple method is described and illustrated. Silk or silkworm-gut is used.

CONDITIONS OF THE CERVIX UTERI.

Profuse Hemorrhage due to a Syphilitic Growth of the Vaginal Cervix.—Wolter [4] records the case of a patient whose husband had been infected with syphilis 15 years before. The patient had been treated with mercurial inunction for 2 years. She had had 9 children born dead, the last dying during labor and showing but few signs of syphilis. One-half year after the birth of this last child she began to have profuse and prolonged menstruation. The hemorrhage finally became so severe that it caused collapse, and had to be controlled by iodoform vaginal tampons. On the right half of the surface of the cervix there was found a growth which extended into the uterine cavity and bled easily when touched. The patient was given potassium iodid, and after 3 weeks the growth disappeared and the hemorrhage ceased.

Endothelioma of the Vaginal Cervix.—Braetz [5] describes a case appearing at the Halle clinic for women which he believed to be an endothelioma. A similar case is reported by Amann in the same journal. The patient was 18 years of age and came complaining of leukorrhea. A tumor 2 cm. in diameter was found growing from the posterior lip of the cervix. It bled easily,

---

[1] The Scalpel, p. 242, Aug., 1896.   [2] Centralbl. f. d. gesammte Therap., Jan., 1897.
[3] Münch. med. Woch., No. 25, 1896.   [4] Ibid., No. 20, 1897.
[5] Arch. f. Gynäk., Bd. ii., 1896.

and the tissue was very friable and easily broken off. Kaltenbach removed the uterus by the vagina. Four weeks after leaving the hospital the patient died. The cause of death was not determined, but very possibly resulted from metastasis. The growth was thought to have originated in the endothelium of the lymph-spaces.

Hypertrophy of the Cervix in a Virgin.—Helme[1] describes a case of hypertrophy of the cervix in an unmarried woman, aged 21 years. The fundus uteri was at nearly its normal level, while the cervix protruded from the vulva, a sound passing to the depth of 4½ in. A modified (high) circular amputation was performed for its removal. The stitches were removed on the 9th day and the patient was discharged at the end of the 3d week. When examined 6 weeks after the operation the canal was patent and the uterus measured 2¾ in.

Stenosis of the Cervix as a Factor in Uterine Disease.—H. P. Newman[2] assigns this condition as a causative factor in much of the gynecic disease that abounds. He claims that it is anything but a rare affection, and most instances may be grouped under the acquired form. Many of the so-called congenital cases are merely the persistence of the normal natal condition, and should properly be called acquired. The stenosis may be situated at the external os, the os internum, or it may include the whole extent of the canal. It causes sterility and dysmenorrhea by offering a mechanical obstruction to the spermatozoa, and by preventing the free discharge of the menstrual fluid. In a uterus that seems to have a fairly free outlet at the cervix, the hyperemia that accompanies the monthly molimen may bring the walls of the cervix so closely into apposition that the flow is materially retarded and the secretions more or less retained; this results in endometritis, metritis, salpingitis, and oöphoritis. Much of this improper development may be prevented by proper attention to the environment of young girls during the developmental period of puberty. [The gynecologic teaching of the day is almost the reverse of the teaching of this paper. True stenosis is a comparatively rare disease—it most often exists in the mind of the physician. The supposed evil effects of this condition are in reality small and unimportant. The great harm done in the past as well as the present is that it draws the attention of the physician away from the real causes of the symptoms.]

Trachelorrhaphy.—A. H. Goelet[3] employs a knife of peculiar construction for denuding the lips of the cervix in the operation of trachelorrhaphy (see Fig. 36). He claims that the operation can be completed in one-half the time that is usually consumed when scissors are employed, and that the surfaces to be approximated are more regular and even. With the knife each lip is denuded with one stroke, and no trimming is required afterward to remove superfluous tissue. The knife, which is a double-edged, pointed blade, set at nearly a right-angle to a firm shaft and handle, is made to transfix the cervix beyond the plug of cicatricial tissue, and cuts it as it is drawn downward, making a clean denudation. For inserting the sutures he employs a round, full, quarter-curved needle, with a flat, spear-shaped point, which penetrates the dense cervical tissue with ease and never breaks. For suture-material he uses silver wire or silkworm-gut only, believing that catgut or any other suture which is not absolutely impervious should not be used in the cervix. The chief advantage of silver wire and silkworm-gut is that the sutures may be left in the cervix for any length of time until complete union has taken place. Catgut is absorbed or loosens too soon, and is liable to absorb septic

---

[1] Brit. Med. Jour., Dec. 26, 1896.   [2] Jour. Am. Med. Assoc., July 25, 1896.
[3] Am. Jour. Surg. and Gynec., vol. viii., No. 10, 1896.

matter from the vagina and convey it along the suture tract. Chromicized catgut may be used for superficial auxiliary sutures. [The knife is infinitely superior to the scissors in the performance of all cervical operations—both as

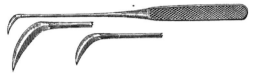

Fig. 36.—Goelet's trachelorrhaphy-knife.

to the result obtained as indicated above and as to the ease of manipulation to the operator.]

W. E. Ashton[1] operates upon all cervical lacerations associated with eversion of the mucous membrane, erosion of the cervix, or cystic degeneration, if local treatment fails, in a reasonable length of time, to effect a cure; also upon all lacerations that are associated with endometritis, uterine retrodisplacement, or subinvolution, if these complications are due to traumatism. [As a matter of fact, the vast majority of cervical lacerations have none of these complications, are entirely harmless to the woman, and need no surgical treatment whatever. The tendency of the day is to attribute too much of the symptomatology to the cervical laceration when most frequently the symptoms are produced by other factors entirely—not infrequently, neuroses.] S. D. West[2] recommends Schleich's fluid in operation on the cervix in patients unable to take an anesthetic. He injects half a dram into both lips with very satisfactory results.

FISTULÆ.

Spontaneous Healing of Fistulæ in the Female Genital Organs.—Boden[3] has searched the literature of medicine for records of cases of fistulæ into vagina or uterus that have healed spontaneously. The result of his effort has an important bearing on the question of operation in such cases, for he was able to collect 235 cases of spontaneous cure. The average duration of treatment before the fistula closed was 3 months, though in some of the cases a much longer period elapsed. The fistulæ were situated as follows in 235 cases: 132 vesicovaginal; 27 vesico-uterine; 3 vesico-enteric; 3 ureteral; 52 rectovaginal; 3 recto-uterine; 9 enterovaginal; 6 entero-uterine.

Vesicovaginal Fistula.—H. A. Kelly[4] describes a new and very rational method of operating upon large and otherwise intractable fistulæ. He begins his operation by a cut similar to the anterior incision in vaginal hysterectomy; he then separates the uterus and bladder up to but not through the peritoneum of the uterovesical space, carrying the separation widely out on both sides; the edges of the fistulæ are then denuded in the usual manner and stitched together from above downward, thus leaving a transverse wound for union. In the case he describes in the article the ureteral orifices were found in the cicatricial tissue on the edge of the fistula, and it was necessary to pass the ureteral catheters through the urethra and into the ureters before stitching the wound together. These were left in place 3 days without evil effect and the patient made a good recovery.

[1] Med. Bull., Feb., 1897.   [2] Med. and Surg. Reporter, Nov. 7, 1896.
[3] Centralbl. f. Chir., No. 38, 1896.
[4] Bull. Johns Hopkins Hosp., vol. vii., Nos. 59 and 60.

W. D. Haggard, Jr.,[1] reports a case of artificial vesicovaginal fistula with subsequent intraperitoneal cystotomy for suppurating papilloma, followed by the formation of a calculus around the dependent portion of a silk suture; the stone was successfully removed and the fistula closed. Baumgartner[2] records a case of pelvic abscess followed by vesical fistula. [The case is interesting as showing the ability of the bladder to resume its normal condition after the removal of irritating discharges which had lasted over seven years.] The source of the pus was not determined.

Rectovaginal Fistula.—Ségond[3] has devised a new method of healing rectovaginal fistulæ with intact perineum. The operation consists of the following steps: 1. Gradual and thorough dilatation of the anus. 2. Circular incision of the mucous membrane 2 mm. above its junction with the skin. 3. Separation of the vagina from the rectum with the finger, and drawing down of the rectum until the fistula is closed. 4. Resection of the portion of the rectum brought down, and suturing of the end to the skin. 5. Suturing of the vaginal opening.

Intestinovaginal Fistula.—Chaput,[4] in a case of intestinovaginal fistula in which the knife and thermocautery had many times failed, applied nitric acid to the edges of the vaginal aspect. The thus cauterized surfaces adhered and the fistula closed.

URINARY ORGANS.

Urethra.—*Prolapse of the Urethra in Female Children.*—Attention is drawn to this accident by Broca,[5] who reports the following case: A girl, aged 6 years, had alarmed her mother through the appearance of blood at the vulva for three days. It was naturally taken for menstruation. The child had been kept in bed for 2 weeks on account of severe bronchitis, with violent coughing; on the day that she arose for the first time the bleeding began. Broca examined the parts, and noted a little red protuberance at the meatus, caused by prolapse of the urethral mucosa. He directed that the everted membrane should be touched with a 2% solution of silver nitrate. The bleeding ceased permanently after the first application, and at the end of 3 days the cure was complete. Broca lays stress on this case, as it shows the extreme importance of early recognition and early treatment of this affection. [In another case the mother suspected rape, but the court ordered a medical examination and the truth was at once made evident. The meatus should be carefully explored in all cases in which blood is found near the child's genitals.]

Tumors of the Urethra.—According to M. Wasserman,[6] *carcinoma* of the female urethra is rare. He has recently collected from medical literature 24 cases. As in other regions, epithelioma of the urethra seems to be often connected with some persistent local irritation. Labor, and especially repeated pregnancy, seem to be the principal etiologic factors, but multiparæ are not exempt. Heredity plays no conspicuous part. Four times the tumor was developed between 29 and 38 years; in all the others from 43 to 72 years. Epithelioma develops mostly around the urethra. The urethrovaginal septum is more frequently affected than the upper wall, but in some cases the roof of the urethra, the clitoris, and even the retropubic tissues are invaded. The growth is at first of a deep-red color, more or less hard in consistence, rugose, nodular, with a granular and easily bleeding surface. Later it ulcerates, and yields

---

[1] Southern Pract., Oct., 1896.　　　[2] Berlin. klin. Woch., May 11, 1896.
[3] Ann. de Gynéc., No. 7, 1896.　　　[4] Gaz. hebdom. de Méd. et de Chir., No. 41, 1896.
[5] Canad. Pract., July, 1896.　　　[6] Ann. de Gyn. et d'Obstét., Apr., 1896.

an ichorous, fetid discharge; then it attacks adjacent parts and forms a large ulcer with cut and indurated edges. In one-third of the cases the inguinal glands are enlarged. The symptoms may be vague at first; later there are painful and frequent micturition, slight loss of blood at the commencement of micturition (sometimes mistaken for menstrual discharge), dull pain in the parts, sometimes lancinating pain radiating down the thighs and toward the abdomen and intense dyspareunia. Rarely a vesicovaginal fistula forms. The treatment consists of free and complete excision of the affected part of the urethra, bleeding being arrested by ligature and by a catheter fixed in the urethra if needed.

C. A. L. Reed[1] records a unique case of melanosarcoma of the female urethra in a single woman 64 years of age, which was cured by urethrectomy. [This is, as far as a reasonably comprehensive research of the literature indicates, the first of the kind to be placed upon record. Sarcoma of even the ordinary varieties, involving the urethra, is exceedingly rare, there being, according to Ehrenderfer, but 2 reported, one by Biegel in 1875, and the other by Ehreuderfer himself. In neither of these cases were melanotic features the distinguishing characteristics.] An absolute cure followed, but the patient died 7 months later from a probable recurrence of the disease in the stomach.

The Bladder.—*Cystitis.*—As regards the etiology of cystitis Kastalskaya,[2] from a bacteriologic study of secretions from the bladder in 12 cases of cystitis, reports the following results: (1) in 1 case he found the bacillus fœtidus liquefaciens mixed with tubercle-bacilli and nonpathogenic cocci; (2) in 5 cases tubercle-bacilli—twice as a pure culture, once mixed with nonpathogenic cocci and bacterium coli immobile, and once with nonpathogenic cocci and the bacillus fœtidus liquefaciens; (3) in 4 cases the bacterium coli immobile, twice as a pure culture, once with nonpathogenic cocci and tubercle-bacilli, and once with streptococcus pyogenes; (4) in 1 case pseudobacterium coli commune as a pure culture; (5) in 1 case bacilli with nonpathogenic cocci; (6) in 1 case streptococcus pyogenes with bacterium coli immobile; and (7) in 1 case a pure culture of pseudostaphylococcus albus.

Wertheim,[3] at a meeting of the Berlin Obstetric and Gynecologic Society, demonstrated a preparation from a case of gonorrheal cystitis which showed the capillary and precapillary veins filled with gonococci, a condition of gonorrheal thrombosis and thrombophlebitis. The cystitis was secondary to a gonorrheal vulvovaginitis and was associated with an infection of both ulnar joints.

In the prophylaxis of the disease W. D. Haggard, Jr.,[4] states that the overwhelming majority of cases result from pyogenic microorganisms introduced from without, although the instrumentality of such causes as exposure to cold, retention and decomposition of urine, calculi, foreign bodies, entozoa, neoplasms, tuberculosis, mechanical injuries, croupous and diphtheritic inflammations, and the secondary infection from rupture of an adjacent pus-collection, is unquestioned. Unclean catheterization must stand the impeached sponsor for the majority of the cases. The extension of septic urethritis, particularly gonorrheal, is another source of infection. The rules (modified) for preparing the catheter, and precautions necessary in passing it, in use in the Woman's Hospital in Nashville are as follows: 1. The catheter is to be boiled in boric-acid solution (4%) for 10 minutes; 2. It must be brought to the bedside in the vessel of solution in which it has been boiled. 3. The parts are to be prepared by washing with bichlorid solution (1 : 3000). 4. The nurse must

[1] Buffalo Med. Jour., Dec., 1896.   [2] Centralbl. f. Gynäk., No. 33, 1896.
[3] Zeit. f. Geb. u. Gynäk., Bd. xxxv., H. 1, 1896.   [4] Jour. Am. Med. Assoc., May 8, 1897.

scrub her hands with brush, soap and water for 3 minutes; the nails and hands are then scrubbed with the brush and bichlorid solution (1 : 1000); she must then not touch anything but the catheter before its introduction. The prevention of extension in gonorrheal urethritis may be secured by daily irrigation of the urethra with a 1 : 20,000 bichlorid solution, which should be preceded by the instillation of a few drops of a 4% cocain solution.

In the treatment of the disease normal sterilized salt-solution (dram to the quart) is the most useful irrigating fluid. The sovereign remedy in the treatment of inflamed mucosæ is silver nitrate, $\frac{1}{10}$ to $\frac{1}{2}$%. In obstinate cases of the disease Escat[1] concludes as follows: 1. A careful examination should be made of the pelvic organs to determine if there is not some extravesical cause for the symptoms. The urethra and kidneys should also receive due attention. 2. After exhausting the usual local methods of treatment (drainage, irrigation, curettage), epicystotomy should be performed, if there are no renal complications. Through the incision the ureters can be catheterized directly, and any diseased portions of the mucosa can be reached with the curet or thermocautery. 3. Vaginal cystotomy is preferable in cases of accompanying renal trouble, or when the patient's general condition is bad. 4. A still more thorough plan of surgical treatment is to follow the epicystotomy and cauterization immediately with a vaginal cystotomy, thus securing perfect drainage. Camero[2] reports 29 cases of painful cystitis treated according to Guyon's method of curettage, with 19 cures and 10 failures. Camero claims that cystotomy should be reserved for the most serious cases, curettage of the bladder by the urethra often effecting a cure.

Gangrenous cystitis with exfoliation of the bladder-wall is rarely attended by recovery; such a case, however, is reported by C. Warren.[3] Under ether "rolls of sloughing tissue" were pulled out by the forceps until a "membrane the size of a small pocket-handkerchief had been extracted from the bladder in a continuous mass." The patient suffered at first from incontinence, but gradually recovered under daily washings out of the bladder with a weak solution of potassium permanganate, and later with a solution of boracic acid. An examination of the specimen removed showed it to be of a character similar to the submucosa of the bladder.

Ureter and Kidney.—*Ureteritis.*—According to E. Reynolds,[4] *ureteritis* is not an infrequent disease. The most characteristic symptoms are frequency of micturition, which is increased by the erect posture, and especially by standing, and is not wholly relieved by recumbency; and a bearing-down pain, which is increased by standing, but is usually completely relieved by a few hours' rest in bed. Severe ureteritis may lead to a palpable enlargement of the ureter, but the physical signs of the milder degree of the disease, obtainable by vaginal examination, are usually limited to the excitation of tenderness and a desire to urinate, by pressure over the vaginal portion of the affected ureter. This tenderness is usually so closely localized as to be easily overlooked; but when it once has been found, its strict limitation to the situation of the ureter is a diagnostic point of great importance. When the micturition is painful it is always best to examine the bladder at once, since in this class of cases both the pain and, to some extent, the frequency can usually be promptly, though not always permanently, relieved by topical treatment of the bladder. The signs obtainable from cystoscopic examination comprise an alteration of the vesical orifice of the affected ureter or ureters,

[1] Ann. des Mal. des Org. gén.-urin., No. 2, 1897.
[2] Gaz. hebdom. de Méd. et de Chir., Sept. 24, 1896.
[3] Boston M. and S. Jour., June 25, 1896.　　[4] Ann. of Gyn. and Pediat., Nov., 1896.

alterations of the vesical mucosa around these orifices, and a very curious alteration of the character of the urine secreted through them. There occur a slight reddening and gaping of the vesical orifice of the inflamed ureter, or there may be an actual eversion of the ureteral mucosa, until in extreme cases the orifice shows a round hole situated on the summit of a little mound of angry-looking mucosa. The vesical mucosa in the vicinity is usually red and injected, or even roughened and eroded. In these cases localized applications of solid silver nitrate give prompt relief of the pain on micturition. When the ulcers or erosions extend into the neighborhood of the urethral opening, or when the nitrate is too freely applied, the application may be followed by a temporary increase of the symptoms; but this increase seldom lasts more than 24 hours, and is then followed by relief. When it is not necessary to approach closely the urethral orifice, and the nitrate is sparingly used, the relief is usually immediate. The regulation of the diet and the ingestion of an amount of bland fluid equal to at least 3 pints of water daily are important adjuncts to the treatment. The diet should be bland, nutritious, and largely albuminous. Asparagus and strawberries should be absolutely interdicted; other fruits should be used but sparingly, and the highly flavored vegetables in general, such as tomatoes, onions, and cabbage, should be tried with caution. General massage is of the greatest benefit, and active exercise, as the use of the bicycle, will be beneficial. As regards medicinal treatment, alkalies and the so-called alterative drugs are indicated, as small doses of potassium iodid with mercury. Acute ureteritis is probably often mistaken for intestinal colic, pain due to renal stone, catarrhal appendicitis, or acute catarrhal salpingitis.

Surgical Injuries to the Ureters.—J. M. Baldy[1] remarks that injuries to the ureters are by no means uncommon accidents, though few of them ever find their way into print. The treatment of the injuries is now practically settled. The adoption of such makeshifts as ligation of the severed ends, formation of a urinary fistula, or nephrectomy, is ancient history. To-day we have but two propositions to consider—*uretero-ureteral anastomosis* and *ureterocystostomy (bladder-implantation)*. Both these procedures have been demonstrated as feasible, first by experimentation (Van Hook, Paoli, and Busachi) upon dogs, and subsequently by various surgeons upon the human subject. There are now on record 7 successful operations of this character. Experience seems to demonstrate more and more that bladder-implantation is applicable to a much larger group than is uretero-ureteral anastomosis; and if any choice must be made between the two methods, this is the method of election. It is necessary for the purpose of performing uretero-ureteral anastomosis that the two ends of the ureter be perfectly free and easily brought together; that the vesical end be more patulous (or capable of being made so) than the renal end; that the injury to the ureter be sufficiently high in the pelvis to enable the surgeon to readily carry out the necessary manipulations. In the case of ureterocystostomy but one point is necessary—that the injury be not too high in the pelvis to enable the kidney-end of the ureter to be approximated with the bladder. Of the 7 operations mentioned, 2 (Kelly and B. Emmet) were of the method of uretero-ureteral anastomosis; 5 (Novaro, Kelly, King, Penrose, Baldy) were of the method of ureterocystostomy. Of these 5 cases in not one was uretero-ureteral anastomosis possible, while of the other 2 cases 1 (Kelly) could have been corrected with equal success by bladder-implantation. If the injury be at or above the level of the ileopectineal line, it is exceedingly difficult, if not impossible, to closely approxi-

---

[1] Am. Gyn. and Obst. Jour., Oct., 1896.

mate the end of the ureter and the bladder. The danger of immediate obstruction in the two operations does not seem to be great. The danger of secondary obstruction after bladder-implantation seems to be absolutely nil, and the dangers of kidney-infection are mythical.

Tuberculosis of the Ureter and Kidney.—H. Kelly[1] describes 3 cases of unilateral tuberculosis of the kidney and ureter which he treated by excision of the kidney and the whole ureter at one sitting (*nephro-ureterectomy*). The three cases were operated upon by three different methods, and represent to his mind three stages in the evolution of the operation. In the first case he opened the abdomen from the front and removed the kidney and ureter. In the second case he removed the kidney by an incision in the back just outside of the quadratus muscle. In the third case the incision was a horizontal or slightly oblique cut between the lower ribs and the crest of the ilium.

A New Method of Obtaining Urine from a Single Kidney.—Rose[2] describes a method of obtaining urine from a single kidney. In order to accomplish this purpose, which is often of great importance diagnostically, various measures have been proposed. Pressure upon one ureter, either bimanually or through the vagina, or by means of a special clamp, is an uncertain procedure. Hegar proposed to cut down upon the ureter through the vagina and stop for a time its flow of urine. This method is certain, but is in itself an operation. By means of the cystoscope it is sometimes possible to determine that the urine from one ureter contains pus or blood, while that from the other is clear. At times this distinction is made with difficulty, or not at all, and in the most favorable cases no information is gained as to the chemie or microscopic condition of the urine. The catheterization, as proposed by Nitze and Kelly, requires considerable practice, expensive apparatus, and often an unpleasant dilatation of the urethra. Rose's procedure is based upon the fact that the bladder of a woman in the knee-chest position, or with the pelvis elevated in the dorsal position, will distend with air if a speculum is introduced through the urethra. Through this speculum it is possible to see by direct or reflected light the openings of the ureters; and if the speculum is cut obliquely, its inner extremity may be clamped over one ureter, while the urine from the other ureter flows down over the posterior bladder-wall toward the umbilicus. When sufficient urine for examination has collected in the speculum it can be drawn into a syringe, the speculum be withdrawn and cleansed, the bladder irrigated, emptied, and again distended with air, and the speculum placed over the mouth of the ureter of the opposite side. In cases of extreme sensitiveness the use of cocain is recommended. As the urethra is not dilated, narcosis is unnecessary, and a resulting incontinence of urine is not to be feared.

MENSTRUATION AND ITS DISORDERS.

Puberty.—[The subject of uterine cardiopathies is very generally overlooked in everyday practice.] Kisch[3] calls attention to the reflex cardiac disturbances observed in women at certain crises in their lives—at puberty, at the menopause, just after marriage, and also during pregnancy and labor. These are palpitation, abnormal acceleration and slowness of the pulse, precordial pains, dyspnea, and sense of oppression. In young subjects with these symptoms the external genitals may be non-developed; menstruation is established with difficulty, and is scanty and irregular. When these women reach

---

[1] Boston M. and S. Jour., Sept. 17, 1896.   [2] Centralbl. f. Gynäk., Feb. 6, 1897.
[3] Gaz. de Gynéc., June, 1896.

the climacteric they have a return of the same phenomena which appeared at puberty, especially if they have been weakened by several previous labors and profuse hemorrhages. Simultaneously with the cardiac disturbances they are troubled with marked gastric irritability. These cardiac neuroses are undoubtedly due to the physiologic changes in the ovaries at puberty and the menopause, though they may be attributed to certain chemic changes which occur during the development and atrophy of the Graafian follicles. The condition is doubtless one of hyperesthesia of the cardiac plexuses. To some extent these cardiopathies seem to be hereditary, and are observed most frequently among the better classes. The treatment recommended is hygienic and moral rather than medicinal.

[The question of *bicycling* for women, whether it be potent for evil or for good, is yet discussed. The discussion is passing through its last stage, and it will take some time yet for it to find its perfect equilibrium.] Evans[1] considers that eventually the use of the bicycle will tend to produce placenta prævia. The author thinks that from the physiology, tissue, and function of the perineum it may be looked upon as a supplementary uterus. Prolonged pressure upon the connective tissue can but lead to " condensation and atrophy," and to increased difficulty of perineal dilatation or more frequent laceration. Turner, in a series of papers in recent numbers of the *British Medical Journal*, has treated the whole matter from all points of view. The conditions under which this exercise should *not* be indulged in appear to be— (1) during menstruation, and if possible for 24 hours preceding and 24 hours after the flow; (2) during pregnancy, although experience has shown that even during the first 3 months of that condition no harm has resulted from resort to the bicycle; (3) pelvic tumors, especially fibroids; (4) recent perimetritis, parametritis, or blood-exudations into the pelvis. [These are naturally only the more important conditions. Each case should be judged on its merits. No woman should ride a bicycle without first consulting her medical man, and she should ride only when suitably dressed.]

E. D. Page[2] believes that the use of the wheel should be conservative. He claims that the principal muscles developed in its use are those of the leg and thigh; that little muscular development of the arms comes from it, as there is comparatively little use for the arms in cycling except in mounting and dismounting, as when one becomes thoroughly master of the cycle very little effort keeps it balanced and guides it, which are the principal uses of the arms in the erect position in which women ride. There is a fascination about bicycling that leads to immoderate exercise, and then it is positively harmful in a general way. As to the advantage to the muscles of respiration, it would appear to be limited and, in a sense, unnatural. These muscles, to receive their fullest benefit, must also have the freedom of action attendant upon the arms being free to move at the side, with the shoulders thrown back or erect; with freedom to take deep inspirations, and with all chest- and arm-muscles free to move in any direction natural to each. With the slight bending forward and the *constant* extending of both arms in grasping the handles, the chest is perforce limited in its freedom; it is bound. The quickened respiration following the exercise of cycling has not, therefore, the benefit claimed for it. The development, if any, would be a cramped, narrower chest, and the training of years of cycling will frequently result in naught else. The plea that those sitting the wheel *aright* would avoid this by keeping the back usually straight and doing all the bending at the saddle or at the junction of thighs and body, is perhaps in a measure true; but the fact remains that the wheel is rarely ridden that way,

[1] Am. Jour. of Obst., Apr., 1896. [2] Brooklyn Med. Jour., Feb., 1897.

it may be more frequently, however, by women. That the abdominal viscera may suffer from cycling is true. Page also claims that the bicycle teaches masturbation in women and girls, and that the saddle causes bruising and chafing of the labia. Also, that abortion is liable to be produced by wheeling, and in young girls there is a liability of narrowing the lateral diameter of the pelvis. [The above is an excellent example of what prejudice opposes to every innovation of any use whatever, and is a fair example of the absurd mistakes made in an attempt to criticise something with which one is not practically familiar. The deductions are purely theoretic and have no foundation in fact. To begin with, all these criticisms are based on the supposition that the woman rides in a leaning-forward (faulty) position, when, as a matter of fact, 9 out of 10 ride in the correct position (upright). The criticism that the chest does not expand properly in riding because the hands and arms are partially extended is theoretically untrue, and practically is answered by the fact that with rare exceptions the chest-measurements are increased after a few months' riding. It is unnecessary to point out to any rider the absurdity of the statement that the arms receive no exercise; it simply needs a trial of the instrument to demonstrate the contrary to be true. The efforts incident to balancing bring all the back-muscles into full play in addition. The pleading for a functionally weak heart is specious. Every experienced rider knows that at first the heart is apt to be overcome by climbing very moderate grades. After short practice these same grades are climbed without the knowledge that they exist, and shortly thereafter considerable hills can be taken with small discomfort. This all means that the weak heart has had constant and increasing judiciously arranged exercise, and is gradually strengthened until it is performing its proper functions easily and with increasing strength and vigor. The same thing may be said of the lungs and the quickened respiration.

Of course, the labia are bruised and chafed at first; but so is any other part of the body under similar experience. A loose shoe, an ill-fitting corset, or even a collar, will produce the same thing in other parts of the body; but in bicycling this is only incident to learning. The parts soon become accustomed to the pressure and the discomfort disappears. As to masturbation, the statement in general is untrue. We have investigated this subject closely and are convinced that it does not result.

The pleading that the perineum is a supplementary uterus and that pressure on it causes placenta prævia is unworthy of discussion, as not a single fact is advanced in support of it. It is merely the unsupported belief of the author.

The bicycle is the most valuable addition to the therapeutics of women of the age. Properly utilized (proper saddle and proper position, with moderation as to speed and distances) it is worth all the drugs in the pharmacopeia together, especially in that class in which it is in some quarters condemned— neurotic, anemic women with functional heart-diseases. In healthy women there is no contraindication.]

Theilhaber[1] recommends cycling in cases of amenorrhea, especially when the uterus is undeveloped. Dysmenorrhea of nervous origin in young girls and sterile women is often relieved. In endometritis the writer has seen no result, either favorable or unfavorable, from this form of exercise; in the hemorrhagic form he advises against it on theoretic grounds. It should be forbidden in chronic as well as in acute gonorrhea, in salpingitis, and in subacute and chronic peritonitis of whatsoever origin. Flexions and versions do not constitute a contraindication; in fact, cycling is often recommended for

---

[1] Münch. med. Woch., No. 48, 1896.

patients with these conditions with the view of relieving nervous symptoms and strengthening flabby muscles rather than actually relieving the displacement. This may account for the good results claimed in some cases of partial prolapsus. The use of the bicycle is inadmissible by patients with fibroid and ovarian tumors. The writer noted rapid increase in the size of fibroids in 2 women who rode contrary to his advice. Bladder-troubles are usually aggravated by cycling, though on this point there is some difference of opinion. Hemorrhoids are sometimes relieved, but are sometimes made worse, especially when improper saddles are used. Such benefit as may be experienced is usually due to the relief of constipation. Women ought not to ride during menstruation, though the writer admits that several of his patients have done so without injury. Pregnancy is a positive contraindication. Two of the patients who disobeyed his injunction aborted, but a third went on to full term, though she had a retroflexed uterus and prolapsed ovaries. In general, he approves of cycling in moderation. H. Macnaughton Jones [1] calls attention to the fact that cycling may have an injurious effect on women at the time of the menopause, and should not be indulged in except on the advice of a physician, especially if the patient is anemic and has functional cardiac trouble. He doubts the propriety of women with retrodisplacements of the uterus riding, with or without pessaries; this applies especially to anemic young girls. Hemorrhoids are aggravated, and coccygodynia may result. The writer recommends a pneumatic saddle, so constructed as to support the ischia, but not to press upon the external genitals or the coccyx ; there should be no projection under the pubes. He approves highly of this form of exercise, which he regards as far superior to massage.

The Influence of Menstruation upon the Excretion of Uric Acid.—At the French Congress of Medicine E. Laval [2] stated that on the second day of menstruation, when the flow is most profuse, the amount of uric acid in the urine suddenly diminishes. On the following day the proportion is slightly increased, and on the fourth day exceeds the normal proportion. Subsequently the rate of excretion resumes its usual course. The effect produced by the menstrual flow is, therefore, comparable to that produced by a true hemorrhage.

Bathing during Menstruation.—Matweieff publishes a series of observations which demonstrate that saline or mud baths, at 25°, 27°, or 28° C., have a favorable influence on menstruation from the point of view of pain, the quantity of blood lost, and the duration of the flow. Mironiff, who made a number of observations to verify this, is in a position to state that alkaline baths at 27° or 28° C., taken during the menstrual period by patients suffering from gynecologic troubles, act as an excellent sedative; the quantity of blood lost is not affected by them, or perhaps slightly diminished. After these results he wished to know the influence of hot baths in the same conditions, for these are what would be, more than anything else, recommended in gynecologic cases. In affections of the uterine appendages the menses are often increased in frequency, as is also the quantity of blood lost. Patients do not use hot baths during this period for fear of increasing the flow, or, perhaps, bringing on severe hemorrhage. His conclusions on this account are interesting. He finds, as a result of 20 observations, that hot baths, taken during menstruation, do not increase the quantity of blood lost ; on the contrary, they often diminish it. At the same time, they soothe the pain accompanying inflammatory affections of the genitals. They are, therefore, of real benefit, not only between the periods, but during the flow.

[1] Med. Press, Nov. 4, 1896.　　　　　　　[2] Med. Bull., Oct., 1896.

Honzel[1] states that most authors are in accord with the opinion that baths are contraindicated during the menstrual period. This opinion may be correct as regards the women of towns, but his personal observation has shown him that the robust and perfectly natural woman is not in a condition bordering on illness during this period. With her menstruation is a purely physiologic act, silently accomplished and accommodating itself to the fatigues and vicissitudes which the necessities of life impose upon her. *Sea-baths*, far from deranging, favor menstruation, prolong the period of sexual activity, and increase her fruitfulness. He has frequently been surprised to see the fisherwomen, poorly nourished, slightly clad, feet and limbs bare, wade into the sea up to the waist, and sometimes up to the armpits, remaining there for hours. In spring and summer, having filled their nets with shell-fish, they come out of the water, and with their wet clothing and the dripping net on their shoulder, traverse the town selling their fish. In the winter they may be seen, in coldest weather, with a heavy basket of mussels on their backs, from which the icy water constantly drops. Sometimes their clothes are completely frozen during menstruation, yet without causing any ill effects whatever. All this may seem surprising, and may by many be attributed to race and habit, but a study of sea-baths and their effect on the uterus easily explains it, and shows that all women, except those with grave lesions of the appendages, might imitate these fisherwomen to great advantage, provided they allow themselves time to receive the benefit of the sea-air and to become accustomed to sea-baths before going into the water during the menstrual period. Of 123 fisherwomen examined by Honzel puberty occurred on an average at the age of 13 years and 10 months, and the menopause at 49 years and 6 months—a difference in their favor, as regards the period of fecundity, of 3 years and 7 months over women not going into the sea. According to Raciborski,[2] the average period of sexual life of the Parisian woman is 31 years and 7 months. [The fear of bathing during menstruation is one of the teachings handed down to us for generations, and is purely fictitious. It is, however, so firmly educated into womankind that it will take a generation or two to remove it. There is no reason why any healthy woman should not bathe during menstruation, with proper precautions against subsequent cold. There is no reason why a woman should allow her person to go unclean at the time of all others it needs cleansing. This is just as true of town women as of country women.]

The Relation between Menstruation and Erysipelas.—Salvy,[3] from a study of 810 cases, found a direct relation between menstruation and erysipelas in only 5.2%. In 1.62% menstruation could be regarded as a direct etiologic factor. In 57 cases of recurrent erysipelas only 3 were due to menstruation. Erysipelas has no appreciable influence on the duration and amount of the flow. On the contrary, menstruation favors the development of erysipelas through its influence on the nervous system. Recurrences during the flow are due to the peculiar nervous state of the patient and to the persistence of colonies of streptococci in the skin and lymph-spaces, whose virulence has not been entirely destroyed.

Precocious Menstruation.—Interesting cases are recorded by J. W. Irion[4] and R. Howie.[5] Irion's case was a baby that menstruated from birth, the flow returning with perfect regularity, and the child being in good health. The skin was fair and clear, the eyes bright and intelligent. The breasts and mons Veneris were considerably developed, and during the flow the breasts

[1] N. Am. Pract., July, 1896.   [2] Traité de la Menstruation.
[3] Gaz. hebdom. de Méd. et de Chir., No. 40, 1896.   [4] N. Y. Med. Jour., Aug. 15, 1896.
[5] Brit. Med. Jour., Sept. 12, 1896.

enlarged and were somewhat sensitive to the touch. The mother's menstrual period was established at the age of 13 years. Howie's case commenced to menstruate when 3 years and 14 days old. During menstruation the child complained of pain in the back, and was languid. The pubic hair was quite well grown, though short. The vulva was well formed and large, and the breasts prominent.

Sterility.—Ashby[1] concludes a paper on this subject as follows: the adjustment of the tube and ovary during ovulation is effected in the human female by the most delicate mechanical arrangement, and may be defeated by trivial mechanical interferences. In animals that habitually have multiple pregnancies a more perfect mechanical provision is made for the reception of the ovum by the tube. The number of ova impregnated seems to bear a close relation to the perfection of the arrangement which is provided for their passage into the tube. Thus, in the bird will be found the most perfect type of mechanical adjustment, in women, the most intricate and difficult. The adjustment of the pavilion of the tube to the ovary may be set aside by the most trivial vices of structure and disease, resulting in absolute or relative sterility. Sterility is due to minor diseases of the tubes and ovaries to a greater extent than has been recognized. In an investigation of the etiology of this condition this fact should be considered in connection with an investigation of other causative influences. The highest aim of surgery is to restore and not to destroy function. In the treatment of minor forms of ovarian and tubal disease this fact should be borne in mind. Organs should not be sacrificed to the rule of expediency, but should be preserved in deference to a law of genuine conservatism. Levy[2] calls attention to the tendency of both physician and patient to ascribe the cure of sterility to some particular method of treatment, either operative or nonoperative. He insists upon the necessity of examining the husband's semen before beginning any course of treatment, even when some obvious pathologic condition is found in the wife. The importance of the psychic factor must never be lost sight of. The assurance given to the patient that she is capable of conceiving may in itself serve to reconcile certain domestic obstacles. In any case the principle *nil nocere* should always be borne in mind, for in performing an operation for the cure of sterility the surgeon may substitute a pathologic for a normal condition.

The Menopause.—W. Armstrong[3] calls attention to the frequency of utero-ovarian irritation at the time of the menopause as a factor in the causation of *rheumatoid arthritis.* This disease is much more common in women than in males, a careful analysis of 180 cases giving the following results: males 34, females 146. Of the latter, 120 suffered from uterine or ovarian derangements or change of function in nearly every case before the onset of the arthritis; and in the few instances in which it was not so, the onset of the pelvic irritation was followed by marked increase of the arthritic troubles. In 58 cases the symptoms came on at or immediately after the climacteric period, and in 62 cases there was distinct uterine or ovarian trouble. As regards treatment, there should be careful attention to uterine and ovarian lesions that may be present; remedies to allay nervous irritation are indicated, as are also general nerve-tonics, and hydrotherapeutic measures and massage, including electric baths.

Reinicke[4] states that *climacteric hemorrhages* are due to arterial sclerosis, in consequence of which the vessels lose their muscular tone and are unable to contract, as they do normally at the time of the menstrual flow; hence the

[1] Brooklyn Med. Jour., Oct., 1896. [2] Frauenarzt, No. 11, 1896.
[3] Brit. Gyn. Jour., xliv., 496, 1896. [4] Arch. f. Gynäk., Bd. 52, H. 2, 1897.

menorrhagia which is so common at the menopause. When the hemorrhages persist in spite of repeated curettement and the administration of ergot (especially if the drug increases the flow), it is safe to infer that these vascular changes are present, especially if endometritis, neoplasms, and disease of the adnexa can be excluded. This diagnosis is confirmed if the uterine body is hard and arterial changes are noted in the extremities. Since these hemorrhages are due to sclerosis of the uterine arteries, no effect can be expected from the use of drugs or electricity—in fact, they are usually aggravated by ergot, which is apt to cause venous congestion rather than arterial anemia. Rest, strict regulation of diet, with the avoidance of alcohol, strong tea and coffee, and the use of laxatives are sufficient in mild cases. Curettement has been advised, but this operation simply opens up the mouths of numerous vessels which are unable to contract, and thus increases the flow. The cause of the hemorrhage is not in the mucosa, but in the muscular substance of the uterus. Dilatation of the cervical canal and intrauterine applications of Monsell's solution are preferable. In obstinate cases in which the patient is really in danger from repeated hemorrhages total extirpation is indicated, the results being quite satisfactory, while the mortality is only a little over 1 %. Castration is not a sure means of relief. This radical treatment should be adopted earlier in the case of workingwomen who cannot rest during the flow.

[Among the most interesting and suggestive of the recent innovations in gynecology stands foremost *ovarian therapy* in the treatment of the phenomena of the menopause, induced or physiologic.]

M. F. Jayle[1] states that this consists in the administration of (1) the ovary in its natural condition; (2) ovarian powder obtained by desiccation or a glycerin-extract. The second in 2-gr. doses a quarter of an hour before the noonday meal is preferred. The indications are against (1) the accidents provoked by castration; (2) certain ovarian lesions; (3) the normal menopause; and (4) Basedow's disease, osteomalacia, and the like. He concludes that (1) the ovary appears to be the source of an internal secretion which is useful to the economy of the woman. (2) This medication appears to be without danger. (3) It is followed by permanent success in the troubles provoked by the artificial menopause. (4) It appears that it can be used to advantage in the different symptoms due to an ovarian lesion (amenorrhea, dysmenorrhea, adiposis, chlorosis). (5) It seems to be useful in certain cases against the symptoms of the natural menopause. Stachow[2] gives an abstract of the mode of experimentation and the results attained by Mainzer, Chrobak, Mond, Krauer, and Fisher as regards animal ovarian preparations and organo-therapy. F. Mainzer[3] used fresh ovarian substance from cows and calves. The patient had had the operation of bilateral oöphorectomy performed, and a few weeks afterward complained of flashes of heat, profuse sweating, also headache, poor appetite, and marked sensations of pressure in the occipital region preceding and during the early part of the menstrual period. Five to 20 gm. of ovarian substance were administered twice a day. The patient improved very much under this treatment; particularly did the attacks of flashes of heat and sweating become less frequent and severe. Chrobak[4] applied the treatment in patients having exaggerated symptoms of the natural or induced menopause. He considered the treatment applied in two ways: (1) through transplantation of ovarian tissue; as in the experiments of Krauer, and (2) through the administration of ovarian tissue by the mouth. In a case (induced menopause through hysterectomy) he gave the fresh ovaries of the calf. He noticed no influence. In

---

[1] Presse méd., No. 71, p. 437, 1896.   [2] Monats. f. Geb. u. Gynäk., Bd. iv., H. 1, 1896.
[3] Deutsch. med. Woch., No. 12, June 18, 1896.   [4] Centralbl. f. Gynäk., No. 20, 1895.

7 other cases (because of severe symptoms during the natural menopause in 1 and the same symptoms in 6 in which the menopause had been induced) he employed pastels made from the dry ovarian substance (cow), each pastel containing 0.2 gm. In the case of the natural menopause and in 3 of the others all the symptoms were very much improved. The remaining 3 cases had not been observed sufficiently long to report results. The treatment causes no symptoms whatever. Mond[1] employed preparations made (tablets of 0.25 gm.— E. Merck) either from the entire ovarian substance, from the precipitate of the follicle-contents, or from the cortical substance of the ovary of the cow. His observations were on 11 patients from whom either part or all of the internal genitalia had been removed; or who complained of symptoms of the natural menopause, or of amenorrhea the result of atrophy of the genitalia, or in cases of rudimentary uterus with a hyperplasia of the ovaries. In 5 of these cases tablets made from the entire ovarian substance were given 3 times a day. The results were generally very encouraging, the symptoms being very much relieved. The urine remained normal. In 5 other cases 10 tablets made from the precipitate of the follicle-contents were given each day. Also in these cases the patient improved very much. In one case, in which the form of preparation is not stated, it was not surely determined that the treatment did good. Krauer[2] reports the following experimentation: he removed the ovaries from 4 rabbits, and then replaced them by suturing part in the mesentery of the horn of the uterus, and part was implanted between the fascia and muscle of the abdominal wall. In 3 of these rabbits at the postmortems, 3, 4, and 6 months after operation, ovarian tissue (proved microscopically) was still found in the mesentery of the horn of the uterus and in the abdominal wall. From this investigation Kraner comes to the following conclusions: (1) that in rabbits the ovaries can be removed and then transplanted in other than their normal position; (2) that they can be attached to peritoneum as well as implanted between muscle-fibers; (3) that the thus implanted ovary is nourished and continues its function. Fisher[3] writes that from the literature and observation it is known that there exists a relationship between the thyroid gland and the genital apparatus in women. As a proof of this he refers to the greater frequency of thyroid disease in women. He then calls attention to the influence of the genital apparatus upon the healthy thyroid gland, as occurs at puberty, during menstruation, birth, the puerperium, lactation, sexual excitement, the menopause, and genital disease. He emphasizes the influence that the removal of part of the thyroid gland has upon the physiologic and pathologic conditions of the female genital apparatus and which investigators have attempted to explain by experimentation. He then considers the changes in the genital apparatus associated with or resulting from goiter, thyroidectomy, hyperthyresis, myxedema, cretinism, morbus Basedowii, and acromegaly. Fisher concludes (1) that certain occurrences influencing the genital apparatus (puberty, pregnancy, fibroid tumor) which cause a distinct change in the metabolism of the entire organism, very frequently cause an enlargement of the thyroid gland; (2) that the deficiency of the normal thyroid secretion (after thyroidectomy in myxedema, cretinism) is often associated with atrophic changes in the genital apparatus. Cheron[4] holds that thyroid extract is an excellent remedy in threatened abortion with hemorrhage, and is valuable in preventing the arrest of uterine involution after childbirth, and that it is potent against the premature return of the monthly periods. Moreover, it is

[1] Münch. med. Woch., No. 14, 1896.   [2] Centralbl. f. Gynäk., No. 20, 1896.
[3] Wien. med. Woch., Nos. 6 and 9, 1896.
[4] Rev. méd.-chir. des Mal. des Femmes, Nov. 25 and Dec. 25, 1896.

a valuable galactagogue. Thyroid extract, in other words, stimulates the mammary secretion, whilst it lessens the functional activity of the uterus. In gynecology it has proved valuable in the control of all forms of uterine hemorrhage, whether this be due to endometritis, tumor, or lesions of the adnexa. The contraindications to the employment of the drug are: tuberculosis, since this seems to be stimulated rather than arrested. In heart-disease, even though thyroidin is strongly indicated, it should be administered with the utmost care, and should be stopped at once upon the first suggestion of tachycardia. The symptoms of thyroid-intoxication are tachycardia, oppression, exophthalmos, and irritability. In certain cases the drug produces rapid emaciation. Sometimes gastric vertigo has been observed. Because of the difficulty experienced in procuring the fresh gland and the repugnance which patients exhibit in consuming it, it is well to administer it in the dry form prepared by druggists— this may be obtained in tablets, pastilles or capsules—in doses of $1\frac{1}{2}$ gr. twice daily before meals. After a month there should be an interval of 8 days during which the drug is discontinued, followed by a 3 weeks' course of the medicine. If indications still exist for its employment, a rest of 2 weeks is given, followed by 2 weeks of the drug. Landau[1] has been employing organotherapy at his clinic for several months, as suggested originally by Mainzer, and subsequently by Mond and Chrobak. Cases were carefully selected, in order to control the experiments, with especial reference to the effect of the remedy upon the characteristic "hot flushes" so common at the menopause, both natural and artificial. The isolation of the active principle of ovarian tissue has not yet been effected. The writer believes that it is probably a nucleo-albumin, or perhaps an albuminous body like spermin. He used the ovaries of cows and pigs, dried at a temperature of 60° to 70° C. for 12 hours, then pulverized and made into tablets, each of which contained $7\frac{1}{2}$ gr. Although not prepared to present any positive results, the writer believes that the remedy does possess the power of modifying the unpleasant phenomena of the climacteric, whether physiologic or anticipated, without producing any evil effects, and deserves careful consideration.

Lissac[2] reviews the various phenomena noted in women after castration, which are more severe in young, neurotic females than in normal subjects who are near the menopause. These are flushing, psychic symptoms, congestions and hemorrhages, disturbances of nutrition, and modifications of the sexual passion. Flushing is a phenomenon that presents wide variations in regard to its appearance and severity. In some women it is noted only once a month, at the time when menstruation should occur; in others it may recur every half-hour or hour during the day or night. Sometimes the face alone is affected; sometimes the entire body seems to be congested and is covered with perspiration. The sensation of heat may be felt during sleep, the patient awaking in terror to find herself bathed in sweat. This symptom may persist for 10 or 15 years. Among the reflex symptoms are headache, insomnia, neuralgia, cardiopathies, and muscular asthenia. Marked changes in the disposition are common, such as irritability, loss of memory, and mental depression, which may persist for many years. Insanity is noted in a certain proportion of cases of castration. Among the congestive phenomena are the irregular uterine hemorrhages and vicarious bleeding from various organs. Increase in adipose has been generally observed, due to profound disturbance of nutrition of vasomotor origin and probable deficient oxidation. The apparent improvement in health, as evidenced by increase in weight, is often misleading. Sexual feelings are more or less changed in about one-half of

[1] Berlin. klin. Woch., No. 25, 1896.   [2] Gaz. hebdom. de Méd. et de Chir., Nov. 15, 1896.

the cases. The effect of administration of ovarian extract upon women after castration has been to modify, in many instances, the before-mentioned disturbances. In 16 cases thus treated by Jayle[1] the flushing was more or less relieved, but returned after cessation of the treatment. Crude ovarian tissue and ovarin were given by the mouth, and ovarian liquid was injected hypodermically. Ovarin was found to be most convenient, though it sometimes caused indigestion. The first effect noted in the case of highly neurotic subjects was that the insomnia from which they all suffered was relieved. Cephalalgia was generally relieved or cured, and many psychic symptoms were ameliorated, especially mental depression. In one instance marked genital hyperesthesia was notably relieved. In 4 cases uterine hemorrhages ceased under treatment. In general, nutrition was improved and the patients expressed themselves as feeling much better; but it must be admitted that the treatment should be continuous. [A careful consideration of this subject, both theoretic and from the reports, forces one to the conclusion that it is destined quickly to follow in the steps of the testicular injections urged several years ago with the object of renewing youth. The late P. T. Barnum is reputed to have said that "the people wanted to be fooled"—he fooled them and grew rich. There seems to be a considerable element of this kind in the medical profession.]

Atrophy of the Uterus following Castration.—Gottschalk[2] concludes that the atrophic changes seen in the uterus after the normal or artificial climacteric are due neither to the diminished blood-supply, nor to nerve-degeneration, as shown by experiments in animals. So long as healthy ovarian tissue is preserved the spermatic vessels on both sides may be ligated without causing atrophy of the uterus; in other words, while ovulation persists this change is absent. The normal size and consistence of the organ are due to periodic vasomotor paralysis. When ovulation ceases, normally or artificially, this periodic increase in the blood-supply does not occur, the vessels lose their tone, and general atrophy results. Gottschalk further states that after removal of the adnexa for disease due to gonorrheal infection the endometrium in the specimens examined by him, as well as the mucosa lining the stumps of the tubes, showed no evidence of such disease. Even when a profuse uterine discharge persisted after castration it contained no specific microorganisms.

Amenorrhea and Chlorosis.—L. G. Baldwin[3] reports a case of amenorrhea due to complete occlusion of the os uteri following labor in a multipara of 33 years. There was no appreciable accumulation of blood in the uterine cavity, though the os was not dilated until 29 months after labor. Heim and Dalcbé[4] land the merit of ragwort as an emmenagogue. They say that groundsel (*Senecio vulgaris*) and ragwort (*S. Jacobœa*) have long been in popular use as emollients in England, and lately as emmenagogues. Two alkaloids, *senecin* and *seniocin*, can be obtained from the plants. The authors, in experiments with extracts, have found that they have no definite effect on the sensory nerves. A small dose of ragwort diminishes the excitability of the motor system, and a large one produces effects like curare; the action of the heart is slowed by a small dose and arrested in systole by a large one. The extract caused no symptoms of gastrointestinal irritation or utero-ovarian congestion in animals. In trying its effects on 15 patients Dalché found reaction absent in 3, and doubtful in 3 others, but the results in the remaining 9 were excellent as regards dysmenorrhea and amenorrhea not depending on

[1] Loc. cit.
[3] Med. News, Nov. 14, 1896.
[2] Arch. f. Gynäk., Bd. 53, H. 2, 1897.
[4] Soc. de Thér. Paris, June 24, 1896.

inflammation of the uterus or adnexa, but otherwise when these organs were affected. Pain was not directly modified. In the discussion Bolognesi stated that he had tried the effect of this drug in 20 cases, 14 cases being amenorrhea from various causes and 6 dysmenorrhea. He had found it a valuable emmenagogue, effective even in small doses and in cases of long standing. It brings on or regulates the catamenia, but must in some cases be repeated at the moustrual periods; it does not modify pain; but never aggravates the causal malady of the amenorrhea, whatever that may be. In large doses it did seem to cause utero-ovariau congestion. Bardet insisted that the drug caused contraction of the muscular tissue of the genital organs, instancing a woman of 38 who some hours after taking the medicine suffered from nausea and such uterine contractions as resembled labor-pains; moreover, it had in a case which he related caused abortion. Blondel agreed as to the dangers of causing abortion; he had found potassium iodid an absolutely safe and effective emmenagogue. As to the etiology of amenorrhea L. Garner[1] says that the normal menstrual flow depends upon the condition of the ovaries, uterus, and tubes; any disorder, either functional or organic, of these organs results usually in amenorrhea. One of the most common causes of this disorder is the non-ripening of the ovules. Again, the menstrual flow may cease in consequence of chronic perioöphoritis, the ovaries being enclosed in a firm mass of exudate. The increased sexuality developed by constant association of young girls with men is largely accountable for amenorrhea and dysmenorrhea, but in most cases the causes may be traced to convalescence from typhoid fever, pneumonia, one of the acute exanthemata, tuberculosis, or generally defective hematosis. Gastric catarrh, fright, great anxiety—especially when of long duration—predispose to amenorrhea. In the treatment of the condition Garner urges the use of apiolin.

The Treatment of Chlorosis with Ovarian Substance.—Spillmann and Etienne[2] state that the ovaries have the following functions: (1) ovulation; (2) through the menstrual hemorrhage organic toxin is removed from the body; (3) they are important in the general nourishment, similar to the testicles in man. If chlorosis is a disease of the ovaries, these functions must be disturbed; if the body is by any method supplied with ovarian substance, these functions must be restored. With this aim the writers have administered ovarian substance, as described by Brown-Séquard. After the first treatment the patients complained of pain in the lower abdomen, discomfort, headache, and muscular pain. Two had fever and rapid pulse. In three patients the result was good; the general health was improved, the anemia disappeared, the number of blood-corpuscles was increased, and the menses returned.

Menorrhagia and Metrorrhagia.—In treating of menorrhagia in virgins Laroyenne[3] distinguishes the majority of cases of profuse menstruation in young girls, which require no local treatment, from a minority in which the use of the curet is advisable. If after long attention to hygiene and a course of suitable tonics menorrhagia persists, interrupted by occasional amenorrhea, granular or fungous endometritis probably exists. This disease is yet more safely diagnosed when the patient has been perfectly healthy and quite free from anemia before profuse menorrhagia appeared, and equally free from evidence of diseased appendages after the local symptoms become marked. When the excessive menstruation causes debility it is right to dilate and use the curet. A single application (immediately after the scraping) of cotton-

[1] St. Louis M. and S. Jour., Mar., 1897.　　[2] Gaz. méd. de Paris, No. 35, 1896.
[3] Lyon méd., June 28, 1896.

wool soaked in equal parts of water and zinc chlorid is sufficient. Repeated cauterizations may easily cause atresia.

G. Foy[1] extols the value of digitalis in menorrhagia; he uses the infusion in half-ounce doses every 3 hours until 8 doses have been taken. He has used the drug in 8 cases with excellent results.

Dysmenorrhea.—A discussion on dysmenorrhea is reported in the *Brit. Med. Jour.*, Oct. 24, 1896. M. Cameron regards the spasmodic variety as by far the most common. For its relief rapid dilatation is preferable. C. Martin states the causes of dysmenorrhea as extrauterine and intrauterine. The treatment differs markedly in the two classes of cases, and what would relieve in the one would be worse than useless in the other. Three factors are concerned in the production of the pain of dysmenorrhea: (*a*) contraction of the muscular fibers of the uterus or Fallopian tubes; (*b*) increased spasm or blood-pressure in the tissues of the uterus or its appendages—congestion; (*c*) neuralgia of the uterus or the appendages. Nearly all cases are benefited by rest at the periods, hot vaginal douches during and between the periods, and, in inflammatory cases, tampons of glycerin and ichthyol, and saline aperients. The drugs he has found most useful are bromids, belladonna, antipyrin, and cannabis indica (in the form of suppositories); both viburnum prunifolium and viburnum opulus are excellent ovarian and uterine sedatives. In cases of dysmenorrhea due to chronic pelvic peritonitis binding down and matting together the uterus, ovaries, and tubes, he recommends conservative operations on the appendages. I. Parsons said that a great many cases occurred in anemic young women, and full doses of iron would cure the anemia, and with it the dysmenorrhea. J. D. Williams believes that the pain of so-called obstructive dysmenorrhea is probably due to irregular abnormal contractions, set up by a diseased condition of the mucous membrane at the seat of flexure. A. Routh in spasmodic dysmenorrhea first treats the constipation, the anemia, or other constitutional state, and then, if need be, examines by the rectum, and if the perimetrium be involved or the ovary enlarged, their state is attended to. As a rule, antispasmodics are very beneficial; the best of these is phenacetin (gr. x) in cachets, antipyrin, and nitroglycerin. J. Connel drew attention to the fact that in sterile married women prescription of abstinence from marital relations for a longer or shorter time, followed by free dilatation immediately before their resumption, would often prove successful in curing dysmenorrhea. He believes in the advantages of cycling, and if growing girls, especially when anemic, were systematically encouraged to practise that exercise in moderation, there would be much less spasmodic dysmenorrhea. G. R. Cadell thought that dysmenorrhea seldom occurred at puberty except in cases of infantile uterus, and that it was often due to some cold or over-exertion, easily cured if taken in time, but, if neglected, extremely intractable. In conclusion, Cameron referred to the marked increase of dysmenorrhea resulting from the too common custom of using preventives against conception. For the form of dysmenorrhea occurring at or soon after puberty J. E. Langstaff[2] injects 10 minims of a 3% mixture of Churchill's tincture of iodin and water into the uterine cavity every 4 or 5 days during the intermenstrual period. This allows about 3 treatments, beginning about 5 days after the flow has ceased and giving the last treatment about 5 days before the next period begins. In cases of dysmenorrhea complicated by pelvic inflammation or by diseases of the ovaries or tubes this treatment is of no value.

---

[1] Va. Med. Semi-monthly, Oct. 23, 1896.   [2] Brooklyn Med. Jour., May, 1897.

UTERINE ANOMALIES.

Interesting cases of **congenital defects** of the female generative organs are recorded by F. J. McCann,[1] Chavannaz,[2] J. W. Leech,[3] R. B. Hall,[4] F. Edge,[5] J. Ramage,[6] and W. L. Burrage.[7] McCann remarks that in reality a so-called malformation is a non-formation of one part involving a relative disproportion. Malformations represent stages of development that have remained permanent. Before an organ has reached the mature or fully developed state, we are enabled to distinguish two processes at work—namely, development and growth. The period of development in the uterus extends up to the time of puberty; the period of growth is much longer, probably lasting until the 20th year. He records a case of rudimentary vagina and uterus, the former measuring $1\frac{1}{2}$ in., and the uterus $1\frac{1}{4}$ in.; there was an associated hernia of the left ovary into the inguinal region. He also reports a case of entire absence of all generative organs, vagina included; the pubic hair was normally developed. He remarks that, owing to their distinct origin, ovaries may be present in the absence of the uterus and vagina. Uterine defects may be grouped as follows: 1. Cases in which no uterus is present, the vagina being a cul-de-sac. 2. Cases in which, at the blind end of the vagina, a nodule is found occupying a central position; this nodule has no canal in its interior. 3. Cases in which the nodule previously mentioned forms the lower portion of a small central body admitting the point of a probe. 4. Cases in which the probe can be passed for a distance of $\frac{1}{2}$ to $\frac{3}{4}$ in. into a body, cord-like or spindle-shaped, occupying a position corresponding to the normal uterus. The last group forms a transitional stage preliminary to what is called the *infantile uterus*, which may persist throughout adult life, and is the normal condition in the female child at full term.

As regards general development, patients exhibiting abnormalities of the genital apparatus may be divided into 3 types: masculine, feminine, and infantile. 1. *The Masculine Type.*—Here there is an approach to the characters distinctive of the male sex. A growth of hair on the upper lip, chin, and cheeks may exist; the voice is masculine; the breasts resemble those of the male sex; nevertheless, well-developed mammary glands are frequently noted. Hair around the nipples is occasionally seen. The pubic hair is continued up the linea alba to the umbilicus, thus resembling the distribution in the male. The shoulders are broad, and the pelvis corresponds to the masculine type. These characters, although possessed by certain females whose genital organs are abnormally formed, are also found when the genitalia are well formed. Many females of the masculine type (with well-formed genitals) bear children despite the popular belief to the contrary. 2. *The Feminine Type.*—Under this head are included those cases in which in appearance and general development there is no departure from that of the human female excepting the abnormality of the genital organs. 3. *The Infantile Type.*—The characters of this type resemble those of the infant, hence the name. There is frequently feeble general development, with smallness of stature. The breasts are poorly developed; the axillary hair is absent, also the hair covering the pubis; the pelvis is small. Burrage records a case of congenital absence of the uterus and vagina in which a plastic operation for artificial vagina was performed, the flaps being taken from the nymphæ and perineum.

[1] Am. Jour. Med. Sci., Oct., 1896.   [2] Jour. de Méd. de Bordeaux, No. 32, 1896.
[3] Brit. Med. Jour., Oct. 10, 1896.   [4] St. Louis M. and S. Jour., Apr., 1897.
[5] Brit. Med. Jour. Oct. 31, 1896.   [6] Lancet, Dec. 12, 1896.
[7] Am. Jour. Med. Sci., Mar., 1897.

Burrage has collected references to 360 cases of absence of the uterus reported by 239 authors from earliest times up to the present; roughly speaking, about 300 cases in the last century. In this number there were but 35 autopsies, 24 of which were on the bodies of adults, 2 on girls 10 and 12 years old respectively, the rest being on monstrosities and fetuses with absence of other organs, making prolonged life impossible. In all of the autopsies on the bodies of adults and girls there were noted in every case rudimentary tissues representing the uterus, generally one or two little knobs of tissue the size of hazelnuts or a thin band between the rectum and bladder. The ovaries were found to be present in all the cases but 6; the tubes were present in all cases except 6, though often without any canal.

The derivation of the hymen is still in dispute. It was formerly held to be formed from the lower end of the vagina, but the many cases of absence of the uterus and vagina in which a well-formed hymen exists would seem to disprove this view. So, also, the absence of smooth muscular fibers in the hymen would tend to show its anatomic dissimilarity to the vagina. Pozzi holds that the hymen is developed entirely distinct from the vagina, and is derived from the urogenital sinus. He accounts for the prolongation of the rugæ and pillars of the vagina on to its posterior aspect as a later developmental change. He thinks that complete atresia of the hymen is generally due to a terminal imperforation of the vagina. It is known that the hymen develops late in fetal life—the nineteenth week, and there seems every reason to believe that it is formed from the same embryonic structure as the vestibular vagina—namely, the urogenital sinus. Ramage reports a case of congenital absence of the ovaries with a rudimentary uterus in a woman of 23 years, who had never menstruated. The uterus measured $1\frac{1}{4}$ in. Edge's case was one of uterus bicornis septus in a woman of 34 years. Leech's patient presented a complete absence of the vagina and uterus. Hall's case was one of double uterus with congenital closure of one cervix, the uterus being distended with menstrual fluid.

UTERINE INFLAMMATION.

Significance of Pelvic Pain.—Dolèris and Pichevin[1] conclude an article on this subject with practical deductions concerning the clinical significance of various pains referred to the pelvis. In *acute metritis* the pain is deep-seated, diffuse, and radiates toward the loins, hips, and hypogastrium. It is principally intrapelvic and is accompanied by vesical and rectal tenesmus. It is most severe in *acute endometritis*, being least in the puerperal form. The pain, however, is only agonizing when the adnexa, peritoneum, or parametrium are inflamed. *Chronic metritis* is characterized by attacks of uterine colic, mostly confined to the menstrual period. In these cases traction on the cervix gives rise to lumbar pains due to stretching of the sacrouterine ligaments. The *pains in retroversion* are of several different types. If complicated by adhesions and disease of the adnexa, the pain is characteristic of these conditions. When retrouterine exudates are present the pain is less severe, except when attempts at replacement are made. It usually radiates toward the rectum, and is often accompanied by severe tenesmus, especially during defecation; this is quite pathognomonic. In simple retroversion the pain may be in the uterus, at the base of the broad ligaments, and in the neighboring organs. The posterior surface of the organ at the fundus is the seat of greatest tenderness, which is to be distinguished by palpation from that caused by pressure of a

[1] La Gynéc., No. 6, 1896.

prolapsed ovary or tube. Lumbar and inguinal pains are often present, due to traction on the sacrouterine and round ligaments. The characteristic pain in *prolapsus uteri* is lumbosacral, from traction on the sacrouterine ligaments, to which are often added painful sensations in the flanks due to dragging on the broad ligaments, and also in the epigastrium from ptosis of the abdominal viscera. Vesical tenesmus is more constant than in retroversion; but rectal tenesmus, on the contrary, is absent. *Carcinoma of the corpus uteri* is often painless until the perimetric tissues have been invaded. Attacks of uterine colic are characteristic of corporeal, as contrasted with cervical malignant disease. *Rapidly growing fibroids* are attended with more pain than are those that develop slowly. Cystic degeneration increases the pain, which is also most marked in connection with multiple growths within the muscular wall of the uterus. The pains are aggravated by the menopause and often disappear temporarily or permanently after the climacteric. Complications—disease of the adnexa, adhesions, and the like—aggravate the distressing symptoms. The painful sensations due to pressure are readily explained. *Cirrhotic ovaries* are most painful, especially when adherent. Attention has often been called to the intermenstrual pain caused by this condition. When both ovaries are diseased the pain often alternates, being on one side in one month, and on the opposite side the following month. The pain in *chronic salpingitis* is twofold, and is due, first, to traction on the nerves within the tube; and, secondly, to distention of the tubal wall, especially during menstruation. The mere presence of adhesions is not sufficient to explain the pain in these cases; the occurrence of an actual infective inflammation is necessary. Pain due to tubal disease is aggravated at the menstrual periods, but the intermenstrual pain noted in ovarian trouble is absent. The pain in *salpingo-oöphoritis* is referred to the lower abdomen and to the affected side, being deep seated and increased by direct palpation. It is usually paroxysmal and lancinating during exacerbations, dull and heavy during the interval between the acute attacks. It is often entirely out of proportion to the extent of the lesions; the amount of displacement of the affected organs rather than the size of the inflammatory mass seems to govern the severity of the pain. [This ingenious attempt to refer certain distinct pelvic pains to recognized pathologic conditions shows keen observation and analysis. Practically, there are so many exceptions to the rules laid down by the writers that they must be regarded as suggestive rather than positive. They are absolutely worthless for diagnostic purposes; in fact, they are dangerous in that they would in 90 % of cases lead astray anyone placing dependence upon them.]

The Condition of the Endometrium following Castration.—Eckardt [1] calls attention to the fact that, while the condition of atrophy of the endometrium following the menopause has been carefully studied, little attention has been paid to the similar atrophy after removal of the ovaries. The difficulty of obtaining suitable specimens from the human subject has compelled investigators to study the subject experimentally in animals. Krukenberg found that in the uteri of rabbits examined 9 or 10 months after castration there were marked atrophy and fatty degeneration of the uterus, with disappearance of the ciliated epithelium. Eckardt had the opportunity of examining a uterus removed from a woman, aged 43 years, whose ovaries had been extirpated 2 years before; transverse section through the organ showed that the endometrium was poor in cells, the ciliated being replaced by cubic epithelium with granular nuclei. In some cases the epithelial was directly continuous with the muscular layer, while in others the mucosa was

[1] Centralbl. f. Gynäk., No 30, 1896.

½ mm. in thickness. The glands were small and often cystic, rarely without external openings; a few were seen in the muscular layer. The latter was atrophied, with an increase in the connective tissue. Neither fatty degeneration nor round-cell infiltration was observed. The openings of the tubes were obliterated. The writer summarizes as follows: the endometrium of the human uterus after castration undergoes retrograde changes, as in senile atrophy, which are indicated by disappearance of the ciliated epithelium, atrophy of the interglandular cells, and destruction or cystic degeneration of the glands.

Classification and Etiology of Endometritis.—Döderlein[1] says that the hitherto general belief that inflammations of the uterus are divided into metritis and endometritis can no longer be considered correct, since it has been shown that the uterus is always diseased *in toto*. The causes of metro-endometritis are very numerous. Up to the present time they can only be separated into 2 chief groups: such inflammations as are caused by the introduction of microorganisms—therefore infectious—and those in which there is no bacteric influence. To the first group belong the septic and saprophytic, gonorrheal, tuberculous, syphilitic, and diphtheritic endometritis. That there is an endometritis that results from fungi or amebæ, the writer believes is not proved. The second group can have its origin in diseases of the tubes and ovaries, in the tumorous growths (fibroid and carcinoma), in nervous irritation and circulatory disturbances, in anomalies in the development of the ovum, or in puerperal subinvolution. From the microscopic anatomic characteristics of the various forms of endometritis nothing definite can be gained regarding their separate causes. It is, however, proved that interstitial endometritis is caused only by infection, and the glandular and hyperplastic forms through various other uterine inflammations.

Pinkuss,[2] from a very exact study of 115 cases, separates the benign changes of the uterine mucous membrane into glandular (24 cases) and interstitial hyperplasia (91 cases). These two changes, however, may be combined in the same mucous membrane. The pure glandular hyperplasia is never caused by inflammation, but through indirect irritation, due to circulatory disturbance. Such irritation is associated with nervohysteria, arises from masturbation or impotence, or is oöphorogenic in origin. Interstitial endometritis is always due to previous infection. Glandular hyperplasia of the endometrium is found in cases of true dysmenorrhea, particularly in those in which there is a mucous discharge, or in which the periods are long delayed and the menstrual hemorrhage slight. Interstitial endometritis causes purulent leukorrhea, which may be associated with hemorrhage. Atrophy of the endometrium is associated with atypical, profuse hemorrhage without leukorrhea.

Heuck,[3] from a microscopic study of portions of endometrial tissue removed by the curet from 70 women, comes to the following conclusions: (1) That except when there exist new-growths or adnexal disease a very important and frequent cause of endometritis is the presence of long-retained portions of chorion and decidua. (2) In cases of long-continued hemorrhage following abortion almost always endometritic processes are to be found, and usually the endometritis is diffuse. (3) In the greater number of cases of hemorrhage after abortion the endometritis antedates the pregnancy. (4) The determination of the presence of chorionic villi is not always possible and not always necessary to prove the etiologic relation between hemorrhage and abortion. (5) In a few cases in which there is a history of hemorrhage and abortion the microscope alone cannot determine a diagnosis. (6) Metrorrhagia is observed

[1] Centralbl. f. Gynäk., No. 45, 1896.   [2] Zeit. f. Geb. u. Gynäk., Bd. xxxiii., H. 2.
[3] Centralbl. f. Gynäk., No. 6, 1897.

both after abortion and when a small portion of chorion or decidua has been retained. (7) In a very large number of cases of hemorrhage after abortion giant cells are to be found for a long time, but they are of no particular pathologic importance.

Gottschalk and Immerwahr[1] have studied the bacteria contained in the female genital canal with special reference to their relations to endometritis. They made bacteriologic examinations in 60 cases of corporeal endometritis. In 21 cases the secretion from the uterine cavity was free from bacteria. In $\frac{2}{3}$ of these cases the secretion was sterile for many months. In 7 eases bacteria were found during the treatment; but they were not pathogenic, and only a few colonies were seen upon the plates; the greater number of these were fungoid endometritis. In 7 other cases (11 % primarily) at the first examination staphylococci were found. Two of these, they conclude, were a particular form of purulent endometritis, since the organism was the staphylococcus pyogenes albus, the pus clinically had a bad odor, and the secretion was now and then bloody—the symptoms thereby having a great similarity to those of gonorrhea. In 4 of the cases the staphylococci were found secondarily, immediately after an acute gonorrheal endometritis. In the remaining 28 cases, which were a chronic catarrhal form of disease, the microorganisms found were not pathogenic; they are known as skin-fungi, since they are found on the skin of the perineum, in the pubic hairs, and in the vulva. Their inflammatory action is explained through their chemotactic influence upon the circulation. If, therefore, diplococci, short bacilli, sarcinæ, and saccharomyces are not found as the primary cause of the inflammation, they can secondarily cause extensive inflammation of the mucosa. Contrary to the investigations of others, the writers found that the bacteria disappeared during menstruation. They, however, explain that this was probably the result of the washing and disinfectant vaginal douching which is their routine treatment during the menstrual period. In 2 cases of endometritis exfoliativa, and in 2 of endometritis hæmorrhagica, occurring as a result of influenza, a bacteriologic examination gave negative results.

Virginal Endometritis.—This condition is discussed by P. F. Mundé[2] and E. A. Benn.[3] Mundé claims that this form of chronic endometritis is undoubtedly of frequent occurrence. As a result of this condition the lips of the external os become so widely separated by the growth of the endocervical mucosa as to present a condition almost identical with that found after well-marked puerperal laceration of the cervix. He suggests that this might be the true etiology of the so-called congenital laceration of the cervix of Leopold, Ahlfehl, Fischel, and Penrose. In some of these cases there is present a profuse, thick, yellow leukorrheal discharge, associated with marked menorrhagia. The curet in these cases may remove an abundant quantity of adenoid vegetations, which would account for the profuse hemorrhages. The treatment consists in excising the hypertrophic cervical mucosa, curetting the whole of the endometrium with the blunt, and the cervical canal with the sharp instrument, and, if the eversion is thought sufficient, of paring the lips and uniting them with silver sutures, precisely as is done for puerperal laceration. After-treatment by intrauterine alteratives may be necessary to effect a permanent euro, as would be the case in ordinary endometritis. According to Latour,[4] endometritis fungosa may sometimes be found in virgins. The clinical symptoms do not differ from those seen during the sexual life of women—fungoid growth

[1] Arch. f. Gynäk., Bd. 50, II. 3, 1896.   [2] Chicago Med. Rec., Sept., 1896.
[3] Physician and Surgeon, Mar., 1897.
[4] Rev. Internat. de Méd. et Chir. prat., No. 18, 1896.

of the endometrium and profuse menstrual hemorrhage. The first character-istic symptoms appear with the first menstruation. Infection with microorgan-isms, masturbation, and traumatisms are, he believes, etiologic factors. The treatment should be ergot, hydrastis canadensis, and hot-water douching. Ordinarily no operation is required, but one should not wait too long before resorting to dilatation, curettement, and the application of zinc chlorid. [The tendency to interfere in virgins is already too great, and the utmost caution should be practised in selecting cases, all doubtful cases being considered non-operative.]

Senile Endometritis.—In speaking of postclimacteric endometritis Mundé[1] remarks that he has for many years noticed that women who have passed the change of life were subject to a certain extent to a disagreeable mucoserous, pungent discharge. which in course of time brought about an erosion of the lips of the cervix and of the vaginal vault, and a chronic vulvo-vaginitis. His explanation of these cases was that, the pelvic organs having undergone a gradual atrophy after the menopause, the nutrition of the various tissues was insufficient, and in consequence there was a breaking-down of the cell-elements in the uterine mucosa and in the vagina, and a serous discharge was the result. He found that not only women who had passed the natural menopause, but also those in whom that condition had been artificially bought on by the removal of the uterine appendages, were subject to senile endome-tritis. In some of these cases the discharge may become bloody, brown or blackish, and yet careful curettage and microscopic examination fail to show any signs of malignancy. The treatment consists in the use of the curet, caus-tics, chiefly nitric acid, followed by a solution of silver nitrate and drainage; and, finally, when the erosion has healed, a contraction of the secreting surface by the frequent application of iodoform and tannin powder. G. E. Herman[2] remarks that the pain in this disease may be so severe as to keep the patient awake at night; there is also sometimes noted wasting. There is little or no tendency to spontaneous cure. If the usual treatment fails, hysterectomy should be performed. [Before such advice is acted upon the opinion of one or more experts should be received in each individual case.] S. E. Shelden[3] remarks that the skin in many cases is dry, harsh, and shrivelled, with the peculiar sallow appearance that indicates malignant trouble. The physical signs as shown by inspection are usually more or less vaginitis and redness of the cervix without much erosion or ulceration; the absence of the epithelium, Nabothian glands, and follicles gives the mucosa a smooth, glistening appear-ance more like fibrous or cicatricial tissue.

Endometritis Decidua Polyposa et Tuberosa.—Bulius[4] reports the case of a primipara, aged 21 years, who gave birth to a dead child in Feb., 1895, and suffered for 6 weeks after with a continuous discharge of blood. The menses then were regular till September. In the beginning of December she again suffered from hemorrhage, and on the 7th experienced pains similar to those of labor, which were accompanied with the expulsion of clots and shreds. Included among these were a fragment of decidua and an ovum surrounded with reflexa. The curet removed more decidua, after which she made a good recovery. Bulius regards the case as one doubtless of hyper-plasia of the decidua vera, which was expelled as an almost quadrangular patch, 6 cm. broad and 11 cm. long.

Endometritis Chronica Malignans.—Under this name J. M. Van

[1] Rev. Internat. de Méd. et Chir. prat., No. 18, 1896.
[2] Treatment, Mar. 11, 1897.   [3] Medicine, Apr., 1897.
[4] Münch. med. Woch., p. 537, 1896.

Cott[1] describes a condition characterized by profuse proliferation of gland-structure, together with a multiplication of capillaries in the endometrium. There is a superficial proliferation merely, and the growth is limited to the tissues of the endometrium. He says that pathologie conditions of the endometrium must be classed under 2 general heads: 1, correlation; 2, coalescence. The former concerns those changes that occur in the form and relation to each other of the component elements of the endometrium. The latter those changes whereby the part has failed of complete development during intrauterine gestation, being fused together or with other tissues. The lesion under consideration is one of correlation. Correlation is a term that embraces two principal conditions in pathology: 1, development in excess—hyperplasia; 2, regressive changes—atrophy. These two conditions are often associated in such a manner that one portion of a complex tissue may be the seat of progressive changes that occur either at the expense of other portions of the same tissue, thus producing atrophy of its elements, or synchronously with primary atrophy. Hyperplastic changes in the endometrium frequently originate as a result of primary inflammatory changes, and it is probable that what may have originated as a simple inflammation may assume all the form of malignancy, and eventually destroy even life itself. True hyperplasiæ endometria, which have lost the characteristics of inflammation, result in multiplication of the gland-elements, or the stroma, or both together, in which latter case the lesion is either a total diffuse hyperplasia, or circumscribed diffuse hyperplasia—polypus. When the glands alone are the seat of the hyperplastic process the stroma often almost totally disappears, giving to the mass an appearance which microscopically resembles closely those new-formations which must be regarded as true neoplasms. The diagnosis between the malignant and non-malignant condition is difficult, and Van Cott regards it the lesser of two evils to remove a uterus in which simple hyperplasia glandularum existed than to leave unoperated upon a uterus in which are the elements of malignancy. There seems to be general agreement that originally harmless glandular hyperplasiæ may retrograde into more lawless growths,—*i. e.*, adenomata. The malignant endometritis has continuous growth and is never metastatic; therefore, it is positively susceptible of radical cure as long as it remains within the confines of the corpus uteri. The uterus is regularly enlarged, somewhat globular, and a trifle soft in consistence.

Treatment of Endometritis.—[The treatment of chronic inflammations of the uterine cavity may be said to include 3 methods of procedure, namely, douching by the vagina and the uterine cavity, topical applications to the endometrium, and curettage and uterine drainage.] As regards hot vaginal douching A. E. Giles[2] remarks that it should be regarded as a temporary measure merely, in order to avoid chronic pelvic congestion which will follow a long continuation of hot douching; as the symptoms improve it should be replaced by tepid, cool, and even cold irrigations. The fluids to be used for vaginal douching fall into 3 categories: 1. *Neutral* or *aseptic solutions:* of these, the first is plain or sterilized water. 2. *Mild antiseptic solutions:* among these we may mention boracic acid or borax, zinc sulphocarbolate, carbolic acid, tincture of iodin, Condy's fluid, kreosol, lysol, mercuric chlorid or biniodid, or chinosol. 3. *Powerful antiseptics:* these are required after operations, in obstetric practice, under septic conditions, and in the treatment of gonorrhea and septic conditions of the vagina and uterus. The most important are: carbolic acid, iodin liniment, mercuric chlorid, and chinosol.

[1] Brooklyn Med. Jour., Sept., 1896. [2] Lancet, May 15, 1897.

In giving hot water vaginal injections J. H. Burtenshaw[1] suggests the following rules: 1. Use a large-sized fountain-syringe, preferably one holding 4 quarts, attached to a support 3 or 4 feet above the body. 2. The patient should always lie upon the back with the hips slightly elevated and the shoulders depressed. 3. Use at least 3 gallons of water as hot as can be borne—at a temperature of 110° F. 4. Give the injection twice daily, morning and evening, except on the 2 days preceding and the 2 days following the menstrual flow.

Breslauer[2] has made a study of the antibacterial action of ointments with particular reference to the value of their constituents as disinfectants. He refers to the work of the Neisser school upon this subject, and the fact, determined by Koch, that carbolic acid in oil is worthless. He says that carbolized oil is now rarely used in obstetrics or by practising physicians. He believes, however, that a combined ointment and disinfectant is often wished for. He concludes that a 1 : 1000 bichlorid lanolin is the most effective disinfectant ointment. Two remedies that have been attracting considerable attention in gynecology are irol and formol. *Irol* has been employed by Högler in more than 2000 cases in the form of powder, gauze, vaselin, collodion, and emulsion. It has been found especially efficacious in the treatment of ulcers and boils. *Formol* is powerfully antiseptic and non-toxic. Legen and Levy state that they have obtained excellent results from these medicaments in the treatment of blennorrhagia. The usefulness of solid glycerin ovules of irol, formol, dermol, aristol, iodol, di-iodoform, ichthyol, microscidin, and thiol commends itself at once to all those whose line of work brings to them many cases of infection of the genital tract. [These form but a few of the innumerable drugs forced on the profession by drug-houses and too-willingly convinced physicians. They are one and all useless for practical work.]

In old inflammatory processes of the genitalia Grammaticatis[3] injects daily into the uterus by means of a Braun syringe a gram of the following liquid: alumnol, 2.5 gm.; tincture of iodin and alcohol, each 25 gm. Each case requires about 40 injections, which should be continued, although the first few injections are followed by a serosanguinous discharge from the uterus. The author has made over 3000 injections without an accident of any kind. The injections, he claims, are indicated in all acute or chronic inflammations of the uterus, adnexa, or pelvic peritoneum. They give the best result in acute cases. The temperature falls, the pain disappears, and resorption takes place rapidly. In cases of pyosalpinx the injections modify the condition of the adnexa so that an operation is performed much more easily and there is no danger of a recurrence. The injections cure completely chronic perimetritis, and the secondary complications, such as retroflexion, are relieved more easily. They also cure the most rebellious cases of endometritis. [It is such tampering as this, especially in acute cases, that causes many subsequent operations, and in no possible manner can it render the operation easier as stated. To follow the author's advice will be to set up many an attack of acute pelvic peritonitis, if not worse.] Sordes[4] recommends the use of vapors medicated with resorcin in the treatment of endometritis. He claims excellent results from their use.

R. C. Norris[5] treats upon the indications, dangers, and technic of uterine

[1] N. Y. Polyclinic, Sept. 15, 1896.
[2] Zeit. f. Hygiene u. Infections-Krankheiten, Bd. 20, H. 2, 1896.
[3] Wratch, Nos. 29 and 30, 1896.   [4] Bull. de l'Acad. de Méd., Nov. 24, 1896.
[5] Univ. Med. Mag., Nov., 1896.

curettage. The indications he groups as follows : A. Curettage of the puerperal uterus : (*a*) incomplete abortion ; (*b*) puerperal sepsis after labor at term ; (*c*) subinvolution. B. Curettage of the uterus uninfluenced by or remote from the puerperal period : (1) Uterine hemorrhages : (*a*) polypoid or fungous endometritis, (*b*) uterine fibromyomata, (*c*) malignant diseases (diagnostic and therapeutic uses) ; (2) uterine discharges (purulent or mucopurulent) : (*a*) acute septic or gonorrheal endometritis, (*b*) chronic septic or gonorrheal endometritis, with or without tubal and ovarian inflammation ; (3) dysmenorrhea and sterility. He states that the curet accomplishes the best results in puerperal sepsis only when it is used early and thoroughly. Clean obstetrics will almost banish the curet from the obstetric bag and from the lying-in hospital. In subinvolution the results of curettage are always brilliant if, when required, mechanical or surgical measures are utilized to correct displacement and to give support to the uterus. The usefulness of the curet decreases in direct proportion to delay. In exfoliative or membranous dysmenorrhea the curet affords the only method of treatment of value [and even it fails, as a rule]. A. Donald [1] insists upon the employment of the flushing curet, a modification of which he has devised.

J. W. Bovée [2] believes that curettage is often a valuable alternative for abdominal section. If pus be present in the adnexa or other surrounding parts, it would be dangerous to curet and leave the pus. If adhesions exist between the uterus and adjacent structures, or if large intrauterine or submucous fibroids be present, curettage is hazardous, on account of the danger of subsequent sepsis. J. D. Emmet [3] remarks that this operation is universally recognized as the best and most efficient agent at our command for the cure of the acute onset of every form of sepsis, for retained placental and other postpartum remains, and for the relief of inoperable carcinoma. As regards packing and draining the uterus after curettage, he believes the two procedures are practically contradictory. If the uterus be properly packed, it cannot properly drain. [The author is evidently at fault : the uterus packed with gauze will most assuredly be drained by capillary action ; in addition, the pressure of the packing will in great part eliminate the throwing out of the serum to be drained.] Only in those conditions that are the immediate effects of the puerperium, in septicemia from traumatism, or in conditions of specific inflammation by continuity, as in gonorrhea, is drainage indicated. He would also drain in simple uncomplicated endometritis. In all other cases in which he curets he does so in order to change the character of the endometrium and to enable its glandular structure to recover its normal anatomic and functional condition ; secondly, in order to effect a local bloodletting for its immediate effect upon the periuterine circulation ; thirdly, he packs the uterus (after thoroughly removing all débris and applying a powerful styptic), in order to produce a counterirritant effect upon the endometrium itself and upon the pelvic circulation outside the uterus. For drainage to be effectual, according to J. H. Richmiller,[4] it must afford a ready exit for the secreted material, and so prevent reabsorption. He recognizes the fallacy of packing the uterine cavity in aseptic cases that have no functional disturbances. Experience has demonstrated that *the average temperature after curettage is lower without than with gauze-packing.* [This statement is somewhat puzzling, as after curettage and packing, *properly* performed, there is practically no temperature other than the normal in the vast majority of cases.] In tamponing, the uterus is stimulated to contraction, tending to expel the gauze through the cervical canal,

[1] Brit. Med. Jour., Nov. 21, 1896.   [2] Va. Med. Semi-monthly, Dec. 11, 1896.
[3] Am. Gyn. and Obst. Jour., May, 1897.   [4] Ibid., Oct., 1896.

and by so doing it presses the gauze over the internal os, forming a plug, which dams back the secretions. The wedge of gauze is always covered with a thick, tenacious mucus, tinged with blood, which resembles uterine catarrhal secretion. This mucus is the result of uterine irritation and inflammation, kindled by the presence of a foreign body. The meshes of the gauze become occluded, and drainage cannot take place; the retained secretions are forced back into the Fallopian tubes, lymphatic sinuses, and blood-vessels, and as a result salpingitis or pyosalpinx develops. *More cases of pyosalpinx are produced from the injudicious use of uterine gauze-tamponade than from the use of the curet.* [These statements *in toto* are absolutely unsupported by facts.] Firm uterine tamponade, on the contrary, is indicated in sterility depending upon flexion of the uterus, in uterine hemorrhage when the muscular walls are flabby and inert, and in some cases with sluggish circulation of the pelvic viscera. The absorption of parametritic exudation is favored by thorough tamponade; likewise phlegmatic nodulations in the broad ligaments, and boggy congestions immediately involving the surrounding structures of the uterus. Capillary drainage, according to R. R. Kime,[1] may be secured by gauze or wicking tubes, or by the use of soft-rubber, hard-rubber, or aluminum drainage-tubes. The strip of gauze drains for a few hours only; the uterine drainage-tube is more efficient. H. Rothstein[2] says that the best time to introduce the tube is about 4 days after the termination of menstruation. The nearer to the termination of a catamenial period the better, as it permits of letting the tube remain longer in the cervix, and consequently favors obtaining a better result. The tube should not remain *in situ* for a longer period of time than 10 days. It may then be removed and reintroduced within a day or two.

UTERINE DISPLACEMENTS.

Anteflexion of the Uterus.—B. Gordon[3] has devised a stem-pessary made of brass gold-plated. It can be sterilized by boiling and can remain in the uterine canal for a long period without becoming corroded. Since there has been no operation yet invented for anteflexions nor for anteverted retroflexion of the uterus, and since many patients absolutely refuse operative intervention, Gordon claims that this instrument is an invaluable addition to the gynecologic armamentarium. [How can an instrument which attempts to correct perfectly normal conditions be of value to gynecology or any other branch of medicine?]

Uterine Prolapse.—Winter,[4] in speaking of the pathology of uterine prolapse, describes 2 forms. One is the result of a relaxation of the peritoneum and ligaments, with retroversion and descent of the uterus (through the latter an inversion of the vaginal walls results); in the other form the prolapse begins with a relaxation and descent of the vaginal walls. In the treatment of the first form, vagino- or ventrofixation is to be considered, while in the second form the various plastic operations of the perineum and vagina are indicated. [Ventrofixation is never of itself to be considered—it must always be accompanied by thorough plastic work in the vagina.]

T. A. Helme[5] reports a case of so-called prolapsus uteri (cervical hypertrophy) in a virgin of 21 years. The treatment adopted was carried out with a twofold object: 1. Removal of the hypertrophic tissues—to reduce the uterus to its normal lenghth; 2. Cutting off of the blood-supply to the cervix to prevent a

[1] South. Med. Rec., Feb., 1897.   [2] St. Louis M. and S. Jour., Apr., 1897.
[3] Am. Medico-Surg. Bull., Aug. 22, 1896.   [4] Univ. Med. Mag., Apr., 1897.
[5] Brit. Med. Jour., Dec. 26, 1896.

recurrence of overgrowth—that is, dissection of the broad ligaments and ligation of the uterine arteries, simple amputation of the cervix being deemed not sufficient.

G. H. Noble[1] reports a case of hypertrophic elongation of the cervix uteri, with complete eversion of the vagina, resulting from a fibroid tumor of the cervix, occurring in a multipara (Fig. 37). A supravaginal amputation of the neck was performed and the everted vagina replaced, the supports being equal to the task of sustaining the parts.

Jacobs[2] recommends the following operation, which he calls "collopexie

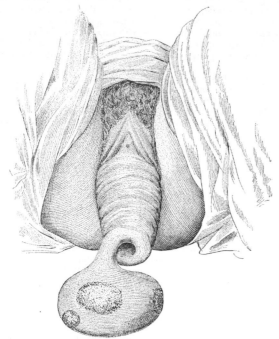

FIG. 37.—Case of cervical hypertrophy and eversion of the vagina, showing tumor and everted vagina before operation (South. Med. Rec., Feb., 1897).

ligamentaire," for prolapse in women of 40 to 50 years, who have been too frequently confined. After disinfection of the vagina and curettage of the cervix the vagina is plugged, and he performs a partial abdominal hysterectomy by amputating the uterus a little above the internal os, not circularly, but by an anterior and posterior flap, leaving enough peritoneum to cover the stump. After applying zinc chlorid to the collum, the flaps are united by a continuous suture and the peritoneum by another. The upper part of the stump is then secured on either side to the upper part of the broad ligament by several sutures, so as to draw the collum well up in the pelvis. In the single instance in which he operated in this way the uterus was sound;

[1] South. Med. Rec., Feb., 1897.　　　　　[2] Centralbl. f. Gynäk., p. 415, 1896.

but if desirable the collum might be amputated before the celiotomy, or after total abdominal hysterectomy the broad ligament might be fastened directly to the vagina. [The operation is almost identical with that devised by Baldy and demonstrated on many patients.]

Prolapse of the Uterus in Young Girls.—Stepkowski[1] reports the case of a woman, aged 25 years, who suffered from complete prolapsus uteri et vagina brought about by vomiting of 12 years' standing. Karczewski[2] cites the case of a girl, aged 13 years, who had complete procidentia of gradual development, due to carrying heavy burdens. Five days before entering the hospital the rectum also prolapsed.

Retrodisplacement of the Uterus.—H. Robb[3] makes mention of the following factors as being concerned in the causation of retrodeviations of the uterus: 1. Congenital defects. A short vagina necessitates a forward position of the cervix; this tends to bring the fundus and anterior surface of the uterus under the direct line of abdominal pressure. The ordinary distention of the bladder, which, as a rule, slightly elevates the fundus, now throws it backward, thus causing a displacement. 2. If extreme distention of the bladder happens often, the malposition is liable to continue. 3. Impacted feces in the rectum change an anteversion into a retroversion. 4. A sudden severe strain put upon the abdominal muscles brings about a retroflexion. 5. Of all causes of retropositions, by far the most frequent is a relaxation of the vaginal outlet. 6. Finally, inflammatory changes in the uterine supports may also cause retrodeviations.

Gottschalk[4] reports several cases to support his assertion that amputation of the uterine neck is resorted to too frequently, since the operation not only often fails to meet the indications, but is even productive of harm by establishing a true pathologic condition. In the 5 cases reported retroflexion afterward developed, the uterus being previously in a normal position. He attributes this condition to the fact that with the removal of the portio the relations between the cervix and corpus uteri are changed, and at the same time cicatrices are formed anterior to the stump, which tend to draw it forward and thus to throw the fundus backward. Unfortunately, these cases cannot be treated by pessaries, and the cicatricial contraction often gives rise to so much disturbance that subsequent ventrofixation becomes necessary.

Treatment of Uterine Retrodisplacements.—[The treatment of this form of displacement is, as it ever has been, the *bête noire* of the gynecologist. During the year there has been made, by its admirers, a very strong attempt to revive the flagging interest in the Alexander operation, while the methods of anterior fixation have commanded considerable space in the various periodicals. The dangers of vaginofixation are more generally appreciated and the operation is practically obsolete, while the limits of ventrofixation have been considerably restricted.] H. A. Kelly,[5] in a comprehensive paper, states that the correct method of dealing with any given case of retrodisplacement will fall under one of the following heads: 1. Cases in which no treatment is required. 2. The use of a pessary. 3. Manual reposition and massage. 4. Operation upon the vaginal outlet. 5. Operation on the uterus at the vaginal vault. 6. Shortening the round ligaments. 7. A suspensory abdominal operation, or ventrofixation. 8. An operation upon the vaginal outlet and a suspensory operation combined.

[1] Gaz. lek in Przegl. Chir.; La Gynéc., No. 1, 1897. [2] Ibid.
[3] Cleveland Med. Gaz., xi, No. 9. [4] Deutsch. med. Woch., No. 18, 1896.
[5] Am. Jour. Med. Sci., Dec., 1896.

No treatment is required when the discovery of the flexion is the accident of an examination and there are no symptoms.

He insists that retroversions and retroflexions are but rarely cured by the use of the *pessary*, and this in spite of the numerous statements to the contrary. In speaking of the mode of action of pessaries J. C. Webster[1] says that the Hodge pessary acts in two ways: (a) It helps to keep up the uterus as a whole, thus tending toward the relief of the congestion of the organ. (b) The upper end of the pessary affords a support over which the posterior vaginal wall pulls on the cervix in an upward and backward direction, the body of the uterus consequently tending to be kept forward. Ring pessaries act merely as a means of support. They lie between the pubic and sacral ligaments, stretching the vagina somewhat transversely. They tend to prevent the vagina and uterus from becoming prolapsed. Ball pessaries act merely by distending the vagina. Vagino-abdominal pessaries keep up prolapsing parts by means of the suspension from an abdominal band. *Manual reposition and massage* may be of service when there is no lateral disease of the pelvis, and when the uterus is movable and the vaginal outlet is not broken down. According to G. T. Harrison,[2] the technic of pelvic massage is as follows: the patient being on her back, 1 or 2 fingers are introduced into the vagina, the cervix is pressed backward, while the other hand above the promontory, executing rotary movements, endeavors to attain between the promontory and fundus to the posterior uterine wall. At the same time the effort is made to enlarge the distance between the uterine fundus and posterior pelvic wall; these efforts should not provoke pain. This maneuver may be practised daily, the object being to relax the adhesions and to lift the fundus and bring it forward. [If adhesions really exist, pelvic massage is utterly useless and harmful.]

Operative Treatment of Retroflexion.—Kuestner,[3] after an exhaustive review of the statistics of various operators, using all the different methods of treatment, arrives at the following conclusions: 1. Although none of the operations for the cure of retroversion restore the uterus and adnexa to an absolutely normal position, the new relation of the pelvic organs is preferable to former displacement. 2. A sharp distinction must be drawn between cases of movable and adherent retroversion. The adhesions must first be separated, after which the treatment in both cases is the same. 3. The abdominal cavity should not be opened for the purpose of separating adhesions unless these are too fine to permit detachment of the uterus by massage or Schultze's method. 4. Celiotomy is preferable to anterior or posterior kolpotomy, since adhesions may be more thoroughly and safely separated by the abdominal route, and, moreover, conservative operations on the adnexa can be carried out more satisfactorily. 5. The test of the value of any given method of fixing the uterus anteriorly is that it should keep the organ in a normal position, and that its functions should not be interfered with. 6. The results obtained by retrofixation and vaginofixation and by Alexander's operation prove that the uterus may be maintained in a good position, but it has been shown that after vaginofixation the functions of the organ are disturbed. 7. The latter operation should, therefore, not be performed in the ease of women who are likely to conceive subsequently; in those who are not liable vaginofixation has given excellent results, especially when supplemented by kolporrhaphy. 8. When the adhesions are extensive the best operation is celiotomy with ventrofixation. Conservatism should be practised as far as possible, especially in young sub-

---

[1] Am. Medico-Surg. Bull., Oct. 10, 1896.   [2] Va. Med. Semi-monthly, Nov. 29, 1896.
[3] Wien. klin. Woch., No. 15, 1896.

jects, in whom a portion of ovarian tissue should be left. If the tubes and ovaries are not seriously affected, it is sufficient merely to separate adhesions. 9. Alexander's operation is preferable in cases of movable retroversion, since it restores the uterus as nearly as possible to a normal position. 10. The indications for the operative treatment of retrodisplacement are furnished by the duration of the trouble, the negative results from the use of pessaries, and the aversion of the patient to palliative measures. A condition of the vagina which prevents the use of pessaries furnishes a positive indication. 11. Since prolapse is generally the result of retroversion, the maintenance of the uterus in a normal position is the essential object to be aimed at. This is best attained by ventrofixation, supplemented by a plastic operation on the vagina. [With the exception of proposition 3 the preceding summary is sound.]

Vaginal Operations.—(*a*) *Kolpotomy, Anterior and Posterior.*—J. Phillips[1] gives the credit of bringing this operation into notice to Dührssen. He has done the operation 4 times successfully. He claims that when practicable this operation appears to have some marked advantages over the abdominal method. These are: (1) Avoidance of the risk of subsequent adhesions of the cicatrix to the omentum or intestines, which so frequently lead to intestinal obstruction; (2) The absence of ventral hernia; (3) There is no post-operative sickness, and the convalescence is much more rapid. The operation is quite unsuitable for large pelvic tumors. It must be remembered that the peritoneum is opened, and hence every precaution should be taken as in the abdominal operation. W. J. Gow[2] says that anterior kolpotomy is performed with one of three objects in view: (1) As a means of exploring the condition of the ovaries and tubes in certain cases when their condition is doubtful; (2) For the purpose of removing the uterine appendages on one or both sides, provided that the diseased appendages are not greatly enlarged or very firmly adherent; (3) For the purpose of overcoming retroversion and retroflexion by means of vaginal fixation. The incision, which may be either transverse or longitudinal, gives great scope for the exploration of the pelvic organs. Steffeck[3] says that anterior kolpotomy is indicated: 1. In small ovarian tumors that lie in the anterior portion of the pelvis; 2. In small interstitial and subserous myomata requiring operation; 3. In diseases of the tubes without suppuration. It is contraindicated: 1. In all diseases of the posterior pelvis; 2. In all adherent ovarian and tubal tumors; 3. In adhesive posterior perimetritis. Posterior kolpotomy is indicated: 1. In small ovarian tumors lying behind the uterus; 2. In adherent ovaries when they lie close to the vaginal vault; 3. In tubal tumors adherent to the vagina, when incision and drainage without extirpation can be accomplished; 4· In adhesive posterior perimetritis. It is contraindicated: 1. In all diseases of the anterior pelvis; 2. In ovarian and tubal diseases in which the organs do not lie close to the vagina.

(*b*) *Vaginofixation.*—A. Dührssen[4] thinks that dystocia following vaginofixation is due to faulty technic, and can be avoided. The fundus of the uterus should be attached to the peritoneum only, and not to the vagina. F. H. Wiggin[5] believes that in all cases thought to require this operation the vesicouterine fold of the peritoneum should be divided, and the exact condition of the adnexa determined by aid of sight as well as by touch. This addition to the original technic does not in any way increase the slight risk of the operation.

(*c*) *Fixation of the Shortened Round Ligaments upon the Anterior Abdom-*

---

[1] Tr. London Obst. Soc., June 3, 1896.   [2] Lancet, July 4, 1896.
[3] Berlin. klin. Woch., Nov. 2, 1896.   [4] Centralbl. f. Gynäk., No. 22, S. 584, 1896.
[5] N. Y. Med. Jour., Aug. 8, 1896.

inal Wall per Vaginam.—The reported cases of dystocia following vaginofixation have resulted in various modifications of the technic. Wertheim and Mandl[1] combine the two procedures for vaginal fixation of the retroverted and prolapsed uterus recently recommended, their method being as follows: a free opening is made in the vesicouterine pouch and the uterus is drawn well downward into the vagina with a volsella, aided by external manipulation. Backward traction on the cervix then enables the operator to see nearly all the posterior surface of the organ, including the tense sacrouterine folds. The intestines are held upward by a gauze compress, posterior adhesions are separated, and the sacrouterine ligaments are drawn backward with forceps until the "slack" is taken up and the fundus is kept well forward; the points at which the ligaments are seized are then united with silk or silkworm-gut to their uterine origins, the amount of shortening varying from $2\frac{1}{2}$ to 3 in. The gauze is removed and the uterus replaced; the round ligaments are exposed by inserting a retractor in the opening, and are drawn down and shortened in the manner already described by the authors. The danger of complications during pregnancy and parturition, noted after Mackenrodt's operation, is not present, since the portio is not directed backward, nor is ascent of the fundus in the pregnant uterus prevented. Vesical and rectal disturbances have not been noted in the cases (3) successfully operated upon by the authors. E. Bode[2] has done this operation 3 times and recommends it. F. Kiefer[3] stitched together a fold of the round ligament through the vaginal incision very much as Mann does through the abdominal incision. Guenther[4] put a silk suture in each round ligament near the uterus and pierced the abdominal wall over each tuberculum ossis pubis with the needles, and thus brought out the threads, pulled the uterus forward by them, and tied them on the skin. H. T. Byford[5] passes two chromicized catgut threads about 1 in. apart through that portion of the peritoneum which lies behind the tubes and attaches the fundus of the uterus to the bladder; the round ligaments are then drawn down until the inguinal ends become taut, when catgut sutures are passed through them as far from the uterine end as possible and secured to the uterus just above the normal uterine insertion. Kocks[6] doubles each broad ligament over the front of the uterus, and then sutures the edge of the one on the left side to that on the right side. Godinho[7] opens the vesicouterine pouch by a transverse incision, after detaching the bladder from the cervix; two fingers are introduced, adhesions are separated, and the uterus is replaced bimanually. A silk suture is then passed through one of the round ligaments near its base, is tied, and is then passed through the same ligament 3 in. below the former point. The same procedure is carried out on the opposite side. The sutures are then tied, thus shortening the ligaments, and with the same needles the resulting loop is sewed together on either side. The wound is then closed.

(d) **Vesicofixation.**—A. Dührssen[8] performs anterior fixation as follows: he opens the anterior vaginal fornix by a transverse incision, dissecting up the tissues until the peritoneum comes into view, then seizing it with artery-clamps and dissecting off the peritoneum from the posterior surface of the bladder. The peritoneum is opened by a sagittal incision, and the upper angles of the peritoneal flap are held by clamps. The uterus is then anteflexed and fastened to the peritoneum of the bladder by 2 catgut sutures. The upper suture passes through the vesical peritoneum $\frac{1}{2}$ cm. above the end of the incision and

[1] Centralbl. f. Gynäk., No. 18, 1896.   [2] Ibid., No. 13, Mar. 7, 1896.
[3] Ibid., Apr. 11, 1896.   [4] Ibid., Feb. 22, 1896.
[5] Med. News, Oct. 31, 1896.   [6] Centralbl. f. Gynäk., Aug. 8, 1896.
[7] La Gynéc., No. 6, 1896.   [8] Centralbl. f. Gynäk., No. 22, 1896.

through the fundus at the level of the insertion of the tubes. The peritoneum is then sewed by a continuous catgut suture and the vaginal incision closed.

Alexander's Operation.—M. C. McGannon[1] reports 91 cases without a death, and 4 subsequent pregnancies with 3 normal deliveries. Kelly[2] states that the disadvantages of the operation are that the ligaments are sometimes found with great difficulty or not at all, and that relapses are not infrequent. To these A. H. Goelet[3] adds the time the operation requires; the doubt about finding the ligaments sufficiently strong in their long overstretched and atrophied condition to bear the strain thrown upon them; the prolonged convalescence necessary before the shortened ligaments can be regarded sufficiently strong to support the uterus; the risk of hernia; and the cicatrices that may become the seat of keloid. Of the 37 patients on whom S. Stocker[4] has performed Alexander's operation, 16 were either single women, widows, or women who had passed the childbearing age. Of the remaining 21, 10—3 of them for the 2d time—have become pregnant. One of these aborted in the 2d month, the other 9 were delivered at term; 7 of the 10 he examined and found the uterus in good position, the 8th was 5 months pregnant for the 2d time; 2 of these women had been sterile for the 2 years of their married life, but became pregnant within 6 months after the operation. From his experience he concludes that Alexander's operation causes no disturbances in the course of future labors, and gives brilliant results in favoring conception.

G. M. Edebohls[5] says that when a round ligament tears in drawing it out the retracted end should be sought for and recovered, if possible, at the internal ring. If this should prove impossible, the peritoneum should be incised at the internal ring and the ligaments sought for and brought out of the abdomen with the aid of a finger or two, assisted, if necessary, by slender forceps. When the ligament tears out of the uterus, or so near the latter as to leave a stump too short to be drawn out and properly fastened, 3 courses are open : the first is to shorten the opposite ligament and trust to one shortened ligament to keep the uterus forward. The second is to open the abdomen in the median line, unite the torn ends of the round ligament, or attach the pulled-out end to the uterus by suture, and complete the operation in the usual way. The third is to substitute immediately the next best retroversion operation. He has operated on 116 cases, with only 4 failures; 12 of the cases became pregnant, with 2 abortions, 6 normal labors, and 4 not yet delivered. Calmann[6] describes the following ingenious procedure: after drawing out the ligament as far as necessary on both sides it is kept on the stretch by an assistant while 2 sutures of fine catgut are passed through it and through the pillar of the external ring on either side. Then sutures are passed on both sides through the aponeurosis, then through either half of the ligament parallel with its long axis, and out through the aponeurosis again near the point of entrance. When tied, these unite the ligament firmly to the aponeurosis without constricting the former. Finally, the redundant portion of the ligament is excised and the distal end is sutured to the stump of the ligament. The wound in the skin is closed with a continuous catgut suture. F. H. Martin[7] performs Alexander's operation without buried sutures as follows : the ordinary incision on either side is extended until the lower ends are about an inch and a quarter apart. After exposing and drawing out the round ligaments, closed, pointed artery-forceps are passed

[1] Am. Gyn. and Obst. Jour., Aug., 1896.   [2] Am. Jour. Med. Sci., Dec., 1896.
[3] Med. Rec., Aug. 29, 1896.   [4] Centralbl. f. Gynäk., No. 21, 1896.
[5] Am. Gyn. and Obst. Jour., Dec., 1896.   [6] Centralbl. f. Gynäk., No. 4, 1897.
                          [7] Am. Gyn. and Obst. Jour., No. 4, 1896.

from the bottom of the lower end of the wound on the right side beneath the
suprapubic tissues to the corresponding point in the lower end of the wound
on the left side ; the left round ligament is grasped and drawn beneath the
skin, fat, and superficial fascia, to the lower end of the right wound.   The
pubic attachments of both round ligaments are then freed, the uterus drawn
well forward, and the 2 ligaments securely fastened by tying them together
with a double knot, as advised by Duret, of Lille.   The wounds are closed
with fine silkworm-gut sutures, allowing every other one to include a small
amount of the ligaments and the edges of the external inguinal rings.   [The
unique feature of this method of operating is the suspension of the uterus by
tying the 2 ligaments together over the symphysis.]

Suspension of the Uterus.— *Ventrofixation.*—In stating the indications for suspensio uteri A. H. Goelet[1] writes that vaginal fixation deserves
condemnation.   Alexander's operation for shortening the round ligaments is
appropriate when the retroflexed organ is freely movable and the adnexa are
not diseased.   In this condition another more simple procedure will accomplish as much in a much shorter time and with less inconvenience to the
patient.   This procedure aims at a cure of the metritis and endometritis, the
maintaining cause of the displacement in a majority of cases in which the
organ is movable.   This places shortening of the round ligaments in the category of unnecessary operations, though there may be certain cases in which it
is appropriate and even necessary.   Ventral suspension should be reserved for
those cases in which the organ is bound down by adhesions, the adnexa are
irreparably diseased and require removal, and the retroflexed organ, though
movable, is prolapsed, and for prolapsus without retroflexion.

E. F. Ross[2] suggests an improvement in the technic of ventrosuspension ;
it consists in the preliminary introduction into the vagina of a plug of absorbent salicylic wool, which pushes the fundus well up out of the pelvis and
keeps it there, so that it becomes unnecessary to use forceps for this purpose.
C. Beck[3] suggests suspending the uterus to the fascia and peritoneum by
means of the round ligaments.

FIBROID TUMOR OF THE UTERUS.

Interesting cases are reported as follows: T. S. Cullen,[4] a case of adeno-
myoma of the round ligament; he states that while adenomyomata of the
uterus are not so rare, similar tumors of the round ligaments have apparently
never been reported.   While admitting the probability of the glands in this
case being due to remains of the Wolffian body, still, from the striking resemblance to those of the uterine mucosa and from the fact that their stroma resembled that of the mucosa, he suggests the possibility that they may be due
to an abnormal embryonic deposit of a portion of Müller's duct.   Hansemann[5]
describes the case of a myoma of the round ligament in an inguinal hernia,
discovered at the necropsy of a woman, aged 66, who died of aortic aneurysm.
Rendu[6] records a case of soft myoma that closely simulated an ovarian cyst,
in a single patient of 40 years.   Depla[7] records a case of death from intrauterine infection of a myomatous uterus by the bacterium coli commune in an
unmarried woman 37 years of age.   The removed tumor was found to be
completely decomposed.   Cultures were made from the tumor, and a pure

[1] N. Carolina Med. Jour., Nov. 5, 1896.   [2] Brit. Med. Jour., Oct. 10, 1896.
[3] N. Y. Med. Jour., Jan. 16, 1897.   [4] Canad. Pract., Aug., 1896.
[5] Zeit. f. Geb. u. Gynäk., vol. xxxiv, Part 2, 1896.   [6] Lyon méd., June 14, 1896.
[7] Sem. gynéc., No. 10, 1896.

culture of the bacterium coli commune was gained. Depla believes the bacteria were introduced into the vagina through defecation; then the uterine cavity was infected, resulting finally in most extensive sloughing of the tumor. Hartmann and Mignot[1] also report a fatal case of general suppuration and necrosis of a uterine fibroid, which they attributed to infection by anaërobic microbes, appearing in the form of short bacilli, frequently joined together, which were found in large numbers on the surface of the uterine mucosa as well as in the pus within the tumor. M. Heurtaux[2] reports a case of myofibroma of the uterus with torsion of the pedicle, cured by operation. E. Van de Warker[3] records a uterine fibroid complicated with adenolymphangitis and phlebitis cured by hysterectomy. J. B. Sutton[4] records a case of large myoma of the neck of the uterus in a sterile woman of 40 years. W. C. Wood[5] records a case of multiple fibroids of the uterus associated with hydrosalpinx cured by hysterectomy.

The Microscopic Relations of the Myometrium in Pathologic Enlargements of the Uterus, with Particular Reference to the Muscle-cells.—Bertelsmann,[6] from a careful microscopic study of 22 enlarged uteri, comes to the following conclusions: hypertrophy of the muscle-cells of the uterine wall is frequently associated with interstitial fibroids. Hypertrophy of the muscle-cells always occurs with submucous fibroids, and in every instance in which the uterine cavity contains an abnormal substance (pyometra and hematometra). Hyperplastic changes, also increase of the connective tissue and muscle-cells, were found, particularly in metritis and in carcinoma and interstitial fibroids. [These results correspond with those of Ritschl and Herczel.]

The Relationship between Myoma of the Uterus and Sterility.—Hofmeier[7] is led to conclude that myoma of the uterus does not in itself cause sterility. He finds in a number of cases that sterility was present during the first 5 years after marriage before a myomatous tumor could be detected. It is only exceptionally that the direct influence of the presence of the tumor in producing sterility can be proved. He reports a number of cases in which the tumor disappeared without interference during the puerperal state.

Indications in Fibroid Tumors of the Uterus.—Kessler[8] says but a short time has elapsed since it was considered advisable to operate upon only a small percentage of the cases of fibroid tumor of the uterus, but that now, on the contrary, one goes so far as to question whether it is not advisable to operate in every instance. It was believed that fibroid tumors, unlike carcinoma and sarcoma, were always benign growths, and, therefore, they were only treated for the hemorrhage, and when this was not present it was thought best to wait for the menopause in the hope that the patient would then be cured. By degrees we have come to know these tumors better. He concludes: (1) It has been determined that the menopause does not always result in a favorable influence, but often the tumor first begins to grow after the menopause. (2) Through continued irritation circumscribed peritonitis is easily developed, and strong and very vascular adhesions are formed. (3) The hemorrhage results in an undermining of the constitution, and particularly in fatty degeneration of the heart-musele, "the fibroid-tumor heart." (4) Frequently gangrene or sloughing of the tumor occurs. (5) Now and then they become telangiectatic and cystic; also more rarely torsion occurs. (6) A fibroid tumor easily degenerates into a

[1] Ann. de Gynéc. et d'Obst., No. 6, 1896.
[2] Bull. de l'Acad. de Méd., Dec. 22, 1896.
[3] Am. Gyn. and Obst. Jour., Dec., 1896.
[4] Brit. Med. Jour., Oct. 31, 1896.
[5] N. Y. Med. Jour., Oct. 10, 1896.
[6] Arch. f. Gynäk., Bd. l., 1897.
[7] Berlin. klin. Woch., No. 43, 1896.
[8] St. Petersburg. med. Woch., No. 19, 1896.

sarcoma. (7) Finally, local compression of neighboring organs occurs. The mortality-statistics of the operation for fibroid tumors have become extrordinarily favorable, and one can now definitely speak of the degree of dager. Kessler believes that all fibroid tumors should be removed as soon as they cause symptoms, at least as soon as the symptoms have a tendency to increase, are pronounced or progressive.

Treatment of Fibroid Tumors. — (a) *Non-operative Treatmet.* — Cheron[1] speaks highly of intrauterine injections of sterilized glycerin in ases of fibromyoma. A little over a dram is slowly injected every two or hree days, the vagina being subsequently tamponed with cotton or gauze satruted with boroglycerid. The effect of the drug is to cause dryness and atropir of the endometrium, and hence diminution of the tumor. A marked decrete in the flow is observed at the following menstrual period. The writer airms that the ease and safety of this method of treatment should recommendt in cases in which operative interference is inadvisable, or is refused.

The use of thyroid extract in the treatment of uterine fibroids is trated of by Jouin.[2] Having had occasion to administer thyroid extract to a tout woman for the purpose of reducing her weight, he noticed that not onlywas the obesity diminished, but a large uterine fibroid which extended abov the umbilicus rapidly lessened in size until it attained only one-fourth (its former dimensions. He accordingly selected 17 cases of fibroids, which ere treated by the internal administration of thyroid, with the following resits : in 12 cases in which hemorrhage was a marked symptom there was a noticrble diminution in the size of the tumor, while the hemorrhage practically cered ; of 5 large tumors, in feeble subjects, 2 were decidedly affected, 2 but sligtly, and 1 not at all. Five other patients with profuse menorrhagia attribute to the climacteric, 2 with bleeding due to carcinoma, and 1 with an intrautrine polypus were treated with the same remedy. The writer concludes that hyroid extract does cause a marked reduction in the size of uterine fibnds, while the symptoms—pain, pressure, general weakness, and especially heiorrhage—are certainly relieved. Moreover, it causes a diminution of the ienorrhagia in women at the climacteric.

(b) *Surgical Treatment of Uterine Fibroids.*—[During the 43 years that hve elapsed since Burnham first successfully removed a uterine fibroid by abdminal section a very large number of operations and modifications of tese have been suggested by surgeons both in this country and abroad.] Accoring to J. Wallace,[3] surgical interference is demanded in : (a) fibrocystic growths b) sarcomata in the early stages if possible (the longer the tumor is left the grerter the risk of recurrence); (c) when the tumor permanently interferes with he action of the bowel or the bladder, with or without pain, and causes inflamation which may give rise to adhesions to superincumbent and pelvic viscera ; d) when ascites is a sequel or when there is overdistention from the size of he growth, and direct or reflex symptoms indicate danger to life (cardiac collare). Hemorrhage alone does not demand extirpation. In the experience of GE. Shoemaker,[4] patients with valvular heart-disease, if without atheroma, whstand operation well, provided there is good compensation in the heart-musle. An irregular or intermittent pulse is a far greater contraindication for opration than a heart-murmur. The use of strychnin and whiskey before the opration, careful preparation of the kidneys and skin, the avoidance of too servre preparatory purgation, the early supply of liquid nourishment by the borel after the operation (*i. e.*, beef-tea or peptonized milk by the rectum in the rst

[1] Rev. internat. de Méd. et Chir. prat., No. 6, 1896.   [2] La Gynéc., June, 1896.
[3] Brit. Med. Jour., Oct. 13, 1896.   [4] Univ. Med. Mag., Aug., 1896.

24 hours) will forestall the failure of a heart which might not otherwise stand a strain. Hysterectomy should not be considered in advanced phthisis. In he incipient stages it may be indicated to remove a drain, and thus enable nature to effect a cure. Chronic coughs not due to phthisis will often disappear marvellously after the removal of abdominal tumors. In hopeless kidney disorganization with purulent urine, large granular casts, and constitutional symptoms, no operation is advisable. It must be remembered, however, that solid abdominal tumors often predispose to kidney-disease by obstructing the ureter or interfering with bladder-drainage, and unless the kidney-lesion is too far advanced relief of pressure and lessened kidney-work may enable restoration to take place.

Methods of Operation.—(1) *Vaginal Ligation of the Uterine Arteries.* —A. H. Goelet[1] states that Martin, the originator of this method, believes that in order to have success in this operation it is very important to include the nerves as well as the blood-vessels in the ligature of the base of the broad ligament. Goelet claims that this is not enough, since permanent obliteration of the vessels is by no means certain ; he contends that in order to secure complete obliteration of the vessels they should be divided between double ligatures. He operates in this manner in suitable cases with considerable success.

(2) *Abdominal Enucleation.*—This method is the enucleation of fibroid tumors of the uterus after abdominal section. According to Témoin,[2] the operation is as follows : after opening the peritoneal cavity the uterus is drawn forward and the broad ligaments clamped and ligated. An incision is then made over the fibroid tumor, and it is enucleated with the fingers, which is very easily accomplished even in the deeper growths. A necessary portion of the uterine tissue is then excised and the wound closed by a deep, superficial, and peritoneal continuous suture. The last suture includes wounds in the broad ligaments. The uterus is then replaced, the peritoneal cavity washed out with warm water, and the abdominal wound closed. When the tumor is very large it is advisable also to include the uterine artery in the clamp. The clamp-blades should be covered with drainage-tube to prevent injury to the tissues. If there are a number of tumors, each one is enucleated, and the wounds treated with a strong carbolic-acid solution before introducing the sutures. Engström[3] strongly recommends this operation. He has performed it in 100 cases in which the tumor varied from the size of a hazelnut to that of an adult head, with but 5 deaths. He believes, with all modern observers, that although these growths may in a few instances remain stationary in the uterine wall without causing symptoms, trouble is apt to develop at any time during life. He believes that the ideal operation is the one that removes the isolated fibroids and allows the uterus, ovaries, and tubes to remain. In his series 63 times there was but 1 tumor, and 37 times multiple tumors ; from 2 to 5, and once 22 growths were enucleated. Tumors which extended into the uterine cavity, intramural, subperitoneal, intraligamentous, and one which distorted and thinned out the cervix uteri, were removed ; also those with marked development of the blood- and lymph-vessels, and those with more or less necrotic or calcareous change ; also those with intestinal and omental adhesions, and sometimes with extensive pathologic changes in the ovaries and tubes. In 3 cases small tumors have since developed. In 113 cases reported by Martin tumors have since been found in 3. This Engström believes is not a contraindication to the operation. Four patients have become pregnant since operation ; 1 aborted at 6 months during an attack of typhoid

---

[1] Med. Rec., Mar. 6, 1897. [2] Arch. provinciale de Chir., No. 7, 1896.
 [3] Monatsch. f. Geb. u. Gynäk., Bd. v., H. 4, 1896.

fever; another in the fourth month; 1 went to term and was delivered of a living and healthy child; and 1 is now in the third month of pregnancy. Of Martin's 113 cases 2 became pregnant; 1 aborted, and the other was delivered of a living child.

(3) *Vaginal Enucleation.*— *Vaginal Myomectomy.*—This method, according to E. C. Dudley,[1] has usually been reserved for the smaller tumors of a size not larger than the capacity of the small pelvis. Latterly, however, the vaginal method has been often and successfully used by certain French surgeons for the removal of much larger tumors, by the operation known as *traction and*

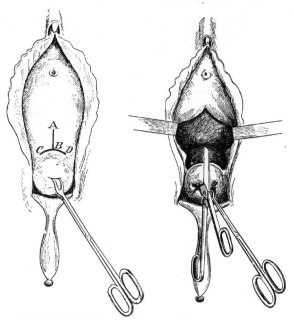

FIGS. 38 and 39.—Dudley's operation (Jour. Am. Med. Assoc., Aug. 15, 1896).

morcellement. One strong contraindication to this operation for large tumors must always be the constant possibility of pus-tubes or ovarian abscesses. The technic of the operation is as follows: the tumor is usually made more accessible and its enucleation or morcellation is facilitated either by dilatation or more frequently by deep lateral (or, what is safer, posterior) incisions of the cervix even to the internal os. These incisions having been made, the cervical lips are drawn well down to the vulva and held widely apart by means of strong double-tooth forceps in the hands of an assistant. Dudley proposes as an improvement on the other method a simple median incision through the anterior wall of the uterus after having made a circular incision in front of the uterus, which shall separate the vaginal wall from the cervix at the uterovaginal attachment in the line *C D* (Fig. 38). The anterior vaginal wall is then incised from the point at the middle of the first incision

[1] Jour. Am. Med. Assoc., Aug. 15, 1896.

for a distance of $\frac{1}{2}$ to $\frac{3}{4}$ of an inch (line *A B*, Fig. 38), care being taken not to invade the bladder and to avoid the ureter on either side. The bladder is dissected up and the anterior wall of the uterus is exposed (Fig. 39), which is then divided longitudinally in the median line by means of scissors to whatever extent may be necessary to render the tumor accessible (Fig. 39). If necessary, the peritoneum may be opened and the incision carried high up into the corpus uteri. With the finger as a guide a long-bladed knife is passed to the highest point of the tumor, and an incision is made parallel with the long axis of the uterus. The mucosa is pushed away from the incision on either side, the myoma seized and firmly held by vulsellum forceps, and traction made as described by Emmet, while the dissection is made close to the capsule. Laceration of the uterine tissue must be avoided as far as possible, because it is apt to give rise to troublesome hemorrhage. If the myoma is too large to remove entire, it is to be done by morcellement. The cervix and uterus may then be sutured.

(4) *Hysterectomy.*—(*a*) *By the Vaginal Route.*—According to F. H. Wig-

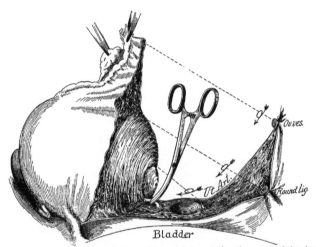

FIG. 40.—Left ovarian vessels tied; left round ligament tied; vesical peritoneum divided and pushed down; left uterine vessels ligated. Cervix amputated and uterus pulled up and out, exposing right uterine artery, which is clamped an inch above the cervical stump. The two following steps are clamping the right round ligament and right ovarian vessels, when the mass is removed (Bull. Johns Hopkins Hosp., Feb.–Mar., 1896).

gin,[1] the selection of the method, whether vaginal, abdominal, or a combination of the two, by means of which the diseased uterus shall be removed, will at the present time depend largely upon the size, benignity or malignity of the tumor, and upon the character of the adhesions that exist in a given case, as well as upon the personal experience and predilection of the individual operator. One of the objections to the operation is, according to H. T. Nelson,[2] that the plastic exudate thrown out upon the surface of the packing which is introduced into the opened vaginal vault for purposes of drainage, as well as to prevent the descent of portions of the abdominal contents, makes a mass of cicatricial tissue in which portions of the bowel are necessarily involved.

[1] N. Y. Med. Jour., Aug. 22, 1896.   [2] Am. Gyn. and Obst. Jour., Nov., 1896.

A certain amount of intestinal adhesion will take place, with the probability of becoming in the future a source of great trouble to the patient. The causes of death after vaginal hysterectomy, as stated by T. Wilson,[1] are: 1. Shock, hemorrhage, and exhaustion; 2. Septic conditions; 3. Cardiac, renal, and other organic complications. He believes that half of the cases of death ascribed to exhaustion and to ileus are due to sepsis. This is also probably a factor in the production of death in some cases ascribed to shock. Intestinal obstruction is a common sequela, immediate and remote, of vaginal hysterectomy. Cases of ileus following soon after the operation are usually due to sepsis. In many cases local signs of infection in the wound are not very marked, and in many cases an exhausted condition of the patient consequent on the length of the operation and hemorrhage is a most important factor in determining reflex paralytic distention of the intestine. Obstruction of the bowel beginning after the first few days following operation is usually due to adhesion of the intestine. Fistulæ connecting the vagina with the bladder, ureter, rectum, or intestine, are common and distressing sequelæ of vaginal hysterectomy.

(b) *By the Abdominal Route.*—Abdominal hysterectomy by amputation, as described in the *Year-Book* for 1897, has, in the hands of skilled surgeons, become the method of selection. The accompanying illustration (Fig. 40) shows far better than could any verbal description the method of procedure. The hysterectomy spud employed in the operation is also shown (Fig. 41).

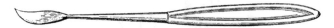

Fig. 41.—Hysterectomy spud. Used instead of a knife for amputating the uterus at the cerviX. The curved blade enables the operator to work easily in a deep pelvis cupping out the stump (Bull. Johns Hopkins Hosp., Feb.–Mar., 1896).

The reasons why the extraperitoneal method of abdominal hysterectomy was so long the only method employed, and why it was so slowly relinquished are, as shown by A. Donald,[2] not far to seek. It possesses two great advantages—the comparative simplicity and the rapidity with which in most cases it may be accomplished. L. Tait[3] still adheres to this method, stating that he now gets runs of success of 30, 40, and even as high as 52 consecutive cases, while with every kind of intraperitoneal treatment of the pedicle which he has tried the mortality has been terrible, and "he is done with it forever." [So many other operators have as good or better results with the supravaginal amputation than Lawson Tait has with the nœud method that the only conclusion to draw from his remarks is that he does not know how to do the amputation operation or his patients die from lack of antiseptic precautions— he is well known to oppose all antisepsis.] However, as Donald points out, the intraperitoneal method, when successfully carried out, does away with many drawbacks attendant upon the extraperitoneal method, as the traction on the stump or broad ligaments, the strangulated and sloughing stump, the pit-shaped wound in the abdominal wall after separation of the necrosed stump, the sinus leading to the pelvis, the adhesions of the stump to the abdominal wall, and the weakness of the abdominal cicatrix at the lower angle where the stump was fixed. It has, on the other hand, the great disadvantage of being a rather complicated operation, requiring a long time for its performance. Its weak point is also the stump.

[1] Birmingham Med. Rev., Apr., 1897.   [2] Brit. Med. Jour., Oct. 24, 1896.
[3] Ibid., Mar. 27, 1897.

Altuchoff and Sengiroff[1] describe their new method of reaching the uterine artery after abdominal section by drawing the round ligament well forward and the Fallopian tube backward, and making a broad triangular space between the two structures. An incision 3 cm. long is then made behind (above) the round ligament and parallel to it. By dissecting down from 12–16 mm. in the loose connective tissue, keeping near the anterior layer of the broad ligament, the artery is easily found and ligated. Sengiroff has ligated the uterine artery 8 times by this method, and in 7 of the cases removed complicated tumors of the uterus and adnexa bloodlessly. Once the ligation was performed for menorrhagia due to fibroids. The ligation is usually performed easily, though large tumors and other complications may greatly increase the difficulty.

Drainage of the Stump in Abdominal Hysterectomy.—Byford[2] says that in 46 cases he turned the uterine stump into the vagina through an opening made into the anterior vaginal fornix. In 18 cases he sutured the stump with chromicized catgut, shutting off the peritoneal cavity and draining through an opening made into the anterior vaginal fornix; in 1 case he did not shut off the peritoneal cavity, but drained the cul-de-sac of Douglas; and in 3 cases he removed the whole uterus and drained the stump through an opening left in the upper part of the vagina. Out of this total of 68, 3 died. It is his opinion that if he had not drained, there would have been at least twice as many deaths. [A mere matter of opinion without a particle of proof accompanying it.] His present method consists in sewing up the stump with catgut and draining through an opening made in the anterior vaginal wall just in front of the cervix.

Doyen's method of abdominal panhysterectomy for large uterine fibromyomata is thus described by F. Edge:[3] A sufficiently large median incision is made, the tumor is fixed by a wire corkscrew of large size, drawn out of the pelvis, and delivered through the incision. Large compresses are placed so as to cover the intestines and each one is held by forceps. The assistant then passes a large pair of forceps into the vagina and up into the posterior fornix; the operator then cuts down in the middle line with scissors upon the elevation in the floor of Douglas's pouch, and having made a free incision into the vagina the anterior lip of the cervix is seized with a volsella and drawn strongly upward. With scissors the mucosa is snipped round the cervix and pushed up in front bluntly with the finger, thus separating the bladder. Having freed the cervix sufficiently all around, the assistant grasps between the finger and thumb of the right hand the base of the broad ligament; starting from behind in the median line the operator cuts upward on the right side so as to leave all the broad ligament with the tubes and ovaries and a free flap of peritoneum and the capsule of the uterine mass. Practically he cuts through the whole broad ligament as near the mass to be removed as possible. The other broad ligament is held by the assistant's left hand and similarly cut through. The tumor is removed, leaving a flap of peritoneum and broad ligament on each side and behind the bladder, on which are the tubes and ovaries. This flap is large enough to easily form the new pelvic floor; the apices of the two flaps are transfixed and doubly ligated, the ovaries and tubes being removed by cutting off the parts beyond the ligatures. The open rectovaginal and vesicovaginal cellular spaces are closed by a continuous catgut suture uniting peritoneum and vaginal walls. The flaps are pulled down over the raw surfaces of the broad ligaments by the ligatures which had been left long after tying off

---

[1] Monatsch. f. Geb. u. Gynäk., Bd. iii, H. 6.   [2] Am. Jour. of Obst., Aug., 1896.
[3] Birmingham Med. Rev., Nov., 1896.

the tubes and ovaries. A continuous catgut suture is now passed, picking up peritoneum all around—*i. e.*, from both flaps and from the rectal and vesical peritoneum. This is tied and pulled into the vagina, and another similar suture, about 1½ in. higher, is passed and tied, absolutely shutting off the peritoneal cavity of the vagina. The abdomen is then closed. Doyen has performed this operation 35 times, with 1 death. A similar operation is done by Le Bec.[1]

MALIGNANT DISEASE OF THE UTERUS.

Etiology of Carcinoma Uteri.—Baccker,[2] from an analysis of 705 cases of carcinoma of the uterus, arrives at the following conclusions with reference to the etiology of the disease: 1. The true origin of malignant disease of the uterus is as yet unknown, nor can it be referred to a specific micro-organism. 2. The indirect cause is endometritis, generally of puerperal origin, which furnishes a suitable nidus for its development. This is shown by the fact that carcinoma is common in women who have borne children, while it is comparatively rare in single and in sterile women, as well as in those who have had gonorrhea. Moreover, in nearly every case of carcinoma there is a chronic catarrh of the endometrium. Endometritis is the primary condition, malignant degeneration being secondary. Hence, the practical importance of treating endometritis actively from the outset as a prophylactic measure.

G. L. Mullins[3] has made a study of carcinoma in New South Wales, and finds that of 585 females who died of cancer, 202 were affected in the uterus. The period of life at which death occurred was between 25 and 85 years, but it was not common before the 40th year. It occurred most frequently between the 45th and the 60th year. The average number of children borne by each female dying of carcinoma of the uterus is 5.07. Two single females died of the disease, and 17 who were married but had no issue. There is no information as to whether any of these women had ever had miscarriages. He concludes : (1) that although New South Wales has one of the lowest death-rates in the world from carcinoma, the disease is undoubtedly increasing in the colony ; (2) the carcinoma-age is from 35 upward ; (3) carcinoma is slightly more prevalent among males than females ; (4) climate appears to have little or no effect on the production of the disease ; (5) the stomach is the organ most affected in males ; the uterus in females ; the stomach is also largely affected in females ; (6) heredity is the chief cause of the production of carcinoma. Chronic irritation is an important factor, but its true significance is still a matter of dispute.

The Origin of Malignant from Non-malignant Uterine Neoplasms.—W. R. Williams[4] remarks that considering the great frequency of both diseases (carcinoma and fibroma) in women of a certain age, one need not be surprised to find them coexisting rather frequently in the same uterus. In 78 uterine carcinoma necropsies he found in 5 concomitant fibroids ; of 45 similar necropsies tabulated by Lebert 6 were associated with fibroids—*i. e.*, in 125 carcinoma patients fibroids coexisted in 11, or in 9%. In the immense majority of cases the two neoplasms are quite separate and independent of one another, the fibroid having sprung from the corpus and the carcinoma from the cervix or portio, so that in these cases there is no question of the latter disease having originated from the former. In the remaining cases the coexisting neoplasms are much more closely associated, most of them arising

[1] Brit. Med. Jour., Oct. 31, 1896.   [2] Arch f. Gynäk., Bd. liii., H. 1, 1897.
[3] Australasian Med. Gaz., Jan., 1897.   [4] Ann. of Surg., Sept., 1896.

in the corpus. A common condition is to find one or more small subperitoneal or intramural fibroids with carcinoma of the adjacent mucosa. Under these circumstances the fibroid is seldom cancerous. Many instances have been recorded of fibroids projecting into the uterine cavity and bearing on their surfaces a cancerous growth or ulcer. In cases of this kind the latter disease usually spreads from the mucosa to the fibroid by way of the perivascular lymphatics. In like manner uterine fibroids projecting into the abdomen sometimes become cancerous through extension of the disease from adherent neighboring organs, as the ovary, intestine, and omentum. There is yet another way in which fibroids may possibly be secondarily invaded by carcinoma, and that is by dissemination from a primary focus elsewhere, as in the lung. In such cases as the foregoing there is no question of the cancerous disease having primarily originated in the fibromyoma. This is, however, an event of such rarity that only about a dozen instances of it have hitherto been recorded; and in most of these the evidence adduced is far from being thoroughly convincing. Uterine fibroids, instead of having any special proclivity to become cancerous, are very much less liable to originate this disease than are the glandular elements of the uterus itself. [The foregoing is contrary to the teachings of the vast majority of textbooks and teachers; it seems to us, however, to be so true that no man can candidly look over his own experience and fail to accept it in great part if not *in toto.*] As to the association of uterine fibroma and sarcoma Williams's analysis of 2649 consecutive cases of uterine neoplasms showed 883 uterine fibromyomata and only 2 sarcomata; while of 205 hysterectomies for fibroids of the corpus, Martin found 4 of the tumors sarcomatous. These figures prove, therefore, that uterine fibroids seldom become sarcomatous, although the occasional origin of sarcomatous disease in uterine fibromyomata has been clearly established. In this connection it must be remembered that fibroids are of composite build, including connective tissue, muscle-elements, blood-vessels, and lymphatics, from either of which the sarcomatous metaplasia may arise; hence corresponding varieties of the disease (myosarcoma, myomyxoma). By far the commonest variety of the disease is the myosarcomatous.

Primary Carcinoma of the Corpus Uteri.—Käpelli,[1] from the investigation of 15 cases at the University of Basel clinic for women, comes to the following conclusions: (1) the frequency of carcinoma of the corpus uteri as compared with cervical carcinoma is 5.3 %; (2) it occurs after the menopause, and perhaps more frequently in unhealthy married than in single women; (3) carcinoma of the corpus uteri can be associated with myoma of the uterus or follow abortion; (4) chronic irritation and inflammatory diseases of the endometrium act as predisposing causes of carcinoma; therefore displacements of the uterus are a relatively frequent cause; (5) the hemorrhage resists treatment and is atypical; pain is present in only a few cases, but its character is pathognomonic; (6) in a typical case it is possible, from the symptoms and clinical examination, to determine the diagnosis. An absolute diagnosis can only be gained through microscopic examination of tissue removed by the curet.

According to H. D. Beyea,[2] the history of primary carcinoma of the uterine body is almost entirely confined to the last 15 years. During the last $2\frac{1}{2}$ years he has seen 7 positive cases. The disease occurs most frequently during the post-climacteric period and between the ages of 50 and 60 years, but it may occur as early as the twentieth year; it is more often found in multiparæ.

---

[1] Dissert., Luzerne, 1896; Centralbl. f. Gynäk., No. 29, 1896.
[2] Therap. Gaz., Aug. 15, 1896.

In Beyea's experience there is a form of malignant uterine disease which primarily appears as a malignant adenoma—or, better, adenoma destruens—and which progresses as an atypical glandular form of disease, which can destroy and perforate the uterine wall, and, if not removed early, will result in the death of the patient. Anatomically, there are 3 forms of growth—that which projects in polypoid masses in the uterine cavity, that which grows diffusely over the corporeal endometrium, and that which appears as a nodule in the uterine wall. Every one of these forms of growth, primarily beginning in the endometrium, must soon infiltrate the endometrial tissue to a greater or less extent. The polypoid and diffuse forms of the disease are by far the most frequent. The only method of diagnosis that can give positive results is that of microscopic examination of tissue removed by the curet.

Adenoma Cervicis Malignum Cysticum.—Knauss and Camerer[1] report the following case of cervical polyp and malignant adenoma of the cervix uteri. A polyp the size of a hazelnut, having a pedicle, was found protruding from the cervical canal and was excised. The woman returned a month later, and at the site of insertion of the pedicle of the previously removed polyp there was found a small round tumor, which proved to be a malignant adenoma. The uterus was removed. Two and a half years later the patient was perfectly well. The microscopic characteristics of the disease are thoroughly described. The writers were able to find only 6 cases of malignant adenoma of the cervix reported in the literature. Smith[2] also reports a case of malignant adenoma of the cervix uteri in an unmarried woman 34 years of age. The diagnosis was made by microscopic examination of tissue removed by the curet. The uterus was removed, and after 6 months there were no signs of a return of the disease. An additional case is recorded by M. H. Richardson.[3]

Carcinoma Uteri in the Young.—Pilliet and Delaunay[4] record a case of cervical carcinoma in a woman of 30 years; Tschop,[5] a case in a girl 19 years of age; and W. L. Little,[6] a case in a girl of 14 years, resulting fatally.

Diagnosis of Uterine Carcinoma.—[The early recognition of uterine carcinoma is probably as difficult as it is important.] W. B. Chase[7] remarks that any escape of blood from the vagina at a period subsequent to the menopause is a matter of deep significance, and, except in rare cases, is the concomitant of malignant disease. An ichorous, foul-smelling discharge, more or less mingled with blood, is almost pathognomonic of carcinoma. If, associated with these symptoms there are those of pain and cachexia, the diagnosis is practically established. Still, according to Masse,[8] it must be remembered that hemorrhagic endometritis, without malignant disease, may arise suddenly in old women 7 or 8 years after the menopause. Most of such cases occur, strange to say, in large and fleshy patients. [Does obesity, which is very frequent after the menopause, cause a modification in the mucosa of the senile uterus? Hermann and Fourneux, while studying this subject, found the muscular tissue lax and pliable, and the vessels atheromatous. Delert has proved the absence of the glands of the mucosa, and this tissue is very vascular in women who have had endometritis. This senile degeneration of the

---

[1] Zeit. f. Geb. u. Gynäk., Bd. xxxiv., H. 3, 1897.
[2] Méd. moderne, No. 60, 1896.   [3] Boston M. and S. Jour., Apr. 29, 1897.
[4] Bull. de la Soc. anat. de Paris. pt. 4, Jan. and Feb., 1896.
[5] Tuschnoruss kaja Medicinskaja Gazata, No. 7, 1896.
[6] New Orl. M. and S. Jour., Dec., 1896.   [7] Med. News, Aug. 22, 1896.
[8] Sem. gynéc., Apr. 7, 1896.

mucosa probably predisposes to the uterine hemorrhages; the etiology, however, is still very obscure. It is evident that they may occur without the presence of a malignant growth or fibroid.] Dorland[1] urges that hemorrhage after the menopause should be regarded as a most ominous sign of grave organic disease, and its cause investigated. Other clinical manifestations of undoubted value are the characteristic sacral pain—a very common symptom—and the offensive and acrid leukorrhea, often resulting in an uncontrollable pruritus. W. R. Williams[2] states that carcinoma is often ushered in by certain vague premonitory indications, as malaise, lassitude, anorexia, uneasy sensations in the lumbosacral and genital regions, and leukorrhea. Physical examination is important, and the condition of the lymph-glands in the groin should be ascertained, for in more than one-fourth of all cases those of one or both sides become obviously enlarged in the course of the disease. This may occur at a comparatively early date, when the disease starts at or near the fundus. The left supraclavicular region should also be examined, as in advanced cases of uterine carcinoma the lymph-glands in this situation are apt to become enlarged (*Troisier's symptom*); it must be remembered, however, that any intra-abdominal carcinoma may cause this adenopathy. Edema of one or both legs—owing to pressure of enlarged glands on the iliac veins—is met with in about 15% of the cases. The symptoms of uterine tuberculosis closely resemble those of carcinoma, but hemorrhage is a less marked feature. In tubercle of the corpus the part is much enlarged, its walls are thickened, and its cavity is distended with yellowish fluid containing curdy, caseous flakes or thick magma. On removing this, irregular patches of rather deep, sharply punched-out ulceration are seen, each ulcer being covered by a deposit of yellowish caseous matter. The adjacent parts are thickened by tuberculous infiltration, in which yellow opaque granules are often noticeable.

To effect an accurate diagnosis, however, in any case resort must be had to the curet and microscope. Gessner,[3] at a meeting of the Berlin Obstetric and Gynecologic Society, on March 13, 1896, read a paper comparing the advantages and worth of curettement, and the microscopic examination of tissue removed, over digital palpation of the uterine cavity in malignant diseases. He says that, although microscopic diagnosis in gynecologic diseases has been known for the last 20 years, the method has not as yet received general acknowledgment. Particularly in England has this method been almost condemned. The only other method of diagnosis of malignant diseases of the corpus uteri which can be considered to compare with this is digital palpation of the uterine cavity. He believes there are 3 factors which a method of diagnosis of these diseases of the corpus uteri must have, as follows: it must be without danger, easily applied, and, most important, it must be positive. In order to digitally palpate the uterine cavity the cervical canal must be dilated. This is always, whether rapid or gradual, dangerous for the patient. Recently, cases have been reported in which death resulted from this procedure. As compared with this, curettement is less dangerous if infection and perforation be isolated. For dilatation and digital palpation, except when rapid dilatation is practised, two sittings and frequently two anesthesias are necessary, while in curettement only one sitting is required. In various complications senile vaginæ, long or constricted cervical canal, ridged pelvic floor, and enlarged myomatous uterus) digital palpation is difficult or impossible, and thus no positive results can be gained. It is also not true that the surface of the endometrium always becomes roughened or nodular in carcinoma. This occurs

---

[1] Univ. Med. Mag., Sept., 1896. [2] Lancet, Oct. 17, 1896.
[3] Centralbl. f. Gynäk., No. 18, 1896.

only when the disease is far advanced. Not rarely carcinoma causes soft polypi which digitally cannot be differentiated from benign polypi. On the other hand, endometritic processes can result in hard growths, as in suppurating myomata. In the cases in which digital palpation gives a positive result a careful curettement in which considerable tissue is removed would also afford a positive diagnosis through microscopic examination. This is also possible in cases in which digital palpation would never have led to any result because the disease was too much localized. In the Berlin University clinic for women, since January 1, 1890, the diagnosis of malignant disease of the corpus uteri has been made and the uterus removed 58 times. In 11 of these cases a carcinomatous, and in 3 a sarcomatous new-growth was directly palpated. In 3 excised polypi sarcoma was diagnosed through microscopic examination. In the remaining 41 cases the diagnosis was made by curettement and microscopic examination alone. During 5 years in this clinic it has never been necessary to employ digital palpation as a means of diagnosis in malignant disease of the endometrium. In 4 cases the carcinoma, although giving the symptoms, was not situated in the corpus uteri, but in the cervix. He therefore believes that the curettement is useful as a method of making an early diagnosis of carcinoma of the cervix. In another case, from the changes occurring in the endometrium, malignant disease of the ovary was diagnosed. He advises that the curettement be done under anesthesia, and the cervical canal be slightly dilated.

Pick[1] describes a rapid method of permanently staining microscopic sections for diagnosis, employed in the Landau clinic. It is as follows : (1) The portions of tissue are washed free from blood and immediately frozen and cut with the small Young microtome. (2) The sections are carried by the finger-tip into a 2% formalin solution, and allowed to remain 2 or 3 minutes (the formalin solution should be made with boiled water). (3) They are then washed for a half minute in water. (4) They are then placed 3 or 4 minutes in a 4% solution of alum carmin. (5) They are washed 1 minute in water. (6) They are placed in 80% alcohol for 10 seconds. (7) They are placed in . carbol-xylol for 1 minute. (8) They are mounted in Canada balsam.

Treatment of Carcinoma.—(1) *Palliative.*—R. M. Stone[2] reports the only case of malignant uterine disease treated by the erysipelas and prodigiosus toxins followed by favorable results. The case was undoubtedly malignant and inoperable, and the patient apparently near to death. The initial dose of the unfiltered toxins was 3 minims, injected between the shoulder-blades; the next day, 3 minims; the next, 10; the next, 14, and the next, 20 minims were injected. The patient's condition was improving steadily. The next day 19 minims were injected into the vagina, the patient shortly falling into collapse, and being saved only by active stimulation. Under a renewal of the treatment the carcinomatous growth entirely disappeared, and the patient made a complete recovery. [This method of treatment has been tried quite extensively, with little or no success. Extreme caution should be observed in its use].

N. G. Bozeman[3] suggests as the indications for treatment in inoperable cases : 1. To keep the seat of the disease in an aseptic condition ; 2. To prevent or counteract any narrowing of the vagina in front of the disease ; 3. When the bladder becomes involved to use effective irrigation and drainage to carry off the urine as soon as it is secreted. E. Duvrac[4] calls attention to the favorable action exerted on malignant neoplasms of the uterus by

[1] Centralbl. f. Gynäk., No 40, 1896.   [2] Med. Rec., Nov. 21, 1896.
[3] Jour. Am. Med. Assoc., Jan. 16, 1897.   [4] Am. Medico-Surg. Bull., Sept. 12, 1896.

the administration of sodium chlorate internally and its simultaneous application to the cervix uteri. Under this treatment the metrorrhagia and fetid discharge decrease and ultimately disappear more or less completely; the pain is alleviated, rendering the use of morphin unnecessary; the puffiness of the cervix subsides, the sores heal, appetite and digestion are restored, and the general condition improves. [It seems necessary periodically to repeat the warning that carcinoma has but one cure—the knife. It is hardly fair to the patient to waste time over will-o'-the-wisps.] M. A. Guinard[1] has employed carburetted calcium (calcium carbid) in several cases of inoperable cervical carcinoma, with good results.

A piece of the material the size of a nut is introduced and placed in contact with the growth. The vagina is then packed with iodoform-gauze, which is left in place for 4 days. After it is removed a vaginal douche is given and the pieces of calcium oxid remaining in contact with the cervix are removed with the fingers. The main objection to this treatment is the moderate amount of pain caused by the application of the drug, but this disappears in a few hours. Although not a curative procedure, the application has a beneficial effect on all of the 3 cardinal symptoms of carcinoma of the cervix—namely, pain, hemorrhage, and fetid discharge. Moreover, the excrescences of the carcinoma dry up and fall off, leaving in their place a smooth, even surface. Calcium carbid, discovered by Moissau, has the property of changing into calcium oxid and acetylen gas, so that one sees the gas bubbling out of the vagina after an application of the drug. The acetylen acts as a hemostatic and the calcium as a caustic, but the fluids of the vagina cause the latter to become hydrated and limit its caustic action.

R. Bell[2] speaks of the treatment of uterine carcinoma and fibroma and certain forms of ovarian disease by means of thyroid, parotid, and mammary gland therapeutics. He asserts that the parotid gland exerts a most powerful influence upon the ovaries, and uterine fibroids are benefited by the employment of mammary glands of healthy animals. He has benefited cases of uterine carcinoma by administering thyroid elixir and palatinoids.

(2) *Radical (Operative) Treatment of Uterine Carcinoma.*—F. W. Johnson[3] has employed Clark's method (see *Year-Book*, 1896) in 10 cases, with the following results: 3 died from the immediate effects of the operation; 3 are alive and in perfect health 16 months after the operation, 1 of these has gained 100 pounds, and at the time of the operation she was the most unpromising of the three; 1 is alive, with no return of the disease, 12 months after the operation; 1 is alive, with no return of the disease, 8 months after operation; in 2 the disease has returned in scar-tissue at the vault of the vagina. [These results speak very ill for such an extensive operative procedure; the removal of the uterus by the usual methods gives far better results. The mortality is something startling, and it would require an exceedingly bold man to continue with the method.]

Supravaginal excision of the uterus by the galvanocautery in place of total or partial hysterectomy is advocated by J. Byrne[4] and W. J. Corcoran.[5] They claim for this method the following: it is aseptic and nearly bloodless; post-operative shock is absent; it has no primary mortality; its ultimate results challenge any and every other method; its action extends beyond the immediate field of operation, thus probably killing or rendering inert the cancer-elements not accessible to the knife. Byrne has employed this method for

[1] Sem. méd., No. 18, 1896. [2] Internat. Med. Mag., July, 1896.
[3] Boston M. and S. Jour., Dec. 31, 1896. [4] Am. Gyn. and Obst. Jour., July, 1896.
[5] Brooklyn Med. Jour., Sept., 1896.

nearly 25 years, and is convinced that *there is positively no place in legitimate surgery for kolpohysterectomy, or high or low amputation in carcinoma of the cervix, except when performed through the agency of the galvanocautery.* Corcoran states that the operation of Byrne is practically painless, there is no such thing as shock, and the convalescence is absolutely afebrile. There is, however, considerable danger of hemorrhage if not properly performed.

Penrose[1] writes that he has performed complete hysterectomy for carcinoma by a combined method of operation through the abdomen and vagina during the last year. In the combined operation, as usually performed, the vaginal part of the operation is done first, the abdominal part last. The method which he has followed was begun through the abdomen and finished by way of the vagina. The advantages claimed for this method of combined operation are as follows: the dirty part of the operation is done last. The septic cervix is withdrawn through the vagina and not through the peritoneal cavity.

[*Vaginal hysterectomy* for carcinoma is not in as great favor as formerly.] As stated by J. H. Croom,[2] for this operation to be successful mobility of the uterus, freedom of the fornices, and, as a result, the possibility of pulling the cervix well down to the vulva, are the essential points. Without these conditions the operation can, of course, be performed; but whether it relieves suffering or prolongs life is questionable. According to J. E. Janvrin,[3] vaginal hysterectomy should be confined to cases in which the disease is limited to the cervix or the cervix and mucous membrane only of the upper part of the vagina, or to those in which the disease, having involved these points, has also begun to develop upon the mucous lining of the uterus itself. To this may be added cases of adenoma and carcinoma uteri in their early stages. In all cases in which there is suspicion of extension of the disease beyond the limits previously mentioned, whether into the parametrium, the folds of the broad ligaments, the ovaries or the cul-de-sac, the combined abdomino-vaginal operation is the most appropriate, if we resort to any radical operation. As to the results of the operation, T. Wilson[4] remarks that of 100 suitable cases of carcinoma of the cervix submitted to vaginal hysterectomy, 40 patients may be reasonably expected to be alive and free from recurrence 2 years after operation. The duration of life after operation in patients dying from recurrence was found by Leopold in 50 cases to average 19.7 months. From the most complete statistics and reports of cases from Great Britain Wilson collects 283 cases of hysterectomy for carcinoma, with 34 deaths (a percentage-mortality of 12). Schramm[5] reports 33 cases of vaginal hysterectomy, with a mortality of 15.1%. He prefers clamps to ligatures for the following reasons: 1. The operation is shorter and easier. 2. Less blood is lost and there is less risk of secondary hemorrhage. 3. In cases of carcinoma the resulting necrosis causes the destruction of the diseased tissue not removed at the time of operation. 4. Even in advanced cases the operation is free from danger. 5. The after-treatment is simpler and there are no ligatures to be removed subsequently. According to Olshausen,[6] in Germany during 1887–1888 only 28% of cases of carcinoma of the uterus were regarded as suitable for a radical operation, while during 1895–1896 the number rose to 40%. The difference is attributed to the greater intelligence of general physicians and the earlier recognition of the initial symptoms. He condemns the sacral and parasacral methods of operation, since they are neces-

[1] Am. Jour. Obst., vol. xxxiv., No. 6, 1896.   [2] Brit. Med. Jour., Aug. 1, 1896.
[3] Am. Gyn. and Obst. Jour., May, 1897.   [4] Birmingham Med. Rev., Feb., 1897.
[5] Arch. f. Gynäk., Bd. lii., H. 2, 1896.   [6] Berlin. klin. Woch., No. 23, 1896.

sary only in cases which he regards as unsuitable for extirpation. In 139 vaginal hysterectomies performed by him since April, 1894, there were only 3 deaths, while in his last 100 cases there was only 1 death, due to pyemia, from which the patient was suffering before the operation. As regards the technic of the operation T. A. Helme[1] prefers, instead of the usual circular incision around the cervix, a barleycorn-shaped or elliptic incision—similar to that usually employed in excision of the breast—which gives more room and greater freedom for subsequent manipulation. The greater diameter of this ellipse coincides with the transverse of the vaginal roof, and its extremities may at times with advantage be prolonged in an outward direction along the lateral fornices. He divides the lateral ligaments gradually and on each side alternately from below upward; delays opening the peritoneal cavity; completely closes the peritoneum after removal of the uterus; cuts short the intraperitoneal ligatures and leaves the others long; partially obliterates the pericervical space by buried sutures; and removes by scissors (if necessary) all ligatures after the third day.

AFFECTIONS OF THE PELVIC VISCERA.

The Diagnosis of Pelvic Disease.—[The ability to properly diagnose affections of the pelvic viscera is by far more important to the general clinician than is a most comprehensive knowledge of the refinements of technic of abdominal or vaginal section. A number of able men have devoted their energies to the perfection of the methods of diagnosis at our command.] Thus Marc See[2] describes a new and very original method of palpating the abdomen, which he names "hydrostatic exploration." It consists in palpation of the abdomen while the patient is in a bath sufficiently deep to cover its surface with water. The relaxation of the parietes thus produced is explained by the fact that, more or less loaded with fat, they tend to rise toward the surface. Thus, this ascending movement, counteracting their elastic and contractile force, which tends to keep them in close relation with the viscera, gives them a laxity which is highly favorable to exploration of the deep parts. The whole of the abdominal organs, even in stout subjects, are thus rendered peculiarly accessible to touch, and the fingers readily make out even the vertebral column and the sacrovertebral angle. Adolphi[3] speaks highly of the Brandt-Dührssen method of examination, which, it is claimed, allows one to practise bimanual examination as thoroughly as if the patient were anesthetized. The essential point is that the thighs should be strongly flexed as the woman lies upon her back, while the examining-finger is introduced under the left thigh, instead of between the thighs. Adolphi employs a low conch, the head and foot of which can be raised by means of screws. The patient lies upon her back with her arms extended, her mouth being slightly open. The physician sits on her left side and places his right hand upon the abdomen, while the left forefinger is inserted into the vulva. If the abdominal muscles are not sufficiently relaxed, the patient is drawn downward and the thighs are flexed still more by raising the lower segment of the table. The symphysis and thorax are approximated and the recti are relaxed, thus favoring the most satisfactory practice of the bimanual method. W. R. Pryor[4] suggests a method of examining the pelvic contents which renders exploratory section unnecessary in inflammatory conditions of the appendages, and in certain other diseased states of the pelvic viscera. It consists in opening Douglas's

[1] Brit. Med. Jour., Oct. 31, 1896.
[2] L'Union méd., No. 25, 1896.
[3] St. Petersburg. med. Woch., No. 43, 1896.
[4] Med. Rec., July 11, 1896.

cul-de-sac by a transverse incision through the vaginal mucosa, downward traction being made upon the cervix; a digital exploration of the pelvic cavity is then made and a knowledge obtained as to the state of affairs. It is in doubtful cases—possible hydrosalpinx, broad-ligament cyst, enlarged ovary with adherent inflamed tube—that there exists the indication for this, as for the abdominal exploratory incision. The advantages of the method are, its rapidity (the cul-de-sac is entered in from 1 to 5 minutes), bloodlessness, and safety. Should a vaginal hysterectomy be indicated the exploratory vaginal incision completes the first step of the radical operation. Should it be deemed wise to open the abdomen the vaginal incision affords the rational drainage-space. [This method is open to all of the objections of the original section, and cannot be recommended as an absolutely safe procedure.]

In considering the value of *rectal exploration in children* G. Carpenter[1] pays considerable attention to the female pelvic organs. The sacrum is almost straight, as is the course of the rectum. The bladder is egg-shaped, with the larger extremity downward; it is almost entirely an abdominal viscus owing to the shallowness of the pelvic cavity. When the girl begins to assume the upright position and walk the bladder tends to sink into the pelvis; at the same time the attachments are so lax that when distended it lies almost completely in the abdominal cavity. This condition exists until puberty. The uterus is almost entirely composed of cervix, the body being very small, and is situated high up in the pelvis. It is found at birth that the ovaries have descended as far as the brim of the true pelvis, while a little later in life there is a further descent. The uterus is 1 in. long and $\frac{1}{2}$ in. broad at the fundus; the Fallopian tubes measure just under 2 in. in length; the right ovary is $\frac{5}{8}$ in., the left $\frac{1}{2}$ in. in length, and both are $\frac{1}{4}$ in. in diameter. As the child approaches puberty the ovary measures $1\frac{1}{2}$ in. in length by $\frac{1}{2}$ in. in breadth. The important anatomic guide to the Fallopian tubes when making a rectal examination appears to be the falciform ligament, or, in other words, the utero-sacral ligaments, which form together a sickle-shaped curve surrounding the rectum, being attached posteriorly to the sacrum and anteriorly to the junction of the vagina and cervix.

Salpingitis.—E. Reymond and W. S. Magill[2] have made an exhaustive experimental study of the pathologic anatomy and bacteriology of salpingo-ovaritis.

The authors assert that the usual classification of salpingitis, although clinically useful, is no more founded upon the successive stages of the affection than upon the different forms of the infection. The *salpingitis productiva vegetans* of Savinoff is the same form as that described by Cornil as *vegetating catarrhal salpingitis;* it is in reality a parenchymatous form, the parenchyma having assumed the preponderance in relation to the other tissues. *Salpingitis papillomatosa* and the *nodular salpingitis* would appear to constitute a special form due to a particular agent of infection. According to Doran, the papillomata invade the salpinx in the same manner as gonorrhea, the contagion being due to direct contact. These papillomata determine a secretion which varies according to its location. The vulva and vagina give rise to a fetid and abundant secretion; in the uterus this affection causes frequent metrorrhagia, sometimes excessive in quantity; in the salpinx the irritation caused by this infection may be so violent as to produce an obliteration of the pavilion, and thus prevent an extension of the affection to the peritoneum; but if the adhesion of the pavilion is not obtained and its permeability persists, there flows into the peritoneal cavity a serous liquid of slight irritating quality, caus-

---

[1] Pediatrics, June 1, 1896.   [2] Ann. of Surg., Sept., 1896.

ing, perhaps, a little ascites, but incapable of provoking adhesions; papillomata of the peritoneum and ovaries may then appear. The nodular variety has two principal characteristics: (1) nodules formed by the muscular tissue itself; (2) culs-de-sac of mucous follicles isolated in this muscular mass. The authors believe that both forms should be united and more advantageously considered as the exaggeration of a usual disposition of the tissue in salpingitis rather than a definite variety. A careful revision of the various elements would seem to explain the formation of the nodulofollicular salpingitis in the following manner: By agglutination of the fringes cysts are formed in the mucosa of the salpinx. The walls of these cysts are very vascular, and this vascular tissue has a strong tendency to transformation in the external coats of the mucosa in contact with the muscular. It may give place to fibrous tissue, but its change into muscular tissue invading the mucosa is often seen. Such transformation would appear analogous to that which Klebs describes for the formation of myomata; the large capillaries first surround themselves with spheric cells that ultimately become fusiform. The cysts included in the wall are crowded out hy the formation of muscular tissue on the inside. These transformations could take place in all points of the salpinx in regular sequence, and in this case the salpingitis would deserve the designation parenchymatous. But in a patient predisposed to fibromata the production of muscular fibers may be so accentuated in a single point as to form a myocystic nodulus; and as the muscular tissue tends toward a transformation into fibrous tissue, a fibrocystic formation would finally be realized in this way.

Under the influence of inflammation the fringes first become enlarged, and their ramifications more numerous, the cellular infiltration distends the connective tissue, separates the epithelial surfaces, tends to obliterate the fine ramifications, and gives the fringe a globular appearance.

In speaking of the symptoms of salpingitis L. G. Baldwin[1] states that it is the general opinion among the profession that pus-tubes spontaneously discharge through the uterus, a cure resulting; and, in case they do not empty themselves, that they may be drained by dilating and curetting the uterus. He would place himself on record as saying that he does not believe that a pyosalpinx ever discharged through the uterine end of the tube into the uterus, either spontaneously or as a result of dilatation and curetting of the uterus. His reasons are, first, the normal size of the lumen of the tube at the isthmus, together with the large amount of muscular tissue it contains at that point, rendering during pathologic conditions narrowing, if not complete occlusion, almost certain as a result of the preceding inflammatory process; and, secondly, the careful observation of a large number of removed specimens in not one of which could pus be squeezed through the uterine end without considerable force being applied. [The author has reached the same conclusion as have a large number of other surgeons in this matter.]

Septic inflammation of the tubes and pelvis is, according to W. Duncan,[2] in the great majority of cases the result of parturition, though a few cases may be due to the use of sponge or laminaria tents or to operations performed on the uterus with dirty instruments. Berntz analyzed 99 cases of peritonitis as follows: 43 occurred in puerperæ; 28 after gonorrhea; 20 during menstruation; and 8 were traumatic. Duncan believes that almost all the cases of peritonitis occurring in women, apart from labor, are most likely secondary to specific infection from gonorrhea. When a purulent collection in the tube leaks into the peritoneal cavity peritonitis follows; and this may be either (a) serous, (b) plastic, or (c) suppurative; it may be quite localized, or affect

[1] Am. Gyn. and Obst. Jour., Nov., 1896.   [2] Lancet, Jan. 2, 1897.

the whole pelvis, or even in very severe cases it may become general. Usually it is limited in extent, the ostium of the tube becoming closed, and the ovary matted to the tube; then ovaritis follows or an abscess may be formed in the ovary. The form most often met with is the plastic, where lymph is thrown out, matting the parts together. The chief symptoms of chronic disease of the tubes and ovaries associated with slight peritonitis are pain, hemorrhage, and yellow discharge. The pain varies; in catarrhal salpingitis it is slight, as there are no pelvic adhesions; but in purulent salpingitis and ovaritis (especially when the ovary and tube are matted together) there is more or less constant pain in the back and iliac fossæ, extending down one or both thighs, and aggravated by coitus, walking, or jolting. Menorrhagia is pretty constant in these cases, with a mucopurulent uterine discharge in the intervals. Deguy [1] records a case of infectious endocarditis following pyosalpinx, and W. R. Lincoln [2] a case of double salpingitis in which lime-salt concretions were found in both tubes.

The Bacteriology of Diseased Adnexa.—Kiefer [3] sought to determine the question as to the presence of bacteria in pyosalpinx; what method of examination is of the greatest practical value, the cover-glass preparation or culture; the proportion of the different species, and the average virulence of the pyogenic bacteria found. He made cover-glass preparations and cultures from 40 cases of pyosalpinx or ovarian abscess, in all of which the pus had soiled the peritoneum during operation. Although cover-glass preparations reveal the presence of bacteria, they do not give information regarding their vitality or degree of virulence. The gonococci were largely in majority, next the bacteria coli, the latter being mainly found in ovarian abscesses. None of the 40 cases died from purulent infection of the peritoneum, which again proves the fact that bacteria confined encapsulated in closed cavities soon lose their virulence; they die from their own products—the toxins. The average time determined from the formation to the sterility of the pus is about 9 months.

Tuberculosis of the Fallopian Tubes.—Cases of tubal tuberculosis are recorded as follows: C. Cone, [4] encysted dropsy of the peritoneum secondary to uterotubal tuberculosis and associated with tuberculous pleurisy, generalized tuberculosis, and pyococcal infection in a colored woman 30 years of age; J. A. Robison, [5] a case of focal tuberculosis in the right Fallopian tube, with general miliary tuberculosis, in a single woman of 22 years; Heydenreich, [6] a case of tuberculous salpingitis in a woman 39 years of age; and G. Carpenter, [7] a case of tuberculosis of the uterus and adnexa in a girl of 9 years, who also had tuberculous peritonitis, and subsequently died of general tuberculosis. [Tuberculosis of the uterus and adnexa is extremely rare in children.] Robison [8] remarks that tuberculosis of the tubes may develop at any age, but rarely before puberty. It is most common during menstrual life, and often arises during pregnancy. It often follows tuberculosis of the genital organs or of the lungs, rectum, and peritoneum. Many authors believe that tuberculosis of the uterus is frequently due to primary tuberculosis of the tubes with extension to the uterus. The diagnosis of tubal tuberculosis is comparatively easy if the abdominal walls are thin and the vagina large, as is taught by Chiari, the tubes being felt as irregular tumors external to the uterus.

Carcinoma of the Fallopian Tubes.—Hennig [9] considers the diffi-

[1] Ann. of Gyn. and Pediat., Aug, 1896.   [2] Cleveland Med. Gaz., Mar., 1897.
[3] Centralbl. f. Gynäk., No. 42, 1896.   [4] Bull. Johns Hopkins Hosp., May, 1897.
[5] N. Am. Pract., Mar., 1897.   [6] Sem. gynéc., No. 15, 1896.
[7] The Practitioner, Oct., 1896.   [8] Ibid.
[9] Centralbl. f. Gynäk., No. 47, 1896.

culty of diagnosis due to the very great infrequency of the disease. When gonorrheal affections are excluded, the diseases to be thought of are sacculated growths, tuberculosis, carcinoma, or abnormal pregnancies. The diagnosis of carcinoma is made more easy than others in that a fluid (increasing in amount) is encapsulated by a ridged wall; sometimes also there is a vaginal discharge of bloody water or cloudy mucus. The statistics regarding its frequency widely differ. Wagner states that in northern Germany 5% of uterine carcinoma are associated with carcinoma of the tube, while Kiwisch, in southern Germany, found the tube carcinomatous 25 times with 100 uterine carcinomata. It very rarely occurs with carcinoma of the cervix, is more frequent with ovarian carcinoma, and most frequent with carcinoma of the uterine body. Primary tubal carcinoma may infect either the uterus or peritoneum, and is most frequently bilateral. Eighteen cases have been reported. *Sarcoma of the tube* is excessively rare—only 4 cases having been reported. The form of carcinoma, according to Sänger, is always medullary; sometimes it is infiltrating, and sometimes villous. The climacteric and catarrhal inflammation are predisposing causes (Sänger). The diagnosis *per vaginam* must be made by exclusion and by rectal and bimanual examination under ether. Cachexia is not present—at least not early. The presence of ascites, disease of neighboring organs, stomachic, urinary, and rectal symptoms are important. When the growth breaks through into the peritoneal cavity marked symptoms result. The appearance of the posterior wall of the bladder is often important. In 6 cases the diseased organ has been removed and the patient provisionally restored. In 4 cases the disease returned—in Thornton's case after 3 years. Doran advises the removal of uterus and both tubes. Four patients died either during or immediately after operation. In the case in which the growth was least advanced the uterus and tubes were removed *per vaginam*. The left tube showed beginning villous carcinoma.

Eckardt[1] reports a case of primary alveolar carcinoma of the tube, the fifth on record. Twelve other reported cases were of the papillary variety. E. Ries[2] reports what he claims is the 7th case of primary papilloma of the tube, and the 20th case of primary carcinoma of the tube, the tables of Doran (in Allbutt and Playfair's *System of Gynecology*, 1896) and Sänger (in Martin's *Krankheiten der Eileiter*, 1896) containing 19 cases. Godart[3] observed a case of papilloma of a Fallopian tube in a sterile woman of 32 years.

Echinococcus of the Tubes.—Doléris[4] reports the case of a multipara, aged 36 years, who had suffered with severe abdominal pain for 11 years. The diagnosis of uterine fibroid was made. On opening the abdomen a tumor was found extending above the umbilicus. It consisted of both Fallopian tubes enormously enlarged and adherent to one another and to the omentum. They contained numerous echinococcus cysts. There were no metastases. The patient was cured. [The formation of a hydatid cyst in the pelvis is very rare. Davaine considered that they formed 7.9% of all cases, but it is probable that this estimate is far too high. The danger caused by their presence in this situation depends to a large extent on their pressure on the surrounding parts, especially on the urinary canals. They may also cause obstruction to delivery in pregnant women. Porak collected a series of 17 cases, in some of which delivery was impossible. No fewer than 6 died. Of the cases recorded in England the majority have been males. Kenwick found 90 cases of the disease recorded in 200 years. The majority appear to have originated

[1] Arch. f. Gynäk., Bd. 53, H. 1, 1897.   [2] Jour. Am. Med. Assoc., May 22, 1897.
[3] Ann. de l'Inst. Sainte-Anne, Brussels, No. 4, Mar., 1896.
[4] Indépendance Méd., No. 22, 1896.

between the muscular coat of the bladder and the peritoneum.]   G. Herman[1] records an additional case forming a retrouterine tumor in a woman of 66 years, and causing retention of urine.   [Pelvic hydatids show a tendency to suppurate, and also to erode and mine the pelvic bones.]

Tuberculous Peritonitis.—Abbé[2] states that the stages of tuberculous peritonitis are divided as follows: There may be (1) an eruption of miliary tubercles on the surface of the peritoneum so acute that acute infectious diseases or even strangulated hernia have been suspected; or there may be (2) an enormous accumulation of ascitic fluid, with rapid wasting, slight pain, and no fever—here a slow deposition of tubercles, widely scattered over the peritoneum, has occurred.   There may be (3) persistent pain or tenderness of the abdomen, with moderate tympanitic distention and irregular areas of dulness, associated with slight afternoon temperature and loss of appetite or flesh, indicating diffuse tuberculosis of the peritoneal cavity without fluid, but with a varying amount of plastic exudate partially sealing its walls together; or there may be (4) wasting of the body with irregular tympanitic distention, fever, anorexia, and sweats, associated with huge cakes of matted lymph and omentum, or sacculated ascites or pus, which illustrates the latest steps of tuberculous development; or there may be (5) the mishaps incident to degeneration of caseating patches ulcerating into the bowel, causing fistulæ or extravasations of feces into the peritoneum, or bowel-obstruction by lymph-adhesions; and, finally, (6) a retrograde course in the life of the bacillus and its products may leave an abdominal cavity partly sealed by atrophied tuberculous elements, which may give the patient years of comparative health.   Abbé believes that the bacillus enters less often through the circulation than through perforation of the intestinal wall or through transmission from the Fallopian tube.

Treatment of Pelvic Disease.—The prevention of pelvic disease is discussed by R. Peterson.[3]   He states that the causes of pelvic disease are: (1) *Imperfect development of the sexual organs.*   At no period of life will prophylactic measures prove of so much avail as during the few years prior to puberty.   Prolonged hours in the school-room and ignorance as to the functions of the generative organs are responsible for much of the disease of later life.   (2) *Gonorrhea.*   (3) *Lacerations due to childbirth.*   The improved obstetrics is doing away with much of the pelvic disease consequent upon unrecognized and unrepaired lacerations of the cervix and perineum.   (4) *Sepsis following childbirth and abortions.*   W. R. Pryor[4] suggests that suppuration may be prevented by curetting the uterus in all cases of acute salpingitis and peritonitis.   He has done this in nearly 100 cases of acute first attacks, and he has never seen failure result from it when early applied.   The causes of failure in the hands of others are the use of strong antiseptics within the uterine cavity, partial removal of débris, and incomplete packing of the uterus.

Abdominal Section.—Interesting cases are recorded as follows: J. H. Galton,[5] a case of successful second ovariotomy at the age of 70 years, the first operation having been performed 12 years before.   [Many instances have been recorded of cases of ovariotomy above the age of 70 years.   J. R. Morison recorded 5 cases, and of these only 1 died.   Homans recorded 12 cases, of whom 3 died.   M. Sherwood collected 38 cases, with 5 deaths.   Spencer Wells's oldest case was 71 years of age, and Keith's 73 years.   Terrier removed both ovaries from a woman aged 77.   Several cases have been recorded

[1] Lancet, Nov. 21, 1896.   [2] Med. News, Nov. 5, 1896.
[3] Jour. Am. Med. Assoc., Dec. 19, 1896.   [4] Med. News, Sept. 5, 1896.
                         [5] Lancet, Aug. 15, 1896.

of ovariotomies on patients over 80 years of age. Schroeder's and Owens's cases were each 80 years old. Edis records a case over the age of 81 years. H. Spencer's case was 82 years 3 months old. Homans's case was 1 month older. J. P. Bush performed an ovariotomy on a patient who had commenced her 85th year. All these patients over 80 years of age recovered from the operation.] G. Carpenter[1] records an ovariotomy on a child 9 years of age suffering with tuberculous Fallopian tubes. [The youngest ovariotomy on record is that reported by Chiene in 1884, on a child aged 3 months.] Carpenter tabulates 35 cases of ovariotomy on children performed for cystic disease, dermoids, fibromyoma, sarcoma, and carcinoma.

The *technic of abdominal section* is discussed by J. G. Clark,[2] T. J. Watkins,[3] and I. S. Stone.[4] The method of preparing sponges at the Johns Hopkins Hospital, as recorded by Clark, is as follows: 1. Reef sponges are pounded with a wooden mallet until freed from gritty particles; 2. They are then immersed in HCl solution (ʒij to Oj) over night; 3. They are then washed in pure water until the latter is perfectly clear; 4. They are immersed for a few minutes in a saturated solution of potassium permanganate; 5. They are transferred from this solution with sterile hands to a saturated solution of oxalic acid, and left there until decolorized; 6. They are then rinsed through sterile water; 7. They are next immersed in mercuric chlorid solution (1 : 1000) for 24 hours; 8. They are transferred to a 1 : 20 solution of carbolic acid, where they are permanently preserved until ready for use.

The *vagina* is carefully cleansed in the following manner: 1. It is thoroughly washed with green-soap and warm water; 2. It is then douched with a 10% creolin solution; 3. It is further washed with sterile water; 4. Finally, it is douched with mercuric chlorid solution (1 : 1000), followed by sterile water.

Sterilization of Ligatures.—Clark and Miller,[5] after a thorough bacteriologic investigation and a practical experience of a year with the cumol method of sterilization of catgut, conclude that it is the most reliable. The sterilization by Krönig's method is perfect, but the transferrence from boiling cumol to benzene is open to serious objection. Clark and Miller have found from this investigation that benzene is not a germicide; also that it cannot be rendered sterile by heat without danger, and, therefore, they have found it necessary to modify the method of Krönig as follows: (1) The catgut, 12 strands, is rolled in a figure-of-8 form, so that it can be slipped into a large test-tube. (2) The catgut is brought up to a temperature of 80° C., and held at this point for 1 hour. (3) It is placed in cumol, which must not be above 100° C.; this temperature is raised to 165° C., and held at this point for 1 hour. (4) The cumol is then poured off, and either the heat of the sand-bath is allowed to dry the catgut, or it is transferred to a hot-air oven, at a temperature of 100° C., for 2 hours. (5) The rings are transferred with sterile forceps to the test-tubes previously sterilized, as in the laboratory. In drying or boiling, the catgut should not come in contact with the bottom or sides of the vessel, but should be suspended on slender wire supports, or placed upon cotton loosely packed in the bottom of the beaker-glass.

Bröse,[6] at the meeting of the Berlin Obstetric and Gynecologic Society on November 13, 1896, advised the following new method for sterilizing catgut. The catgut, wound on glass rollers, is first placed in juniper oil or tur-

[1] Practitioner, Oct., 1896.   [2] Therap. Gaz., Dec. 15, 1896.
[3] Med. News, Aug. 8, 1896.   [4] Jour. Am. Med. Assoc., July 25, 1896.
[5] Bull. Johns Hopkins Hosp., Nos. 59 and 60, 1896.
[6] Centralbl. f. Gynäk., No. 52, 1896.

pentine, in a vessel having a stopper that will not allow steam to enter. The vessel is then placed on a water-bath (the water being cold) and heat is applied for one-half hour. These ethereal oils, which boil at a temperature of from 155° to 160° C., reach a temperature of from 99° to 100° C. in the half hour. In these thus heated ethereal oils all bacteria, including the anthrax-bacillus, are destroyed. This the writer proved by a thorough bacteriologic investigation. The catgut retains the strength, and, besides, it is free from fat and water. These oils are also strong disinfectants. Since catgut taken directly from the oil would be difficult to handle, and, again, since the oil would irritate the tissue, he advises that the catgut be placed, just before operation, in a 1 : 1000 alcoholic solution of the mercuric chlorid. Bröse has employed catgut thus prepared for 3 months with perfect satisfaction. Schaffer, in the discussion, stated that only fresh juniper oil should be employed, as this alone has the power to disinfect.

Tretrop[1] has been experimenting with formol as a means of sterilizing catgut and other ligatures. Soaking in a 2% solution for 24 hours will kill all bacteria except staphylococci. A 5% solution (by volume) rendered catgut, silk, silkworm-gut, and rubber tubing absolutely sterile. The experiments included tests with streptococci, staphylococci, anthrax, bacterium coli, Löffler's bacillus, and the bacillus pyocyaneus. The sterilized material was kept in common alcohol (94%), and was found to be sterile after 4 weeks. An experiment on a dog showed that the catgut was completely absorbed after 4 days, so that no trace remained of No. 4 gut.

Closure of the Abdominal Wound.—In discussing this subject before the International Congress at Geneva[2] Bantock offered the following conclusions: 1. Suppuration of the abdominal wound is due, not to the presence of bacteria, but to foreign bodies or to strangulation by tight sutures. 2. In many cases simple through-and-through sutures are sufficient. 3. In stout patients it is better to close the peritoneum separately and the remaining layers of the wound with 1 or 2 series of sutures. 4. Silkworm-gut is the best for interrupted sutures and catgut (*not* chromicized) for buried sutures. Le Torre thinks that it is not sufficient to unite the fascial edges alone; the edges of the muscle should also be included in the sutures. Howitz believes that just as little of the peritoneum as possible should be included; in fact, he approves of the plan of some operators not to suture the peritoneal edges at all, but to allow them to unite toward the abdominal cavity. Patients should not be allowed to leave their beds until 3 weeks have elapsed. Condamin recommends a tier-suture in the form of corset-lacing, especially in large wounds.

At the Johns Hopkins Hospital[3] the following method is employed: 1. Continuous catgut sutures to the peritoneum; 2. Silver mattress-sutures, which are passed only through the aponeurosis of the separated recti muscles, and closely twisted 5 times. The wires are cut smoothly with dull scissors, and the point turned down upon the aponeurosis of the recti muscles, projecting neither upward nor downward; 3. Continuous catgut to the fat; 4. Subcutaneous catgut suture. No. 24 sterling silver wire is used. It is sterilized by boiling with the instruments. After the abdominal dressing is applied the patient is elevated to the medium high Trendelenburg posture, and a liter of warm salt-solution (0.6%) is injected well up into the sigmoid flexure. In order that the patient may retain the enema *she must yet be under the anesthetic when it is given*, otherwise the bowel will not tolerate such a large quantity of fluid. This means of alleviating thirst was first employed 2

[1] Centralbl. f. Gynäk., No. 15, 1896.   [2] Ann. de Gynéc. et d'Obstét., No. 9, 1896.
[3] Clark, Loc. cit.

years ago and has proved remarkably effective. Goelet[1] unites the peritoneum by a continuous suture of fine (No. 0) chromicized catgut, which is made to include the muscle as well. Next, deep interrupted sutures of silkworm-gut are inserted about $\frac{1}{2}$ or $\frac{3}{4}$ in. apart and $\frac{1}{2}$ in. from the margin of the wound. They include skin, fascia, and muscle, and are not tied at once. The

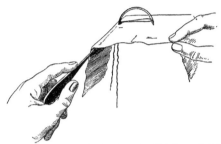

FIG. 42.—Shimonek's figure-of-8 ligature (Jour. Am. Med. Assoc., Sept. 26, 1897).

fascia is then united separately by means of a continuous suture of the same size chromicized catgut as before. The interrupted silkworm-gut sutures are now tied. C. P. Noble[2] has employed the buried silkworm-gut suture in 297 abdominal sections; of these cases suppuration occurred in 7, or 2.3%. The silkworm-gut should be carefully selected, and should be light in weight and

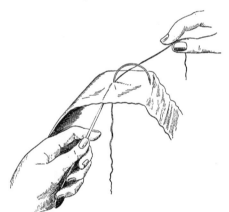

FIG. 43.—Shimonek's figure-of-8 ligature (Jour. Am. Med. Assoc., Sept. 26, 1897).

absolutely aseptic. To secure the best results the abdominal incision should pass through one rectus muscle rather than through the linea alba. F. Shimonek[3] describes a new figure-of-8 ligature. An armed needle is passed through the pedicle, as shown in Fig. 42. That part of the ligature passing through the eye of the needle is withdrawn from it, as shown in Fig. 43. We

[1] Clinical Record, July, 1896.   [2] Am. Gyn. and Obst. Jour., Dec., 1896.
[3] Jour. Am. Med. Assoc., Sept. 26, 1897.

now have the needle and ligature passing through the same opening in the pedicle, and yet they are independent of each other. Take that part of the

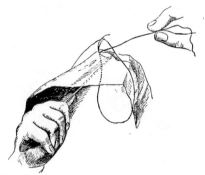

FIG. 44.—Shimonek's figure-of-8 ligature (Jour. Am. Med. Assoc., Sept. 26, 1897).

ligature corresponding to the handle of the needle, carry it half-way around the pedicle, and pass it through the eye of the needle, as shown in Fig. 44.

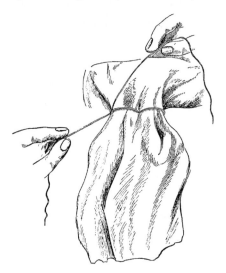

FIG. 45.—Shimonek's figure-of-8 ligature (Jour. Am. Med. Assoc., Sept. 26, 1897).

Now withdraw the threaded needle from the pedicle, thereby forming a loop upon one side of the latter; the ends passing and crossing through the same opening appear upon the other side and may be tied, as shown in Fig. 45; or, in a very broad pedicle that cannot be securely tied with one figure-of-8, the needle may be passed through the pedicle at a distance of $\frac{1}{2}$ in. or more, threaded with one of the free ends, then unthreaded at that end and again threaded with the other one, and so on, until the entire pedicle is encompassed and the free ends tied.

Schaffer[1] writes that silk as a suture-material has greatly replaced the smooth, hard silkworm-gut and silver wire because of its flexibility, elasticity, and strength. The reason why silkworm-gut and silver wire are still frequently employed is that when silk is employed stitch-hole abscesses are apt to result. The great trouble which every one has experienced in the sterilization of the silk suture, chemical as well as physical disinfection, has continually become less and less ; also the physical quality of the silk itself is now considered—the construction of the Ihle silk suture-carrier, which has the object of exposing each strand directly to the sterilization. As experimentation has shown, these methods are sure enough in rendering the bacteria in suture-material unharmful, except as regards catgut, which sometimes contains an irritating toxin which will develop in water, but not in the preparing alcohol or ether. He says that in order to prevent the invasion of the stitch-canal with bacteria two conditions must be considered : (1) the site of introduction of the suture must be free from bacteria, and (2) the suture-material should not absorb fluids, so that the stitch-canal remains dry ; no bacteria are then introduced as, at least, a favorable culture-medium is not prepared. This, however, is not usually attained, for during the manipulation of the wound and skin the suture-material is saturated with fluid. The first condition is prevented, or, at least, greatly prevented through thorough mechanical (the brush, soap, water, and alcohol) and chemical (mercuric chlorid) disinfection. The mechanical disinfection not only removes a large amount of fat, but also partially empties the glands of the skin. The second condition as regards the silk suture is not gained ; for, although sterile, it is very hygroscopic. If the silk suture is introduced in the abdominal wall in the ordinary manner, particularly in fat women, it is very easily removed, and Ihle believes this is true of the figure-of-8 ligatures in the abdominal cavity. The silk ligature absorbs the wound-matter and continues saturated, and such saturated suture at the body-temperature constitutes a most favorable culture-medium for pus-organisms which may have been introduced from the skin-surface or its glands. Considering this factor as important, the writer sought to get a silk suture which would act as a capillary drain, and therefore now advises the use of silk suture-material which is impregnated with gutta-percha, prepared by Evens and Piston, of Kassel. Its advantages are that it is as soft, elastic, strong, and as easily sterilized as before ; it receives a satin luster, a proof that it has the consistency of vessels ; if dry, ordinary and impregnated portions be placed in water, the impregnated is unchanged while the other becomes soft and saturated ; and if the end of each be placed in colored water at the body-temperature, the impregnated remains dry and the surface only is slightly discolored.

T. J. Watkins[2] performs abdominal salpingo-oöphorectomy without leaving a pedicle. This is done by passing a ligature under the infundibulopelvic ligament just deep enough to include the ovarian artery ; the suture is tied, the short end is cut off near the knot and the long end is left to suture the broad ligament. The tube and ovary are then separated from the broad ligament by dividing the latter close to the tube from a point just external to the tube and ovary, and by continuing the division until the uterus is reached, when the tube is excised flush with the uterus. The wound is then closed

[1] Centralbl. f. Gynäk., No. 46, 1896.   [2] Med. News, Aug. 8, 1896.

with the long end of the suture by the glover's stitch. The advantages of this method are : (1) no pedicle is made ; (2) the entire tube and ovary can be excised ; (3) very little tissue is included in the suture and very little tension is made on the broad ligaments ; (4) little or no raw surface remains to form adhesions or cicatrices ; (5) absorbable sutures may be used without fear of hemorrhage ; (6) blood-vessels are ligated while in normal location, which protects against retraction and hemorrhage ; (7) when the broad ligaments are friable hemorrhage can be more easily controlled by suture than by ligature *en masse ;* (8) bleeding points in the posterior surface of the broad ligament are more accessible after suturing than after the broad ligament has been puckered by ligature. In order to remove pus-tubes without rupture, I. S. Stone[1] prefers to make a longer incision, tie the ovarian and ovaro-uterine arteries and free the specimen at one or both ends or sides before attempting enucleation.

Drainage.—Baldy[2] remarks that the tendency of the day is to as much as possible eliminate drainage, and experience is daily proving that this procedure is less and less necessary in abdominal surgery. He has drained very little of late and has not seen a fistula occur, nor does he know of but 1 or 2 hernias during the past 3 years' work. Not over 5% of cases require drainage. J. G. Clark[3] endorses the postural method of draining the peritoneal cavity after abdominal operations. The method consists in introducing 500 to 1000 c.c. of salt-solution into the peritoneal cavity after thorough irrigation ; the patient is then returned to her room, and the foot of the bed elevated about 20°, which gives sufficient inclination of the posterior pelvic wall to assist the flow toward the general peritoneal cavity. This posture should be maintained for 24–36 hours, after which the bed may be lowered. This method of drainage is offered as a prophylactic measure against postoperative peritonitis, but *not as a curative measure* after the peritonitis is established. It should, therefore, not be employed when an operation is performed for the relief of purulent peritonitis or for inflammatory conditions associated with general peritonitis. According to Watkins,[4] drainage should be employed : (1) when general septic peritonitis exists ; (2) when septic matter has escaped into the general peritoneal cavity ; (3) when necrotic or septic tissue is left in the pelvic cavity ; (4) when hemorrhage exists which cannot be readily controlled by ligature, suture, or temporary pressure ; (5) when an intestine has been so injured that fecal fistula is liable to occur.

After-treatment of Abdominal Section.—According to Clark,[5] thirst may be controlled by saline enemata ; if, however, the fluid is expelled, as is occasionally the case, water in small sips, cracked ice, or small saline enemata may be used to alleviate it. For the *vomiting,* a mustard-plaster over the epigastrium, hot or cold water bags to the nape of the neck, 20 drops of a 5% solution of cocain, cerium oxalate in 1 gr. pill, or chloroform-water may be tried. Rectal feeding must be the only means of alimentation. The treatment of *tympanites* consists in the free administration of purgatives, usually calomel or salts, large high enemata, and the insertion of a rectal tube well up into the colon. The very light application of the Paquelin cautery to the abdominal surface has been of the greatest value in many cases. The platinum point is heated to a dull red and so lightly applied that it makes not a distinct burn, but a decided erythema ; this is accomplished by just touching the tips of the short hairs on the abdomen.

---

[1] Med. News, Aug. 8, 1896.   [2] Am. Gyn. and Obst. Jour., May, 1897.
[3] Bull. Johns Hopkins Hosp., Apr., 1897.   [4] Loc. cit.
                         [5] Therap. Gaz., Dec. 15, 1896.

Complications during and after Abdominal Section.—1. *Stitch-hole Abscesses.*—Clark [1] employs large flaxseed poultices made up with 1 : 1000 mercuric chlorid solution until localization of the pus occurs, when the abscesses are freely opened. Subsequently the abscess-cavity is kept clean with boric-acid irrigations and hydrogen peroxid. W. E. Ashton [2] employs a snare of silkworm-gut to remove infected ligatures from sinus-tracts in the abdominal wall.

2. *Phlebitis.*—Clark [3] lightly touches the line over the inflamed vein with a Paquelin cautery, after which the leg is elevated and enveloped in rolls of cotton and a gauze bandage.

3. *Parotitis.*—W. S. Morrow [4] reports 3 cases occurring during the course of pelvic disease and W. Krusen [5] 2 cases following abdominal sections. [Paget has collected 101 cases of parotitis following injury to the abdominal or pelvic organs, and due not to pyemia, but to reflex nervous action. Fifty of these were due to slight injuries, as a blow or the introduction of a pessary. It may occur during pregnancy. In 78 of the cases 45 were suppurative and 33 resolved without suppuration.]

4. *Peritonitis.*—Michoux [6] during the last 3 years has employed the intravenous injection of serum in 25 to 30 cases of septic peritonitis, obtaining very good results, even though the symptoms were severe, as when there existed tympanites, small and rapid pulse, and subnormal temperature. The serum was that advised by Hayem, and when this could not be procured he employed boiled water containing 105 to 150 gr. of sea-salt to the quart. The quantity of serum used was usually 32 to 48 oz., but in 2 cases 80 and 96 oz. The amount of urine was always very much increased. With this treatment he combines hypodermic injections of ether, caffein, and alcohol. Monod, in 7 patients with septic peritonitis, practised intravenous injections of serum, with the result that 4 died and 3 recovered.

5. *Pulmonary Embolism.*—Gessner [7] believes that the production of thrombosis and the resultant pulmonary embolism is always brought about through the concomitant action of several causes. The origin of the thrombosis is inflammatory disease acting either directly within the blood-channel, or the inflammatory process arises in the tissue surrounding the blood-vessel, and then it extends to the blood-vessel wall. Further important factors that favor thrombosis are the presence of anemia and changes in the heart. These last conditions are most often found with fibroid tumors, which accounts for the greater number of instances of thrombosis and pulmonary embolism associated with this disease. Besides fibroid tumors the malignant new-growths may predispose the patient to thrombosis. The writer considers mechanical causes to be of very little moment. The characteristic increase of the pulse-frequency which Mahler has described in these cases Gessner has not observed in all cases. The careful observation of the pulse after operation is always of the greatest importance. He agrees with Mahler and Wyder that in fatal pulmonary embolism the thrombosis usually occurs in the large pelvic veins. The separation of emboli is without doubt mechanical. The treatment should be chiefly prophylactic. If, in spite of this, pulmonary embolism does occur, the patient is best treated with hypodermic injections of ether and elevation of the upper part of the body. For the subjective symptoms morphin hypodermically has a favorable influence.

[1] Therap. Gaz., Dec. 15, 1896.   [2] N. Y. Med. Jour., Apr. 24, 1897.
[3] Loc. cit.   [4] Montreal Med Jour., Mar., 1896.
[5] Am. Gyn. and Obst. Jour. Nov., 1876.   [6] Gaz. hebdom. de Med. et de Chir., No. 5, 1896.
                [7] Centralbl. f. Gynäk., No. 6, 1897.

6. *Psychoses.*—Jacobs[1] believes that mental derangements that appear immediately after operation offer a more favorable prognosis than those that develop after a considerable lapse of time.

7. *Emphysema of the Abdominal Wall.*—Heil[2] reports this interesting case, 9 others having been recorded : on the third day after a Porro operation (the abdominal incision having been closed with deep and superficial sutures) emphysema developed along both edges of the wound. By the eighth day it had disappeared on the left side, but on the right it extended to the iliac region, when it gradually subsided, no trace of it remaining 4 days later. Madlener affirms that Trendelenburg's position favors the development of emphysema, as air is drawn into the abdominal cavity by the upward movement of the intestines and diaphragm ; hence he advises that the sutures should not be tied until the patient has been lowered to a horizontal posture. Gräfe advises that the abdomen should always be compressed by an assistant before sutures are tied. However, in cases reported by Leopold and Brosin the patient remained in the horizontal position throughout the operation. The writer believes that emphysema is due entirely to imperfect approximation of the deeper layers of the abdominal wall, with firm union of the skin. This he demonstrated clearly by experiments on rabbits. To avoid emphysema, he concludes, as well as hernia, exact approximation of the recti and their sheaths is all-important, the position of the patient being a minor consideration.

8. *Opening of the Abdominal Wound.*—Switalski[3] reports a case in which the wound opened a week after operation as a result of severe and persistent coughing. The suture-material employed in the primary operation was catgut, 3 separate layers being introduced. [This accident is very rare ; Rosner has been able to collect but 31 cases during the last 3 years.]

Vaginal Prolapse.—Baldy[4] describes a method of preventing vaginal prolapse after abdominal hysterectomy. He includes both the ovarian artery and the round ligament in the first ligature on either side ; this ligature is placed as near the pelvic wall as possible, so as to leave but a small amount of broad ligament behind with the stump ; one ligature is placed on each side of the uterus, including the uterine artery, with as little other tissue as possible ; this leaves both broad ligaments open ; the uterus is amputated as low on the cervix as possible. The sutures employed are of heavy silk, and include both the ovarian and uterine stumps, deeply placed well back of the ligatures ; they include the sides of the cervical stump, and when tied lift this together with the vagina and bring it in close approximation with the ovarian stumps, doubling the open broad ligaments together, between which folds firm adhesions take place.

Hysterectomy for Suppurative Disease of the Pelvic Organs.— R. Peterson[5] suggests that after 3 years' work in this line it would be well to pause and ask ourselves not, How many uteri have been removed during this period ? but, How much has been learned from careful microscopic and bacteriologic examinations of these removed organs ? In other words, do the pathologic lesions found in the ablated uteri confirm the correctness of the reasoning of those who, mainly upon clinical grounds, advocate hysterectomy in certain inflammatory pelvic diseases ? He claims that the surgeon has no right to remove the uterus after removal of the appendages unless he is convinced that the organ is diseased beyond the hope of cure by less radical methods.

---

[1] La Policlinique, No. 4, 1896. [2] Arch. f. Gynäk., Bd. lii., H. 3, 1897.
[3] Monats. f. Geb. u Gynäk., Bd. v., H. 4, 1897. [4] Am. Jour. Obst., Jan., 1897.
[5] Jour. Am. Med. Assoc., Aug. 8, 1896.

He believes that the prediction of Baldy made 2½ years ago that uteri would be removed that might safely be left has proved true to a far greater extent than one could have predicted. F. H. Martin[1] gives some reasons why the uterus should not always be removed with bilateral disease of the appendages. In the first place, he believes that many of the cases of apparently incurable diseases of the appendages can be cured without mutilation if time be given, stimulated by rational treatment, for the organs to exert their own powerful natural reparative capabilities. Frequently macroscopically, and, reasoning from analogy, microscopically, the uterus appears absolutely healthy when a septic process has destroyed the integrity of the appendages. Here he would remove the appendages thoroughly and institute a course of treatment for the uterine cavity. In the next place, it is not consistent to remove the body of the uterus and not the cervix, which is the portion most liable to be infected with the primary disease—in its deep glands—and which is also most liable to be infected with carcinoma. The removal of the cervix, however, causes a considerable shortening of the vagina from cicatricial contraction, and, thereby, interferes with the marital relations. In the third place, the nervous phenomena during convalescence from hysterectomy are far greater than from simple removal of diseased appendages.

Hysterectomy in Puerperal Sepsis.—J. H. Croom[2] believes that vaginal hysterectomy for other than malignant disease is much more limited than the present literature of the profession would lead us to believe, for 3 reasons: 1. That in acute septicemia the onset is so sudden and the general systemic infection so rapid that no purely local measures are of any avail. 2. In those cases in which the absorption from septic foci is slow satisfactory results may be obtained by antiseptic irrigation or by curettage. 3. The conditions under which puerperal hysterectomy is undertaken must always be unfavorable, since the woman is exhausted by labor and sepsis. [Practically, there has been no change in the status of this question during the past 2 years and the conclusions advanced in the 2 preceding volumes of the *Year-Book* hold good at the present time.]

Vaginal Incision for Pelvic Disease.—[Those advocating the vaginal methods of operating have during the past year notably receded in their claims and in many instances are returning to the abdominal methods.] Coe[3] states that the *abdominal method* is to be elected in: (1) neoplasms or obscure enlargements which are situated in the abdominal cavity, or have risen above the pelvic brim, especially if such be more or less adherent; (2) ascites of doubtful origin, more particularly when tuberculous or malignant disease is suspected; (3) disease of the adnexa in which the latter are situated near or above the pelvic brim, as established by bimanual palpation; (4) when the history and symptoms point to general intestinal adhesions, and, above all, when appendical complications are suspected; (5) ectopic gestation before rupture, when the sac is high up, at the side or in front of the uterus, instead of in Douglas's pouch; (6) intractable pelvic and abdominal pain of obscure origin, including the so-called neuroses. On the other hand, *explorative vaginal section* is preferred in: (1) cases in which the presence of pus within the pelvis is suspected, as in pyosalpinx, pelvic abscess proper, suppurating dermoids and cysto-adenomata, and hematocele; (2) small intrapelvic tumors situated in the pouch of Douglas, or at least readily accessible from below; impacted ovarian cysts, dermoids, and fibroids belong to this category; (3) adherent adnexa situated in

[1] N. Am. Pract., June, 1897. [2] Brit. Med. Jour., Aug. 1, 1896.
[3] N. Y. Polyclinic, No. 6, 1896.

the true pelvis ; (4) unruptured ectopic sacs in the same locality ; (5) circumscribed exudates and indurations in the broad ligaments or behind the uterus, especially when associated with displacement and fixation of the latter organ. Fehling,[1] in spite of the ease with which the vaginal operation can be performed, and the absence of an external cicatrix and subsequent hernia, regards it as unsatisfactory, since one must always be prepared to perform abdominal section or even to remove the uterus. He believes that anterior kolpotomy for the removal of diseased adnexa must have a limited application. I. S. Stone[2] gives as the most suitable cases for vaginal operation the following : (1) when the patient demands the vaginal extirpation ; (2) when she has borne several children and has a roomy pelvis and vagina ; (3) when the case is of very serious nature, the pulse weak, and the surgeon is in doubt as to her ability to withstand the greater shock of the abdominal operation ; (4) when the sigmoid and rectum are thought to be greatly involved. W. D. Haggard, Jr.,[3] gives as the especial indications for vaginal section : (1) early cases of acute suppurating salpingitis ; (2) incipient post-puerperal peritonitis ; (3) large pyosalpinx and true pelvic abscess.

DISEASES OF THE OVARIES.

Position of the Normal Ovary.—Waldeyer[4] states that the ovary lies normally in a triangular fossa formed by the round ligament, umbilical artery, and ureter. Hernial protrusion of the fossa with the ovary may occur either at the greater ischiatic foramen, or beneath the pyriformis muscle, and in the lesser ischiatic foramen.

The Internal Secretion of the Ovary.—Curatulo[5] publishes the following conclusions in regard to this question : 1. The ablation of the ovaries exercises a considerable influence on metabolism. 2. The quantity of phosphates eliminated by the urine is notably diminished after removal of the ovaries. 3. The curve of nitrogen, after ovariotomy, ascertained either by Kjeldahl's method or by Yvon's, presents a slight oscillation, without a very distinct tendency to elevation or to lowering. 4. After oöphorectomy the quantity of carbonic acid eliminated by the respiration, and that of the oxygen absorbed, diminish considerably up to a certain limit, from which time it remains stationary. 5. In animals from which the ovaries have been removed the curve of the weight is progressively elevated until it attains considerable proportions from five to six months after the operation. 6. When a certain amount of ovarian juice is injected subcutaneously into sluts deprived of the ovaries the quantity of phosphates eliminated by the urine, which diminishes considerably soon after the operation, tends to increase and even to become superior to that which was ascertained before the operation ; when still larger amounts are injected the quantity of phosphates increases in a very marked degree. Hysterectomy performed in conjunction with oöphorectomy does not seem to cause modifications other than those ascertained after simple removal of the ovaries. [This fully accords with observations on the human subject.] The author advances the following theory : the ovaries, like other glands of the animal economy, have, according to Brown-Séquard's general doctrine, a special internal secretion. These glands continually throw into the blood a peculiar product, the chemical composition of which is completely unknown, and the essential properties of which tend to favor the oxidation of phosphor-

[1] Centralbl. f. Gynäk., No. 30, 1896.   [2] Va. Med. Semi-monthly, Nov. 13, 1896.
[3] Am. Gyn. and Obst. Jour., Mar., 1897.   [4] Centralbl. f. Gynäk., No. 30, 1896.
[5] Ann. di Ost. e gin., No. 10, 1896.

ized organic substances, of carbohydrates, and of fatty substances. It results therefrom that, when the function of the ovaries is suppressed, whether because oöphorectomy has been practised or because these organs do not act, as is the case before puberty and after the menopause, there should be produced, on the one hand, a more considerable retention of organic phosphorus, whence there is a greater accumulation of calcareous salts in the bones, and, on the other hand, the very manifest corpulency which is ordinarily seen after oöphorectomy or after the menopause.

Cystomata.—According to J. Fabricus,[1] the following are the different varieties of cysts that occur about the female genitalia: 1. In the broad ligament, about the middle of the tube, is usually found a small cyst not larger than a pepper-corn, which evidently belongs to the broad ligament, as it is not connected with the tube. 2. The hydatid of Morgagni, a cyst usually about the size of a cherry, which is attached to one of the fimbriæ of a tube. Embryologically, this comes from the upper end of Müller's duct. 3. Cysts in the broad ligament between the tube and Gärtner's canal. These cysts have the same characters as those described under 1. They do not seem to have any connection with the epoöphoron. 4. Cysts from the tubes of the parovarium. These cysts always develop interligamentously, but may reach such a size that they press out the peritoneum, and may finally become pedunculated. They are usually not larger than a bean. They are lined on the inside with ciliated cylindric epithelium, and contain a thin serous fluid. The cysts often reach a large size. Kossmann has recently pointed out that the cysts of the broad ligament do not all come from the parovarium, but a great many of them originate from secondary tubes (*Nebentuben*), which may be situated anywhere in the broad ligament. The cyst-wall gives no indication as to the origin of the cyst, as muscular tissue occurs in the walls of both parovarian cysts and those from the secondary tubes. The fimbriæ of the secondary tubes become adherent and form little pedunculated cysts which Kossmann calls *hydroparasalpinx*. Cysts may also originate from the epoöphoron. The different tubes of this organ are often separated widely from one another by the development of the broad ligament, and cysts originating from them occupy different positions. 5. There are also cysts found in the broad ligaments, uterus, or vagina which owe their origin to the Wolffian or Gärtner canals. The termination of these canals has not been definitely determined. Some claim they terminate at the uterus, others think they end at the cervix, while still others believe they extend down the vagina. 6. Cysts are often found between the layers of the broad ligament, which reach the size of a pigeon's egg. They are often symmetric—*i. e.* situated in both ligaments— and are situated near the larger vessels. They are lined with a simple layer of endothelial cells. The author believes them to be merely dilated lymphspaces, while Pozzi considers them cysts of the Wolffian ducts. According to Brigidi,[2] such women are apt to be sterile, because of the frequency with which both ovaries are found in an abnormal position. 7. Chiari has described some little cysts which he has seen about the uterine end of the tube. They were evidently diverticula of the mucous membrane of the tube, caused by a chronic catarrh which had destroyed the muscular coat of the tube. 8. Zedel has described a cyst the size of an apple, into which the right tube opened. The cyst was probably formed by a growing together of the layers of peritoneum about the tube, forming a peritoneal sac into which the tube opens. 9. In addition to the above, the author has found another kind of cyst situated under the serosa of the tube, always multiple, and placed along the whole

[1] Arch. f. Gynäk., v., No. 3, S. 385.　　　　[2] Ann. di Ost. e Gin., No. 3, 1896.

length of the tube. Two cases were observed. In both the cysts were about the size of an oat, and were lined with cylindric epithelium, which was often found undergoing degeneration.

The author thinks that they are formed by a folding in of the serous covering of the tube due to inflammatory processes. The process is exactly similar to that which takes place in the ovary in the formation of Graafian follicles. The flat epithelium of the tube is changed to cylindric epithelium under the influence of the inflammation. This change can readily take place, as is declared by several observers. Thus Paltanf has seen a similar change take place in the pericardium after a pericarditis.

Burckhard[1] has investigated the origin of *multilocular* ovarian cysts, and concludes that all arise in the germinal epithelium, or from Pflüger's tubes. The cysts appear to develop in fetal life as a true malformation. Burckhard cannot find any evidence that a cystoma may develop in a normally formed adult ovary. The cutting off of the cysts from the epithelial tubes is brought about by the underlying connective tissue, and not by an active growth of the epithelium. When a cyst is already developed it does not increase by the pressure of its contents, but by active hyperplasia of its connective-tissue wall with a similarly secondary growth of the epithelial elements.

T. Wilson[2] treats of intermittent cysts of the ovary, those in which there occurs a more or less periodic bursting of the cyst-wall. In some cases after bursting the cyst may be permanently cured. In this event a permanent breach in the wall is supposed to allow the cystic fluid to escape as it is formed into the peritoneal cavity, whence it is at once absorbed by the lymphatics and discharged by the kidneys. In by far the majority of cases the hole in the cyst-wall becomes closed and the fluid re-collects, sometimes in a few weeks, or it may be not for 6 or 8 years.

Semb[3] concludes that the true *papillary cystoma* is a distinct growth, to be separated from the papillary cysto-carcinoma, and also from the papillary colloid cystoma. They are most benign new-growths; the epithelial covering of the papilla is always infiltrative, never shows atypical growths; they do not cause cachexia; never give metastasis; are not destructive, are free from return, and are only dislodged and implanted. The implantation on the peritoneum is also benign. Semb says that carcinomatous degeneration of papillomatous cystoma has never been proved. Usually the papillary growths arise from the superficial epithelium. In one of the cases investigated by the writer the papilloma appeared to develop from the primary follicles. The prognosis in the disease after operation is always good; the remaining papillary growths on the peritoneum disappear. If the growths are extensive, they always follow the course characteristic of benign growths. In elderly persons the writer removes both ovaries, as sometimes a similar growth later develops in the remaining ovary which appears healthy. Frequently the disease is bilateral, and often they grow intraligamentous. Dirner[4] reports a case of ovarian papilloma which on microscopic examination was found to be histologically innocent. Elischer considered that these innocent papillomata are more frequent than is generally suspected. Tauffar insisted that some papillomatous growths of the ovaries are essentially innocent, others distinctly malignant. J. Oliver[5] records a case of pelvic cyst containing cholesterin, and remarks that cholesteatomata originating in the pelvis have evidently no very decided malignant tendency. H. Cripps[6] records a case of ovarian cyst communicating

[1] Virchow's Archiv, vol. cxliv., H. 3, June, 1896.   [2] Ann. of Sur., May, 1897.
[3] Centralbl. f. Gynäk., No. 11, 1896.   [4] Ibid., No. 28, 1896.
[5] Edinb. Med. Jour., July, 1896.   [6] Brit. Med. Jour., Jan. 2, 1897.

with the rectum ; W. H. Baker,[1] an ovarian cyst of 12 years' duration, having a wall 1 in. in thickness ; and Ehrendorfer,[2] a tuberculous ovarian cyst.

Doran[3] points out the anatomic difference between real and apparent encapsulation of ovarian cysts, and shows how important it is for the operator to recognize the true condition before beginning the enucleation of the sac. In the case of an intraligamentous cyst the capsule consists entirely of the mesosalpinx, presents a dull-red appearance, and moves freely over the cyst-wall. After tapping, the sac can be drawn out readily and a pedicle can be obtained without enucleation. This is to be distinguished from false encapsulation, in which the cyst is firmly adherent to the floor of the pelvis and to the posterior layer of the broad ligament, and is covered with a pseudocapsule, with the tube apparently lost on its surface, as in the former case; but here the uterus is flattened against the anterior aspect of the tumor, instead of being pushed over to the opposite side. The anatomic relations are apparently identical with those in the former case, and the surgeon often finds out his error only after removing the cyst and finding that no capsule remains, while the tube and mesovarium are intact. The important practical point is that if the intraligamentous development of the growth is recognized at the onset, the surgeon can begin the process of enucleation cautiously, working between the folds of the broad ligament, and thus avoiding important structures, instead of lacerating the peritoneum and injuring ureters or larger veins by trying to tear up a cyst which he erroneously supposes is bound down in Douglas's pouch. Moreover, the after-treatment of the true capsule (by suturing or drainage) will be entirely different from that of a case of false encapsulation.

Suppuration of Ovarian Cysts.—Bouilly,[4] in a clinical paper on this subject, devotes considerable space to the question of etiology. Owing to the infrequency of tapping at the present day, it is rare that a cyst becomes infected from without. Infection usually comes from an adjacent septic focus, either through the lymphatic channels or bloodvessels, or by direct continuity through the medium of new-formed adhesions. In cases of suppuration of the cyst-contents following labor septic germs are doubtless conveyed through the lymphatics of the broad ligaments from the infected endometrium. The writer has never observed a case of suppuration that could be attributed to coitus during menstruation, as suggested by Mangold. Infectious general diseases may serve as etiologic factors. Two cases of suppuration following typhoid have been reported by Werth, in one of which the characteristic bacilli were found in the cyst-contents. Here the infection is doubtless through the medium of the circulation. In many cases the cause of the suppuration is unknown, especially in dermoids, so that Mangold has advanced the hypothesis that it may result purely from chemical changes in their contents. Infection of ovarian cysts may be distinguished as saprophytic, due to the presence of saprophytic staphylococci, bacterium coli, and similar germs, and septic, caused by pyogenic microorganisms, as the streptococcus pyogenes, gonococcus, bacterium coli commune, and typhoid- and tubercle-bacilli. The clinical symptoms and prognosis are much graver in the latter case, being those of general, as contrasted with those of local, infection.

Rupture of Ovarian Cysts.—Causes of rupture of ovarian cysts may, according to M. Storer,[5] be divided into (1) those arising within the tumor itself, and (2) external causes. The first produce the spontaneous ruptures of frequent observation. In the advancing growth of a proliferating cystoma,

[1] Boston M. and S. Jour., Nov. 19, 1896.   [2] Wien. klin. Woch., No. 15, 1896.
[3] Brit. Med. Jour., Apr. 18, 1896.   [4] La Gynéc., June, 1896.
[5] Boston M. and S. Jour., Nov. 19, 1886.

as the walls of the daughter-cysts are absorbed they may rupture outwardly as well as inwardly. So, too, papillary excrescences, as they impinge against the inner wall of a cyst, may cause pressure-necrosis and perforation. External causes of rupture all come under the general head of traumatism. Storer makes a study of 108 cases collected from literature. In about 30% rupture occurred as the result of sudden, constrained, or violent movement. Rupture may follow torsion, and it has frequently been seen associated with labor. Tapping may cause it.

Torsion.—M. Storer[1] has made a special study of this accident. He states the frequency of rotation as from 25% to 35% of all ovarian tumors and of torsion 8% to 11%. Bilateral rotation is not uncommon. Dermoid tumors are especially liable to the accident. The seat of the torsion is usually in the middle of the uterine third. Sometimes there are 2 or more distinct points of strangulation. The number of twists depends upon the length of the pedicle.

Dermoid Cysts of the Ovary.—Saut Anna[2] records a dermoid cyst in an infant 1 year old; it weighed 2 pounds. Nine other cases are reported in which the ages of the patients varied from 20 months to 7 years, 4 terminating fatally. C. S. Kalb[3] records a case in a girl 3 years 10 months old, and Dandois[4] one in a girl of 5 years; it weighed 15 pounds. E. Knauer[5] records a case in which the sac was filled with perfectly symmetric spheres, surrounded by a yellowish, turbid fluid, and a coil of hair. The balls varied in size from a pea to a nut; were soft, friable, and of a smooth, shining surface. Microscopically they were found to consist of epithelial cells with a small amount of fat interspersed. [This spheric formation of dermoid cyst contents is rare, but 4 similar cases having thus far been described—2 by Rokitansky, 1 by Routh, and 1 by E. Fränkel.] S. Keith[6] records an ovarian dermoid weighing over 100 pounds successfully removed, and W. R. Williams[7] one containing about half a gallon of thick pea-soup fluid with large masses of putty-like substance in which balls of hair were imbedded, the whole being the size of a large football. Rendu[8] removed a dermoid cyst from the round ligament.

Solid Ovarian Tumors.—H. M. Jones[9] and H. Briggs record cases of ovarian fibromata; Gessner,[10] a pure myoma of the ovarian ligament; and G. Seymour[11] a sarcomatous ovary, forming a hernia in the right inguinal region.

D'Urso[12] concludes as follows a comprehensive study of 21 observations of ovarian tumors, most of them personal: 1. In the cortical substance of the normal ovary there are remains of germinal epithelium in the form of cystic formations, which sometimes present the appearance of modified sweat-glands. 2. The Kobelt tubes of the mesosalpinx in the adult have sometimes irregular and papillary outlines. 3. The tubes of the epoöphoron penetrate into the hilus and the medullary substance, and produce cavernous papillary formations, besides the isolated tubule. 4. There are also found in the mesosalpinx, altogether at the abdominal end, small knobs of epithelial tubes, which proceed from the remains of the Wolffian body. 5. The cysts of the ovaries and broad ligaments can be classified into : (*a*) cystic adenoma, glandular neoplasms formed from the epithelial remains of the cortex ; (*b*) simple Wolffian

[1] Boston M. and S. Jour., Nov. 7, 1896.   [2] Sem. méd., No. 18, 1896.
[3] Med. Sentinel, Mar., 1897.   [4] Arch. de Gynéc. et de Tocol., Mar., 1896.
[5] Wien. klin. Woch., June 18, 1896.   [6] Brit. Gyn. Jour., part 44, p. 466, 1896.
[7] Brit. Med. Jour., Oct. 10, 1896.   [8] Ann. de Gynéc. et d'Obst., July, 1896.
[9] Lancet, Aug. 1, 1896.   [10] Zeit. f. Geb. u. Gynäk, vol. xxxiv., part 2, 1896.
[11] Med. News, Feb. 20, 1897.   [12] Centralbl. f. Chir., Apr. 10, 1897.

cysts; (c) papillary Wolffian cysts, developing from the epithelial remains in the hilus and mesosalpinx, without glandular formations. 6. Malignant papillary cysts present a peculiar proliferation of the epithelium, contrary to malignant papillary Wolffian cysts. 7. Dermoid cysts show evidences of transformation from simple cysts to true teratomas. Some can be traced to fetal contents, others probably to embryonal development from the ovum cell. 8. Ovarian fibromas can develop in the connective tissue of the corticalis, independently of the corpora lutea and the regressive metamorphoses of the Graafian follicles. 9. Among the simple, connective-tissue ovarian tumors, endotheliomas often occur, not infrequently malignant, which cannot be explained by peculiarities in the histologic structure. He has nothing to say in regard to the histogenesis of alveolar sarcoma and endothelioma except the query whether the theca folliculi may not be the matrix. 10. There is a simple true epithelioma of the ovary; it develops very slowly and probably originates in the epithelium of the papillary embryonal remains of the hilus.

Angiodystrophia Ovarii.—Bulius[1] refers to a chronic diseased condition of the ovaries in which there is no very distinct enlargement; the pathologic anatomy shows nothing of importance; there are definite functional disturbances and other phenomena. The characteristics of these changes are: (1) Macroscopically, enlargement of the ovaries, particularly in their greatest diameter, the formation of deep furrows on the surface, remarkable density of the entire organ, and the formation of cysts. (2) Extensive disease and increase in the number of blood-vessels. The arteries and capillaries are separated in the medulla and cortex. The disease is an extensive thickening and hyaline degeneration of the walls with obstruction of the lumen. (3) Marked reduction in the primary (developing) follicles; developing to the completely developed follicles are seen, with small cystic degeneration of the Graafian follicles; decisive pathologic occurrences in the retrograde metamorphosis of the misplaced, augmented, and destroyed follicles. The clinical symptoms, which are dependent upon the amount of anatomic changes, are very profuse menstrual hemorrhage, lasting sometimes 3 weeks; and pain in the abdomen and back, occurring paroxysmally, the paroxysm often being so long that the patient is free from pain only a few days. Also there are severe nervous symptoms. Endometritis is constantly associated. There is comparatively little change in the remaining genital organs. Bulius believes the changes in the ovaries must be regarded as primary. As to the cause of the disease nothing definite up to the present time has been determined. The results after oöphorectomy in 4 cases were good, in 3 others the hemorrhage ceased and the pain disappeared. Herff, in the discussion of this paper, stated that he doubted the belief that the disease is primary in the ovaries. The fact that patients had not been improved through oöphorectomy seemed to prove that it is a neurosis. Bulius replied that in only one of his cases could the disease possibly be considered a neurosis, and therefore it must be primary in the ovary.

Tuberculosis of the Ovaries.—Wolff[2] concludes an elaborate article on this subject by denying the probability of primary infection of the ovaries, since the changes in the ovisacs are so slight as compared with the advanced degeneration in other organs. He believes that there is direct infection of the peritoneal covering of the ovaries, transmitted either through the tubes or from the pelvic peritoneum. It is, of course, impossible to exclude as an etiologic factor the entrance of bacilli, carried through the blood-vessels from distant organs, though this mode of infection must be exceptional. In all the writer's cases there was no doubt as to the fact of direct infection. The ques-

---

[1] Centralbl. f. Gynäk., No. 44, 1896.   [2] Arch. f. Gynäk., Bd. lii., H. 2, 1896.

tion of the transmission of tuberculosis from the mother to the fetus through the medium of the infected ovum is an interesting one. Although it must be admitted that the development of such an ovum is arrested, it is possible that the tubercle-bacilli from an infected Graafian follicle after the rupture of the ovum may, together with the latter, enter the uterus and infect it during the development of the ovum.

The Anatomy of the Ovaries in Osteomalacia.—Heyse,[1] from a careful microscopic study of ovaries removed from osteomalacic women, decides that there is no reason to infer that there is a marked decrease in the number of primordial follicles. This is also proved by the well-known fertility of these subjects. He believes that the ovarian nerves play an important part in the process, and that future investigations will disclose pathologic changes in them; but whether these changes are primary or secondary is not clear. Unfortunately, ovaries have not been examined in an early stage of the disease.

Hernia of the Ovary in an Infant.—Lockwood[2] reports the following interesting case : a female infant, aged 6 months, suddenly became ill, drawing up its legs as if suffering from severe abdominal pain. Two days later a swelling was noticed in the right inguinal region, tender, and disappearing on pressure. When brought to the hospital an examination of the little patient showed a tense, oval swelling, 3 in. long and 1½ in. broad, the skin covering it being inflamed. There was no impulse on crying. Obstinate constipation and occasional vomiting were present, but flatus and later fecal matter were passed. The diagnosis of strangulated inguinal hernia was made. On incising the swelling a quantity of dark grumous fluid escaped, and a mass appeared which was at first supposed to be the cecum, but proved to be the fimbriated end of the Fallopian tube and a hemorrhagic ovary, the pedicle of which emerged from the internal abdominal ring being twisted half around its axis, but not constricted at the ring. The pedicle was transfixed and tied, the tube, ovary, and sac excised, and the stump attached beneath the internal oblique and transversalis muscles. The inguinal canal was sutured and the external wound closed with silkworm-gut. The patient's convalescence was normal. The cause of the torsion was obscure, but was probably due to the fact that, as the ovary and tube slipped through the internal ring, the ovary lay in front of and above the tube and slipped down in front of it, thus producing the twist. A similar case has been reported by Owen.

[1] Arch. f. Gynäk., Bd, liii., H. 2, 1897.　　　　[2] Brit. Med. Jour., June 13, 1896.

PEDIATRICS.

By LOUIS STARR, M. D., AND THOMPSON S. WESTCOTT, M. D.,

OF PHILADELPHIA.

The Year's Work.—It is almost impossible to single out any one department of pediatrics for special mention, with the advance that has been made along the whole line. The fields in which there was greater room for work and in which, perhaps, more was accomplished, were those of etiology and pathology. In these lines the contagious diseases offer abundant opportunity, and we need only refer to the investigations on pertussis and parotitis to indicate the activity that is being shown. The success which has attended serum-therapy in diphtheria has been a great stimulus to all methods of treatment, but especially in the same line, although we do not expect a second antitoxin to be developed (we are considering only pediatrics, and therefore exclude tetanus and its antitoxin) until the etiology and pathology of the different diseases are more thoroughly worked out. With reference to the antitoxin of diphtheria, its value is so well established that we have not deemed it necessary at this time to go into the question of statistics as thoroughly as before. Those that have been given in the preceding issues of the *Year-Book* should convince any unbiassed reader that it has value ; and if he will then observe the effects of a proper dose given in the early stages of a severe ease of the disease, he will be convinced that no case of diphtheria should be allowed to run its course without the injection of antitoxin. In our review we have noticed only one article opposing its use, not because there have been no others, but because they are merely reiterations of what had been mentioned in the preceding issues, and seem to consider the antitoxin an empiric remedy rather than a specific, as it is in almost the highest sense of the term. As J. McFarland stated in the discussion before the American Medical Association, a definite amount of antitoxin (a) will render inert a certain amount of toxin (t); n times a will render inert n times t. The fact that some cases of diphtheria die after injections of antitoxin is no argument against its use. The activity in pediatrics has not been limited to the field as covered by the articles in the journals. Many treatises on pediatrics or some of its branches have appeared ; and while it is impossible to mention all that deserve it, the following are some of the noteworthy ones: in Germany Baginsky's *Lehrbuch der Kinderkrankheiten* is in its fifth edition, and Henoch's *Vorlesungen über Kinderkrankheiten* is in its ninth. In France A. B. Marfan has written a book on artificial feeding, and J. Grancher, J. Comby, and A. B. Marfan are editing a *Traité des Maladies de l'Enfance* in two volumes. In this country we must go back beyond the past year to mention A. Jacobi's *Therapeutics of Infancy and Childhood*, and J. L. Smith's *Diseases of Childhood;* during the past year L. E. Holt's *Diseases of Infancy and Childhood* has been published.

605

INFANT-FEEDING. ·

Bunker's Modification.—H. A. Bunker[1] suggests a method of increasing the digestibility of the proteids of cow's milk which seems to be similar to that originally recommended by Jacobi in 1876, to boil milk with dilute hydrochloric acid. The method of procedure is simple : a solution of hydrochloric acid in milk is secured by adding from 20 to 30 drops of a 10% acid to 1 pint of water and then mixing thoroughly with 1 quart of milk. The mixture is then boiled, with constant stirring, for 20 minutes, or is kept at a boiling temperature for that length of time in an Arnold sterilizer. If the milk shows decided activity to litmus, the milk-acids should be neutralized with lime-water before further preparation. The loss by evaporation in boiling in an open vessel may be made up, if desired or found necessary, by a fresh addition of water ; or further dilution may be made to meet the demands or limitations of any special case. No addition of sugar is necessary except when heavily sweetened foods, like condensed milk, have previously been used, and under these circumstances the amount can be rapidly lessened. His experience has been that such milk is easily digested and gives full nutrition after failure with plain sterilization or partial peptonization. L. Grant Baldwin,[2] who has made use of the method, considers it far superior to any artificial food he has tried. [In the discussion Golding stated that the method was proposed by Ruddisch, one of Jacobi's assistants, but was abandoned because no milk in the market could be found sufficiently fresh to remain uncoagulated.]

Infant Foods Compared.—R. H. Chittenden[3] has made a careful comparative analytic study of a number of the most widely known manufactured infant foods, standardizing their products as prepared for the nursing-bottle in accordance with directions for infants of 6 months ; and these are compared with the analysis of mother's milk, according to Leeds. The table is of considerable interest :

	Mothers' milk.	Malted milk.	Nestlé's milk food.	Imperial granum.	Mellin's food.	Peptogenic milk powder.
Specific gravity	1031	1025	1024	1025	1031	1032
Water	86.73	92.47	92.76	91.53	88.00	86.03
Total solid matter (by direct determination). .	13.26	7.43	7.24	8.47	12.00	13.97
Inorganic salts.	0.20	0.29	0.13	0.34	0.47	0.26
Total albuminoids	2.00	1.15	0.81	2.15	2.62	2.09
Soluble albuminoids . . .	2.00	1.15	0.36	1.67	2.62	2.09
Insoluble albuminoids . .	0	trace.	0.45	0.48	0	0
Fat.	4.13	0.68	0.36	1.54	2.89	4.38
Milk-sugar	6.93	1.18	0.84	2.71	3.25	7.26
Cane-sugar	0	0	2.57	0	0	0
Maltose	0	3.28	trace.	trace.	2.20	0
Dextrin	0	0.92	} 0.44	0.58 {	0.53	0
Soluble starch	0	0			0	0
Starch	0	0	1.99	1.22	0	0
Reaction	alkaline.	alkaline.	alkaline.	alkaline.	alkaline.	alkaline.

If, as Chittenden observes, mother's milk is to be accepted as the standard, it will be seen from the table that cow's milk, modified by the addition of water, cream, and peptogenic milk powder, offers a product containing to the full extent all of the proximate principles present in human milk and wholly free

[1] Brooklyn Med. Jour., Nov., 1896.　　[2] Ibid.　　[3] N. Y. Med. Jour., July 18, 1896.

from extraneous admixtures. The process of modification takes into account the radical difference between cow's casein and human casein, and affords a method by which the former can be modified to a closer resemblance to the latter without the addition of any substance that will permanently interfere with the purity of the final product. [Partial peptonization by this method may be quite satisfactorily employed with milk mixtures of other proportions, according to the methods of laboratory modification, and also with cream and condensed milk mixtures in the rare cases in which condensed milk seems to be the only form of milk that can be borne.]

Dufour[1] gives the following method for **humanizing cow's milk:** put the quantity of milk suitable for one day at the child's age into a large graduate with a corked spout at the bottom. Set aside tightly covered and at proper temperature for about 4 hours to allow the cream to rise. Draw off one-third the lower milk and add the same amount of water. Add 35 gm. milk-sugar and 1 gm. of salt per liter. Shake and pour into sterilized bottles.

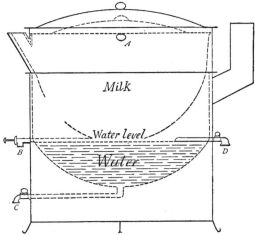

FIG. 46.—Aymard's milk-sterilizer, large size.

If the child's gain in weight is unsatisfactory, add a teaspoonful or two of cream to the whole amount of milk. [The replacement of one-third of the bulk of milk by an equal quantity of water reduces the proteids and salts of the milk, but does not reduce the proteids of the cream.] More definite results are obtained in the wholesale manipulation advised by Dufour, in which the milk is diluted with one-third of water, and to each liter of mixture are added 15 to 20 gm. of fresh cream, 35 gm. milk-sugar, and 1 gm. sodium chlorid. The amount of cream here added produces 4% or more of fat. This preparation is used in all cases, the amount at a feeding alone varying with the age of the child.

Aymard's Sterilizer.—One of the recent additions to sterilizing apparatus is Aymard's,[2] two sizes of which are here pictured. It differs from the usual form in having the receptacle for the milk shut off·tightly from the

[1] Rev. mens. des Mal. de l'Enfance, Sept., 1896.   [2] Brit. Med. Jour., Oct. 10, 1896.

steam-chamber, though exposed partly to the air by a narrow spout. In the small sizes about 10 minutes are required to raise the milk to a temperature of 200° F., after the water has begun to boil. It is claimed that there is no separation of cream or formation of scum on the surface, which is partly accounted for by the fact that the milk-chamber is entirely closed during heating and cooling, thus keeping the whole bulk of milk at an equable temperature. There is said to be but slight alteration in the taste and smell of the milk, and the loss by evaporation is reduced to a minimum. It is not claimed to produce absolute sterilization by this apparatus, and it is not adapted to purposes of storage; but it can be counted upon to destroy all adventitious pathogenic microorganisms. Larger sizes of the apparatus are made for use in institutions.

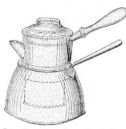

FIG. 47.—Aymard's milk sterilizer, small size.

An Improvement of the Dresden Modification.—Hesse[1] describes in detail an improvement on the so-called Dresden modification, a description of which from an English observer, Worcester, was given in the *Year-Book* for 1897 (p. 749). Using Lehmann's analyses of human milk and cow's milk, Hesse demonstrates that if to 1 liter of 9.5% cream 1½ liters of water are added, and to this 105 gm. of milk-sugar, and fresh egg-albumin (enough to represent 9.5 gm. dried albumin), a mixture is produced yielding 1.2% casein, 0.5% albumin, 3.8% fat, 6% sugar, and 0.3% ash. To insure sterilization, however, he has found better results can be obtained by drying and pulverizing the paste of albumin and sugar; and the similarity to human milk is more closely approached by adding to this in process of manufacture a certain amount of lacto-saccharate of iron. The resulting sterile powder is readily soluble in water, and when added to the diluted cream produces a mixture very closely resembling mother's milk in all its ingredients. In practice it was found that a reduction of the fat-percentage to 3, and of the sugar-percentage to 4.5, gave a more readily digested mixture. In a series of cases fed from birth for 1 to 5 months, the average monthly gain was 13 oz. [Not a very encouraging showing under conditions most satisfactory for testing a new process of feeding.]

Use and Limitation of Condensed Milk in Infant-feeding.— C. G. Kerley[2] recognizes the inadequacy of dilutions of condensed milk as an infant diet, and states that fully 95% of the many hundred marasmic and rachitic children observed had been fed on the meal foods or on condensed milk. At the same time he feels constrained to use condensed milk in many cases among the poor, the ignorant, and the careless, making up the deficiency in fat and proteids by the addition of cream or, in dispensary practice, of cod-liver oil. With the latter cases the dose of oil varies with the age of the baby, the ability to digest it, and the season of the year. Ten drops to a dessert-spoonful, 3 or 4 times daily after feeding, are usually prescribed. During very hot weather the dose must be reduced or suspended if there are evidences of gastrointestinal disturbance. The low proportion of proteids may be increased by adding a meat-broth prepared by boiling 1 pound of lean beef in a quart of water till the liquid is reduced to 1 pint. Such a broth contains 0.8% proteids, so that 1 part of condensed milk to 12 of broth will give 0.5% fat, 1.4% proteids, and 4% sugar, which with cod-liver oil will suffice till the age of 6

---

[1] Berlin. klin. Woch., July 27, 1896.   [2] Med. News, vol. lxx., No. 23, 1897.

months, when 1 part of condensed milk to 9 of broth may be used with the oil till the 8th or 9th month.

Sterilization.—Referring to the danger of scurvy from the use of sterilized milk J. K. Barton[1] states that comparatively or temporarily sterilized milk may be administered for any length of time without fear, but that sterilized milk that is put into hermetically sealed vessels, and which can thus keep fresh for several or many days, will produce scurvy unless some fresh food is administered daily. One meal of fresh whey daily will achieve this in younger infants than those who may have fresh vegetables, meat, or fruit.

Low-temperature Pasteurization.—R. G. Freeman's[2] later studies have led him to recommend a lower temperature for pasteurization than was previously considered necessary. From his previous studies he concluded that the tubercle-bacillus was the most resistant organism found in milk, and could not be certainly destroyed by a lower temperature than 75° C. More recent experiments, however, by various competent observers have given him strong reason to believe that a temperature of 65° C. for 15 minutes is amply sufficient to kill tubercle-bacilli. He has accordingly modified his pasteurizer in order to fit it for this lower temperature. If the milk introduced has a temperature of 10° C. (50° F.), the resultant temperature will be about 68° (155° F.); while if the milk has a temperature of 20° C. (68° F.), the resultant temperature will be about 69½° C. (157° F.). The improved apparatus is shown in the accompanying cuts (Figs. 48, 49).

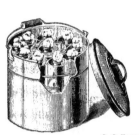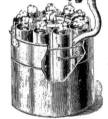

R. G. Freeman's pasteurizer.

FIG. 48.—Showing the apparatus arranged for heating the milk before the pail is covered.

FIG. 49.—Showing the apparatus arranged for cooling the milk.

Breast-milk Variations in Prematurity.—V. and J. S. Adriance[3] present a clinical report of the chemical examination of milk from 200 mothers, which especially emphasizes the fact that in every case of prematurity the variations of the colostrum-period are present, but are exaggerated in the proteids. This increase in proteids extends over a longer interval than in ordinary colostrum-milk, and is not easily dispelled; it consequently taxes the delicate digestive organs of the untimely born infant for a longer period than usual in term-infants. In these cases it is difficult to say how long the disturbance will persist, and it is often wiser to give the child to a wetnurse whose milk has been demonstrated to be good by its effect upon her child and by analysis. In the meantime the mother's breast should be pumped and kept active for future use.

Analysis of Colostrum-milk.—George Woodward[4] has made a series

[1] Brit. Med. Jour., Jan. 2, 1897.
[3] Ibid., Feb., 1897.
[2] Arch. of Pediatrics. Aug., 1896.
[4] Jour. Exper. Med., Mar., 1897.

39

of analyses of human colostrum-milk from 6 cases, which has been carried out with great care and accuracy. He concludes that colostrum-corpuscles are not always found in so-called colostrum-milk; but when they are present the percentage of proteids is higher, and as they disappear the percentage falls. The color of colostrum-milk is yellow, especially marked in negroes' milk; its reaction is alkaline, and its sp. gr. varies from 1024 to 1034, this variation being chiefly due to variation in the amount of fat. The fat varies from 2% to 5.3%, the proteids from 1.64% to 2.22%, and the ash from 0.14% to 0.42%. The total solids vary from 10.18% to 13.65%. An average colostrum-milk contains fat 4.00, proteids 1.9, lactose 6.5, ash 0.20, making the total solids 12.5. Two of the cases confirmed the observation of Townsend, that the infants of multiparæ do not lose as much weight in the colostrum-period of lactation as the children of primiparæ, and the 4 other cases showed results which agreed with those of the same observer—that the shorter the period of colostrum-milk the smaller is the so-called physiologic loss of weight in the newborn.

INFECTIOUS DISEASES.

Diphtheria.—Etiology.—In a discussion on "Diphtheria in Town and Country," before the British Medical Association,[1] interesting facts were mentioned, but nothing definitely established to account for epidemics of diphtheria. J. C. Thresh advanced the opinion that the proper field for investigation is the origin of sporadic cases, as their study will be more likely to lead to valuable etiologic conclusions than the investigations of extensive epidemies. He studied the statistics of the county of Essex, and found that the only positive point favoring the spread of cases was the overcrowding of population in the tenement-houses of towns. The quality of the water-supplies, presence or absence of drainage, the character of the soil and subsoil, seemed of trifling importance. The curve of the number of cases shows a depression in the early part of the year (February or March) and a marked rise in October. The time of the summer vacation seems to exclude the schools from playing any part in outbreaks, unless possibly a restraining influence.

For London, F. A. Dixey[2] showed that there is a decrease in the number of cases during the summer vacation for each year. He gave the figures for the case-mortality during the past 3½ years, and concluded that it is difficult to see what cause can have been at work to produce the marked diminution from 23.8 to 20.2 (representing the annual saving of some hundreds of lives), unless it be the treatment by antitoxin. Gordon Sharp[3] gave the results of his studies as to the relation of soil to diphtheria and its organism. He was able to obtain from a peaty surface-soil (rich in organic matter) over a hard subsoil, an organism which in morphology and cultural peculiarities was indistinguishable from the diphtheria-bacillus. Diphtheria had been prevalent some years before in that district in a very fatal form, and still occurred up to recent times. His conclusions are: 1. Diphtheria would appear to be endemic in certain districts. Soils organically laden are dangerous, but much may depend on the nature of the subsoil. Where the subsoil is porous a neighborhood may be free. Where the subsoil is impervious the surface at certain seasons of the year may be a favorable breeding-ground. 2. Deep drainage renders soils innocuous which would be otherwise sources for spreading the disease. 3. A large amount of air in the surface-soil has a beneficial effect, and

[1] Brit. Med. Jour., Aug. 22, 1896.   [2] Ibid.   [3] Ibid.

the contrary holds. This may be accidental. A moist rather than a water-laden soil seems to be the home of the organism of diphtheria.

DeBlasi and Russo-Travali[1] examined cultures from 234 cases of membranous angina, with the following results: 1. In 26 cases, with a mortality of 3.8 %, the diphtheria-bacillus was absent. 2. Pure cultures of the diphtheria-bacillus were obtained from 102 cases; mortality, 27 %. 3. The bacillus was associated with the staphylococcus pyogenes in 76 cases; mortality, 33 %. 4. The bacillus was present with the streptococcus pyogenes and Fränkel's pneumococcus 7 times; mortality, 43 %. 5. The bacillus was present with the streptococcus pyogenes 20 times; mortality, 30 %. 6. In 3 cases the bacterium coli was associated with the bacillus, the mortality being 100 %, which tends to show that the addition of the bacterium coli increases the severity of the disease. The virulence of the bacterium may be increased relatively by the action of the diphtheria-germ in lowering the vital resistance or directly as a result of the association of the two germs. [If the cultures in this last instance were taken shortly before death, it would of course be necessary to consider agonal infection as perhaps the cause for the appearance of the colon-bacillus.]

C. L. Wilbur[2] gives a statistic study of diphtheria and croup in Michigan with reference to age and sex incidence. He finds that the two forms of the disease are distinctly separated by their age and sex incidence, and also by their monthly and seasonal prevalence. Under 5 years of age males furnish a higher death-rate from diphtheria than females, while the reverse holds after 5 years of age, the reason for which is not clear. He suggests that it would be better to ascertain the death-rates for diphtheria and croup in terms of the susceptible population, under 15 for diphtheria, and under 5 for croup.

G. Homan[3] has also studied the relations of diphtheria and croup as shown by the statistics of the city of St. Louis.

Pathology.—H. B. Biggs[4] (in connection with the bacteriologic laboratory of the Health Department of New York City) investigated the virulence of the diphtheria-bacilli found in some cases of simple acute angina not presenting the clinical features of what is usually called diphtheria. In 48 such cases there were non-virulent bacilli in only 3. Out of 450 primary cultures made from April 1st–28th only 239 were true diphtheria. One hundred and seven cases reported as diphtheria to the department were excluded from that list by the bacteriologic examination, while during the same period only 80 cases considered to be false diphtheria or of doubtful nature were found to be due to the diphtheria-bacilli. [These rather important figures are the only ones which have come to notice tending to throw doubt on the oft-repeated claim that the bacteriologic diagnosis of diphtheria would in itself tend to lower the mortality of diphtheria by including a greater number of mild cases than it would exclude.] The author contends that the anatomic conception of diphtheria (an inflammation associated with the formation of a false membrane) is insufficient, and "that all inflammations of mucous membranes due wholly or in part to the Klebs-Löffler bacillus should be included under the name 'diphtheria' without reference to the site or extent or intensity of the inflammatory process or the character of the exudate."

B. M. Bolton's[5] observations in Philadelphia bear out Biggs with reference to the effect of bacteriology on the total number of diphtheria cases. Of 557 cases diagnosed as diphtheria, the bacilli were present in 507, or 90.2 %. Of 148 cases which were not considered by the attending physician to be diph-

[1] Riforma med., No. 170, 1896.   [2] Jour. Am. Med. Assoc., Aug. 15, 1896.
[3] Med. Mirror, No. 3, 1896.   [4] Am. Jour. Med. Sci., Oct., 1896.
[5] Med. and Surg. Reporter, June 16, 1896.

theria, bacilli were present in 40. The total number of true diphtheria cases, then, was reduced to 547.

Loos[1] experimented on animals with the blood-serum of healthy and diphtheric children, and found that in severe cases of diphtheria the blood can be shown to contain the toxin. Antitoxin is found in the blood not immediately, but some time after an attack. It is also found after a curative, but not after an immunizing dose of antitoxic serum.

Wassermann,[2] working on a similar line, found that the blood-serum of some individuals had strong antitoxic properties, while that of others had none, explaining the difference in the liability of individuals to diphtheria. It is of interest in this connection to refer to Fischl and Wunscheim's investigations on the blood of newborn infants (see *Year-Book* for 1897, p. 727).

J. Love[3] also studied the blood-serum of healthy and diphtheric children with regard to the diphtheria toxins and antitoxins. In order to determine whether an injection of the healing serum would cause the serum of the individual to acquire antitoxic properties, a boy of 3 years was bled, and the serum found to have no antidiphtheric qualities. An injection of Behring's serum equal to 2000 units was then made, and 14 hours later the same blood not only delayed death in guinea-pigs, but actually prevented it. Five cases were next tested to determine whether a prophylactic injection could be recognized, 150 units being employed. The results were negative, and as a further proof of their slight utility 1 of the children under observation actually had an attack of diphtheria—a very mild one, however. By good fortune, a child, whose serum had been previously examined and found to contain no antitoxic qualities, suffered an attack of diphtheria. Fifteen days after recovery its serum manifestly delayed death in the guinea-pigs under experimentation, and at 60 days it had a distinct antitoxic influence. Love explains the lesser activity of the 15th day's serum by supposing that the reabsorbed toxins counteract, to a certain extent, the action of the antitoxins. In 2 cases where serum had not possessed any antitoxic properties during the course of the disease antitoxins appeared after recovery, at least in sufficient quantity to delay death. In 1 case strongly antitoxic serum was found during the course of the disease; but as in this instance cocci were found in the membrane and desquamation of the skin appeared, it was considered one of scarlet fever. In 2 instances virulent diphtheria-bacilli were found in the mouths of healthy children, and in both cases their serum was found to have strong antitoxic properties. On the other hand, toxins were found in the blood of a child suffering from a severe attack of diphtheria, that had failed to react to the serum-treatment. Love believes that this case indicates the limitation of the value of Behring's serum, as it shows that where patients are attacked in whom no antitoxin exists the poison can produce so much injury to the organs that recovery is impossible. Finally, investigation upon 2 children suffering from indifferent diseases showed that human blood-serum may retain its antitoxic properties unaltered for a long series of weeks.

G. S. Engel[4] has made a number of observations on the blood in diphtheria, finding but one feature which seems to have value from a prognostic point. If the myelocytes (large, mononuclear, neutrophilie leucocytes) are present in 2% or more, the case will terminate fatally. The reverse of this does not always hold good, as 8 fatal cases were observed which showed no increase in these cells.

[1] Jahrb. f. Kinderh., B. 42, H. 3 and 4.   [2] Zeit. f. Hyg., Bd. 19.
[3] Wien. klin. Woch., May 28, 1896, ref. in Internat. Med. Mag., Aug., 1896.
[4] Deutsch. med. Woch., Feb. 18 and 25, 1897.

Symptoms.—O. Vierordt,[1] on the clinical features of diphtheria and diphtheroid anginas, remarks that it must always be the aim of clinical medicine to be able to establish a diagnosis in the simplest way possible and at the sick-bed. While methods of precision, examinations with the microscope and chemic reagents, may make the diagnosis of a disease clear, they are not sufficient for forming a judgment of an individual case, and individual patients are the objects of treatment rather than a " disease-form." He discusses then the clinical features of different forms of anginas and the bacteriologic investigations. He lays stress upon a point to which Koplik (*Year-Book* for 1897, p. 758) in this country has called attention, namely, that typical lacunar anginas may be of bacillary (Klebs-Löffler) origin. Such a tonsillitis may be follicular throughout its course, or it may develop after a few days into clinical diphtheria. On the other hand, there are anginas which resemble diphtheria in the formation of pseudomembrane, but differ from it in the absence of the specific bacillus. A feature of this group is its tendency to relapses. He recommends, to describe this class, the term suggested by Heubner—" diphtheroid " [which is much better than the term at present rather loosely used in this country to describe the same condition—" diphtheritic "]. For the other groups lacunar diphtheria and simple lacunar tonsillitis will be accurately descriptive. Unfortunately, these cannot always be separated clinically, and therefore bacteriologic investigation is greatly to be desired in each case. He describes 2 cases of necrotic angina, due to the staphylococcus pyogenes, setting up rodent ulceration.

Paralysis.—Goodall[2] has contributed a valuable paper analyzing the statistics of 1071 cases of diphtheria, occurring in preantitoxin days, with special reference to the occurrence of paralysis. The mortality-rate was 33.8%. Of the 709 survivors, 125, or 17.6%, became paralyzed, and 17 succumbed to the sequel. 22% were under 10 years of age, which is contrary to Gowers' statement that adults furnish the largest proportion of paralysis after diphtheria. The appearance of paralysis varied from the 7th to the 49th day, in the majority of cases not occurring until after the throat had cleared. The palate alone was first affected in 66% of the cases, and in combination with other muscles in 12% more. In a little over half of the cases the paralysis was limited, while it was generalized in about 12%. In no case did facial, glossal, vesical, or rectal paralysis occur. Sensory disturbances were common, manifested by tingling and numbness in the fingers and toes. The paralysis, which was not permanent in any case, varied from 1 to 15 weeks in duration. Contrary to Henoch and Gowers, Goodall, with de Gassicourt, found that the probability of paralysis increased with the severity of the attack of diphtheria. Goodall divides the modes of heart-failure into 3 groups, as follows: 1. That occurring when exudation is still present on the fauces, before other symptoms of paralysis have appeared, and being due to the direct action of the toxins on the nervous mechanism. 2. That occurring, after disappearance of the membrane, but during the other symptoms of paralysis, and being due to disturbed innervation or fatty changes of the heart-muscle, such as occur in fevers. 3. That occurring in convalescence, some time after the membrane has disappeared, and resulting from a degeneration either of the muscle or of the vagus. The symptoms usually present in the latter condition are: (*a*) alteration in the action of the heart; (*b*) paresis or paralysis of the intrinsic muscles of the larynx and alteration in the rhythm of respiration; (*c*) vomiting.

[1] Berlin. klin. Woch., No. 8, 1897.
[2] Brain, 1895; ref. in Buffalo Med. Jour., Oct., 1896, from Jour. of Nerv. and Ment. Dis., July, 1896.

Otto Katz[1] gives a valuable "contribution to the study of diphtheric paralysis." He has found the ganglion-cells always affected by one of two morbid processes, the more severe and uncommon of the two being necrosis or direct local death of the cell, which causes death of its processes, especially the axis-cylinder. The other process, less severe, is manifested by the appearance of fat-granules in the cell, and causes a degeneration of the nerve-fibres, not, like the first, an irreparable damage. That the neuron is only diseased and not destroyed, in this lighter affection, is seen in the greater difficulty in swallowing that patients experience, after a night's rest, than later on in the day, when the repeated attempts have, through irritation, made the reflexes more active. The same effect is seen when different substances are swallowed, a bland fluid like milk being harder to swallow than an alcoholic beverage. Katz believes that, aside from the true symptoms of paralysis, the other symptoms in convalescence, the weakness, loss of energy, anorexia, etc., are dependent upon central nervous disturbances. The cases under observation showed that the medulla oblongata was affected earlier and more severely, as a rule, than the rest of the cerebrospinal axis, but the greater prominence of symptoms depending on affection of the medulla is partly due to the importance of the nerves arising from it. The reason for the weaker resistance of the medulla to the action of the toxin is probably physiologic rather than anatomic, and depends upon the ceaseless activity of the centers of life with a consequent greater demand upon the circulation, and, therefore, a greater amount of toxin to resist.

A. Levi[2] reports a case of cerebral hemiplegia in the course of diphtheria, and reviews the literature of the subject. The causes, in the order of their frequency, are embolism, hemorrhage, and thrombosis. The complication is most frequent among older children, from 8 to 15 years, and the prognosis is grave, both for life and for restoration of function of the paralyzed limbs.

Diagnosis.—E. L. Vansant[3] thinks that fewer cases of clinical diphtheria would give negative bacteriologic results if cultures were taken from the nasal cavities as well as from the pharynx, illustrating the statement by notes of 2 cases.

Koplik,[4] in referring to the urgent need for a rapid method of bacteriologic diagnosis of diphtheria, states that if the culture be put in the incubator at a temperature of 37°–39° C. and examined in 2½ to 3 hours, the bacilli, if present, will be more easily detected than if the culture be not examined until several hours later.

Treatment.—E. M. Sutton[5] recommends, as a useful adjunct to any other line of treatment, the use of a 1% or 2% solution of cocain atomized on the fauces and tonsils as often as seems necessary. One great advantage is that nourishment can be taken in greater amounts and more frequently because of the lessened discomfort in swallowing.

W. L. Pyle[6] suggests the intravenous injection of mercuric chlorid, because of the safety of this method of administration and the increased efficiency of the drug when given in this way in other diseases in which its use is indicated.

Pinet[7] uses a 0.5% solution of resorcin as a prophylactic against diphtheria, claiming that it is more powerfully antiseptic than boric acid.

H. Wickers[8] applies to the pseudomembrane once or twice a day a mix-

[1] Arch. f. Kinderh., Bd. 23, H. 1-3.   [2] Ibid., Bd. 22, H. 1 und 2.
[3] Jour. Am. Med. Assoc., Feb. 20, 1897.   [4] N. Y. Med. Jour., Aug. 1, 1896.
[5] Jour. Am. Med. Assoc. Jan. 16, 1896.   [6] Med. News, July 15, 1896.
[7] Pharm. Centralbl., 37, p. 385.   [8] Lancet, vol. 23, p. 1562.

ture of equal parts of glycerin and a saturated solution of sodium hyposulphit, finding that the membrane disappears after three or four applications, general treatment being, of course, used.

Antitoxin.—M. P. Haushalter,[1] in discussing the indications for the use of antitoxin, attaches importance to the morphology of the Löffler bacillus, considering the short bacillus to be nonvirulent (*cf.* Klein, *Year-Book* for 1897, p. 758), and its presence to be a coincidence without relation to the development of the pharyngeal inflammation. In case the pseudomembrane is white and bacteriologic examination shows strepto- or staphylococci with the short bacillus, the use of antitoxin may be deferred unless laryngeal symptoms arise. In a mild, localized angina without marked general symptoms, the result of the bacteriologic examination may be awaited, as these cases usually recover, even if due to the long bacillus, but a single injection will hasten the exfoliation of the deposit. Antitoxin should be given immediately, without waiting for the result of the bacteriologic examination, if the pharyngeal deposit is extensive, or if there are laryngeal symptoms, whether there is membrane elsewhere or not. If the bacillus is associated with the streptococcus, the antitoxin should be given in large and frequently repeated doses. In cases of croup it is recommended to inject 20 c.c. [number of units not stated], to be repeated every 12 hours until relief. Intubation or tracheotomy may be deferred as long as the pulse and color are good. Attacks of dyspnea warn against delay. With reference to immunization, Haushalter thinks that it is not wise, under ordinary circumstances, to submit a healthy organism to the possibilities of serotherapie accidents, however rare and slight they may be. The indication for preventive injections is a persistent fatal epidemic of diphtheria which cannot be controlled by ordinary hygienic measures.

The *Medical News* (Dec., 1896) investigated the different makes of antitoxin on the market with reference to the **strength in antitoxin-units,** the results being shown in the following tables:

TABLE I.—*Shows the Results of the Examination of Nineteen Samples.*

Serum number.	Times tested.	Immunizing units per c.c.	Number of c.c. of serum in original flask.	Total number of immunizing units in each flask.
1	12	350	10	3500
2	14	350	9.9	3465
3	6	150	11.2	1680
4	10	250[2]	2.8	700[2]
5	6	70	9.25	647.5
6	6	150	9.2	1380
7	14	350	18.4	6440
8	6	150	4.2	630
9	7	50	3.55	177.5
10	5	100	9.7	970
11	7	Less than 20	3.6	Less than 72
12	4	100	9.7	970
13	7	100	3.45	345
14	13	350	9.1	3185
15	8	Less than 50	8.2	Less than 410
16	8	70	9	630
17	4	100	9.7	970
18	4	100	9.1	910
19	10	200	9.3	1860

[1] Gaz. hebdom. de Méd. et Chir., Aug. 16, 1896.
[2] The serum in flask No. 4 was exhausted before this test could be carried higher.

TABLE II.—*The Advertised Strength as shown on the Labels.*

Serum number.	Immunizing units per c.c. Claimed.	Number of c.c. of serum in original flask. Claimed.	Total number of immunizing units in each flask. Claimed.
1	50	Not stated.	Not stated.
2	150	10	1500
3	Not stated.	Not stated.	1500
4	Not stated.	Not stated.	1500
5	100	10	1000
6	100	10	1000
7	"Dose 5 to 30 c.c."	20	Not stated.
8	"Dose 5 to 20 c.c."	5	Not stated.
9	Not stated.	Not stated.	1000
10	Not stated.	10	Not stated.
11	Not stated.	Not stated.	1000
12	Not stated.	10	Not stated.
13	100	5	500
14	Not stated.	Not stated.	600
15	Not stated.	Not stated.	1500
16	20 "estimated."	10	200
17	100	10	1000
18	100+	10	1000+
19	100	10	1000

A. Monti[1] maintains that the **proper classification of diphtheria** is not merely into mild, severe, and grave forms, but into three groups on a pathologic-anatomic and bacteriologic basis, the terms mild, severe, and grave then being applied according to the clinical picture produced by the diphtheria-toxin. His three groups are: 1. A fibrinous form, in which the diphtheric products are only placed upon the mucous membrane. Virchow, Weigert, and Cohnheim call this the croupous form. 2. A mixed form, called also diphtheritic croup or the phlegmonous form, in which the fibrinous exudates lie deep in the tissues as well as upon the upper layers of the mucous membrane. 3. A septic, gangrenous form, in which a fibrinous pseudomembrane is formed in the deep tissues of the mucous membrane, the process really consisting of a necrosis of the tissues and a mingling of the dead particles with the diphtheric products. In the first form, death, when it occurs, is usually due only to the mechanical obstruction; in the second form both the obstruction and the action of the diphtheria-toxins may cause a fatal termination; while in the third form it results from the joint action of the diphtheria-toxins and pathogenic bacteria. According to Sidney Martin, there are two classes of diphtheria-toxins. The first is found in the diphtheric membrane, causing the local and general symptoms of diphtheria. When a sufficient amount of this toxin is taken up into the circulation it changes the albuminous bodies of the tissues into "tissue-poisons." There are two varieties of these, one belonging to the class of digested proteids—albumoses; the other, an organic acid belonging to the non-proteids.

The specific action of the albumoses is in small doses to produce fever, and, if the action is long continued, paralyses; in large doses, they cause prostration, with fatty degeneration of the heart and kidneys. The antitoxin can neutralize only the toxin formed in the pseudomembrane, and cannot neutralize the "tissue-poisons," which explains why the sequels of diphtheria continue to appear after the use of antitoxin [and why an early injection of antitoxin is very desirable]. The pathology, then, of diphtheria necessarily

[1] Arch. f. Kinderh, Bd. xxi., H. 1–3, 1896.

conditions several clinical pictures of the disease, rendering it impossible to group all cases together in estimating the value of a therapeutic agent.

In 1895 Monti treated 104 cases of diphtheria with antitoxin, of which 72 belonged to the fibrinous form, 26 to the mixed form, and 6 to the gangrenous form. An exhaustive analysis is made, including classifications according to the location, extent, and duration of the membrane, ages of the children, and the degrees of severity.

In the *fibrinous form* there were 31 mild, 12 severe, and 29 grave cases. In all the grave cases the larynx was involved, there being a high degree of stenosis in 25, of which 3 died. "In none of the earlier methods of treating diphtheria have I been able to point in such severe diphtheric infections of the larynx to so favorable a result, and in this regard I must consider the results obtained by serum-therapy as brilliant." Of the 12 severe cases 3 died, all being artificially fed newborn infants. All of the 31 mild cases recovered, but it is to be taken into consideration that this result might not have occurred without serum-therapy, and that with other methods of treatment the diphtheric process would have shown a much greater tendency to involve other mucous membranes, or, through the formation of tissue-poisons, to produce sequels which might endanger life. The 72 fibrinous cases gave a general mortality of 6% to 8%. In one case there was a slight paralysis of accommodation and deglutition appearing 2 days after the injection, which, owing to its short duration, was attributed to the toxic working of the albumin-bodies in the horse-serum. In another case there was a light transitory albuminuria, also considered as due to the serum.

With regard to **dosage**, Monti recommends in tonsillar diphtheria with a thin pseudomembrane and mild constitutional symptoms a dose of 600 units as sufficient to limit the process and bring about rapid recovery. 1000 units are to be used if the general symptoms are more severe, or if the membrane is thicker or extends to the uvula, mouth, or post-pharyngeal wall. If at the end of 24 hours the symptoms are aggravated or stationary, the number of units was not enough to free the system from the toxin, and the dose should be repeated. Should the pseudomembrane, when first seen, extend over the tonsils, fauces, and pharynx, the initial dose must range from 1500 to 2000 units, depending upon the character of the membrane, the fever, and the duration of the disease before injection. A repetition of the dose is indicated if there is no improvement in 24 hours. If the pseudomembrane is situated both on the nasal and on the pharyngeal mucous membranes, 2000 to 3000 units should be given at once, and repeated as above. Laryngeal cases will need from 1000 to 1500 units if there is a slight degree of stenosis and a slight tonsillar deposit. This must, however, be repeated in 12 hours, if signs of improvement have not appeared. When the laryngeal obstruction is marked, large doses (2000 to 3000 units) should be given at once, and repeated in full or half doses, according to circumstances, every half hour. In the course of a single case it may be necessary to give as many as 5000 units. If the deposit on the tonsils and pharynx is extensive and thick, and the stenosis of high degree, the first dose should be not less than 2500 units. If the diphtheria is simultaneously nasal, pharyngeal, tonsillar, and laryngeal, even larger doses (3000 units) are to be used, with repetitions of 2000 units at intervals of 12 hours, until a bettering is noticed. Monti is of the firm opinion that other observers' more unfavorable results than his are due to too small amounts of antitoxin, and that in the fibrinous form of diphtheria serum-therapy causes a more rapid decline of the disease than any other method of treatment could bring about.

If sufficient antitoxin is used at the beginning of an attack, an improvement is always noticed within 24 to 36 hours, a constant criterion being a normal temperature.

Monti saw 26 cases of the phlegmonous form (also called diphtheric croup), of which 3 were relatively light, 9 were severe (mittleschwer), and 14 were very grave (absolutschwer), the local conditions in all being extensive and severe. 10 of this group died, a mortality of 37%, which "shows that the action of the heilserum in the phlegmonous form of diphtheria is uncertain." The reason why all of these cases are really grave is because the sudden development of the pseudomembrane on several mucous membranes leads to a rapid and abundant formation of toxins, which, on account of the changes in the deeper tissues, are quickly absorbed, and, as quickly, set up extreme intoxications and degenerative processes, which, of course, cannot be restored by an antidote to the causative poisons; therefore serum-therapy, in spite of the use of large doses, will be unable to save as many of these cases as of the fibrinous form. Further investigation is, accordingly, necessary to perfect serum-therapy for the phlegmonous form.

Six cases of the gangrenous, septic form [which probably corresponds to the malignant form of other writers] were observed, with 1 recovery—83% mortality. This series, although small in number would seem also to make further investigation necessary. With the failure of other methods of treatment, and with little to be hoped for from the antitoxin, it is, however, well to begin at once with large doses, and occasionally a case may be saved. In the 104 cases, one-third showed sequels due to the albumin-bodies of the serum, the frequency of their appearance being dependent upon the amount of serum used; therefore Monti urgently recommends the use of serum of high potency.

F. Ganghofner[1] has contributed an exhaustive article on **the serum-treatment of diphtheria.** Justice cannot be done to the pamphlet in a brief review, but perhaps the most interesting chapters are those on the nature, mode of action, and limitations of the antitoxin. Ganghofner has given the views of the different investigators very fully, with their reasons for their theories. He quotes Behring as considering the antitoxin a specific product of the immunized animal body. Buchner and others think that the toxin introduced in the process of immunization contains specific cell-substances of the bacteria, which are modified and rendered harmless in the animal organism. The blood of a healthy animal has been shown to have a bactericidal action (due to proteid bodies, alexins), a globulicidal action (dissolving blood-corpuscles of another species), and an antitoxic action, all of which processes Buchner looks on as similar in nature, and considers any antitoxic serum to act by increasing the normal capabilities of the blood in a specific direction, artificial immunization, therefore, being the combination of alexin and antitoxin-action. Emmerich thinks that the bacterial poisons unite with the globulin of the blood to form substances which he calls "immuntoxinproteins." Roux's vitalistic theory supposes that the poisons exert a stimulating influence upon certain cells, probably the phagocytes. Buttersack maintains that the cells of the body can only produce what they have always produced, and that the toxin acts through the nervous system, increasing the quantity of the products, but making no qualitative change.

While all of this is theory, it has been definitely shown by Brieger and Boer that the antitoxin is an albuminous body, capable of being separated

[1] First supplementary volume to the Handbook of Special Treatment of Internal Diseases. G. Fischer, Jena, 1897.

from the serum. However, speculation is still rife as to its mode of action. Behring thinks that a neutralization occurs of the toxin by the antitoxin, the artificial or passive immunity being more quickly obtained than the active, but being of more transitory duration. Buchner opposes the neutralization-theory because a mixture of the antitoxin and toxin of tetanus which gave no symptoms when injected into mice, produced tetanus in guinea-pigs. It has also been shown that some antitoxins will protect against other than their special toxin; thus, antitetanus-serum protects against snake-venom. Therefore, Buehner holds that the antitoxin acts, not on the toxin to neutralize it, but on the animal body to render it resistant to the action of the toxin. Max Gruber holds the same view, but emphasizes the share of the animal's own serum in reacting to the antitoxin. Gabritschewsky explains the healing of the local process in diphtheria by the local leukocytosis, sequestration of the necrotic mucous membrane, and the phagocytosis of the leukocytes. The necrotizing power of the diphtheria-virus paralyzes the phagocytic action of the leukocytes, while the antitoxin tends to maintain this action, by rendering the cells less susceptible to the poison, thus explaining the rapid disappearance of the pseudomembrane after antitoxin injections. Schlesinger found that the leukocytosis which accompanies diphtheria tends to disappear as the case approaches recovery, but persists in those cases that are to result fatally. Following the injection of antitoxin there is a marked diminution in the number of white cells, and then a slow increase, not, however, reaching the earlier height. This he considers to be a favorable action of the antitoxin, either directly upon the blood-cells or indirectly upon them through the blood-making organs. The general consensus of opinion seems to indicate the leukocytes as furnishing the ultimate protection through their products, nuclein and spermin.

After discussing other theories and also Smirnow's method of obtaining the antitoxin by electrolysis, and considering objections to the acceptance of the Klebs-Löffler bacillus as the cause of diphtheria, Ganghofner asserts that all these theories cannot change the fact that the diphtheria-antitoxin obtained by Behring's method is the best remedy by far for diphtheria that has been brought out up to the present time.

With regard to the limitations of the action of antitoxin, it is generally agreed that it is of great value if used before the third day, but that after that time the result is more uncertain. In the so-called septic cases its value is also lessened, and some discussion has arisen as to the nature of the septic diphtheria. Heubner and Ranke maintain that it is not always a mixed infection, as bacteriologic examination sometimes gives a pure culture. Ranke found, however, that even in septic cases the antitoxin gave good results when used early, and he, therefore, concludes that "either Behring's serum antagonizes streptococci also, or else the so-called septic diphtheria is not a true septic infection secondary to the diphtheria, but a high degree of general infection with the diphtheria process itself."

With regard to **local treatment,** Ganghofner advises it only in severe cases where the deposit is extensive, or the infection a mixed one. In early cases not far advanced he considers it unnecessary.

Lennox Browne[1] has become more strongly opposed to **the antitoxin treatment** than before. He gives a list of clinicians in different parts of the world who are "either definitely adverse to the treatment, or who deprecate the extravagant enthusiasm of some of its advocates." He makes an epitome of his objections (which are practically the same as those advanced by other

[1] Jour. Laryngol., Rhin., and Otol., Dec., 1896.

opponents of the treatment, and are therefore given *in extenso*) as follows:
1. Objections to the claims for antitoxin do not come from one or two writers,
but from authorities in all parts of the world; 2. The basis of comparison of
the new treatment with the old, as adopted by enthusiasts, is unfair; 3. Percentage-mortality is also misleading; 4. The gross mortality from diphtheria
in this [London] and other large cities has not decreased; 5. To the increased
attention given to the subject by the introduction of serum is the improved mortality mainly due, for the death-rate of cases treated with seru n is out of all proportion greater than that of cases treated without it in the same hospitals. 6.
This is especially true in the case of children attacked under 5 years of age,
the period of life at which diphtheria is admittedly most fatal; 7. The value
of immunizing-injections of antitoxin with a view to prevent diphtheria is
but slight, and cannot outweigh the dangers of the procedure; 8. The scientific basis on which the treatment is founded cannot be sustained by any practical test, especially since internal medical and local treatment, as formerly
adopted, is still continued; 9. The benefits, equally with the dangers, of the
antitoxin are due to the albumin in the blood-serum, and not to any special
antidotal element; 10. The assertion that the comparative failure of antitoxin
in this country is due to insufficient dosage is not sustained by the figures now
available. [In view of the publications of Biggs and others, objection 4 is
scarcely tenable at present, and objection 8 is answered by the American
Pediatric Society's investigations with regard to croup. If objection 9 is
true, then the serums relatively high in antitoxin units are of less value than
the more dilute.]

Sidney Martin[1] emphasizes the effect of the antitoxin in limiting the
growth of the membrane, and urges that the initial dose should be large (4000
units in one injection) and given as early in the course of the case as possible.

The compilation showing the greatest **number of cases treated with
antitoxin** has been made by Loddo,[2] who collected official statistics of 86
hospitals in Europe, America, Australia, and Japan. They include 10,000
cases, with an average mortality of 18%. Seven thousand of these cases,
showing a mortality of 20%, were compared with preceding cases, which had
a mortality of 44%. Guerard[3] collected reports of 3760 cases treated in
private practice, giving a mortality of 7.8%.

E. M. Goodall[4] reports the use of antitoxin for diphtheria in 2 patients
who were affected at the time with **post-scarlatinal nephritis,** the nephritis not being in any way unfavorably influenced. In a third case in
which the nephritis had subsided, it relapsed 10 days after the diphtheria
attack and 4 days after the appearance of an antitoxin-urticaria which was
accompanied by fever. Recovery was prompt.

Fourrier[5] has used the diphtheria-antitoxin with great success in a number
of severe cases of **scarlet fever.** Dotti[6] recommends it in pertussis, having
seen the paroxysms in a case complicated by diphtheria cease after the injection
of antitoxin.

Adamkiewicz[7] attributes the **deaths following antitoxin-injections**
to a disturbance of the self-regulating apparatus which protects the system
against noxious influences within certain limits. This adaptive mechanism of
the organism is disturbed first by a forcible injection, and secondly by the
specificity of the substance injected.

[1] Lancet, Oct. 11, 1896.
[2] Riforma Med., July 11, 1896; ref. in Brit. Med. Jour., Sept. 5, 1896.   [3] Ibid.
[4] Lancet, Nov. 21, 1896.   [5] Rev. mens. des Mal. de l'Enfance, June, 1897.
[6] Ibid.   [7] Wien. med. Presse; ref. in Arch. of Pediatrics, Dec., 1896.

A. King [1] reports convulsions with disturbed respiration and a slow, weak pulse in an adult, after 2 separate injections of 1 c.c. each of antitoxic serum.

A. Possett [2] reports in detail on **59 cases of diphtheria** treated in the Innsbruck Hospital. It is interesting to note that cerebral embolism occurred in one of the fatal cases. The antitoxin was found to act very favorably in a great number of cases, but in some cases its use seemed to be without effect, the explanation for which, the author thinks, cannot be given until further researches are made on the antitoxin characteristics of human blood-serum.

P. Bernheim [3] reviews his **statistics of diphtheria** for the past 20 years, seeing a fall in the death-rate of 12%, from 19.9% to 7.7%, which he attributes to an absolute diminution in the number and severity of cases. He has apparently used the antitoxin but little, seeing no specific action from it.

E. Rosenthal [4] reports his own results in **intubation** before the introduction of antitoxin, and collects the reports of other observers, showing not only the lowered mortality, but the marked shortening in the time during which it was necessary to leave the tube in the larynx.

The Committee of the American Pediatric Society appointed to investigate the **value of antitoxin in laryngeal diphtheria** reports that 1704 cases were collected, giving a mortality of 21%. The mortality of 637 intubations was 26%; of 20 tracheotomies, 45%; of 11 tracheotomies subsequent to intubation, 63%; of 1036 nonoperated cases, 17%.

It is emphasized: first, that before the use of antitoxin it was estimated that 90% of laryngeal diphtheria cases required operation, whereas now, with the use of antitoxin, 39.21% require it; second, that the percentage-figures have been reversed, formerly 27% approximately representing the recoveries, while now, under antitoxin-treatment, 27% represents the mortality.

J. Herald [5] reports 100 cases treated with antitoxin in the Kingston General Hospital (Ontario), without a death. In 12, intubation was necessary.

M. Tschlenow [6] reports on the use of antitoxin in **102 cases** of diphtheria in his practice among the Cossacks of Southern Russia. The mortality of 15.6% is wonderfully good, considering the poverty of the people, who opposed the treatment at first, but were soon so impressed by its value that they brought cases over 25 miles for treatment. No other treatment was adopted.

M. Gornow [7] also reports on **130 cases** treated only with antitoxin—mortality 13.8%. During 1 month when no antitoxin was obtainable the mortality rose to 52%. Of the 112 recovered cases, 2.8% were subsequently affected with palatal paralysis, 1 with paraplegia, and 1 with hemiplegia.

J. H. Moore [8] reports a case of diphtheria in which **3 relapses** occurred in a few weeks, the membrane disappearing each time after the use of antitoxin. The bacilli persisted until all mercury by the mouth was stopped and 500 units of antitoxin injected night and morning for 5 days. During the 4 weeks of treatment 16,500 units were given without any untoward result.

The **insusceptibility of nurslings** to diphtheria makes interesting the report of a family epidemic by D. G. Sanor, [9] one of the patients being an infant 9 days old. Injection of 750 units in two doses was followed by rapid recovery.

[1] Boston M. and S. Jour., Sept. 24, 1896.
[2] Wien. med. Woch., No. 45, 1896.
[3] Therap. Monats., June, 1896.
[4] Med. and Surg. Reporter, lxxiv., 1896.
[5] Brit. Med. Jour., June 5, 1897.
[6] Arch. f. Kinderh., Bd. 23, H. 1.
[7] Ibid.   [8] Med. Rec., Apr. 17, 1897.
[9] N. Y. Med. Jour., June 26, 1897.

A. J. Turner and L. N. Ashworth[1] report on the **use of antitoxin** in the Brisbane Children's Hospital. Their experience was so favorable, especially in laryngeal cases, where the mortality was reduced from 60 % to 13 %, that they believe that, with rare exceptions, no child. ought to die of diphtheria, provided that a sufficiently large dose of antitoxin be given at the start.

H. M. Biggs and A. R. Guerard[2] report on the use of antitoxin by the N. Y. City Health Department, and include an exhaustive *résumé* of the published statistics from all quarters. The Health Department provided antitoxin free for the poor, and the cases treated were, therefore, as a rule, among the very poorest classes and in the most unfavorable surroundings. Over 1200 cases were injected, with a mortality of 15.8 %, or, excluding moribund cases and those dying in 24 hours, 10 %. In the same way the mortality of the laryngeal cases was 30.4 % or 22 %. Kossel is quoted extensively, in his collection of statistics, which show that there has been a decrease not only in the mortality-percentage, but also in the absolute number of deaths. [Without quoting figures further, those interested in seeing how decided a fall there has been in the number of deaths are referred to Biggs and Guerard's paper.]

W. H. Seibert[3] gives a similar table for cities of the United States.

J. Lewis Smith[4] reports favorably on 5 months' use of antitoxin in the N. Y. Foundling Asylum, attributing the unsatisfactory results obtained earlier to the quality of serum used.

I. M. Snow[5] finds that Buffalo is an exception to the general rule for other cities in that the number of deaths from diphtheria has not been lessened, although the percentage of deaths has been lowered.

Glaser[6] gives the **statistics** of the Hamburg General Hospital with reference to diphtheria for the 19 years from 1872–91. In the whole town there were 52,000 cases, with a mortality of 14 %. Over 4000 cases were treated in the hospital, with a mortality of 36 %. Of those admitted before the fourth day of the disease, 37 % died; of those admitted later, 50 % died. Of 1768 tracheotomies, 20 % recovered.

Prophylaxis.—C. Fränkel's exhaustive address at the Kiel Congress on the prevention of diphtheria is reported thoroughly by G. Sobernheim.[7] The importance of the subject is fully emphasized by the figures for the death-rate of the disease in Prussia for the 12 years from 1875 to 1886, which show that over half a million human beings died from diphtheria in that time, a rate of 165 deaths to 100,000 population. For the whole of the German Empire the figures were first obtained in 1892 and 1893, with a rate of 118 and 158 respectively. The almost incredible statement is made and verified that between the ages of 2 and 15 years 98 % of deaths are due to diphtheria. Since the discovery of the diphtheria-bacillus the preventive measures do not have to be aimed in the dark, but can be directed with a purpose. After a discussion of the mode of propagation of the disease by individuals and contaminated objects (rarely by dust, as the bacilli do not survive desiccation for any length of time), the points are mentioned on which immunity and susceptibility rest: local conditions, especially of the mucous membranes of the upper air-passages, and general conditions, as the presence or absence of antitoxins, "those natural protecting substances of the body which are found in the blood in the majority of human beings, but are absent in many." One class of protective measures

---

[1] Intercol. Med. Jour. of Australia. Oct. 20, 1896.   [2] Med. News, Dec. 12, 1896.
[3] Jour. Am. Med. Assoc., Mar. 6, 1897.   [4] Med. News, Mar. 6. 1897.
[5] Buffalo Med. Jour., May, 1897.   [6] Zeit. f. klin. Med., Bd. 30, H. 3.
[7] Berlin. klin. Woch., Oct. 5, 1896.

has for its aim to put the individual in a condition to resist infection, the other class attempts to confine and destroy the infection. In the first class are all hygienic products, both of local antisepsis and of constitutional measures, such as cold bathing, which will tend to build up the individual and also to improve the resisting power of the mucous membranes; also other hygienic measures which tend to uplift the lower classes and to foster cleanliness. With regard to immunizing-injections, while Fränkel does not believe that the causal connection has been definitely proved in the 6 or 7 fatal cases collected by Gottstein,[1] yet he says that many physicians will hesitate before recommending a not absolutely harmless measure against a not absolutely certain infection. The concentrated serums are, however, rendering the risk so slight that it may be scarcely considered.

The second class of protective measures is covered by thorough isolation and disinfection. The former can only be obtained in a hospital, and should be continued as long as the bacilli remain on the affected mucous membranes.

Measles.—W. Moeller[2] studied the **statistics of epidemics of measles,** especially that of Munich in 1887, and arrived at the following conclusions: 1. There is no fixed periodicity in the recurrence of epidemics of measles. 2. For an epidemic of measles to arise it is necessary that there be the contagium acting on unprotected individuals. The intervals between epidemics is being continually shortened by the increase of commerce and of population. 3. There are certain factors still unknown, varying from time to time, which favor the spread of epidemics. Whether the warmer seasons exert their lessening influence upon the number of cases of measles directly because of the higher temperature, or indirectly through the dilution of the contagium by the better ventilation of rooms, cannot be determined. 4. An average for 20 years in Munich shows the mortality for measles to have two maximal periods, a slight one in December and a much greater one in May and June. 5. The mortality from measles in Munich for the first, and still more for the second, half of the 80's was nearly 3 times that for the decade from 1870 to 1880. The first half of the present decade shows a marked decline in the rate. 6. No age shows immunity to the infection, but nurslings are less susceptible than others. 7. Children under 5 years furnish almost all the fatal cases, and the majority of these are under 2 years of age. 8. In Munich the relative mortality for children under 1 year of age is 55 times, and for children between 2 and 5 years is 12 times that for children over 5 years. 9. Although the average number of cases is less, owing to the shorter intervals between epidemics, yet in Munich the average age of the fatal cases has not been lowered. 10. Both sexes, in Munich, show about an equal number both of cases and of deaths. 11. The absolute rate of mortality, like the relative, shows for the different divisions of Munich constant and important variations, and falls and rises with the birth-rate, the evident reason for this being imperfect care and nursing. 12. Primary thoracic rachitis increases threefold the disposition of a measles patient to catarrhal pneumonia and doubles the danger of this complication.

Diagnosis.—H. Koplik[3] asserts that small, irregular spots of a bright-red color with a minute bluish-white speck in the center of each, appearing on the mucous membrane of the mouth and lips, provide a constant and pathognomonic sign of measles. He has always found them present in measles and never in any other disease. They occur at the beginning of the disease, when the diagnosis is doubtful, increasing in intensity to reach their height

---

[1] Therap. Monatsh., May, 1896.　　　　[2] Arch. f. Kinderh., Bd. 21, H. 4.
　　　　　　　　[3] Arch. of Pediatrics, Dec., 1896.

and to fade when the skin eruption appears. Robet[1] reports varieties of eruptions preceding the measles-rash, considering them to be due to streptococcus infection, with entrance through the inflamed mucous membranes. Bernard,[2] in a discussion on the prodromal and secondary exanthems (preceding or following other infections), thinks that they are not always due to the streptococcus, but sometimes depend on the virus of the infectious disease in the case.

Relapse.—Chauffard and Lemoine[3] have observed 11 cases of relapse after measles, 8 of which occurred in one family. The relapses occurred from 11 to 14 days after the primary attack and none was serious. Eonnet[4] reports 4 relapses after measles, all occurring within 20 days after the previous attack. In 1 case the child had had measles for the first time 3 years before. He also reports several attacks occurring in 122 of 300 cases which had been under his own observation, and insists upon the frequency of recurrence. Gottstein[5] reports the case of a girl of 10 who had measles with marked eruption and slight respiratory symptoms. Two years later she had another attack, in which the catarrhal symptoms were pronounced, the eruption late and slight. He believes that the case supports Schleich's theory of acquired immunity, and that in the first attack the skin became immunized and was therefore but little affected in the subsequent attack.

G. J. Dudley[6] notes the seeming occurrence of **measles during convalescence from scarlet fever.** The measles-eruption appeared 4 days after desquamation from scarlet fever began. The child had had no opportunity for infection by measles for 14 days, so that the incubation-period must have been at least that long. [The diagnosis of the measles is a matter of some doubt, owing to the possibility of a post-scarlatinal accidental rash.]

Complications and Sequels.—T. M. Allison[7] records a case of **hyperpyrexia** in measles with bronchopneumonia, the axillary temperature reaching 109° at least twice. The issue was fatal. Wunder[8] observed as a rare sequel to measles **gangrene of the soft parts** of the thoracic wall. Recovery ensued. W. A. Ellison[9] saw **acute ascending myelitis** occur from the fifth to the seventh day of measles in a boy of 14 years, the postmortem temperature being 42.9° C. (109° F.). Ed. Mackey[10] reports fatal **septic phlebitis** of the arm occurring during an attack of measles. There was no bacteriologic report. Rouger[11] describes 2 forms of **hemorrhagic measles,** 1 a true hemorrhagic form in which there as visceral as well as subcutaneous hemorrhages with a grave state, the other form including infectious purpuric erythemas, the infection being of buccal, pharyngeal, or bronchial origin, and occurring either in the course of measles or subsequently. The eruptions become hemorrhagic usually from the second to the fourth day, taking 10 to 15 days in which to fade. The prognosis is good unless there is marked dyspnea from laryngeal or pulmonary involvement. Méry and Lorrain[12] made a bacteriologic examination of **gangrene of the lung,** complicating measles, and found streptococci and bacilli resembling the Klebs-Löffler bacillus and some resembling streptothrix. M. Mosets[13] reports 3 cases of **nephritis,** occurring in one instance with the appearance of the measles-rash, in

[1] Thèse de Paris, 1896.   [2] Münch. med. Woch., No. 34, 1896.
[3] Gaz. méd. de Paris, tome iii., No. 1, 1896.
[4] Gaz. hebdom. de Méd. et de Chir., Oct. 29, 1896.
[5] Münch. med. Woch., No.13, 1896.   [6] Brit. Med. Jour., Jan. 16, 1897.
[7] Ibid., Jan. 9, 1897.   [8] Münch. med. Woch., May 18, 1897.
[9] Lancet, Oct. 17, 1896.   [10] Brit. Med. Jour., Dec. 19, 1896.
[11] Rev. mens. des Mal. de l'Enfance, June, 1897.
[12] Ibid.   [14] Vereinsbl. d. pfälz. Aerzte, Sept., 1896.

the others several days later. Two other cases of nephritis were observed at the same time which were considered to be of measles origin, although there was no eruption. F. Bezold[1] found either mucopurulent or **purulent secretion in the temporal bone** in all cases dead of measles. The otitis media is not due to extension from the Eustachian tube, but to general systemic infection. Perforation of the drum-membrane rarely occurs, and the prognosis of the local condition even then is usually favorable.

Scarlet Fever.—Myositis as a complication of scarlet fever is reported by M. Bruck,[2] who has seen 3 cases. The muscles became tender from 2 to 3 weeks after the eruption had appeared, and the temperature rose to 38.5° C. (101° F.). The symptoms subsided in a few days with the use of the salicylates. Goodall,[3] reports a case of scarlet fever dying in convulsions, the condition being found, postmortem, to be **thrombosis** of the veins of Galen. M. Alexeieff[4] reports 2 cases of **hemiplegia** in scarlet fever, 1 recovering completely, the other presenting postmortem a thrombus in the left middle cerebral artery. M. N. Ingerslen[5] reports 3 cases of **surgical scarlet fever** in which the eruption started around a wound in the skin. The throat in each case was red, but there was no pseudomembrane except in one case, when it was slight. Amitrano[6] reports a case of **typhoid fever** developing in convalescence a scarlatiniform eruption with fever, which was followed by desquamation. After this fever had subsided marked meningeal symptoms appeared for a few days. These disappeared, and after desquamation was complete a second intense erythema appeared, which was also followed by desquamation, after which recovery ensued. Weisbecker[7] has treated cases of typhoid fever, scarlet fever, pneumonia, and the bronchopneumonia of measles with **blood-serum** from patients who had recovered from the corresponding disease, without any marked effect in shortening the course, but apparently making the patients more comfortable. **Warm baths** (35° C.) have been used by J. Schill and G. Schellenberg,[8] in many cases of scarlet fever, all of the cases assuming a mild type in a short time. Varnali[9] reports a case of scarlet fever complicated with **diphtheria,** running an afebrile course. The records[10] of **2000 cases** of scarlet fever admitted to the Bagthorpe Fever Hospital showed that relapse, with sore throat, fever, and a rash lasting from 1 to 4 days, occurred in 14 cases. Accidental rashes were excluded. Depasse[11] reports a case of **hyperpyrexia** in scarlet fever. On the 12th day a temperature of 107.5° F. was reached and maintained for 70 hours following, in spite of antipyrin and cold baths. Decline of temperature and good recovery ensued. W. P. Northrup[12] among **details of the treatment** of scarlatina at the Willard Parker Hospital notes the use of douches of **hot saline solutions to the throat** to relieve the local symptoms and to prevent ear complications and cervical abscess. A wet-pack, Dover's powder, and nitroglycerin are relied upon for nephritis, while for hyperpyrexia tub-bathing is insisted upon as the most efficient means of reducing the temperature and of combating the attendant nervous symptoms. The temperature of the bath is to be regulated by the urgency of the case. Marsden[13] has investigated the **joint-affections** occurring during or subsequent to the course of scarlet fever and divides them as fol-

[1] Der Kinderärzt, No. vii., 1896.   [2] Arch. f. Kinderh., vol. xxi., H. 5, 1897.
[3] Rev. mens. des Mal de l'Enfance, June, 1897.   [4] Dietsk. Med., No. 5., 1896.
[5] Zeit. f. klin. Med., Bd. xxxi., 1.   [6] Riforma med., No. 146, 1896.
[7] Zeit. f. klin. Med., vols. 30 and 32.   [8] Rev. mens. des Mal. de l'Enfance, June, 1897.
[9] Arch. f. Kinderh., Bd. xxi., p. 358.   [10] Quart. Med., vol. xxv., No. 2, June, 1896.
[11] Rev. mens. des Mal. de l'Enfance, June, 1896.   [12] Arch. of Pediatrics, Nov., 1896.
[13] Med. Chron., Aug., 1896.

lows : 1. Scarlatinal synovitis, which occurs in 7% of cases, nearly always appearing from the 4th to the 10th day ; in 72% of cases affecting the wrists. It has no relation to the severity of the throat-symptoms or to rheumatism, and seems caused by the scarlatinal poison. 2. The septic form, occurring in 0.75%, often connected with fatal cases and closely related to severe throat-symptoms. This is probably due to mixed infection. 3. Rheumatic, less frequent and occurring usually in convalescence. 4. Tuberculous—occurs late, and the previous disease only affords the predisposition to the tuberculosis ; orchitis, a rarer complication, probably arises from a mixed infection from the throat.

Typhoid Fever.—J. O'Malley [1] records a **family epidemic** of typhoid fever. Both parents and three children became infected at about the same time, and in all the disease ran the typical course. J. P. Crozer Griffith [2] reports a positive **Widal reaction** with the blood of an infant 7 weeks old. The child was born when the mother was in the third week of typhoid fever, and it had been entirely well itself. He thinks it was probably a case of fetal typhoid, though admitting the possibility of the agglutinative principle having reached the child's blood through the placental circulation. The mother's milk had not been tested. Mossé [3] reports that he obtained the Widal reaction from the blood of a newborn infant whose mother had passed through typhoid fever in her sixth month of gestation. The mother's milk and placental blood also gave the reaction. [While the Widal reaction will be of great value in deciding as to the nature of intestinal infection in infants, and will perhaps increase to a considerable extent the number of recognized cases of typhoid fever under 2 years of age, yet such cases as the above must be carefully investigated to determine how long the infant's blood will give the reaction after the breast-nourishment has been removed. This question and the full value of the Widal test will undoubtedly be settled in time.] S. S. Adams [4] reports 4 cases of **temporary insanity** following typhoid fever in children. G. N. Acker [5] reports a case of typhoid fever in a boy of 8 years, terminating fatally with **gangrene of the lungs.** The typhoidal lesions had begun to heal.

Varicella.—P. Bolognini,[6] in an epidemic of 15 cases of varicella, found 12 complicated with a **staphylococcus and streptococcus infection,** which caused the vesicles to pustulate and form blebs. One case, resulting fatally from abscess of the kidney, gave a pure culture of streptococci. Von Stark [7] observed a case of general **anasarca,** without other symptoms, in a boy of 2 years, just recovered from varicella. The edema disappeared in 10 days, and was attributed to the preceding infection. [This seems reasonable, until more light is thrown on the etiology of angioneurotic edema.] Löhr [8] reports two cases of varicella terminating fatally, one from **miliary tuberculosis,** the other from septic infection. J. P. C. Griffith [9] records a case of **varicella gangrænosa.** Gangrenous ulcers ranging from the size of a split pea to that of a quarter-dollar developed from the vesicles. The distribution was universal, and death resulted. J. Comby [10] observed in a case of varicella a **scarlatiniform rash** [probably streptococcic].

Pertussis.—Etiology.—Kohn and Neumann[11] made bacteriologic studies without arriving at any definite conclusions, having found in 20 out of 25

[1] Univ. Med. Mag., June, 1897.   [2] Med. News, May 15, 1897.
[3] Progrès méd., Mar. 13, 1897.   [4] Arch. of Pediatrics, Nov., 1896.
[5] Ibid., Sept., 1896.   [6] La Pediatria, Mar., 1897.
[7] Deutsch. Arch. f. klin. Med., v. lvii., 1896.   [8] Deutsch. med. Woch, June 18, 1896.
[9] Univ. Med. Mag., Aug., 1896.   [10] Rev. mens. des Mal. de l'Enfance, June, 1897.
              [11] Arch. f. Kinderh., vol. 17, 1895.

cases a streptococcus, to which they did not attach any importance. Koplik[1] has isolated **a motile bacillus,** growing on hydrocele-fluid, and of very small dimensions, 0.8μ long and 0.3μ broad. It will not produce the symptoms of pertussis in the lower animals.

E. Czaplewski and R. Hensel[2] have worked out a method which has not failed, in every case of pertussis thus far examined, to show a **characteristic bacillus in the sputum.** The more severe and more advanced the case, the more numerous are the bacilli. The method consists in washing the sputum in a test-tube containing peptone water, putting it through at least three washings to free it from superficial contamination with other germs. The more solid lumps are then taken for the smear-preparation, which is fixed and stained with dilute carbol-fuchsin. The bacillus is oval, with rounded ends which sometimes stain deeper than the center, giving the appearance of a diplococcus. It resembles the influenza-bacillus but differs in its ability to grow on the ordinary media. It is polymorphous, the completely developed organism being only two or three times as long as it is broad.

Incubation.—Léon[3] reports a case of pertussis in which the **period of incubation** could be exactly fixed at 11 days. The contagion was derived from a child in whom the diagnosis was only established 4 days later, showing that the disease is contagious in the early stages.

Symptoms.—Guérin,[4] in a study of the temperature in pertussis, finds in many cases an irregular temperature, intermittent, sudden in onset and subsidence, and reaching as high as $40°$ C. He considers it to be due to the disease, and not to any complication. [We have observed in several cases a similar condition with nothing to account for the febrile paroxysm.]

J. Fröhlich[5] found in all of 55 children with pertussis a marked **lenkocytosis,** which kept pace proportionately with the number of kinks.

Bernhardt[6] reported to the Society of Internal Medicine, Berlin, a case of pertussis in a child of 5 years, in which a **paraplegia** occurred, which he attributed to capillary hemorrhage in the spinal cord. In the discussion Furbringer upheld an infectious origin for the hemorrhages, while Leyden considered them mechanical. Baginsky thought the paralysis was hysteric.

At the Frankfort Congress Ritter[7] gave the results of his observations in epidemics including **1163 cases** of whooping-cough. Seasonal influence could not be noted, but strong children seemed more disposed than weak ones. Five children had second attacks, and 37 who were exposed to the disease at one time without taking it, contracted it at a subsequent exposure. In the sputa of 147 patients Ritter's diplococcus tussis convulsivæ was found in every instance. For treatment he prefers bromoform, and has seen no bad results. Sonnenberger,[8] with Kassowitz, prefers antipyrin, but thinks that extreme care should be used in giving it. Neumann[9] has found Ritter's diplococcus in only 1 out of 18 cases.

Theodor[10] notes 2 cases of **hemiplegia** occurring during pertussis. Both regained power completely. In 1 case chorea minor appeared 4 months after the hemiplegia, which he attributes to hemorrhage at the time of the hemiplegia—probably in the basal ganglia. The chorea disappeared after 4 months. He also notes a case of recurrence of pertussis.

[1] Jour. Am. Med. Assoc., Sept. 18, 1897. [2] Deut. med. Woch., Sept. 9, 1897.
[3] Jour. de Méd. de Bordeaux, Oct. 25, 1896.
[4] Rev. mens. des Mal. de l'Enfance, June, 1897. [5] Jahrb. f. Kinderh , vol. 44, 1897.
[6] Rev. mens. des Mal. de l'Enfance, June, 1897.
[7] Arch. f. Kinderh., Bd. xxi., H. 5 and 6. [8] Ibid. [9] Ibid.
[10] Arch. f. Kinderh., Bd. xx., H. 3 and 4, 1896.

Tuberculosis.—K. Szegö[1] discusses the present status of our knowledge on the **inheritance** of tuberculosis, and concludes "that the transmission of tuberculosis is either bacillary or predisposing (perhaps toxic). Transmission does not exclude contagion, but, on the contrary, the predisposed furnish the most receptive soil. It is difficult to say which form of transmission predominates. It may result from infection of the semen or of the ovum, or it may occur through the placenta. An affection of the respiratory passages or of the glands near the mouth and nose points to contagion, while tuberculosis of the brain, bones, joints, and abdominal viscera suggests a congenital origin. The inherited germ of tuberculosis can remain latent in the system for an indefinite period until the vital resistance is lowered, when it is then able to become pathogenic."

Lymphatic Tuberculosis.—Starck[2] calls attention to the frequency of the occurrence of **enlargement of the cervical glands** in children that have carious teeth. In 113 children with enlarged cervical lymph-glands he found that 41 % had carious teeth, and, in the absence of other apparent causes, he concludes that the swollen glands resulted from the defective teeth. The two conditions corresponded in situation and in time of development, the enlargement of the glands being upon the same side as the diseased teeth, and the anterior glands being enlarged when the incisor teeth were involved, the posterior when the molars were involved. He holds that the disease is tuberculous in quite a number of these cases, and reports 2 interesting examples. One, a boy of 18, who had always been healthy, had caries of the molar teeth on both sides, with enlargement of the cervical glands. The glands were excised and the teeth extracted. Tubercle-bacilli were found in cover-slip preparations from two of the teeth, while the glands were tuberculous. The second case was that of a girl aged 14, one of whose molar teeth on the left side was carious; there was an enlarged gland below the ramus of the jaw. Between the diseased molar and the adjacent tooth, and forming the floor of the cavity in the tooth, were characteristic nodules with typical giant cells. The gland was tuberculous. [These observations are of considerable interest; that tuberculous adenitis of the cervical group may occur with disease of the teeth and mouth seems well established. We cannot, however, refrain from calling attention to the unreliability of the statistical evidence which he adduces showing the frequency of carious teeth in children with enlarged cervical glands. The author fails to state the frequency of carious teeth without enlarged glands.]

Marfan and Apert[3] note the ease of a child which showed the **first signs of glandular tuberculosis** at 9 months; after death at 17 months extensive intestinal, mesenteric, bronchial, and cervical tuberculosis was found. The occurrence of cervical adenitis with ulcers of gums as the initial lesion, and the facts that the mother had healed glandular tuberculosis, and that two other children had had tuberculosis, led the authors to think it probably a case of infection by the mother's milk, though cow's milk had been occasionally used.

Kossel[4] found the **pulmonary lesions** and those of the adjacent glands most important in 22 cases which died of tuberculosis, and in 14 other children who presented tuberculous lesions after death from other causes. The digestive system was affected with a frequency next to the respiratory. The author considers that the absence of older foci in the liver in any of these cases speaks strongly against intrauterine infection.

[1] Arch. f. Kinderh., Bd. xxi, II. 5 and 6.   [2] Rev. de la Tuberculose, July, 1896.
[3] Rev. mens. des Mal. de l'Enfance, June, 1896.   [4] Der Kinder-Arzt, vii., 19, 1896.

L. E. Holt[1] records the presence of tuberculosis in 102 of **1045 post-mortems** at the New York Infant Asylum and the Babies' Hospital. The lungs were affected in 99%, the bronchial glands in 96%, the spleen in 75%, other organs less frequently. He thinks 3 cases were infected in utero. In one this probability seemed especially strong, since the 20-days-old child of a tuberculous mother had cheesy glands. The frequency of pulmonary lesions points to infection by the respiratory tract, and the comparative infrequency of lesions in the digestive tract leads him to remark that isolation and such sanitary measures will produce more good than milk and dairy inspection, although these also must be continued.

Maas[2] notes the rarity of **tuberculosis of the genital organs** in children, and adds another to the 7 cases recorded. There was tuberculous ulceration of the mucosa of the uterus and tubes, and nodules in the walls of his case. The probable exclusion of other sources and a line of old fibrous tubercles in adhesions extending inward from the umbilicus led him to consider the navel the avenue of infection.

Labbé[3] adds 2 cases of **tuberculosis of the myocardium** to the 36 previously reported. The first occurred in a boy of 6 years, whose cardiac symptoms were increased area of dulness, pain, irregular pulse, and edema. At autopsy tubercles were found in numerous organs; the pleuræ were adherent to the pericardium, which was thickened and contained cheesy nodules. The hypertrophied heart-muscle was lardaceous and hard, especially at the apex. The second subject died with pulmonary tuberculosis in other organs as well, and in the myocardium was a cheesy tubercle which showed through the pericardium. Tubercle-bacilli were found in both specimens.

Syphilis.—E. Welander[4] reports the case of a child with **congenital syphilis** in which the infection seemed to be post-conceptional, as the father developed chancre 8 weeks before the child was born and infected the mother at that time, both subsequently showing secondary symptoms. He believes placental disease, such as hemorrhagic necrosis of the endothelium, may result in infection of the child, which would not occur were the placenta healthy. Zappert[5] relates a case of hereditary syphilis in which the only manifestations were **divergent squint** of the left eye, paralysis of the iris, and ptosis of the eyelid. Specific treatment brought about entire cure. He thinks the condition due to neuritis of the oculomotor. G. F. Harding[6] records the case of a child who developed **secondary syphilis at 3 years** of age. Although both parents were infected shortly before the conception of the child, it showed no signs until 3 years old, and then a probable chancre appeared on the arm, followed by a secondary eruption. The author thinks that a short course of mercurial treatment taken by the mother early in the disease had prevented infection in utero, and that infection came from subsequent contact with the mother at a time well defined in the history, the child having lived apart from the mother for the first 3 years of life.

Glandular Fever.—J. P. West[7] records an epidemic of 96 cases of what is now called glandular fever, occurring in a hamlet of 100 inhabitants and in the surrounding country. The ages of those affected varied from 7 months to 13 years, although both older and younger children were exposed. The duration averaged 16 days. But one death occurred, and there were no recurrences

[1] Med. News, Dec. 12, 1896.   [2] Arch. f. Gynäk., vol. xii., part 2, 1896.
[3] Rev. mens. des Mal. de l'Enfance, June, 1896.
[4] Nordiskt. Medicin. Arkiv., Mar., 1896; Am. Gyn. and Obst. Jour., vol. x., No. 5.
[5] Arch. f. Kinderh., Bd. xix., S. 161.   [6] Boston M. and S. Jour., July 23, 1896.
[7] Arch. of Pediatrics, Dec., 1896.

or sequelæ. The most marked symptom was the swelling of the carotid lymph-glands, which was nearly always double, though often beginning on one side. In three-fourths of the cases either the post-cervical, axillary, or inguinal glands were enlarged. In 37 cases the mesenteric glands could be felt; while enlarge-ment of the liver was noted in 87 cases, and of the spleen in 57 cases. There was no ear-trouble nor coryza, and no abnormal pulmonary signs were discov-ered. All but one case occurred between Oct. 1 and June 1. There was no definite period of incubation, but 7 days after exposure was the average time of appearance of the attack. Convalescence began in the severe cases with a thin greenish mucous diarrhea, and diarrhea was present in almost all the mild cases. Treatment was of no influence in shortening the disease. No case of mumps occurred during the epidemic; 57 of the children had had or have since had mumps in the ordinary way. The cases sprang up in families isolated from each other, and there seemed to be no house-to-house infection. Dawson Williams [1] reports 3 cases of glandular fever in the same family. About a week elapsed between the development of the first and second cases, and the same interval between the second and third. In all the affection was uni-lateral. No acute disease of the throat was present, but there was chronic granular pharyngitis. T. E. Sandall [2] records a case of the same affection in an infant of 6 months. The glandular swelling was limited to one side. Alex. McPhedran [3] reports a case in a boy of 4 years. The child passed through an attack of mumps a few weeks later. S. M. Hamill [4] reviews the literature, in reporting several cases.

Pneumonia.—E. Schlesinger [5] analyzes 173 cases of croupous pneumonia in children, occurring in the K. and K. Friedrich Children's Hospital. The monograph is an interesting and valuable one. J. P. C. Griffith [6] discusses the varying features of pneumonia in children. Comba [7] records the case of a child who died on the sixth day of life after presenting, clinically, aphonia, diffuse sclerema, and general weakness. The autopsy showed serous infiltration of the skin and of the muscles, and foci of bronchopneumonia in the lungs. There was general cloudy swelling of the liver and kidneys, and occasional areas of fatty degeneration were seen. Bacteriologic examination of the blood and lung-tissue showed a bacillus resembling in its characteristics the bacillus of Friedländer. The infection seems to have occurred from the foci in the lungs.

Peritonitis.—Brun,[8] after observations on 3 new cases, reasserts his earlier claim that peritonitis from the pneumococcus may be distinguished from that of other forms. It begins as sub-umbilical peritonitis, and after the subsidence of the acute symptoms suprapubic tumefaction appears, which is sometimes distinctly fluctuating. This sign, together with pouting or fistuliza-tion of the umbilicus, he considers almost pathognomonic. The prognosis is less grave than in other forms of purulent peritonitis. Eleven cases out of 14 recovered. It is more frequent in girls, and since the pneumococcus has been found in the walls and cavity of the uterus it seems probable that the tubes and the uterine lymphatics are the sources of infection in some cases at least.

Mumps.—Michaelis and Bein [9] have found in 7 cases of mumps a **diplo-coccus** 1μ in size and resembling the biscuit-shaped meningococcus in appear-ance. The microorganism was obtained in all cases in the fluid from Steno's

[1] Lancet, Jan. 16, 1897.
[2] Ibid., Feb. 13, 1897.
[3] Canad. Pract., May, 1897.
[4] Arch. of Pediatrics, May, 1897.
[5] Arch. f. Kinderh., Bd. xxii., H. 3-6.
[6] Med. News, Dec. 5, 1896.
[7] Lo Sperimentale, Fasc. 2, 1896.
[8] Presse méd., Feb. 27, 1897.
[9] Deutsch. med. Woch., suppl. 1, page 93, May 13, 1897.

duct; in 1 case from the pus of an abscess. It stained with Löffler's methylen-blue, was decolorized by Gram's method, and grew on all the usual culture-media. They think it bears etiologic relation to the disease.

P. M. Mecray and J. J. Walsh[1] found a **microccus,** usually in the form of a diplococcus, in Steno's duct in all cases of mumps examined. The same microorganism was found in pure culture in the blood of 3 of 8 cases thus examined. In 3 other cases cultures from the blood gave this microorganism mixed with others. Two were sterile. In 5 healthy children the microorganism was never found. The diplococcus showed the same characteristics as that described by Laveran and Catrin.

F. L. Benham[2] records a case of **mumps with severe orchitis,** in which there was high temperature for about a week, sometimes reaching 104.8°, and part of this time accompanied by stupor and other severe cerebral symptoms. The rare cases of mumps exhibiting cerebral symptoms he divides into those showing (1) high fever and delirium, (2) insanity—both of these due to excessive poisoning of the disease, and (3) paralysis—probably due to thrombosis or embolism. These are conjectures, since pathologic records are wanting.

Other Infectious Diseases.—F. M. Crandall[3] records epidemics of **influenza** in 3 families. In the first, 7 of a family of 9, including 3 children, developed the disease, the mother and a boy of 2 years escaping. Seven cases occurred in the second family, and of those, 3 were below puberty. In the third family, of the 10 members but 3 escaped; 4 children were among those affected. Follicular tonsillitis was noticed at the same time in many of the cases.

Haushalter[4] records a case of **gonorrheal rheumatism** in a newborn male child who had gonorrheal ophthalmia. The left wrist and right knee became swollen in the 4th week of life, and cultures from the fluid removed from the joints showed gonococci, as did the examination of the pus from the conjunctivæ. As in the 10 similar cases reported, the duration of the joint-disease was short (1 week) and recovery ensued.

Griffon[5] records the case of a newborn infant with double purulent ophthalmia, in which **purulent arthritis** of the right hip and wrist afterward developed. During life, in liquid from the hip-joint, staphylococci and probably gonococci were found; the vaginal secretion showed the same, and the conjunctival pus contained both these microorganisms and a bacillus. Examination of the blood was negative. Pus taken after death from the affected joints showed probable gonococci; all cultures showed only staphylococci and the bacillus mentioned.

G. A. Turner[6] quotes from Arthur Mitchell the frightful previous mortality of 67.2% from **tetanus neonatorum** among all children born on the island of St. Kilda. The newborn were wrapped in blankets, with no dressing to the umbilicus. Turner had antiseptic dressings of iodoform applied and carefully changed daily, and no deaths from tetanus have occurred since among the children thus treated.

A thorough *résumé* of the European literature for 1896 on **vaccination** is given by L. Voigt.[7]

E. Kronenberg[8] records a case of infection from **vaccinia.** A few days after washing his face with a sponge used by a child with vaccinia an 8-year-

[1] Med. Rec., Sept. 26, 1896.   [2] Lancet, Jan. 30, 1897.
[3] Arch. of Pediatrics, Dec., 1896.   [4] Arch. Clin. de Bordeaux, vol. iv., No. 11, 1896.
[5] Presse méd., No. 15, 1896.   [6] Brit. Med. Jour., Oct. 24, 1896.
[7] Arch. f. Kinderh., Bd. 22, H. 3 and 6.   [8] Deutsch. med. Zeit., xviii., 283, 1895.

old boy developed an eruption of vesicles on the cheeks, eyelids, and nose, and in the mouth. After inoculation from the contents of one of the pustules the father developed typical vaccinia.

Krasnobajew [1] exhibited a boy, 8 years old, with **actinomycosis of the intestine.** The diagnosis was made by finding the ray-fungus in the pus from one of the fistulæ. Improvement was marked under persistent use of potassium iodid.

R. Abrahams [2] reports as **rheumatism of the newborn** the cases of 3 infants whose mothers had all had attacks of rheumatism in the later months of pregnancy. The father, also, of one child was rheumatic, and there was a history of rheumatism in the family of another. Two of the children were found within the first day of life to have swollen, red, and tender joints, and the third had the cardiac murmur of aortic insufficiency. In one child suppuration occurred later in some of the joints, while the second case which presented joint-trouble recovered under the use of salicylate of sodium, and an endocardial murmur which was at first present disappeared.

GENERAL NONINFECTIOUS DISEASES.

Rachitis.—J. P. West [3] records rachitis in a breast-fed infant of 4 months, seemingly due to the demonstrated deficiency of fat in the mother's milk. J. L. Morse [4] publishes the results of the examination of the blood of 20 rachitic infants, and concludes from these and other publications that most cases are accompanied by anemia of a severity generally proportionate to the severity of the process. The anemia may be of any form, but usually the hemoglobin is relatively and absolutely decreased. Leukocytosis is more frequent when splenic tumor exists, and any of the forms of leukocytes may be increased. There is nothing distinctive of the disease in the condition of the blood. J. Thomson [5] describes the case of a rachitic boy of 13 months, who had convulsions, laryngismus stridulus, facial irritability, and head-nodding. Changing the diet from a weak dilution of condensed milk to a milk-and-cream mixture was followed by distinct improvement, but the condition persisted in lessened intensity. About a year later, after a fit, he had convulsive laughter, and shortly afterward died in a general convulsion. No autopsy was allowed.

Scurvy.—D. Lichty [6] records a case of infantile scorbutus with such marked tumefaction of the gums as almost to cover the incisor teeth. S. E. Leard [7] records a case of the same disease. A. H. Bogart [8] notes 2 cases in which the lesions were subperiosteal, with no mouth or skin symptoms. J. Leidy [9] records 9 cases, 7 of which were seen in dispensary practice. Six of the infants had been fed upon one or other of the proprietary infant's foods and 3 upon sterilized milk. A. H. Burr [10] records a case with marked swelling of the femur and scapula and suppuration of the hemorrhagic cutaneous lesions. C. W. Townsend [11] records 12 cases, in 1 of which there was hematuria. Three had moderate rickets. W. F. Cheney [12] saw 1 case associated with marked rickets.

Status Lymphaticus.—Galatti [13] records a case in which death occurred

[1] Arch. f. Kinderh., Bd. 23, H. 1–3.   [2] Med. Rec., Oct. 17, 1896.
[3] Cincin. Lancet-Clinic, vol. xxxvi., No. 15, 1896.
[4] Boston M. and S. Jour., Apr. 22, 1897.   [5] Arch. of Pediatrics, Oct., 1896.
[6] N. Am. Practitioner, Aug., 1896.   [7] Med. Rec., May 8, 1897.
[8] Brooklyn Med. Jour., May, 1897.   [9] Boston M. and S. Jour., Oct. 29, 1896.
[10] Jour. Am. Med. Assoc., Nov. 7, 1896.
[11] Boston M. and S. Jour., vol. cxxxiv., No. 21, 1896.
[12] Med. News, vol. lxviii., No. 9, 1896.   [13] Wien. med. Blätter, Dec. 10, 1896.

in a child with status lymphaticus 10 hours after an injection of diphtheric antitoxin, and in which the rapidly fatal issue seemed due to the lymphatic condition. He insists upon a guarded prognosis and treatment of these cases.

Biedert[1] found an **enlarged thymus** as the cause of death in a case which had presented, during life, the symptoms of croup, and for which intubation and then tracheotomy had been performed without benefit. Death was caused by pressure on the trachea and by obstruction to the venous circulation. The enlargement of the gland was due to round-cell infiltration and increased vascularity.

T. Escherich[2] emphasizes the danger of using certain procedures which are usually harmless, such as **hydrotherapy,** in children with status lymphaticus. As an instance of this danger, he relates the case of a 2-year-old boy who went into collapse while in a wet-pack of salicylic-acid solution used for prurigo, and death occurred the next day. He further considers the relation tetany and laryngospasm bear to the lymphatic constitution, and details a case with marked laryngospasm in which the other main symptoms of tetany were present, though latent, and in which case sudden death occurred during a laryngeal attack. Postmortem the thymus and numerous other glands were found enlarged. He suggests that here we may have an indication of the pathogeny of tetany and of laryngospasm, and mentions the possibility that the thymus may be related to these spasmodic attacks as is the thyroid to exophthalmic goiter.

Diabetes Mellitus.—Josias[3] points out that we cannot use opiates in diabetes in children as in adults. Of medicinal remedies, he recommends Fowler's solution in full doses, and, to diminish the sugar, antipyrin in daily doses of 10 to 20 gr. The infrequency of diabetes mellitus **in infancy** makes it of interest to refer to a case in a child $2\frac{1}{2}$ years old, reported by L. Rosenberg.[4]

Arthritis Deformans.—W. Stowell[5] reports a case of arthritis deformans in a girl of 9 years. The disease was of 3 years' duration, and the child was nearly helpless from ankylosis of the shoulders and elbows and extreme flexion of the head on the chest. Massage benefited her greatly.

F. G. Finley[6] records the case of a girl of 11 years with **chronic polyarthritis.** Nearly 4 years before, the affection began in the right ankle, with swelling and stiffness, and was then considered tuberculous. Subsequently the right knee, the metacarpophalangeal articulations, the wrist, left knee and left ankle became affected, and the legs drawn up ; the patient had been bedridden for 2 years. The swelling left the joints 2 years previous to the report, but they remained almost without motion and useless. There was some crepitation on movement. The soft parts of the joints were thickened, and the skin over them was tense and glossy. The bodily organs were normal. No Heberden's nodosities were present, and there was no history of rheumatism or tuberculosis in the family. Tonic treatment and manipulation had resulted in marked improvement.

DISEASES OF THE ALIMENTARY TRACT.

F. Forchheimer[7] contributes a suggestive paper on **elimination as an etiologic factor** of diseases of the alimentary canal, pointing out that as

[1] Berlin. klin. Woch., June 29, 1896.   [2] Ibid., July 20, 1896.
[3] Jour. des Praticiens, Aug. 6, 1896.   [4] Münch. med. Woch., May 18, 1897.
[5] Arch. of Pediatrics, Oct., 1896.   [6] Montreal Med. Jour., vol. xxv., No. 2, 1896.
[7] Arch. of Pediatrics, Jan., 1897.

the absorptive function of any part of the tract lessens as compared with another, its eliminative capabilities probably increase. The value of lavage and purgatives in the different diseases is in part due to their removing not only the irritants, but also the toxalbumins and other substances that have been eliminated from the circulation into the canal.

Beco[1] describes as **diphtheroid stomatitis** an affection of infants which has often been confused with aphthous stomatitis. It occurs in the form of discrete plaques on the middle of the lower lip, dorsum and edges of the tongue, and, more rarely, on the gums. These are not preceded by vesicles, are adherent, and detachment leaves a bleeding ulcer. The affection is parasitic and due to several microorganisms, of which those most frequently found are the staphylococcus aureus and the streptococcus pyogenes. When plaques have formed the disease may be transmitted. Ghika[2] describes a similar affection of staphylococcic origin, first vesicular and then becoming membranous.

F. Fede[3] describes a **disease of the mouth** seen in Lower Italy, and affecting children shortly after the eruption of the lower incisors. The appearance is somewhat like that of an aphtha situated on the frenum and under surface of the tongue—a raised, gray swelling, which is at first papillomatous and later of the nature of a granuloma. There are 3 types of the disease : one in which the general health is good ; a second, in which the local condition has lasted for some time and some intercurrent disease, like tuberculosis, sets in ; and a third, a severe form, which may terminate fatally. The local treatment is excision and cauterization. [Of the terms suggested for the condition, Riga's disease and aphtha cachectica are the best.]

S. S. Adams[4] records a case of **pharyngo-esophageal stenosis** in a child of 4 months. Until 2 weeks before admission it had been well, since which time, and until its death 2 weeks after admission, it had regurgitated all food which it attempted to swallow. A catheter and the examining-finger were arrested below the epiglottis. Postmortem the pharynx was found to end in a wide cul-de-sac, with only a pinhole-opening into the esophagus, and this perhaps artificial. There was no evidence of inflammation from any cause.

A. Clopatt[5] considers that the cause of acute **retropharyngeal abscess** is usually to be found in affections of the skin, or of the mucous membranes of some of the cranial cavities, with infection through the lymphatics leading to the postpharyngeal glands. Sometimes enlargement of the cervical glands in the acute infectious diseases may lead to the condition. He records 6 cases, 3 of which were under a year of age, 2 under 2 years, and 1, 2 years old.

Diarrheal Diseases.—A. F. Plicque[6] recognizes : 1. Simple diarrhea, for which he uses ordinary treatment ; 2. Green bilious diarrhea, in which the green color is recognized as due to bile by the nitric-acid tests, and for which alkalies (sodium bicarbonate) are essential ; 3. Green bacillary diarrhea, for which the most important medication is lactic acid ; 4. Cholera infantum, in which he insists upon continued feeding in spite of vomiting, stimulation, and the use of lactic acid, hydrochloric acid, and laudanum.

A. Baginsky[7] contributes a valuable monograph on the **pathology of the diarrheal diseases** of childhood, with the following conclusions : 1. The summer-diarrheas of children are in the beginning only functional dis-

[1] Arch. de Méd. expér. et d'Anat. path., p. 433, July, 1896.
[2] Jour. de Clin. et Thérap. inf., No. 11, 1896.   [3] Arch. f. Kinderh., Bd. xxi., H. 5 u. 6.
[4] Arch. of Pediatrics, Oct., 1896.   [5] Progrès méd., vol. xxxviii., Jan. 16, 1897.
[6] Presse méd., July 1, 1896.   [7] Arch. f. Kinderh., Bd. xxii., H. 3–6.

turbances of motion and secretion with abnormal chemistry of digestion ; later the intestinal wall undergoes severe anatomic changes. 2. These changes may range from catarrh to necrosis of the mucous membrane. 3. The follicular changes are peculiar and independent of the catarrhal, although if they are of long duration the two coexist ; the follicular changes often lead to ulceration. 4. The causes of the inflammation are not specific germs, but the ordinary saprophytic bacteria which inhabit the intestinal canal and take on a special virulence. 5. Under some circumstances, other bacteria, not ordinarily present, may gain access to the intestinal tract and cause disease with severe anatomic changes. 6. These bacteria may penetrate into other organs, especially the kidney, and set up inflammation even to suppuration ; the metastasis rarely occurs through the blood-vessels. 7. The most severe disturbances are caused by the products of bacterial metabolism, which are either of the nature of acids or products of albumin-decomposition, which may have proceeded as far as ammonia or its compounds ; these act as powerful irritants in the intestine and so injure the wall as to gain access through the circulation (blood and lymph) to more remote organs, and throw such a strain upon the eliminative organs as to destroy them. 8. Through the influence of this intoxication the whole organism loses its power of resisting the many forms of hostile microbes, and disposition to disease is shown in the occurrence of many complications.

O. Reinach [1] reports the use of **sterilized cow's serum for gastroenteritis.** Of 15 infants, 11 showed marked improvement of circulation, digestion, and general appearance. The 4 other cases died—2 of lobar pneumonia, 2 of severe follicular disease of the intestine. The favorable action of the injections is attributed to the fluid added to the blood, the stimulating action on metabolism of the salts of the serum, and to the nutriment in the albumin of the serum. No unfavorable effects were noted, except slight fever in 2 cases and an eruption like measles which appeared in 1 case 2 weeks after the injection. From 10 to 26 c.c. were used in one injection.

Lesage [2] has treated 52 children with grave diarrheas with **serum obtained from asses** after injecting colon-bacilli from virulent milk or stools. 26 children had no marked symptoms after 48 hours, 14 were improved, 12 unimproved. In all cases where the stools were green the color disappeared after the injections. The serum obtained after treating asses with the colon-bacilli normally present in stools did not give these results.

Watu [3] advocates the treatment of infantile diarrhea with **cooled boiled water** given in small portions, while food is excluded for from 8 to 24 hours. This is said to promote recovery by diluting and flushing out the intestinal contents, and by carrying out with them the dissolved toxins.

K. Szegö [4] made a **bacteriologic study of the intestinal discharges in infants,** some of whom were healthy, while others had "dyspepsia," which term was not used to include the diarrheas, but to cover those cases in which there were sour-smelling acid stools, containing mucus and curds. Many bacteria were found, the bacillus coli communis being the predominant form. There was no bacterial distinction between the two groups of cases, so the dyspepsias were considered to be merely changes in the chemistry of digestion.

W. Soltau Fenwick,[5] in a report on the **pathology of infantile marasmus,** drawn from observations on 16 cases, shows that the failure of nutrition is due to organic and often incurable changes in the mucous membrane of the

[1] Münch. med. Woch., xliii., 42. 1896.   [2] Rev. de Thérap. Med.-Chir., No. 24, 1896.
[3] Thèse de Paris, No. 40, ii., 1896–97.   [4] Arch. f. Kinderh., Bd. xxii., H. 1 and 2.
[5] Brit. Med. Jour., Sept. 26, 1896.

stomach and intestines (see Plate 2). By means of test-meals and lavage the condition of gastric digestion may be ascertained and the prognosis made.

L. E. Holt[1] reports a case of **appendicitis in a child** 2½ years old. There was persistent vomiting, with moderate constipation and considerable fever. Examination under chloroform failed to reveal anything in the abdomen suggestive of intussusception or appendicitis. Signs of peritonitis were marked on the following day, and death occurred 5 days after the initial attack of vomiting. At the autopsy the appendix was found to contain a hard concretion just above a perforation, which was an inch from the distal end.

The maximum length of time at which it is justifiable to continue enemata to reduce an **intussusception** is not yet clearly defined ; but those who favor the medical rather than the surgical treatment will find encouragement in the reports of W. P. Northrup[2] and M. H. Brown,[3] the former reporting 1 and the latter 2 cases in which the persistent use of enemata accomplished reduction. In one of Brown's cases 2 days had elapsed after the onset, and in the other fecal vomiting had set in. Fifteen injections in all were required in the latter case.

Th. Hecker[4] records a case of **congenital intestinal occlusion.** Vomiting began soon after birth, and continued uninterruptedly. There were jaundice and distended abdomen. A catheter passed only 6 cm. into the rectum. The stricture could not be reached per rectum, however, so an artificial anus was made in the groin. A feculent fluid flowed from the opening. The child died on the 6th day of life. Postmortem there was found old and recent fetal peritonitis, and two separate tracts of intestine were discovered. The lower began blindly above at the cecum and continued as a collapsed, cord-like body extending to the anus. The other began at the pylorus, and ended at the pelvic brim. The separation seemed due to torsion, and this to either fetal peritonitis or volvulus. The mother had suffered from slight abdominal trauma at the 4th month of pregnancy, but this scarcely bore any relation to the condition.

DISEASES OF THE CIRCULATORY SYSTEM AND BLOOD.

Congenital Defects.—J. P. C. Griffith[5] calls attention to the difficulty and sometimes impossibility of diagnosing **congenital cardiac defects** intra vitam. He reports a case of perforate septum ventriculorum in a child of 4 years, in which the diagnosis was reasonably well established during life, and was confirmed at the autopsy. A. Caillé[6] reports **transposition of the great arteries of the heart** in an infant of 6 weeks. The aorta arose from the thick-walled right ventricle and the pulmonary artery was given off from the left ventricle, the walls of which were of moderate thickness. T. M. Rotch[7] records an unusual congenital **malformation of the heart** of an infant which seemed perfectly well and had normal heart-sounds until 16 days old, when it became cyanosed, dyspneic, and cold, and died next day. Postmortem the heart was found hypertrophied, and the foramen ovale open ; the interventricular septum was incomplete, and the aorta arose from the right ventricle, the pulmonary artery from the left ventricle. The latter vessel was dilated into a pouch, from which were given off the right and left pulmonary and a third vessel which seemed to be the ductus arteriosus, and which took the place of the arch and descending aorta and supplied the trunk and lower extremities. The aorta supplied the head and arms.

[1] Arch. of Pediatrics, Jan., 1897.   [2] Med. News, Dec. 12, 1896.
[3] Arch. of Pediatrics, Aug., 1896.   [4] St. Petersburg. med. Woch., N. F. xiii., No. 45, 1896.
[5] Arch. of Pediatrics, Sept., 1896.   [6] Ibid., Oct. 1896.   [7] Ibid., Dec., 1896.

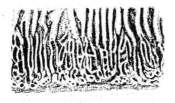 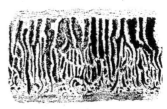

FIG. 1.—Drawing of the mucous membrane of the stomach of a healthy infant (× 65).

FIG. 2.—Drawing of the mucous membrane of the stomach in the first stage of chronic catarrh, showing the exudation of round cells between the gastric glands (× 65).

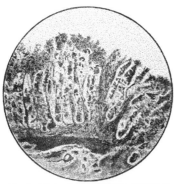 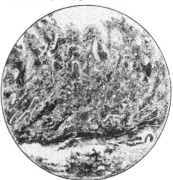

FIG. 3.—Photomicrograph of the stomach in a case of marasmus, showing the formation of fibrous tissue between the glands—second stage of interstitial gastritis (× 65).

FIG. 4.—Photomicrograph of the stomach in a case of marasmus, showing complete cirrhosis of the mucous membrane, with obliteration of the glands—third stage of interstitial gastritis (× 65).

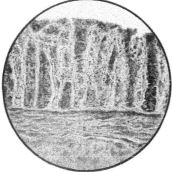 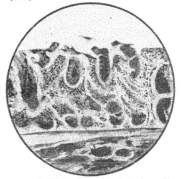

FIG. 5.—Photomicrograph of the cecum, showing the effects of chronic inflammation upon the glands of the mucous membrane (× 65).

FIG 6.—Photomicrograph of the descending colon from a case of chronic marasmus, showing partial obliteration of the glands of the mucous membrane (× 65).

(Fenwick, in Brit. Med. Jour., Sept. 26, 1896.)

Myocarditis.—Weill and Barjon[1] decide from their examination of the hearts from 4 children who died with endocarditis that parenchymatous myocarditis occurs in childhood, especially in the course of a chronic endocarditis. These hearts showed an excessive development of the protoplasm of the muscle-eells, while the contractile substance suffered. The elementary fibrils were thinned and separated, the nuclei proliferated and enlarged, and the muscular striæ were diminished, while vascular and interstitial changes were absent. Three of the cases died during or soon after recurrent attacks of rheumatism, with evidences of a general febrile infection, and from this they conclude that the myocarditis seems to come from infection due to rheumatism. Erysipelas and probably other contagious diseases are also active. The condition manifests itself by asystole, lasting some days to several months, without change in the cardiac rhythm.

Adhesive Pericarditis.—L. E. Holt[2] records the case of a child of 16 months in which adhesive pericarditis with complete obliteration of the pericardial sac was found after death. The family history bore no relation to the condition and it had not been suspected during life. There was acute pneumonia and extensive pleural adhesions were present on both sides. G. M. Swift[3] reports 4 cases at the ages of 4, 6, 10, and 14 years.

Endocarditis.—A. J. Wood[4] records the case of a girl who had rheumatic endocarditis at 12 years of age. Compensation was established, but this broke down at puberty and the child died. He considers puberty an especially trying time for children with damaged hearts.

Malignant Endocarditis.—J. H. Fruitnight[5] reports a case and discusses the etiology, pathology, symptoms, and treatment. Its infrequency in children is mentioned, a point also emphasized in the discussion by W. P. Northrup, L. E. Holt, and Wm. Osler. Wood[6] records a case of malignant endocarditis in a girl of 5. Severe paroxysms of pain in the head, fever, cough, and weakness of the right side were the early manifestations. Right-sided complete hemiplegia also existed. The heart was somewhat enlarged, and there was a loud systolic murmur. The spleen was enlarged, the urine albuminous, and petechiæ appeared. Optic neuritis and retinal hemorrhages were present. The temperature reached 104° F. and a convulsion preceded death in coma. A history of rheumatism was not obtainable. At the autopsy the anterior mitral valve was much thickened and infiltrated, and a large ante-mortem clot hung from the valve. There were infarcts in the spleen, kidney, and brain, and petechial hemorrhages throughout the body. No primary cause was discovered, except possibly old pleurisy. The records of the Children's Hospital at Melbourne furnish but 1 other case in 10 years.

Hematoma of Valve.—V. Kahlden[7] reports a hematoma of the posterior leaflet of the mitral valve, with a diameter of 12 to 14 mm., in the heart of a child 1 year of age which had apparently presented no cardiac symptoms during life. It caused a spherical, hollow tumor projecting mainly from the upper surface of the valve and bounded by the upper and end surfaces of the leaflet. The vessels of the valves were thickened and the lumen narrowed. The hollow portion of the tumor contained some fibrin. The commonly favorable course of hematoma of the valves seemed interfered with in this case by the large size of the tumor. Death was caused by miliary tuberculosis secondary to infected bronchial glands.

[1] Rev. mens. des Mal. de l'Enfance, Dec., 1896.   [2] Arch. of Pediatrics, Oct., 1896.
[3] Ibid.   [4] Intercol. Med. Jour. of Australasia, Jan. 20, 1897.
[5] Ibid., Sept., 1896.   [6] Intercol. Med. Jour. of Australasia, July 20, 1896.
                        [7] Ziegler's Beiträge, Bd. xxi., H. 2, 1897.

Arteriosclerosis.—Seitz [1] reports 3 cases of arteriosclerosis in children, with hypertrophy of the left ventricle. Preceding infectious diseases seemed to be the only causes.

Anemias.—A. Baginsky [2] reports 2 cases of **pernicious anemia** in children aged $3\frac{1}{2}$ and 10 years. The bacterium coli was found in the blood, and may have been of etiologic significance. F. Theodor [3] tabulates 45 cases of acute leukemia, 6 of which occurred in children under 10 years. He reports a case in a boy of 4 years, ending fatally in 6 weeks. The proportion of white to red cells approximated 1 to 3. Cultures from the blood on different media remained sterile. A family history pointing to syphilis was considered to have some etiologic bearing.

Purpura.—E. A. T. Steele [4] records a fatal case of **purpura hæmorrhagica** probably due to "scurvy rickets," and with the rare complication of pemphigus. The disease began with epistaxis and bleeding gums. Later purpuric spots appeared on the face and limbs, and in the center of many of these were large bullæ filled with dark serum. The wrists and ankles were swollen and the child cried if moved. Death occurred the day after admission, in hyperpyrexia and coma. Autopsy showed many small hemorrhages in the lungs, a decolorized clot in the superior longitudinal sinus, soft and porous bones, and enlarged ends of the ribs. Claude [5] notes a case of **infectious purpura** occurring as the eruption of measles was disappearing and while the child was in a second attack of bronchopneumonia. The issue was fatal. Another case was apparently toxic, as it came on during violent poisoning from tainted meat and bacteriologic examination was negative.

Melæna Neonatorum.—The literature of this disease is reviewed by J. W. Smuck,[6] who reports 2 cases, one of them recovering. F. M. Crandall [7] reports an unusual case, the hemorrhages appearing first on the 15th day after birth. Recovery ensued under rest, small doses of paregoric, and abstinence from food for a short time. J. L. Morse [8] also records a case remarkable for the severity of the symptoms and for the recovery. A fatal case is reported by R. H. Shaw.[9] J. v. Chrzanowski [10] reports 2 fatal cases in which cultures of the blood during life were negative. He discusses at length the different theories with regard to the etiology.

Hemophilia.—E. Berggruen [11] reports a case of hemophilia in a girl of 9, developing cerebral apoplexy, hematuria, and pernicious anemia, but recovering under the use of tablets of bone-marrow. Cultures of the blood were taken, with negative results. Comby [12] records the case of a girl, aged 11 months, in whom from the third week of life there had been continuous and spontaneous hemorrhages from the nose, mouth, and rectum, and into the substance of the skin, without, however, impairing in any manifest way the child's development. There was a history on the father's side of hemophilia, but not on the maternal side. The patient was the only living one of their children; there had been two other girls, who had died in infancy, but had not shown any signs of hemophilia.

[1] Arch. f. Kinderh , Bd. xxi., H. 5 and 6.   [2] Ibid., Bd. xxi., H. 1–3.
[3] Ibid., Bd. xxii.. II. 1 and 2.   [4] Lancet, Apr. 17, 1896.
[5] Rev. mens. des Mal. de l'Enfance, No. 3, 1896.   [6] Canad. Pract., Mar., 1897.
[7] Arch. of Pediatrics, Sept., 1896.   [8] Ibid.
[9] Brit. Med. Jour., Nov. 14, 1896.   [10] Arch. f. Kinderh., Bd. xxi., H. 5 and 6.
[11] Ibid., Bd. xxi., H. 1–3.   [12] Bull. de la Soc. méd. des Hôp., June 25, 1896.

DISEASES OF THE LIVER, SPLEEN, AND GENITO-URINARY SYSTEM.

Lewin[1] discusses briefly simple **hypertrophy of the spleen**, describing 2 cases not depending on rachitis or syphilis, one of the patients being cured by arsenic, the other by electricity. S. M. Hamill[2] exhibited a boy of 6 years with an enlarged spleen reaching several inches below the costal border, syphilis being suspected as the cause.

Lancereaux[3] protests against allowing children **alcoholic beverages.** He details the condition of a child of 13, whose father died of alcoholic cirrhosis of the liver, while the mother was living, but intemperate, and had allowed the little girl since her third year about half a liter of wine every day. The child was extremely small, pale, and had an enormous liver and spleen, and the urine contained considerable amounts of albumin. A second child had taken from half a liter to a full liter of wine each day since its second year, and at 14 years of age had had for several years severe night-terrors and symptoms of neuritis. This child also was very ill-developed, and had enlargement of the liver and spleen, albuminous urine, muscular atrophy, weakness and some loss of sensation in the limbs. Both cases had uremic attacks.

J. A. C. Kynoch[4] records the case of a child that had **jaundice**, vomiting, distended abdomen, and white stools from birth, with progressive emaciation. After death at the age of 3 months the **liver** was found enlarged, while the common duct was narrowed a little below its commencement, and toward its lower end it was so small as to appear like a small cord. No orifice could be readily found in the papilla, but bile flowed through the entire duct, though slowly and with some difficulty. The case resembled congenital obliteration of the bile-ducts. There was no family history of syphilis, and the child exhibited none of the signs of specific disease. **Acute yellow atrophy of the liver** has been observed by F. Lanz[5] in a boy 4 years old, and by Aufrecht[6] in an infant 6 days old.

Sohön[7] found **cyclic albuminuria** in 2 sisters, both the subjects of **chlorosis.** Since fatty degeneration of blood-vessels and consequent edema by transudation occur in chlorosis, the author suggests that cyclic albuminuria may have the same cause.

Thomas[8] remarks upon the frequency of **hematuria or albuminuria in infantile scurvy,** and records a case in which these conditions were the earliest and most marked symptoms. He considers the cause an irritant in the blood, and thinks the diagnosis might be early secured in suspected cases by examining the urine. Hematuria may be sometimes the only symptom of the disease.

Simmonds[9] examined the kidneys in 60 athrepsic infants who had presented no digestive or respiratory disturbances. All showed **parenchymatous nephritis.** After excluding other causes, he attributes the nephritis to purulent otitis media, which was present in all of these cases and in 128 of 133 cases dead of athrepsia. Many bacteria were found in cultures of the exudate from the middle-ear and the same microorganisms were found in the kidneys.

E. Cacace[10] reviews the literature of **renal sarcoma** in children, reporting

[1] Arch. f. Kinderh., Bd. xxi., H. 5 and 6.   [2] Arch. of Pediatrics, July, 1897.
[3] Bull. de l'Acad. de Méd., Oct. 13, 1896.   [4] Edinb. Med. Jour., July, 1896.
[5] Wien. klin. Woch., No. 30, 1896.   [6] Centralbl. f. innere Med., No. 11, 1896.
[7] Jahrb. f. Kinderh., Bd. 41, S. 307, 1896.   [8] Boston M. and S. Jour., Sept. 3, 1896.
[9] Deutsch. Arch. f. klin. Med., Bd. 56, S. 385, 1896.   [10] La Pediatria, Feb., 1897.

a case in a girl of 7 years. Durante [1] reports a similar case in a girl of 2 years.

Steinmetz [2] reports a case of **primary sarcoma of the urinary bladder** in a child $2\frac{3}{4}$ years of age. But 31 other cases of primary tumor of the bladder are recorded, most of which were sarcomatous, and 23 occurred within the first 5 years of life. Hematuria is an infrequent symptom, while symptoms of stone are common. Prognosis is fatal—only 1 of 15 operated cases lived. Death usually occurs in from 10 weeks to 3 months.

Trumpp [3] describes a primary and a secondary form of **cystitis** due to the colon-bacillus, both occurring more frequently in girls than in boys. In the primary form the bacilli gain entrance, either directly through the walls of the rectum and bladder, or through the urethra, and this form may be mild or of severe type with grave complications. The secondary form is usually consequent to follicular enteritis. Of 17 cases of intestinal disease, 14 showed colon-bacilli in the urine. Treatment consisted of lysol irrigations and salol internally.

Various pathologic conditions of the **kidneys** are described by A. Baginsky, [4] including pyelonephritis, lymphomatosis, and sarcoma. He has also [5] studied the metabolism of a child with diabetes mellitus.

P. Sommerfeld [6] examined the urine from 70 cases of **scarlet fever** and 30 cases of diphtheria, testing for albumoses, but with negative results. The cases included all types of the diseases, and Sommerfeld concludes that, if albumoses occur in the urine in these diseases, no prognostic significance can be attached to them.

H. Hellendall [7] reports 2 interesting cases of **hereditary contracted kidney** occurring in sisters, one 12 years old, the other 6 months. There was no family history of syphilis, but the mother had been under treatment for chronic nephritis, which, from the history, evidently began when she was pregnant with the first of the 2 children. Both children died with bronchopneumonia and enteritis, and the kidneys were found very atrophic and granular, and in the younger child the cortex of the kidney showed areas of cartilage.

DISEASES OF THE NERVOUS SYSTEM.

J. Zappert [8] gives a thorough discussion of the **etiology of nervous diseases in childhood.** He groups the causes in 4 main divisions—traumatic, infections or toxic, hereditary or family, and psychic—and considers them in order in their relations to diseases of the peripheral nerves, cord, and brain, and to diseases with no discoverable anatomic basis.

F. A. Packard [9] records a case of **endothelioma of the cerebral membranes,** with the interesting symptom of wasting of the paralyzed muscles which has been noted in but 7 previous cases, which are reviewed. The patient, a 14-year-old girl, had had mental disturbance and headache for a year, and 5 months before death a left-sided convulsion. Subsequently blindness, at first temporary, but afterward permanent, appeared with choked disk. Paralysis of the left arm and leg with atrophy of these members came on, and she had numerous attacks of Jacksonian epilepsy affecting the paralyzed limbs. There was a conical, sessile, hard tumor, an inch in diameter, which was firmly

[1] La Pediatria, Aug., 1896.   [2] Deutsch. Zeit. f. Chir., xxxix., 313, 336, 1896.
[3] Münch. med. Woch., xliii., S. 1008, 1896.   [4] Arch. f. Kinderh., Bd. xxii., H. 3–6.
[5] Ibid.   [6] Ibid., Bd. xxiii., H. 1.   [7] Ibid., Bd. xxiii., H. 1 and 2.
[8] Wien. med. Woch., May 15, 1897.   [9] Arch. of Pediatrics, Sept., 1896.

attached to the calvarium, just back of the vertex. Postmortem there was found a growth continuous with this external growth, lying on the cerebral surface of the parietal and posterior portions of the frontal region, not extending to the lateral aspect, but running down into the great longitudinal fissure. It involved the upper portion of the Rolandic fissure and the ascending parietal and frontal convolutions, while the supramarginal and angular gyri escaped. Microscopically it was found to be an endothelioma. There was no descending degeneration of the pons, medulla, or upper cord.

H. D. Chapin[1] details a case of **multiple tuberculous brain-tumor.** There were symptoms of tumor during life, and lumbar puncture had been performed and the fluid examined for tubercle-bacilli, without result. Autopsy showed 3 tumors about the size of walnuts, one on the basal surface of the left cerebellar lobe, one at the head of the right caudate nucleus, and one in the substance of the anterior and posterior quadrigeminal bodies. The author has had fluid obtained by lumbar puncture in several cases of tuberculous meningitis examined, and tubercle-bacilli were never found. S. S. Adams[2] also reports a case of tuberculous abscess of the brain, with firm, cheesy masses in the right hemisphere.

M. P. Jacobi[3] records the interesting clinical history of a girl of 11, who had had, about 6 months before coming under observation, an attack of what was probably **cerebrospinal meningitis.** Following this there was a varied complex of symptoms, chief among them being ataxia, absence of knee-jerks, vomiting in the nature of gastric crises, and disturbances of tactile and heat sensibility. After a thorough discussion of the case the author concludes that the most probable lesions were those of a disseminated meningitis affecting especially the meninges of the cerebellum.

Wentworth[4] draws the following conclusions from the use of **lumbar puncture** in 29 cases: 1. The normal cerebrospinal fluid contains neither cells nor fibrin, and is perfectly clear. 2. In cases of meningitis the cerebrospinal fluid is invariably cloudy when withdrawn. The degree of cloudiness is to some extent proportionate to the amount and character of the exudation in the meninges. 3. The cloudiness is caused by cells. The character of the cells differs with the variety of meningitis. After withdrawal more or less fibrin is formed in the fluid. The presence of these cells and fibrin is pathognomonic of inflammation in the meninges. 4. The cloudiness is oftentimes so slight that close observation is necessary to detect it. 5. The operation is not difficult to perform on infants and children. It is not dangerous, if strict cleanliness is observed. 6. The differential diagnosis between the various kinds of meningitis can be made by microscopic examination of the sediment, by cultures taken from the fluid, and by inoculation-experiments. 7. Inoculation-experiments afford the surest means of determining tuberculous meningitis. They are of value to distinguish between the varieties of meningitis in order to determine if tuberculous meningitis is recovered from. 8. In the normal fluid a faint trace of albumin is usually present, about 0.02 %, or less, by quantitative analysis. In meningitis the amount of albumin is increased, and has varied from 0.03 % to 0.1 %. 9. In one case a diagnosis of general infection with the staphylococcus pyogenes aureus was made from cultures taken from the cerebrospinal fluid. A. Caillé[5] reports 21 cases of lumbar puncture in which the fluid was examined for sugar, albumin, and bacteria. Tubercle-bacilli were found in 5 of 7 cases of tuberculous meningitis; 1 case of cerebrospinal meningitis showed

[1] Arch. of Pediatrics., Feb., 1897. [2] Ibid., Aug., 1896.
[3] Med. Rec., May 29, 1897. [4] Boston M. and S. Jour., Aug. 6, 1896.
[5] Arch. of Pediatrics, Aug., 1896.

pneumococci ; 2 cases of acute hydrocephalus showed sterile fluid with a trace
of albumin ; 1 case of brain-tumor, sterile fluid with 0.2 % of sugar.   In 2
cases he attempted the local treatment of tuberculous meningitis by means of
lumbar puncture, injecting in one case a solution of sodium salicylate, and in
another iodoform in water.   The autopsies showed extensive lesions, and the
author suggests a more radical and thorough irrigation by combining with the
lumbar puncture a trephine-opening in the skull.

M. Nicoll 1 gives the clinical notes and postmortem findings in a case of
acute **ependymitis,** the choroid and pia being unchanged.

J. Grósz [2] reports on the clinical features and postmortem findings in a case
of **congenital cerebral diplegia.**   The child was the product of ectopic
gestation, delivered by Cæsarean section, and lived 4 months.   At first only
the right arm and leg were spastic, showing some improvement, but during
the second month the left side began to stiffen and athetosis was present in
both hands.   The child died of inanition, and the brain was found to be compressed, the pressure on the right hemisphere having been prenatal and due to
the position of the fetus ; the membranes over the left hemisphere were the seat
of an internal chronic hemorrhagic pachymeningitis.

Romme [3] reviews the claims of various authors as to the **etiology of
tetany,** and concludes that the views of Kassowitz and his school (that it is a
manifestation of rickets) and those of others who would ascribe the condition
to any especial primary disease, are incorrect, as there are no constant postmortem findings in tetany, and it occurs with various diseases.   Clinical and
pathologic studies tell us only that the main symptoms are evidences of mechanical or reflex hyperexcitability of the cord and peripheral nerves due to a
diversity of causes.

At the Frankfort Congress (1896) there was an interesting discussion [4] on
laryngismus stridulus, with papers by Loos and Lange.   The former has
seen 164 cases, 14 of them ending fatally, and most of them being complicated
by tetany.   Lange's paper was on the relation of laryngeal spasm to rickets,
especially to craniotabes, and the connection between the two was shown to be
very slight.   With reference to the etiology of spasm of the glottis and tetany,
Fischl thinks that we have still much to learn, the infections or epidemic origin
being difficult of proof, and digestive disturbances occurring in greater amount
in summer-time, when tetany and laryngismus are rare.   Biedert [5] thought
that this might be explained by the difference in the nature of the digestive
disturbances, the acute carrying off the toxic materials, while the chronic,
which occur in cooler weather, allow a greater chance for the absorption of
toxic substances.   Lewin [6] reports a case of laryngismus stridulus which
depended upon indigestion set up by the use of a certain infant's food.   The
attacks ceased with a change of diet, to return again when the " kindermilch "
was used, and to disappear when it was discontinued.   J. Abercrombie [7] states
that in his experience facial irritability is always present in tetany, but he has
changed his belief that it is to be found only in tetany, as he has never failed
to find it present in a case of laryngismus stridulus.   He has also seen it in
about 20 cases of rickets, none of which presented signs of laryngismus or
tetany.

Among the nervous symptoms of **rachitis** A. Jacobi [8] classes insomnia,
night-terrors, hyperidrosis of the head, Chvostek's facial phenomenon, laryn-

---

[1] Arch. of Pediatrics, Oct., 1896.   [2] Arch. f. Kinderh., Bd. xxii., H. 1 and 2.
[3] Gaz. hebdom. de Méd. et de Chir., Jan. 24, 1897.
[4] Arch. f. Kinderh., Bd. xxi., H. 5 and 6.   [5] Ibid.   [6] Ibid.
[7] Arch. of Pediatrics, Nov., 1896.   [8] Ibid.

gismus stridulus, general convulsions, hydrocephalus, Trousseau's symptom, tetany, nystagmus, and spasmus nutans. He explains the ability of some rachitic children to sleep when held erect in the arms as due to the lessened hyperemia of the brain, and their arousing when laid down as due to the increase in cerebral congestion. He thinks that the coexistence in a rachitic child of Chvostek's and Trousseau's signs is not a sufficient basis for the diagnosis of "latent tetany."

L. Braun[1] advances the view that **pavor nocturnus** is not a disease *sui generis*, but a neurasthenic symptom due to inflammatory, parasitic, and other affections of the gastrointestinal tract and of the external genitalia, to insufficient sleep, and other causes. The prognosis is favorable if these causes be sought for and removed.

A. Stengel[2] reports a case of **arsenical neuritis** in a boy of 5, to whom Fowler's solution had been given in increasing doses until a maximum dose of 10 drops 3 times a day was reached. The physiologic action was then noticed, and the drug discontinued. Three weeks later it was seen that he did not use the right foot properly, and 2 weeks after this the gait suggested poliomyelitis or neuritis. The paralysis increased for a time, and the diagnosis of neuritis was made by the almost completely symmetric character of the paralysis, the absence of decided wasting, the preservation of reflexes, the distinctly tottering and ataxic gait, and the disturbance of station. Recovery ensued. As elimination does not keep pace with administration even when moderate doses are given, the author advises that the remedy be discontinued from time to time for periods of a week or two.

L. S. Somers[3] reports a case of **rumination** in a boy of 5 years. The child had had convulsions when 3 months old, and seemed intelligent as an infant. When 3 years old he had measles and lost his hearing, after which he could not speak intelligibly, and 6 months before the rumination began it had been noted that his head was hydrocephalic. The rumination occurred usually 15 to 20 minutes after meals, sometimes at other periods, when he would regurgitate, remasticate, and again swallow his food. Treatment and training brought about decided improvement. A maternal uncle and cousin had been unable to speak until 6 years old.

Epstein[4] reports 8 cases of **catalepsy in rachitic children,** all of whom presented evidence of imperfect or arrested development of the intellect, which with their general weakness recalled the condition of patients exhibiting catalepsy after grave diseases like typhoid fever. In the cases he reports a limb that was raised or otherwise moved kept the new position for 15 minutes or longer. There was no tremor during this time, and the reflexes of the cataleptic member were diminished.

C. W. Townsend[5] reports 5 cases of **thigh-friction,** a form of masturbation, in infants under 1 year of age, all of whom were females.

Collignon[6] gives as the diagnostic points of **migraine** in children of 4 or 5 years, recurring attacks of vomiting lasting 3 or 4 days, attended not with marked headache, but with considerable prostration, contracted pupils, pallor, slight fever, rapid respiration, and sensibility to light and sound. The individual attack may begin suddenly with palpitation or epistaxis, and may also end suddenly.

W. Osler[7] gives the French classification of the tic or **habit-move-**

[1] Jahrb. f. Kinderh., Jan., 1897.   [2] Arch. of Pediatrics, Mar., 1897.
[3] Med. Rec., Apr. 17, 1897.   [4] Rev. mens. des Mal. de l'Enfance, Jan., 1897.
[5] Arch. of Pediatrics, Nov., 1896.   [6] Ibid., Aug., 1896.
[7] Ibid., Jan., 1897.

ments, as follows : 1. Simple tic or habit-spasm, including mainly the common cases of spasmodic movement, chiefly of the facial muscles, which are, to a certain extent, under the control of the will. 2. Tics with superadded psychic phenomena, *maladie de la tic convulsif,* or Gilles de la Tourette's disease, in which, in addition to the simple tic, there are explosive utterances and imperative ideas. 3. Complex, coördinated tics, which include actions more extended and involved than simple tics, and also such conditions as head-nodding or swaying, and other bizarre movements. 4. Tic psychique, in which the imperative idea is the psychic equivalent of, and has an origin similar to, the motor tic.

W. Osler[1] describes a case of **head-swaying** in a girl of 5. At times there would be a rhythmic swaying of the head from side to side to the extent of a foot from the median line. The condition had existed from infancy, and the only point in the history that seemed to have any bearing was that other members of the family were nervous.

Osler[2] also reports 2 unusual types of night-terrors in boys aged 7 and 11 years. The attacks in the first case consisted in incoherent muttering, were more in the nature of night-mare than night-terrors, and ceased when the hypertrophied tonsils and adenoid growths were treated. A third case was related in which the attacks came on during waking-hours. Chloroform-inhalation seemed to control them.

John Thomson[3] reports the case of a girl who, from the age of 7 until menstruation became established at 13, had a **sensory hallucination of worms** crawling beneath the skin and of dryness of the palms and soles.

TUMORS.

E. Neuhaus[4] gives an extensive report of a case of **congenital sarcomatosis** of the skin, the child dying at the age of 2 months. The author reviews the literature of the subject.

A. Johannessen[5] reports a case of **sarcoma of the pelvis** in a girl 11 months old.

I. M. Snow[6] records the case of a boy of 13 months in whom **multiple laryngeal papillomata** developed after an attack of tracheobronchitis. The main symptoms were complete and persistent aphonia, stridulous breathing, recession of the chest, and attacks of dangerous dyspnea. Tracheotomy caused relief for 50 days, when a fatal attack of diphtheria occurred. At autopsy 3 cauliflower growths were found almost completely occluding the lumen of the larynx.

E. Berggruen[7] reports a case of **neurofibromatosis** in a boy of 11 years, involving the cerebrospinal axis as well as the peripheral nerves. He gives an exhaustive report of the case, introducing it with a review of the literature on neurofibromatosis.

G. N. Acker[8] records a **sarcoma of the thymus gland** and bronchial glands. The most conspicuous symptom during life was great edema of the left side of the face and of the left arm. A large growth of the thymus, involving part of the left lung and compressing the left subclavian vein, a large tumor in the left axillary space, and a smaller mass in the right axillary space, all sarcomatous, were found after death.

[1] Montreal Med. Jour., No. 12, 1896. [2] Ibid., No. 10, 1896.
[3] Arch. of Pediatrics, Apr., 1897. [4] Arch. f. Kinderh., Bd. xxi., H. 5 and 6.
[5] Jahrb. f. Kinderh , Bd. xliv., II. 1. [6] Arch. of Pediatrics, Oct., 1896.
[7] Arch. f. Kinderh. Bd., xxi., II. 1-3. [8] Arch. of Pediatrics, Dec., 1896.

THERAPEUTICS.

M. Jewnin[1] used **warm baths** (30°–35° R.) in 5 cases of cerebrospinal meningitis, all of which ended in recovery. Renant[2] advocates the use of warm baths in bronchitis in infants. Three or four baths at 100° F., if the rectal temperature of the child reaches 102°, combined with cold to the head and stimulants, are said to cause rapid improvement and prevent extension to the fine bronchioles. C. J. Rix[3] uses as a routine treatment for measles the full bath at 90° to 100° F., and continued for about 10 minutes. The first bath is given as soon as the disease is suspected, repeated every 12 hours, or oftener if necessary to bring out the rash, and continued twice daily until the temperature is normal. He claims that this treatment shortens the disease and almost entirely prevents renal and pulmonary complications and sequelæ.

L. Maestro[4] concludes from the use of **ichthyol** in pills ($\frac{3}{4}$ to 3 gr. in 24 hours, rapidly increasing the dose to 10 to 15 gr. in the day) that it is one of our most valuable remedies in whooping-cough. No untoward action was noticed, and the attacks decreased rapidly in number and severity, while the duration of the disease was shortened.

Vargas[5] has found his best results from the use of **phenocoll hydrochlorate** in a daily dose of from 0.07 gm. to 2 gm. It seems to act as a sedative rather than a germicide.

Maisend[6] uses nasal **insufflation in pertussis** of a powder of equal parts benzoin and salicylate of bismuth with $\frac{1}{5}$ part of quinin sulfate. The attacks were said to become less severe and more infrequent, and the cure was rapid.

Ferreira[7] ascribes to **bromoform** both a sedative action on the nervous system and a direct action on the pathogenic microorganisms when used in pertussis. In doses of 3–6 drops at 1 year of age and in corresponding quantity to older children he claims that a cure usually ensues in 6–12 days.

Lable and Oudin[8] report 22 cases of whooping-cough treated exclusively by **ozone.** This seemed to act through its antiseptic properties, and, they consider, reduced with rapidity the violence and frequency of the attacks, the dyspnea and cyanosis, and shortened the duration of the disease.

Staas[9] especially recommends **antispasmin** for whooping-cough in infants under a year, in whom bromoform may cause serious symptoms. It is also recommended in the spasmodic cough of measles. The dose, under a year of age, is $\frac{1}{6}$ to $\frac{1}{4}$ gr.

Moncorvo[10] used **analgen** in doses of 0.25 to 1 gm. in 24 hours in 33 cases of malaria in children, and considers it a useful adjuvant to quinin, and a substitute when the latter cannot be administered, as analgen is tasteless and not depressing. It also seemed of use in other diseases, especially in acute and subacute tuberculosis for the fever and cough.

Oppenheimer[11] thinks that the value of **oxygen-inhalation** in pneumonia is due to its being a very powerful heart-stimulant.

M. Goriatchkine[12] strongly opposes the use of **alcohol** by prescription in all cases except in acute diseases with heart-failure, and combats any tendency of parents to give it to children, lest the habit be formed. He states that of

[1] Arch. f. Kinderh., Bd. 23, H. 1.
[2] Med. Rec., xlix., 636. 1896.
[3] Brit. Med. Jour., Nov. 7, 1896.
[4] Med. Week., iv., 1896.
[5] Therap. Woch., Jan. 5, 1896.
[6] Jour. de Méd. et de Chir. prat., Aug. 10, 1896.
[7] Bull. gén. de Thérap., June 30, 1896.
[8] Bull. méd., x., No. 3, 1896.
[9] Nouv. Rèm., xii., p. 232, 1896.
[10] Bull. de l'Acad. de Méd., Nov. 10, 1896.
[11] Arch. f. Kinderh., Bd. xxi., H. 5 and 6.
[12] Vratch, No. 15, 1896; Gaz. des Hôpitaux, Aug. 11, 1896.

ments, as follows : 1. Simple tic r habit-spasm, including mainly the common cases of spasmodic movement chiefly of the facial muscles, which are, to a certain extent, under the contr of the will.   2. Tics with superadded psychic phenomena, *maladie de l tic convulsif,* or Gilles de la Tourette's disease, in which, in addition to t simple tic, there are explosive utterances and imperative ideas.   3. Comple, coördinated tics, which include actions more extended and involved tha simple tics, and also such conditions as head-nodding or swaying, and othr bizarre movements.   4. Tic psychique, in which the imperative idea is the psychic equivalent of, and has an origin similar to, the motor tic.

W. Osler[1] describes a case of **had-swaying** in a girl of 5. At times there would be a rhythmic swaying of the head from side to side to the extent of a foot from the median line The condition had existed from infancy, and the only point in the history tat seemed to have any bearing was that other members of the family were ervous.

Osler[2] also reports 2 unusual tyes of night-terrors in boys aged 7 and 11 years. The attacks in the first ca: consisted in incoherent muttering, were more in the nature of night-mare tan night-terrors, and ceased when the hypertrophied tonsils and adenoid groths were treated. A third case was related in which the attacks came on durg waking-hours. Chloroform-inhalation seemed to control them.

John Thomson[3] reports the ce of a girl who, from the age of 7 until menstruation became established a 13, had a **sensory hallucination of worms** crawling beneath the ski and of dryness of the palms and soles.

TUMORS.

E. Neuhaus[4] gives an extensive eport of a case of **congenital sarcomatosis** of the skin, the child dyig at the age of 2 months. The author reviews the literature of the subja.

A. Johannessen[5] reports a case **sarcoma of the pelvis** in a girl 11 months old.

I. M. Snow[6] records the case of a bov of 13 months in whom **multiple laryngeal papillomata** develop after an attack of tracheobronchitis. The main symptoms were complete an persistent aphonia, stridulous breathing, recession of the chest, and attacks odangerous dyspnea. Tracheotomy caused relief for 50 days, when a fatal attac of diphtheria occurred. At autopsy 3 cauliflower growths were found almst completely occluding the lumen of the larynx.

E. Berggruen[7] reports a case **neurofibromatosis** in a boy of 11 years, involving the cerebrospinal ais as well as the peripheral nerves. He gives an exhaustive report of the ase, introducing it with a review of the literature on neurofibromatosis.

G. N. Acker[8] records a **sarcom of the thymus gland** and bronchial glands. The most conspicuous symtom during life was great edema of the left side of the face and of the left rm. A large growth of the thymus, involving part of the left lung and capressing the left subclavian vein, a large tumor in the left axillary space, anc smaller mass in the right axillary space, all sarcomatous, were found after deth.

[1] Montreal Med. Jour.. No. 12. 1896.   [2] Ibid.. No. 10. 1896.
[3] Arch. of Pediatrics. Apr.. 1897.   [4] Arch. f. Kinderh.. Bd. xxi.. H. 5 and 6.
[5] Jahrb. f. Kinderh.. Bd. xliv.. H. 1.   [6] Arch. of Pediatrics. Oct.. 1896.
[7] Arch. f. Kinderh. Bd.. xxi.. H. 1-3.   [8] Arch. of Pediatrics. Dec. 1896.

THERAPEUTICS.

M. Jewnin[1] used **warm baths** (30° 35° R.) in 5 cases of cerebrospinal meningitis, all of which ended in recovery. Renaut[2] advocates the use of warm baths in bronchitis in hants. Three or four baths at 100° F., if the rectal temperature of the child reaches 102°, combined with cold to the head and stimulants, are said to cause rapid improvement and prevent extension to the fine bronchioles. C. J. Ki[3] uses as a routine treatment for measles the full bath at 90° to 100° F., an continued for about 10 minutes. The first bath is given as soon as the disease is suspected, repeated every 12 hours, or oftener if necessary to bring on the rash, and continued twice daily until the temperature is normal. He eims that this treatment shortens the disease and almost entirely prevents real and pulmonary complications and sequelæ.

L. Maestro[4] concludes from the use of **ichthyol** in pills (¾ to 3 gr. in 24 hours, rapidly increasing the dose to 10 to 15 gr. in the day) that it is one of our most valuable remedies in whooping-cough. No untoward action was noticed, and the attacks decreased rapidly in number, while the duration of the disease was shortened.

Vargas[5] has found his best results from the ... **chlorate** in a daily dose of 1m 0.07 gm. to 2 gm. ... sedative rather than a germicie.

Maisend[6] uses nasal **insufation in pertussis** of ... parts benzoin and salicylate of bismuth with ¼ part of quinin ... attacks were said to become less severe and more infrequent, and ... rapid.

Ferreira[7] ascribes to **bromoform** both a sedative action on the system and a direct action on he pathogenic microorganisms when ... pertussis. In doses of 3–6 dros at 1 year of age and in corresponding tity to older children he claims hat a cure usually ensues in 6–12 days.

Lable and Oudin[8] report 2 cases of whooping-cough treated exclusively by **ozone**. This seemed to at through its antiseptic properties, and, t consider, reduced with rapidity he violence and frequency of the attacks, t dyspnea and cyanosis, and shortened the duration of the disease.

Staas[9] especially recommens **antispasmin** for whooping-cough in infants under a year, in whom bromoform may cause serious symptoms. It is also recommended in the spasmodic cough of measles. The dose, under a year of age, is ⅙ to ¼ gr.

Moncorvo[10] used **analger** in doses of 0.25 to 1 gm. in 24 hours in 33 cases of malaria in children, and considers it a useful adjuvant to quinin, and a substitute when the latter canot be administered, as analgen is tasteless and not depressing. It also seemed of use in other diseases, especially in acute and subacute tuberculosis for the feer and cough.

Oppenheimer[11] thinks that the value of **oxygen-inhalation** in pneumonia is due to its being a ery powerful heart-stimulant.

M. Goriatchkine[12] strongly opposes the use of **alcohol** by prescription in all cases except in acute diseas with heart-failure, and combats any tendency of parents to give it to childn, lest the habit be formed. He states that of

[1] Arch. f. Kinderh., Bd. 23, H.
[2] Brit. Med. Jour., Nov. 7, 1896.
[3] Therap. Woch., Jan. 5, 1896.
[4] Bull. gén. de Thérap., June 30 896.
[5] Nouv. Rém., xii., p. 232, 1896.
[6] Arch. f. Kinderh., Bd. xxi., 1 5 and 6.
[7] Vratch, No. 15, 1896; Gaz. d Hôpitaux, Aug. 11, 1896.
[8] Med. Rec., xlix., 636. 1896.
[9] Med. Week., iv., 1896.
[10] Jour. de Méd. et de Chir. prat. Aug. 10, 1896.
[11] Bull. méd., x., No. 3, 1896.
[12] Bull. de l'Acad. de Méd., Nov. 10, 1896.

1671 children from 1 to 12 years of age, seen at Saint Olga's Hospital in Moscow, 506 took alcohol either as the result of environment or by advice of a physician. He cites the case of a child with night-terrors and restless sleep, and with enlarged liver and spleen, whose habit it was to take 2 glasses of port and a teaspoonful of cognac daily.

M. L. Brown[1] has used **potassium bromid** with great satisfaction in cholera infantum, considering it to be a specific, or physiologic antidote to the toxins which cause the disease.

A. Salter[2] reports rapid cure of ringworm of the scalp by 4 applications (daily or every second day) of a 40% solution of **formaldehyd.**

Senfft[3] uses **lactophenin** as an antipyretic in children, claiming that it does not disturb the stomach nor depress the heart.

A. Dobrowsky[4] used **desiccated thyroids** in cases of parenchymatous goiter, obesity, prurigo, and idiocy, with improvement in all except the last condition. Thyroid-feeding is of great value, in his opinion, in those patients who, through idiosyncrasy, cannot tolerate the iodin preparations. To a child with chorea, who was passing about 300 c.c. of urine daily, and who was receiving no apparent benefit from large doses of arsenic, D. I. Wolfstein[5] gave thyroid-extract, with the result that the flow of urine immediately increased to normal and the choreic movements disappeared, so that the child was perfectly well in a month's time.

J. F. Hartcop[6] recommends **phosphorus** for the chronic headaches of children, whether dependent upon rachitis or not.

TOXICOLOGY.

Anthony[7] records a case of **creolin-poisoning.** Inhalation of the drug had been ordered for pertussis, and ℥j was given internally to the 5-year-old boy by mistake. The symptoms most marked were coma, contracted pupils, muscular relaxation, weak and irregular pulse and respiration. Atropin $\frac{1}{100}$ gr., followed by $\frac{1}{50}$ gr. hypodermically, caused rapid improvement, and after large doses of magnesium sulfate recovery ensued.

L. Fischer[8] saw grave **bromoform-poisoning** in a child of 2½ years. Forty drops of the drug were ordered in a mixture, and, being heavy, it probably sank to the bottom, and the child received the whole amount in one dose. The author therefore advises against the use of the drug in mixtures. W. F. Cheyney[9] records a case of bromoform-poisoning in a child of 3 years. The drug had been prescribed in a mixture with alcohol, syrup, and water, and the symptoms of poisoning—laughing intoxication, followed by vomiting and coma—came on after the last dose, so that the bromoform had probably been swallowed nearly or entirely in one portion. An emetic and strychnin hypodermically brought recovery. Czygan[10] saw a child of 2½ years accidentally poisoned by 5 to 7 gm. of bromoform. Coma ensued quickly, and the symptoms persisted, though somewhat lessened in intensity after hypodermics of ether, excitation of the skin, and artificial respiration. Injections of 1.5 gm. of tincture of nux vomica within an hour restored the reflexes, and complete recovery after 5 hours' coma ensued upon the application of the faradic current.

[1] Boston M. and S. Jour., Dec. 3, 1896.   [2] Brit. Med. Jour., Sept. 12, 1896.
[3] Wien. med Presse, No. 50, 1896.   [4] Arch. f. Kinderh., Bd. xxi., H. 1-3.
[5] Arch. of Pediatrics, Oct., 1896.   [6] Sem. méd., No. 23, 1896.
[7] Med. Rec., Mar. 27, 1897.   [8] Ann. of Gyn. and Pediat., June, 1897.
[9] Arch. of Pediatrics, Feb, 1897.   [10] Sem. méd., Dec. 30, 1896.

H. Conrads[1] reports a case of **petroleum-poisoning** in a child of 1¾ years. An unknown quantity had been swallowed, immediately after which the gait became ataxic. The child became semi-unconscious, as if thoroughly drunk, the pulse rapid and irregular, the respirations very rapid, and the temperature subnormal. The symptoms improved rapidly after lavage. Next day there were signs of bronchitis, and the respirations were 120 to the minute, but these symptoms soon subsided. Five. other cases have been reported, in all of which consciousness was befogged and the pulse weak and rapid. The respirations were in several cases very rapid, due, he thinks, to hyperemia of the lungs. The pupils were very variable, as was the temperature. The diversity of some of the symptoms he attributes to the various kinds of petroleum which caused the poisoning.

. MISCELLANEOUS.

Precocious Maturity.—J. L. Morse[2] reports a case of precocious maturity in a girl infant, menstruation beginning at 9 months. He reviews the literature of the subject, arriving at the following conclusions : Precocious maturity is a physiologic congenital anomaly of development. Menstruation is never the first symptom, but is always preceded and accompanied by others. Menstruation most often appears in the first two years ; it is accompanied by ovulation. The attributes of maturity are not all acquired before the age of 7 or 8 years. Sexual desire is soon developed. Pregnancy may occur early. Menstruation may continue as long as when it begins at the normal time. The etiology of precocious maturity is unknown. The relation to precocious menstruation is obscure. There is no medical treatment. As the mental development of the unfortunates afflicted with this condition is usually far less than the sexual and physical, they must be carefully guarded against voluntary or involuntary intercourse. Wladmiroff[3] records a case of precocious adolescence in a rachitic girl of 6½ years.

Superficial Gangrene.—B. K. Rachford[4] details a case of superficial gangrene in an infant of 7 months. A spot of dry gangrene of the skin of the left buttock, 3 by 3½ in. in size, appeared suddenly, accompanied by pain but no fever, and preceded by no indisposition. The gangrenous skin separated after 17 days, and the remaining ulcer healed after about 3 months, during which time there were none but the local symptoms. The baby had suffered no injury and had been in good health, and there was no family history bearing on the case except the fact that the father had probably had syphilis. M. Cailland[5] discusses at length a similar condition under the term "infectious disseminated gangrene of the skin."

Transposition of the Viscera.—Reefschlager[6] reports a case of transposition of the viscera in a child who died at 23 months. The position of the stomach, intestines, liver, and spleen was the reverse of the normal, as was that of the heart, lungs, and great vessels. There was but one cardiac ventricle which communicated by the usual orifice with the right auricle, but was closed to the left auricle. The blood-current was from the venæ cavæ into the left auricle, thence through several interauricular foraminæ into the right auricle, thence to the ventricle, and finally into the aorta and pulmonary

[1] Berlin. klin. Woch , Nov. 2, 1896.   [2] Arch. of Pediatrics, Apr., 1896.
[3] Arch. f. Kinderh. Bd. xxi., H. 5 and 6.   [4] Arch. of Pediatrics, Dec., 1896.
[5] Rev. mens. des Mal. de l'Enfance, Jan. and Mar., 1897.
[6] Berlin. klin. Woch., Jan. 25, 1897.

artery. Emaciation, some cyanosis, and clubbing of the fingers and toes were the only signs during life. Death was caused by tuberculous meningitis.

Insolation.—H. A. Lafleur [1] records a case of insolation in an infant of 13 months. The temperature reached 108° F., but was controlled by cold full baths, and the child recovered completely. In the discussion, Fruitnight, Seibert, Griffith, and Adams spoke of cases of insolation in infants seen by them. In one mentioned by Griffith the temperature reached 110° F.

Hospitalism.—O. Heubner [2] has noted that the same infants did better outside of institutions than within them, even when cared for in like manner. He examined bacteriologically the cleansed nipples and the nurses' hands, and found quantities of living colon-bacilli. To prevent infection from child to child from the sources mentioned and many others, he recommends that children in institutions be put in wards containing not more than 8 beds, and that separate nurses have charge of the feeding and of the bodily care of the children in those wards.

H. D. Chapin [3] refers to hospitalism as most likely to affect infants under one year of age, and says that admission should therefore be made only for acute illnesses, discharge not being delayed for more than two weeks after convalescence has begun. The hospitalism is first manifested by the child's weight remaining stationary; then a loss in weight occurs, associated with hydremia, dryness of the skin, and wearing off of hair from the occiput. There is also a tendency for latent, hypostatic pneumonia to set in. Female children are apt to develop vaginitis. As soon as signs of hospitalism appear the child should be promptly discharged, because, if the atrophic tendency becomes well started, recovery will be impossible even under new and favorable hygienic surroundings.

[1] Arch. of Pediatrics, Dec., 1896.   [2] Berlin. klin. Woch., May 24, 1897.
[3] Arch. of Pediatrics, May, 1897.

PATHOLOGY.

By JOHN GUITÉRAS, M. D., AND DAVID RIESMAN, M. D.,

OF PHILADELPHIA.

Resume of the Year's Progress.—Among the problems in general pathology the etiology of tumors is still *facile princeps*. The researches of the year in this field have not brought a definitive solution, although the investigations of the Italian school seem strongly to point to blastomycetes as the cause of cancer. Pathologists, however, have been made cautious by the collapse of the erstwhile much-acclaimed "protozoan theory," and there now exists a conservatism that demands indisputable proof before acquiescing in a new doctrine. Another interesting question is that raised by Rosenfeld, namely, as to the existence of fatty degeneration as a morbid process. His experiments are on the surface very convincing; whatever fallacy, if any, there may be in them, will no doubt be soon brought to light. In bacteriology the subject of agglutination is absorbing a great deal of attention. The phenomenon is now viewed, especially by Widal, as not related to immunity; its true significance is not yet established, nor is its specificity definitely proved. Of importance are also the cumulative observations on the virulence of the gonococcus, which is shown to be capable of producing grave secondary lesions—endocarditis, pleurisy, pyemia, peritonitis—as well as diverse morbid processes in the female pelvic cavity. The various fundamental problems connected with the subject of antitoxins still await solution; there is as yet no union of the opposing schools. In pathologic technic the growing popularity of formalin as a preserving and fixing agent, and of thionin as a nuclear and bacterial stain, is to be noted. In the domain of special pathology, the nature of Graves' disease is one of the most interesting problems; considerable space is given to it in this section. Reference is also made to certain important researches in pneumonokoniosis, a subject that in American literature has not received much attention. In the pathology of the nervous system the interesting observations of Marinesco on the effects of infectious diseases merit special mention. The experiments of Goldscheider and Flatau on the influence of the toxins and antitoxins of tetanus are important, both in themselves and in their bearing on the problems of acquired immunity. Cirrhosis of the liver receives considerable attention in this present section—the theory of Aufrecht is briefly given; we are constrained to withhold our opinion on it for the present. Under the subject of "the urinary organs" some reference is made to the alloxur-bodies; space forbade us entering at greater length into the questions connected with the origin of those interesting nitrogenous compounds. In this same section Councilman's excellent article on nephritis is also abstracted. Various interesting subjects, such as the study on terminal infections by Flexner, the experiments of Abbott on the effect of alcohol on resistance to infectious diseases, Virchow's latest views on inflammation, as well as numerous other matters, will be found treated in the final section entitled "miscellaneous."

THE BLOOD AND BLOOD-MAKING ORGANS.

The Properties of the Extravascular Blood.—M. Hahn [1] finds
that the diastatic ferment in blood and blood-serum (discovered by Majendie)
is, unlike the globulicidal and bactericidal agents, not destroyed at 55°
C., but only at between 65° and 70° C. Light, which causes the globulicidal and bactericidal agent quickly to disappear, has but little effect
on the diastatic ferment. The bactericidal agent and the ferment were
also proved to be entirely independent. The lipolytic property of serum
is destroyed at 60° C. (Hanriot, Camus). Hahn was also able to confirm
the earlier observation of Röden, that the contact of blood inhibits the
action of the labferment, pepsin, and trypsin. The action is not a simple
chemic one, for by heating the serum to 65° C. the inhibitory property is destroyed, and the serum is promptly digested by trypsin. These facts are suggestive in connection with the old problem why the stomach or the pancreas does
not digest itself. Some studies were made on the glycolytic property of the
blood, which is not connected, as some have claimed, with the coagulation of
the blood, being in this respect analogous to the bactericidal agent. Like the
latter, it is destroyed by a temperature of 55° C., and, like it, is augmented in
hyperleukocytosis. Nevertheless, the two are not identical, for the serum is
bactericidal but not glycolytic. The observations, however, show that there
is an intimate relation, though not an identity, among the globulicidal, the
bactericidal, and the glycolytic properties of the blood, and that these are
connected with the active albumins in the sense of Buchner, as is especially
shown by their slight resistance to trifling physical influences. On the other
hand, the ferment-destroying substance, the diastatic and the lipolytic ferments do not seem to be united to such labile bodies. [These researches,
though in a sense physiologic, are of great interest to the pathologist, and
suggest experimental studies in diabetes, obesity, and other diseases, as well as
offering pegs on which to hang new theories.]

A New Morphologic Constituent of Blood.—Wernicke [2] has made
some observations on the blood that are of interest in relation to Müller's subsequently published discovery of the hemakonia (see *Year-Book*, 1897, p. 671).
In addition to the well-known morphologic elements, the blood contains yet
another constant constituent, in the form of minute spheric bodies, the number
of which increases in preparations not fresh. Diverse studies have shown that
these small motile bodies are nothing more than dispersed granulations of the
neutrophiles or myelocytes, which become free when these cells disintegrate.
For this reason it is not permissible to attribute any pathologic or diagnostic significance to such bodies. Larger motile granules ($1-2\mu$) may be : (1) eosinophile
granulations (most frequently) ; (2) γ-granulations (very rare, except in leukemia) ; (3) Laveran's " corps sphériques "—*i. e.*, young, unpigmented malarial
parasites ; or (4) very small, pale microcytes and poikilocytes. For purposes
of differentiation staining is indispensable. The author employs the following solutions : (*a*) Saturated watery solution of methylen-blue, 100 ; eosin
(French, soluble in water), 1.5 ; absolute alcohol, 132 ; distilled water, 168 ;
20 % NaOH solution, 16 drops. After standing 10 days and then filtering,
the solution is used warm (heating on cover-glass). (*b*) Distilled water, 100 ;
glacial acetic acid, 2 drops ; $\frac{1}{2}$% eosin solution, 1.0 ; concentrated solution of
orange, 3 drops. This is used for decolorization (a few seconds only) ; the

[1] Berlin. klin. Woch., June 7, 1897.
[2] Przeglad Lekarski, Mar. 7, 14, 21, 1896 ; ref. in Centralbl. f. allgem. Path. u. pathol.
Anat., Mar. 1, 1897.

cover-glass is then washed in water, dried, and mounted in balsam. Normal red corpuscles will be rose-colored, poikilocytes poor in hemoglobin a bluish-red, small lymphocytes uniformly dark blue, eosinophile granulations bright red, δ-granulations dark blue, and γ- (basophile) granulations dark bluish-red. Plasmodia become steel-gray-bluish. The protoplasm of the neutrophiles and blood-plaques remains unstained.

The Action of Drugs on the Leukocytes of the Blood.—George Wilkinson[1] injected various drugs—potassium iodid, pilocarpin nitrate, camphor, antipyrin, quinin hydrochlorate, salicin, and sodium salicylate—into animals, and studied the changes in number and structure of the leukocytes in the blood. The general results of the experiments may be stated thus : the first effect of the drug-injection was to cause a diminution in the number of leukocytes per c.mm. The degree and duration of the diminution varied with the drug employed, but with all those mentioned above, unless the dose was very small, its occurrence was recognized when the blood was examined sufficiently early. As a rule, it was not of long duration ; but a notable exception occurred in the case of one of the experiments with quinin hydrochlorate. A large dose (0.7 gm.) of this drug caused the death of the animal 2 days after the injection ; the blood was examined frequently between the time of injection and its death, and on every occasion the scantiness of the leukocytes was very striking. Coincidently with the diminution in the total number of leukocytes there was a distinct increase in the proportion of the uninuclear to the multinuclear varieties. Following the diminution there was observed in the case of all the drugs employed an increase in the number of leukocytes per c.mm. This change did not occur in the above-mentioned experiment, in which a very large dose of quinin was administered ; but with smaller doses of this drug its occurrence was noted, although, as with salicin and salicylate of sodium also, the degree of increase was slight in comparison with that which followed the injection of the other drugs. With nearly all of them the increase was a much more evident phenomenon than the preceding diminution, and was of much longer duration. It was further constantly distinguished by the fact that the multinuclear leukocytes were relatively more increased in number than the uninuclear forms. Regarding structural changes, it was found that repeated doses of pilocarpin caused a disappearance of the granules in the small oxyphile leukocytes. Neither the large oxyphile cells with coarse granules (Ehrlich's eosinophile cells) nor the red corpuscles showed any change.

The Effects of Repeated Hemorrhages on the Blood.—A. H. Hill[2] tabulates the results obtained by bleeding dogs. From a study of his table we learn that repeated venesection produces a steady reduction in the specific gravity and a reduction in the solids, and an increase in the amount of fibrin. There is a diminution in the amount of ash, of hemoglobin, and of red corpuscles, and an increase in the number of leukocytes. This increase affects chiefly, if not altogether, the multinuclear elements.

Post-phlebotomic and Post-revulsive Hyperleukocytosis.— Maurel[3] found on the day following a venesection a genuine hyperleukocytosis which continued for several days. Such an augmentation of leukocytes may be of value in infectious diseases. Regarding the effects of revulsants (cauterization, punctures, mustard, cantharides, and ammonia), Maurel found that during the first few hours following their application there is a hyperleukocytosis, but it is only apparent, and depends on a transportation of the leukocytes along the vessel-walls into the circulatory stream. After about the 4th day of the application a true leukocytosis dependent on newly formed leu-

[1] Brit. Med. Jour., Sept. 26, 1896.   [2] Ibid.   [3] Gaz. des Hôpitaux, Aug. 13, 1896.

kocytes is observed, and it is possible that this leukocytosis is useful to the organism in bacterial infections. We may see in this a justification of the popular use of revulsives in these diseases.

The Influence of Baths on the Alkalinity of the Blood.—A. Strasser[1] found that cold baths increased and warm baths decreased the alkalinity of the blood; likewise of the urine.

The Changes in the Blood in Jaundice.—v. Limbeck[2] states that icteric blood is deficient in sodium chlorid. This depends on a lack of NaCl and a reduction in the volume of the serum. The latter is produced by an increase in the volume of the red corpuscles, which in turn is due to the presence of bile-salts in the plasma.

Blood-coagulability and Serous Hemorrhages.—A. E. Wright,[3] whose researches on blood-coagulability are well known, in the present paper takes the stand that certain conditions of serous transudation are to be considered as depending on deficient blood-coagulability. *E. g.*, he names : 1. *Serous hemorrhages into the skin—i. e.*, urticaria—particularly those following (*a*) the injection of diphtheria-antitoxin ; (*b*) the eating of acid fruits ; (*c*) the eating of crabs or shellfish ; probably also the urticaria following the ingestion of rhubarb and the administration of soap-enemata is due to the same cause, both producing an abstraction of lime-salts. (2) *Serous hemorrhages into the subcutaneous and muscular tissues,* the best example of which is the serous hematomata seen in hemophilia ; chilblains may also belong here. 3. *Serous hemorrhage into the tubules of the kidney*—cyclic albuminuria. 4. *Serous hemorrhage into joints and serous cavities.* Joint-effusions are a prominent symptom of hemophilia, but some pleural and pericardial effusions are also probably due to diminished blood-coagulability, a belief which the author thinks is substantiated by the association of mucous-membrane hemorrhages and signs of defective clotting of the blood in the large vessels often seen postmortem. 5. *Serous hemorrhages into the intestinal canal.* The diarrheas of hemophilics and those seen in purpura hæmorrhagica, also the diarrhea occurring after croupous pneumonia at a time when peptone (albumose) is being excreted in the urine, are referable to diminished blood-coagulability. The author also thinks that the non-irritant hydragogue cathartics owe some part of their efficacy to their power of diminishing blood-coagulability, while the constipating action of lime-salts is due to the opposite effect. In like manner, the notoriously constipating effect of a milk-diet may be in part due to the large percentage of calcium-salts contained in cow's milk. This last inference is to some extent confirmed by the fact that obstinate infantile constipation will often disappear when the child is put upon a diet of citrated milk ; *i. e.*, milk which has been deprived of its excess of lime-salts by an addition of $\frac{1}{100}$th of citrate of sodium. The general conclusion is then postulated that a defect of blood-coagulability tends to manifest itself, not only in "actual hemorrhages," but also (according to the particular idiosyncrasy of the patient) in some one or more of the forms of "serous hemorrhage" which have been described.

Although the question of treatment does not belong to this part of the *Year-Book,* we shall, for completeness' sake, append the author's words on that topic : methods of treatment which augment blood-coagulability will be methods of treatment that will be appropriate, not only to the prevention and treatment of "actual hemorrhage," but also to the prevention and treatment of "serous hemorrhage." The more important of these therapeutic measures

---

[1] Wien. med. Presse, Nos. 22 and 23, 1896.   [2] Centralbl. f. innere Med., No. 33, 1896.
[3] Lancet, Sept. 19, 1896.

appear to be the following : (*a*) the exhibition of calcium chlorid (or other soluble lime-salt) in suitable quantities; (*b*) the avoidance of such vegetable acids as citric, malic, tartaric, and oxalic, which form insoluble salts with lime ; (*c*) the concentration of the blood either by diaphoretics or by such purgatives as do not owe their efficacy to a power of reducing blood-coagulability ; (*d*) the restriction of the amount of fluid ingested ; (*e*) the increase of the amount of carbonic acid in the blood, either by direct inhalation of the gas or by other methods ; and (*f*) the avoidance of alcohol. Some experiments are then cited illustrating the effect of treatment on local edema. [The author's reasoning appears to us somewhat theoretic. He leaves out of consideration the influence of the vessel-wall on transudation, an influence that is not passive, but probably active—"lymphagogue." The fact that the serous hemorrhages are localized, points to a local factor, and if a general one like lessened coagulability does exist, it can probably only play the part of a predisposing factor.]

The Blood in Pernicious Anemia.—Cabot,[1] from a study of 50 cases of pernicious anemia, concludes that the points most typical in the blood of this disease are : 1. A reduction of the number of red cells to about 1,000,000 ; 2. The absence of leukocytosis ; 3. Possibly a relatively high percentage of hemoglobin in some cases ; 4. Increase in average diameter of the red cells ; 5. The presence of large numbers of polychromophilic red cells ; 6. The presence of nucleated red cells, a minority being normoblasts ; 7. The presence of myelocytes ; 8. A relatively high percentage of small lymphocytes at the expense of the polymorphonuclear cells. Postmortem examination in 8 cases brought out nothing not already well known. Fatty degeneration and pallor of all organs were noted in all ; the "tiger-lily" heart in 6 ; and pericardial and peritoneal ecchymoses in 4. The spleen was slightly enlarged in 2 ; no enlargement of lymphatic glands was observed. The marrow was examined in 5 cases, showing in all a notably red color in the shaft of the long bones. No microscopic appearances were recorded.

Peculiar Blood-changes in Purpura Hæmorrhagica.—Bensaude[2] confirms Hayem's observation of the absence of retraction of the blood-clot and of the formation of serum in 16 cases affected with various forms of purpura hæmorrhagica, all of which presented large cutaneous ecchymoses and hemorrhages from the mucous membrane. Purpuras in which the hemorrhages were small did not present the blood-anomaly. The author has succeeded, though the researches are not yet completed, in producing the blood-lesion and hemorrhages in animals by the injection of the blood of a purpuric patient. [We may add that Müller and Denis have observed absence of blood-plaques in cases of Werlhof's disease.]

The Relation between Leukemia and Pseudoleukemia.—Martin and Mathewson[3] point out the close relation between these two diseases, and quote examples in which, together with well-marked lymphatic hyperplasia, a variable blood-picture as regards the leukocytes existed, and are of opinion that leukemias in their various manifestations, acute and chronic, lymphatic, splenic, and myelogenous, the similar varieties of Hodgkin's disease, and all such like affections characterized by a hyperplasia of the lymph-gland structures, when no primary focus can be found, are for the present to be classed in one group.

The Leukocytes in Splenic Leukemia.—Maurel[4] in 4 cases of splenic leukemia noted that the leukocytes were more voluminous than the normal ; that their activity was less; and that they were less resistant to extreme temperatures. They died at 44° C., and lost their movements at 32°

[1] Boston M. and S. Jour., Aug. 6, 1896.   [2] Sem. méd., Jan. 20, 1897.
[3] Brit. Med. Jour., Dec., 1896.   [4] Sem. méd., July 28, 1897.

C., whilst normal leukocytes die only at 46° C., and lose their movements only toward 25° C.

Apparent Crystallization of Eosinophile Granulations.—A. J. Patek,[1] in some cover-glass preparations of blood from a case of suppurative axillary adenitis, found peculiar eosinophilous sheaf-like crystals, which he believes originated from the eosinophile granulations of the leukocytes.

Acute Leukemia.—Benda[2] describes the anatomic lesions observed in 7 cases of acute leukemia. The hemorrhages into the tissues and the regional adenopathies were characteristic. The splenic tumor differed from that of acute infectious diseases in being less soft and not so large. A peculiar lesion of the veins was also constantly observed—the walls were permeated by numerous lymphomatous nodules, which, however, did not seem to lead to thrombosis. The chief blood-change was the increase of uninuclear elements.

Differential Count of the Leukocytes.—Jolly[3] writes as follows: 1. In estimating the variations in the proportion of the different forms of white corpuscles accurate results can be obtained only when preparations of dried blood are examined which have been fixed with care and always by the same process. 2. It is not possible to conclude with certainty concerning the increase or diminution of a given variety of leukocytes by a simple examination without counting; this is particularly the case when a variety which is normally present in small numbers is under consideration. 3. If the leukocytes are divided into two classes, a total of at least 300 should be counted; if the leukocytes are divided into three classes, a total of at least 400 should be counted; this method will yield results which are nearly accurate, with a maximum error of about 4 in each 100; this classification allows for large and small uninuclear elements and for multinuclear elements, but excludes eosinophiles. 4. It is also necessary to allow for the possible unequal distribution of the different forms on the cover-glass as the count is made.

A New Method of Determining the Alkalinity of the Blood.—Berend[4] recommends the following method: After cleansing the pulp of the finger a prick is made with a sticker or needle. The blood is drawn into the mixer up to the mark 0.1, and the latter then emptied into a centrifuge-tube (see Fig. 50) containing 5 c.c. of a 1% neutral NaCl solution, and washed out by repeatedly sucking up this solution. The latter is then at once centrifuged, and the clear serum-solution poured into a glass vessel. To the corpuscular mass remaining 10 c.c. of water (neutral) are added, and the mixture placed aside. The serum-solution is mixed with litmus so that it is not too highly colored, and titrated with an acid solution, and back with sodium hydrate. The mean of the two figures is taken as the result. The corpuscle-mass is then poured into a porcelain dish, the tube rinsed with 5 c.c. of water, and litmus added until the red color is completely obscured. To the bluish-green, opaque mixture the acid solution is added in excess; after stirring, the mixture is titrated with sodium-hydrate solution, drop by drop. Sufficient has been added when the solution loses its red color and is again opaque. The last drop (0.05 c.c.) is deducted, and the difference between the acid and the alkali used determined. The sum

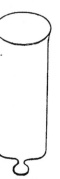

Fig. 50. — Centrifuge-tube. The spheric projection ought not to have a capacity of more than 0.20 c.c.

[1] N. Y. Med. Jour., Oct. 17, 1896.   [2] Centralbl. f. innere Med., June 26, 1897.
[3] Arch. de Méd. expér. et d'Anat. path., July, 1896.
[4] Zeit. f. Heilk., xvii., H. 4, p. 351; Univ. Med. Mag., Mar., 1897.

of the estimations of the serum and the corpuscles represents the total alkalinity. The double titration referred to above is performed by first titrating with a centinormal sulphuric-acid solution; an excess of acid is then added, and the solution titrated back to the blue color with a $\frac{1}{50}$ normal sodium-hydrate solution.

The Pathology of the Lymphadenoid Structures.—W. G. Spencer[1] deals in an admirable manner with this subject, particularly as far as the physiologic aspects are concerned. The papers scarcely admit of abstracting; we would only refer to his treatment of lymphadenoma, a term which applies to a growth of lymphadenoid tissue closely resembling in structure that of a lymphatic gland. He classifies the lymphadenomata as follows: 1. Local lymphadenoma: (*a*) simple or benign, and (*b*) malignant. 2. Generalized lymphadenoma or lymphadenomatosis: (*a*) benign, and (*b*) malignant. The terms in common use—leukocythemia or leukemia, pseudoleukemia, Hodgkin's disease, and lymphosarcoma—are greatly confused and employed differently by different authors. The only rational way at present of grouping the various cases of lymphadenoma is by taking the point of origin in each case. The various localities in which lymphadenomatous growths may occur are then considered.

THE CIRCULATORY SYSTEM.

Tuberculosis of the Intima of the Aorta.—Victor Hanot and Levy[2] report the case of a man, aged 61, in whom there was a distinct tubercle on the upper portion of the intima of the thoracic aorta. The tubercle was about the size of the head of a pin, and its nature was proved by the finding of the tubercle-bacillus.

Perforation of the Vena Cava.—S. Flexner[3] reports 2 instances of perforation of the inferior cava in amebic abscesses of the liver.

The Sequelæ of Pericardial Obliteration.—Heidemann[4] finds that in certain cases presenting ascites and hydrothorax, without edema of the legs, there is a general chronic inflammation of all the serous membranes. The pericardial adhesions lead to myodegeneration of the heart, and the stasis resulting from this to ascites, because the peritoneal vessels are more pervious on account of the chronic peritonitis. The cirrhotic processes observed in the liver are produced by extension inward of the inflammatory irritant from the capsule of the liver and by the chronic hyperemia of the organ. Through hyperplasia and contraction of the fibrous tissue upon and in the liver the stasis and ascites are increased.

Myocardial Changes in Diphtheria.—Scagliosi[5] describes the results found by him in the hearts of cases of diphtheria that had died in from 3 to 10 days after the onset of the disease. The sequence of phenomena is as follows: 1. The poison first acts on the vessel-walls, especially on the small arteries; 2. It diffuses into the tissues, being aided in this by the changes in the vessel-walls, and causes degenerative changes in the muscles; 3. Around the altered vessels and muscle-fibers small-cell infiltration may occur, but this is never a primary phenomenon. Regarding the vascular changes, the intima may be swollen, the endothelial cells bulging into the vessel-lumen and often showing some loss of staining-power. The middle coat may undergo hyaline changes, and some leukocytic infiltration may be found in the adventitia. All these changes occur early, preceding the degeneration of the muscle-fibers.

[1] Lancet, Mar. 6, 13, 20, 1897.   [2] Arch. de Méd. expér. et d'Anat. path., Nov., 1896.
[3] Am. Jour. Med. Sci., May, 1897.   [4] Berlin. klin. Woch., Feb. 1 and 8, 1897.
[5] Virchow's Archiv, Oct., 1896.

Capillary congestion is usually well marked, and there may be small hemorrhages. In the muscle the earliest change is a loss of striation and a granular degeneration, the latter affecting groups of fibers irregularly in patches or portions of individual fibers. A further stage, seen in those fibers in which the change is advanced, is the fusing together of the granular matter into a hyaline and highly refractive substance. The changes in the muscles occur first in the columnæ carneæ and beneath the endocardium. In the later stages fatty degeneration also occurs. From these observations the author concludes that the primary effect of the diphtheria-toxin is to produce a parenchymatous inflammation which corresponds in the mode of its production with the changes described by him and Perenice in the central nervous system in diphtheria—first, alteration in the vessel-walls, and then degenerative changes in the nearlying nerve-cells.

Pulmonary Complications of Aortic Aneurysm.—A. Fränkel[1] refers to the pulmonary complications of aortic aneurysm, among which he names fibroid pneumonia, croupous pneumonia, and pulmonary tuberculosis. All of these are contingent on a narrowing of the trachea or bronchus, special factors operating to bring about now one and now another process. Among the causes of aneurysm syphilis plays, in his opinion, a very important part; it had existed in 11 out of 30 cases (over 36 %).

Infectious Endocarditis in Typhoid Fever.—W. T. Connell[2] reports a case of this rare complication of typhoid fever; vegetations were found on the mitral and tricuspid valves. Microscopic examination of the vegetations showed the staphylococcus.

Calcareous Degeneration of the Heart.—J. J. Hanley[3] found at the autopsy on a tuberculous subject a calcified plate 8 cm. long, from 3 to 5 cm. wide, and 5 mm. thick, situated mainly on and in the posterior wall of the left ventricle of the heart.

THE NERVOUS SYSTEM.

Ascending Degeneration, and the Changes in Nerve-cells Consequent Thereon.—Rob. A. Fleming[4] has made a large series of nerve-sections, and from examination of the central ends concludes—1. That in process of time a slow atrophy of "motor" fibers occurs. 2. That certain "sensory" fibers degenerate centrally, possibly because severed from their peripheral trophic centers. 3. That the minute fibers found in a normal nerve undergo very marked change. 4. That distinctive connective-tissue increase occurs. The fine fibers mentioned in 3, as Gaskell has pointed out, are probably designed for the supply of vessels, and they mostly leave the cerebrospinal axis in certain regions alone, pass to the sympathetic ganglia, and from them return to peripheral nerves. These fibers, scattered all through the funiculi in which they occur, seem to find their way to the periphery of a fasciculus at different levels, and probably do so near their points of distribution. The bulk of these vasomotor nerves is medullated. The author is at present engaged in determining how far these fine fibers degenerate after division of a nerve. The changes occurring in the nerve-cells—in those of the ganglia on the posterior roots and those of the anterior horns—are summarized as follows: 1. The cells of the ganglia on the posterior nerve-roots undergo definite changes as the result of nerve-section or ligature, and do so at a much earlier period than the multipolar cells in the cord—beginning probably as early as the 4th

[1] Deutsch. med. Woch., Nos. 6 and 7, 1897.　　[2] Montreal Med. Jour., Aug., 1896.
[3] Medical Council, Aug., 1896.　　[4] Brit. Med. Jour., Oct. 3, 1896.

day and certainly by the 7th day. 2. That one of the very first changes observed in the cells of the ganglia and anterior cornu is a diminution in the size of the nucleus—in proportion to the size of the cell, and that sometimes, but not in all cases, nucleoli also become smaller, and very frequently the nuclei take up an eccentric position, sometimes even bulging the cell-wall. 3. That in both sets of cells the chromatic granules are either smaller in size, fewer in number, and scattered through the cell-body, tending to be most numerous around the nucleus, or else they are grouped together in large masses round the nucleus, leaving the periphery of the cell quite clear. 4. That pericellular lymph-spaces may become enlarged, especially in the ganglia-cells, and where the enlargement is very marked the cells become proportionately smaller in size—although actual atrophy may also occur. In several specimens the author found large vacuoles—not the vacuoles described by many writers as occurring in the cells of the cord and cerebral cortex, which are probably to some extent artificial—but big vacuoles, more resembling distended pericellular lymph-spaces. They differ, however, inasmuch as they are surrounded by the remains of cell-protoplasm containing chromatic granules. 5. That in the multipolar cells not merely are there these changes in position and size of nuclei, and arrangements and number of chromatic granules, but there is, as a later phenomenon, marked disintegration of cell-protoplasm. This disintegration has been described by Marinesco as occurring in certain cord-lesions in man. It consists of patches, which with toluidin-blue and eosin are whitish in color and surrounded by masses of chromatic granules. In conclusion, the author points out that after a lesion of axis-cylinder processes those trophic cells suffer first the processes of which conduct stimuli toward the cell.

Changes of the Central Nervous System in the Course of Infections.—Marinesco[1] has examined the spinal cords and brains of a number of individuals that had succumbed to infectious diseases, such as pneumonia, bronchopneumonia, typhoid fever, smallpox, erysipelas, miliary tuberculosis, etc., and found lesions in the majority of cases. The changes in the cells varied greatly in intensity, and showed gradations from partial chromatolysis to degeneration of the cytoplasm. The same variability existed in the interstitial and vascular changes. In some cases (pneumonia, bronchopneumonia, etc.) he noted a genuine meningitis, with extensions along the pial trabeculæ and the presence of diplococci. Besides a well-marked leukocytic infiltration he also observed instances in which interstitial nodules of neuroglia-cells were situated at times in the gray, at times in the white matter. Although there was great variability, it seemed as if diseases attended with leukocytosis provoked especially vascular changes. [The author, to our surprise, includes miliary tuberculosis among the diseases characterized by leukocytosis.] Other infections, by reason of their toxins, exert a harmful influence on the nerve-cell. The age of the patient, the duration of the disease, the height of the temperature, are other important factors. But whatever the factors may be, it is evident that the more intense the nervous phenomena, the greater the interstitial and parenchymatous lesions in the nervous system.

Action of the Influenza-bacillus on the Central Nervous System.—A. Cantani,[2] Jr., was able to produce striking nervous phenomena in rabbits by injecting cultures of the influenza-bacillus directly into the brain. It seems that the latter is a *locus minoris resistentiæ*. The bacilli produce an intracellular poison, the first action of which is on the central nervous system.

Brain-lesions in Acute Yellow Atrophy of the Liver.—C. W.

[1] Sem. méd., July 28, 1897.   [2] Zeit. f. Hyg. u. Infektionskrank., xxiii., H. 2, Oct., 1896.

Burr and A. O. J. Kelley [1] describe the brain-lesions in a case of acute yellow atrophy of the liver in a man aged 40. In sections stained by Lenhossek's method changes were found in the nucleolus, nucleus, and cell-body. The nucleolus was situated variably, as in normal cells, but was of somewhat irregular contour, though but slightly, if at all, increased in size. The nucleus was distorted in shape. Owing to the excessive staining-tendency of the finer chromophilic granules, the two or three chromophilic bodies normally seen were not visible. The karyoplasm also evinced an abnormally great affinity for the stain. The cell-body was most intensely affected, the changes varying from slight implication to almost complete destruction. In some cells only a few chromophilic granules had disappeared; in others the cell-body was almost devoid of these granules, a few perhaps remaining at the periphery of the cell. In some instances the nucleus and cell-contents had been entirely destroyed, or the nucleus had dropped out of the cell. In many of the cells not so excessively affected there was an appearance suggestive of fat-globules and detritus. The protoplasmic processes, as a rule, showed no deviation from the normal. In sections stained by Berkeley's method swelling and atrophy of the processes, probably stages of one process, were observed. The lesions described by the authors were parenchymatous, affecting the nerve-cells primarily, and were not secondary to vascular changes. In all probability they were the result, as suggested by the writers, of the action of a poison.

Lesions Induced by the Action of Certain Poisons on the Nerve-cell.—H. J. Berkley [2] has studied the brains of three guinea-pigs that died after injections of diphtheria-toxin. In all, moniliform swellings were found on the dendrites, with denudation of the gemmules. Some of the psychic cells showed alterations in their outlines, while the neuroglia presented advanced swelling. The axons and collaterals appeared well stained. The cerebellar cells showed less change than those of the cerebrum. From studies conducted on the cerebra of hydrophobic and diphtheric guinea-pigs it would appear that all severe infections are followed by brain-cell degeneration of an order not dissimilar to that found in the cells of the abdominal viscera under similar conditions—a degenerative process unaccompanied by inflammatory reaction and a tendency to atrophy and necrosis.

Degenerative Changes in the Spinal Roots, and their Intraspinal Prolongations in Consequence of Cerebral Disease.—A. Pick [3] reports a case of tumor of the left hemisphere, one of softening, one of osteosarcoma with compression of the brain, one of glioma, and one of cerebral hypertrophy, in all of which he found a more or less marked degeneration of the posterior roots, at times also of the anterior roots. In view of the ease of cerebral hypertrophy, the author thinks the degeneration is probably an effect of cerebral pressure.

Effect of Tetanus-toxin on the Ganglion-cells.—Goldscheider and Flatau [4] found, by using Nissl's stain, that disintegration of Nissl's chromatophilic elements took place within a short time after the intoxication. Tetanus-antitoxin given at the proper time after the toxin prevented the changes; when injected after the production of the latter it was capable of causing restitution of the ganglion-cells to the normal. [The antidotal effects of antitoxin could not be more clearly shown, and the discoveries seem to strengthen the view of the Behring school, that toxin and antitoxin neutralize each other. Another subject to which Goldscheider also referred in a discussion on the aims of

[1] Jour. Nerv. and Ment. Dis., Nov., 1896.   [2] Bull. Johns Hopkins Hosp., Feb., 1897.
[3] Prag. med. Woch., 36 and 37, 1896.
[4] Centralbl. f. allg. Path. u. path. Anat., July 15, 1897.

modern therapeutics is suggested by these observations—namely, that there is really no antagonism between the humoral and the cellular theories—toxins and antitoxins act on the cell.]

The Pathology of Epilepsy.—Joseph Collins[1] reports the findings in the portion of cortex excised from the brains of 2 epileptics, one a youth of 20, the other, a married woman of 30. In the first case the area for the right hand was cut out; on microscopic examination the excised piece showed: (1) meningo-encephalitis; (2) marked obliteration of the blood-vessels of the pia and cortex; (3) slow degenerative changes in the ganglion-cells; (4) softened areas at junction of gray and white matter; (5) replacement of the softened area by true neurogliar tissue. In the second case the area in which the left leg-center is situated was removed and examined by Nissl's method. The ganglion-cells were found much altered, staining more deeply than normal cells, and presenting shrunken and attenuated protoplasmic processes. In addition there was a great scarcity of cells.

Pathologic Changes in Dementia Paralytica.—Boedecker and Juliusburger[2] report the clinical histories and anatomic findings in 3 cases of paralytic dementia. We reproduce, in condensed form, the pathologic changes discovered. In the first case, a man of 45, without history of syphilis, alcoholism, or trauma, the pia was turbid, but easily peeled off, except in the region of the right posterior central convolution, where it was adherent, and carried bits of the brain with it on removal. The cortex in this region had a grayish-red color, and was marked by a granular striation. The ependyma was distinctly granulated. Macroscopically, the spinal cord showed no changes. In microscopic examination of brain-sections the pia was found adherent and thickened over the right central gyrus; blood-vessels were abundant, but showed no thickening; pigment-masses were present, especially about the vessels of the pial trabeculæ. Compared with the corresponding region of the left side, the right showed a great excess of blood-vessels. The stratification of the cells of the cortex was no longer visible; instead, a dense cell-accumulation was noted. The pyramidal cells were smaller and shrunken; many were devoid of processes and stained intensely. Evidently, the changes consisted of an extraordinary increase of the interstitial tissue, with diminution in number and degenerative changes of the ganglion-cells. In addition, a degeneration of the pyramidal tract was, by means of Marchi's method, found extending from the right central convolutions down into the lumbar region of the spinal cord. The second patient, a painter, had had syphilis and lead-poisoning, and had also suffered a trauma. At the autopsy chronic leptomeningitis and granular ependymitis were found. The cortex of the right posterocentral convolution and its transition into the paracentral lobule were diminished in comparison with the left side. In the third patient, a bookkeeper, aged 54, the macroscopic lesions consisted in a granular ependymitis and atheroma of the basilar vessels. In both the second and the third cases stained alcoholic preparations of the brain-cortex from the right motor area showed hyperplasia of the neuroglia and diminution of the ganglion-cells; but neither the vessels nor the pigment seemed to be increased. The pyramidal tracts in both cases were the seat of degeneration, rendered visible by Marchi's stain. The interesting features in these 3 cases are, first, the involvement of a localized cortical area; secondly, the degeneration of the pyramidal tracts, showing, as has already been noted by others, that there are cases of paralytic dementia in which the primary cortical disease leads to secondary degeneration in the spinal cord. Finally, the coexistence of sensory and motor disturbances in the

[1] Jour. Nerv. and Ment. Dis., Oct., 1896.   [2] Neurol. Centralbl., Sept. 1, 1897.

limbs tributary to the affected brain-areas seems to corroborate Wernicke's view that every cortical region constitutes the central projection-field for the entire sensibility and motility of the corresponding part of the body. The old contention as to which is the primary process, the vascular changes or those in the nervous elements, is passed over by the authors. They think that the two are practically inseparable.

Typhoid Meningitis.—L. Kamen [1] reports another case of typhoid fever complicated with fibrinopurulent meningitis due to the typhoid bacillus, and points out the fact that he was the first to call attention to the occurrence of typhoid meningitis.

Serous Meningitis.—For the best and the first exhaustive exposition of this subject we are indebted to Quincke.[2] The pathology of the condition is still in dispute, although the general belief is that it is an inflammation, a meningitis or ependymitis of serous character, analogous to serous pleuritis, synovitis, or pericarditis. Three cases, with autopsies in two, are reported by Morton Prince.[3] The disease occurs at all ages, usually causes an internal hydrocephalus, and may be acute or chronic. The etiologic factors are trauma, mental strain, alcoholism, otitis media, and acute infectious diseases. Microscopic examination of the ependyma in one of Prince's cases showed only a slight increase in the neuroglia lying beneath the ependyma, and no evidence of any inflammatory change.

Serous Meningitis due to the Pneumococcus.—Levi[4] reports 2 cases of serous meningitis which were due to the action of the pneumococcus, and in which that organism was found in the exudate. The first case was in an infant aged 3 months and 3 days. At autopsy there was a double bronchopneumonia and a thick serofibrinous exudate beneath the arachnoid. The cerebrospinal fluid and the pneumonic areas in the lungs contained pneumococci. The second case occurred in a child, aged 6½ months. At autopsy there was a double bronchopneumonia, ventricular hydrocephalus, and a serous exudate beneath the arachnoid. The pneumonic areas in the lungs and the hydrocephalic fluid contained pneumococci. The author concludes as follows : 1. The pneumococcus is capable of producing a meningitis which is characterized by a serous exudate between the meninges and a marked vascular congestion. These lesions, of an infectious origin, are usually due to the microbic toxins (pseudomeningitis) ; but they frequently result from the presence of the microorganism itself, and, from this point of view, the pneumococcus acts like the bacillus typhosus, the microorganism of grippe, the streptococcus, and probably also the bacillus coli communis. 2. These cases of meningitis, as toxic lesions, may have a tendency to recover. They indicate, as a rule, an attenuated infection which the phagocytes are able to conquer; whilst purulent exudates indicate the victory of the microorganisms over the phagocytes, which are degenerated into pus-corpuscles. It is probable that certain cases of meningeal accidents (pneumonic meningitis) are lesions of this nature. 3. It is not proper to say that a given cerebrospinal fluid is sterile when cultures have been made on the ordinary media only. A pneumococcus of weak vitality may not grow, but the inoculation of a mouse may demonstrate its existence. In case this inoculation is negative it will, perhaps, be possible to prove that the trouble was due to toxins by a certain immunization which the injection will convey to the mouse in respect to virulent inoculations.

[1] Centralbl. f. Bakteriol., Parasiten. u. Infektionskrank., Apr. 6, 1897.
[2] Volkmann's Sammlung, No. 67, 1893.   [3] Jour. Nerv. and Ment. Dis., Aug., 1897.
[4] Arch. de Méd. expér. et d'Anat. path., Jan., 1897.

4. These lesions may leave permanent trouble behind them, and may probably be the cause of persistent hydrocephalus or of cerebral scleroses.

On Certain Toxic Lesions of the Posterior Columns of the Spinal Cord.—Redlich[1] presents a critical digest of the spinal lesions in various intoxications. In cases of *ergot-poisoning*, in which psychoses of different kinds, epileptiform attacks, and phenomena resembling those of tabes are the chief symptoms, the principal lesion found was sclerosis of the posterior roots and posterior columns. In *pellagra*, a disease produced by the ingestion of spoiled maize, the lesions found by Tuczek resembled those of a combined sclerosis, and were most intense in the upper part of the cord, gradually diminishing lower down. Neither the posterior roots nor the gray matter was involved. The symptoms, if we might allude to them here, were chiefly of a paralytic and spastic nature; disturbances of sensation, ataxia, and myosis were absent. Regarding lesions of the posterior columns in *infectious diseases*, the observations are surprisingly few, but they suffice to show that, as in the other cases, the posterior system-tracts have a special vulnerability to the influence of toxic agents. So far, such lesions have been found positively only in diphtheria This is important and interesting, since it has been customary to ascribe all the nervous complications of that disease to multiple neuritis. Lesions of the posterior columns are also met with in *chronic intoxications* and in *polyneuritis*, and the author cites cases of the latter affection (some dependent on alcohol, others on lead) in which sclerosis of the posterior columns was found. The question as to the relation of the spinal lesion to the affection of the peripheral nerves cannot be answered positively. Some maintain that the former is secondary, either by direct extension of the process along the sensory nerves through the spinal ganglia into the cord, or in other ways. Redlich, however, believes that the two lesions are co-ordinate; in other words, that the same noxious agent acts on the peripheral nerves and on the posterior root-system of the cord; that there is, in short, a lesion of the entire sensory neuron. The author next considers the changes in the posterior columns in *pernicious anemia, leukemia, etc.* Since Lichtheim first called attention to these changes quite a large number of cases have been reported, and a study of these leads to the conclusion that grave anemias of different etiology may produce similar cord-lesions. These lesions are focal degenerations in the posterior columns, which may coalesce and lead to ascending degeneration; the posterior roots and the fibers in the gray matter escape. The process is not strictly symmetric, involves the cervical cord more than the other parts, and presents histologically acute degeneration of the nervous tissue with secondary hyperplasia of the neuroglia. The anemia is not directly the cause of these changes; the latter are probably due to toxic substances circulating in the blood. The last subject dealt with is the lesions of the posterior columns in *diseases of metabolism and constitutional diseases.* Sandmeyer, Leyden, and Williamson describe cord-changes in diabetes mellitus; Lubarsch, in 6 cases of gastric cancer, found changes in the posterior columns, once also small foci in the lateral tracts, and is inclined to attribute them to the absorption of decomposed gastro-intestinal contents. Fleiner describes macroscopic changes of a doubtful nature in the posterior columns in 2 cases of Addison's disease. From the foregoing facts we can draw the conclusion that there are poisons of exogenous and of endogenous origin that are capable of producing a primary degeneration of the nervous structures, especially of the posterior columns. From the point of view of the localization two groups are recognizable—one, exemplified by the lesions in

[1] Centralbl. f. allg. Path. u. path. Anat., Dec. 15, 1896; Univ. Med. Mag., Mar., 1897.

pernicious anemia, presents disseminated foci of degeneration ; in the other, as, e.g., in ergot-tabes, the degeneration is systemic, affecting the posterior roots and their tracts. But it is to be noted that in no case was any reference made to diseases of the spinal ganglia which could explain the involvement of the posterior roots. In concluding, Redlich points out that these facts may have an important bearing on our conception of tabes, and implies that in them we may perhaps find support for the theory of the toxic origin of that disease.

The Spinal Cord in Pernicious Anemia.—C. Eugene Riggs[1] reports a case of pernicious anemia with marked spinal changes. Patches of sclerosis were present in nearly all the columns, but none, except possibly the left direct cerebellar and the right direct pyramidal, had all their fibers involved. The scleroses were, the author thinks, probably vascular in origin. (See Plates 5, 6).

J. Mitchell Clarke[2] describes the cord-changes in 2 cases of pernicious anemia. In the first, a woman of 46, the changes consisted in fairly complete degeneration of the posterior columns, extending the whole length of the cord and the lower dorsal and upper lumbar regions, and a small area of degeneration in the posterior part of the left lateral column. The internal posterior root-zone escaped, and this explained the preservation of the knee-jerk. With Golgi's stain a marked hyperplasia of the neuroglia in the degenerated areas was demonstrated. In the second case, a laborer, aged 38, the gray matter of the cord was particularly affected—the vessels were intensely injected and there were numerous microscopic hemorrhages distributed chiefly about the central parts of the gray matter. Small areas of sclerosis were also noticed. Some of the nerve-cells of the anterior horns showed degenerative changes. The walls of the small vessels appeared thickened ; the central canal was blocked. All the changes were most marked in the upper dorsal region.

The Spinal Cord in Tetanus.—Walter K. Hunter[3] reports studies in 3 cases. In the cord of the first, a lad of 12, he found dilatation of the vessels, especially in the gray matter, and minute hemorrhages. There were no signs of round-cell infiltration. Regarding the ganglion-cells, the only change noticed (on comparing with normal cords) was that the plasma stained more diffusely, and showed none of the normal differentiation of its substance. The second had been successfully treated with antitoxin, but developed exfoliative dermatitis, to which he succumbed in 5 days, 15 days after the onset of the tetanic convulsions. No hemorrhages were found, and the hyperemia was scarcely more marked than in a normal cord. The ganglion-cells presented an appearance similar to that of the first case. The third case was a child of 4, which died in spite of an injection of antitoxin. The *bacillus tetani* was cultivated from the wound. The cord, including the ganglion-cells, was normal. From these cases the author concludes that the hyperemia (noted in Cases I. and II.) is probably the same as that seen in the other organs, and results from the spasm of the muscles of respiration. Its absence in the third case is difficult to explain ; possibly the child died from syncope rather than from asphyxia. The changes in the ganglion-cells in two of the cases the author brings in line with those experimentally produced by Marinesco in guinea-pigs, and looks upon them as early signs of degeneration, the result of the toxins, though it is possible that the toxin is a powerful stimulant, and that the degeneration is the consequence of overuse.

The Pathology of Bulbospinal Atrophospastic Paralyses.—Hoche[4] used Marchi's method for the study of the nervous system of a typical

[1] Internat. Med. Mag., Sept., 1896.   [2] Brit. Med. Jour., Aug. 7, 1897.   [3] Ibid.
[4] Neurol. Centralbl., Mar. 15, 1897 ; Univ. Med. Mag., May, 1897.

case of amyotrophic lateral sclerosis with progressive bulbar palsy in a man, aged 52, who died with symptoms of vagus-paralysis a year and a half after the beginning of the disease. The designation in the title is employed in accordance with the suggestion of Senator.[1] The patient had presented spasticity of the upper and lower limbs, with exaggerated reflexes, some atrophy of the interossei of the hands, fibrillary twitching, *main-en-griffe* of the left hand; the pupils and external ocular muscles were normal; the tongue showed no anomaly; sensory or sphincter disturbances were absent; mimic movements were normal; there was progressive impairment of swallowing and of speech, and toward the end persistent acceleration of the pulse. The gross morbid findings were unimportant. In Marchi's (and Weigert's) preparations the following was noted: a degeneration of the entire motor pathway and slight changes in the ganglion-cells; in addition, extensive degeneration of the fiber-systems that unite the motor nuclei, both of the cranial and of the spinal nerves—viz., the posterior longitudinal bundle and the short tracts of the anterolateral columns. It was apparent from a combined study of Marchi's and Weigert's sections that the degeneration in the pyramidal tracts had progressed from below upward; it could be traced through the corona radiata to the central convolutions. In the nuclei of the cranial nerves but little degeneration of the ganglion-cells was noted; in the cord the number of cells was reduced in the cervical portion, apparently not at all in the dorsal, while in the lumbar region the fibrillar network of the anterior horns plainly showed degenerative changes. In marked contrast with these rather insignificant cell-changes were the degenerations of the root-fibers of the oculomotor, pathetic, abducens, facial, glossopharyngeal, vagus, hypoglossus, and spinal accessory nerves. The involvement of the ocular nerves was interesting in view of the absence of clinical symptoms referable to the eyes, while those in the facial, hypoglossus, and spinal accessory were more marked than had been expected. The chief interest of the case lies, however, in the involvement of the two commissural tracts. Marie was the first to call attention to this degeneration in the anterolateral tracts, and Brissaud went so far as to consider amyotrophic lateral selerosis a primary disease of the supplemental or commissural fibers. While withholding his full approval of this theory, the author believes that the changes demonstrated in the posterior longitudinal bundle in his case accord very well with it, for this bundle is for the motor cranial nerves what the short tracts of the cord are for the nuclei of the different spinal segments. The pathologie anatomy of amyotrophic lateral sclerosis (bulbospinal atrophospastic palsy) may be summed up as follows: 1. Destruction of the motor cortical neurons—degeneration of the pyramidal tracts to their terminations. 2. Destruction of the peripheral motor neurons—motor pathway from the nuclei of the cranial and spinal nerves to their terminations—the muscles. 3. Destruction of the commissural cells and fibers in the cortex, the posterior longitudinal bundle, and the anterolateral tracts of the cord. Of the clinical phenomena which correspond to the disappearance of the commissural tracts we know practically nothing.

THE DIGESTIVE TRACT.

Tuberculous Occlusion of the Esophagus with Partial Cancerous Infiltration.—W. Pepper and D. L. Edsall[2] report a case of tuberculous occlusion of the esophagus, with partial cancerous infiltration of the strictured portion of the gullet. This rare case forms the text for an ex-

---

[1] Deutsch. med. Woch., 1894.   [2] Am. Jorr. Med. Sci., July, 1897.

haustive paper on tuberculous occlusion of the esophagus and on the association of tuberculosis and cancer. The authors consider that in their case the tuberculous lesion preceded the development of the cancer.

The Infectious Origin of Certain Perforating Round Ulcers of the Stomach.—Widal and Meslay,[1] in the body of a patient dead of staphylococcic pyemia secondary to a suppurating corn of the sole of the right foot, found a liter of pus in the pericardium, and abscesses in the kidney, the epididymis, and the lung. Gastric pain, vomiting, and hematemesis had been absent. On opening the stomach a punched-out ulcer was found, the base being formed by the subperitoneal tissue; about the ulcer the mucosa and submucosa were considerably edematous and vascularized. Staphylococci were, however, not found in the sections. But despite their absence the acute ulcer should be attributed, Widal and Meslay believe, to the infection. They hold that a small abscess or erosion was produced by the staphylococci, and that the gastric juice rapidly transformed a small loss of substance into a large ulcer. Primarily microbic, the ulcer later became peptic, the bacteria disappearing with the spread of the lesion. The first stage of ulceration is sometimes found in cases dead of septicemia, as, *e. g.*, in women that have perished of puerperal infection. In animals dead of experimental infections these early stages of ulceration are frequently encountered, and even true ulcers, though more rarely, may be seen. In endeavoring to settle the infectious origin of ulcers we cannot depend on the finding of the pathogenic microorganism, for the latter is only discoverable in the beginning stages, in the region of the specific ulceration; when the round ulcer has once been formed the organisms are no longer found—the ulcer has lost all signs of its specific etiology. [Nauwerck[2] has reported 2 cases of such mycoticopeptic ulcers, one in connection with endocarditis of rheumatic origin, the other in a case of scarlet fever. The edges of the first showed masses of streptococci and diplococci; those of the second, streptococci. He believes that many gastric ulcers begin as hemorrhagic erosions, and that some of these were microbic in origin.]

Congenital Hypertrophy and Stenosis of the Pylorus.—F. Schwyzer[3] reports a case of this kind in a female child 3 months old, that had died with symptoms of chronic gastritis. The pylorus formed a distinct tumor, 2.4 cm. in length, and 2.1 cm. in width. On microscopic examination the hypertrophy was found to depend chiefly on a hyperplasia of the circular layer of muscle-fibers.

Cancer of the Stomach with Unusual Metastasis.—Israel[4] reports a case of gastric cancer in a man 57 years old, in which the stomach was no larger than a small fist, the lesser curvature being greatly shortened and occupied by a deep gangrenous ulcer. The metastasis had spared the organs usually involved in cancer of the stomach—namely, the liver, lung, spleen, and kidney. Secondary nodules were, however, found in many other localities—the retrogastric, mediastinal, and retroperitoneal lymph-glands; both suprarenals, the tail of the pancreas, the left testicle, and both tonsils; also the mucous membrane of the jejunum and colon, and the rectum, in which the lowest metastasis was situated 2 cm. above the anus. The mesenteric glands were but slightly affected. During life a left-sided recurrent paralysis had existed. At the autopsy it was found that one of the mediastinal glands at the side of the trachea had become as large as a hazelnut on account of cancerous infiltration. A cancerous periadenitis had fixed the left recurrent laryn-

[1] Sem. méd., Mar. 17, 1897.
[2] Münch. med. Woch., Sept. 17, 1895; Year-Book, 1897, p. 692.
[3] N. Y. Med. Jour., Nov. 21, 1896.   [4] Berlin. klin. Woch., Jan. 25, 1897.

geal between the gland and the trachea; the nerve, for a distance of a little less than 1 cm., was infiltrated. The distribution of the secondary growths indicates that metastasis took place both along the lymph-paths and the arterial system.

A Case of Myosarcoma of the Small Intestine.—Babes and Nanu[1] report a case of myosarcoma of the small intestine. The specimen was obtained, by operation, from a man aged 30, and was as big as two fists. Microscopic examination showed that the growth took its origin from the muscularis, and was produced, the authors believe, by a sarcomatous transformation of the muscle-cells. Diagnostically important is the fact that this form of tumor in the present case and in 3 others recorded occurred in the fourth decennium, cancer being more frequent later in life. Metastasis usually takes place early in sarcoma of the small intestine.

Cirrhosis of the Liver.—H. D. Rolleston and W. J. Fenton[2] publish a study of 114 cases of cirrhosis of the liver abstracted from the autopsy-records of St. George's Hospital, London. We give their more important conclusions: 1. There is a high rate of mortality from tuberculosis in cases of cirrhosis, and in fatal cases of cirrhosis pulmonary tubercle, often obsolete, is found in 21.2%; while in latent cases of cirrhosis, death occurring from other causes, pulmonary tubercle was less frequent, being present in 14%. 2. Taking all the cases, cirrhosis is commoner in males, 5:2, but it is more often latent than in females. 3. Cirrhosis is fatal to women earlier in life (3 years 8 months, or at the age of 46.6 years) than in males (50.3 years). 4. There is little or no difference between the average ages of persons dying from cirrhosis and those dying from other causes but with cirrhotic livers. 5. Alcoholic cirrhosis is fatal earlier (3 years 4 months on the average) than nonalcoholic cirrhosis; this is more especially so in females. 6. Cirrhotic livers are, on the average, considerably increased in weight (65.49 oz.). 7. The livers of cases dying from nonalcoholic cirrhosis are very much lighter (weighing 41 oz.) than the livers of cases dying from alcoholic cirrhosis (67.7 oz.). 8. Alcoholic cirrhosis is commoner than nonalcoholic cirrhosis. 9. There is a marked difference (20 oz.) between the weight of the nonalcoholic livers in cases fatal from cirrhosis and in cases with cirrhotic livers dying from other diseases. 10. In cases fatal from cirrhosis the heavier livers are found at an earlier age than the lighter ones. 11. Malt-liquors and spirits may both give rise to enlarged cirrhotic livers. The author's figures, though scanty, are opposed to the view that beer necessarily or usually gives rise to an enlarged and spirits to a contracted cirrhotic liver. Fatty change was more marked, contrary to expectation, in spirit-drinkers' livers. 12. Fatty change occurs equally in large and small cirrhotic livers; half of the large livers (weighing over 60 oz.) did not show any fatty change. 13. In cases fatal from cirrhosis the liver weighs less than normal in 23% of the cases. 14. Of cases fatal from cirrhosis, 80% were alcoholic, 12.7% nonalcoholic, and in the remainder there was no evidence either way. 15. In women dying from the effects of cirrhosis a large liver associated with head-symptoms and with little or no ascites is more frequent earlier in life, while later a small liver and ascites are more often met with. 16. Ascites and hemorrhages were commoner in males than in females dying from cirrhosis. 17. In both sexes the decade between 50 and 60 years of age is the one in which most deaths result from cirrhosis. 18. In patients with latent cirrhosis the liver was generally much enlarged, weighing on an average 67.19 oz. In only one group—cases fatal from granular kidney—was this not so. The weight of the liver in fatal granular

[1] Berlin. klin. Woch., Feb. 15, 1897.   [2] Birmingham Med. Rev., Oct., 1896.

kidney approaches the normal weight. 19. Taking the average weight of the normal spleen as 7 oz., it is increased in the cases fatal from cirrhosis; whereas it appears that latent cirrhosis does not, apart from complications, lead to splenic enlargement. 20. The average weight of the spleen is heavier in alcoholic than in nonalcoholic cases of cirrhosis. 21. In cases fatal from cirrhosis there is no constant relation between the weight of the liver and that of the spleen. This appears to be true also of all cases of cirrhosis.

T. N. Kelynack[1] has collected 121 cases of common cirrhosis of the liver from the postmortem records of the Manchester Royal Infirmary. Those secondary to cardiac and other chronic affections have been omitted; likewise syphilitic, biliary, and hypertrophic cirrhosis. From a study of the 121 undoubted cases the author draws the following conclusions: 1. Common cirrhosis cannot conveniently be divided into alcoholic and nonalcoholic varieties. Most examples met with in hospital occur in alcoholic subjects. 2. Nearly 50% of the cases die directly from the effects of the hepatic cirrhosis. 3. Over 12% die from active tuberculosis. Tubercle of the peritoneum occurs in a little over 9%. Either active, latent, or obsolete tubercle is met with in nearly 24% of all cases. 4. Cirrhosis appears commonest in males, the proportion being about 2 to 1. 5. The average age at death is—for males, 45½, and females, 42 years; that is to say, cirrhosis is fatal to women earlier than to men by 3½ years. 6. Ascites occurs in 56% of all cases. It is usually less extensive in females than males. 7. Ascites constantly occurs in association with hematemesis, and they are not to be considered as mutually exclusive. 8. The weight of the liver averages—in males, a little over 53 ounces; in females, nearly 54 ounces. 9. The liver is increased in size in nearly 33% of all cases, diminished in about 61½%, and normal in size in about 5½%. 10. The liver varies in size between its antemortem and postmortem conditions. 11. Typical "hobnailed" livers are not common at the present day, although evidence of alcoholism is constantly being met with. 12. The spleen in hepatic cirrhosis weighs on the average in males 14¼ ounces, in females a little over 11½ ounces. 13. The spleen is enlarged in 83%, normal in size in nearly 9½%, diminished in 7¾%. 14. The "cyanotic" spleen of hepatic cirrhosis is larger and heavier than that met with in "cardiac" cases. 15. Renal "cirrhosis" only occurs in association with hepatic cirrhosis in a little over 18½% of all cases.

Experimental Cirrhosis of the Liver from Phosphorus.—Aufrecht[2] has administered phosphorus hypodermically to rabbits and has studied the changes produced in the liver, employing Biondi-Heidenhain's stain. He was able to produce a typical cirrhosis, but is of the opinion that this was never the result of an interstitial inflammation, but was due to an inflammation of the liver-cells at the periphery of the acini; the apparently newly formed tissue is nothing more than the morbidly altered peripheral cells of the hepatic acini. This is, he maintains, also true of human cirrhosis, to which the experimental is completely analogous.

The Condition of the Gall-bladder in Persistent Obstruction of the Ductus Choledochus.—Ecklin[3] finds that in cases of stone the gall-bladder is usually atrophied (in 110 out of 172 cases); in other cases of obstruction (121 out of 139) it is generally dilated. The contraction may be brought about by inflammation of the gall-bladder or the bile-ducts.

Primary Sarcoma of the Liver.—Bramwell and Leith[4] report an

[1] Birmingham Med. Rev., Feb., 1897.
[2] Deutsch. Arch. f. klin. Med., Bd. lviii., H. 2 and 3, 1897.
[3] Centralbl. f innere Med., No. 5, 1897.   [4] Edinb. Med. Jour., Oct., 1896.

enormous primary sarcoma involving nearly the whole of the right lobe and part of the left lobe of the liver in a married woman of 25 years. A large blood-cyst developed in the tumor and simulated hepatic abscess. The tumor was a spindle-cell sarcoma, probably arising from the cells lining the perivascular lymphatics of the intralobular capillaries of the liver. On account of its numerous blood-vessels, the growth deserved the name of angiosarcoma. [It is interesting that there was no metastasis whatever.]

Cancer of the Pancreas with Dilatation of the Stomach.—V. H. Taliaferro[1] records a case of cancer of the head of the pancreas, with infiltration entirely around the duodenum close to the pylorus, causing constriction at this point and dilatation of the stomach.

Primary Sarcoma of the Tail of the Pancreas.—F. J. E. Ehrmann[2] reports a primary round-cell sarcoma of the tail of the pancreas in a woman 56 years of age. The growth had given metastasis to the liver.

" Fremdkörpertuberculosis " of the Peritoneum.—De Quervain[3] describes a case of what the Germans call " Fremdkörpertuberkulose " of the peritoneum, the result of rupture of an echinococcus-cyst. At the operation, a few weeks after the rupture, a piece of the omentum containing small nodules closely resembling tubercles was removed. The nodules consisted of giant cells, epithelioid cells, and small round cells, and contained in their center a distinct piece of echinococcus-membrane. Some of the larger nodules showed caseation. Quervain considers the condition a benign process analogous to that developing about every aseptic foreign body.

The Etiology of Dysentery.—W. Janowski[4] gives an exhaustive *résumé* of the literature of the etiology of dysentery, summing up his conclusions in the following words : Dysentery is etiologically not a single disease, and is probably never caused by a single parasite, but by the conjoined action of several varieties. The data of literature permit us to say that the ordinary dysentery is caused by a bacterial association ; tropical dysentery, however, is probably produced by the association of " definite species of ameba with bacteria."

THE RESPIRATORY TRACT.

Fibrinous Bronchitis.—Klein[5] examined the coagula chemically and microchemically, and found that they were composed of mucin, not of fibrin, and suggests as a better name for the disease *bronchitis pseudofibrinosa vel mucinosa.*

Experimental Researches on Pneumoconiosis.—Claisse and Josué[6] have made a study of this subject under the following heads : simple anthracosis, influence of anthracosis on morbid states, and influence of morbid conditions on anthracosis. They conclude: 1. That experimental anthracosis, even after inhalations of long duration (280 administrations), produces neither ·true anatomic lesions nor functional disturbance of the respiratory apparatus. It may, therefore, be affirmed that the different acute or chronic inflammatory, sclerotic, or ulcerous lesions described in human pathology, in the chapter on pneumoconiosis, are not due to the direct action of the dust, but rather to the infectious processes which are superadded. Any of the microorganisms which habitually infect the bronchi may become the pathogenic agents of these secondary infections. This is particularly true of the tubercle-bacillus. It

---

[1] Med. Brief, Dec., 1896.   [2] Jour. Am. Med. Assoc., Dec. 12, 1896.
[3] Centralbl. f. Chir., p. 1, 1897.
[4] Centralbl. f. Bakteriol., Parasiten. u. Infektionsk., Jan. 30, Feb. 6 and 15, Mar. 5, 1897.
[5] Wien. klin. Woch., No. 31, 1896.   [6] Arch. de Méd. expér. et d'Anat. path., Mar., 1897.

will be useful to revise the pathologic anatomy of human pneumoconiosis, employing modern histobacteriologic methods. The experiments show that bronchitis, phthisis, and sclerosis of an anthracotic, siderotic, or like origin do not exist in the strict sense; but that lesions due to the streptococcus or to the tubercle-bacillus, etc., occur in patients who are subjects of anthracosis, siderosis, etc. 2. That the influence of pneumoconiosis upon the evolution of morbid states may be neglected when the inhaled dust-particles are very small in size. The migration of such dust across the alveolar wall and through the pulmonary tissue is made without incident. On the other hand, voluminous dust-particles having angular surfaces may become lodged in the bronchioles; they act under such circumstances as foreign bodies in the air-passages. The local traumatism produced by the presence of these bodies prepares a soil upon which inhaled microorganisms may develop, and thus excite acute or chronic secondary affections which must have considerable influence upon the evolution of a preexisting morbid state. 3. That morbid states have no appreciable influence on the evolution of pneumoconiosis if they are of short duration, but favor its development if they are prolonged. This increase of anthracosis is thus explicable in certain of the author's experiments in which lesions of the lymph-nodes or of the pneumogastric nerves were present. The lesions of the lymph-nodes increase pneumoconiosis by impeding the circulation and the elimination of particles of dust by the lymphatics. Pneumogastric lesions act by destroying the defence of the upper bronchial passages, thus permitting the penetration of an abnormal quantity of dust even into the alveoli. Pneumogastric lesions also act, possibly, by the vasomotor troubles which they produce. The marked increase of anthracosis produced by vagotomy renders directly appreciable the role of the pneumogastric nerve in the protection of the air-passages, not only from inert and insoluble dust, dangerous simply by its accumulation, but also from living, microbic, infecting dust.

Primary Carcinoma of the Pleura.—Benda[1] reports a massive primary tumor of the left pleura in a man of 54. Nearly the entire pleura was affected; microscopically, the growth consisted of epithelioid cells and stroma. The author looks upon the tumor as a carcinoma, taking the view that the cells lining the pleural cavity are epithelial. [As the majority of pathologists adopt Thiersch and Waldeyer's theories of the origin of tumors, they cannot agree with Benda in classing his tumor as carcinoma, and would probably designate it as endothelioma, meaning thereby a peculiar connective-tissue tumor belonging to the sarcomas. But it seems to us that the best basis of classifying tumors, as long as the causal one is not available, is the morphology; and according to that, any tumor that presents the histologic features of a carcinoma, no matter what its "Provenienz," is a carcinoma. Hausemann, in his recently published book,[2] is of the same opinion.]

Charcot-Leyden and Calcium-oxalate Crystals in Sputum.— D. Riesman,[3] in the sputum of an asthmatic patient, found, in addition to Charcot-Leyden crystals, crystals that appeared to be calcium oxalate. He refers to a similar observation made by Ungar, and calls attention to Cohn's studies,[4] by which it seems to be established that Charcot-Leyden crystals are not octahedra, but hexahedra.

Albuminous or Serous Expectoration.—West[5] reports the occurrence of albuminous or serous expectoration following paracentesis thoracis.

[1] Centralbl. f. innere Med., No. 10, 1897.
[2] "The Mikroskopische Diagnose der bösartigen Geschwülste."
[3] Phila. Polyclinic, Sept. 12, 1896.   [4] Arch. f. klin. Med., 54, p. 515, 1895.
[5] Clinical Society Trans., xxix, p. 169, 1896.

After 40 ounces of fluid had been withdrawn with a siphon the patient began to cough; expectoration commenced in 10 minutes, and in 3 hours the patient brought up a pint of frothy fluid. The fluid divided into 3 layers on standing; it was rich in mucin and poor in albumin. Its production is ascribed to edema of the lungs.

THE THYROID AND THYMUS GLANDS.

The Physiology and Pathology of the Thyroid Gland.—Victor Horsley[1] reviews the work of the last few years on these subjects. He believes, with Gley, that the parathyroid is a gland *sui generis*, and has a specific function related to that of the thyroid; and holds further, with the majority of writers, that while myxedema and cretinism result from simple loss of the function of the thyroid gland, exophthalmic goiter depends on a perversion of that function.

Hemorrhagic Cysts of the Thyroid Gland.—W. I. Bradley[2] points out that there is a form of cystic enlargement of the thyroid gland not generalized, but localized, in which the enlargement is not due to multiple retention-cysts, but to the development of large isolated cystic swellings, either solitary or not exceeding 3 or 4 in number. These cysts appear to be essentially of hemorrhagic origin, and are probably due to rupture, traumatic or otherwise, of some of the vessels of the organ.

The Pathology of Exophthalmic Goiter.—An interesting discussion on this subject took place at the Carlisle meeting of the British Medical

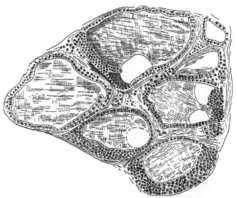

FIG. 51.—Normal thyroid gland (Brit. Med. Jour., Oct. 3, 1896).

Association.[3] G. R. Murray, basing his views on the paucity of lesions in Graves' disease apart from those of the thyroid gland, the similarity of the histologic changes between compensatory hypertrophy and exophthalmic goiter, the apparent antagonism between myxedema and this disease, the transformation of cases of exophthalmic goiter into myxedema by the development of fibrosis in the thyroid, and, finally, the effects of overdoses of thyroid extract, adopts the theory that in exophthalmic goiter there is an excessive formation and

[1] Brit. Med. Jour., Dec. 5, 1896.   [2] Jour. Exper. Med., July, 1896.
[3] Brit. Med. Jour., Oct. 3, 1896.

absorption of thyroid secretion, which may or may not be normal in character, and that the symptoms of the disease are due to the presence of this excess of

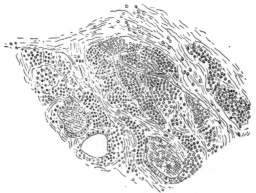

FIG. 52.—Fibrosis of thyroid gland from case of myXedema (Brit. Med. Jour., Oct. 3, 1896).

secretion in the blood, and to its action upon the tissues and especially upon the nerve-centres in the medulla. The practical conclusion from this is that

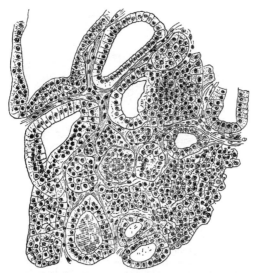

FIG. 53.—Compensatory hypertrophy of thyroid gland of monkey (Brit. Med. Jour., Oct. 3, 1896).

we should endeavor to improve our methods of treating the diseased thyroid gland. We want to be able to induce a moderate degree of fibrosis, and so imitate the natural process of recovery. Removal of a portion of the gland, though most successful in some cases, has proved to be a dangerous operation in others. Possibly injections of iodin, electrolysis, or some similar means of starting a limited fibrosis, may help us to attain the object we have in view without danger. Victor Horsley was also of the opinion that the functional disturbance appeared to be a perversion of the secretion of the thyroid.

The objections to the thyroid theory of Graves' disease were stated by Walter Edmunds, and they were presented so clearly that we reproduce them almost in full. The changes in the thyroid are practically identical with those found in an hypertrophied portion of the gland; in an animal after excision of a portion of the thyroid the remaining part hypertrophies; these changes in animals, then, are due to compensating hypertrophy. In Graves' disease, too, the changes in the thyroid are due to compensating hypertrophy; in other words, the change in the thyroid is not the primary lesion. This, too, tells against the view that the disease is due to an excessive secretion of normal thyroid juice, because if it were, there would be no occasion for a com-

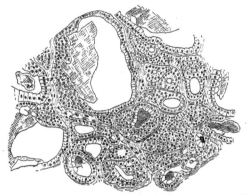

FIG. 54.—Thyroid gland, exophthalmic goiter (Brit. Med. Jour , Oct. 3, 1896).

pensating hypertrophy. It is certainly very natural to conjecture that, as myxedema is due to a decrease of thyroid secretion, Graves' disease is due to an excess; but there are objections to this theory. First, although the contrast between the symptoms of Graves' disease and those of myxedema is well marked in the chronic forms, in the acute form (as seen in dogs) it is not at all marked—indeed, the two affections resemble one another. In both there are well-marked tremors and occasional attacks of dyspnea. Secondly, the theory of excessive secretion will not explain the exophthalmos; the injection, subcutaneously, of thyroid extract in large quantities into monkeys does not produce exophthalmos in these animals, although the condition can be readily enough produced in them by the injection of cocain. Thirdly, the theory will not explain why in many recorded cases the exophthalmos was on one side, or mainly on one side, and the enlargement of the thyroid more marked on that side. Fourthly, the not uncommon occurrence of myxedema following Graves' disease seems to support the secretion-view; but the theory would require an interval of good health in the transitional stage. One finds mention of cases in which the two diseases appeared to coexist. Edmunds recently saw a case in which this condition possibly existed and which improved while taking thyroid extract. Finally, against the secretion-theory is the effect of thyroid-feeding; different results have been obtained, and the majority of observations seem to show that the treatment does no good, but it does not seem to do harm with the certainty that might be expected were the symptoms due to an excess of thyroid-secretion. The secretion of the enlarged thyroid of Graves' disease is probably abnormal, but its physiologic effect has not been recorded; it would certainly be desirable when the opportunity presents to determine this point by experiment. Besides the thyroid being enlarged, the thymus is also enlarged; if this condition occurs in a considerable number of cases, it has some important bearing on the pathology. Microscopically the enlarged thymus contains—(1) a large number of lymphocytes; (2) the concentric corpuscles of Hassell seem to be enlarged and in an active condition, somewhat inconsistent with the view that they are fœtal remains with no part to play in the organism; (3) here and there numerous eosinophile corpuscles are found. The pathology of the disease must be partly nervous and partly humoral; the exophthalmos must be produced in some way through the nervous system, and, on the other hand, it is difficult to see how removal of a portion of the enlarged thyroid gland can act directly on the nervous system. It is possible that the primary lesion is a derangement of the metabolism of the body. J. G. Adami and J. Hill Abram, on the whole, agreed with Murray.

The thyroid-theory was also strongly opposed by Robert Hutchison, who maintained that two of the arguments in favor of the thyroid theory, (1) the contrast between the symptoms of myxedema and those of exophthalmic goiter, and (2) the alleged fact that cases of exophthalmic goiter are aggravated by thyroid-feeding, were entirely fallacious. Any disease characterized by an exaggerated rate of metabolism would present a similar contrast to a disease such as myxedema, in which general metabolism was abnormally slow. It would be found on consideration that the general symptoms of fever were just the opposite of most of the symptoms of myxedema. It had been proved by experiment that thyroid-feeding caused an increased metabolism in the tissues, and it was not to be wondered at if it should exaggerate the symptoms of such a disease as exophthalmic goiter, in which metabolism was already too rapid. No one would expect fever to be benefited by thyroid-feeding. Hutchison was inclined to regard the disease exophthalmic goiter as consisting essentially in a specific change in tissue-metabolism, probably due to a functional alteration in the central nervous system, the relationship of the enlargement of the thyroid to these changes being as yet undetermined, but not to be regarded as their primary cause. [The question of the pathology of Graves' disease is still unsettled, but it seems that Möbius' view of the thyroid origin of the symptoms is the most satisfactory. That, however, there must be a cause for the thyroid-changes no one can deny; and to discover that ultimate cause is a task of the future.]

Eulenburg[1] is of the opinion that the assumption merely of an increased secretory activity of the thyroid gland does not explain Graves' disease, but that we must assume also a qualitative change, the latter depending on primary modifications in the blood supplied to the gland. The toxic action of the altered secretion is expended chiefly in the nervous system, on the higher psychic centers especially, and thus gives rise to the hysteroneurasthenic nature of the disease.

John Hill Abram,[2] from an examination of the thyroid gland in 4 cases of exophthalmic goiter, is led to reiterate an earlier statement made by him,[3]

[1] Centralbl. f. innere Med., June 26, 1897.   [2] Liverpool Med.-Chir. Jour., July, 1896.
                          [3] Lancet, Nov. 16, 1895.

that the goiter in Graves' disease is not a vascular one. The microscopic changes are summed up as follows: absence of colloid; duct-like character of the alveoli; hypertrophy of the epithelium.

Metabolism in Exophthalmic Goiter.—Matthes[1] was able to confirm the fact that there is in Graves' disease an increased destruction of albumins. After strumectomy this destruction gradually suffered a diminution, which was coincident with an increase in body-weight.

The Pathology of the Thymus Gland.—Ernst Siegel[2] reports a most interesting case that seemingly settles affirmatively the question as to the existence of the so-called *asthma thymicum*. In a boy 2½ years old, suffering from dyspnea, in whom tracheotomy gave no relief, the thymus was elevated and stitched to the fascia over the sternum, with the result that the threatening dyspnea disappeared; the child eventually made a good recovery. The author also has reviewed the literature, and finds a considerable number of cases recorded in which dyspnea, generally fatal, was caused by an enlarged thymus. The manner in which the thymus hyperplasia produces dyspnea is still *sub judice*. Direct pressure on the trachea alone seems hardly sufficient, for Scheele has shown that in dead children a weight of 1000 gr. is necessary to compress the trachea so that air cannot pass. For the purpose of demonstrating compression of the trachea it is best to remove the latter together with the thymus, and then to divide both by transverse section. [The pathology of the thymus as a whole, and that of hyperplasia in infancy in particular, demand careful attention. Friedleben maintained that the thymus could not cause laryngismus, and that there was no asthma thymicum, a view also adopted by Robert H. Harvey,[3] in a paper dealing with the literature on the constitutio lymphatica. Arnold Paltauf explained the sudden deaths in which the thymus was found enlarged (most of them recurring during swimming) as connected with a pathologic state that he designated the constitutio lymphatica, characterized by hyperplasia of the entire lymphatic system, including the thymus gland, and often by a hypoplasia of the vascular system, and in females of the generative organs. The relief given in Siegel's case by operation points, it seems to us, to some influence exercised by the thymus. The whole question, however, still requires answer. We have ourselves seen a case from the Maternity of the Hospital of the University of Pennsylvania in which an enlarged thymus was apparently the cause of death.]

Primary Epithelioma of the Thymus.—Paviot and Gerest[4] report a case of primary epithelioma of the thymus in a woman aged 52. Histologic examination of the growth showed masses of cells which were so arranged that they formed little spheres, the so-called concentric bodies of Hahn and Thomas. These bodies are the essential element in the histologic diagnosis of epithelial tumors of the thymus. These bodies are more easily seen if sections are cut from the periphery of the fresh tissue.

THE URINARY TRACT.

Uric-acid Excretion in Croupous Pneumonia.—Dunin and Nowaczek[5] report 5 cases of croupous pneumonia in which they estimated the uric-acid elimination throughout the course. In all the cases the amount of acid began to increase the day before the crisis set in, and after the crisis suddenly increased so markedly that the quantity eliminated was threefold

[1] Centralbl. f. innere Med., June 26, 1897. [2] Berlin. klin. Woch., Oct. 5, 1896.
[3] Chicago Med. Rec., Dec., 1896. [4] Arch. de Méd. expér. et d'Anat. path., Sept., 1896.
[5] Zeit. f. klin. Med., Bd. xxxii., H. 1 and 2, 1897.

43

that excreted during the febrile stage. This "uric-acid crisis" lasted 3 or 4 days. Dunin and Nowaczek did not count the number of leukocytes, and as the leukocytes usually fall to normal at the time of or near the crisis, it cannot be said that there was actually an association in their cases between the uric-acid eliminated and the number of leukocytes. But the authors believe that their results substantiate Horbaczewski's view that the uric-acid elimination is dependent on the nuclein derived from the destruction of leukocytes.

The Urine in Myxedema.—Hertoghe and Masoin [1] found the urine feebly toxic in myxedema.

The Urine in Hypertrophic Osteoarthropathy.—Guérin and Étienne [2] report a case in which the urine of the patient contained, on an average, 0.328 gm. of lime, 0.140 gm. of magnesium, 20.831 gm. of urea, and 1.737 gm. of phosphoric acid, every 24 hours. This hypophosphaturia clearly shows that the decalcification of the osseous system is effected only at the expense of the carbonate of lime, and this decalcification, which occurs only in the initial stage of the disease, explains the accompanying deformities.

The Alloxur-bodies in Gout and Granular Kidney.—Kolisch has announced the opinion that there is in gout an increased elimination of alloxur-bodies, and that the quantity of uric acid is lessened in proportion to the extent of involvement of the kidneys; for in nephritis the alloxur-bases are increased. Rommel [3] found only average quantities of alloxur-bodies eliminated in a case of chronic gout following lead-poisoning, and despite advanced granular kidney the uric-acid elimination was normal. In a non-gouty case of granular kidney, on a diet free from large quantities of nuclein, and in the absence of leukocytosis, Rommel found an elimination of alloxur-bodies above the normal. These high values of uric acid in advanced Bright's disease go to show that the theory making the kidneys the only source of uric acid cannot be true.

Alloxur-bodies and their Relation to Gout.—Malfatti, [4] in a case of gout, found an increase of alloxur-bodies above the quantity eliminated before the attack, but the amount did not exceed normal limits. This would disprove Kolisch's theory that gout is a disturbance of metabolism in which the nuclein-content is increased beyond the normal. The author adopts the view that gout is a process in which the normal metabolism is altered in such a way that the nitrogen-equilibrium is destroyed, and that periodically nitrogen is either eliminated in excess or retained in the body.

Influence of Ingestion of Albumin on Alloxur-bodies.—Hess and Schmoll [5] found that the ingestion of albumin and paranuclein (egg-albumin and yolk of egg) had no influence upon the excretion of alloxur-bodies in the urine. The quantity of those bodies in the urine seems entirely to depend, first, on the quantity of nuclein (food or body-nuclein) broken up, and, second, on the degree of further oxidation.

Elimination of Methylen-blue in Renal Disease.—Achard and Castaigne [6] have found that in cases of renal disease the elimination of methylen-blue injected under the skin is retarded as compared with the elimination in a normal subject. If a healthy man receives a hypodermic injection of 0.25 gm. of methylen-blue, the urine will become feebly tinged in half an hour; in an hour the blue color is distinct, and increases up to the 4th or 5th hour. After remaining at its maximum several hours, it diminishes, and disappears between the 35th and 50th hour. In an individual with improperly functionating kidneys the blue color appears in the urine much later—not until 1, 2, 3, or even

[1] Rev. Neurol., Aug. 30, 1896.　　[2] Arch. de Méd. expér. et d'Anat. path., July, 1896.
[3] Zeit. f. klin. Med., Bd. xxx, H. 1 and 2.　　[4] Wien. klin. Woch., No. 32, 1896.
[5] Arch. f. exper. Path. u. Pharmacol., Bd. xxvii., p. 242.　　[6] Sem. méd., May 5, 1897.

more hours have elapsed; the duration of elimination may be diminished or prolonged; in these persons nearly all of the methylen-blue is retained in the organism. If the urine contains very little methylen-blue, it may be shaken in a tube with a little chloroform, which takes up the coloring-matter. Voisin and Hauser,[1] in connection with this subject, point out that the methylen-blue is eliminated really in two forms—as a colored substance and in the form of a colorless compound. Sometimes, when the urine is not colored by the methylen-blue, boiling will cause the blue tint to appear, showing that the substance is present in the form of a colorless compound.

Fibrinuria.—Klein[2] reports a case of fibrinuria in which the autopsy revealed atrophy and amyloid degeneration of the kidneys. What relation, if any, existed between the amyloid disease and the fibrinuria remains unrevealed. Klein also observed coagula in the urine of a case of cystitis; chemie examination showed them to be composed of nucleo-albumin surrounded by an envelope of mucin.

Formation of Urobilin.—Joffé, in 1868, first noted the occurrence of urobilin in the urine of febrile patients; 10 years later Gerhardt described a urobilin-icterus in which the skin, instead of having the greenish-yellow color of ordinary jaundice, has a dirty yellow color, and the urine gives no reaction with Gmelin's test, but shows a marked increase in urobilin. Vaughan Harley[3] reviews the various theories propounded for the explanation of the origin of urobilin; we shall merely name them, not having space for a detailed account: hepatogenous, hematogenous, nephrogenous, histogenic, and enterogenous. Harley adopts the last, which was first advanced by Maly, but does not deny the possibility that under certain pathologic conditions urobilin may be formed in the tissues or the blood.

According to the enterogenous theory, urobilin is formed in the intestines out of bile-pigment, probably by the action of bacteria. Its place of formation is chiefly the large intestine. The author has also investigated the visible color-changes in the feces in various parts of the intestinal tract, and has endeavored to determine the nature of the staining of the intestinal walls seen postmortem. The general conclusions are as follows: 1. Bile-pigment present in the upper part of the small intestine during its passage along the alimentary canal is converted into some colorless chromogen, to be again converted in the lower part of the small intestine into pigment. 2. Urobilin is, as a rule, formed in the large intestine below the ileocecal valve, and only rarely in the small intestine; that is to say, only in those parts where intestinal putrefaction is most active. 3. The staining of the wall of the cecum and large intestine with urobilin is due to postmortem diffusion, and is not any indication of the absorption of urobilin in the living animal. Why in some cases it is most marked in the cecum and just below the cecum, and not in the rectum, can only be explained by the fact that those parts are generally found in the postmortem room more decomposed than the rectum. 4. The increase of urobilin in the urine, as well as having pathologic significance—as has been already recognized in cases of internal hemorrhages, such as cerebral, peritoneal, or hemorrhagic infarctions, and extrauterine pregnancy, and probably when red blood-corpuscles are being destroyed, as in infectious fevers, scurvy, and pernicious anemia—points also in favor of increased intestinal putrefaction, and may be a useful chemie test for such purpose.

W. B. Ransom[4] enumerates the following conclusions: 1. "Pathologic" urobilin is "normal" urobilin present in increased amount. Some of its supposed properties are (as Hopkins has shown) due to admixture with hematoporphyrin.

[1] Gaz. hebdom. de Méd. et de Chir., May 27, 1897.   [2] Wien. klin. Woch., No. 31, 1896.
[3] Brit. Med. Jour., Oct. 3, 1896.   [4] Ibid.

Urobilin in the urine is probably always derived from the bile, being absent when all the bile escapes from the body. It was found especially abundant in cases of hepatic congestion or cirrhosis, in some cases of jaundice without white stools, in some cases of typhoid fever, even after subsidence of the temperature to normal, and in a case of Graves' disease with severe diarrhea but no fever. It was not found increased in pernicious anemia, nor in a case of hemophilia with extravasations. 2. The pigment of the feces (apart from that of food) consists of various and varying reduction-products of bile, some of which give no bands in the spectrum. One, stercobilin, is identical with a concentrated solution of urobilin and is usually present. In one case of pernicious anemia hydrobilirubin, with two bands (λ 480 to λ 510, and λ 590 to λ 610), was found in its stead. 3. Urobilin in urine is probably mainly derived from stercobilin absorbed from the intestines. The fact that it was found in ascitic fluid in cases of portal obstruction, but was not found in the fluid of pleural effusions, supports this view. In cases of hepatic disorder and of slight jaundice without white stools it is possible that the urobilin of the urine may have its source in bile which has not reached the intestine, but has been reduced in the liver. In the discussion Harley agreed that there were as many if not more cases of pernicious anemia with pale urine, but he thought that even in these the urobilin was increased.

Nephritis.—In a scholarly paper, W. T. Councilman[1] describes his researches into the subject of the forms of nephritis, their anatomic characters, and bacteriology. He proposes the following classification : 1. *Acute Diffuse Nephritis.*—(*a*) Acute degenerative nephritis ; (*b*) acute glomerular nephritis ; (*c*) acute hemorrhagic nephritis ; (*d*) acute interstitial nephritis. 2. *Subacute Glomerular Nephritis.* 3. *Chronic Diffuse Nephritis.*—(*a*) Chronic glomerular nephritis ; (*b*) chronic arteriosclerotic nephritis ; (*c*) chronic degenerative and interstitial nephritis. 4. *Senile Nephritis.* 5. *Amyloid Nephritis.*

Nephritis due to the Diplococcus Lanceolatus.—Michelle[2] reports the occurrence in children of parenchymatous nephritis due to the diplococcus lanceolatus. In 18 out of 19 cases of nephritis he found the organism in the kidneys. Not rarely the nephritis is a primary lesion, the organisms probably reaching the kidney through the blood.

Interstitial Nephritis in Children.—Bernhardt[3] reports 2 cases of chronic interstitial nephritis in children, one a boy suffering from pulmonary phthisis, the other a case in which the nephritis was an accidental discovery. One of the kidneys of the latter case was filled with calculi.

Congenital Cystic Degeneration of both Kidneys.—Burckhardt[4] reports the case of a male infant, born after a tedious labor and dying 25 minutes after birth. On opening the abdomen 2 large tumors were found, $6\frac{1}{4}$ x $3\frac{1}{2}$ x $3\frac{1}{2}$ in., which were the cystically degenerated kidneys.

Colon-bacillus and Infection of Urinary Tract.—Max Melchior[5] concludes a literary study with the statement that the colon-bacillus is the most frequent cause of cystitis and purulent affections of the urinary organs.

TUMORS.

The Origin of Tumors.—Ribbert,[6] in further elucidation of his theory

---

[1] Am. Jour. Med. Sc., July, 1897.
[2] Morgagni, Aug., 1896 ; Centralbl. f. innere Med., No. 22, 1897.
[3] Centralbl. f. innere Med., No. 10, 1897.
[4] Indiana Med. Jour., Mar., 1896 ; Medicine, July, 1896.
[5] Centralbl. f. d. Krankh. d. Harn - u. Sex.-Org., Bd. viii., H. 5.
[6] Deutsch. med., Woch., No. 30, 1896.

of the origin of tumors (see *Year-Book*, 1897, p. 706), points out that a study of the margin of a tumor can give no proper clue as to the mode of the original development; especially can no reliable conclusions be drawn from an examination of the growing edges of a gastric or intestinal cancer. The proofs so far offered in favor of the view that cancer spreads by a direct downward growth of the epithelium are entirely inadequate. Regarding the question whether, in addition to the separation of the cells from their physiologic connections, an increased proliferative tendency is necessary, the author is of the opinion that the proliferation consequent on the separation is sufficient, and that an augmented power of growth or a diminished resistance of the surrounding tissues need not be assumed.

Malignant Growths.—E. Klebs[1] does not believe in the parasitic origin of malignant growths; neither coccidia nor blastomycetes have anything to do with the propagation of tumors. The only characteristic of malignancy is metastasis, and this is brought about by the transport of cells from the original growth: he would employ the term implantation. We frequently see a dissemination of normal epithelium, as in the multiple adenomas; but here it does not produce carcinoma. The malignancy of tumors, the faculty of spreading by its elements, is due to a modification of the tumor-cells. The embryonic condition of any part of the body can only be regarded as one of the causes of tumor-formation, but not of the malignancy of the tumors. As to the origin of the modification of cell-life giving rise to cancerous growth, the author, as already stated, refuses to accept the microbic theory, and holds that one of the strongest arguments against it is the fact that cancer nearly always originates as a secondary metamorphosis of proliferating tissue. He then refers to the well-known instances of the development of cancer in lupous or tuberculous ulcerations of the skin, in adenomatous, papillomatous, and polypoid vegetations of the neck of the uterus, etc. Regarding the true features of cancerous proliferation, it is found by the author in a *hypermitosis* of the cells, a feature to which Hansemann so strongly called attention. This hypermitosis is associated with the penetration of leukocytes into the epithelial cells; the leukocytes feed the epithelial cells. The author finally sums up the phases of carcinomatous metamorphosis as follows: The first stage is that of chronic irritation or inflammation, originated by microbes or by mechanic, or probably also by chemie influences producing a chronic state of hyperplasia, the so-called benign growths composed of all normal tissues constituting the part. This development can lead to diffuse hyperplasia or tumor-formation. The second stage commences with new emigration of leukocytes and progressive development of certain cells, losing through the hypermitotic production the faculty of normal tissue-formation. The excessive proliferation and the possibility of living in a strange medium promote the formation of metastasis, the true feature of carcinoma.

The Role of "Rests" in the Origin of Tumors.—W. Roger Williams[2] is an ardent advocate of Cohnheim's theory of the origin of some, but not of all, tumors. He, however, widens the concept of rests as originally laid down by Cohnheim, who thought they consisted solely of embryonic tissue, which, after sequestration, lay dormant in the body without undergoing further developmental changes. The "rests," as we now know them, always present indications of having undergone more or less development. The author limits himself to a consideration of mammary and uterine neoplasms springing from rests. The former may arise from embryonal or postembryonal glandular sequestrations, or from heterotopic rests. Many cases in illus-

---

[1] Jour. Am. Med. Assoc., Mar. 27, 1897.   [2] Brit. Med. Jour., Oct. 10, 1896.

tration are cited from the literature. In the case of the uterus it has been shown that islets of cylindric epithelium or embryonic remnants often persist in the portio, and it is from such residual elements that, the author believes with Ruge and Veit, the great majority of the primary cancers of this part originate. If the current views as to the origin of the deciduoma malignum are correct, the part played by rests in its origin would be very interesting. The author also thinks that the proneness of uterine fibroids to calcification probably depends on the inclusion of osteogenic elements sequestrated from adjacent parts during early embryonic life. Besides arising from rests, malignant and nonmalignant tumors may originate wherever undifferentiated cells are present, and they are most prone to arise where such cells most abound.

On the Presence of Nerves in Tumors and of other Structures in them as Revealed by a Modification of Ehrlich's Method of "Vital Staining" with Methylen-blue.—H. H. Young[1] was able to demonstrate by means of a modification of Ehrlich's method of vital staining by methylen-blue the existence of definite nerve-fibers in 5 out of 10 tumors, none of them developing from nerves nor being true neuromata. In the case of the sarcomas he believes that the nerves are integral parts of the growth as much as are the sarcomatous blood-vessels. As to their function, no definite statement can be made; a part at least may be connected with the vasomotor system. Regarding the nerves found in carcinoma, the author is of the opinion that they represent normal structures that have been surrounded by the invading cancer-cells; but it would not be surprising if subsequent investigations should prove the presence, at least in the stroma of cancers, of nerves which may properly be considered actual parts of the new growth. Many *mastzellen* were found in the tumors by the methylen-blue method, the cells evidently possessing a special affinity for the dye. They were observed in both sarcomata and carcinomata. Numerous blue-staining cell-inclosures were found in two of the tumors, both sarcomas of bone; their nature was doubtful. In the sections of sarcoma and carcinoma treated by the modified Ehrlich method a considerable number of fibrils having a special affinity for the blue dyes were encountered. They bear no resemblance to nerve-fibers, are often very long, and as a rule straight; their significance is undetermined. [These researches are interesting and suggestive, and open a profitable field in onkology.]

Deciduoma Malignum.—Julia Cook[2] reports a case of deciduoma malignum in a woman aged 30, who had been confined 3 weeks before admission to hospital. Death occurred about 5 weeks later, and at the autopsy an oval mass, 2 in. by 1 in., was found growing from the posterior wall of the uterus, projecting forward and filling the cavity. It had an irregular, pinkish, somewhat granular appearance. Secondary nodules were found in the lung and ovary. Microscopically, the growth showed: 1. Large irregular spaces filled with blood, fibrin, and leukocytes. 2. Protoplasmic masses, the so-called syncytia, in which were imbedded nuclei of varying shapes and sizes, staining irregularly and containing one or more nucleoli. In some parts the syncytial masses were vacuolated or split into elongated cavities, which gave the appearance of a coarse network. Where new tissue was being invaded the syncytium appeared to advance by means of narrow, finger-like processes. 3. Epithelioid cells, occurring singly or in groups of two or three or in larger masses adhering together. Some of these cell-masses were free in the blood-spaces; in parts they adhered to the syncytia, or blocked off one blood-space from another. No blood-vessels were seen, and no intercellular substance was detected in the

---

[1] Jour. Exper. Med., Jan., 1897.   [2] Brit. Med. Jour., Dec., 1896.

growth. Without expressing an opinion as to the true nature of the deciduoma, whether it is sarcoma or cancer, the author adopts the view that it is a distinct pathologic entity, a disease arising from the products of conception.

The Nature of Chloroma.—Paviot and Gallois[1] believe that chloroma (*cancer vert* of Aran) is constituted by enlarged lymphatic glands of the temporal, orbital, and occipital regions, which are due to leukemia.

Pathology of Rodent Ulcer.—H. Muir Evans[2] thinks that rodent ulcer arises in abortive lacrimal glands upon the face, corresponding with the sites in which these glands exist in many of the higher mammalia.

Teratoma of the Tunica Vaginalis.—Koslowski[3] reports an interesting teratoma of the tunica vaginalis removed from a boy 1 year and 9 months old. The tumor had no connection with the testicle, was surrounded by a fibrous capsule, and had attained the size of a plum. Microscopic examination showed the presence of cysts and tubules lined by columnar epithelium and resembling the tubules of the rectum; cysts with ciliated epithelium; and cyst-like spaces, the walls of which had the structure of the skin, showing epiderm, hair and hair-follicles, sebaceous and sweat-glands. Parts were also found resembling more complicated organs, as, *e. g.*, a chambered structure suggesting the heart. Cartilage and nerve-cells arranged in the form of ganglia were likewise present. The tumor represents an embryo, the parts of which have, so to say, been mixed and have remained in the earliest developmental stage. [This tumor is well explained on the " parthenogenetic " theory of Wilms.]

Leydenia Gemmipara Schaudinn, a New Rhizopod found in Ascitic Fluid.—Von Leyden and Schaudinn[4] found in the ascitic fluid of a patient suffering from ascites, edema, aortic insufficiency, and multiple abdominal tumors (detected after abdominal puncture) a large number of round cellular elements, filled with fat-like drops and yellowish pigment-granules, and occurring in nest-like groups. In a number of cells the formation of pseudopods was observed. In a second case, one of cancer of the stomach, these same cells, with the formation of bristles or bead-like projections from the periphery, could be noted. Some of the cells seemed to present a formation suggesting budding. Schaudinn, a competent zoologist, pronounced the bodies a species of rhizopods, and gave them the name of Leydenia gemmipara, the latter term expressive of the mode of reproduction by budding. A connection between the amebæ and the carcinoma is considered possible, and it is striking that the small buds projecting from some of the amebæ bore a close resemblance to the parasitic enclosures in cancer-cells described by Sawtschenko.

THE BLASTOMYCETES.

F. Sanfelice,[5] in a further communication, gives the results of inoculations of saccharomyces neoformans into animals. 1. *Mus musculus.*—Ten mice inoculated in the peritoneal cavity died in 8 days. Miliary nodules were found in the omentum and, not always, small gray spots in the spleen, and kidney. Saccharomycetes were found in the organs and several times in the blood. 2. *White rats.*—Of 2 inoculated under the skin 1 died in $1\frac{1}{2}$ the other in 2 months. At the point of inoculation both showed a growth the size of a hazelnut; miliary nodules were found in the omentum; there was swelling of the

[1] Compt. rend. de la Soc. de Biol., No. 20, 1896.   [2] Brit. Med. Jour., Dec. 12, 1896.
[3] Virchow's Archiv, cxlviii., H. 1, p. 36; Univ. Med. Mag., June, 1897.
[4] Centralbl. f. innere Med., Nov. 14, 1896.
[5] Ann. d'Igiene Sperimentale, vol. vi., nuova serie, Fasc. iii., p. 265, 1896; Centralbl. f. Bakteriol., Parasitenk. u. Infektionskrank., Feb. 6, 1897.

spleen and mesentery, and small gray specks were found on the kidney. Saccharomycetes were observed in the organs, but not as numerous as in mice. 3. *Rabbits.*—Subcutaneous inoculation in 4 was unsuccessful. Of 8 animals inoculated in the peritoneal cavity, 2 died in from 1 to $1\frac{1}{2}$ months, with swelling of the inguinal and axillary glands and nodules in the spleen and kidney. In the organs blastomycetes were not as numerous, but the new formation of cells was more abundant than in mice and rats. 4. *Dogs.*—Of 30 dogs inoculated in various ways, only 2 inoculated in the mammary gland showed tumors at the point of injection and in various organs (the one dog was killed in 2 months, the other died after 10 months), of the slut that died in 10 months, Sanfelice calls the tumors epithelioma. 5. *Chickens.*—Of 8 chickens only 3 presented new formations of saccharomyces neoformans.

Blastomycetes and Cancer.—R. Binaghi,[1] a pupil of Sanfelice's, in an enthusiastic and well-written article, maintains both the parasitic nature of carcinoma and the theory that blastomycetes are the etiologic agents of these growths. In 40 out of 53 carcinomas he was able to demonstrate the presence of these parasites (see *Year-Book*, 1897, p. 708). The exceptions he attributed to faulty fixation and to the fact that it is not always possible to find the parasites by examining a few sections only, and it is probable that another part of the tumor might show them. The method of preparing and staining sections is as follows: the tissue is fixed in absolute alcohol or in Müller's fluid, being, when the latter is used, hardened in alcohol up to absolute. From absolute alcohol it is transferred, for purposes of clearing, to xylol, and then is imbedded in paraffin. After the sections have been mounted with albumin, and freed from paraffin by means of xylol, they are placed in a dish of absolute alcohol. The sections are then stained for from 5 to 15 minutes in Ehrlich's solution, washed in distilled water, and treated for from 2 to 5 minutes with Gram's solution; again washed in water, and then dipped for from 2 to 3 minutes in a 1% watery solution of safranin, and washed in water. They are then carried through three dishes of absolute alcohol, until clouds of color cease to be given off. After clearing in xylol, they are mounted in balsam. The parasites are violet or of a shining blue, the tissues red. The parasites appear both free and enclosed in the neoplastic cells; they are also found among the cells of the round-cell infiltration. In answer to the contention that the so-called parasites may be the result of degeneration, the author offers the testimony of the "chemie reaction." When sections containing the parasites are treated with sulphuric acid the cell-elements are gradually dissolved, while the parasites remain and become more highly refractive. When alkalies are employed instead of the acid the results are even more striking—the tissue-cells disappear entirely, but the parasites remain. These reactions the author seems to consider as proof of the cellulose character of the bodies. The final conclusions are as follows: 1. In cancer there occur constantly parasitic forms which differ from the elements of the tissues and from other accidental elements. 2. The parasites are, as far as their morphologic properties, their specific behavior toward stains, and their reactions with chemie agents are concerned, identical with the blastomycetes. 3. They are not found in other pathologic nor in normal tissues. 4. In view of their relation to the cells of the neoplasm and their regular and definite distribution, the assumption that they are accidental may be excluded, and the conclusion that they are the real cause of carcinoma is justified.

D. B. Roncali[2] believes that the etiologic relation of blastomycetes to can-

[1] Zeit. f. Hygiene, xxiii., H. 3. p. 283.
[2] Centralbl. f. Bakteriol., Parasitenk. u. Infektionskrank., Nos. 9 and 10, 1897.

Fig. 1.—Epithelioma of the orbit (Oc. 3, Obj. $\frac{1}{12}$ Zeiss). Multiple infection of Soudakewitch. In one cell the very young parasites are stained homogeneously; in the other there are, besides these forms, several with an intensely stained nucleus.

Fig. 2.—Epithelioma of lingual frenum (Oc 3, Obj. C, Zeiss). Parasites in the columns of lymphoid cells, which are at the point of being transformed into epithelioid cells. In the Malpighian cells no parasites are seen.

Fig. 3.—Epithelioma of orbit (Oc. 3, Obj. $\frac{1}{12}$ Zeiss). Two groups of young parasites in the columns of lymphoid cells, which lie between two bands of epithelial cells.

Fig. 4.—Epithelioma of stomach (Oc. 3, Obj. $\frac{1}{12}$ Zeiss). Two free and one intracellular parasite. All three have a refractive, intensely stained capsule, and a homogeneous, paler center.

Fig. 5.—Epithelioma of orbit (Oc. 3, Obj. $\frac{1}{12}$ Zeiss). Groups of very young, young, and adult parasites lying free among the lymphoid cells.

Fig. 6.—Epithelioma of uterus (Oc. 3, Obj. $\frac{1}{12}$ Zeiss). Group of parasites, the center of which is stained, and which are surrounded by an unstained halo.

Figs. 7, 8, 10.—Epithelioma of lip (Oc. 3, Obj. $\frac{1}{12}$ Zeiss). Multiplying parasites.

Fig. 9.—Epithelioma of penis (Oc. 3, Obj. $\frac{1}{12}$ Zeiss). Group of parasites formed of a central adult and numerous peripherally situated very young individuals.

Fig. 11.—Epithelioma of mamma (Oc. 3, Obj. $\frac{1}{12}$ Zeiss). Parasites with halo of varying width, and very young forms without halo. One in stage of budding.

(Zeit. f. Hyg. u. Infectiousk., xxiii., Heft 3.)

PLATE 3.

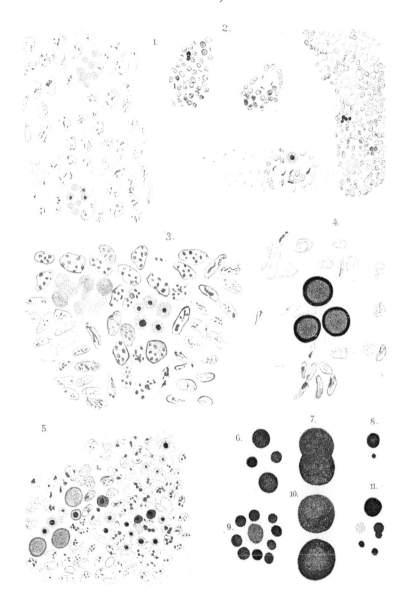

cer is established, (1) because of the morphologic proofs, from a study of the histology of the tumors; (2) because of the successful isolation of the products (ferments) of malignant neoplasms in man; (3) because of the production of malignant new growths in animals by the inoculation of the isolated blastomycetes. The blastomycetes are morphologically identical with the so-called coccidia; they resist concentrated acids and alkalies, and are rarely found in other pathologic conditions [not at all (Binaghi)]; they are found in tumors at the points of active growth, not in the center, where degeneration is in progress. They are found either in the cell-protoplasm, rarely in the nucleus, or between the bundles of fibrous tissue; they react to specific stains and give the cellulose-reaction with iodin. The lesions produced by inoculation in lower animals are variable; the higher mammals (dog) are less susceptible than the lower (guinea-pig, mouse, rabbit, rat, etc.). Some of the blastomycetes produce lesions of a neoplastic and not of an inflammatory character. In dogs new growths may be produced which spread along the lymphatics to various organs, and kill the animals by cachexia. Some parasites, inoculated into the milk-glands of sluts, produce new growths of an epithelial nature. [This is apparently a very strong array of facts which almost compels acquiescence in the theories of the Italian school, but the failure of the protozoan theory, which was so enthusiastically received, to maintain itself, has made nearly all men cautious in the acceptance of new doctrines.]

The Protective Means of the Organism against Blastomycetes. —G. Jona,[1] using saccharomyces opiculatus, found that injected in large numbers into the blood, the peritoneal cavity, or the subcutaneous tissue of rabbits, the organisms were always promptly destroyed, chiefly through the action of the fluids, and always in the region inoculated—*i. e.*, in the blood, the peritoneal cavity, or the subcutaneous tissue.

TUBERCULOSIS.

Concerning New Preparations of Tuberculin.—Robert Koch,[2] in the introductory part of this important article, dwells on the subject of immunity, and contrasts the two distinct forms—*i. e.*, the one against the bacterial toxins (*e. g.*, tetanus) and that against the microorganisms (typhoid fever, cholera). The ideal type of immunity is that against both these noxious agencies. In the case of tuberculosis, on account of its prolonged course, one is disinclined to believe in the existence of an immunity, and persons who have recovered from an attack of the disease are not immune; indeed, they seem more liable to a new invasion. But there are facts which seem to indicate that tuberculosis can carry with it a certain degree of immunity. This is observed in miliary tuberculosis in man and in the experimental tuberculosis of the guinea-pig. There is a period in those affections when the bacilli, which previously propagated actively, become very scarce. Unfortunately this condition supervenes too late to be of use. In miliary tuberculosis of man and in experimental tuberculosis of the guinea-pig there is a rapid general invasion of the organism with bacilli, and it appears that we must look to this phenomenon for the explanation of the period of immunity accompanying the disease. In the ordinary form of human tuberculosis the bacilli present are too few and their absorption too restricted for the production of immunity, which seems to be contingent on the dissemination of the bacilli through the entire system, as in miliary tuberculosis. Efforts to obtain an artificial immunity with living

[1] Centralbl. f. Bakteriol., Parasitenk. u. Infektionskrank., Feb. 6, 1897.
[2] Sem. méd., Apr. 7, 1897; Univ. Med. Mag., June, 1897.

or dead bacilli failed ; abscesses were invariably the result ; if bacilli were injected into the circulation of rabbits, they set up nodules in the lung, in which they were found unabsorbed and unaltered. Unmodified bacilli proving thus inefficacious, Koch endeavored to render them absorbable by chemie means. Treatment with dilute mineral acids or alkalies facilitated absorption ; but, evidently through destruction of the active agent, immunity was not produced. The next attempt was to secure immunity with extracts prepared from the bacilli themselves, and resulted in the discovery of tuberculin, which has the property of evoking a reaction in individuals affected with tuberculosis, a property that renders it a useful diagnostic agent, particularly in pearl-disease of cattle. In referring to this subject, Koch takes occasion to deny emphatically that a mobilization of bacilli occurs during the use of tuberculin. The continned injection of tuberculin is capable of inducing an immunity, but this extends only to the bacillary toxin, not against the bacillus itself. Another unfortunate circumstance is the loss of reaction to tuberculin before a complete cure has been attained ; relapses occur during which the reaction returns. The necessity of finding an antibacterial substance thus remained. By treating the bacilli with a 10% sodium-hydrate solution Koch obtained an alkaline extract (T A) which produced reactions very similar to those of tuberculin, except that they were briefer in duration, while the reactive power of the organism persisted longer ; the results, too, were more constant. But the preparation possessed the disadvantage, dependent on the presence of the bodies of dead bacilli, of producing abscesses. On removing the bacilli by filtration the substance approached tuberculin in its action, but being less staple was inferior to the latter.

Koch next conceived the idea of mechanically reducing the bacilli to a detritus capable of absorption by the tissues. He had found that the bacilli contained two fatty acids which constituted a protective envelope and prevented absorption. The first essential was the destruction of this fatty substance. This was secured by triturating the bacillary mass in an agate mortar with an agate pestle ; it was then taken up with distilled water and submitted to centrifugation. In this way an upper opalescent but transparent layer (T O) and a muddy residue were obtained. The latter was dried, triturated, and centrifuged ; the residue from this was similarly treated. By this process a series of clear fluids, which from the second onward presented no difference, was obtained. These fluids were collectively termed T R (residual tuberculin). Both preparations are readily absorbable, and neither produces abscesses. Further researches demonstrated that T O contains the substances soluble in glycerin, T R those insoluble, whence the former resembles tuberculin, and especially T A, but is only feebly immunizing, while T R possesses marked immunizing power. In employing it, it is not necessary, as in the case of tuberculin, T A, or T O, to produce a reaction, but it is important cautiously to render the patient rapidly insensible to progressively larger doses. T R contains all the immunizing factors of cultures of the tubercle-bacillus, the proof being that the subject immunized with it no longer responds to large doses of tuberculin or T O. For the preparation of T R it is necessary to use young, highly virulent cultures. The immunizing substances are conserved by the addition of 20% glycerin. Administration and dosage are simple. The injections, as in tuberculin, are given beneath the skin of the back. The fluid contains 10 mgm. of solids per c.c., and before using is diluted with saline solution ; the inaugural dose is $\frac{1}{500}$ mgm. The injections are repeated every second day, and the dosage is gradually increased. Koch has generally pushed it to 20 mgm. He succeeded in rendering guinea-pigs so completely immune that they were able to withstand inoculations of virulent bacilli. The point of inoculation presented no changes; the neighboring lymph-glands were generally normal, and even when slightly swollen were free from bacilli. Immunization required from 2 to 3 weeks. In infected animals treated with T R regressive changes were always observable in the tuberculous foci. In the case of human tuberculosis the remedy is of little use in advanced stages or in those in which secondary infection has occurred.

In lupus, Koch has always seen a more marked improvement than that yielded by ordinary tuberculin or by T A. It is too early, however, to speak of "cure." Violence in reaction, infiltrations in the region of the pulmonary lesions—common phenomena under the use of tuberculin—were not observed. The only local alteration consisted in a transitory increase of crepitant rales; a very favorable influence was exercised on the fever. In conclusion, Koch states his belief that everything that is possible of attainment with cultures of the tubercle-bacillus can be attained with these preparations. It is possible, however, that combinations of T R with T O, or serums derived from T O or T R, in the preparation of which he is at present engaged, may give better and more rapid results. [The therapeutic results obtained so far seem to have been unsatisfactory.]

The Earliest Stages of Experimental Tuberculosis in the Rabbit's Cornea.—F. Schieck[1] has endeavored to settle the dispute still existing between the school of Metschnikoff and that of Baumgarten relative to the part taken by the fixed cells in the formation of the tubercle. The former, as is known, refers all cellular elements of the tubercle to the leukocytes, while the latter holds that they originate chiefly from the fixed cells, a leukocytic infiltration occurring as a later and secondary feature. Schieck confirms Baumgarten's theory of the participation of the fixed cells, but shows that the number of leukocytes depends on the character of the region of inoculation, and the quantity and quality of the bacilli. As in Baumgarten's experiments the eyes were kept constantly under the influence of atropin, which retards leukocytic immigration, that observer necessarily obtained different results regarding the participation of the white cells from those of Schieck.

Histologic Alterations of the Liver and of the Kidneys produced by the Tuberculous Toxins (Tuberculin).—Carrière[2] injected large doses of tuberculin into animals, and found the following lesions in the liver and in the kidneys:—

Liver: 1. Tumefaction of the cells of the periphery of the lobule, particularly in those cases in which the doses of tuberculin were very large. 2. A special necrosis of the centrolobular cells, characterized by fragmentation and by a reticular condition, vacuolization of the protoplasm, and fragmentary and granular degeneration of the nuclei. 3. Endothelial lesions of the portal vein in cases in which large doses of tuberculin were injected into the veins. 4. Vasodilatation of the centrolobular capillaries and areas of interstitial hemorrhage. 5. Endarteritis in the cases in which tuberculin was injected in large doses; slight periarteritis in the opposite cases. 6. Absence of fatty or amyloid infiltration.

Kidney: 1. Glomerular hyperemia or glomerulitis, more pronounced when the experiments were continued for a long time. 2. Tumefaction and necrosis of the epithelial cells of the convoluted tubules and of the ascending limbs of Henle's loops. This necrosis, as that of the hepatic cells,

[1] Ziegler's Beiträge zur path. Anat. u. allg. Path., xx., H. 2, 1896; Centralbl. f. Bakteriol., Parasitenk. u. Infektionskrank., Jan. 20, 1897.
[2] Arch. de Méd. expér. et d'Anat. path., Jan., 1897.

was characterized by the fragmentary degeneration and vacuolation of the protoplasm and the fragmentary disintegration of the nuclei. 3. Simple tumefaction of the lining epithelium of the other portions of the uriniferous tubules, which were often obstructed by granular casts. 4. Slight endarteritis, hyperemia, and interstitial hemorrhages in animals that had received large doses; slight periarteritis in those that had received small doses during long periods of time. 5. Neither fatty degeneration nor amyloid infiltration was found.

Tuberculin, therefore, contains substances which are capable of producing profound modifications in the structure of the liver and the kidney.

Tuberculosis of the Tonsils in Children.—E. Schlesinger,[1] as the result of the examination of the tonsils in 17 cases of tuberculosis, concludes that pulmonary phthisis is almost always accompanied by tonsillar tuberculosis, and, conversely, in tuberculosis of the tonsils pulmonary phthisis is never absent. In trivial tuberculous lesions of the lungs the tonsils are free from tuberculous changes.

G. Gottstein[2] describes primary tuberculosis of the adenoid vegetations of the nasopharynx and the pharyngeal tonsils.

Miliary Tuberculosis secondary to Tuberculosis of a Mesenteric Gland.—D. Riesman[3] reports a case of acute miliary tuberculosis, affecting especially the liver and lungs, originating from a single large caseous mesenteric gland.

Tuberculosis of Small Animals.—Cadiot,[4] supported by the results of numerous careful autopsies, opposes the prevalent opinion that tuberculosis is rare in dogs. Within a few years he dissected no less than 205 that had the disease. [Tuberculosis in a St. Bernard dog is also reported by U. G. Houck.[5]] Of 9 tuberculous cats, one had a cervical fistula, another ulcerations about the nose. Such external forms of tuberculosis he found to be very frequent in parrots. Of special significance is the fact that the tuberculosis of the latter animals is transmissible to mammals. While mammalian tuberculosis is harmless for chickens, it can be inoculated into parrots; human tuberculosis is also transferable to these birds. These facts show that the tuberculosis of our domestic animals is justly to be feared as a source of human tuberculosis.

Tubercle-bacilli in Feces from a Nontuberculous Intestine.—R. B. Shaw[6] reports the case of an old tuberculous patient who had suffered from diarrhea for 6 months. In the feces a moderate number of tubercle-bacilli were found. At the autopsy no intestinal tuberculosis was discovered. The source of the bacilli was evidently the sputum. The case was interesting in other ways—the blood showed 400,000 red corpuscles and 8% hemoglobin. There were also found at the autopsy meningeal hemorrhage and a prominence in front of the various cerebelli.

DIPHTHERIA.

Cultivation of the Diphtheria-bacillus on Nonalbuminous Media.—N. Uschinsky[7] has succeeded in growing the diphtheria-bacillus on his albumin-free medium (containing iron). The unfiltered culture is almost as toxic as bouillon-culture, the filtrate from 6 to 10 times weaker. He was unable to precipitate the toxin by Brieger and Boër's method.

Glycerin-media for Diphtheria-bacillus.—A. M. Gossage[8] recom-

[1] Berlin. Klinik, H. 99, 1896. [2] Berlin. klin. Woch., Nos. 31 and 32, 1896.
[3] N. Y. Med. Jour., Apr. 17, 1897. [4] Sem. méd., p. 462, 1896.
[5] Veterin. Mag., No. 3, p. 183, 1896. [6] Montreal Med. Jour., Jan., 1897.
[7] Centralbl. f. Bakteriol., Parasitenk. u. Infektionskrank., Feb. 6, 1897.
[8] Lancet, Aug. 15, 1896.

mends the use of a medium containing a large percentage of glycerin for the cultivation of the diphtheria-bacillus. He prefers glycerin-serum containing 9 % of glycerin. By means of this medium he claims that it is possible positively to distinguish, in stained specimens, the diphtheria from the pseudodiphtheria bacillus, the former showing, when stained with methylen-blue, metachromatism, the latter not. [It seems to us that in view of the slender dividing-line between the diphtheria-bacillus and forms resembling it, such a fundamental difference as that pointed out by the author, which is " so characteristic that the merest tyro could recognize it," cannot exist. Kanthack [1] also strongly opposes Gossage's statements.]

The Influence of Carbon Dioxid on the Growth and Toxin-production of the Diphtheria-bacillus.—N. P. Schierbeck [2] found that a weakly acid medium through which CO_2 is passed (air containing 8 % CO_2) constitutes the best medium for the production of the diphtheria-toxin.

The Differences between the Xerosis-bacillus and the Diphtheria-bacillus.—J. Eyre [3] sums up the differences between these two organisms as follows: 1. After inoculation of the secretion upon the blood-serum colonies of the xerosis-bacillus do not appear within 36 hours; those of the diphtheria-bacillus appear in from 16 to 18 hours. 2. When grown in neutral bouillon or milk, the xerosis-bacillus never gives rise to an acid reaction; the diphtheria-bacillus invariably does. 3. When grown upon potato the xerosis-bacillus rapidly degenerates and dies; the diphtheria-bacillus grows with more vigor and to a greater size than on any other medium. 4. When grown upon 10 % gelatin colonies of the xerosis-bacilli are not visible to the naked eye within 48 hours; the colonies of diphtheria-bacilli can be recognized in from 12 to 24 hours. 5. The invariably innocuous nature of the bouillon-cultures of the xerosis-bacillus when inoculated into the subcutaneous tissues of animals susceptible to the bacillus of diphtheria. As to the exact nature of the xerosis-bacillus—whether it be a nonvirulent and slightly altered species of the bacillus diphtheriæ, or a totally separate and distinct bacillus—it is impossible at present to decide.

Diphtheria-bacillus in Normal Throats.—H. W. Gross [4] examined 314 normal throats and noses for the Klebs-Löffler bacillus, and found it present in 7.9 % of the cases examined.

The Production of Antitoxin by the Passage of Electricity through Diphtheria-cultures.—B. M. Bolton and H. D. Pease,[5] continuing the researches of Smirnow and others, were able to produce antitoxin by electrolysis of diphtheria-cultures. The antitoxin was produced over the positive pole, and the strongest obtained was such that 2 c.c. neutralized 10 times the minimal fatal dose for guinea-pigs.

The Production of Potent Diphtheria-antitoxins.—G. E. Cartwright Wood [6] secured very potent diphtheria-antitoxin (in the case of one horse the serum contained 1000 immunity-units in 1 c.c.) by injecting the horses with Martin's diphtheria-albumose. After a fortnight the animals could tolerate large quantities of ordinary toxin, and a high degree of immunity was rapidly developed.

Antitoxin in the Blood of Normal Horses.—B. M. Bolton [7] found antitoxin in the blood of 3 out of 12 horses tested previous to the injection of diphtheria-toxin.

[1] Lancet, Aug. 22, 1896.
[2] Arch. f. Hyg., xxvii., H. 4; Centralbl. f. Bakteriol., Parasitenk. u. Infektionskrank., Feb. 5, 1897. [3] Jour. of Path. and Bacteriol., July, 1896; Medicine, Dec., 1896.
[4] Univ. Med. Mag., Oct., 1896. [5] Jour. Exper. Med., July, 1896.
[6] Lancet, Oct. 24, 1896. [7] Jour. Exper. Med., July, 1896.

TYPHOID FEVER.

Atypical Forms of Typhoid Fever.—Chiari [1] believes that there are forms of typhoid fever without intestinal and mesenteric lesions, such cases deserving the name typhoid septicemia. In the cases seen by him Widal's test had been obtained, yet at autopsy the characteristic lesions were absent, but the typhoid-bacillus was shown to be present by bacteriologic examination. Such cases must be distinguished from those in which, in the absence of lesions in the intestines, a diagnosis can be based on the characteristic changes in the mesenteric glands, and in which the finding of the bacillus confirms the diagnosis. [The existence of typhoid septicemia was pointed out some years ago by Italian writers. The knowledge of the occurrence of this form of typhoid infection ought to help pathologists in clearing up certain obscure cases that clinically present themselves as typhoid fever.]

THE GONOCOCCUS.

II. Heiman [2] publishes further studies on the **biology of the gonococcus** (see *Year-Book*, 1896, p. 1001). The organisms were obtained for cultivation by centrifugalizing the urine. It was found that the purulent sediment was acid, while the pus, which was obtained by means of a platinum-loop from the urethra, was neutral or alkaline. The author's more important conclusions are as follows : 1. In the examination of secretions from urethritis the employment of the centrifuge not only is the most convenient method, but also gives the best and most reliable results. 2. The medium employed by Hammer, consisting of albuminous urine plus glycerin-agar, does not give so good results as chest-serum agar. 3. Fractional sterilization of serum should be continued longer than 6 days, and after an interval of 2 or 3 days it should be sterilized again on 3 consecutive days. 4. Fermentation-broth (Theobald Smith's) plus liquid chest-serum, Dunham's peptone-solution plus liquid chest-serum, nutrient broth plus liquid chest-serum, are recommended as liquid media for the gonococcus. 5. Gonorrheal pus submitted to centrifugalization and kept moist at room-temperature contained living gonococci after 48 hours, as proved by culture. 6. In gonorrheal pus which had been smeared on linen the gonococcus was demonstrated morphologically by Gram's method after 49 days on cover-glass. 7. The gonococcus was demonstrated after 29 days in cover-glass preparation made from pus which had been dried on glass. 8. In chronic urethritis, culture-media alone are to be recommended for the detection of the gonococcus. 9. In 34 examinations of gonorrheal threads with cover-glass alone, by Gram's method, 7 cases showed the gonococcus. 10. Of 61 cases of gonorrheal threads examined with cover-glass and culture-media, 13 gave positive results with cover-glass and 14 with culture-media. 11. For the collection of the secretions and threads for planting at least 2 specimens of urine must be obtained ; first, that which washes out the urethra ; second, that which contains threads of the posterior urethra and secretion expressed from the prostate. 12. A urethra may contain gonococci which lie dormant and may be innocuous in that person for years, but which may at any time excite an acute gonorrhea in another person.

Culture of the Gonococcus.—Wassermann [3] employs the following medium : 15 c.c. of hog-serum, 30–35 c.c. of water, 2–3 c.c. of glycerin, and 0.80 gm. of Salkowski's nutrose (sodium phosphate and casein). The mixture is

---

[1] Centralbl. f. allg. Path. u. path. Anat., Oct. 15, 1897. [2] Med. Rec., Dec. 19, 1896.
[3] Sem. méd., July 28, 1897 ; Berlin. klin. Woch., Aug. 9, 1897.

sterilized by boiling from 20 to 30 minutes over an alcohol-flame. At the moment of using an equal part of liquefied 2% peptonized agar is added and the whole poured into a Petri dish. Wassermann found in the cultures of the gonococcus an active toxin which produced an inflammation at the point of injection, as well as fever and muscular and articular pains. The toxin is contained in the bodies of the bacteria, and not in the filtrate of the cultures. All efforts to produce immunization failed.

Internal Localization of the Gonococcus.—D. N. Eisendraht[1] reviews the literature on the subject of the internal localization of the gonococcus from the time of the discovery of the bacterium.

Fatal Systemic Infection from Gonorrhea.—J. M. Robinson[2] reports the case of a hotel-clerk, aged 32, who presented signs of septicemia, complicated shortly before death with swelling of numerous joints, for which no cause could be discovered. At the autopsy an old urethral stricture was found; the urethral pus contained gonococci. The author thinks the posterior urethritis was the source of the pyemia. [This is probably correct, although we should be inclined to think that the ordinary pyogenic organisms were to blame, and not the gonococcus itself.]

THE STREPTOCOCCUS.

The Specificity of the Erysipelas-streptococcus.—Petruschky[3] discusses this question, and comes to the conclusion, which, of course, is not new, and has been accepted by most recent writers, that there is no specific erysipelas-streptococcus. The particular morbid condition produced by streptococcus-infection depends on—1. *The seat of infection.* Dermal erysipelas, *e. g.*, arises only when the infection is in the lymph-spaces of the skin or mucous membranes. 2. *The virulence of streptococcus for man.* This is by no means equal to the virulence of the same streptococcus for mice or rabbits. 3. *The individual resistance* of the infected person. 4. *The influence of existing diseases* which modify the resistance of the individual. In tuberculosis, diphtheria, scarlet fever, small-pox, typhoid fever, and influenza the resistance is lessened; in carcinoma and sarcoma it is not lessened, but perhaps increased.

Nonidentity of the Streptococcus of Marmorek and the Streptococcus of Erysipelas.—J. Courmont[4] maintains that the streptococcus of erysipelas and the streptococcus of Marmorek are two different species. [The reasons given are not cogent.]

The Question of the Homology of the Streptococci.—C. Zenoni[5] found a very large streptococcus in the false membranes of a case of peritonitis secondary to an old gonorrhea. The question arose as to the identity or nonidentity of the organism with the ordinary streptococcus. As the bacterium after successive cultures and on various media changed its form to that of the other, and as immunity could be produced against it with Marmorek's serum, it must be considered identical with the other forms of streptococcus.

The Value of Chrysoidin in the Diagnosis of Cholera.—Blachstein[6] claims that chrysoidin is of diagnostic value with respect to cholera-cultures, producing in the turbid bouillon a flocculent precipitate with clearing of the medium. Walter Engels[7] shows that other vibrios respond in the

[1] Chicago Med. Rec., Sept., 1896.
[2] Med. News, Aug. 29, 1896.
[3] Zeit. f. Hyg., xxiii., H. 1.
[4] Sem. méd., July 28, 1897.
[5] Centralbl. f. Bakteriol., Parasitenk. u. Infektionskrank., Jan. 9, 1897.
[6] Münch. med. Woch., Nos. 44 and 45, 1896.
[7] Centralbl. f. Bakteriol., Parasitenk. u. Infektionskrank., Jan. 30, 1897.

same manner, whence it follows that chrysoidin has but little diagnostic value and cannot be used as a substitute for the serum-reaction.

The Cause of Rabies.—E. Marx [1] doubts the fact that Bruschettini has found the cause of rabies, believing that the latter has probably cultivated a contaminating organism. Furthermore, paralytic rabies is not so clearly characterized that it might not be simulated by another infection attended with paralysis. He himself has examined nearly 60 cases of rabies, and only once found a bacterium resembling Bruschettini's rabies-bacillus. He does not believe that bacteria have anything to do with the etiology of the disease.

The Influence of the Röntgen Ray on the Poison of Rabies.— E. Frantzius [2] found that the x-ray acting for not less than an hour on the spinal marrow of rabbits dead of rabies influenced the poison in such a manner that in animals inoculated with it a distinct prolongation of the incubation-period was noticeable, but death was not prevented. The hope that the Röntgen ray would prevent a fatal termination of the disease must, therefore, be abandoned.

A Pathogenic Streptothrix.—Scheele and Petruschky [3] presented at the Fifteenth Congress of Internal Medicine at Berlin cultures of a streptothrix variety which they had found in the sputum of a man who, after an attack of influenza, developed pleuropneumonia, cystitis, pyelitis, and multiple cutaneous abscesses. The bacteria were also cultivated from the abscesses. This is the first time that a pathogenic streptothrix has been found *intra vitam.*

Virulent Pneumococci in Dust.—Netter [4] demonstrated, after the manner of Cornet, the presence of virulent pneumococci in the dust of a hospital-ward.

The Smegma-bacillus.—A. S. Grünbaum [5] examined 50 specimens of urine from 47 individuals for the smegma-bacillus, by centrifugalizing the urine, spreading the sediment on cover-glasses, and staining in the usual way with Ziehl-Neelsen's and Gabett's solutions. In no case was the bacillus found in the urines of men, but it was present in 59 % of the urines from women. It was never found in urine obtained by catheter from either women or men. The author succeeded in growing on milk a bacillus from the smegma which stained red with carbol-fuchsin, and was not decolorized in 2 minutes by Gabett's solution.

Pertussis.—Julius Ritter [6] found in all cases of pertussis examined the diplococcus described by him in 1892, and in 3 fatal cases was able to demonstrate its presence on the inflamed bronchial mucous membrane.

The Cause of Mumps.—At a session of the Verein für innere Medicin of Berlin, held on March 29, 1897, Michaelis [7] described the microorganism found last year by von Leyden in the parotid-saliva, obtained by catheterization of Stenon's duct, and reported researches carried on by him (Michaelis) and Bein. The organism is morphologically and culturally characteristic; it is a motile diplococcus, resembling in form, position in cells, and staining-properties the gonococcus. It grows on ordinary media, also on ascitic fluid and milk, which last is curdled by it. Inoculation of animals, even direct injections into the parotid and testicle, was unsuccessful. The coccus possesses a very slight virulence.

---

[1] Centralbl. f. Bakteriol., Parasitenk. u. Infektionskrank., Nos. 22 and 23, 1896; No. 5, p. 205, 1897.   [2] Ibid., Mar. 5, 1897.

[3] Centralbl. f. innere Med., June 26, 1897.   [4] Sem. méd., June 2, 1897.

[5] Lancet, Jan. 9, 1897.   [6] Berlin. klin. Woch., Nos. 47 and 48, 1896.

[7] Ibid., Apr. 12, 1897; Univ. Med. Mag., June, 1897.

The Bubonic Plague.—M. Ogata[1] made careful studies during the pest-epidemic in Formosa, from which he has drawn the following conclusions: 1. In the tumefied lymph-glands of pest-sufferers and in the organs and blood of cadavers a pathogenic bacillus is found that in experimental animals produces a disease resembling the plague. 2. The plague-bacillus is not found constantly in the blood of patients suffering from the disease; not even in grave cases. 3. The bacillus may be found in the bile and the urine. 4. The bacillus is transported from wounds by insects, such as fleas and mosquitoes. 5. In the lymph-glands, blood, and internal organs of rats falling ill spontaneously or after artificial inoculation, the same bacillus as that of human plague is found. 6. The fleas found on rats suffering with the plague likewise contain virulent plague-bacilli and are capable of spreading the disease after the death of the rats. 7. In the blood, lymph-glands, and internal organs of pest-sufferers or cadavers other bacteria in addition to the plague-bacillus may be found. 8. The plague-bacillus is but feebly resistant against antiseptics. 9. In the floors of the pest-houses the bacillus was not found. [To these conclusions the author, whose scientific method speaks volumes for the thoroughness of the Japanese, appends some valuable suggestions regarding the prophylaxis of plague-epidemics. Of interest to us in the United States is his advice thoroughly to disinfect rags, wools, etc., coming from plague-stricken countries; ships from such regions should be inspected and quarantined.]

The Bacillus of Yellow Fever.—J. Sanarelli[2] describes a bacillus that he found in cases of yellow fever studied by him as director of the hygienic laboratory at Montevideo. The organism is a small rod with rounded ends, 2 to 4 μ long, occurring in pairs in culture and in groups in the tissues. It was never found in pure culture in the cadaver, and its isolation was possible in only 58 % of cases. Strange as it may appear, it is not found in the gastrointestinal tract, but in the blood and tissues. It is facultative anaerobic, stains by Gram's method, and is very resistant to drying. Pathogenic for nearly all animals, its chief properties are: (*a*) steatogenic [causing fatty degeneration]; (*b*) congestive and "hemorrhagiparous;" and (*c*) emetic. The filtered toxin produces analogous consequences. Injections of filtered cultures in man give rise to typical yellow fever. [It would seem as if Sternberg's bacillus *X* and Sanarelli's bacillus were identical; nevertheless the latter's discovery, which he has followed up with efforts toward the preparation of immunizing and curative substances, deserves attention. The studies and experiments should be repeated; unfortunately, the opportunity for the work has been very good in the United States.]

Hospital-gangrene.—Vincent[3] obtained in 47 cases of hospital-gangrene from the membranous pulp covering the ulcers a bacillus of from 4 to 8μ long, 1μ broad, not coloring by Gram's method, but staining well with thionin, and displaying a great resisting-power to antiseptics. In 40 out of the 47 cases a spirillum was also found, usually in small numbers and most abundant just beneath the pseudomembrane. Vincent considers this spirillum the true cause of hospital-gangrene. It produces a necrotic and hemorrhagic process, but its action is mainly local. Cultivation of neither organism succeeded. Inoculation of the pus into artificial wounds of animals gave no results, except in a rabbit suffering from general tuberculosis—in which an unhealthy wound was produced; similar results were obtained by injecting the bacillus with cultures of streptococci, colon-bacilli, etc. Two factors seem necessary to the production of hospital-gangrene: a condition of inanition in the patient and an association of the specific agent with other microorganisms.

[1] Centralbl. f. Bakteriol., Parasitenk. u. Infektionskrank., June 24, 1897.
[2] Sem. méd., July 7, 1897.   [3] Ann. de l'Inst. Pasteur, Sept. 25, 1896.

Chronic Glanders in Man.—Buschke[1] describes a case of chronic glanders localized to one extremity. It is the fifth recorded case, and, like the others, was characterized by a remarkably chronic course, the presence of intramuscular, subcutaneous, and subperiosteal abscesses, and a localization at the nares. The diagnosis can only be made after bacteriologic examination and by getting Straus's reaction (see *Year-Book*, 1897, p. 716), which is to be supplemented by cultures from the testicular pus. Mallein may perhaps be of use in the diagnosis.

The Thrush-fungus.—Max Steiner[2] finds that rabbits inoculated with pure cultures of the thrush-fungus (Soorpilz) die in from 5 to 10 days, a considerable number presenting paresis, chiefly of the hind limbs. In the microscopic sections (nearly all organs were affected) he noted well-marked round-cell infiltration about the fungus-colonies.

Pathogenic Spirillum in Schuylkill Water.—A. C. Abbott[3] describes a pathogenic spirillum isolated from the Schuylkill River water at Philadelphia. The organism (Vibrio schuylkiliensis) is pathogenic to pigeons, guinea-pigs, and mice, and is closely allied to the Vibrio Metschnikovi. Pigeons rendered immune to Vibrio schuylkiliensis were also immune to V. Metschnikovi.

Influence of Sunlight on the Bacteria of Street-dust.—Wittlin[4] found that sunlight had a distinctly bactericidal action on the bacteria of street-dust, but that sprinkling of the dust favored the growth of bacteria.

PROTECTION AND IMMUNITY.

The Bacteriologic Contamination and the Preservation of Vaccine-lymph.—G. H. Weaver,[5] in a study of this subject, arrives at the following conclusions: 1. Vaccine-lymph in a fresh, pure state almost always contains bacteria, and often pathogenic forms. 2. Pure vaccine-lymph after being kept in a fluid state, or dried upon ivory points as now prepared, is unfit for use and often dangerous. 3. Vaccine-lymph diluted with pure glycerin or equal parts of glycerin and distilled water, becomes sterile in about 2 weeks, and should not be used sooner. 4. All animals used for propagating vaccine-lymph should be tested with tuberculin before being used. 5. All vaccine establishments should be regularly inspected by properly qualified officials, and samples of virus from each lot of vaccine examined bacteriologically by a competent person, and the result certified before it is placed upon the market. 6. Each package of vaccine-lymph should be so marked that the date on which it is taken, and, if fluid, what has been added, shall be shown.

Self-protection of the Organism against Bacterial Infection.—A. J. Kondratieff[6] has prepared from the adrenals and spleen of the horse (which is susceptible to tetanus) a substance (*atoxogen*) which protects white mice against an otherwise positively mortal dose of tetanus-toxin, so that 50% of the animals survive. The protective substance resembles the enzymes, and is chemically allied to the antitoxins and toxins, which, as Brieger has shown, are nonalbuminous bodies. The author then expounds this theory of tetanus-immunity (based on Courmont and Doyon's), which briefly is as follows: after its entrance into the organism the tetanus-poison forms a nontoxic combination

[1] Arch. f. Dermat. u. Syph., Bd. xxxvi., H. 3 ; Centralbl. f. Bakteriol., Parasitenk. u. Infektionskrank., May 10, 1097.
[2] Centralbl. f. Bakteriol., Parasitenk. u. Infektionskrank., Mar. 30, 1897.
[3] Jour. Exper. Med., July, 1896.   [4] Wien. klin. Woch., No. 52, 1896.
[5] Jour. Am. Med. Assoc., Dec. 26, 1896.
[6] Centralbl. f. Bakteriol., Parasitenk. u. Infektionskrank., Mar. 30, 1897.

with the proteids of the cell-protoplasm, which combination at the end of the incubation-period decomposes in one of two ways : either the toxin is split off from the albumin and poisons the nervous system, or harmless products are split off—in susceptible animals antitoxin, in naturally immune animals other nontoxic compounds. Similar combinations can be formed by antitoxin and atoxogen, and it is the presence of atoxogen (always found in the normal body) and of antitoxin that promotes the reaction whereby the poison is transformed into antitoxin (or other nonpoisonous products). The active immunity remaining after recovery from tetanus can be explained by the existence of specific changes of the proteids which result after combination with the toxins.

The Mechanism of Reaction to Peritoneal Infection.—Durham [1] has undertaken a study of the factors concerned in the reaction of the peritoneum to infection. For the inoculation young agar-cultures of various bacteria were employed, the dose being regulated by a standardized loop. Within a variable period peritoneal fluid was withdrawn, and examined in hanging-drop and fixed preparations on cover-slips. At the autopsy on the animal the various membranes and organs involved were also examined. The different cells concerned in peritoneal inflammation are the following : (*a*) *Hyaline cells.* (*b*) *Coarsely granular oxyphile cells*—the *a*-granulation-cell of Ehrlich, for which the author proposes the not very euphonious term megoxyphile cell or megoxycyte. Contrary to the usual belief, Durham holds that this cell can be phagocytic, though it is much less so than the hyaline and other cells. (*c*) *Finely granular oxyphile cells* (microxyphile cell or microxycyte)—cells containing fine oxyphile granules and a more or less pigmented nucleus. They do not occur in the normal peritoneal fluid of man or the guinea-pig, and probably not in that of the rabbit. (*d*) *Macrophage.* This appears within 20 hours after an easily recoverable inoculation. Its nucleus is pale, large, and oval or round, and the protoplasm stains with basic dyes. The cell has an extraordinary capacity for ingesting microxyphile cells, bacteria, etc., and is apparently derived from the endothelial cells of the omentum and the peritoneal covering of the various organs. (*e*) *Basophile cell.* This was not observed in the peritoneal fluid, but was found adherent to the mesentery, omentum, parietal peritoneum, etc.

The changes following peritoneal infection are divided by the author into five stages : 1. Stage before leukopenia ; 2. Leukopenic stage ; 3. Microxyphile stage ; 4. Macrophage stage ; 5. Recovery to normal.

1. Among the changes occurring in this stage are the " balling" together of the cells, apparently due to increased stickiness of their surfaces. This increased surface-stickiness also facilitates phagocytosis. When the bacteria are extremely virulent they swim about and hit all forms of cells with perfect impunity, none remaining adherent. If many nonvirulent individuals are present, some become adherent to the hyaline cells, producing at times a " hedgehog" appearance of these cells. A preliminary attack of the megoxyphile cells, and a subsequent phagocytosis by the hyaline cells, as described by Kanthack and Hardy, were never observed. Microbes adhering to the hyaline cells immediately lose their motility, but contact with the megoxyphile (eosinophile) cells is not harmful to them. 2. The leukopenic stage is due to the combination of several factors: (1) attachment of the cells to the membranes lining the peritoneal cavity, especially the omentum ; (2) removal of cells by the lymph-paths ; (3) entanglement in clots ; (4) actual destruction of cells ; (5) in sexually mature female animals removal by the Fallopian tubes. Of these the first is the most important. Bacteria also become adherent to the

[1] Jour. of Path. and Bacteriol., Mar., 1897.

omentum, and in cases in which the peritoneal fluid is entirely sterile cultures from the omentum may show abundant bacterial growth. This is most readily demonstrated after Pfeiffer's reaction. This proves that microorganisms continue living among multitudes of phagocytic cells upon the omentum and on pseudomembranes, while the peritoneal fluid becomes absolutely sterile. In regard to chemotaxis, the author is very sceptical, and considers the phenomena ascribed to it as largely physicochemic in nature. 3 and 4. *The Microxyphile and Macrophage Stages or Stages of Leukocytosis.* The microxyphile cells appear in all cases whether virulent or nonvirulent microorganisms or solutions are used, the number depending on the virulence and quantity introduced. If the infection is highly virulent or toxic, only a few cells appear; if mild, they are found in increasing numbers. In the former case the cells disintegrate rapidly and phagocytosis is slight. By acting upon the microorganisms with bactericidal serum a good deal of phagocytosis may be observed. As to the source of the microxycytes, the author holds that they emigrate from the blood-vessels. Regarding the macrophages, which are actively phagocytic, their origin is probably not hemal, but local. In all animals that recover from peritoneal infections there is constantly a very considerable microxycyte leukocytosis, followed by the appearance of macrophages. These phenomena appear essential to recovery. As to the nature of the resistance, the author believes that intracellular (phagocytosis) and extracellular processes run hand in hand, and that probably neither alone is sufficient.

Changes in the Microorganisms after Inoculation.—The bacteria assume a coccus-like or spheric condition; the more virulent the infection, the more difficult it is to discern these extracellular degeneration-forms. These bodies, which are formed without direct interference on the part of the cells, are ingested by phagocytes.

Conclusions and Summary.—1. By means of cellular changes which occur after peritoneal infections in guinea-pigs the following stages may be recognized: (*a*) preliminary stage; (*b*) leukopenic stage; (*c*) microxyphile stage; (*d*) macrophage stage; (*e*) return to normal. 2. The peritoneal fluid, membranes, and lymph-paths must be examined in order to obtain complete and accurate notions of the processes. 3. The nomenclature megoxyphile cells, or megoxycytes, for coarsely granular eosinophile cells, and microxyphile cells, or microxycytes, for finely granular eosinophile cells, is suggested. 4. The megoxycytes take a minimal share in the processes of bacterial destruction. They may be very scanty during the leukocytic period. 5. Important changes are to be observed upon the peritoneal membranes; of these the omentum is especially to be noticed. 6. Pure cellular and pure humoral theories fail to account for many of the phenomena of bacterial destruction in the peritoneal cavity. Both are of importance. A compromise between the two seems the most satisfactory for the explanation of the facts. Alexocyte theories of secretion, etc., are at present not entirely satisfactory, as all the other possible factors have not yet been eliminated or defined. 7. Extracellular degeneration of microbes can always be detected in normal animals, even in the face of the most virulent and toxic infections. It is especially well seen in actively and passively immunized animals and in animals to which temporary resisting power has been given. 8. The observations of Issaeff on the period of general increased resistance are worthy of careful notice in discussing the theory of immunity. Issaeff's period of resistance promises to be useful clinically as an aid to the surgery of the peritoneum. 9. The general phenomena of reaction of the peritoneal infection resemble those occurring in the blood after intravascular and in connective tissue after subcutaneous infection. 10. The general phenomena after peritoneal infection in rabbits and guinea-pigs are not widely dissimilar from those occurring in man.

Concerning the Augmentation of the Natural Resistance by the Production of Hyperleukocytosis.

—Hahn[1] refers to the fact that Buehner more than two years ago discovered that pleural exudates rich in leukocytes, obtained by the injection of sterilized aleuronat-emulsion into the pleural cavity of animals, were more bactericidal than the blood or blood-serum of the same animals. The greater power was proved to depend on the leukocytes or on some secretory product furnished by them. The thought then suggested itself that it might be possible by increasing the number of leukocytes in the blood to augment the natural resistance of the individual. Two courses lay open for the accomplishment of this purpose: either the quantity of bactericidal substances could be increased by the introduction of fluids rich in leukocytes obtained from other animals, or a hyperleukocytosis could be produced by artificial means. The first course seemed unproductive, since Buehner had shown that the alexins of different animal species are mutually destructive. The second gave better results. Hyperleukocytosis was secured by the injection of nuclein or nucleinic acid. When dogs were used it was found that the blood obtained during the stage of hyperleukocytosis was decidedly more bactericidal than the normal blood of the same animal. But the author points out that the favorable effect of hyperleukocytosis cannot be expected in cases in which the bacteria are localized and do injury by their poisons, but only in those in which they are actually circulating in the blood. For the purpose of studying the effects of hyperleukocytosis in man the blood of a patient receiving tuberculin-injections was employed. It was found that leukocytosis followed the injections, but only when the number of white cells reached 13,000 or 14,000 was any increase in bactericidal power observed. This indicates, however, that the bactericidal properties of human blood depend in the main on the number of leukocytes. Yet it is not likely, as already indicated, that hyperleukocytosis will exert a favorable influence on all bacterial infections. We know, for example, that in diphtheria progressive increase in the leukocytes is not a favorable symptom. This will probably be found true of all infections in which the bacteria remain localized and act by virtue of poisons which they elaborate. In such cases the point is not so much the destruction of the bacteria as the neutralization of their toxins, and the antitoxin-treatment will be of chief use.

Alkalinity of the Blood and Infection.

—Fodor and Rigler[2] have continued their researches on this subject, and in their present essay deal among other things with the *influence of protective inoculations* on the blood-alkalinity, finding that the injection of anthrax and schweinerothlauf vaccine causes an increase in the alkalinity. Rabic virus produces a rapid fall of alkalinity, but when an animal inoculated with such virus is treated antirabically there is only a very slight diminution of alkalinity. The *influence of toxin and antitoxin-injections* was also tested. The injection of diphtheria-toxin is followed by a rapid fall of alkalinity, after which there is a slight rise, and then a gradual decline until death. Between the quantity of toxin on the one hand, and the depression of the alkalinity, the rapidity of this depression, and the period from the injection to the death of the animal, on the other, there is a noticeable, though not rigid, parallelism. Antitoxin-injections increase the alkalinity, but, differing from that following vaccination, the increase is only transient, lasting scarcely 48 hours. When antitoxin and toxin are simultaneously injected at

---

[1] Berlin. klin. Woch., Sept. 28, 1896.
[2] Centralbl. f. Bakteriol., Parasitenk. u. Infektionskrank., Feb. 6 and 15, 1897.

opposite points the alkalinity-depressing action of the latter is neutralized ; there is even a slight increase. The resistance of the animals runs parallel with the increase in alkalinity. When antitoxin was injected first and toxin afterward, there was just as great a reduction of alkalinity as if the antitoxin had not been injected, and the animals died. This result differs markedly from that observed in the case of vaccines—an injection of virulent anthrax after an antecedent immunizing injection of anthrax-vaccine caused no diminution in alkalinity. Maragliano's tubercle-antitoxin produced a rise in alkalinity, likewise transient as that from diphtheria-antitoxin. Laborious investigations were made to determine the cause of the changes in alkalinity. It seems that the increase in alkalinity is brought about chiefly through organic substances, which are increased in the blood during immunization and antitoxin-treatment, and diminished in consequence of infection or the introduction of toxins. The organic substance raising the alkalinity is not furnished by the injected fluid, nor is it produced by any chemic transformation of the latter, for the degree of alkalinity bears no regular relation to the quantity of fluid introduced. Everything seems to point to the theory that the injections act as *specific excitants* of a vital reaction in the body, in response to which the body—*i. e.*, the leukocytes—produces specific substances with bactericidal and antitoxic properties. This reaction of the body Fodor terms *cytochemism*. The variations in alkalinity after injections, etc., are a sign and even a measure of this vital reaction. Whether the alkaline substance found in the animal after immunization and antitoxin treatment is identical with that which protects an infected animal against infection or toxin, and, if so, how the substance is formed, are questions that must be solved in the future. [The careful researches of Fodor and Rigler must impress every one as deserving weighty consideration ; they serve to confirm the observations of Calabrese (*Year-Book*, 1897, p. 727). The authors do not distinctly state that the organic substance upon the presence of which the variations in alkalinity are said to depend is also the protective substance, though it seems to us as if their leanings were in that direction. Whatever the outcome of future investigations may be, they have shown by their experiments that the alkalinity is an index of the state of the battle of the organism against infection. Perhaps this fact may in time be utilized by the clinician.]

The Role of Iron in the Phenomena of Motion and Degeneration in Cells and in the Bactericidal Action of Immune Serum. —In a somewhat obscure and highly theoretic preliminary communication N. Sacharoff[1] propounds the hypothesis that the bactericidal action of the serum of immunized animals is conditioned on a combination of the substance of the microorganisms with an iron-containing body, which by transmitting oxygen kills the bacteria. This hypothesis he bases (1) on the fact discovered by Metschnikoff and Bordet, that the formation of the bactericidal substance takes place in the protoplasm of the neutrophile leukocytes ; (2) on the transformation of bacteria englobed by leukocytes into an eosinophile substance before their destruction, this substance containing iron which serves as a mordant for eosin ; and (3) the fact, discovered by him, that the granulations of the neutrophile leukocytes contain iron. An attempt to prove this hypothesis by chemic means failed, so the author had recourse to histologic studies. The basis of these was an artificial vacuolization by which important facts in cellular biology have revealed themselves to the author. To produce vacuolization in the cells of the blood he employs a concentrated solution of picric acid in absolute alcohol. Under the influence of this reagent the red corpuscles become

---

[1] Centralbl. f. Bakteriol., Parasitenk. u. Infektionskrank., Mar. 5, 1897.

vacuolated, and bodies resembling blood-plates appear in the vacuoles. In thick parts of the blood-film dark or black bodies are seen that gradually assume a crystalline form. The bodies and crystals are the picrate of hematin or of a hematin-like body. As the nuclei of erythrocytes and hematoblasts and the eosinophile granulations also become vacuolated under the same conditions as the red cells, the author infers that this is likewise produced by the splitting off of hematin contained in these cells. The same thing is true of the neutrophile granulations. The hematin in all these cells is united with a larger or smaller quantity of proteid bodies. The molecule of nuclein in the granulations has, it may be inferred, the property of splitting up in various ways, a fact of great significance for the theory of immunity. As proteids are not capable of direct oxidation, chemists have assumed the existence of a living proteid. This latter, the author believes, is identical with the iron-containing paranuclein-substance of the blood and the tissue-cells. Upon the molecular attraction of the iron-containing granulations for oxygen depends the motility of leukocytes, as probably also that of muscles, spermatozoa, bacterial cilia, pulsating infusorial vacuoles, centrosomes, etc. Degeneration of bacteria (as of other cells) is due to the too rapid transformation of the nuclein of the microorganisms into the iron-containing paranuclein-granules, and the further oxidation and destruction of the latter. The author has shown that the nucleoli (metachromatic bodies) of bacteria contain iron. The degeneration of cholera-vibrios in the bodies of leukocytes is explained on the theory that the iron in the cells unites with the nuclein of the bacteria. In the decomposition of the paranuclein of the leukocytes a simpler substance is formed which resembles the bactericidal substance. The author considers the iron-containing body split off from the paranuclein and acting on the microorganisms the bactericidal substance. In the mode of formation of this substance, which must be different for each species of bacteria, he sees the cause of the specific action of immune serums. Many facts show that the bactericidal substance passes out of the leukocytes into the serum, where it collects in the immunizing process It probably consists of two parts: an iron-containing and an iron-free body; the former undergoes destruction in the union of the bactericidal substance with the microorganisms. The presence of dissolved paranuclein in very fresh serum proves that this substance can also be formed outside of the leukocytes. This fact serves to reconcile the views of Metschnikoff and his opponents. The action of fresh cholera-serum on cholera-vibrios (in Pfeiffer's phenomenon) is brought about by the same iron-containing substance as that which destroys the intracellular vibrios. The specificity of action of the agglutinating substance is explained by the meeting of two substances which only have the ability to unite and agglutinate when their chemie composition is similar. One of these substances is the bacterial protoplasm (formed by the paranuclein-bodies of the bacteria), the other is the agglutinin, which is the iron-free element of the bactericidal substance. The agglutinin itself is incapable of destroying the bacteria; for that purpose it must be conjoined with the iron-containing part of the paranuclein.

The Presence of Bactericidal Substances in Leukocytes.— Schattenfroh[1] has made some experiments with the purpose of proving Buchner's theory that the alexins are products of the leukocytes. By means of the injection first of aleuronat-suspension and then of physiologic salt-solution he obtained an exudate very rich in leukocytes. The repeatedly frozen and thawed exudate possessed an extraordinary bactericidal power, which greatly

[1] Münch. med. Woch., No. 1, 1897; Centralbl. f. Bakteriol., Parasitenk. u. Infektionskrank., Mar. 30, 1897.

surpassed that of the unfrozen exudate. The bactericidal substances obtained had almost no influence on cholera-vibrios, but acted energetically on staphylococcus pyogenes aureus and bacterium coli. If coagulation occurred in the exudate, it was less active than that free from cells. The author believes in that case more nutritive and less bactericidal substances are extracted.

The Action of Antitoxins.—Ehrlich,[1] by means of an interesting experiment, shows that a toxalbumin can be neutralized by its antitoxin, without any participation of cell-activity. Ricin, it has been shown, produces in the extravascular blood as well as in the living animal a peculiar coagulation, in which the red corpuscles agglomerate and are thrown down. Ehrlich filled 6 test-tubes with 10 c.c. of a mixture of 95 c.c. normal saline solution, to which 0.5 % sodium citrate and 5 c.c. of rabbit's blood had been added. One c.c. of a 2 % ricin solution promptly precipitated the corpuscles from this mixture. Ehrlich now treated 1 c.c. of the ricin solution with 0.3, 0.5, 0.75, 1.0, and 1.25 c.c. of antiricin-serum diluted one-half. Test I. behaved like the control-tube; with 0.5 and 0.75 c.c. of serum the coagulation was retarded, and was incomplete with 0.75 c.c. With 1.0 c.c. only a trace of coagulation showed itself. The same ricin and antiricin mixtures were now used for animal-experiments. Six mice were inoculated with 0.4, 0.5, 0.6, 0.7, and 0.8 c.c., respectively, of the 6 mixtures. Mouse I. died in 18 hours; mouse II. in 30 hours; mouse III. showed moderate infiltration; the others remained healthy. The animal-experiment thus confirmed the conclusions drawn from the test-tube experiment—namely, that, as far as ricin is concerned, toxin and antitoxin influence each other by direct chemie action.

Influence of Nerve-section on Local Resistance.—Charrin and Nittis[2] found that when they cut the sciatic nerve of a rabbit on one side, and immunized the animal with antiproteus-serum, and then inoculated the same quantity of a proteus-culture into each hind foot, the abscess attained a larger size in the foot deprived of nervous influence than in the other, or, if the immunity was high, developed only in the former foot.

The Influence of Acute Alcoholism on the Normal Vital Resistance of Rabbits to Infection.—A. C. Abbott[3] was entrusted by the Committee of Fifty to Investigate the Alcohol Question with the investigation of the influence of acute and chronic alcoholism on resistance. His conclusions as to the influence of acute alcoholism are as follows : The normal vital resistance of rabbits to infection by streptococcus pyogenes (erysipelatos) is markedly diminished through the influence of alcohol when given daily to the stage of acute intoxication. A similar, though by no means so conspicuous, diminution of resistance to infection and intoxication by the bacillus coli communis also occurs in rabbits subjected to the same influences. While in alcoholized rabbits inoculated in various ways with staphylococcus pyogenes aureus individual instances of lowered resistance were observed, still it is impossible to say from these experiments that in general a marked difference is noticed between alcoholized and nonalcoholized animals as regards infection by this particular organism. It is interesting to note that the results of inoculation of alcoholized rabbits with the erysipelas-coccus corresponded in a way with clinical observations on human beings addicted to the excessive use of alcohol when infected by this organism. In the course of the work an effort was made to determine if, through the oxidation of alcohol in the tissues to acids of the corresponding chemie group, the increase of susceptibility could be referred

[1] Fortschr. d. Med., xv., No. 21, 1897 ; Centralbl. f. Bakteriol., Parasitenk. u. Infektionskrank., Mar. 30, 1897.
[2] Sem. méd., Jan. 13, 1897.　　　　　　　　　　[3] Jour. Exper. Med., July, 1896.

to the diminution in the alkalinity of the blood as a result of the presence of such acids. The number of experiments thus far made on this point is too small to justify dogmatic statements, but from what has been gathered there is but little evidence in support of this view. Throughout these experiments, with few exceptions, it was seen that the alcoholized animals not only showed the effects of the inoculations earlier than did the nonalcoholized rabbits, but in the case of the streptococcus-inoculations the lesions produced (formation of miliary abscesses) were much more pronounced than are those that usually follow inoculation with this organism. With regard to the predisposing influence of the alcohol, one is constrained to believe that it is in most cases the result of structural alterations consequent upon its direct action on the tissues, though in a number of the animals no such alteration could be made out by macroscopic examination. The author believes, however, that closer study of the lesions of the animals would have revealed important structural changes. [An interesting result of these experiments is the fact that rabbits bear really enormous quantities of pure ethylic alcohol—7.5 to 10 c.c.; equivalent doses for a man of 150 pounds would be represented by from $\frac{2}{3}$ to $\frac{5}{6}$ of a pint of absolute alcohol.]

Immunization against Typhoid Fever.—Pfeiffer and Kolle [1] injected typhoid-culture, sterilized at 56° C. (1 dose agar-culture in 1 c.c. bouillon) under the skin of the back of persons that never had had typhoid fever. Within 2 or 3 hours chilliness, vertigo, malaise, and pain at the point of inoculation set in, and the temperature rose by evening to 38.5° C. All phenomena subsided on the following day. The blood obtained by cups on the 11th day showed features which it did not possess before the inoculation. The serum presented the same degree of bactericidal properties as that of typhoid convalescents. The authors hope that their method may be made applicable in typhoid epidemics, especially among armies in the field.

Immunity to Hog-cholera.—E. A. de Schweinitz [2] has succeeded in conferring immunity against hog-cholera upon guinea-pigs by injecting them with serum from an immune hog. He also noted the fact observed in some other diseases that an animal may remain immune to hog-cholera while its serum has lost the power of conferring immunity upon other animals. The author also found that swine-plague serum had no protective power against hog-cholera, nor hog-cholera serum against swine-plague infection.

Toxins and Electricity.—Marmier [3] has repeated the experiments of Smirnow and of d'Arsonval and Charrin of producing antitoxins from toxins by means of the electric current, but failed entirely to confirm them. Smirnow's method of electrolysis with weak currents does produce a destruction of toxin, but the formation of antitoxin is only apparent, for during electrolysis hypochloric salts are formed which, as Martin's not yet published results show, have a certain degree of curative action in diphtheria.

Antistreptococcic Serum.—Merieux and Miemann [4] tested three specimens of antistreptococcic serum and found "Lyon-Vaise" the strongest. Bornemann [5] likewise made experiments with various brands of antistreptococcic serum, including one of his own. The results were not at all satisfactory, and Petruschky,[6] in reviewing both of these papers, remarks that they do not offer any grounds for applying the serum in the treatment of disease in man.

[1] Deutsch. med. Woch., No. 46, 1896; Centralbl. Bakteriol., Parasitenk. u. Infektionskrank., Jan. 30, 1897.
[2] N. Y. Med. Jour., Sept. 5, 1896.   [3] Ann. de l'Inst. Pasteur, t. x., No. 8.
[4] Berlin. klin. Woch., No. 49, 1896.   [5] Wien. klin. Woch., No. 51, 1896.
[6] Centralbl. f. Bakteriol., Parasitenk. u. Infektionskrank., Mar. 30, 1896.

He thinks that there is as yet no positive proof of the production of a specific transmissible immunity to streptococcic infection.

The Production of Streptococcus-antitoxin by means of Electricity.—Bonome and Viola[1] have succeeded in converting virulent streptococcic toxin into antitoxin by means of the alternating electric current.

Cholera Immunity.—Kolle[2] has immunized 3 persons by Haffkine's method: first, $\frac{1}{12}$ of a 24-hour agar-culture killed with chloroform, in 5 days the same quantity of living culture, and 5 days later $\frac{1}{8}$ culture, injected into the back. Eleven persons received only $\frac{1}{10}$ dead agar-culture; finally, he inoculated 3 persons with $\frac{1}{10}$ dead culture that had been preserved four weeks. In all cases a painful infiltration and fever ensued.

The results were confirmatory of Haffkine's experiences that immunity sets in about the 5th day after the injection, reaches its height on the 20th, and then diminishes, although it is still demonstrable for a year afterward. He, furthermore, corroborated his own previous assertion that the blood of immune persons contains bactericidal but not antitoxic substances. An important fact brought out by Kolle is that dead cultures give just as good results as living cultures, and are, of course, considerably safer.

Antibodies in Milk.—Rudolf Kraus[3] found that the milk of goats immunized to typhoid, cholera, or colon-bacillus, produced Pfeiffer's phenomenon when injected into the peritoneum of guinea-pigs, together with the typhoid, cholera, or colon-bacillus, and also caused agglutination of the organisms on the concave slide or in the test-tube. In regard to the cholera-goat the relation of the strength of the serum to that of the milk was as 10 : 1, and resembled that found by Ehrlich and Wassermann for the antitoxins of serum and milk. It appears then that the excretion of antibodies in milk is analogous to the excretion of antitoxins.

Antivenomous Serum.—A. Calmette[4] showed before the Conjoint Board of the Royal College of Physicians (London) and Surgeons (England) the efficacy of antivenomous serum in protecting animals against venom, and curing them when injected in time after the administration of the venom.

Limitations of Antitoxins.—T. R. Fraser[5] calls attention to the limitations to the antidotal power of antitoxins, in particular of antivenene, believing that an estimation of this power by experiments *in vitro* will lead to fallacious conceptions. He also reiterates his theories of the mode of action (chemic antidote) and the origin of antivenene (from the venom itself, in part, at least, being normally one of its constituents). Calmette[6] takes issue with Fraser, and is of the opinion that antivenene is a physiologic antidote rendering the body-cells immune, and that it is not produced from venom.

Death from Antitoxin.—The sudden and sad death of Prof. Langerhans' son after an injection of antitoxin has given rise to considerable polemic literature. Prof. Strassmann, who, at the request of the State, made the autopsy, came to the conclusion[7] that death probably took place from inspiration of food during an act of vomiting. Prof. Langerhans[8] vehemently opposes this view, and contends that death was due to poisonous effects produced by the antitoxin, which, as Bischoff, Ehrlich, and Strassmann have shown, was normal.

Cause of Death from Serum-injections.—Chas. T. McClintock[9]

[1] Centralbl. f. Bakteriol., Parasitenk. u. Infektionskrank., Nos. 22 and 23, p. 843, 1896.
[2] Deutsch. med. Woch., No. 1, 1897.
[3] Centralbl. f. Bakteriol., Parasitenk. u. Infektionskrank., May 10, 1897.
[4] Lancet, Aug. 15, 1896.   [5] Brit. Med. Jour., Oct. 3, 1896.   [6] Ibid.
[7] Berlin. klin. Woch., No. 23, 1896.   [8] Ibid., No. 27, 1896.
[9] Jour. Am. Med. Assoc., Feb. 27, 1897.

does not believe that the injection of air in hypodermic medication, as in serum-injections, is responsible for some of the sudden deaths recorded, but would class the phenomena observed, varying from slight faintness to death, as shock.

Contribution to the Theory of Agglutination.—E. Levy and H. Bruns[1] have studied bacterial agglutination, comparing the observations of Gruber, Durham, Pfeiffer, and Kolle, and others. They noted the phenomenon in connection with the cholera, typhoid, colon, and pyocyaneus bacillus, and also with proteus. In all these cases the animals yielding the serum had been treated with dead cultures of the bacteria. The authors now hit upon the thought that it might be possible to endow the serum with agglutinating properties by injecting the soluble metabolic products of the bacteria, although Gruber, the discoverer of the *agglutinins*, had held that these, the agglutinins, were formed from the constituents of the bacterial bodies. Levy and Bruns injected filtered cultures of typhoid and cholera into rabbits, and, indeed, found that the serum developed typical agglutinating power. It was also observed that this did not occur immediately, but that several days ($3\frac{1}{2}$–5) were required. Then, however, it seemed as if the reaction appeared all at once.

Widal[2] is of the opinion that the agglutinating property of blood-serum is not a protective phenomenon of the organism.

Transmission of the Agglutinating Substance by the Breast-milk.—Widal and Sicard[3] found that mice, the serum of which they had endowed with the agglutinating property, transmitted it to their young, while guinea-pigs and cats did not. The ingestion of strongly agglutinating goat's milk by man does not transmit the reaction to the blood. These differences in the transmissibility of the agglutinating substance by way of the digestive tract is at present not explicable. The authors are not prepared to discuss the hypothesis of the digestive chemism, but recall the fact that agglutinating milk coagulated naturally or by the action of an acid, such as acetic or hydrochloric acid, loses only a small part of its agglutinating power.

Serum-diagnosis by Means of Dried Blood-samples in (experimental) Cholera.—Wyatt Johnson and E. W. Hammond[4] obtained Pfeiffer's reaction with the dried blood of animals $3\frac{1}{2}$ days after infection with virulent cholera-culture.

The Agglutinating Property of the Blood-Plasma.—Achard and Bensaude[5] have undertaken a series of experiments which are designed to show whether the agglutinating property of the blood is dependent upon the blood-corpuscles, or whether it is a characteristic of the blood-plasma. They have shown that blood-plasma which has been deprived of all formed elements possesses the agglutinating power perfectly. They have also shown that the presence of very large numbers of white and red corpuscles does not increase the agglutinating power of the plasma to an appreciable degree. They have concluded that living leukocytes which have been separated from the primitive plasma do not retain the agglutinating property. They think that the differences in the agglutinating property of the different fluids of the body are not to be accounted for by the presence of white corpuscles; but rather are dependent upon the elective action of the living membranes—glandular epithelia in particular—which are concerned in the transudation of the agglutinating substances. Their experiments have also shown that the blood always contains the largest quantity of the agglutinating substances, and that the agglutinating substances are preserved for the longest time in the blood.

---

[1] Berlin klin. Woch., June 7, 1897.
[2] Centralbl. f. allg. Path. u. path. Anat., Oct. 15, 1897.   [3] Sem. méd., July 28, 1897.
[4] N. Y. Med. Jour., Nov. 28, 1896.   [5] Arch. de Méd. expér. et d'Anat. path., Nov., 1896.

He thinks that there is as yet no positi? proof of the production of a specific transmissible immunity to streptococcicnfection.

The Production of Streptococus-antitoxin by means of Electricity.—Bonome and Viola[1] have succeeded in converting virulent streptococcic toxin into antitoxin by means of the alternating electric current.

Cholera Immunity.—Kolle[2] hc immunized 3 persons by Haffkine's method: first, $\frac{1}{12}$ of a 24-hour agar-cuure killed with chloroform, in 5 days the same quantity of living culture, a 1 5 days later $\frac{1}{8}$ culture, injected into the back. Eleven persons received on $\frac{1}{10}$ dead agar-culture; finally, he inoculated 3 persons with $\frac{1}{10}$ dead cultui that had been preserved four weeks. In all cases a painful infiltration and fever ensued.

The results were confirmatory of Iaffkine's experiences that immunity sets in about the 5th day after the injecon. reaches its height on the 20th, and then diminishes, although it is still de on-trable for a year afterward. He, furthermore, corroborated his own prev us assertion that the blood of immune persons contains bactericidal but not antoxic substances. An important fact brought out by Kolle is that dead cultres give just as good results as living cultures, and are, of course, considerab safcr.

Antibodies in Milk.—Rudolf Kaus[3] found that the milk of goats immunized to typhoid, cholera, or colon-bcillus. produced Pfeiffer's phenomenon when injected in the peritoneum of inea-pigs, together with the typhoid, cholera, or colon-bacillus, and also cated agglutination of the organisms on the concave slide or in the test-tube. In regard to the cholera-goat the relation of the strength of the serum to iat of the milk was as 10 : 1, and resembled that found by Ehrlich and Wassermann for the antitoxins of serum and milk. It appears then that the excetion of antibodies in milk is analogous to the excretion of antitoxins.

Antivenomous Serum.—A. Cmette[4] showed before the Conjoint Board of the Royal College of Physicns (London) and Surgeons (England) the efficacy of antivenomous serum in otecting animals against venom, and curing them when injected in time afterhe administration of the venom.

Limitations of Antitoxins.—T.R. Fraser[5] calls attention to the limitations to the antidotal power of antitoxn-, in particular of antivenene, believing that an estimation of this power y experiments *in vitro* will lead to fallacious conceptions. He also reiteras his theories of the mode of action (chemie antidote) and the origin of ativennc (from the venom itself, in part, at least, being normally one of it con-tituent-). Calmette[6] takes issue with Fraser, and is of the opinion th: antivenne is a physiologic antidote rendering the body-eells immune, and hat it is not produced from venom.

Death from Antitoxin.—The sddcn and sad death of Prof. Langerhans' son after an injection of antitoxin ias given rise to considerable polemic literature. Prof. Strassmann, who, a the request of the State, made the autopsy, came to the conclusion[7] that dcth probably took place from inspiration of food during an act of vomit.g. Prof. Langerhans[8] vehemently opposes this view, and contends that dcth was due to poisonous effects produced by the antitoxin, which, as Bischof Ehrlich, and Strassmann have shown, was normal.

Cause of Death from Serum-njections.—Chas. T. McClintock[9]

[1] Centralbl. f. Bakteriol., Parasitenk. u. Infeionskrank., Nos. 22 and 23, p. 843, 1896.
[2] Deutsch. med. Woch., No. 1, 1897.
[3] Centralbl. f. Bakteriol., Parasitenk. u. Infetionskrank., May 10, 1897.
[4] Lancet, Aug. 15, 1896.   [5] Brit. ed. Jour., Oct. 3, 1896.   [6] Ibid.
[7] Berlin. klin. Woch., No. 23, 1896.   [8] Ibid., No. 27, 1896.
[9] Jour. Am. Med. Asc.. Feb. 27, 1897.

does not believe that the injection of air in hypodermic medication, as in serum injections, is responsible for some of the sudden deaths recorded, but would class the phenomena observed, varying from slight faintness to death, as shock

Contribution to the Theory of Agglutination.—E. Levy and H Bruns[1] have studied bacterial agglutination, comparing the observations of Gruber, Durham, Pfeiffer, and Kolle, and others. They noted the phenomenon in connection with the cholera, typhoid, colon, and pyocyaneus bacillus, and also with proteus. In all these cases the animals yielding the serum had been treated with dead cultures of the bacteria. The authors now hit upon the thought that it might be possible to endow the serum with agglutinating properties by injecting the soluble metabolic products of the bacteria, although Gruber, the discoverer of the *agglutinins*, had held that these, the agglutinins, were formed from the constituents of the bacterial bodies. Levy and Bruns injected filtered cultures of typhoid and cholera into rabbits and, indeed, found that the serum developed typical agglutinating pow[ers] observed that this did not occur immediate, but that several [days were] -uired. Then, however, it seemed as if th[e] reaction appeared all a..

Widal[2] is of the opinion tht the agglutinating property is not a protective phenomenon of the organism.

Transmission of the Agglutinating Substance by milk.—Widal and Sicard[3] found that mice, the serum of which endowed with the agglutinating property, transmitted it to their you guinea-pigs and cats did not. Te ingestion of strongly agglutinatin milk by man does not transmit te reaction to the blood. These diff in the transmissibility of the agglutinating substance by way of the dig tract is at present not explicable. The authors are not prepared to discuss hypothesis of the digestive chensm, but recall the fact that agglutinat milk coagulated naturally or by te action of an acid, such as acetic or hyd[ro] chloric acid, loses only a small pa of its agglutinating power.

Serum-diagnosis by Meas of Dried Blood-samples in (experi mental Cholera.—Wyatt Jonson and E. W. Hammond[4] obtained Pfeiffer's reaction with the dried blood of animals 3½ days after infection with virulent cholera-culture.

The Agglutinating Property of the Blood-Plasma.—Achard and Benaude[5] have undertaken a series of experiments which are designed to show whether the agglutinating property of the blood is dependent upon the blood-corpuscles, or whether it is characteristic of the blood-plasma. They have shown that blood-plasma which has been deprived of all formed elements possesses the agglutinating power perfectly. They have also shown that the presence of very large numbers o white and red corpuscles does not increase the agglutinating power of the plasma to an appreciable degree. They have concluded that living leukocytes which have been separated from the primitive plasma do not retain the agglutinating property. They think that the differences in the agglutinating property of the different fluids of the body are not to be accounted for by the presence of white corpuscles; but rather are dependent upon the elective action of th living membranes—glandular epithelia in particular—which are concerned i the transudation of the agglutinating substances. Their experiments have also shown that the blood always contains the largest quantity of the agglutinating substances, and that the agglutinating substances are preserved for the longest time in the blood.

---

[1] Berlin. klin. Woch., J. e 7, 1897.
[2] Centralbl. f allg. Path u. path. An., Oct. 15, 1897.   [3] Sem. méd., July 28, 1897.
[4] N. Y. Med. Jour., Nov. 28, 1896.   [5] Arch. de Méd. expér. et d'Anat. path., Nov., 1896.

Distribution of the Agglutinating Substance in the Body of Typhoid-fever Patients.—Courmont[1] has examined the comparative agglutinating power of the blood of the general circulation and of that from various organs in 7 autopsies on cases of typhoid fever. In 3 cases an exact quantitative estimation was made. While the blood of the heart, of the lung, of the kidney, of the thyroid gland, and of the ovary exhibited a very marked agglutinating action, like that of the blood during life, the blood of the liver and spleen, the bile, and the juice of the mesenteric glands gave a reaction, on an average, ten times less intense; in some cases it was entirely absent. The liquid of serous cavities produced an intense reaction, most frequently when there was an acute effusion due to the presence of another microorganism. This is not true of pleural effusions due to the typhoid-bacillus (Ménétrier).

TECHNIC.

Preservation of Museum-specimens.—T. L. Webb[2] recommends the following method of preserving gross specimens for museum-purposes :
1. Soak the object in Jores' fluid for from 1 to 3 days, the fluid being changed once or twice. 2. Wash specimen in 95 % alcohol; Webb places it in methylated spirit for half an hour. 3. Place in alcohol and leave there until the normal color returns, but no longer. Here, too, he uses methylated alcohol. 4. Preserve in glycerin and water, equal parts. It is well to change this fluid once after about a week's immersion. Jores' fluid is prepared by Webb as follows: sodium chlorid, ℥ss; sodium sulfate, ℥j; magnesium sulfate, ℥j; water, ℥l. These are mixed, and from ℥ij to ℥v of formalin added.

Conservation of Gross Morbid Specimens in their Natural Colors.—C. Kaiserling[3] places the organ in an abundant quantity of a solution of: formalin, 750 c.c., distilled water, 1000 c.c., potassium nitrate, 10 gm., and potassium acetate, 30 gm. In 24 or 48 hours the specimen is transferred, after allowing the solution to drip off, to 80 % alcohol, when the original color will reappear. After 12 hours it is placed for 2 hours in 95 % alcohol, and finally conserved in a mixture of equal parts of water and glycerin, with the addition of 30 parts of potassium acetate. Delicate objects, as intestine, remain in this only 1 or 2 days, and are then transferred to equal parts of glycerin and water plus absolute alcohol (1 : 10).

The Preparation of Anatomic Specimens by the Formalin-alcohol-glycerin-potassium-acetate Method.—Melnikow-Raswedenkow[4] gives the details of a method, already published in abstract, by which anatomic preparations can be preserved in their natural color. The specimens are treated first with formalin, then with alcohol, and finally with glycerin and potassium acetate. The author has devised the following schema of his method :
STEP I.—*Fixation of Specimen ; Change of Color.*—(1) *Dry Method.*—Cotton saturated with undiluted formalin.

(2) *Moist Method.*—Cotton soaked in 10 % formalin with the addition of—
(*a*) Gases: (1) H_2O_2; (2) H_2S. (*b*) Reducing-substances : (1) hydrochinon; (2) hydroxylamin ; (3) pyrocatechin. (*c*) Reagents rich in oxygen—*e. g.*, potassium chlorate. (*d*) Acetates: (1) potassium acetate; (2) sodium acetate; (3) aluminum acetate; (4) ammonium acetate ; (5) calcium acetate ; (8) magnesium acetate ; (7) strontium acetate ; (8) nickel acetate ; (9) barium acetate ; (10) manganese acetate. (*e*) Various combinations of reagents of groups *b* and *c*

[1] Sem. méd., Feb. 24, 1897.   [2] Birmingham Med. Rev., June, 1897.
[3] Berlin. klin. Woch., Aug. 31, 1896.
[4] Centralbl. f. allg. Path. u. path. Anat., Feb. 10, 1897.

with those of group *d;* the best is—sodium acetate, 4%; potassium chlorate, 0.5%.

STEP II.—Restoration of color by means of alcohol, 50%, 75%, and 95%.

STEP III.—Preservation of color in glycerin containing an acetate. Small organs or pieces of organs are immersed in the fixing-solution and then into alcohol; in the case of large organs injection first of a fixing-solution, then of alcohol, is recommended.

Explanation of the Schema.—The organ, without previous washing in water, is laid on cotton saturated with pure formalin. This method is especially valuable when it is desired to preserve mineral or mineral-like deposits,—*e. g.*, urie-acid infarcts of the kidney. The specimens preserve an almost natural color for more than a year. In the moist method cotton is saturated with 10% formalin containing any one of the reagents under *a, b, c,* or *d,* and is then wrapped completely around the specimen. When 10% formalin, with 3% sodium acetate and 0.5% potassium chlorate, is employed, about 48 hours are required for fixation. In the second step the cotton already used is squeezed out, and then weak alcohol, 60%, poured on. After 3 or 4 days alcohol of about 80% is substituted, and at the end of a week the strength is raised to 95%. Afterward the specimen is transferred to a conserving solution (glycerin, 20; potassium acetate, 15; distilled water, 100), in which it can remain perpetually. All the fluids employed in this method can be used a second time.

At the conclusion of his paper the author offers an explanation of the mode of action of his method, which, however, it is not necessary to reproduce here.

Preparation of Frozen Sections by Means of Methyl and Ethyl Chlorid.—H. W. Cattell[1] recommends a very simple method of preparing frozen sections. The tissue, prepared by Hamilton's,[2] Orth's,[3] or Plenge's[4] method, is placed with some formol and gum acacia fluid upon the specimen-bolder of the microtome, and a small stream of ethyl chlorid, methyl chlorid, or anestile (a mixture of these two agents), is played from above directly upon the specimen. The tube containing the ethyl chlorid is held about a foot from the specimen, and moved from place to place until the specimen is firmly attached to its base of support, and the upper portion is coated with a few crystals of ice. These crystals are extremely small and delicate, and, therefore, do not injure the tissue so markedly as in some other of the freezing-methods. The specimen is readily frozen in from thirty seconds to a minute. Sections are then cut and placed in water or 50% alcohol, and mounted in the usual way. Excellent stained preparations may be prepared in 15 minutes or less from the time that the tissue is removed from the body.

A Rapid Method of Preparing Permanent Sections for Microscopic Diagnosis.—L. Pick[5] recommends the following method: the excised or curetted material is freed from blood and coagula by dipping in water and then brought directly on to the freezing-plate of the microtome and frozen. In order that the freezing should be rapid and not too severe it is important that the mass be laid flat, and be not thicker than 2 or 3 mm. The breadth is immaterial up to 1 cm. square, or even greater. The ice block so obtained in a few seconds must be merely firm, not stone-hard; the knife must cut through lightly and without grating. Particles from curettage may be laid on the plate, a half dozen or more at once, and sections obtained from all at one time. The sections as they are cut are wiped from the knife-blade by the finger-tip, floated onto a 4% aqueous formalin-solution, and left there

[1] Internat. Med. Mag., Dec., 1896.   [2] Text-Book of Pathology, vol. i., p. 58.
[3] Berlin. klin. Woch., No. 13, 1896.   [4] Virchow's Archiv, cxliv., p. 409.
[5] Brit. Med. Jour., Jan. 16, 1897.

4 minutes to harden and fix the cell-plasma and intercellular substance. The use of the huger in place of a brush is to allow the warmth of the former to thaw the section before it reaches the solution, avoiding in this way the formation of air-bubbles in the tissue, which are often very annoying. From the formalin-solution the section is carried directly into a 4% alum-carmin solution (4 gm. carmin boiled three-quarters of an hour in 100 gm. 5% aqueous alum-solution, cooled, filtered), and left from 3 to 5 minutes, staining a deep red. For transport-ing the sections from one liquid to another up to absolute alcohol a glass rod is used, about which the section is rolled, obtaining a flat and even specimen much more quickly and conveniently than with a spatula. The section taken from the carmin-solution is rinsed in pure water to remove the superfluous stain, using the glass rod as before, and then dehydrated by bringing it for 15 seconds each into 80% alcohol and absolute alcohol. Finally it is placed in xylol-carbol to clarify, and mounted and conserved in Canada balsam. The microtome employed is the Jung-Heidelberg Hobel (carpenter's plane).

The Preparation of Blood for Microscopic Examination.— Henry G. Piffard[1] lays down a number of rules dealing with some important points in technic for the guidance of hematologists. He prefers the Zeiss glass slide 76x26 mm.; in cover-glasses he condemns emphatically the square variety, by means of which, he thinks, good smears cannot be obtained. Cover-glasses should be tested as to thickness, and only those approaching 0.17 mm. should be employed. He advises battery-fluid (water, 9 oz.; potassium bichromate, 1 oz.; sulphuric acid, 1 oz.) for purposes of cleansing. The cover-glasses are left in this 24 hours, then rinsed in water, then placed in distilled water, and from this transferred to pure methylic alcohol, where they are kept until needed. A straight surgical needle (the author uses one made of an alloy of iridium and platinum) should be employed for making the puncture. The cover-glasses are held in forceps; one of these should be of the self-closing variety, the other any sort that will hold the cover nicely. Heating is pre-ferred as a method of fixation, the author employing an electric heater con-trolled by a rheostat. The ordinary staining-methods are recommended, especially eosin and methylen-blue. The author prefers to examine the cover-glasses mounted dry, and prepares his permanent preparation, not with bal-sam, which he cannot condemn strongly enough, but by placing the covers in a ring of cement. A few words as to choice of condenser conclude the paper. [We are glad that there is a medical man in the United States who is not averse to dealing with the difficult mechanical problems of optics, but cannot follow him in all the innovations he suggests. For routine-work mounting with cement and by means of a turning-table is too time-consuming, and it is not likely that the convenient balsam-method will be abandoned.]

In another communication, Piffard[2] gives some valuable suggestions as to stains and technic. In the first place, he recommends oil of cinnamon (cassia) as superior to balsam; still better is his naphthalin-amber (see *Year-Book*, 1896, p. 973). He also points out a common error, viz., the use of the word methyl-blue when methylen-blue is intended; the former is an acid, the latter a basic stain. He is partial to thionin as a nuclear stain; in this we fully agree with him. As to eosin, only that soluble in alcohol should be used. He also recommends Grübler's neutral red as a beautiful basic and nuclear stain. [We have found a combination of eosin and thionin to give the most beautiful results. Thionin is especially useful for staining Ehrlich's mastzellen. The best effects are obtained when the section is first stained in a strong solution of eosin, and then, after washing in water, is placed in thionin.]

---

[1] Med. Rec., Oct. 17, 1896.   [2] Med. Rec., Feb. 13, 1897.

A Method of Fixing and Staining Blood.—G. Lovell Gulland[1] recommends a new method of fixing and staining blood-films. In its most rapid form the process is as follows: a small drop of blood, drawn in the usual way, is taken up on the center of a cover-glass held with forceps, and distributed evenly between that and another cover. The utmost care must be taken to avoid all pressure, as the after-appearance of the red corpuscles depends almost entirely upon the way in which this maneuver is carried out. The covers are then gently and rapidly slid off one another, and dropped with the wet side downward into the fixing-solution. This is made up of: absolute alcohol saturated with eosin, 25 c.c.; pure ether, 25 c.c.; sublimate in absolute alcohol (2 gm. to 10 c.c.), 5 drops (more or less). The quantity required for use at one time, which may be 5 to 10 c.c. for 4 cover-glasses, should be poured into a wide-mouthed bottle or flat dish, and may be used several times over if it be preserved from evaporation. The fixation of the elements is practically instantaneous, but the cover-glasses should be allowed to remain in the solution for at least 3 or 4 minutes, to fix the film to the cover. They are then taken from the solution with forceps (steel forceps will do), and washed rapidly but thoroughly by waving them to and fro in a small basin of water. They are then stained for 1 minute (not longer) in a saturated watery solution of methylen-blue, and again rapidly washed in water. Next they are quickly dehydrated in absolute alcohol, which at the same time removes the excess of methylen-blue, cleared in xylol, and mounted in xylol-balsam on a slide. The method is no less useful for fixing pus, sputum, and anything else which can be spread in a film; only with these it is generally advisable to prolong the fixation.

Yolk of Egg as an Addition to Culture-media.—A. Capaldi[2] finds the addition of yolk of egg to culture-media of great value. A fresh egg is broken, the white allowed to escape, and the yolk with the adherent white placed in a sterile Petri dish. In order to get rid of any bacteria on the outside of the yolk (the yolk itself is always sterile), it is burnt at one point with a glass rod. With a platinum needle the charred part is removed and 3 or 4 drops of the yolk are added to the agar, which has previously been melted and allowed to cool to 45° or 47° C. Plates are then prepared, or the agar is allowed to solidify in the tubes. The medium may be used for diphtheria-bacilli, which grow upon it as rapidly and as well as on blood-serum; and the tubercle-bacillus does this also. The yolk may be added to bouillon; in such yolk-bouillon the diphtheria-bacillus produces a stronger toxin than in ordinary bouillon.

A New Method of Staining Bacteria, especially the Gonococcus.—L. Pick and J. Jacobson[3] recommend the use of a mixture of two basic dyes. The combinations that can be employed are numerous. For the gonococcus they suggest the following method: 1. Spread pus on cover-glass or slide, and dry. 2. Pass thrice through flame. 3. Stain at the most for from 8 to 10 seconds with distilled water 20 drops, carbol-fuchsin 15 drops, concentrated alcoholic solution of methylen-blue 8 drops. 4. Rinse in water; dry. 5. Mount in Canada balsam.

Culture of Amebæ.—O. Casagrandi and P. Barbagallo[4] were unable to obtain pure cultures in liquid media. Of solid media, egg-albumin, well sterilized by Tyndal's method, mixed with peptone, and alkalinized with

[1] Brit. Med. Jour., Mar. 13, 1897.
[2] Centralbl. f. Bakteriol., Parasitenk. u. Infektionskrank., xx., Nos. 22 and 23, 1896.
[3] Berlin. klin. Woch., Sept. 7, 1896.
[4] Centralbl. f. Bakteriol., Parasitenk. u. Infektionskrank., May 10, 1897.

sodium carbonate, is a very efficient medium. Agar is not reliable; much better is Fuscns crispus (5%) of Celli and Fioca (see *Year-Book*, 1897, p. 738). With respect to the reaction of the medium, amebæ can live in an alkaline as well as in a neutral medium, but they can also adapt themselves to an acid reaction. Of interest are the authors' observations on the presence of organized substances. They find (*a*) that protozoa are not necessary for the propagation of amebæ; the two can live side by side in cultures without the one swallowing the other, although parasitic amebæ have the habit of ingesting trichomonads, etc. (*b*) Bacteria are also not necessary, though by some authors a symbiosis of the two has been assumed. The authors hold that the ameba coli is only a commensal in the human bowel, and has nothing to do with the production of catarrhal affections, the latter being caused by bacteria. (*c*) Fungi and (*d*) blastomycetes are likewise contaminations, and are not essential to the growth of amebæ in culture-media. The authors divide amebæ into cultivatable and noncultivatable forms. Those living free—*i. e.*, nonparasitic— are cultivatable; all parasitic amebæ found in feces and all those not possessing a contractile vacuole or a multinuclear cyst are noncultivatable.

MISCELLANEOUS.

The Role of the Vessels and the Parenchyma in Inflammation.

—In a masterly address delivered at the Twelfth International Congress, at Moscow, on the " Role of the Vessels and the Parenchyma in Inflammation," Virchow[1] sums up as follows: 1. Inflammation, as at present definable, is not a uniform process with constant characteristics. 2. According to their nature, four varieties of inflammation are distinguishable: the exudative, the infiltrative, the parenchymatous, and the proliferative. Each of these furnishes different products. 3. The necessity to group these under one name is less a scientific than a practical and diagnostic one. It is the desire to distinguish the inflammatory infiltrates, exudates, metamorphoses, and new formations, from the noninflammatory. 4. The diagnostic interest is heightened by therapeusis, inasmuch as the different varieties of inflammation demand a certain uniformity of treatment. 5. The condition of the vessels and of the local circulation presents not inconsiderable differences in the various forms of inflammation. While the inflammatory hyperemia appears as a prime factor in exudative and infiltrative inflammations, it occupies only a secondary part in the metamorphosing and proliferating forms. 6. The conditions of the parenchyma are no less varied. The exudative inflammations produce the least, the proliferative and metamorphosing the greatest alterations. The infiltrations are similar to the exudations. There is, however, no inflammation in which the parenchyma is entirely unaffected. In some cases the participation is chiefly passive; as an example may be mentioned the greater friability of the lung-tissue in exudative pneumonia (hepatization) and the destructive action of many infiltrations. In other cases, as in the secretion of mucus, the parenchyma furnishes the chief part of the exudate. 7. The common character, in the narrower sense, of inflammatory changes in the vessels and in the parenchyma consists in that the cause of the changes in each case is to be found in an irritation which evokes certain activities (actions, reactions). The primary consideration in diagnosis, therefore, is whether the process is really irritative. 8. The irritation involves both the nerves and the vessels, and the specific as well as the nonspecific parenchyma. It varies with the constitution of the irritated parts and the nature of the acting irritant. The irritants are at times

[1] Centralbl. f. allg. Path. u. path. Anat., Oct. 15, 1897.

mechanic, more often chemie in nature. The irritative action of many bacteria depends likewise on chemie products. 9. The not improper comparison of inflammations with fever, which is based on the temperature-rise in the external parts, is not valid for inflammation as a whole, but only for the increased fluxion to the inflamed part, in as far as such a comparison is possible. Indeed, it can be said that the modern opposition against the essentiality of fever is in line with that, as yet poorly developed, against the unity of inflammation. There are febrile diseases and inflammatory diseases, but neither fever nor inflammation has a separate existence. [Despite the stupendous labors expended on the investigation of the process of inflammation, it is evident, and is clearly pointed out by the Nestor of pathologists, that no comprehensive definition can be framed. It is particularly the so-called parenchymatous inflammations that are stumbling-blocks, for it is often next to impossible to say to what extent the parenchyma-changes are part of the inflammatory process, and to what extent they are purely degenerative. In the kidney, especially, does this question confront us often.]

Inflammation.—Paul Grawitz,[1] whose views as to the origin of the cells in inflammation have not met with general acceptance, endeavors in the present essay to answer his opponents by an appeal to biologic data. He denies, in the first place, *in toto*, the leukocytic nature of the cells—*i. e.*, their derivation from the blood—claiming that there is no observation on record sustaining the Cohnheimian view. As for the proliferation-theory of Virchow, he is willing to let it stand, but cannot consider it the only source of the cell-accumulation. His own view, "the Schlummerzellen-theory," is that the cells originate from cell-particles and from the intercellular substance. He combats the teachings of Senftleben and Leber, who interpreted the cells found in supposedly dead cornea introduced into the tissues as immigrated cells. In the first place, he shows that the corneal tissue employed was not dead, for (*a*) the removal of the cornea from an animal dead for several days, or (*b*) the heating to 80° C. for $\frac{1}{4}$ hour, or (*c*) the drying of the tissue, is not sufficient to kill it, so that under favorable conditions it is incapable of manifesting certain signs of life. If such pieces of cornea are introduced, *e. g.*, into the lymph-sac of a frog, they will become pervaded by wandering-cells, which, however, are not immigrated cells, but are derived from the still-living corneal tissue. This is proved by the fact that in absolutely dead cornea (killed by heating to 52° or 55° C. or by immersion in sublimate solution) no wandering-cells are found when it has been kept in a frog's lymph-sac. The corneal wandering-cells are readily distinguished from the adhering lymph-cells of the frog by the fact that the former take the gold stain, the latter not. Pieces of cornea from a hare, removed 10 or 12 days after death, and kept 1 day in the lymph-sac, still showed gold-staining wandering-cells, although mould had already formed on the corneal surface. All wandering-cells found in a transplanted recuperable cornea originate from the living tissue itself; their formation is intimately connected with the preservation of vitality, and ceases at a degree of temperature which by no means corresponds to the coagulating-point of albumin, and also disappears under the influence of sublimate and similar noxious agents which kill the protoplasm. Arguments are also brought forth to show that the usual evidence relied upon to prove that the intercellular substance is dead, is fallacious. Whether the newly formed cells arise solely from cell-particles or from the matrix, must be left to the future to decide. [Grawitz's experiments admit, it seems to us, of other interpretations than those he has given.]

Is there a Fatty Degeneration?—Rosenfeld[2] has tried to solve in an

---

[1] Wien. med. Woch., Jan. 23, 1897.   [2] Centralbl. f. innere Med., June 26, 1897.

45

interesting manner the question whether there is such a thing as fatty degeneration, and has arrived at the conclusion that there is no such process. The differentiation of fatty processes into two—infiltration and degeneration—was based on the hypothesis of the origin of fat from albumin, which hypothesis, the author tells us, has been disproved by Pflüger. He (Rosenfeld) has investigated many of the conditions in which fat is apparently formed from albumin, as the fatty liver of phloridzin- and phosphorus-poisoning, and the formation of milk. In fasting animals receiving phloridzin fat to the amount of 75% is stored in the liver. But this fat cannot be derived from the albumins of the hepatic cells, for the quantity of albumin in the liver is not materially diminished. The fat has been carried from the "fat-depots" to the liver, as may be observed in dogs that, having through long starvation become devoid of fat, are then fed with a foreign fat—*e. g.*, sheep-tallow. When such sheep-tallow dogs are given phloridzin the sheep-fat is carried from the subcutaneous tissue to the liver, in which nearly 50% of such fat may then be found. In phosphorus-poisoning the fat is also only infiltrated, for in totally fat-free animals phosphorus-poisoning is not able to produce fatty liver, because the fat-depots are empty. If the fat originated from albumin, it is difficult to understand why it is not formed from the abundant albumins present. If the sheep-tallow dog is poisoned with phosphorus, the fat is carried from the depots to the liver, which may store as much as 40% sheep-tallow. That the fat in the milk is not derived from albumins was shown by the following experiment: a sheep-tallow slut was allowed to become pregnant; and then received only the leanest meat. The fat in the milk was sheep-fat, and hence it cannot have been formed in the body of the animal, for then it would have been dog-fat, but must have been conveyed to the mammary glands from the fat-depots. The theory of a fatty degeneration, the author insists, must be entirely relinquished; in its stead is to be placed that of an albuminous degeneration of the cell; this injury to the cell is followed by the infiltration of fat as a reparative attempt. The fat of the organism consists of the fat of the food and that formed from the carbohydrates.

Terminal Infections.—It is a common experience to see patients that have suffered from chronic diseases succumb to some form of acute infection. Simon Flexner[1] has undertaken a study of this subject, based on a large series of carefully investigated autopsies made at the Johns Hopkins Hospital. He found 255 cases of chronic heart- or kidney-disease, or of both combined, in which bacteriologic examination had been sufficiently complete to make them of use for this study. Of these 255 cases, 213 gave positive and 42 negative results. Negative results, as the author clearly states, do not afford positive proof of the absence of microorganisms—a number of factors may prevent development of cultures.

Bacteriologic study of cases of chronic Bright's disease showed in 32 cases unassociated with cardiac or other chronic disease 29 positive and 3 negative results. Similarly, of 112 cases of combined chronic renal and chronic cardiac disease, 85 yielded positive and 27 negative results. In a considerable number of cases of chronic Bright's disease other chronic diseases were present. These consisted of tumors, such as carcinomata, sarcomata, and myomata, of cirrhosis of the liver and lungs, chronic proliferative peritonitis, etc. Of 54 cases of combined chronic Bright's disease, bacteriologic examination gave 51 positive and 3 negative results.

A similar study of the cases of chronic heart-disease yielded the following: the number of cases of heart-disease alone in which bacteriologic examinations

---

[1] Jour. Exper. Med., July, 1896.

were made was 41, of which 32 were positive and 9 negative. The number of cases of chronic heart-disease associated with other chronic diseases than chronic Bright's disease was 22, of which 16 gave positive and 6 negative results. The cases of combined chronic heart- and kidney-diseases are the same as are given with the summary relating to the latter organ.

The infections may be local or general, the former being much more common. In the general infections, in contradistinction to the local infections, no special group of bacteria is present. At times the point of entrance of the microorganism cannot be made out at the autopsy. In the series of chronic kidney-diseases 38 cases of general infection are included. The microorganisms causing these infections were the streptococcus pyogenes, 16 cases; staphylococcus pyogenes aureus, 4 cases; micrococcus lanceolatus, 6 cases; gas-bacillus, three times alone and twice combined with the bacillus coli communis; the gonococcus, anthrax-bacillus, bacillus proteus, the last combined with the bacillus coli, the bacillus coli alone, a peculiar capsulated bacillus, and an unidentified coccus, each in one instance. What is striking in this list is the preponderance of the usual pyogenic cocci. These may occur without association with abscess-formation. In a large proportion of the cases of septicemia visible focal lesions within the organs were not present at the autopsy. The usual conditions found were acute splenic tumor and more or less severe parenchymatous degeneration of the viscera, with sometimes microscopic necroses of tissue-cells as well.

Of the 16 instances of streptococcus-infection the infection-atria into the general circulation were believed to be as follows: cellulitus, erysipelas, leg-ulcer, bedsore, 7; phthisical cavity, 1; laparotomy, 2; tapping abdomen, 1; acute pleurisy, peritonitis, or pericarditis, 3; sloughing angiosarcoma, 1; necrosis of placental attachment in uterus, 1. Of the 4 cases of staphylococcus aureus septicemia there were: acute pericarditis following diphtheria, 1; operation upon the perineum and cervix uteri, 2; undetermined (generalized melanotic sarcoma), 1. Of the 6 cases of micrococcus lanceolatus infection, acute pneumonia claimed 4; acute endocarditis and acute pericarditis, and pleuritis, 1 each. The 5 gas-bacillus cases gave aneurysm of the aorta opening externally, amputation of arm, each 1 case, and intestine 3 cases. The 2 proteus cases took their origin, one in a sloughing bedsore and the other from a chronic diphtheric colitis. The capsulated bacillus gained entrance from an ascending pyelonephritis; the anthrax-bacillus from an anthrax-edema of the face.

The number of local infections was much larger—127 among the cases of chronic Bright's disease, of combined heart- and kidney-disease, and of kidney and other chronic diseases. The bacteria were for the most part the same as those met with in the general infections. Certain bacteria appeared with such frequency in certain organs that these may be inferred to offer better opportunities for their growth. Thus the colon-bacillus was commonly found in the kidneys and lungs, and the streptococcus in congested and edematous lungs.

Regarding the infection-atria in the local infections, the intestine was found to be the portal of entry not only of many of the bacteria found in the inflamed peritoneum, but also of some of those present in the pleura, upon the heart-valves, and within the organs.

In cases of heart-disease uncomplicated with kidney-disease terminal infections were often encountered. Of 41 cases of arteriosclerosis and chronic valvular disease cultures showed in 32 the presence of bacterial infection, while in 22 cases of cardiovascular disease, associated with some other chronic condition than Bright's disease, positive results were obtained in 16. In these 48 positive cases the distribution of the bacteria was general in 14 instances. The microorganisms associated with these septicemias were streptococcus pyogenes, 9 cases; micrococcus lanceolatus, 2 cases; staphylococcus pyogenes aureus, 1 case; staphylococcus albus and streptococcus, 1 case; bacillus coli communis, 1 case.

An interesting point brought out by the author's studies is the fact that the bacillus pyocyaneus is, like the more common pyogenic organisms, capable of producing distinct and widespread lesions. He has met with several instances in which extensive necrosis, associated at times with ulceration, had been caused by it in the gastrointestinal tract.

It being evident from all these observations that chronic diseases predispose to infection, it becomes important to determine whether there is a demonstrable difference in the bactericidal power possessed by the body-fluids and cells. Some experiments were made by the author in this line, primarily to estimate the relative bactericidal power of normal blood-serum and that from individuals suffering from chronic diseases. Normal serum was in 2 out of 3 cases (the author is in doubt whether the exceptional case should be included) found to be strongly bactericidal to the staphylococcus aureus, while of 9 samples of blood taken from persons suffering with some form of chronic disease, no appreciable effect was exerted upon this microorganism in six.

The author recognizes the importance of the antitoxic substances as an additional factor in establishing and preserving immunity, and expects to deal with that phase of the question in a future communication. [The studies which the author has begun deserve to be extended to a wider field, for the question of terminal infections is not so very different from that of infections in apparently healthy subjects. We find that the same diseases which carry off the cardiac and renal sufferer attack other persons.]

Histologic Changes Produced by Ricin and Abrin Intoxications.—Simon Flexner[1] has made a careful histologic study of the changes produced in animals by repeated doses of ricin and abrin. We have not space to describe these in detail, but a comparison with the changes found in many forms of bacterial infection and toxemias discloses their essential similarity. The chief and characteristic lesions are degenerative and focal in character—are especially focal necroses. The toxins exert their influence upon individual cells, but not all the cells of the body show the same susceptibility to their action, lymphoid cells suffering to a greater degree than epithelial cells. Furthermore, the various organs do not suffer to an equal extent; thus, the liver-cells are more affected than those of the kidney and adrenals. Finally, in highly differentiated cells, not all parts of the protoplasm need be equally affected by the poison.

There is evidence to prove that the extent of cell-injury in any particular organ is in a measure proportionate to the functional activities exerted in dealing with the particular poison. It is not easy to account for the focal character of the lesions in the organs, assuming the action to be due to a soluble substance contained within the circulating blood and fluids of the body. The author would elucidate it by reference to the part played by the circulation of the blood in the affected organs. The action of the poison has been shown to be exerted in part upon the capillary walls, causing necrosis and fragmentation of the endothelium, and nowhere is the injury to the capillary parietes greater than in the areas in which the necrosis is found. This fact suggests the possibility that in certain capillaries in which the circulation was much diminished or was temporarily at a standstill at the time when the irritant acted with the

---

[1] Jour. Exper. Med., Mar., 1897.

PLATE 4.

FIG. 1.—Focal area of necrosis of liver-cells and single cell-necroses. Karyolysis to be seen in the center and pyknosis and karyorrhexis in the periphery of the nodule. A few fragments of nuclei are also present in the central portion. Methylen-blue and eosin staining. (Objective No. 3; eye-piece No. 3.)

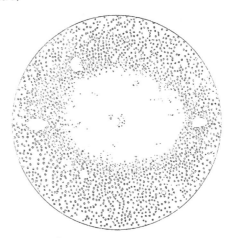

FIG. 2.—A focal area of necrosis similar to Fig. 1. Magenta staining to show the alterations in nuclei and protoplasm. Karyorrhexis is more marked than in preceding figure. (Same magnification as Fig. 1.)

(Jour. of Exp. Med., March, 1897.)

greatest intensity, so much damage was done to the vessel-wall that a freer transudation than occurred elsewhere took place into the tissues in the neighborhood, resulting in the destruction of cell-groups. Reference is also made to intracapillary thrombosis as a possible factor in the local necrosis. [The great significance of these observations appears to lie in the light they shed on focal necrosis in various organs in man. In animals that survived a long time the author was able to note reparative changes, and the replacement of the necrotic areas by new tissue—by a scar; in other words, a form of cirrhosis developed. It is especially the chronic changes that will prove of interest in the study and interpretation of fibroid changes in man. We append an illustration (Plate 4) showing focal necrosis of the liver.]

Echinococcus-cyst of Rectovesical Space.—Nuyens [1] describes an echinococcus-cyst between the bladder and the rectum, and collects 32 cases from the literature with the view of establishing a general symptomatology of the condition.

Multiple Echinococcus-cysts.—W. C. Keyes and F. C. Busch [2] report the case of a German, aged 53, in whose body at the autopsy were found a large hydatid cyst of the right kidney, a cavity at the base of the right lung, and two cavities below the diaphragm, one of which communicated with that in the lung. All these cavities had a calcareous lining. Neither hooklets nor scolices were found in the 3 cavities, so that their nature remained in doubt. The authors refer to 2 other cases of echinococcus-disease that have occurred in Buffalo, in the practice of Roswell Park, which have not yet been reported. [Echinococcus-disease appears to be more frequent in the United States, possibly only because the cases observed are published more often than was the custom formerly. We have ourselves observed a case of echinococcus-cyst of the liver and possibly of the lung in a negro from Delaware.]

Sarcosporidia.—Pluymebs [3] has studied the action of the sarcosporidium on the tissues of its host, and concludes: 1. These organisms are usually inoffensive parasites. 2. Exceptionally they become the cause of more or less extensive inflammatory lesions, with destruction of the muscular tissue, and may cause death if the organ attacked is essential to life (heart or diaphragm). 3. The inflammatory lesions appear only after the complete development of the parasite and after the rupture of the capsule which contains it. 4. The inflammation always terminates by the organization of the infiltrating tissue.

The Relation of the Specific Gravity and the Amount of Albumin in Pathologic Fluids.—Ott [4] has estimated the amount of albumin in pathologic fluids (by means of Kjeldahl's method, and multiplying the percentage of N by the factor 6.25) for the purpose of determining (1) the amount of albumin in the various diseases; (2) the relation of these amounts to the specific gravity. In the first table, containing 25 examinations, 11 appertain to the fluid in cancer of the peritoneum—the albumin was about 4% on an average. The amounts differed in the same case at different punctures. In peritoneal tuberculosis it was 6.558%; in hepatic cirrhosis from 2.006% to 6.887%; in echinococcus-cyst of the liver 0.360%; in ovarian cysts from 1.818% to 5.435%; in pyopneumothorax from 8.281% to 8.928%; in hydrocele the amount was usually high, but varied greatly, from 0.737% to 7.851%. The general conclusion from these figures is that there is no definite amount of albumin for any one disease. A study of the specific gravity in the light of the albumin-content of the fluids showed further that the former—*i. e.,* the spe-

---

[1] Centralbl. f. Bakteriol., Parasitenk. u. Infektionskrank., Feb. 15, 1897.
[2] Buffalo Med. Jour., Aug., 1896.   [3] Arch. de Méd. expér. et d'Anat. path., Nov., 1896.
[4] Zeit. f. Heilk., xvii., H. 4, p. 283.

cific gravity—does not permit any conclusion as to the quantity of albumin
in pathologic fluids, and that it is of no diagnostic value. For example, the
fluid from a case of cancer of the peritoneum and that from an echinococcus-
cyst had the same specific gravity, 1009, yet the former contained 2.6 % albumin and the latter only 0.36 %.

**The Significance of the Leukocytes in Exudates and Transu-
dates.**—Winiarski [1] confirms the assertion of Korczynski and Wernicki that
in serous exudates which neither show a tendency to pass into suppuration nor
are due to malignant disease the lymphocytes, especially the small ones,
numerically preponderate. When the neutrophiles are in the majority the
case is either one of neoplasm (carcinoma) or suppuration is going to take
place. The presence of eosinophiles and of red corpuscles is without significance. The author found in all pleural and peritoneal transudates almost
exclusively lymphocytes; in the purulent pleural exudates only neutrophiles;
in all serous inflammatory effusions, where new growths were not present,
lymphocytes were practically found alone. None of the last group ever
passed into suppuration, although the number of lymphocytes rose at times
as high as 6230 per cb. mm. In a case of metapneumonic serous pleurisy in
which the number of leukocytes was small, but in which neutrophiles were
chiefly present, suppuration developed later. All this is true of peritoneal
exudates. In the serous pleural exudates the number of leukocytes varies
from 270 to 9270 per cb. mm., in the transudates from 60 to 300. In peritoneal
effusions the numbers are smaller. During the absorption of exudates and
transudates the number of leukocytes increases; during the formation of fibrinous deposits it diminishes.

Pigmentation from Injection of Suprarenal Gland Extract.—
Charrin [2] produced pigmentation in dogs by the injection of aqueous glycerin-
extracts of suprarenal glands from guinea-pigs.

Toxicity of Human Sweat.—Arloing [3] found the human sweat toxic
for animals. If the intravenous injections did not produce a fatal termination
in from 1 to 3 days, the animals died later in a cachectic state. The toxicity
varies with the circumstances that accompany or precede sweating, with the
individual, the mode of preparing the extract, and the susceptibility of the
experimental animals.

[1] Kronika Lekarska, No. xii.; ref. in Centralbl. f. allg. Path. u. path. Anat., Mar. 1, 1897.
[2] Sem. méd., July 28, 1897.   [3] Ibid., p. 209, June 2, 1897.

NERVOUS AND MENTAL DISEASES.

By ARCHIBALD CHURCH, M. D.,

OF CHICAGO.

Introductory Epitome.—In the department of nervous diseases the past year has seen considerable activity. A great deal has been written about meningitis, and there is a very general belief that a form of acute serous meningitis may now be differentiated. This matter, however, is still under consideration, as it is recognized that meningitis is a disease of heterogenetic origin. The subject of cerebritis is a growing one. Cases of acute primary hemorrhagic cerebritis are being reported from all parts of the world, and it is likely that the clinical differentiation of the disease will be made possible by the accumulation of abundant material. Operative interference in hydrocephalus under new methods promises better results, and puncture of the lateral ventricles, when puncture of the lumbar cord is not productive of relief in cerebral pressure, is gaining adherents. The do-nothing attitude in the face of cerebral hemorrhage is likely to give way to more active interference when the differential diagnosis is sharply made between the condition of hemorrhage and thrombosis. Attention may also be called to the treatment of the hemiplegic state, so commonly neglected. A number of very important and interesting cases of cerebellar tumor, with and without operation, leads to the belief that surgical invasion of the posterior fossa has a larger field than had been supposed. The relation of the anterior gray matter of the spinal cord to peripheral neuritis is more and more well established by recent investigations. The subject of neuralgia has received important contributions, and the disorder apparently is a common one. The literature of syringomyelia is rapidly growing. The condition is now recognized as very far from rare, and cases are being reported on every hand. Cord-changes following the pernicious anemias, including leukemia and the like, are well represented in the literature of the year. It is now evident that such changes are not confined to the white matter, as was at first supposed, but that they are heterogeneous in distribution and multiform in character. Material and experiments are bringing forward the fact that myelitis is usually the result of arterial disease or of infection reaching the cord by the arterial route; in other words, that it is a softening rather than an inflammation. The frequency of spinal and cerebral hemorrhages in the newborn has received additional importance from the investigations of Schäffer. An important contribution is made to the joint-changes in locomotor ataxia, independent of so-called arthropathies. The anesthesias of tabes have been well worked out, and the important group of symptoms dependent thereupon has become general property. In the treatment of the disease a new method of stretching, which actually stretches the cord, is described, and the exercise-treatment to restore muscular control, as devised by Fränkel, which is herein outlined, has received decided support.

In the treatment of tetanus, antitoxin has been frequently tried during the past year, but the results are about the same as quoted in the *Year-Book* for

1897. Material is rapidly accumulating to show the relation of tetany to infection, especially infection arising from the gastrointestinal tract. The post-mortem findings in acromegaly almost uniformly include a pituitary tumor. Such cases now number nearly a score. A great deal of work has been done on the subject of exophthalmic goiter, and the value of the thymus treatment has been pretty well established as being slight. Treatment by ablation of the cervical sympathetic is gaining adherents, especially in France. The intimate, if not identical, relations of myxedema, cretinism, and goiter have developed during the past year. Some valuable contributions have been made to the literature of epilepsy from the Craig Colony in New York. Nothing partien-larly new in regard to the treatment of this neurosis has been forthcoming. Less value than formerly is attached to operative treatment in partial epilepsies.

In mental diseases importance attaches to the views regarding the bed-treatment of acute cases, and to the further elaboration of the subject of toxins and insanity. A number of notable papers on senile mental disturbance have appeared. Among the most interesting contributions to the subject of paretic dementia are the findings of Piccinnino, who, in several instances, claims to have discovered Lustgarten's bacillus of syphilis in fluid drawn from within the cranium. Studies on the subject of idiocy have been unusually numerous.

DISEASES OF THE CEREBRAL MENINGES AND CRANIAL NERVES.

Non-tuberculous Posterior Basic Meningitis in Infants.—J. W. Carr[1] calls attention to what he considers a special variety of meningitis; 11 cases were observed in Victoria Hospital, Chelsea, all of them occurring in previously healthy infants under 1 year of age. The onset was gradual in some, sudden in others; but in all the most characteristeric symptoms were severe vomiting, extreme head-retraction, and stupor passing into coma of several weeks' duration or more, with retracted head to the last. The cases all terminated fatally in from 5 weeks to 3 months; 10 necropsies were had, demonstrating inflammation of the pia-arachnoid in a very definite area at the base of the brain, with hydrocephalus and in some cases closure of the openings between the fourth ventricle and subarachnoid space. No tubercular disease was discovered in the cranial cavity or elsewhere. In two of the cases tapping of the lateral ventricles was done, in one with distinct improvement. In two other cases trephining proved rapidly fatal, apparently from too rapid escape of fluid. The nature of the infection was not determined, though it was supposed to have some relation to the epidemic cerebrospinal form.

Pachymeningitis Hæmorrhagica Interna.—Adolf Meyer[2] gives the findings in 21 cases showing hemorrhagic laminated membranes, 4 being in senile dementia, 7 in general paralysis, 1 in chronic mania, 1 in acute mania, 6 in terminal dementia, and 2 in epilepsy. In cases in which the membrane was single and the condition simple the deposit was found to be due to hemorrhage arising from the surface of the dura, and in a number of other cases membrane arising at this point secondarily involved the pia, and was even associated with pial hemorrhage in one instance. All of the cases, according to the writer, may be denominated vascular dural exudation. [This is at variance with some recent dogmatic statements to the effect that pachymeningitis is a misnomer, and that the condition arises from the soft membranes, and would better be called meningeal hemorrhage.]

[1] Brit. Med. Jour., Apr. 17, 1897.
[2] Path. Report Ill. East. Hosp. for the Insane, 1896.

Acute Serous Meningitis.—G. Boenninghaus, in a critical monograph [1] upon this subject, bases his conclusions upon 27 recorded cases, with an additional case under his personal care and treatment. The author divides acute serous meningitis into external and internal or ventricular, and acknowledges that the internal form may be secondary to the external. The ventricular form is the less serious, and death usually occurs at a much later period than in the external variety. In the majority of cases recorded the cause of the meningitis was middle-ear disease. This of itself throws some doubt on the diagnosis, especially in those cases that were not sectioned. The 5 cases operated on with recovery are interesting, but the evidence is not conclusive that the disease was serous meningitis; 3 of these were also secondary to ear-disease. In one of the remaining cases spinal puncture was done, and in the other trephining and puncture. [It must be admitted that the acute serous meningitis is extremely infrequent, although many good observers believe in its existence. A suppurative focus as a primary source of infection cannot be excluded without the most systematic and rigid examination of every portion of the body, and those who are doing the largest amount of postmortem work rarely fail to find some such primary origin for what appears to be a serous meningitis.]

Epidemic of Cerebrospinal Meningitis.—F. H. Williams and W. T. Councilman [2] reported an epidemic of cerebrospinal meningitis in a paper read before the American Medical Association, June, 1897. By lumbar puncture fluid was withdrawn from a little below the spinous process of the second lumbar vertebra and then studied by Dr. Councilman, who found organisms in 77 cases, including staphylococci, streptococci, and diplococci. The spleen was enlarged in some cases. Similar organisms were found in the nasal sinuses and once in an abscess of the tonsil. The most common bacterium found was the diplococcus intracellularis meningitidis (Jäger).

An Early Symptom of Meningitis.—Simon [3] states that tubercular meningitis always presents during the early period a disharmony in the respiratory movements of the diaphragm and thorax.

Atrophy of the Optic Nerve from Inflammatory Causes.— Wilder [4] gives the report of a case of optic atrophy, due perhaps to cerebral meningitis, in which the ocular fields were greatly reduced and vision was much obscured, but in which notable improvement was obtained, as shown by perimeter charts, after the subconjunctival injection of mercuric chlorid, and vision raised from $\frac{20}{120}$ to $\frac{20}{40}$ after 4 injections practised within a month. References to this method of procedure, especially as carried out by Derier, will be found in the same article.

Sallard [5] calls attention to the claim of Valude for the use of antipyrin in the treatment of optic atrophy by subcutaneous injections. Jeffrois had also tried the method in 10 cases, injecting the antipyrin deeply under the muscles of the back. Injections were continued daily for 5 months, with amelioration in 3 cases, but no modification of the visual field in any. The author gives preference to strychnin.

Congenital External Ophthalmoplegia.—Gourfein [6] reports 6 cases of this condition in the members of one family, the father and 5 sons. The mother of the first patient was also said to have suffered from the same condition, and a half-sister, daughter of this mother, had a convergent squint; 2 daughters were free from defect. There was no trace or evidence of syphilis.

---

[1] Published by J. F. Bergman, 1897.   [2] Med. Rec., June 5, 1897.
[3] La France méd., Mar. 29, 1895.   [4] Medicine, Dec., 1896.
[5] Rev. de Thér., Sept. 15, 1896.   [6] Rev. méd. de la Suisse Romande, No. 12, 1896.

In these cases ptosis was marked, the superciliary arches were flattened, and there was rotary nystagmus, but no protrusion of the eyeball. There was more or less amblyopia, but no false projection. He believes that the condition consisted in a congenital defect of the muscles, and that it was not of nuclear origin.

W. M. Leyzinski[1] reports a patient 4 years of age, of German parentage, born at full term after normal labor, without asphyxiation. Primary dentition commenced at 8 months, but owing to large size and great weight the child did not walk until he was 14 months old. There were no convulsions, the health being especially good—even the infectious diseases were escaped. No injuries. The child had always been bright and talkative, slept well, and was free from nocturnal disturbances. At the end of the first year he began to draw his head backward, and it was then noticed that the eyes turned inward. Upon examination there was found a convergent strabismus, more pronounced in the left eye. Neither eye could be turned beyond the middle line. Pupils normal. The author quotes the literature of the subject, and reports eases to show that associated malformations are frequently found. In the few postmortem examinations there has been found complete absence of the muscles in question, or they have been present but ill-developed or attached to the eyeball in abnormal position. Whether the nuclear condition is primary or secondary to the muscular loss is not yet determined.

Treatment of Trifacial Neuralgia.—William M. Leyzinski,[2] after defining what he means by trigeminal neuralgia, says of the treatment that the most efficient therapeutic measure is rest of the organs of mastication and articulation, and quite often complete bodily rest in bed. Conversation and solid food are forbidden. Nourishment, which is important, is maintained by semi-fluid or fluid food, sometimes introduced through the nasal tube. He also finds morphin, opium, aconitin, the coal-tar derivatives, cocain, nitroglycerin, and the fluid extract of ergot useful. The only form of aconitin that has proved valuable in his hands is the crystallized aconitin of Duquesnel, and this often succeeds when other aconite preparations fail. In conclusion, he says, "As there is a possibility—nay, even great probability—of relief in most cases of tic douloureux or chronic trigeminal neuralgia without surgical operations, the latter should be seriously considered only as a *dernier ressort*, or after all available resources have been exhausted.

C. L. Dana[3] makes an additional contribution to this subject, adding 5 cases that have been treated by large doses of strychnin hypodermically, to the 8 cases formerly reported and mentioned in the *Year-Book* for 1897. Of the first 8 eases 6 were relieved and 2 were not relieved. In the last 5 cases 4 have been successfully managed by this method. Dana discourages surgical operations, and believes that this line of treatment, which, it will be recalled, embraces rest in bed, should be persistently tried.

Tiffany[4] gives an analysis of 108 eases of facial neuralgia treated by intracranial operation. Of these cases 24 were fatal. In the discussion of the cases the author states that intracranial resection of the branches of the fifth nerve relieves pain for the time and perhaps permanently, but pain may recur in the same or neighboring territory. Recurrence of pain after known **removal of the Gasserian ganglion** is not recorded, but he doubts the expediency of removal of the entire ganglion. Marchant and Herbert[5] report 2 cases of extirpation of the Gasserian ganglion for the relief of rebellious facial neuralgia.

[1] N. Y. Med. Jour., Feb. 27, 1897.   [2] Med. Rec., Mar. 27, 1897.
[3] Ibid., May 1, 1897.   [4] Ann. of Surg., Nov. 18, 1896.
[5] Rev. de Chir., Apr. 10, 1897.

They analyze 93 additional cases collected from the literature. In these there were 17 deaths.

Sewill[1] relates 2 cases of trigeminal neuralgia which he considered **due to the loss of the teeth.** He found that, all teeth being gone, the approximation of the jaws put the maxillary articulations in an abnormal position, and perhaps served to make traction upon the lower branch of the fifth. In both cases the neuralgia was confined to this portion of the trifacial. Relief was given by introducing proper dental plates, and the condition could be reproduced by having them removed for a few days.

Facial Hemiatrophy.—Schlesinger[2] reports a man of 23, who complained of pain on the right side of the neck, difficulty of swallowing, and disturbance of vision of the right eye. Later there were paralysis and atrophy, with fibrillary contractions of the right side of the tongue and difficulty in pronunciation; still later, complete paralysis of the vocal cord, wasting of the right side of the face, disturbance of gait, vertigo, and anxiety. The previous history of the patient was free from notable incident. The facial atrophy was very pronounced, involving the bones of the head. A tumor could be felt on the right side of the pharynx, and it was supposed to be the cause of the cerebral symptoms, and that the facial atrophy was a basal affection connected with this tumor. [Additional cases tend to show that facial atrophy is due to disease of the fifth nerve, and it is to be hoped that this case will eventually come to autopsy and that others may be added, to make the matter plain.]

E. S. Yonge[3] reports a case following intense facial neuralgia of 6 months' duration and publishes a photograph.

Paralysis of the 5th Nerve.—Sidney Phillips[4] presented a woman before the Clinical Society of London with paralysis of the left 5th nerve. The following symptoms were present: anesthesia and analgesia of the left side of the cheek and of the hard and soft palate; insensibility of the teeth to pressure and loosening of several of them; loss of sensation on the left side of the tongue, and loss of sense of taste over the posterior third, as well as the anterior two-thirds, strychnin, sugar, and salt being unrecognized; anosmia of the left nostril, with a constant sanious, ichorous discharge and frequent epistaxis; a left conjunctival injection with an area of cloudiness of the surface of the cornea unless the eye was kept constantly protected by a watch-glass, and even with this protection a tendency to growth of loops of vessels over the cornea, which was kept in check by atropin; sight on the left side was defective, nothing smaller than 14 Snellen being read; there was no optic neuritis, but there was pallor of the disk.

Facial Paralysis.—F. Schultze[5] asserts that in peripheral facial paralysis the base of the tongue on the affected side occupies a lower level than on the sound side when the organ is lying in the floor of the mouth, and that this may be noticed also upon protrusion. He thinks it is due to the fact that paralysis of the facial nerve also involves the stylohyoid muscles and the posterior belly of the digastric.

Solitary Tubercle of the 7th and 8th Cranial Nuclei.—Manasse[6] exhibited a specimen of this sort removed from a tuberculous patient, 43 years of age, who had become deaf in the left ear and presented left facial palsy with reaction of degeneration. The autopsy revealed in the posterior part of the pons, on the left side, a tumor the size of a hazelnut, containing a cavity filled with friable cheesy material. Both the 7th and 8th nerves were im-

[1] Brit. Med. Jour., Jan. 16, 1897.
[3] Brit. Med. Jour., Mar. 6, 1897.
[5] Münch. med. Woch., June 8, 1897.
[2] Wien. klin. Woch., No. 20, 1896.
[4] Ibid., Jan. 30, 1897.
[6] Arch. f. Ohrenh., vol. xli., p. 62.

bedded in the mass. The vagus, glossopharyngeal, and accessory nerves were firmly adherent to a tumor of the same sort, and other tubercles were found in the cerebellum and right occipital lobe.

Anton[1] reports a fibrosarcoma of the auditory nerve. The patient was seized with headaches and blindness of the right eye and three hours later with blindness of the left eye. There were vomiting, and ringing, hissing sounds in his ears and difficulty of hearing. Bilateral optic neuritis and right facial paralysis appeared. Death occurred 8 months later. The autopsy revealed a tumor the size of a hen's egg situated between the pons and cerebellum. [Both of these cases show the vulnerability of the auditory group, which, of all the cranial nerves, is the most commonly affected by new growths.]

Spasmodic Torticollis.—Richardson and Walton[2] make a further contribution to the study and treatment of spasmodic torticollis, and report upon some of the cases appearing in a former paper by them, giving three additional ones. They properly look upon the disease as often based upon a neurotic foundation and as constituting a tic, in some instances a mental tic. They point out that all operations in such instances may be followed by improvement through the effect of the operation *per se*, and also find that the same influence may be accomplished by massage, electricity, gymnastics, and hypnotism. They would reserve surgical measures until everything else has been tried or unless the case was too well established and severe to justify delay. De Quervain[3] strongly advocates Kocher's method, which consists in division of the sterno-cleido-mastoid and of the cervical muscles at the back of the neck, including the splenius and the greater and small rhomboids, and subsequently the inferior oblique, avoiding the great occipital nerves that pass near this point. The author believes that the operation produces not only palliation, but sometimes a cure.

J. S. Risien Russell[4] reports an experimental investigation of the cervical and thoracic nerve-roots in relation to the subject of wry-neck that is of great surgical importance. The experiments were carried out upon monkeys, and the cervical roots were stimulated by electricity. The movements of the head resulting on extension of the anterior spinal nerve-roots were as follows : *First Cervical Root.*—The movement characteristic of an excitation of this root is a well-marked lateral inclination of the head onto the shoulder of the side excited. *Second Cervical Root.*—Excitation of this root produces a movement of the head closely resembling that which resulted on excitation of the first root—*i. e.*, a lateral inclination of the head to the side stimulated, by which means the side of the head and face are approximated to the shoulder. *Third Cervical Root.*—The movement which predominates is distinctly one in which the head is drawn backward, and the occiput being drawn to the side excited, the chin is directed upward and to the opposite side. *Fourth Cervical Root.*—There is still less of the lateral inclination of the head so characteristic of the first and second roots, while the backward movement of the head, in which the occiput is drawn to the side stimulated, is still more pronounced than in the third root. *Fifth Cervical Root.*—The little movement that results consists in a slight drawing of the occiput backward and to the side stimulated. *Sixth Cervical Root.*—The movement corresponds in all respects to that represented in the fifth. *Seventh Cervical Root.*—The movement which results on excitation of this root is decidedly more pronounced than that observed in connection with the fifth and sixth roots. *Eighth Cervical Root.*—As in the case of the seventh, movement of the head appeared to be entirely one indi-

[1] Arch. f. Ohrenh., vol. xli., p. 62.   [2] Am. Jour. Med. Sci., July, 1896.
[3] Sem. méd., Oct. 14, 1896.   [4] Brain, 1897.

rectly induced by the vigorous drawing down of the scapula by the latissimus dorsi. *First Thoracic Root.*—The movement of the head obtained by excitation of this root depends largely on whether the latissimus dorsi is represented in it or not; when it is so the representation is only slight, so that the resulting movement of the head, while resembling that produced by excitation of the seventh and eighth cervical roots, is very much smaller in amount. *Second Thoracic Root.*—The movement is a lateral curving of the spine by the action of the erector spinæ, and the head is slightly tilted laterally toward the opposite side.

Angina Pectoris.—Osler[1] in a number of able lectures gives a very full consideration of this neuralgic disorder, and in the final lecture[2] advises, in its *general management*, an investigation of the exciting causes of the attacks. The use of exercise within the limits of the individual's abilities is to be systematically adopted, and the diet regulated strictly to the requirements of the patient and his personal peculiarities. As to general medical treatment, he directs attention to underlying conditions, such as gout and syphilis, against which vigorous measures should be adopted. The persistent and intelligent use of the iodids, colchicum, and the nitrites is insisted upon. He cordially indorses the use of nitroglycerin, and urges that its dosage be pushed to the requirements of the case, preferring nitrite of amyl to meet the paroxysms. Commencing with doses of nitroglycerin of $\frac{1}{100}$ gr. three times a day, he increases until the patient takes four or five or even more times as much three times a day—care being taken to select an active preparation, and being guided by the flushing of the face and throbbing of the head as to its activity. Arsenic also comes in for a share of praise.

In regard to the *treatment of the attack*, he urges that gastrointestinal disturbance should be particularly guarded against, and the moment the patient feels any difficulty in the stomach Hoffman's anodyne, spirits of camphor, peppermint-water, or hot whiskey should be taken with a carminative draught to remove the difficulty. For the paroxysm itself he lists three remedies: nitrite of amyl to be inhaled, morphin hypodermically, and chloroform by inhalation if the first two do not succeed. He states that he has never seen any dangerous effects from the careful use of chloroform, even in persons with very weak hearts, and that the vigorous and continued use of the nitrites—in the form of trinitrin—never gives rise to any disturbance.

DISEASES OF THE BRAIN PROPER.

Acute Nonsuppurative Encephalitis.—Data regarding this recently differentiated disease is accumulating in all quarters. J. J. Putnam[3] reviews this subject, adds a case, and gives a synopsis of Oppenheim's reported 6 cases.[4] The case reported by Putnam followed several weeks after the mumps. Most other cases that have been of record have followed influenza, though Brie's case was in a dement, without known antecedent acute infection. Putnam's case was a healthy boy 13 years of age, who had passed through an attack of mumps with apparent recovery for 10 days, when he woke up feeling badly, and complained of a squint in his eye, but followed his usual occupations. Next morning he had a partial ptosis of both lids, but more on the right side, and impairment of motion of the right eye, which turned inward. He also became slightly hard of hearing, complained of pain in the forehead, which developed into intense, persistent headache, and he manifested dulness and drowsiness,

[1] N. Y. Med. Jour., Nov.-Dec., 1896.   [2] Ibid., Dec. 19:
[3] Jour. Nerv. and Ment. Dis., Jan., 1897.   [4] Deutsch. Zeit. f. Nervenheilk. for 1895.

passing into lethargy, from which he could not be aroused. Two days later his temperature was 100°, the paralysis of the eyes and deafness had increased, and he grew steadily worse with delirium; but generally his consciousness was good when he was fairly roused. Sensations of numbness referred to the left arm and leg were complained of, and these limbs were weaker than on the right side, though there was no paralysis. The temperature ranged from 99° to 100°, and pulse from 70 to 90. Ophthalmoscopic examination showed double optic neuritis. He would not respond to questions. The knee-jerks and wrist-jerks were absent on both sides. As far as could be judged, in the comatose condition of the patient, the sensibility of the skin of the entire left side of the body, and the left extremities, was less than on the right. Under expectant treatment, with rather large quantities of nourishment and full doses of strychnin, the case made a gradual recovery. The fever disappeared in about 10 days, but the hearing and sight continued as before. He continued to improve gradually, and 3 months later sight was still defective, with double vision. The boy then had epileptiform attacks, which at first occurred many times during the day, lasting 5 to 15 seconds, with twitching of the right arm and right side of the face. These attacks grew less frequent. About a year after the attack his hearing was practically normal, but the diplopia was still present. The epileptiform seizures had ceased, but there seemed to be some loss of mental vigor. [It will be seen that the symptoms often closely resemble those of meningitis, for which it has no doubt been frequently mistaken. The treatment would be practically the same in either case.]

W. W. Murawjew[1] reported a case to the Neurological Society of Moscow. J. Feinberg[2] reports a case following influenza and terminating favorably, but with persisting slight paresis of the right upper extremity.

Hydrocephalus.—Henle[3] calls attention to a surgical plan introduced by Mikulicz in cases of hydrocephalus, the purpose of which is to secure continuous drainage, at the same time preventing infection. The first case was a child of 6½ months, who had a purulent periostitis of the upper portion of the thigh-bone, from which an acute hydrocephalus developed. In the absence of persistent communication between the ventricles and the subdural spaces Mikuliez introduced a gold tube into one lateral ventricle communicating with the scalp. The purulent cerebrospinal fluid was readily drained, and after 50 c.c. had been withdrawn the scalp was closed over the end of the gold tube, which had been furnished with a plate to prevent its slipping within the cranium. Owing to the suppuration of the stitch-hole the small tube was discharged 25 days later. After 12 days the tube was again introduced in the opposite lateral ventriele, and the fluid evacuated was clear and free from infectious microbes. The child died 6 days later. At the autopsy 2 large abscesses were found in the lower portion of the left hemisphere, one the size of a billiard-ball, the other as large as a walnut. Henle also calls attention to the ease of Troje, reported at the German Surgical Congress of 1893, in which Mikulicz's glass-wool drainage had been similarly introduced into the lateral ventricle. Two years after this operation the drainage remained in place and the child had improved in speech and in gait. The hydrocephalus was trifling in amount and showed no tendency to increase.

[Previous to Mikulicz's first suggestion, as carried out by Troje, a similar operation was devised by L. L. McArthur, of Chicago. A child of 6 months, with subacute hydrocephalus, was operated on in such a manner as to introduce a metallic tube into the descending horn of the lateral ventricle, the tube being

[1] Neurolog. Centralbl., June 1, 1897.   [2] Ibid., July 15, 1897.
[3] Centralbl. f. Chir., Sept. 5, 1896.

fitted with a collar which rested upon the surface of the skull at the margin of the drill-hole which had been used to penetrate the cranium. Improvement in all symptoms promptly appeared. Six months later the corresponding side of the head was reduced in size, but the hydrocephalic condition increased and persisted on the opposite side of the head, apparently from obliteration of Monro's foramen. A second case, in a child of about 4 years, in whom the hydrocephalic condition had reached an extreme degree and the head measured 25 in. in circumference, was similarly operated. This operation was also followed by benefit and disappearance of the convulsions and of the comatóse attacks. A third case of subacute hydrocephalus was operated on by Christian Fenger, of Chicago. Within 3 hours the temperature suddenly ran up to 107° and the child died the same day. The purpose of the operation is to place the ventricular cavities in permanent communication with tissue-spaces from which absorption can readily take place, and avoid a fistulous tract along which infection would be propagated.]

Puncture of the Lateral Ventricle.—Von Beck[1] reports 3 cases of puncture of the lateral ventricle. He maintains that puncture of the ventricle will often be preferable to Quincke's spinal puncture, as in many instances the fluid cannot be withdrawn by the spinal route, while puncture of the ventricle through a small trephine-opening, the needle being introduced into the ventricle through the lateral portion of the cortex, is easily accomplished and presents no greater dangers than spinal puncture.

Large Brain-tumor Successfully Removed from the Left Frontal Region.—Thomas and Keen[2] report the ease of a boy 17 years old, well developed, who presented no symptoms until a few months before the operation, which was done March 27, 1896. He was seen by Drs. Osler and Starr, the latter of whom made the following report:

"The general symptoms and course of the case make it evident that Mr. de B. is suffering from a tumor of the brain. The existence of a right facial paralysis, a thickness of speech, a protrusion of the left eyeball, with greater degree of optic neuritis in the left eye, and very marked change in mental characteristics and mental activity, the hebetude and indisposition to move about, with some decided instability in motion, point to the left frontal lobe as the seat of this tumor. The slowly progressive character of the symptoms, with lack of great variability in their character, and the absence of headache and tenderness on percussion, make it seem probable that the tumor is of a hard, sarcomatous character rather than a vascular glioma, and make it open to operation. Such an operation is necessarily exploratory, and it seems likely that the best point for exploration will be over the second frontal convolution about its middle, the probable situation of the tumor being subcortical within the white matter of the frontal lobe, pressing backward upon the motor tract and upward toward the cortex of the posterior part of the second frontal convolution. It is the absence of epileptic attacks which leads specially to the idea of the tumor being subcortical. If exploratory operation is undertaken, I suggest that the method employed be that of a large bony flap, in order that the surface exposed may be as large as possible. If, after the opening of the dura, nothing is found at the spot indicated, and palpation at the bottom of the deepest fissure accessible fails to reveals any growth, I suggest that the base of the frontal lobe over the orbit be investigated, if possible, by lifting the entire lobe and exploring with the finger beneath. From the fact that destructive lesions of the forward tip of the frontal lobe appear to give rise to few symptoms, I think it would be justifiable to make an incision into the frontal lobe

[1] La Tribune méd., No. 13, 1896.　　　　[2] Am. Jour. Med. Sci., Nov., 1896.

for the purpose of exploring the white matter in case the tumor is not found at either of these two positions."

Finally, after a thorough trial of mercury and iodid had been made without effect, an operation was done and a large tumor removed. Its position corresponded accurately to the expectations, being subcortical, located in the frontal lobe, and protruding through the cortex at a point corresponding to the second frontal convolution. The tumor was $7\frac{1}{2}$ cm. long, $5\frac{1}{2}$ cm. broad, and 4 cm. deep, weighed $2\frac{1}{2}$ oz., and is among the largest that have been removed. It was shelled out without much difficulty, but its lower portion invaded the lateral ventricle, which was widely opened. Subsequently the cavity left by the enucleation of the tumor was packed with gauze which extended into the lateral ventricle. An uneventful recovery occurred, and in view of the fact that the tumor was of a noninfiltrating character, being a firm sarcomatous mass, there is a fair probability of the result being permanently good. [The opening and packing of the lateral ventricle are novel and instructive, showing that even these spaces may be invaded.]

Intracranial Aneurysm.—Macleren[1] reports a case of a domestic servant aged 40, who had been suddenly seized with pain in the left side of the head and left eye, at the same time becoming aware of a rushing noise in the left side of the head. Shortly afterward the eye felt weak and watery and the eyelid swelled. Upon examination the eyeball was found pushed forward, both lids on the left side swollen and edematous, with congestion of the conjunctival vessels and almost complete paralysis of the external rectus, but the pupil was active and vision normal; the fundus and disk were normal. On auscultation a loud systolic bruit was heard over the cranium, extending a short distance down the back of the neck, being loudest over the left temporal region. Upon pressure of the left common carotid the murmur disappeared, and was not influenced by pressure on the right side. Everywhere the arteries were atheromatous, the heart large, and the apex-beat two inches to the left of the middle line. There was considerable albumin in the urine. The common carotid was tied, and improvement began at once; the swelling disappeared slowly, the bruit instantly. Patient was discharged from the hospital seven weeks after the operation, the condition of the eye being then perfect.

Disease of the Anterior Lobe of the Brain.—Durante[2] reports the case of a man who had suffered for some time with pains in the head, which at first were improved by antisyphilitic treatment. Later, prominence of the left parietal region, exophthalmus, and amblyopia appeared, memory was diminished, and the patient became melancholy and unsociable and had hallucinations. Three hard syphilitic gummata were removed from the frontal lobe. The next day vision and memory returned, and eight days later the man's intellectual and moral faculties recovered their normal condition. Six months later he had an attack of Jacksonian epilepsy. The second case was a woman who had loss of memory for words and things, altered moral sense, etc. On operating an adherent fibrous body was found and removed from the frontal lobe. The patient changed as if by magic, and speedily recovered her intellect and moral faculties. [These cases, while reported too briefly to be very valuable, emphasize the importance of moral and mental disturbance as symptoms of lesions of the frontal lobe.]

The Treatment of Cerebral Hemorrhage.—Byron Bramwell[3] points out that at the commencement of the attack of cerebral hemorrhage the first

[1] Brit. Med. Jour., Jan. 2, 1897.
[2] Sup. al Policlinico, Oct. 31, 1896; Brit. Med. Jour., Jan. 2, 1897.
[3] Treatment, July, 1897.

indication is to arrest the bleeding and limit the extravasation. To this end he raises the head and shoulders, places an icebag to the head, warmth to the feet, leeches behind the ears, and gives a drop or two of croton oil to produce a brisk watery evacuation and determine the blood to the intestines. Venesection, bleeding from the temporal artery, compression of the common carotid artery, and ligating the carotid artery on the side of the hemorrhage, are other measures which may be recommended. Bleeding is contraindicated in those cases in which the pulse is feeble, rapid, or weak, the heart dilated or weak, and the patient very old or debilitated. If there is retention of urine, the bladder should be emptied by catheter, and the patient must be kept dry in case of incontinence. The author is doubtful whether any internal remedies have influence in arresting the bleeding. Ergot has been recommended, but it is of no utility. The nitrites, including nitrite of amyl, may be useful in some cases in which the pulse is hard and tense, but venesection is better. Aconite has also been recommended in cases of full, bounding pulse. In cases in which the coma gradually becomes deeper, the pulse slower and slower, the respiration more and more affected, and evidence of progressive hemorrhage is marked, trephining and tapping the hemorrhagic cavity to prevent rupture into the lateral ventricles should be considered. Fortunately, such cases are rarely met with. The second indication is to attend to the condition of the bladder and take means to prevent, if possible, the formation of a bed-sore. The third indication is to sustain the vital powers by appropriate feeding, and, if necessary, by the administration of cardiac tonics and stimulants. If the patient recovers from the state of coma, the next effort is to allay the secondary cerebritis. At this stage the author commences the administration of potassium iodid 5 gr. 3 times a day. If symptoms of secondary cerebritis, consisting in a rise of temperature, headache, muscular twitching, delirium, return of coma, develop, a brisk purge is again administered, an ice-bag applied to the head, and potassium bromid or bromid and chloral added to the iodid. When the secondary cerebritis subsides the bromid and chloral are discontinued, and complete rest is enjoined until the acute changes around the clot have subsided. The author postpones attention to the paralyzed limbs, except such as is necessary for the comfort of the patient, until he has reason to suppose that acute changes have subsided in the neighborhood of the clot—namely, 6 weeks or 2 months. In the recovery of motor control he lays great stress upon the value of frequently repeated systematic voluntary efforts by the patient to use the paralyzed limbs. In the prevention of subsequent attacks a great deal can sometimes be done by removing exciting causes ; blood-pressure should be kept down, sudden efforts, mental excitement, exposures, straining at stool, must be avoided, and a quiet, routine life must be led. The diet should be light and nutritious, and gouty or kidney conditions must be under constant surveillance.

Treatment of the Hemiplegic State.—Archibald Church[1] discusses the treatment of this common condition, urging that in the treatment of a case of hemiplegia, from whatever source arising, the paralytic members should be carefully massaged from the first, and all joints put through their full range of motion, even during the period of coma following the stroke. This is essential to prevent the tendency to joint-changes and the rigidity and limitation of joint-motion which sometimes develop very early, and to maintain the functional sensitiveness of the muscles to any slight cerebral impulses which may reach them. After a week or ten days very decided massage and electric treatment should be used and applied to the muscles which ordinarily are overbalanced in the hemiplegic attitudes. These measures consist principally, in

---

[1] Chicago Med. Recorder, June, 1897.

46

the majority of cases, in faradizing and massaging the extensors of the shoulder, arm, wrist, and fingers, while in the lower extremity attention must be given to prevent foot-drop; the anterior leg-muscles require the most treatment. After the first week or ten days the patient should be encouraged to attempt motion in the paralyzed members, and his courage maintained in the face of apparent helplessness. At this time advantage may be taken of the phenomena of associated movements, and the patient urged and repeatedly encouraged to make double-sided movements, firmly fixing his attention upon the paralyzed side. As movements return in the limbs from above downward, first appearing in shoulders and hips, then in elbows and knees, and last of all in hands and feet, this order should be followed in directing voluntary movements. The erect position and attempts at walking may be advised much earlier than is ordinarily done. It is important to insist early upon the step being taken in a proper manner, and to this end elevation of the toe with light orthopedic apparatus or an elastic band is strongly advised. As soon as secondary rigidity sets in, which takes place in from a few weeks to 3 months after the stroke, the difficulties are greatly increased and progress is much retarded. It is important to secure all possible advantage before this appears, and to delay its appearance as far as possible by the judicious use of massage and electricity. As long as the limbs can be kept supple there is room for hope.

S. Erben[1] teaches the patient the proper position of the feet at each step; then insists upon his duplicating them, instead of merely swinging the paralyzed limb in advance of the sound one and then bringing up the sound foot to or a little in front of the affected one.

Cerebral Syphilis.—Kuh,[2] in a very capable article, discusses the subject of cerebral syphilis. He gives preference to the use of mercury, but believes that the iodid should not be omitted, and prefers inunctions as a means of administering the metal. After a month's use of inunctions the mercury is stopped and iodid substituted, and the inunctions again resumed after another month, with or without the iodid, according to the gravity of the case.

Sunstroke.—Alexander Lambert,[3] in a very admirable article, gives a history of numerous cases of sunstroke, and statistics regarding insolation in New York. Of the utmost importance are the findings of Ira Van Gieson as to changes in the nervous system in 3 of the cases. A fuller report is expected to follow later. Sections were examined from the spinal cord, cerebellum, and various portions of the cerebrum, and all showed more or less pronounced changes in the chromophile plaques of the ganglion-cells. These were sometimes changed in shape and reduced in number, at other times they were broken into fine dust, and in others had entirely disappeared. The nucleus is stained more deeply with methylen-blue than normal, and abnormal spheric granules appear. It is supposed by Van Gieson that these conditions show an acute autointoxication, and that this may be considered the basis of insolation.

Later Results of Fractures of the Skull.—W. N. Bullard[4] reports 70 cases of cranial fracture passing through the Boston City Hospital, the diagnosis depending upon the case-records and evidences in the patient. The fractures occupied the base, frontal, parietal, temporal, and occipital regions, and embraced both sexes and all ages. The time elapsing between the injury and investigation varied from 9 months to 47 years. In 15 of the cases trephining had been done. His conclusions are as follows: 1. Out of 70 persons with fractures of the skull, 37 presented no symptoms when examined some

---

[1] Neurolog. Centralbl., Feb. 1, 1897.   [2] Am. Jour. Insan., Jan., 1897.
[3] Med. News, July 24, 1897.   [4] Boston M. and S. Jour., Apr. 29, 1897.

time later. 2. Seven persons only presented serious symptoms, and in at least 4 of these it is doubtful whether the symptoms were due to the injury. 3. The most frequent consequences found were headache, deafness, dizziness, and inability to resist the action of alcohol on the brain. 4. Out of the 15 cases in which operation (trephining, etc.) was performed, 12 had no symptoms; in 1 it was doubtful whether the symptoms present were due to the injury; in another the symptoms were slight (headache rare, tension over wound while lying in bed); the other was deaf, but had no other trouble. We are justified, therefore, in concluding, so far as our statistics lead, that those cases in which trephining was performed have shown much better results, as far as the symptoms discussed were concerned, than those in which no operation was performed.

Tumor of the Cerebellum.—Thomas, Barker, and Flexner[1] had a patient, a school-teacher of 30, who complained of difficulty in walking, deafness, and difficulty in seeing. The symptoms extended over 3 years, commencing with fainting, and severe headaches brought on by excitement, especially by laughing. The pain was very severe, but was momentary, and there were momentary losses of vision, especially in the left eye and sometimes in both. Difficulty in walking then appeared; at times she staggered as if she were drunk, and finally walking became impossible. There was a tendency to fall to the left and there was some tremor in the legs. She also complained of tingling in the feet and numbness in the nose and mouth; deafness occurred in the left ear, and was subsequently followed by right-sided deafness. There was some slight jerking of the eyeballs, which later became a well-marked nystagmus, increased toward the left. Fields of vision were at first contracted; the colors were seen in their normal order; then vision was lost in the left eye and afterward in the right eye, the neuroretinitis being followed by atrophy. Sensation objectively was undisturbed, and there was no paretic condition aside from that in the eyes. The deep reflexes were active, and as long as she could stand she had a tendency to fall to the left if unsupported. There were also some pain and drawing at the back of the neck, and at times vomiting. A diagnosis was made of tumor involving the corpora quadrigemina. At the autopsy, made by Flexner, the tumor was found occupying the left lobe of the cerebellum, measuring 6x4x4 cm., attached to the periosteum in the floor of the cerebellar fossa. It had exerted lateral pressure on the left corpora quadrigemina, but there was no growth directly into these bodies. The left half of the pons was also flattened almost to the median line, the left crus was pressed upon, and the left superior peduncle of the cerebellum completely flattened. The middle and right lobes of the cerebellum were free from tumor and the effects of direct pressure. Upon microscopic examination the neoplasm was found to be an alveolar sarcoma.

Joseph Collins and G. E. Brewer[2] report a case of subcortical cerebellar tumor, in part removed, with death $2\frac{1}{2}$ months later. The patient was 26 years old, an unmarried laborer, without notable family history or personal antecedents of any significance. On Oct. 20, 1896, headache suddenly developed, the pain being principally in the back part of the head, of a boring, agonizing character, and soon after dizziness occurred, aggravated by movement. In a few weeks the gait was uncertain and staggering. Later on, vomiting occurred repeatedly, and the headaches then became generalized and often were located in the frontal region. When seen he was apathetic, remained in bed, and was disinclined to talk. At that time the special senses were not altered, nor was there any cranial nerve disturbance. The right

[1] Bull. Johns Hopkins Hosp., Nov., 1896.   [2] Med. Record, May 15, 1897.

knee-jerk was lively, the left diminished, and the patient did not hear as acutely in the right ear as in the left: no difference in strength on the two sides of the body, and sensation of touch and position showed no disturbance. There was a moderate degree of choked disk in both eyes, but more marked on the left side. The condition remained unchanged for a month, with the exception that sleeplessness was added. On Feb. 10, 1897, the knee-jerks were very much diminished on both sides, and the gait was simply asthenic. There was some loss of hearing on the right side. A diagnosis, or rather a guess, was made that there was a cerebellar tumor, probably situated subcortically on the right side close to the middle lobe. The patient eagerly accepted operation, and after the dura was opened the cerebellum appeared normal. The finger, however, introduced into the substance of the right lobe a distance of 1¼ in. detected a nodule ¾ in. in diameter. The position of the tumor was quite close to the 4th ventricle and necessitated great care. It was removed by the finger and Volkmann's spoon. The patient's condition became critical, but be rallied, with immediate improvement in all his symptoms. He did not vomit after the operation nor complain of headache. Two months later his eyesight was nearly normal, and he had gained 30 pounds. During this time he presented two peculiar symptoms: a continuous salty taste in the mouth and a notable increase in the secretion of the urine. During the first month he ordinarily passed 100 ounces of urine in 24 hours, and one day passed 196 ounces. He then presented a pleural effusion with slight temperature only. A clear fluid was withdrawn, which upon examination was found negative as to microorganisms. He suddenly failed and became stuporous with fixed pupils. The vomiting recurred and he was in extremis. The symptoms pointed to rapidly increasing intracranial pressure. Under restoratives, but without an anesthetic, the wound was opened and showed a comparatively healthy condition. The finger carried into the substance of the cerebellum impinged upon a large hard mass, irregular in outline and firmly fixed. A gentle effort was made to get the finger beneath it, when instantly the patient stopped breathing and was dead. Upon postmortem examination 24 hours later the right cerebellar hemisphere was found about one-fourth smaller than the left and in its substance, in close proximity to the ventral surface, in the neighborhood of the vernis, there was a hard, irregular mass, the same that had been felt on the operating-table. It measured when removed 4.5 cm. in length, this diameter lying transversely in the brain; 3.5 cm. in width, anteroposteriorly; 2.5 cm. in thickness. It was irregular in form and almost fibroid in hardness. When laid open it was a pale yellowish caseous-looking mass, and was in every respect, as well as by subsequent proving, a tubercle. The ventricles of the cerebral hemispheres were distended and enlarged, containing a corresponding amount of fluid, due apparently to the pressure of the tumor upon the lower exit of the ventricular passages. [This case is interesting as showing the ability of surgery to invade the cerebellum and actually remove a tumor, or a portion of a tumor, as it is not clear whether the mass removed was a part of the larger growth subsequently found or an independent mass. The immediate improvement after the removal of the tumor was also of the most satisfying nature, and life might have been continued for an indefinite time, as far as the intracranial condition was concerned. It is possible that the active interference served to rapidly increase the tuberculoma and led to internal hydrocephalus and death. At the postmortem extensive tubercular changes in the pleural cavity and in the lungs were also detected. This case, with perhaps the exception of that reported by Stewart and Anandale, is the only one in which a cerebellar tumor has been removed without

early fatal termination, though a number of cerebellar cysts have been evacuated with immediate and permanent benefit.]

Agusto Murri,[1] in a report to the Medico-Chirurgica Society of Bologna, describes the clinical history of a youth of 17 who presented the majority of symptoms of cerebellar tumor. An operation was done by Dr. G. Bendani, who extracted from the left half of the cerebellum a part of the tumor, which the microscope showed to be fibrosarcomatous. Total removal was impossible. One month later the boy was still alive and rather better than worse.

Cerebellar Hemorrhage.—Robert E. Peck[2] gives an account of 4 cases of this rather rare accident, and tabulates the symptoms in these 4 cases and in 20 others published in the literature. The most constant symptoms occurring in this outline were: vomiting, 55 %; paralysis, 45 %; headache, 30 %; vertigo, 35 %. The headache was usually occipital, sometimes severe, generally preceding the onset of the more serious symptoms by a longer or shorter period varying from a few days to several weeks, and in one instance there was severe headache for 2 months prior to the attack. Paralysis occurred in 9 out of 20 cases. In 4 cases it was confined to the left side, in 2 cases to the right side, opposite the lesion. In one instance the upper extremities were free and the lower limbs paralyzed. Unconsciousness is an inconstant condition which developed in all but 4 cases at some time before death; in 3 cases the patients were semicomatose, and in 1 instance the patient remained conscious to the end.

Huntington's Chorea.—J. Mitchell Clarke[3] gives the history of an instance of this family affection, and reports postmortem examinations upon 2 cases. He sums up the morbid changes as consisting " in a widespread but partial degeneration of the cells of the cerebral cortex, especially the cells of the second and third layers, most marked in the frontal and motor convolutions, together with an increased amount of interstitial tissue and number of neuroglia-cells."

DISEASES OF THE SPINAL MENINGES AND SPINAL NERVES.

Ascending Degeneration of the Nerves and the Changes in the Nerve-cells Consequent Thereon.—Fleming[4] first goes over the contributions to this subject. The differences of opinion which have been expressed he attributes some to the manner of operating upon the peripheral nerves and others to the technic employed. In his own series of experiments he used boiled water only, rejecting all antiseptics. He rejects all cases in which union was not by first intention, thus avoiding infection-cases and the changes of the nerve dependent upon it. He also calls attention to the differentiation of nerve inflammation and the Wallerian degeneration. His results were, briefly, that in the process set up by division or ligation of a nerve there was a slight atrophy of motor fibres, with certain sensory fibres degenerating centrally, possibly because separated from their peripheral trophic cells; that the minute fibres found in a normal nerve undergo very marked change; that a distinctive connective-tissue increase occurs. By comparing the normal with the operated side he was able to check up his findings, many of which he was thus able to distinguish as mainly artificial.

In the cells he noted the following changes: " 1. The cells of the ganglia on the posterior nerve-roots undergo definite changes as the result of nerve section or ligation, and do so at a much earlier period than the multipolar cells

[1] Lancet, Jan. 30, 1897.
[3] Brain, 1897.
[2] Yale Med. Jour., June, 1897.
[4] Brit. Med. Jour., Oct. 3, 1896.

in the cord—beginning probably as early as the fourth day, and certainly by the seventh day. 2. That one of the very first changes observed in the cells of the ganglia and the anterior cornu is a diminution in the size of the nucleus, in proportion to the size of the cell, and that sometimes, but not in all cases, nucleoli also become smaller, and very frequently the nuclei take up an eccentric position, sometimes even bulging the cell-wall. 3. That in both sets of cells Nissl's granules, otherwise known as the chromatic granules, are either smaller in size, fewer in number, and scattered through the cell-body, tending to be most numerous round the nucleus; or else they are grouped together in large masses round the nucleus, leaving the periphery of the cell quite clear. 4. That pericellular lymph-spaces may become enlarged, especially in the ganglion-cells; and where the enlargement is very marked the cells become proportionately smaller in size, although an actual atrophy may also occur. In several of my specimens I found large vacuoles; not the vacuoles described by many writers as occurring in the cells of the cord and cerebral cortex, which are probably to some extent artificial, but big vacuoles, more resembling distended pericellular lymph-spaces. They differ, however, inasmuch as they are surrounded by the remains of cell-protoplasm containing chromatic granules. 5. That in the multipolar cells not merely are there changes in position and size of nuclei, and in arrangements and number of chromatic granules, but there is, as a later phenomenon, marked disintegration of cell-protoplasm, well seen in some of my specimens. This disintegration has been described by Marinesco as occurring in certain cord-lesions in man. It consists of patches, which with toluidin-blue and eosin are whitish in color and surrounded by masses of chromatic granules.

"In no case did I find any evidence of degeneration in the anterior roots, and I wish to hold over the description of the posterior roots till the full details of my experiments are published, as it would add greatly to the length of this paper. The abdominal sympathetic ganglia show also changes similar in certain respects, but of them I cannot yet speak with confidence. The diminution in size of the nuclei is a point not previously recorded, and yet it is a result upon which it is possible to count with considerable certainty. If, however, there is any inflammation, pus, etc., at the site of lesion, the nuclei may swell up, becoming greatly distended. This appearance is by no means common in my experiments. When examining the cord of a case of peripheral neuritis in which the one arm was much more paralyzed than the other, the nerve-cells in the anterior cornu on the affected side showed diminished size of nucleus and cells as compared with those on the less affected side, and the whole nucleus had a crenated appearance. It is extremely interesting to find the same changes in the multipolar cells in at least one case of peripheral neuritis as after experimental ligation or section. [The importance of this line of investigation and its bearing on the cord-changes in peripheral neuritides, so called, and in the genesis of posterior scleroses of the cord, cannot be overestimated.]

The same author[1] gives a detailed report of 2 cases of peripheral neuritis terminating fatally, in which he found the following spinal changes: "The tracts of white matter show practically nothing. The nerve-cells in the cord, although fixed in Müller's fluid, and therefore not so capable of showing nuclear changes, still demonstrate certain interesting facts, because the multipolar cells on the two sides of the cord show distinct differences. On the left side the cells are practically the nerve-cells of a normal specimen hardened in Müller's fluid. On the right side we find great shrinking of the cells as a

---

[1] Brain, 1897.

whole. The nuclei are much smaller, and in place of having a distinctly rounded contour their outline is jagged and totally irregular. On the left side the cells show a clear, distinct nucleolus and endonucleolus, and a rich, refractile chromatin network. On the right side the nucleus stains more deeply and homogeneously, the nucleolus is with difficulty made out, and it is sometimes impossible to distinguish the endonucleolus. There are one or two healthy cells in each cell-group of the right anterior horn; there are rather larger numbers of degenerated cells on one side, and the apparently normal cells on the other are quite characteristic. A nilin blue-black reveals further that the affected cells possess fewer processes."

Brauer[1] discusses a case of fatal multiple neuritis occurring in a syphilitic patient treated by mercury. The only cause for the neuritis was the syphilis and the mercurial poisoning. The author is inclined to attribute it mainly to the mercury, in spite of the rarity of such action, but thinks the specific poisoning contributed to the wide involvement of nerves. [We have seen a case of multiple neuritis caused by quarter-grain doses of the green iodid given t. i. d. for several months immediately get well upon the discontinuance of the mercury.]

Erythromelalgia.—Contrary to the views of Nonne, Dehio[2] considers that erythromelalgia is a special disease with a special pathology of its own. He believes that the hand- and foot-symptoms in his case were due to lesion of the lumbar and cervical portions of the spinal cord, but limits it to the posterior horn of the gray matter. Headache, dizziness, vomiting, and facial symptoms he attributes to intracranial lesion. He thinks the disease is central rather than peripheral, and may be gliomatous in nature.

Henry L. Elsner[3] reports a case of this disease in which Raynaud's condition was clearly present, and resulted in amputation of the thumb by dry gangrene. The author calls attention to the rarity of the association of these two conditions, and to the fact that despite the absolute independence of them, as asserted by Mitchell and others, they may be combined and the differential diagnosis rendered difficult or impossible. T. W. Prentice[4] reports 2 cases in women, in both of which the hands were affected, and in one of which the thumb was at one time so cyanotic as to lead to the fear of gangrene. Both patients were of a neurotic temperament, and other evidences of general nervous instability were present. [The majority of writers are inclined to follow Mitchell in his later expressions that in this condition we are dealing with one of the many phases of polyneuritis.]

Paralysis following Anesthesia.—An editorial[5] calls attention to the palsies that follow anesthesia, and to the article of Vautrin read at the meeting of the French Medical Congress of 1896, in which he related 3 cases of post-anesthetic palsy, one involving the deltoid, biceps, and brachialis anticus; another involving the deltoid and the long supinator, and a third affecting the face. It is usually the right brachial plexus that seems to be affected, but the face and tongue may be affected, accompanied by ocular troubles, such as dilatation of the pupil, amaurosis, etc. The palsy is sometimes noticed immediately after waking from the anesthesia, or it may be several hours or days afterward. These palsies come on irrespective of the anesthetic employed. Two forms are recognized—one peripheral, the other central in origin; the first being the more frequent and the arm the part usually affected. They are to be attributed to pressure on the brachial plexus, especially when the arm is elevated to facilitate operations on the breast and abdomen. Traction on the shoulder in arti-

[1] Berlin. klin. Woch., Mar. 29, 1897. [2] Ibid., No. 37, 1896.
[3] Med. News, June 19, 1897. [4] Med. Rec., July 10, 1897.
[5] Ibid., Oct. 17, 1896.

ficial respiration may have the same effect. Vautrin also suggests that other cases may be due to the toxic conditions provoked by long anesthesia. The palsies of central origin are due to cerebral accidents, especially hemorrhages, which are favored by the struggles of the patient during the period of excitement. Garrigues[1] reports 5 cases of paralysis following anesthetics, in his service, adds 9 cases from the paper of Buedinger,[2] and refers to Vautrin's paper. [The writer has recently seen a case of sciatica due to the lithotomy position employed for two hours in a hysterectomy operation, with weakness in the leg and some loss of sensation about the toes, and a large amount of pain. The most sensitive point was at the sciatic notch and behind the neck of the femur.]

Intradural Section of the Spinal Nerves for Neuralgia.—Abbe[3] collected 7 cases of this operation, 3 of which were by himself, and from these cases he draws the following conclusions : a comparatively new and interesting field of work is opened by these few cases. Thus far, even in weak patients, the operation has been devoid of risk. It is sound in theory, and has yielded enough results to show that it may become a meritorious operation. It should be resorted to early in cases of ascending neuritis, which have heretofore been subjected to successive nerve-stretching and resection and finally amputation, uniformly without benefit. The experimental and practical evidence shows that two additional roots higher up than the apparent origin of pain should be included. There ought to be no risk in severing the posterior roots of the third and fourth cervical, as well as those to the brachial plexus, simply because they supply the phrenic, inasmuch as that needs motor supply only, and at best it has the opposite phrenic in reserve.

Meralgia, or Paresthesia of the External Femoral Region.—John C. Shaw[4] reports 3 cases, giving diagrams of the paresthetic areas. These cases conform closely to those of Roth and Bernhardt. He points out that advanced age, or at least middle life, has some relation to the condition. As a rule, one leg only is affected ; but it may be both. Bernhardt considered the symptoms due to degenerative neuritis of the external cutaneous, and was inclined to attribute it to infection and toxic states. It has been suggested by others that it might be due to compression of the nerve by the fascia as it emerges from the pelvis. For this claim there is no foundation. It is increased by awkward positions during the attacks of tingling, but not otherwise. Roth attributes it to disorders of the venous circulation of the nerve, but this does not explain the selection of this particular nerve. The author is inclined to attribute it to toxic infectious causes, in spite of the fact that, as a rule, it has a unilateral distribution. Osler[5] proposes the term paresthesia meralgia. T. H. Benda[6] reports a case that complained of this disturbance in the distribution of the external cutaneous nerve for over 30 years. C. Dopter[7] reports a case. He thinks that in some cases, at least, neuralgia and neuritis may both be excluded, and attributes the condition to congestion of the veins in and about the nerve, as was first suggested by Roth.

DISEASES OF THE CORD PROPER.

Syringomyelia.—Hinsdale[8] furnishes an essay on this subject which re-

[1] Am. Jour. Med. Sci., Jan., 1897.   [2] Arch. f. klin. Chir., 1894.
[3] Boston M. and S. Jour., Oct. 1, 1896.   [4] N. Y. Med. Jour., Feb. 13, 1897.
[5] Jour. Nerv. and Ment. Dis., Mar., 1897.   [6] Neurolog. Centralbl., Mar. 15, 1897.
[7] Gaz. hebdom. de Med. et Chir., June 12, 1897.
[8] Internat. Med. Mag., Dec., 1896, and Jan., 1897.

ceived the Alvarenga Prize for 1895. It contains a bibliography of 514 references, and is the most complete *résumé* of the subject available to the English reader. It is also published as a monograph.

Dercum and Spiller[1] report a case of syringomyelia limited to one posterior horn in the cervical region, with arthropathy of the shoulder-joint and ascending degeneration of the pyramidal tracts. This is a case reported upon several times, and appears as an illustration in a number of books. The confirmation of the diagnosis by autopsy, with exact lesions, makes it a valuable one.

Astie[2] calls attention to the **boat-shaped deformity of the thorax** which has been met with in some cases of syringomyelia. It consists in a characteristic depression of the central portion of the anterior wall of the chest above the lower margins of the pectoral muscles, on either side of which the chest-wall rises, so that the shoulders appear to be brought forward. This depression has no resemblance to any hitherto-described deformity, and is not a consequence of atrophy of the pectoral muscles nor of scoliosis, but seems to be a trophic lesion analogous to those in other parts of the skeleton. It does not cause any functional trouble. He gives 4 cases, illustrated by photographs.

G. Marinesco[3] calls attention to the vasomotor disturbance of syringomyelia, with especial emphasis upon edema of the hands, for which he uses the somewhat fantastic designation of *main succulente*.

At a *séance* of the Société médicale des Hôpitaux de Paris, Feb. 12, 1897,[4] Marinesco and Jeanselme presented a report on 3 cases of Morvan's disease, with autopsies. Marinesco's report was on a case frequently used by Charcot in illustration of his lectures. Jeanselme reported the necropsies of 2 cases in Bretagne, where Morvan first recognized the disease. In all 3 cases cavities occupying the region of the gray matter of the cord were found, while careful examinations for the bacillus of leprosy and other forms of bacterial life, both in the cord and in the peripheral lesions, were negative.

Progressive Muscular Atrophy of the Duchenne Aran Type.— J. B. Charcot, son of the late Professor J. M. Charcot, in a brochure entitled *A Contribution to the Study of Progressive Muscular Atrophy of the Duchenne-Aran Type*, Paris, 1895, takes up the controversy between those who discard the autonomy of this type and the classical teaching of his father on the subject. He is enabled by searching the literature and by bringing forward the material at his disposal in La Salpêtrière to produce two or three cases only in which the lesion was confined with practical completeness to the anterior horn. [It must be evident to one who is not wedded to special names for diseases that the contention is one of words and not of conditions. The progressive atrophies showing spinal lesions take on the pure atrophic atonic wasting, or the spastic tonic atrophy, as the anterior gray is primarily affected or is affected secondarily, in point of time, to the pyramidal tracts. The process practically is one and the same, usually reaching from the motor cortex to the muscular terminals, and it is conceivable that in some cases it may be limited to the lower motor neuron, producing the so-called Duchenne-Aran type. Involvement of the pyramidal tract, if occurring early enough to produce symptoms through the lower motor neuron, gives rise to the amyotrophic lateral sclerosis variety.]

Treatment of Progressive Muscular Dystrophy by Physical Exercise.—Alfred Wiener[5] reports a case that appears to be one of the myopathic dystrophies, in which great benefit followed persistent exercises calcu-

---

[1] Am. Jour. Med. Sci., Dec., 1896.   [2] Thèse de Paris, No. 225, 1896–97.
[3] Nouv. Icon. de la Salpêt., Mar. and Apr., 1897.   [4] Med. News, Mar. 27, 1897.
[5] Am. Jour. Med. Sci., Oct., 1896.

lated to develop the muscles which had wasted and were greatly weakened. After two years of exercise-treatment the man was able to execute readily every possible muscular motion, but still showed weakness in some of the groups, and the wasting, while it had improved, had not entirely disappeared. The muscles of the face had not improved, and these were the only ones that had not been exercised. The lordosis was lessened and the scapulæ projected less, the patient being able to put on his coat, collar, and shirt without assistance, which he formerly was unable to do. He could turn about in bed and walk great distances without exertion, and was able to ride 40 miles on a bicycle in one day. The gait, formerly waddling, had become normal. The author urges others to try this line of treatment, and expresses the hope that some of these cases are not inherently beyond improvement.

Epidemic of Acute Poliomyelitis.—Altmann[1] gives an account of 14 cases occurring within 2 months, only 1 isolated case having appeared in the community 8 years previously. In 2 instances 2 members of the same family were attacked in rapid succession. Pasteur[2] reported an epidemic of poliomyelitis in 7 children in one family. [The reader is also referred to the Vermont epidemic reported by Caverly, and outlined in the Year-Book for 1897.]

Pernicious Anemia and the Spinal Cord.—In special literature during the last two or three years a great deal has appeared regarding the spinal cord in cases of pernicious anemia. Lichtheim was the first contributor. Nonne examined 17 cases, in 7 of which the findings in the spinal cord were negative, in 3 lesions were clearly defined in the neighborhood of vessels, and in 7 there were spinal cord lesions of pronounced character. These he attributod to vascular disturbance, either hemorrhagic or by diffusion, similar to the changes which appear in the retina in some cases of pernicious forms of anemia. C. Eugene Riggs[3] reports a case at some length, and furnishes illustrations of cross-sections of the cord at every segmental level from the first cervical to the fifth lumbar (Plates 5, 6). The clinical history of the case is rather meager, but indicates a pronounced anemia. Unfortunately, there is no statement of the condition of the brain aside from the fact that the arteries of the circle of Willis showed thickening of the middle coat. In the spinal cord he noted degenerations in the anterior pyramidal tract, the direct cerebellar tract, the crossed pyramidal tract, the column of Lissauer, the column of Burdach, the posterior external field of the posterior column, and the column of Goll. All other columns were normal throughout their entire extent. The gray matter appeared normal throughout. The arteries wherever present showed thickening of the endothelium, and here and there an inward projecting growth of new connective tissue. [Clinically these cases sometimes present symptoms which lead to their being mistaken for locomotor ataxia or multiple neuritis. A close examination should enable the physician to exclude both of these conditions, and if he is aware of the association of cord-lesions of the indiscriminate vascular type with the pernicious anemias, it will not be difficult to clear the diagnosis]

K. Petran[4] in 9 cases of pernicious anemia found changes in the nervous apparatus in all. Teichmueller[5] reports a case of pernicious anemia with arteriosclerosis, paresthesia, chronic enteritis, and increased knee-jerk. Postmortem, small hemorrhages were found in the corpora striata and corpora quadrigemina. Microscopic examination revealed such changes as have been described by others, especially by Nonne, in the posterior columns, and

---

[1] Australas. Med. Gaz., Apr. 24, 1897.   [2] Brit. Med. Jour., 1897.
[3] Internat. Med. Mag., Sept., 1896.   [4] Nordiskt Medicinskt Arkiv, No. 7, 1896.
[5] Deutsch. Zeit. f. Nervenheil., viii., H. 5 u. 6 ; Am. Jour. Med. Sci., Feb., 1897.

PLATE 5.

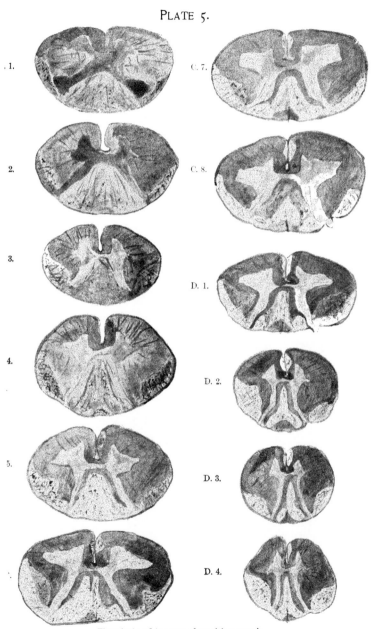

The spinal cord in a case of pernicious anemia.
(Int. Med. Mag., Sept., 1896).

PLATE 6.

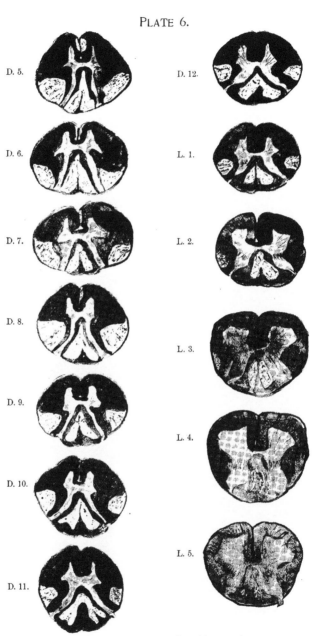

D. 5.

D. 6.

D. 7.

D. 8.

D. 9.

D. 10.

D. 11.

D. 12.

L. 1.

L. 2.

L. 3.

L. 4.

L. 5.

The spinal cord in a case of pernicious anemia
(Int. Med. Mag., Sept., 1896).

hemorrhages in the anterior and lateral columns as well as in the gray matter. The author does not believe that these changes constitute a combined-system disease, but attaches much importance to the lesion of the gray matter. Bastianelli[1] reports a case marked by clinical evidences of disturbance in the lateral columns, especially by increased reflexes and some loss of power, in which changes were found in the posterior lateral columns, but none in the gray substance. In a second case spinal symptoms antedated the recognition of the pernicious anemia. A third case presented changes in the gray substance of the cord in addition to the posterolateral variations.

M. Nonne[2] investigated the changes in the nervous system, especially in the cord, consecutive to splenic **leukocythemia.** From the literature he finds that 2 cases have been reported in which there were changes in the cranial nerves. These were reported by Eisenlohr and Müller, who found multiple hemorrhages in the sheath and substance of the nerves, with lymphoid elements similar to those found in other organs in this disease. Kast and Alt have also reported 2 cases in which paralysis on the part of the cranial nerves was due to changes in their nuclei in the medulla. Aside from the 2 cases reported by Nonne in this connection, Müller has reported a case in which there was a slight sclerosis of Goll's and Burdach's columns in the upper portion of the cord in a case of splenic leukocythemia. Nonne's first case was a man 59 years old, who presented an enormous splenic tumor and great enlargement of the liver, with the usual blood-count and all the clinical features of splenic leukocythemia. He showed no symptoms on the part of the nervous system, but at the autopsy, and subsequently, Nonne found in the dorsal and cervical cord, and also in the lumbar cord, small spots of acute myelitic changes in the nerve-substance, confined to the white portion of the cord, the gray substance being entirely spared. The roots, ganglia, and meninges were normal. In the cervical cord there was a clearly marked sclerosis of Goll's columns. In the second case, a male of 31, with well-marked clinical evidence of splenic leukocythemia but who presented no objective symptoms on the part of the nervous system, similar spots of myelitic softening were found, particularly in the direct and crossed motor tracts. In this case there was no sclerosis of Goll's or Burdach's columns. Nonne suggests that the changes in leukemia are considerably like those in pernicious anemia, to which subject he has already made notable contributions, and he expects similar changes in other fatal anemias. He believes it likely that the majority of cases of splenic leukocythemia will present these changes, just as is the case in pernicious anemia, with or without clinical symptoms of involvement of the nervous apparatus. A plate showing the areas of the cord involved and the microscopic character of the myelitic spots, as well as the sclerotic portions of the cord, accompanies the article.

Dr. Abrams[3] had a patient who had Hodgkin's disease and locomotor ataxic symptoms. [The ataxic symptoms were probably due to the cord-changes secondary to the leukemia.] J. Michell Clarke[4] reports two cases, in one of which the changes in the cord were confined to the white matter, especially the posterior columns with a small tract of degeneration in one lateral column. In the other case the gray matter was notably involved.

Toxic Lesions of the Posterior Column of the Spinal Cord.— Redlich[5] gives a *résumé* of the spinal lesions in various intoxications associated with psychoses of different sorts, epileptiform attacks, and phenomena

[1] Bull. del R. Accad. Med. di Roma, xxii., 1895–96.
[2] Deutsch. Zeit. f. Nervenheil., H. 3, Bd. 10.   [3] Med. Rec., Aug. 7, 1897.
[4] Brit. Med. Jour., Aug. 7, 1897.   [5] Centralbl. f. Allg. Path., Dec. 15, 1896.

resembling those of tabes. In ergotism the principal lesions found were sclerosis of the posterior roots and posterior columns. In pellagra, due to the eating of spoiled maize, the lesions were those of combined sclerosis of the posterior and lateral portions of the cord, or practically the posterior half of the cord, and were most intense at the upper levels, gradually diminishing below. Neither the posterior roots nor gray matter was involved. The symptoms are paralytic and spastic, with disturbance of sensation, ataxia, and contracted pupils. In chronic intoxications, polyneuritis and lesions of the posterior columns of the cord are also met with, and the author gives a number of instances of the latter affection dependent upon alcohol, etc., in which sclerosis of the posterior columns was found. The relation of the spinal lesion to the peripheral affection in the nerves, according to Redlich, is a coördinate one, some agents acting on the peripheral nerves and the posterior root-system of the cord at the same time. The changes in the cord due to pernicious anemia present a number of lesions, from which Redlich draws the conclusion that grave anemias of different origin may produce cord-lesions. These are focal degenerations in the posterior columns, which may lead to descending degeneration of the posterior roots, and the fibres of gray matter may escape. The process is indiscriminate, and inclined to affect the cervical cord more than the other portions. The anemia is the indirect cause of the change, which is due, apparently, to toxic substances circulating in the blood. [It thus appears that from a variety of poisons arising from within the body or absorbed from extraneous sources, and from a number of blood-states, sclerotic processes of systemic or indiscriminate distribution may be set up in the cord.]

Myelopathia due to Acute Endarteritis.—E. Biernacki[1] gives the full history and complete anatomic investigations in 3 cases that presented the clinical appearance of acute transverse myelitis. In all 3, under a proper technic, acute softening was found variously distributed in white portions of the cord, in most instances in the shape of triangular infarcts with the base toward the pia, and, most important of all, in all cases in anatomic association with such foci there was found an obliterating pial endarteritis the starting-point of the cord-lesion, in two instances apparently attributable to syphilis, in one, without known cause unless due to exposure to cold. [That acute myelitis is frequently due to endarteritis, and is in effect a thrombotic softening, there can be no doubt. Even embolism may act in this way, as shown by the following:] Prof. Singer[2] found, through the injection of embolic substances into the vertebral arteries, that he could produce in the cervical and upper cord a cross-myelitis corresponding in all particulars to the clinical type.

Lumbar Puncture.—Furbringer[3] notes a case in which lumbar puncture several times repeated secured no fluid, although there was every evidence of intracranial distention. The autopsy showed tuberculosis at the base of the brain, with great ventricular dilatation. The base of the brain was converted into a gelatinous and very edematous mass, which extended into the spinal canal, filling the dura and completely plugging the passages. [It is not unlikely that this condition will be found with considerable frequency in tubercular meningitis of the base, the usual location. It is also well recognized that disease of this character may obstruct the passage from the ventricles into the subarachnoid spaces, and consequently lumbar puncture will fail to secure fluid from the intracerebral chambers. The importance of lumbar puncture, from a diagnostic standpoint, must be limited to the cases in which positive evidences are obtained. In such instances the value and practicability of ventricular puncture

¹ Deutsch. Zeit. f. Nervenh., H. 3, Bd. 10.   ² Deutsch. Zeit. f. Heilk., Bd. 17, 1897.
³ Deutsch. med. Woch., No. 45, 1895.

should be kept in mind. Ventricular puncture in one case at St. Luke's Hospital, under the writer's care, furnished tubercle-bacilli, where no fluid could be obtained by the spinal method.]

Tumors of the Spinal Cord.—L. Bruns[1] records 2 cases of spinal tumors, with operation. The first case was a woman of 24, of good heredity. She first complained of pains in the region of the sacrum, radiating into the lower members and into the hypogastrium. Paraplegic symptoms followed, corresponding to a lesion appearing to be located at the junction of the dorsal and lumbar cord, and later the lumbar enlargement seemed to be invaded, the bladder and rectum being paralyzed. A diagnosis was made of fibrosarcoma of the spinal cord beginning in the pia mater and the arches of the right side of the lumbar enlargement, finally compressing the cord from the fifth lumbar pair to the last dorsal segment. Operation followed. No tumor was found. Fourteen months later the patient died, and at autopsy multiple sarcomas of the meninges and of the spinal roots were discovered, especially in the lumbar cord. The tumors penetrated the pia mater along the roots and invaded the cord-substance. The entire lumbar cord was transformed into a compact sarcomatous tumor as large as a small apple and the sarcomatous degeneration extended along the pia mater and the roots as high as the middle of the dorsal cord.

The second case was a man of 18, without heredity, who had already undergone several operations for tumors, teratoma of the abdominal cavity, sarcomas of the subclavicular glands and of the testicle. Cutting-pains developed near the left nipple, and total motor and sensory paraplegia followed, extending to this level. A metastatic tumor of the meninges, located between the 3d and 4th dorsal roots, with extension to the 2d dorsal pair, was the diagnosis made. Operation discovered a tumor outside the dura mater, surrounding the posterior portion of the cord, involving the roots of the 2d to 5th pairs. Partial extirpation was accomplished. Much blood was lost, and the patient died the same day. Upon examination postmortem the tumor was found to extend to the 5th and 6th dorsal roots, and at the point where it exerted most pressure extended around the cord to the posterior surface of the vertebral bodies. The anterior surface of the dura mater was not invaded. The tumor was found to be a metastatic sarcoma located in the extradural fat, the internal surface of the dura mater, the pia mater, and the cord being intact as far as tumor-infiltration was concerned. The spinal cord was completely softened and practically divided for the length of $1\frac{1}{2}$ cm. at the point of greatest compression, and was much diseased between the 2d and 7th dorsal segments. The lumbar cord was normal except for descending degenerations in the pyramidal tracts.

Joseph Collins and G. W. Blanchard[2] describe a case of tumor of the spinal pia at the first cervical segment, which during life was considered a case of cervical pachymeningitis. The symptoms, briefly recapitulated, were as follows: 1. Pain, at the onset, in the back of the neck, later extending into the side of the face and into the upper extremities, and later into the lower extremities. 2. In the beginning the pain was continuous, and of a dull, irritating character; later it occurred paroxysmally, and was of a lancinating nature. 3. A feeling of tension and spasticity in the cephalic extremity, and, to a less degree, in the upper extremities, more particularly in the left arm. 4. Progressive loss of strength in the left upper extremity, and, to a less degree, in the left lower extremity. 5. Exaggeration of the deep reflexes. In the beginning this exaggeration was of the left side alone, but later increased myotatic irritability was universal. 6. Progressive flaccidity of the parts

[1] Arch. f. Psychiat., Bd. 28, H. 1, 1896. [2] Med. News, July 10, 1897.

which had previously shown a state of tension or spasticity. 7. Progressive and uncontrollable diarrhea. 8. Symptoms referable to deranged intracranial circulation, pressure, and delirium. During the delirium the patient died, apparently of exhaustion, and the autopsy was held within a few hours. On opening the spinal canal nothing noteworthy was encountered until the pia was reached. This was found to be distended, and upon puncture in the dorsal region a considerable quantity of clear fluid escaped. The distention subsided. Some small white calcareous flakes were found in the dorsal and lumbar regions. On opening the skull and upper portion of the spinal canal a tumor of the pia was found lying upon the cord from the upper margin of the foramen magnum downward 2.1 cm. It was about 2 cm. in its widest measurement. The tumor had the appearance of a sarcoma, was dark reddish in color, and very firm to the touch. Upon microscopic examination it showed the structure of a spindle-celled sarcoma with very large blood-vessels and evidence of small hemorrhages from the degenerated vessels. Foci of cheesy degeneration were also found. The cervical cord at the point which had been subjected to pressure showed degeneration in the crossed pyramidal tracts and the posterior columns.

W. E. Cladek [1] reports a case in which the symptoms were for a long time misleading and obscure. Rather suddenly, he lost power in the lower extremities, with rectal and vesical incontinence, sensation was dulled, and he gradually sank and died 6 months after the original injury, having lost sensation and motion from the waist down. A bedsore had formed. On opening the spinal canal the arches of the vertebræ were found softened, and a growth covering the dura, from which it seemed to spring, completely filled the spinal canal and crowded out through the spinal openings. The growth extended from the second lumbar to the ninth dorsal vertebra, and the cord was not directly involved except by pressure, no adhesions being present. The growth proved to be a spindle-celled sarcoma.

Spinal Hemorrhages in the Newborn.—Schäffer [2] makes report upon cases observed in the Heidelburg clinic. In 100 autopsies of newborn infants he found that 1 in every 10 had blood extravasated in the vertebral canal, while cerebral extravasations were twice as frequent. In 17 cases the vertebral hemorrhage followed the use of forceps or extraction by the breech. Some of the children perished at birth, others at varying periods subsequent to birth ; 64 of the children died of birth-injury. He observed that premature children most often sustained birth-injury, while those born at term developed the postpartum diseases. The most frequent location for the bleeding was in the cervical and dorsal regions, less frequently in the neighborhood of the medulla and in the lumbar cord. He believes that Schultze's manipulations in asphyxiated children may cause spinal hemorrhage. [The etiologic relation of such hemorrhages to spastic paralyses and to syringomyelia has been affirmed by many writers.]

Caisson-disease.—A. Hoche [3] describes 2 cases of spastic paraplegia following exposure in caisson-work in the building of the Rhine bridge at Kehl. He then proceeds to the discussion of the disease, with a review of the literature on the subject, and accepts the gas-theory as set up by Catsaras, and experimentally proved by him, as well as by P. Vert. He speaks of the congestion-theory, ordinarily emphasized by American and English writers only to condemn it. When a large amount of gas occurs in the aorta the passage of such gaseous collection into the pulmonary circulation may terminate in

[1] N. Y. Med. Jour., Aug. 14, 1897.   [2] Arch. f. Gynäk., Bd. liii., H. 2, 1897.
[3] Berlin. klin. Woch., May 31, 1897.

PLATE 7.

1

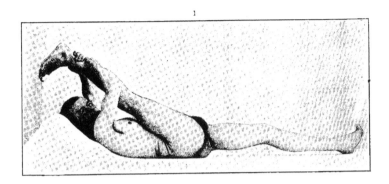

2

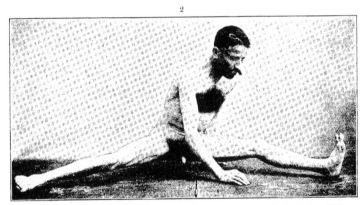

Unusual range of motion in tabes hypotonus (Nouv. Icon. de la Salp., July and Aug., 1896).

sudden death, and this occasionally occurs in the history of caisson-disease. In the same way it may produce fatal cerebral conditions. The tendency of the gas-emboli to absorption explains the temporary manifestations in lighter cases. The gas that is produced by the removal of increased pressure in the blood is mainly nitrogen, but oxygen and carbox dioxid are also thus liberated, and may separately or in combination act as emboli. He accounts for the usual gradual onset of symptoms by the progressive liberation of the gases. Incidentally he speaks of the liability of employers for injuries of this character arising through neglect to take sufficient time in passing the men through the locks, as it has been very fairly proved that time proportionate to the numbers of atmospheres of difference will protect against accidents arising from the change in air-pressure. Snell [1] also adopts the gas-theory, but thinks carbon dioxid is probably the pernicious agent, and lays much stress on the ventilation of such works.

Joint-changes in Locomotor Ataxia without Arthropathies.— Frenkel and Maurice Faure,[2] in a beautifully illustrated article, give the results of their investigations into the range of joint-motion in locomotor ataxia, and find that, as a rule, all joints have an increased range of extension and flexion, more especially of extension. They selected 33 cases of tabes, and afterward compared with them a number of cases of hysteria and neurasthenia. For purposes of investigation they selected the position secured by hyperflexion of the lower extremity upon the chest, as shown in Plate 7, Fig. 1, and noted the angle formed by the two extremities. In this number of tabetics the angle thus obtained averaged about 110°, sometimes reaching the extraordinary angle of 150°. This was obtained without the slightest pain to the patient, and was maintained for a considerable length of time without difficulty. Among normal individuals, often embracing children and females, an angle of 65° to 70° was ordinarily obtained, and only exceptionally did it exceed 80°, but this was accomplished with considerable pain in the posterior portion of the flexed thigh. The observation was also checked by similar examination of hysterics and neurasthenics, in whom muscular tone is comparatively reduced, and here an average of about 85° was noted. The same condition was also observed in other joints, as in the ankle-joint, where the range of movements in inversion, shown in Plate 7, Fig. 2, largely exceeds that which could be secured in a normal foot. They explain this over-range of motion by the lowered tonus in the muscles, and call attention to the fact that this lack of tone had been formerly pointed out by Debove.

Bailey [3] takes up the subject of the **effect of early optic atrophy upon the progress of tabes,** and gives a history of 12 cases which he examined. From them he draws the following conclusions: 1. In about 75% of the cases of tabes in which optic atrophy is an early symptom some of the other tabetic symptoms may be late in appearing, or may not develop at all. This is especially the case in respect to the lightning-pains and the incoördination of movement. The loss of knee-jerk in such cases is very constant. 2. The most distressing symptoms may develop simultaneously with or immediately succeed the blindness. 3. The association with the optic atrophy of oculomotor palsies is without prognostic significance. 4. The subject will receive its best elucidation by the observation over long periods of time of patients with "primary optic atrophy." [In this article, which is prepared with great attention to detail, there is no mention made of the occasional recession of ataxia after the appearance of optic atrophy, a fact insisted upon by Benedict.

[1] Compressed-air Illness. London, 1896. [2] Nouv. Icon. de la Salpêt., July and Aug., 1896. [3] Med. Rec., Nov. 14, 1896.

and which does undoubtedly occur as in a case now under observation in which there were extreme ataxia and the characteristic gait, which completely disappeared when vision was reduced to counting fingers at three feet. At present the man can walk with eyes closed with as much precision if not more than the ordinary individual.]

H. T. Patrick,[1] after calling attention to the early investigations of trunkal anesthesia in locomotor ataxia described by Laehr, publishes a number of cases of **tabetic anesthesia,** with diagrams showing in almost every instance a close relation in the distribution of the anesthesia to the segmental areas that have been mapped out by Thorburn, Starr, Head, and others. Often there is an area of hyperesthesia above the anesthetic band, and the anesthesia is not complete, but is more pronounced for tactile impressions than for painful stimulation. The usual location affected is a band about the body, level with the nipple, sometimes being confined to a patch over the pectoral muscles, from which it is likely to spread in a girdle about the entire trunk. This anesthesia may appear early, but is usually only found when the ataxia is well marked.

A. B. Bonar[2] gives as the result of an investigation of **the anesthetic areas** in 21 cases of locomotor ataxia a confirmation of the evidence of Laehr and Patrick.

Bettman[3] gives his observations of **Fraenkel's exercise-treatment** of ataxia and the rules Fraenkel lays down for the employment of this means. " There are two classes of exercises, those performed in bed and those performed out of bed. In bed, the patient is called upon to flex, extend, abduct, and adduct each leg separately, and then both simultaneously. The knees and hips are likewise exercised. The patient is asked to place the heel of one foot on the big toe of the other foot. Place the heel upon knee of the other leg and then slowly travel from the ridge of the tibia toward the ankle. Exercises are made alternately, first with one leg, then with the other one, with open and with closed eyes. These exercises are attempted over and over again, every morning a half-hour, with frequent rests between times. The patient is encouraged to persevere until he succeeds. The exercises are repeated twice a day, a half-hour in the morning and again a half-hour in the afternoon. 1. Patient is placed with his back to a chair, heels together; then seats himself slowly in the chair, and is then made to rise in the same careful manner. No cane is used. If patient cannot stand, an attendant is placed at either side of him to support him if necessary. 2. One leg is placed at an ordinary walking-step in front of the other, and then placed with great exactness back into its original position. Same exercise is then performed with other leg. The patient, if necessary, supports himself with a cane or otherwise. 3. Walks three paces slowly and with precision. 4. Rest in standing position, one foot before the other ; with hands placed akimbo he flexes his knees and slowly raises himself again. 5. Patient, as in exercise No. 2, advances one foot, then returns it to its original position, and then puts it one step behind the other one. This exercise is usually a very difficult one, requiring as it does a great deal of balancing power. 6. Walk twenty steps as in exercise No. 3. 7. No. 2, performed without a cane. 8. Stand without a cane, with feet placed together and hands on hips. 9. Stand without a cane, feet separated ; various movements with the arms, grasping objects, forcing back outstretched hand of physician, etc. 10. Maintain same position as in No. 9, flexing trunk forward, backward, to the right and to the left. 11. Exercise No. 9, with feet.

[1] N. Y. Med. Jour., Feb. 6, 1897.   [2] Med. Rec., May 22, 1897.
[3] Jour. Am. Med. Assoc., Jan. 2, 1897.

together. 12. Exercise No. 10, with feet together. 13. Walk along a painted line on the floor, patient supported by a cane. 14. Same without a cane. Exercises for the fingers and arms are also employed, based on the above-mentioned principles." [This method of treating ataxia is extremely valuable, and will often serve to keep patients on their feet, perhaps for years, when otherwise they might become bedridden, and it will sometimes succeed in getting patients on their feet who have not walked for a long period of time.]

Tourette and Chipault[1] have investigated, and during the past 4 years put into operation, **a plan of stretching the spinal cord.** They first determined by suspending a cadaver in a Sayr apparatus, without the arm-pieces, that the cord was not influenced mechanically by the procedure; on the contrary, by seating the cadaver upon a table with the lower limbs extended and forcibly bending the trunk forward, the result in 5 bodies was that the cord was actually elongated, as was proved by measurements, the vertebral arches and dura having been removed. The greatest stretching of the cord took place below the middorsal region, and was about equally divided between the cord and the cauda, amounting all together to from 1.1 cm. to 2. cm., the stretching of the cord proper being tolerably uniform, the variation occurring in the cauda. This finding was then applied to the treatment of cases of locomotor ataxia, for which purpose a small low table with a slight headboard was provided. By a waistband the patient is secured to the headboard, and by a circingle about the shoulders to which are attached cord and pulleys playing through a sheave, placed between the thighs close to the body, the trunk is forcibly flexed anteriorly. The method was used in 47 cases selected with some care, the early and practically stationary cases of mild degree not being included, and the late cachectic cases also being excluded as well as the cases of acute and very rapidly progressing form; 22 of these 47 patients showed improvement in all their symptoms; especially was there amelioration of the pains and the various visceral crises, as well as improvement of the sensibility. Renal troubles, particularly retention, were improved. Impotence was favorably affected. Twelve of these 22 cases were markedly incoördinate, and in 10 the gait presented some improvement. Ocular and palpebral symptoms were not modified, which the authors rather incline to attribute to the fact that the stretching of the cord only affects the lower portion of it. Fifteen other of the 47 cases received some slight benefit; 10 secured no benefit whatever. The patients received from 15 to 20 *séances*, usually every second day, lasting from 8 to 12 minutes; and the authors advise that the method should be used from 3 to 4 months consecutively, say for 40 or 50 *séances*, when an interval of a month or two should follow. In conclusion, they state that, based upon their experiments, extending over 4 years, and their experience they consider spinal flexion as the only means of attaining elongation of the cord exempt from the dangers of suspension, and obtaining twice as much benefit as by the earlier method.

Friedreich's Ataxia.—Zabludowski[2] presents a case which was considerably improved by massage.

William G. Spiller[3] reports a case of **cerebellar hereditary ataxia, with autopsy.** Death occurred from tuberculosis.

Hodge[4] reports 4 cases of **family ataxia** in one family. They correspond closely to the cerebral type of Marie. Pauly and Bonne[5] describe three

---

[1] Nouv. Incon. de la Salpêt., May–June, 1897. [2] Brit. Med. Jour., Oct. 24, 1896.
[3] Brain, 1896. [4] Brit. Med. Jour., June 5, 1897.
[5] Rev. de Méd., Mar. 10, 1897.

47

brothers of 26, 23, and 12 years, who between the ages of 5 and 15 developed rigidity in the lower extremities, nystagmus, difficulties of speech, increased knee-jerks, ankle-clonus, and other evidence of lack of development in the motor tracts or in the cerebellar control. The cases closely conform to those of the hereditary cerebellar type.

Little's Disease.—The French are inclined, following Brissaud, to regard as cases of Little's disease only the congenital spastic forms of diplegia which are due to lack of development of the pyramidal tracts of the cord. This condition is commonly the result of premature birth or the birth of a child of very small dimensions, at term. Embryologically it has been shown that the lateral motor tracts in the cord are the last to develop, and the fibres only become myelinated at the 9th month and not fully developed until several months after birth. Joseph Collins, in an editorial,[1] quotes Van Gehuchten and others to the same effect, and states that this author contends that absence of the myelin-sheaths of the corticospinal fibers constituting the pyramidal tract is attended by the same clinical phenomena as the degeneration of the fibers. In both conditions there is an absence of the inhibitory action of these fibres upon the ganglion-cells of the anterior horns.

Family Spastic Paraplegia.—C. Achard and H. Fresson[2] report a family presenting 2 cases of this disease. It seemed stationary, and consisted of a pure spastic paraplegia. The first symptoms were noticed under 16 months of age—that is, as soon as the children commenced to walk, which is rather younger than in most of the reported cases, in some of which it appeared as late as 20 years, and at 56 years in Strümpel's case. As in most other reported cases, the disease seems to have been incited by an acute infection, the exact nature of which, however, in the present instance, is not clear. The family history contains nothing notable from a neuropathic standpoint except an epilepsy in a sister of one of the patients. Syphilis is excluded. Newmark[3] gives a description of two families in which the children were afflicted with a spastic condition of the lower extremities. Jendrassik[4] throws doubt upon the degeneration of the pyramidal tracts as beginning primarily in the cord-fibers in cases of spastic paraplegia. He believes the process may commence at the cells of origin, either in the brain, in the bulb, or in the spinal cord, and would speak of diplegia cerebralis, bulbaris, or spinalis, according to the location of the commencing cellular lesion. The author does not believe in the explanation that the pyramidal tracts fail to develop normally in prematurely born children, and thereby cause the typical form of Little's disease, in which he is at variance with the authors already quoted.

Multiple Spinal Sclerosis.—Eichhorst[5] records a case of multiple sclerosis in a child. The disease was congenital and inherited. The boy was born two years after symptoms of multiple sclerosis had appeared in the mother. Slight tremor on voluntary movement was the only symptom noticed until the boy reached 8 years, when tremor on voluntary movement, nystagmus, optic atrophy, scanning speech, and exaggerated tendon-reflexes appeared. He died shortly afterward. Microscopic examination showed sclerotic islets in all parts of the cord, but none in the pons or brain. In the mother, who died a few years later, the sclerosis had the same limited distribution.

[1] Med. News, Feb. 6, 1897.   [2] Gaz. hebdom. de Méd. et de Chir., Dec. 24. 1896.
[3] Med. News, Jan. 16, 1897.   [4] Deutsch. Arch. f. klin. Med., vol. 58, p. 137.
[5] Virchow's Archiv, Nov., 1896.

NEUROSES FOLLOWING INFECTION.

Chorea.—The vexed question of the **relationship between rheumatism and chorea** that has had warm advocates on both sides since its early conception by Kirks, is illuminated by the examination of 552 cases of rheumatic fever and 157 cases of chorea, made by T. Churton, and summarized in the *Brit. Med. Jour.* of Sept. 19, 1896. From these cases and a study of the current literature on the subject he adduced the following conclusions: 1. The postulated toxin (*x*) being accepted as an essential element in the causation of rheumatism, depressing conditions (*y*) determine the first position or locus of the disorder—that is, what cells or tissues (*z*) the toxin shall strike. (There is probably a quite separate and independent causation for (*x*).) In 91 cases of rheumatism in which the incidence of the chill, strain, etc., was recorded with precision, and also the joints or parts first affected, it was seen in every case—or with very few, and doubtful, exceptions—that the part receiving the impact of the conditioning cause was the first to become disordered by the toxin—for example, wetting of feet always caused arthritis first in the lower extremities; of shoulders, in the upper extremities. 2. If (x) and (y) are given, the position of (z) can be stated within certain limits. 3. If (y) is a fright, shock, or intense excitement, (z) will be the nervous system; in the developing brain of a child the result is usually chorea; in adults it may be delirium or coma, perhaps hyperpyrexia. 4. Arthritis or endocarditis may follow the nervous disorder, since the symptoms themselves may become causes of depression of tissues, and thence of multiplication of microorganisms and toxins. 5. Similarly, chorea may follow arthritis; but, 6, arthritis is never the first result of fright; and 7. Chorea is never the first result of chill, unless fear or brain excitement accompanies the chill. 8. A man who, being rheumatic, and having no other known disease, is accidentally subjected to strong excitement—a quarrel—and in a few hours develops chorea, is an "experiment devised by Nature" to prove that the essential cause of the two disorders is the same, and that only the conditioning (localizing) causes are different. In non-rheumatic persons, even young children, brain-disturbance does not cause chorea.

H. L. K. Shaw [1] has been observing the **knee-jerk in chorea**, and with certain London observers believes in the "choreic knee-jerk," the characteristic feature of which is its irregularity. On striking the patellar tendon the reflex is manifested in several ways: the foot may be jerked upward a slight distance, stop a moment, then complete its course and return, or it may be stopped several times in its upward excursion. More commonly these stops occur in the descent of the foot, the ascent being normal, or the foot may remain stationary at the height of the upper excursion for a second or more, and then descend normally or in an irregular manner, as above described. These jerky movements may occur in both the ascent and descent of the foot. The reflex itself is not exaggerated, and is often slightly diminished. It is sometimes necessary to use Jendrassik's method of reinforcement to bring out the choreic knee-jerk. Its intensity bears no relation to the severity of the chorea.

Habit-chorea.—Wharton Sinkler [2] discusses the subject of habit-chorea, basing his paper upon 141 cases that have passed through the Philadelphia Infirmary for Nervous Diseases. The author is disposed to follow in the footsteps of Weir Mitchell, and considers habit-chorea as identical with or closely allied to Sydenham's chorea, and believes that similar lines of treat-

[1] Albany Med. Ann., May, 1897. [2] Am. Jour. Med. Sci., May, 1897.

ment are of advantage in both. [There can be no question that in some instances habit-chorea partakes closely of the nature of Sydenham's chorea, but the majority of cases which can be properly called habit-chorea are, as insisted by Gowers and as reiterated and confirmed by French observers, a form of tic. It is a mental habit, and the mental factor is the important one in it. Arsenic without the addition of moral suasion—in other words, mental treatment and constant suggestion and encouragement—is practically of no value whatever. Aside from its tonic qualities it is doubtful that it ever accomplishes any good in true habit-chorea. It would be advisable that the term habit-chorea be entirely dropped, and the term habit-spasm, or, better, spasmodic tic, be employed.]

Chorea in the Aged.—Riesman[1] reports a case of chorea in a man of 75, affecting the limbs on the left side, especially the hand; he concludes that: 1. True Sydenham's chorea may occur in advanced life and may run a short course, terminating in recovery. 2. The majority of cases of chorea occurring late in life run a chronic and progressive course. 3. At the commencement of the disease it is, as a rule, impossible to say whether it will terminate favorably or become chronic. 4. The movements are generally most marked in the arms; they may begin in the lower extremities, and rarely may remain confined thereto. In 20% of the cases in the table they were unilateral. 5. The mind is normal in three-fifths of the cases in which no hereditary element exists. 6. Rheumatism holds a very subordinate relation to the chorea of late adult life. 7. Endocarditis is comparatively rare, having occurred in only 12.3% of the cases collected in the table. 8. The anatomic lesions in the fatal cases are not characteristic. [While it is certain that Sydenham's chorea in extremely rare instances appears after the age of 40, a close scrutiny of the cases in the above, coupled with the fact that rheumatism is usually absent, cardiac lesions wanting, the onset gradual, recovery exceptional, and the movements of an athetoid character, there is much ground to doubt that many of these cases are those of true chorea. In view of the advanced age, the existence of senile arterial changes, the variations in the postmortem findings, and the hemiplegic distribution, it is much more than likely that they are due to organic changes in the cerebrum, usually of vascular origin.]

Tetanus and its Treatment.—Alexander Lambert[2] makes a careful study of this subject, in which he gives special emphasis to the localization of tetanus in the body, principally at the point of infection, a fact having important bearing upon the treatment. Under this head he discusses the local and the general measures. Locally, reliance must be placed upon disinfection and antitoxic measures; that is, those calculated to destroy or arrest the toxic products. Against the spores it is practically impossible sufficiently to saturate the tissues with antiseptics, as they are resistant to the action of such agents; but by the addition of a little hydrochloric acid, especially with carbolic acid, they may be readily killed. Silver nitrate and the iodin preparations, as, for instance Gram's solution and Lugol's solution, are also of advantage. He therefore advises that the tetanus-wound be thoroughly cleansed, the most active antiseptics used, and in addition the iodin preparations. Regarding amputation he speaks guardedly, but rather favors it. General treatment consists in, first, speedy elimination of the poisons; second, administration of physiologic antidotes; and, third, the use of chemic antidotes, which change the poison by destroying it or rendering it inert. The elimination of tetanus-poisons is managed through the kidneys, and to this end the author advises active diuresis and the ingestion of large quantities of fluids. Physiological

[1] Am. Jour. Med. Sci., Aug., 1897.   [2] N. Y. Med. Jour., June 5, 1897.

antidotes of the most value are chloral, bromids, physostigmin, and perhaps also antimony, suggested by Bross, who employed it successfully in 5 acute cases, giving it in doses of $\frac{1}{8}$ to $\frac{1}{6}$ gr., with an equal amount of morphin, every two hours. Chemic antidotes in the form of hypodermic injections of corrosive sublimate and carbolic acid, as by Baccelli, have been recommended; but there is doubt of their being efficacious, as the toxin is operative in the presence of a $\frac{1}{2}\%$ solution of carbolic acid, which indeed is used in the laboratory for the purpose of preserving it. Antitoxic serum seems to be of value. This, the author believes with Tizzoni, does not act by neutralizing the active principles of the infection, but by immunizing those parts of the body not already tetanized, thus limiting the tetanus locally. In estimating the value of the antitoxin the author accepts 80% as a fair statement of the fatality usual in tetanus. He analyzes a total of 114 cases, which presented a mortality of 46% under the antitoxin treatment, and recognizes (as has been pointed out in previous issues of the *Year-Book*) that cases which appear after prolonged incubation, or appear after a short period of incubation but in a mild form, usually get well without any treatment, and so eliminates a large number of these cases. He found that in acute cases developed within 8 days of the injury 31 recovered under antitoxin, or 38.71%, as compared with 80%, shown by former statistics, and calls attention to the fact that there are certain cases of tetanus of such short incubation and such rapidity of onset that in spite of all treatment they die within 24 to 36 hours after the first symptoms appear. These cases he still considers hopeless, as at least 24 hours are required to secure full saturation of the system with the antitoxin. With Bazy, Nocar, and others he is inclined to advise preventive inoculations of antitoxin in animals and men presenting grimy and dirt-laden wounds, such as sometimes are followed by tetanus. This recommendation is especially based upon Roux's statement, amply proved by experiment, that the toxin can be readily neutralized at the time of infection, but that a very short time afterward it requires doses thousands, and even hundreds of thousands, of times larger to accomplish the same purpose.

Hendley[1] reports a case of tetanus treated with corrosive sublimate, with recovery. Poli[2] reports the case of a boy of 16 who was kicked on the foot by a horse, and 5 days later developed symptoms of tetanus. Bromid and chloroform were given internally and injections of a 1% carbolic solution every 2 hours. In 12 days the patient was practically well, but the injections were continued every 2 hours for another 2 weeks; 500 in all were given, with no bad results. Hoefling[3] relates the case of a lad of 17 who developed tetanus about a week after a crushing injury to the little finger; 5 days after the onset he was unable to open his mouth; 8 days after the onset 5 gm. of dry antitoxin, dissolved in 45 c.c. of sterilized water, were injected, without much improvement; 2 days later there was difficulty in breathing, and a second injection produced immediate improvement, from which point the patient steadily got well.

Tetany.—Gustav Singer,[4] in a paper taking up the subject of **autointoxication**, refers to a case of tetany in a man 41 years of age, who was attacked with diarrhea and weakness after eating roast pork. Three days before admission to the hospital constipation set in, and this was followed within 24 hours by typical tetany. The urine contained no albumin, but indican, diacetic acid, acetone, and aromatic sulfates were present. Under treatment with calomel and purges, followed by iodoform internally, the tetany entirely disappeared

[1] Brit. Med. Jour., Jan. 16, 1897.   [2] Gaz. degli Ospedali, Mar. 14, 1897.
[3] Deutsch. med. Woch., Apr. 1, 1897.   [4] Wien. med. Presse, No. 12, 1897.

and the urine became normal. [The ease seems to be a very conclusive one regarding the source of tetany, at least in some instances, from intestinal intoxication.] Oddo[1] rejects the view that in childhood tetany is merely a manifestation of **rickets,** although admitting the frequency of rickets. He accepts the view that the essential cause of the nervous symptoms is a toxemia due to the absorption of poisonous bodies produced in the gastrointestinal canal. This is usually attended by dilatation of the stomach and long retention of food in that viscus. He believes that tetany in the adult is essentially the same, and the result of gastric indigestion marked by hypersecretion of gastric juices containing an excess of hydrochloric acid. The changes in the anterior gray matter of the spinal cord noted by Weiss and others he considers are due to a toxin circulating in the blood. In the treatment of tetany the two indications are the expulsion of toxic substances and the prevention of their formation. Both are met by calomel, which he recommends to be given in doses of $\frac{3}{4}$ gr. every other day, or in larger doses, depending upon the age of the patient. The stomach is to be washed out, a measure to be used with discrimination, however, owing to the risk of exciting laryngeal spasm. The diet must be carefully supervised, and a deficiency of acids in the gastric contents supplied to check decomposition in the intestines. He also recommends in some instances to wash out the large intestine with a boric-acid solution, and the use of vermifuges where there is a suspicion of worms. For the immediate relief of the spasms warm baths are the most effective agents, and of drugs, chloral, which may be given by enema. As a sedative in the continuance of the tetanic state he prefers bromid of strontium, and in some cases has resorted to inhalations of chloroform. A sponge soaked in very hot water applied to the front of the neck often relieves laryngeal spasm, and it may be necessary to follow it by the inhalation of chloroform carefully administered in very small quantities, as at first it may have a tendency to aggravate the spasm.

Cassel[2] has made an analytical study of 6822 cases, with special attention to determining the nature of tetany and its **relationship to rickets and laryngeal spasm.** There were 60 cases of tetany. The nutrition was good in 14, moderately good in 13, poor in 23, and bad in 10. All presented spontaneous intermittent spasm, which could be induced by pressure upon the large nerves and vessels of the affected parts. In all but three the facial phenomenon was present. Only two had laryngeal spasm, and both of these presented craniotabes in addition to other symptoms of rickets. Without exception the children were nervous and slept badly. Fourteen presented temperature, in 9 the result of complicating conditions, and in the remainder without apparent cause. In 21 cases digestive disturbance preceded or accompanied the tetany, in 5 there was chronic dyspepsia, in 43 digestive disorder, in 6 obstinate constipation, in 4 habitual vomiting. Rickets was present in 52 of the 60 cases; in only 8 was there no trace of rickets. Tetany was seen throughout the entire year, although the largest number appeared to occur in the spring and late autumn. There was no suggestion of an epidemic occurrence of the disease, nor was there any relation as to frequency between tetany, rickets, laryngeal spasm, and craniotabes. He concludes that tetany is neither a complication of rickets nor of digestive disturbance, but is dependent upon unfavorable conditions of living, improper nutrition, and bad air. Kassowitz[3] reports a case of latent tetany and rickets, recovery from the tetany following the administration of phosphorus. He discards the gastrointestinal origin of tetany,

[1] Rev. de Méd., June-Sept., 1896.   [2] Deutsch. med. Woch., Jan. 28, 1897.
[3] Neurol. Centralbl., Mar., 1897.

and insists upon the association with rickets, having never seen tetany occur with gastrointestinal catarrh in the absence of rickets, and points to the seasonable variation of tetany, which is opposed to that of gastrointestinal disorders. J. B. McConnell[1] reports a case in which well-marked tetany came on during convalescence from scarlet fever. The condition improved under the use of sodium bromid and potassium salicylate and disappeared within a week.

Tetany and Mental Disease.—F. Schultze[2] reports a case of a girl of 16, presenting a classical type of tetany, in whom, after a week of disease, during which time she was given doses of iodothyrin, mental disturbance appeared in the form of mild mania, during which she was uneasy, restless, and more or less destructive. He refers to the case recorded by Fränkl-Hochwart in 1891, and a subsequent case by Hochhaus, in which there were epileptic attacks in addition to the mental disturbance. [Osler is inclined to believe that mental features in tetany are not purely accidental, but may be considered, perhaps, as a part of the manifestation of the disease.]

Endemic Paralytic Vertigo of Japan, or Kubisgari.—Miura[3] gives a report of this disease, which prevails in Northern Japan. It occurs from May to October among laborers of both sexes and all ages, coming on in paroxysms, with ptosis, diminished vision, double vision, optic hyperemia, motor disturbance of the tongue, lips, and muscles of mastication, and paresis of the muscles of the neck, body, and extremities. The involvement of the neck-muscles and the ocular symptoms are the most common. There may be increased reflexes, lachrymation, increase of saliva, and nasal secretion. In the intervals the patients are free from the symptoms, or after severe attacks may retain a mild degree of ptosis. The attacks seem to be brought on, in patients subject to the disease, by the stooping posture. They also present some weakness of the neck-muscles during the intervals between the paroxysms. There are likewise weakness and depression, loss of appetite, and headache. Miura calls attention to the resemblance of this disease to Erb's asthenic bulbar paralysis [a sketch of which was given in the *Year-Book* for 1897], but points out that it most resembles the paralyzing vertigo described by Gerlier, which is epidemic in certain parts of Switzerland. The disease seems to be due to an infection, and is associated with the habits of life, hard work, and close quarters with cattle that obtain in both Japan and Switzerland. P. Lucas-Championnière[4] gives a similar description of this paralytic vertigo and indicates its infectious character.

TROPHONEUROSES.

Acromegaly.—Vinke[5] reports a case of acromegaly, photographs of which appear in the *Year-Book* for 1897. He collects from the literature 12 recorded autopsies in which the pituitary gland was found enlarged or disorganized. [A number of other autopsies showing pituitary tumors are noted in the following paragraphs.] Rathmell[6] gives the clinical history and postmortem findings in a case of acromegaly showing some peculiarities. For a period of months previous to the patient's death there was projectile vomiting of everything introduced into the stomach, necessitating rectal alimentation. He was also troubled with attacks of dyspnea, in which the respiration was of the marked Cheyne-Stokes character, and finally died from apnea. On postmortem the

[1] Mont. Med. Jour., Sept., 1896.
[2] Berlin. klin. Woch., Mar. 1, 1897.
[3] Mitt. der Med. Fac. der Kaiserl.-Japan Univ. zu Tokio, Bd. iii., No. 3, 1896.
[4] Jour. de Méd., May 25, 1897.
[5] Med. Rec., Nov. 28, 1896.
[6] Jour. Am. Med. Assoc., Mar. 20, 1897.

costal cartilages were found ossified, the lungs speckled with calcareous particles, all the bones of the skeleton characteristically enlarged. A number of
sharp-pointed spinous projections, on the inner surface of the skull, pressed on
the dura. There was a tumor of the pituitary, weighing 476 gr. after it had
been immersed in alcohol for a number of weeks, and about the size of a hen's
egg, and a very tortuous posterior cerebral artery on the left side, resembling a
string of beads. Harlow Brooks[1] reports a typical case of acromegaly, with
full autopsy. The pituitary fossa was enlarged and contained an ovoid, red
mass measuring 1.5 cm. by 0.7 cm., attached to the lower portion of the pituitary body. It pressed on the left optic tract posterior to the chiasm. The
hypophysis was also enlarged to about five times its ordinary dimensions.
The thyroid gland was symmetrically enlarged. The thymus was found persistent and symmetrical in form. The sympathetic ganglia were large and
distinct. Microscopic examination of the enlarged pituitary demonstrated an
apparently simple hyperplasia of the lymphadenoid portion of the body.
R. Roxburgh and A. J. Collis[2] report a case of acromegaly in a woman of
35, in whom symptoms had occurred several years before. At the necropsy,
43 hours after death, a large thymus gland, measuring 3.5 in. long and 1.5 in.
wide, was found. The thyroid gland appeared normal. The skull presented
enormously dilated frontal sinuses, some signs of meningitis were detected,
and the pituitary body was the size of an English walnut, very soft and vascular. The microscopic characteristics of the growth were midway between
those of glioma and round-celled sarcoma, but from their description and the
drawing it is not unlikely that it was a disintegrated adenoma. Hansemann[3]
describes a case of acromegaly, recognized postmortem, with the usual pituitary tumor. In reviewing the literature of the subject he finds records of 15
cases going to section, 12 of which presented enlargement of the pituitary
gland. The 3 not showing this condition embraced at least 2 cases that
properly could not be called acromegaly and the third case was doubtful.
E. Comini[4] report 3 cases, in one of which postmortem was obtained. In
this the hypophysis was also enlarged. Von Schwoner[5] reports a case of
acromegaly in a woman of 50 whose mother had also presented the disease at
about the same age. T. A. Tamburini[6] reports a case; postmortem discovered a tumor of the hypophysis with enlargement of the sella turcica.

Prof. W. Uhthoff[7] reports 3 cases, in 2 of which the full picture of acromegaly was established, and in 1 of these a sarcomatous enlargement of the
hypophysis was found after death.

Acromegaly and Gigantism.—Walker[8] reports, with a number of
photographs, a case of acromegaly of the giant type in a boy of 16, admitted
to Cook County Hospital. At that age he presented a weight of 245 pounds
and a stature of 6 ft. 5¼ in. The hands and feet were enormously enlarged and
of the typical pattern. The superciliary ridges were hypertrophic, but the lower
jaw was proportionate to the head. He was noticed to commence to grow very
rapidly at the age of 6, but at birth weighed 13 pounds, his brothers and sisters averaging 9 and 10 pounds. Marinesco[9] secured skiagraphs in 3 cases of
acromegaly of the common massive type and in 1 of the giant variety. In all
the cases of acromegaly the lateral aspect of the last phalanges appeared to be

[1] N. Y. Med. Jour., Mar. 27, 1897.   [2] Brit. Med. Jour., July, 1896.
[3] Berlin. klin. Woch. May 27, 1897.   [4] Arch. per le scienze Med., xx., 21.
[5] Zeit. f. klin. Med., Bd. xxxii., 1897.
[6] Riv. sperim. di Fren. e di Med. legale, vol. xx.
[7] Berlin. klin. Woch., May 31, 1897.   [8] Jour. Am. Med. Assoc., Jan. 23, 1897.
[9] Compt. rend. de la Soc. de Biol., No. 21, 1896.

excavated, probably as the result of the very considerable enlargement of the epiphyses of these bones. The case of gigantism showed an increase in the direction of length.

George R. Murray [1] reports, with plates and skiagraphs, 2 cases of acromegaly, the first of which also presented exophthalmic **goiter,** and the second cystic goiter. The association of acromegaly with exophthalmic goiter is, therefore, including this case, on record 5 times. The presence of goiter in acromegaly has been more frequently noted. Rolleston [2] reported to the Medical Society of London a case of acromegaly in which the disease had been present over 2 years. For 4 or 5 months the patient had been under treatment by pituitary and thyroid extracts, and had shown great improvement, which had been maintained after she left the hospital.

Exophthalmic Goiter.—Gerhardt [3] calls attention to the distended condition of the arteries of the body generally in this disease, especially the aortic branches, but finds similar conditions in the arteries of the extremities, as in the palmar arches and the crurals. He also notes capillary pulsation, and pulsation of the spleen, of the liver, and even of the kidneys. [This calls attention prominently to the fact that vasomotor disturbances of the disease are not limited to any particular part.] Tricomi [4] reports 3 cases of Graves's disease, with marked improvement after partial resection of the lateral lobes of the thyroid.

James A. Spalding [5] reports a case of goiter in which the protrusion of the eyeballs successively required their **enucleation** because of the purulent choroiditis and hypopyon which had destroyed sight. In a search of the literature he can find but one other case in which the exophthalmus was of this grade. This was reported in Mooren's " Fuenf Lustren."

H. C. Wood [6] advocates the use of **splenic extract** in the treatment of this disease, and reports a case with satisfactory result. The remedy is rather disagreeable, causing dyspepsia, pain, and vomiting. Used hypodermically it causes great local irritation and even suppuration.

Thymus-feeding in Exophthalmic Goiter.—Owen [7] has collected the reports of Mikulicz, Cunningham, Eads, Solis Cohen, McKie, Maude, Todd, and Williams who have all had more or less good results in this disease from the therapeutic use of the thymus gland given in a manner similar to that used in thyroid-feeding, and in somewhat similar doses. He says: " Some facts also suggest the possibility of an antagonism between the thymus and thyroid in their relationship to the nervous system." Mackenzie [8] gives the details of 15 cases of exophthalmic goiter treated with thymus gland, as reported by others. He then adds 20 cases in which he himself had employed the thymus. Of these 20 cases, 1 died, in 6 no improvement was observed, and in 13 there was some improvement. In none did he observe any such decided effects on the symptoms or progress of the disease as would justify him in concluding that the thymus has any great therapeutic activity. As a matter of comparison, he then adds 20 similar cases treated on general principles and by other methods, and in final conclusion states that he finds " the thymus gland has no specific action in Graves's disease. In most cases it had no effect on the heart, or on the goiter, or on the exophthalmus, but at the same time did seem to have some value in improving the general condition." He would rank it with cod-liver oil. The dose varied from a few grains to several

[1] Edinb. Med. Jour., Feb., 1897.
[2] Brit. Med. Jour., Apr. 17, 1897.
[3] Centralbl. f. Chir., Sept. 5, 1896.
[4] Il Policlinico, No. 3, 1896.
[5] Med. News, July 10, 1897.
[6] Am. Jour. Med. Sci., May, 1897.
[7] Brit. Med. Jour., Oct. 10, 1896.
[8] Am. Jour. Med. Sci., Feb., 1897.

as found that thyroids controlled the tremor and cachexia as powerless. Robert Hutchinson[5] refers to former article that the chemistry of the thyroid furnishes two proteids, a colloid matter. The extractives include creatin, xanthin ... of other organs, but include, according to Fränkel ... an important part in the activity of the gland is to be ... these three varieties of products. Hutchinson experi ... reached the conclusion that the pure colloid matter wa ... of the gland, a position which is confirmed by th ... and others, that the athyroidal state is proportionate to ... material in the gland. Hutchinson advises the us ... which has a uniformity of activity and is capable of ...

... the *Boston Medical and Surgical Journal*, June 24, 1897 on goiter and cretinism, the results of his investiga ... the Committee of Twenty-five Physicians. More thar

... 12, 1897.   [2] Lyon méd., Feb. 7, 1897.
June 12, July 1, 1897.
..., de Chir., p. 582, June 24, 1897.
... 22, 1896.   [6] Brit. Med. Jour., Jan. 23, 1897.

76,000 school children between the ages of 7 and 16 were reviewed, with their parentage and antecedents. The investigations were principally made in the Canton of Berne, Switzerland. The formulated results may be briefly stated as follows: the female is more frequently the victim of goiter than the male. In children between the ages of 9 and 14 years goiter reaches its highest degree of frequency, and rarely appears before they are sent to school, where the position of the head in reading and writing gives a tendency to the ailment. There is, therefore, a school-goiter. The secondary changes in the thyroid are proportionate to the advanced age of the individual. Congenital goiter is extremely rare. A still greater exception is congenital atrophy of the thyroid. Kocher noted that the districts supplied with water from the fresh-water sandstone showed a prevalence of goiter, while in the districts in which the water originated from salt-water sandstone goiter was infrequent. He concluded, however, that the prevalence of goiter depended upon the abundance of organic elements in the water rather than upon its source, and that neither deficient nourishment, unhealthy dwellings, nor wretchedness and poverty are a direct causation. Often the districts rich in goiter are separated by narrow limits from those free from the disease, and he discovered in goiter-laden localities oases free from goiter. He also found that there were actual goiter-fountains, the water of which almost invariably produced goiter in the children that drank it. On the other hand, in localities where goiter was prevalent families who had a private water-supply were sometimes free from the infection. Brooks and rivers and long, open conductors of water were unfavorable.

As to cretinism, Kocher, referring to heredity, finds that strong, healthy parents who in regions free from cretinism had begotten normal children, moving into a cretinoid district produced cretins. In these cases, however, the parents, one or both, had previous to the birth of the cretinoid children developed goiter. Such parents upon returning to their former place of residence have again had healthy children. In Kocher's opinion, whenever goiter or cretinism appears in children one of the parents will be found to have goiter; that cretinism arises only and solely when by degeneration of the thyroid gland, due to goiter or some other injury to the gland, its function is impaired or destroyed. Goiter is, therefore, the first stage of cretinism either occurring in the individual or through the parentage. He goes further, and declares that congenital inherited cretinism is derived from the mother alone, while inherited cretinism that appears after the lapse of a few months or years is derived from the father alone. This is explained by the fact that the fetus is supplied with normal thyroid conditions if the mother be not in an athyroidal state, and the inherited tendency from the father may be corrected during intrauterine life and even during lactation by the mother's condition, and only appears when the maternal source of thyroid products is cut off. The reports closes with the injunction to boil the drinking-water, thereby destroying the organic matter, the source of goiter in parents and of cretinism in the offspring.

Grünfeld[1] tried **thyroantitoxin** in 3 cases of exophthalmic goiter, 4 of obesity, 2 of bronchocele, and 1 of simple psoriasis. The drug induced loss of body-weight in 7 of the cases within a few days, subsequent loss of weight being very gradual. In one case of exophthalmic goiter the body-weight rapidly increased, in another it remained stationary. In one case of exophthalmic goiter there was rapid improvement at first, followed by relapse; the other two improved markedly, but were improving when the drug was commenced. In all cases the thyroid tumor softened without diminishing in size. In two cases the perspiration was decreased. In one there was decrease of

---

[1] Wien. med. Bl., Nos. 49 and 50, 1896.

ounces 3 times a day. He would place the usual dose at 1 to 2 drams a day of the fresh gland or its equivalent in the extracts and powders.

Resection of the Cervical Sympathetic for Exophthalmic Goiter and Epilepsy.—Jonnesco[1] has performed complete and bilateral resection of the cervical sympathetic nerve in Basedow's disease. In both cases the operation was followed by the disappearance of prominence of the eyes and lessening in the size of the goiter. The tachycardia was relieved in one case, but persisted in the other. Jaboulay[2] reports 3 new cases in which he has followed Jonnesco's plan. The first patient was reported cured in a few days; the second case presented immediate relief as to the goiter, rapid heart, and tremor; the third patient was better from the time of operation, and ultimately much improved. The author would also apply the operation to ordinary cases of large goiter, as it seems invariably to diminish the size of the gland, removing the danger from extirpation or pressure. Valençon[3] refers to the cases of Jonnesco, Jaboulay, and Marchant. In the case operated upon by himself the sympathetic was divided upon both sides, and the patient left the hospital 9 days later cured of her exophthalmia. Reclus and Faure[4] have reported a case. Medical treatment had been without benefit and electricity brought only passing amelioration. The cervical sympathetic was readily resected on either side through an incision along the posterior border of the sternomastoid muscle, and improvement speedily ensued. By the 7th day the exophthalmos had almost entirely disappeared, and the ulceration of the cornea had cicatrized; the swelling of the neck had diminished; the pulse was reduced to 90; the trembling was less marked; and the general condition was greatly improved.

Myxedema.—Notkin[5] divides the symptoms following the removal of the thyroid into two marked groups, those of tetany and those of myxedema. Myxedema he considers the resultant of an albuminous substance, probably "thyreoproteid," whereas tetany depends upon autointoxication of the thyroidectomized animal with products of metabolism which are not of a proteid nature. While thyroidless men and animals are restored to perfect health by the administration of thyroid substance, and the albuminous poisons causing myxedema are neutralized by Baumann's iodothyrin, this preparation has no antitoxic property in respect to the poison inducing tetany. In a number of experiments on dogs he found that thyroids controlled the tremor and cachexia, but that iodothyrin was powerless. Robert Hutchinson[6] refers to former articles in which he showed that the chemistry of the thyroid furnishes two proteids, a nucleo-albumin and colloid matter. The extractives include creatin, xanthin, etc., and resemble those of other organs, but include, according to Fränkel, amido-bodies, to which an important part in the activity of the gland is to be ascribed. Separating these three varieties of products, Hutchinson experimented with each, and reached the conclusion that the pure colloid matter was the essential constituent of the gland, a position which is confirmed by the statements of Horsley and others, that the athyroidal state is proportionate to the absence of the colloid material in the gland. Hutchinson advises the use of the colloid material, which has a uniformity of activity and is capable of scientifically adjusted doses.

A correspondent of the *Boston Medical and Surgical Journal*, June 24, 1897, gives Kocher's views **on goiter and cretinism,** the results of his investigations as chairman of the Committee of Twenty-five Physicians. More than

[1] Centralbl. f. Chir., Jan. 16, 1897.   [2] Lyon méd., Feb. 7, 1897.
[3] Gaz. des Hôpitaux, June 19, July 1, 1897.
[4] Gaz. hebdom. de Méd. et de Chir., p. 592, June 24, 1897.
[5] Wien. klin. Woch., Oct. 22, 1896.   [6] Brit. Med. Jour., Jan. 23, 1897.

76,000 school children between the ages of 7 and 16 were reviewed, with their parentage and antecedents. The investigations were principally made in the Canton of Berne, Switzerland. The formulated results may be briefly stated as follows: the female is more frequently the victim of goiter than the male. In children between the ages of 9 and 14 years goiter reaches its highest degree of frequency, and rarely appears before they are sent to school, where the position of the head in reading and writing gives a tendency to the ailment. There is, therefore, a school-goiter. The secondary changes in the thyroid are proportionate to the advanced age of the individual. Congenital goiter is extremely rare. A still greater exception is congenital atrophy of the thyroid. Kocher noted that the districts supplied with water from the fresh-water sandstone showed a prevalence of goiter, while in the districts in which the water originated from salt-water sandstone goiter was infrequent. He concluded, however, that the prevalence of goiter depended upon the abundance of organic elements in the water rather than upon its source, and that neither deficient nourishment, unhealthy dwellings, nor wretchedness and poverty are a direct causation. Often the districts rich in goiter are separated by narrow limits from those free from the disease, and he discovered in goiter-laden localities oases free from goiter. He also found that there were actual goiter-fountains, the water of which almost invariably produced goiter in the children that drank it. On the other hand, in localities where goiter was prevalent families who had a private water-supply were sometimes free from the infection. Brooks and rivers and long, open conductors of water were unfavorable.

As to cretinism, Kocher, referring to heredity, finds that strong, healthy parents who in regions free from cretinism had begotten normal children, moving into a cretinoid district produced cretins. In these cases, however, the parents, one or both, had previous to the birth of the cretinoid children developed goiter. Such parents upon returning to their former place of residence have again had healthy children. In Kocher's opinion, whenever goiter or cretinism appears in children one of the parents will be found to have goiter; that cretinism arises only and solely when by degeneration of the thyroid gland, due to goiter or some other injury to the gland, its function is impaired or destroyed. Goiter is, therefore, the first stage of cretinism either occurring in the individual or through the parentage. He goes further, and declares that congenital inherited cretinism is derived from the mother alone, while inherited cretinism that appears after the lapse of a few months or years is derived from the father alone. This is explained by the fact that the fetus is supplied with normal thyroid conditions if the mother be not in an athyroidal state, and the inherited tendency from the father may be corrected during intrauterine life and even during lactation by the mother's condition, and only appears when the maternal source of thyroid products is cut off. The reports closes with the injunction to boil the drinking-water, thereby destroying the organic matter, the source of goiter in parents and of cretinism in the offspring.

Grünfeld[1] tried **thyroantitoxin** in 3 cases of exophthalmic goiter, 4 of obesity, 2 of bronchocele, and 1 of simple psoriasis. The drug induced loss of body-weight in 7 of the cases within a few days, subsequent loss of weight being very gradual. In one case of exophthalmic goiter the body-weight rapidly increased, in another it remained stationary. In one case of exophthalmic goiter there was rapid improvement at first, followed by relapse; the other two improved markedly, but were improving when the drug was commenced. In all cases the thyroid tumor softened without diminishing in size. In two cases the perspiration was decreased. In one there was decrease of

[1] Wien. med. Bl., Nos. 49 and 50, 1896.

pigmentation. Doses of 2 gr. a day were administered in some cases, though usually less. Grünfeld considers the preparation to have a certain therapeutic importance and one distinct from Baumann's iodothyrin.

Hyperostosis Cranii.—Putnam[1] writes on the subject of hyperostosis cranii, for which Starr proposed the term megalocephalic, and adds a number of cases (see Plate 8). The disease appears to develop early in life, often as the result of injury or of local inflammatory processes, and consists in an ostitis with deformities. Frequently there are osteophytic outgrowths on the exterior and the interior of the skull, giving rise to symptoms of cerebral tumor in the latter locality. Involvement of the cranial nerves at their exits is a common feature, and the patients usually perish as a result of the encroachment upon the cerebral structures. Dr. Edes[2] adds an additional case of this disease. Several of the cases mentioned by Putnam and the one by Edes, as well as the one reported by Starr[3] some months previously, were treated, without advantage, by the administration of thyroids. The suggestion that the disease is analogous to acromagaly does not seem to be borne out by the facts, as this disease is confined to the bones of the skull, especially the anterior portion, and the upper part of the face, and in most instances does not involve the extremities. Hinsdale[4] reports a case that occurred under the observation of Dr. Herwirsch, of Philadelphia.

Raynaud's Disease.—Aitken[5] reports a case of Raynaud's disease associated with uremic symptoms, marked by vascular spasm. The uremia reached the point of producing convulsions, which occurred sometimes in rapid succession, and during these periods the patient passed an extraordinarily small amount of urine with a gradually diminished output of urea. Death finally followed from uremic coma. This case, taken in connection with the numerous cases of Raynaud's disease marked by hemoglobinuria and the cases showing cerebral symptoms from vascular spasm, indicates the widespread nature of the vascular disturbance and the secondary symptoms which might arise from derangement of parenchymatous organs. Osler[6] reports three cases of Raynaud's disease in which there were notable **mental symptoms,** and refers to other instances in the literature in which it has been noted in asylum cases or under other conditions. There seems to be nothing uniform in the mental features associated with Raynaud's disease; sometimes there are maniacal disturbances, at others depression.

PSYCHONEUROSES.

Neurasthenia.—Knapp[7] discusses the mental symptoms in 150 cases of neurasthenia, 100 of which were observed in hospital and the remaining 50 in private practice. The commonest mental symptom he finds to be a simple depression, which existed in 27 cases to a degree sufficient to warrant complaint. He finds this more common in private patients than in those entering general hospitals. In some cases the depression passes beyond physiologic bounds and enters the realm of melancholia, the line of division being an indefinite one. Ideas of suicide occasionally result from the depression, and usually occur under conditions of more or less pain, the sight of lethal weapons, or opportunities for self-destruction. These impulses are usually fully described by the patient, unlike those which occur in melancholia and which often show the result of prolonged premeditation. He considers them analo-

[1] Am. Jour. Med. Sci., July, 1896.　　　[2] Ibid.　　　　　　　　[3] Ibid.
[4] Jour. Nerv. and Ment. Dis., Dec., 1896.　　[5] Lancet, Sept. 26, 1896.
[6] Am. Jour. Med. Sci., Nov., 1896.　　　[7] Boston M. and S. Jour., Oct. 22, 1896.

PLATE 8.

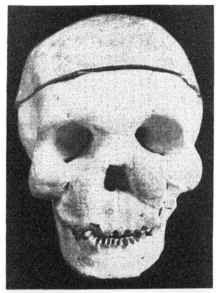

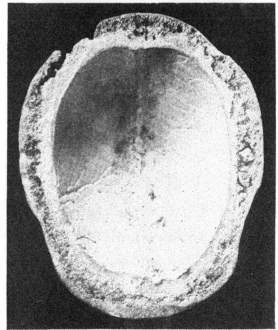

Hyperostosis cranii (Am. Jour. Med. Sci., July, 1896).

gous to the vague suicidal impulses that are common in mental health, in which people think of jumping in front of a train or from a height, or shooting themselves, or taking poison, but which impulses are controlled promptly and with readiness. Aside from simple depressions, the largest mental manifestation of neurasthenia may be classed under the head of imperative ideas and morbid fears. These he finds, as might be expected, more common among his private patients than in the hospital cases, mental disturbance being in some relative proportion to the mental development, education, and experience of the patient. He noted such morbid ideas in 21 cases out of his 50 private patients, 15 times in the form of fear, and 6 times in the form of imperative ideas. In the severe forms of neurasthenia, in which the chronic character of the trouble and the failure of various forms of treatment lead to despondency, these fears may persist, and out of them grow delusions which carry the patient into the field of insanity. This is either in the direction of melancholia, or these patients will discuss their morbid fears with the greatest readiness and dwell minutely upon all the circumstances, without a corresponding amount of dejection. The ideas becoming fixed, the condition approaches paranoia, into which it may eventually pass.

Epilepsy.—H. Higier[1] reports a case of **epileptic paroxysmal paralysis** which is closely related to the Jacksonian variety of epilepsy. A boy 6 years of age, of sound parentage, like his sister had convulsions in infancy, which were attributed to the teeth, and was rachitic from the age of 2 years until brought under observation. From the age of 3 he had grown well and developed both physically and mentally. At about the age of $5\frac{1}{2}$ he had experienced a convulsion with loss of consciousness and other evidences of an epileptic character, including the tonic and clonic phases. A week and a half later he complained of prickling, tickling sensations below the right knee, and at the same moment felt such a complete weakness of the limbs that he scarcely had time to seek the bed. Since that time, nearly every day, sometimes 15 or 20 times a day, he has experienced similar attacks. Under personal observation the paresthesia and loss of power seemed to affect the lower extremities without subjective feeling of cramp or contracture. There was no alteration of the patellar reflexes or sensibility.

Clark[2] makes a study of **mental automatism in epilepsy,** either following an epileptic attack or taking its place, and recites several cases in which the automatism lasted several hours and even several days, during which time the patients acted in a practically normal way, and their automatism was only determined by comparison with their more natural moods. In one case a female patient had a severe attack the night before admission to the Craig Colony. After three weeks of automatism the patient became conscious of where she was, and partially conscious of what had occurred since her admission. In another case a first attack was followed by maniacal disturbance lasting for some days. Three years after this first attack the patient, on his way home from work as a railroad engineer, stopped in the way-station, threw out both operators, and sent a message by telegraph to the central station and received the reply. After doing so he locked the door of the station and went on his way home. He only became aware of what he had done by finding the key of the station in his pocket the next morning. In both these cases the return to consciousness was rather sudden. In another instance the patient, in an automatic state, carried packages about the colony and conversed rationally upon any subject suggested. During the day he made but one mistake in carrying messages and packages, and the same day received letters and

[1] Neurol. Centralbl., Feb. 15, 1897.   [2] Boston M. and S. Jour., Jan. 14, 1897.

papers from his friends. The following morning he was entirely oblivious of their receipt and of all the occurrences of the previous day. The same author [1] tabulates 9545 epileptic seizures arranged to show the number of attacks occurring in each hour during the day. He finds that they were about evenly divided, the greatest number, 537, occurring between 4 and 5 A. M., and the least number, 224, between 7 and 8 P. M. The author points out that these particular patients being under bromid and chloral, the early morning hours would be the furthest removed from the last bromid dose, and the low tone of the nervous system in the early morning hours may in addition predispose to the frequency of the fits at that hour. Clark [2] also gives a brief account of 3 cases of epilepsy presenting psychical attacks substituting the fits. Regarding the prognosis in these cases, he considers it unfavorable as to recovery, but of better prognosis as to life than is usual in the cases showing more pronounced motor storms.

A. M. Bleile [3] reports on **examinations of urine** carried out at the Epileptic Colony at Gallipolis, Ohio, the purpose of which was to seek for poisonous bodies, ptomains or toxalbumins, and variations in the ordinary constituents of the urine. The examination covered a period of 30 days, embracing 12 patients. Consideration was given to the specific gravity and amount, urea, uric acid and its relation to urea, phosphates, sulfates, and indol. As to specific gravity and quantity, the epileptic attacks cause, according to this series, no definite variation in either direction. It was found that very generally there was a diminution of the total phosphates, and that there was usually an increase of alkaline phosphates in the ratio existing between the alkaline and earthy forms. This variation, however, is supposed to be no greater than would be occasioned by muscular exercise of equal violence and duration to that produced in the motor phenomena of the fit. Sulphuric acid was investigated as total sulfates, both in the form of ethereal and preformed. The ethereal sulfates embraced the aromatic series, phenol, indol, skatol, etc. The greatest importance was attached to the ethereal, as showing the amount of putrefaction going on in the organism, and its increase, absolute or relative to the preformed sulfates, was considered an index of putrefactive activity, though it is admitted that forms of putrefaction or fermentation may occur without the formation of these bodies, as is claimed by Herter and Smith. For the whole period it was found that in all cases the total amount of sulfates remained below the average normal, this, with other similar findings, being attributed to the diminished quantity of meat in the dietary of these patients. As a general result, it was noted that the putrefactive sulfates were absolutely and relatively decreased below the quantities found in ordinary health and upon an ordinary diet. The author, however, inclines to the view that putrefaction in the economy might go on in certain directions without increasing the ethereal sulfates, but would be indicated perhaps by the production of different bodies, still to be discovered. The search for indol or indican shows practically the same thing as the investigation for the ethereal sulfates in general. In regard to urea, nothing in particular was found, the sum total being usually below 30 gm. of the normal amount, owing to the restricted diet. The same was true of uric acid; but as to the ratio between uric acid and urea the writer finds, contrary to the assertion of Haig and in agreement with Herter and Smith, that the proper proportions were not overpassed at any time by their epileptic patients. In a general way, Bleile anticipates that some toxic substance will be discovered in epilepsy, probably in the uric-acid

[1] Med. Rec., July 31, 1897.   [2] Ibid., Feb. 20, 1897.
[3] N. Y. Med. Jour., May 8, 1897.

group similar to the paraxanthin found by Rachford in migraine. The toxicity of the urine was determined by injections of the ethereal putrefactives into frogs and rabbits, and showed that in epilepsy it was increased.

Medical Treatment of Epilepsy.—Mairel and Bose[1] have reported their experiments with pituitary extract in 21 epileptics. Its administration was followed by a slight elevation of temperature and increase in pulse, but no effect upon the epilepsy was produced. In some instances a slight delirium was occasioned.

Féré[2] gives a *résumé* of a number of cases treated by **borax,** showing that very little importance is to be attached to the remedy.

Spratling, Superintendent of the Craig Colony for Epileptics, in his third annual report to the State Board of Charities of New York, October 13, 1896, states regarding the treatment of epileptics under his care that **the Flechsig treatment** was tried in 12 carefully selected cases. In 3 the opium produced great stupor and had to be withdrawn, bromid being at once substituted. The others had the full course of opium, and then bromid was administered. The results were at the time of the report: 1 had had no attacks, 2 were greatly improved, in 3 the attacks were reduced to one-third of their former frequency and severity, and 6 showed no improvement. *Thyroids* were administered in 5 cases, and resulted in benefit in 2 cases; 2 others were slightly benefited, and 1 derived no benefit. The changes induced related to the physical and mental state of the patients, and no modification of the epilepsy was observed. A great majority of the cases were treated by *bromid and chloral,* in addition to which importance is attached to the *dietetic management,* the purpose being to reduce the overconsumption of meat so characteristic of the neurosis, and to furnish outdoor labor, with resulting good physical conditions. He observed that 131 out of 145 cases admitted showed the various *stigmata of degeneracy* in the ear, palate, face, and cranium. Valuable tables showing the character of the aura, the character of the attack, the time of its occurrence, and the assigned causes, with other data related to the disease, are appended.

Henry P. Frost[3] reports upon the use of **sulfonal and trional** in the management of these cases. The patients invariably felt well under the influence of the medicine, and disturbances among them in the way of assaults and altercations were less frequent. The dose varied from 5 gr. twice daily to 10 gr. three times a day, the object being to obtain a slight effect only, and the larger dose was rarely continued more than a few days in any case. In one case the heart was seriously depressed even by a very moderate dose of sulfonal.

Flechsig[4] reviews the unfavorable results of the **Flechsig treatment** with the combination of opium and bromids, as reported by several recent writers. He believes that the fatal cases on record have no relation to the treatment, pointing out that a fatal result is common enough in status without any treatment or under any treatment. In his own experience, in treatment by increasing doses of opium, 6 cases out of 50 have had no recurrence. All of the cases treated were severe, of many years' duration, and had resisted all previous treatment. When the opium is used the patient must be treated as one who is seriously ill, and kept under skilful medical attendance and observation.

Operative Treatment of Partial Epilepsy.—[The question of operation in epilepsy is one that has called for very much attention during the last few years. The optimistic outlook of 6 or 8 years ago has unfortunately not

[1] Arch. de Physiol., No. 3, 1896.   [2] Nouv. Icon. de la Salpêt., July and Aug., 1896.
[3] State Hospitals Bull., Oct., 1896.   [4] Neurol. Centralbl., Jan., 1897.

been substantiated by results, and there is a tendency to go to the opposite extreme.] A conservative estimate of operation in epilepsy is furnished in an article by Sachs and Gerster,[1] of New York, in which the following conclusions are reached : 1. Those cases of partial epilepsy are suitable for operation in which at most 1 to 3 years have elapsed since the trauma or the onset of the disease. 2. In depression of the skull or in other injuries to the skull operative interference is indicated even after years. The prognosis, however, is less good the longer the elapsed time since the original injury. 3. Simple trephining may suffice in many cases ; this is especially true if one is concerned with skull-injury, or with cyst-formation. 4. Excision of the cortical lesion is advisable, if the epilepsy is of short duration and referable to an exactly localizable portion of the brain. 5. Since such lesions are often only visible microscopically, excision should be undertaken even if the diseased part macroscopically appears normal. Still one should, however, use the greatest caution, in order that the proper portion be excised. 6. Surgical interference in epilepsy occurring in connection with infantile cerebral paralysis is permissible, if it occurs not too long after the onset of the paralysis. 7. In old cases of partial epilepsy, in which very probably an extended degeneration of association-fibers has taken place, surgical interference is entirely useless.

Brauu[2] has reported a successful case, the patient remaining free from recurrence during a period of 6 years since the operation. In addition, an analysis is given of 22 cases treated by removal of the motor center from which the epileptic attack had started. In 14 of these cases treatment had been completely successful, but in only 5 had the interval between the operation and report exceeded a year. [Braun is inclined to be more hopeful regarding the advantages of operation in traumatic Jacksonian epilepsy than in any other form, which corresponds with the experience of competent writers the world over.]

Beach[3] calls attention to his early use of **gold foil placed within the dura** to prevent adhesions between the meninges and the cortex. The operation was done in 1892, with favorable results regarding the epileptic attacks, which had returned subsequent to a previous operation done in the ordinary manner. He refers to a case seen by Oliver, of Cincinnati, who had the opportunity of making a postmortem examination, and found that adhesions had been prevented. Sachs and Gerster, in an article already referred to, make the same recommendation. [This measure has everything to commend it.]

Hysteria.—Kattwinkel,[4] in a careful examination of 104 cases of hysteria, found that in 100 there was abolition of the pharyngeal reflex, and concludes that the disappearance of this reflex is a very satisfactory stigma of hysteria, and must be so recognized.

Prince[5] relates several cases in which sensory impairment on one side was associated with **monocular blindness.** His cases prove that a high degree of binocular vision is absolutely consistent with hysterical monocular blindness.

P. Ricker and A. Sougues[6] give the history of a case of **male hysteria** in which the principal symptom was contracture of the anterior and posterior muscles of the trunk, producing a rigid, semiflexed position of the body, which could not voluntarily be extended dorsally nor further flexed anteriorly (see Fig.

[1] Deutsch. med. Woch., Aug. 27, 1896; also Am. Jour. Med. Sci., Oct., 1896.
[2] Centralbl. f. Chir., No. 44.   [3] Boston M. and S. Jour., Mar. 25, 1897.
[4] Deutsch. Arch. f. klin. Med., Bd. 57, Sept. 5 and 6, 1896.
[5] Am. Jour. Med. Sci., Feb., 1897.   [6] Nouv. Icon. de la Salpêt., Mar. and Apr., 1897.

55). Over one shoulder-blade and about a portion of the chest there was a zone of hyperesthesia containing a hysterogenetic spot that made the diagnosis certain. This hysterical spasm was the result of traumatism, and, as in other cases, such as those of P. Janet, referred to in the *Year-Book* for 1897, and the cases published by Duret and by Vich, was solely dependent upon the fixed idea of dorsal injury. [It is not unlikely that many cases of so-called traumatic lumbago and of rigidities of the spine after traumatic conditions may be of this same nature.]

Karplus[1] reports a case of hysteria in which there was **absence of the pupil-reflex.** The diagnosis was confirmed by Krafft-Ebing, and the symptom was also recognized by Bernheim, the ophthalmologist. An observation by Féré constitutes with this the only two in the literature in which hysteria served to paralyze the pupil. To these we now add the following: V. Jez[2] reports a case of hysteria in a male who presented the full clinical features of Charcot's grande hystérie ; but in addition there was paralysis of the facial, of the hypoglossus, and of the third cranial pairs, causing complete ophthalmoplegia, etc., with loss of hearing, all of which passed away under general treatment of the neurosis.

Arthur Van Harlingen[3] takes up a consideration of **hysterical neuroses of the skin,** and gives an extensive bibliography. The different affections of the skin which have been described as occurring in the course of hysteria he lists as follows : erythema, dermatitis, urticaria (including dermographism), hyperidrosis, edema, urticaria bullosum, pemphigus, herpes zoster, eczema, gangrene, pigmentation, vitiligo, lichen, chromidrosis, ecchymosis, hematidrosis. He then describes them in detail. These, the author states, belong to one category marked by erythema, which may go on to urticaria and

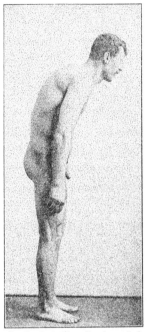

Fig 55 —Contraction of trunk-muscles in traumatic hysteria (Nouv. Icon. de la Salp., Mar. and Apr., 1897).

edema. In a further stage there are vesicular and bullar formations, and finally gangrene. Side by side with these are noted alterations in pigmentary deposit and disturbances of sweat-secretion. They make up a group of vasomotor neuroses. Other disturbances of the skin, such as those found in erythromelalgia, Raynaud's disease, Morvan's disease, disturbances of the hair and nails, are probably more commonly coincidences than due to the hysteria.

MENTAL DISEASES.

Pathologic Studies in Insanity.—Adolf Meyer[4] reports on 192 autopsies in the two years, 1893 to 1895. In a large number of senile dements he finds that the fundamental cause consisted in atheromatous

---

[1] Wien. klin. Woch , No. 52, 1896.   [2] Ibid., Aug. 1, 1896.
[3] Am. Jour. Med. Sci., July, 1897.   [4] Path. Report, Ill. East. Hosp. for the Insane, 1896.

degeneration of the cerebral blood-vessels and in the frequently resulting atrophy of the brain. These anatomical changes stand as the basis of senile dementia. In 25 cases of epilepsy a large variety of organic lesions are recorded; 15 of the 25 showed some lesion of the nervous system, and the author is at a loss often to decide whether the lesion was primary or secondary. In one case only does he note sclerosis of the cornu ammonis. Among the other conditions found were a small foci of softening, hemorrhagic pachymeningitis, tubercle, cerebral hemiatrophy, diffuse cortical sclerosis, etc. In general paralysis the pia in all cases presented more or less edema and opacity which almost invariably involved the ependyma of the ventricles. Regarding the syphilitic etiology of the disease, the detailed histories are not competent. It is noted only 8 times in 41 cases. The groups of cases denominated acute mania or acute delirious mania will be found interesting to those who are inclined to look upon acute psychoses as of toxic or septic origin. Lesions of the body-organs, usually of an infectious character, were commonly present.

Anatomic Changes in the Brain in Paranoiac Insanity.—Feist,[1] as the result of an examination of the brains and nervous systems of four paranoiacs, reports one case showing peculiar punctate, mesh-like growths in the neuroglia of the posterior columns of the cord, apparently due to degenerated axis-cylinders. There was also a neuroma on one of the dorsal nerves. In another case there was an ascending degeneration of the posterior 6th cervical root, with hyperplasia of the neuroglia of the posterior columns. A third case presented a disappearance of fibres in the gray matter of the cord and a small spot of softening in one anterior horn, due to vascular sclerosis, degeneration of the white matter, and atrophy of the cerebral cortex. A fourth case gave hyaline areas in the gray matter of the cord and some degeneration of the posterior columns. The most constant change was in the posterior columns, in the form of degeneration of the nerve-fibres and diffuse hyperplasia of the neuroglia. The relation of these changes to paranoia is as yet unexplained. They may have something to do with the anesthesia and indifference to traumatism, inflammation, etc., so common in such cases. [The indifference to cutaneous sensibility is not confined to paranoiacs, but reaches its highest degree in the demented, and is a very common finding in paresis. The changes in the cord cited above are not sufficiently marked or widely distributed to account for these particular symptoms. Their value consists in showing the tendency of the nervous system to break down, though the four cases mentioned were all advanced in years, and some of these changes may be of senile origin merely.]

Intestinal Autotoxis and Insanity.—A. McL. Hamilton,[2] after discussing the possible relation of intestinal autointoxication to mental disturbance, reaches the following conclusions, which are based largely upon his investigations of evidence of putrefaction, as shown by the condition of the urine, and particularly by the presence of the ethereal sulfates in that excretion, as they are taken as an evidence, and to some extent as an indication, of the amount of putrefaction occurring within the economy: 1. Urines rich in indican contain very little or no preformed sulphuric acid, and are toxic. 2. When the sulfate ratio is materially changed, it is likely to indicate autotoxis in connection with an increase in the amount of combined or ethereal sulfates. 3. Such indications are generally found with acute insanities, in which rapidly developing symptoms occur. 4. Fugacious and changing illusions and hallucinations, unsystematized delusions, confusion, and verbigeration in connection

---

[1] Virchow's Archiv, Bd. 138, p. 443. [2] N. Y. Med. Jour., Nov. 14, 1896.

with insomnia, pallor, intestinal indigestion, constipation, and rapid exhaustion, are due to autotoxis. 5. Paranoiac states, or those in which concepts are the features, chronic stuporous conditions and certain forms of dementia have little to do with the formation of intestinal products of putrefaction. 6. Various postfebrile, traumatic, alcoholic, or drug insanities are those in which autotoxis is most constant. 7. The variations in the excretion of combined sulfates keep pace with the changes in the progress of an established insanity, acnes and epileptoid attacks being directly connected with the putrefactive processes. 8. The most successful treatment consists in lavage, intestinal douches, gastric and intestinal antisepsis by means of hydrochloric acid, borax, sodium salicylate, charcoal, guaiacol, or naphthalin in small, repeated doses, and the administration of a combination of the red marrow from the small bones, blood, and glycerin.

W. von Jauregg,[1] basing his statements upon clinical and chemical facts, supposes that many acute psychoses are dependent upon autointoxication from gastrointestinal derangements. These are shown by acetone, diacetone, and butyric acid in the urine, and he corroborates von Jaksch's observations of acute mental trouble, such as amentia and postepileptic and postalcoholic deliriums following upon acetonuria. His treatment is based upon calomel and iodoform to empty and disinfect the gastrointestinal canal.

Masturbation and Insanity.—Goodner[2] reports 4 cases of young males in whom insanity, which caused them to be brought to the Illinois Southern Hospital for the Insane, was attributed to masturbation. In 3 there was the stuporous form of melancholia. In the fourth a diagnosis of acute melancholia was given. Although the author is inclined to believe that hereditary tendency is a much stronger factor than masturbation itself, in these 4 cases no such element existed, and he thinks that onanism acted as the sole exciting cause of the insanity. [The cases are not reported with sufficient fulness, and the history is not sufficiently complete to enable the reader to decide for himself whether masturbation played any part or not.]

Mania following Orchotomy ; Successful Treatment with Testiculin.—Cabot[3] reports a case in which during a crushing-operation for stone the surgeon removed both testicles, in a well-preserved man of 75. He had, however, showed some slight mental disturbance previous to the operation. Following recovery from the anesthetic there was confusional mental disturbance with exacerbations of a maniacal sort. The wound healed kindly and the prostate became considerably reduced, so that a month after the operation the patient passed some urine voluntarily. With care to prevent suggestion and without informing the patient or his friends, testiculin was employed for about two weeks, under which a practically complete improvement of the mental symptoms appeared. [This is perhaps the first case in which the substitution of an organic extract for these removed organs has been tried. We hope to have later accounts of the case and of other cases of a similar nature which now are falling into the hands of surgeons who do orchotomy for enlarged prostate. The possibility of the increased mental disturbance being due to the anesthetic, and not to the orchotomy, must be kept in view.]

Typhoid Fever in Insanity.—R. A. Goodner[4] discusses the influence of typhoid fever in the production of insanity, and its effect upon insanity when occurring during mental disease. He reaches the following conclusions: Typhoid does not cause insanity nearly so often as is believed and

[1] Wien. klin. Woch., No. 19, 1896.   [2] Med. News, Feb. 27, 1897.
[3] Ann. of Surg., Sept., 1896.   [4] Medicine, Feb., 1897.

taught. If typhoid causes insanity, it is usually indirectly the result of the great general physical enfeeblement. Typhoid often results in mental recovery, by renovating and improving the condition and functions of the intestines. The melancholias are most likely to be benefited by or to recover after typhoid, as they commonly originate in derangement of the gastrointestinal tract. A valuable lesson to be drawn from a study of the effects of typhoid on the insane is that in treating the insane or those predisposed to mental trouble we should give special attention to the intestinal tract. [Taking into account the relation of acute infections and confusional mania there is little reason to doubt the causative relation of typhoid to many cases of acute mania. It is also true that it is often the inciting cause, a predisposition existing. With the author's conclusions as to the effect of typhoid when occurring in the insane we can agree, but as to the mechanism the case is not proved.]

Insanity in Women.—Rohe[1] takes up this subject again, and continues his plea for gynecological work among insane women. He is inclined to discredit the number of cases showing mental disturbance after gynecological operations, and believes that the mental disturbances following pelvic operations are analogous to those of climacteric insanity, except where they come on within a few days of the operation, when they are usually in the nature of septic delirium.

Endemic Insanity.—Laffan[2] describes an area of four square miles in County Meath, Ireland, with a population of about 300 persons. One-half of the families have one or more insane, suicidal, idiotic, or goitrous members. This he attributes to consanguinity and heredity, as the conditions under which the people live and their agricultural employment neither account for the endemic nor serve to limit it.

Influence of Tobacco on Nervous and Mental Disorders.—Buccelli,[3] after some experiments with tobacco and observations upon its use, reaches the following conclusions: 1. Tobacco is a poison, which, perhaps more than any other, though having little effect in health, has, on the other hand, the most pronounced action in diseased conditions. 2. Tobacco is especially a poison to the subcortical and bulbar nerve-centers, as is demonstrated by the phenomena developed in individuals affected with serious morbid processes of the cortical centers. 3. Being thus capable of producing disastrous effects in convalescent cases who were given to its use before their disorder, and had then suffered no disadvantages, we should be very cautious as to permitting the resumption of its use in such cases, especially in asylums.

Morphinism.—Erlenmeyer[4] advocates the chemical treatment of morphinism. He has abandoned the method of simply rapidly cutting off the morphin, which method he formerly most vigorously advocated, and now finds superior results in what he calls the chemical treatment. He noticed that the sudden withdrawal of the drug was associated with symptoms of hyperacid dyspepsia, and upon investigation found that the suffering caused by the discontinuance of morphin was attended by the presence of an excess of hydrochloric acid in the stomach. This accords with the fact that morphin is eliminated through the stomach after having been absorbed, and one habituated to the drug, being deprived of the regular sedative effect of the morphin upon the glandular apparatus of the stomach, is placed in a condition of overgastric activity, excess of acid is poured out, with symptoms of gastric dis-

[1] Am. Jour. Obst., Dec., 1896.   [2] Brit. Med. Jour., Sept. 26, 1896.
[3] Rivista di Patologia. I Fasc., Oct. 10, 1896; Am. Jour. Insan., Jan., 1897.
[4] Progrès méd., Aug. 1, 1896.

order and reflex disturbance. To counteract this, Hitzig washed out the stomach and introduced a solution of Carlsbad salts. Erlenmeyer, on the other hand, aims at the neutralization of the acid by means of Fachingen water, which contains a considerable portion of sodium bicarbonate. Thirty cases have been treated in this manner with an entire absence of gastric or nervous symptoms, but the craving for morphin remains unappeased, and it must be gradually withdrawn.

Magnan's Sign in Chronic Cocainism.—Ribakoff[1] has observed Magnan's sign as a predominant symptom of cocain-addiction in 2 cases. This sign consists in an hallucination of cutaneous sensibility characterized by a sensation of foreign bodies under the skin, which are described as inert and spherical, varying in size from a grain to a nut, or as living organisms, worms, bugs, etc. It seems peculiar to intoxication by cocain, and is of considerable differential value. [In the case of a physician, falling under the writer's notice, this hallucination was attributed to "little bugs" that dug deeply into the tissues. He was a mass of scars and wounds where he had proceeded with a scalpel to eject the invaders. In this case there was also hallucination of sight, as he claimed to be able to see the bugs, and asserted that he had watched them boring through the marble top of the washstand. Another physician addicted to cocain had precisely the same ideas.]

Bed-treatment and Isolation in Acute Insanity.—Heilbronner[2] draws the following conclusions on this subject : 1. In institutions that receive a large number of excited patients the association of the same in large observation-halls is accompanied with serious disadvantages. 2. These disadvantages can be relieved : *a.* By a separate observation-room for the extremely disturbed cases, and, eventually, a third for quiet and orderly patients, separate from the receiving-ward properly so-called ; *b.* By a subdivision of the observation-ward, and, finally, by removing the most affected patients into single rooms of a homelike appearance. 3. By suitable architectural arrangements permitting this separation into single rooms, together with thorough watching and care, and the use of the treatment in bed ; isolation in this form is to be considered as a valuable therapeutic method. 4. Isolation for other than therapeutic reasons can in this way be reduced to a minimum, but cannot as yet be altogether dispensed with. For certain cases rooms of a stronger construction should be provided.

A. Berustein[3] reports the results of this method for the acutely insane, as shown in a year's experience in the psychiatric clinic at Moscow. He finds it practicable beyond expectation, and that under this method of treatment the manifestations of the mental disorder become less intense, the motor excitement is reduced to a minimum, the intellectual excitations diminished, and the delirium is milder and monotonous. He deduces from this no general conclusions, and leaves the future to decide whether the contraction, so to speak, of the intellectual horizon, tends to repose of the brain or to mental decadence. The experience of the Moscow clinic proves only one thing, viz., the negative finding that recovery is not more prompt and frequent than under the former methods with all their disadvantages. In this he admits that he is in disagreement with some others who have reported on the results of this treatment elsewhere, but he appeals, apparently with reason, to their own statistics in support of his opinion. He deprecates the zeal for this new method which would make it a routine treatment, disregarding the individual needs of every patient, but believes it an advance, as aiding to do away with

---

[1] Gaz. degli Ospedali e delle Clin., Aug. 4, 1896.   [2] Am. Jour. Insan., Apr., 1897.
[3] Ann. Médico-Psychologiques, iv., No. 1, Jan., 1897.

seclusion, untidiness, and destructiveness, and the costly and objectionable appliances hitherto employed to meet these requirements.

Clark Gapen,[1] describing this method at Kankakee, speaks very highly of the results obtained by bed-treatment. According to him, "nearly every new case is given bed-treatment under nursing-care for a month, more or less, according to circumstances." He seems to precede the treatment with massage and flushing of the colon, and a steam or vapor bath, after all which "the patient is both weary and thirsty." Then he is put to bed under the care of the female nurse and food administered. The patient usually goes to sleep as soon as he has partaken of the food, and generally awakes quieter. This is described as the routine treatment, and is applied as well to irritable epileptics as to violent maniacs. Gapen is enthusiastic in favor of female nurses, and says that in no case has there been any indignity offered them, though it was feared this might happen. He finds this class of patients are much more quiet in the hands of women than men. His system requires a specially fitted ward, in which are four trained female nurses and three orderlies, who have charge of never more than 11 cases. It is spoken of, nevertheless, as "taking all the troublesome cases off the other wards."

Senile Insanities.—Ralph Lyman Parsons[2] treats this very important subject in a careful article. Perhaps senile insanity falls as often under the immediate care of the general practitioner as any other form of mental aberration, and very many of these cases can be properly cared for at home if their circumstances are such as to enable them to have the proper liberty and supervision. The author considers the causation of senile insanities as those so remote as to have been beyond control; those in action in earlier periods of life; and those in action when senility is impending. Under the second class, which are within the range of medical direction, are principally the causes of vascular change and premature senility of the arteries. These are chronic alcoholism, syphilis, gout, rheumatism, venereal excesses, great and prolonged physical strain, intense and long-continued mental application, with anxiety or worry and lack of self-control, as indulgence in the passions of grief or anger. Causes in operation at a more advanced period of life are some of those above enumerated; others are due to advanced physical feebleness and the associated mental decay. At this time many men attempt to maintain a youthful habit which their powers does not justify. This pride may lead them to physical or mental excesses. On the other hand, cases are encountered in which the patient is inclined to yield too readily to the feeling of feebleness, and here needs encouragement. A lack of sufficient food and of digestive ability is one of the prominent causes of the invasion of mental disturbance late in life. This is usually associated with insomnia or with disturbed and inadequate sleep, which is often pieced out by a nap during the day. The indications are clearly for full attention to the digestive apparatus and the securing of a proper amount of sleep at suitable intervals. The prophylactic management of these various items will at once suggest itself. In case of actual insanity the question at once arises whether the patient shall be treated at home or in a sanitarium, hospital, or asylum. This must be determined by the individual circumstances of each case and the character of the mental disturbance. The manias usually require institution-management. The depressed features and the demented forms can be readily cared for at home. The author points out very forcibly, in case lay attendants or kind neighbors assume charge of the patient, that they must be individually instructed by the physician most thor-

---

[1] N. Am. Pract., Feb., 1897.   [2] Med. Rec., Oct. 10, 1896.

oughly in all the details of watchfulness and nursing, and that it is never safe to trust anything to their appearance of intelligence.

Shäfer [1] calls attention to **the mental state of the aged,** opening with the statement that old age is the period of normal decline, an intermittent stage between growth and death. It is a physiological process presenting a special aspect, which is the consequence of complicated atrophic processes, and may be considered as a particular phenomenon of cellular life. From a mental point of view the evolution of old age may be divided into three periods, with numerous variations. The first period is characterized especially by a change of temperament, and of instinctive manifestations, sometimes badly controlled. In this stage the old man remains the master of his faculties, but with difficulty acquires new ideas. The second period is prefatory to dementia, and is characterized, first, by the gradual disappearance of mental faculties; second, by the gradual disappearance of affective faculties and the sentiments; third, by the return of instinct. Disappearance of faculties and sentiments occurs in inverse order to their acquisition, the most complex and most elevated first subsiding. The weakness of intellect and of sentimental life always creates a disharmony in their ideas and judgment eminently likely to produce erroneous interpretations and the perpetration of reprehensible acts or leading to action under sudden impulse. In this way the author explains the frequency of suicide among the aged, acts of immodesty and exhibitionism. The artistic acquisitions do not follow the law of recession laid down by Herbert Spencer, often remaining to the last. The third period is the period of senile dementia. The aged reach it gradually, or sometimes suddenly after a period of physical or intellectual overactivity. In certain of the aged, physical decay is not accompanied by intellectual degradation. Regarding responsibility, the author states that it is practically complete in the first period of senility, partial or limited in the second, and *nil* in the third. Certain of the aged grow old with great suddenness—they are precociously senile. This seems to be due to heredity or acquired diathetic influences, such as infections or intoxications. Melancholia is the psychosis most frequently observed in the aged, and all the psychoses are usually manifest in exaltation of the sentiment of personal preservation and preservation of property, frequently with erotic tendencies.

Paretic Dementia.—Piccinnino,[2] an assistant of Prof. Bianchi, reports five examinations of paretic brains in the laboratory of the Institute Psichiatrico of the University of Naples. These cases of paresis had clear syphilitic histories in some instances, in others it was suspected or denied. With the greatest precautions portions of the meninges and brain were removed through small trephine-openings, to prevent contamination by the removal of the calavarium, and culture-experiments gave absolutely negative results. Slightly modified staining-methods of Lustgarten for his syphilis-bacillus, on the other hand, revealed a great abundance of this bacterium in all the tissues, especially in the perivascular spaces. The same method employed in a number of brains of other varieties of insanity met with a negative result. [It is to be hoped that these findings will be at once confirmed or refuted, as in case they are true it definitely fixes the syphilitic etiology of paretic dementia.]

Gross[3] discusses **the early diagnosis of paretic dementia,** and maintains that the differential diagnosis in the early stage of general paresis mainly concerns neurasthenia, and he further points out the important consideration that the ordinary hydrotherapeutic treatment of neurasthenia is very likely to aggravate general paresis. He bases his statements upon the

---

[1] Lyon Thesis for 1896, abstracted in Arch. de Neurol., June, 1897. [2] Ann. di Neurologia.
[3] Heidelberg Allg. Zeit. f. Psych., H. 3, Bd. 2.

observation of 189 cases. In only 10 of these was a very acute onset noted; in all the rest neurasthenic or pseudoneurasthenic conditions marked the early stage. He would base the differential diagnosis, even before motor symptoms and intellectual enfeeblement appear, upon the modifications of character, certain expansive phenomena, cerebral excitement, and spasmodic activity. He calls especial attention to the modifications of character which show themselves in a tendency to brutishness, with the occasional appearance of mental confusion, shown by tardiness of conception and enfeeblement of thought, with a diminution of memory. The abnormal acts of general paretics are traceable to the loss of elevated sentiments and an impairment of judgment. These acts, often considered as the cause of neurasthenia, are really the symptoms of the general paresis, and embrace heedless speculation, absurd conduct, and all sorts of excesses. He admits, however, that there is a considerable series of cases in which the differential diagnosis is impossible. Here he considers the age to furnish certain useful indications, stating that neurasthenia is a constitutional affection that nearly always shows itself during youth, while, on the contrary, paretic dementia is a disease of adult life. In his 189 cases only 3 appeared before the age of 30. He believes that when neurasthenia shows itself between 30 and 50 years of age, in a man up to that time of normal health and not neuropathic, that very fact should weigh for something in raising a suspicion of general paresis. In the same way, the appearance of psychical trouble for the first time in adult age has some significance, and apparent recovery is not sufficient to upset the diagnosis. In regard to remissions, he cites a number of interesting and important cases in which the periods of depression, with ideas of persecution and the hypochondriacal delirium, have, even after many months or years, during which there was apparent health, recurred with the full train of somatic conditions common to paresis. He has noted remissions of from 2 to 10 years between the first and second manifestations of the disease, and in many of these cases the first attack was not at the time recognized as belonging to the malady.

August Hoch[1] reports **general paresis** in sisters aged 16 and 19 years respectively, with the autopsy in one case. He makes the following summary, in which especial attention may be called to the luetic history of the father: " It is evident that the two sisters, who were in apparently good health previous to the onset of their disease, gradually developed the symptoms of general paralysis, the one beginning at the age of 10, the other at the age of 15 years. There is a neuropathic heredity, inasmuch as the father was prematurely senile, the mother very nervous. Besides, it is probable that the father has had lues, and we have seen that a luetic heredity is very common in such cases. [It may be said to be invariable.] The clinical course in both sisters was that of a simple progressive dementia, lasting in one case for 6 years, in the other, so far, 4 years. We see from the literature that this simple demented form is the most common in these juvenile cases. The autopsy in the younger sister proved the diagnosis. The lesions in the cerebral cortex were those commonly seen in general paralysis. Similar changes were found in the basal ganglia. In the cerebellar cortex was seen a more or less pronounced degeneration of many Purkinje cells, with great increase in the neuroglia of the cortex and marked diminution in the thickness of the cortex. In the cord the anterior and lateral pyramids were affected. This degeneration could be followed into the pons, but was apparently lost in the crura. From the upper dorsal cord upward there was a degeneration in Gowers' tract, the field of degeneration becoming best marked in the high cervical region and at the be-

[1] Jour. Ment. and Nerv. Dis., Feb., 1897.

ginning of the medulla oblongata. This degeneration is probably due to changes in the gray matter of the cord, which we find in the upper portions in the center of the gray matter on either side. We have finally concluded that while we have every reason to regard the cases which Homen described as differing in their essential disease-process from general paralysis, it may be impossible to differentiate the two diseases clinically." Alzheimer[1] has collected the recorded cases of general paralysis of the insane occurring in children and young persons; 38 cases have been reported, and to these the writer adds 3 cases observed by himself, 1 beginning at the age of 9 years. Unlike the disease in adults, it occurs with equal frequency in the two sexes. The onset in 8 cases was in the 13th or 14th year, in 11 cases it was in the 15th or 16th year, while other cases began a little later. In 28 out of 34 cases hereditary syphilis was certain or probable, and in more than half the cases there was some neurotic heredity. The symptoms and pathology were the same as in adults, and the duration of the disease was about $4\frac{1}{2}$ years in most of the cases, but in some was more than 7 years.

Kleptomania.—A. Lacassahne[2] calls attention to this variety of mental disturbance, and endeavors to classify the subjects of the tendency to steal when this tendency is due to some mental disturbance rather than a manifestation of vice. He points out that kleptomaniacs have usually been considered as individuals who steal absolutely for the sake of stealing, but he does not take that view of it. In his estimation kleptomania has a special place, and is a morbid manifestation that may appear in a number of neuroses and manias, and is also in all these forms a manifestation of vicious and feeble natures. Kleptomaniacs are criminals by opportunity, and merit some consideration, for often there is no premeditation, but an absence of all desire and a struggle against the inclination to steal, which in them is rarely a result of morbid impulse. He pertinently remarks that the majority of kleptomaniacs of late have been arrested in the large department stores, and that they are inclined to confine their operations to these exciting and fashionable places of business, and that therefore kleptomania at present is most common in the large cities. The author states that in London the police and the proprietors of these places have a list of kleptomaniacs which numbers over 800, with only about a dozen men on the list. When a merchant misses some article, if he can recall the recent presence in his shop of any of the kleptomaniacs on the list, their friends are notified. In some cases the price of the article is returned from as many as a dozen different sources, as often the kleptomaniacs can give no account of themselves and cannot deny the implied charge. In the large bazaars of Lyons and Paris the proprietors state that there are more losses from kleptomaniacs than from thieves. The author points out that thieves usually attempt to sell or dispose of their plunder, while the kleptomaniac secretes and preserves it, and usually, in an individual case, the kleptomaniac confines herself to a certain sort or list of articles, which are taken in great number, but without any possibility of usefulness. Kleptomaniacs frequently become so habituated that they appear at regular hours, and in some places are regularly expected.

Lacassahne would divide them into three categories: First the collectors, who gather articles, apparently for the pleasure of possession. The author likens them to the bibliomaniacs, who, although they buy their books, derive a certain morbid pleasure in merely having them at hand. In the kleptomaniac the formality of the buying is dispensed with, and perhaps there is an additional excitement in executing the theft. In this group he recognizes certain elements

[1] Allg. Zeit. f. Psychiat., lii., fasc. 3.   [2] Jour. de Méd. de Paris, Oct. 25, 1896.

of dementia and feebleness of will, and believes that a modified punishment usually serves as a salutary lesson for the future with them.

His second class contains those of unstable makeup, who are unable to resist the temptation to steal, and who usually have behind their thefts some motive, such as vanity or coquetry. In certain instances they degenerate into regular thieves, greatly enjoying the excitement and anxiety of the acts of theft.

In the third class he places those actually diseased, such as maniacs, imbeciles, and paralytics, who steal without knowing what they do, their thefts representing internal evidence of their mental disturbance.

In regard to prophylaxis, he points out that these stores present a temptation truly diabolical, and that the plan of supervision now secretly maintained should be superseded by a system of uniformed inspectors, so that the prospect of being apprehended would constantly serve to restrain the kleptomaniac, who is too often inclined to steal under the impression that it may be done without detection. Further, that when kleptomania has once become established such people should be compelled to stay away from places in which their inclination is likely to overcome their self-control.

Walter Channing[1] makes a study of **palatal deformities in idiots**, reviewing the subject and adding many observations of his own. He disagrees with the statements of Clouston and discredits his observations. In his own studies he follows the plan of Talbot, and reaches the following conclusions : 1. Two-fifths of the palates of idiots are of fairly good shape. 2. Palates of normal individuals may be deformed. 3. In the idiot it is a difference in degree, and not in kind. 4. In either case it shows irregular development anatomically. 5. Palates of average children and idiots under 8 years of age probably do not in the majority of cases markedly differ. 6. There is no form of palate peculiar to idiocy. 7. The statement that a V-shaped or other variety of palate is a "stigma of degeneracy" remains to be proved.

W. L. Andriezen,[2] in a paper entitled **"The Pathogenesis of Epileptic Idiocy and Epileptic Imbecility,"** takes up the subject of the fine anatomic changes in these conditions. The observations extended over 14 cases of epileptic idiots or imbeciles and several cases of epilepsy, 1 being a case of typical epilepsy in a child, operated on by Horsley. After giving the changes found in the nerve-cells and the neuroglia in detail, he says that the morbid process in the brain underlying epileptic idiocy and imbecility may be briefly stated, as follows : " There is a sclerotic overgrowth of the neuroglia fibre-cells (diffuse or focal, and in the latter case often corresponding to a particular vascular territory), with corresponding slow irritation, destruction, and final atrophy of the nerve-cells and fibres in the same area." Then taking a bird's eye view of all the cases reported and examined, he says " the type of lesion present in the before-mentioned cases was as follows : " (*a*) A diffuse sclerosis or overgrowth of the neuroglia fibre-cells in the brain-substance. (*b*) A coextensive change in the nerve-cells. This change was of two kinds —namely, negative and positive. The negative changes consisted in a defective development (fewness and slenderness) of protoplasmic processes— imbecile type of nerve-cell ; while the positive changes consisted of an increase in amount and diffusion of pigment throughout the cell-body, especially its basal part, and a displacement of the nucleus toward the apex of the cell. Later changes were a gradual destruction and atrophy of the nerve-cell processes consequent upon or coextensive with the further outgrowth of the glia (sclerosis) until whole groups or islands of cells might be so destroyed.

[1] Jour. Ment. Sci., Jan., 1897.   [2] Brit. Med. Jour., May 1, 1897.

" There is thus a common pathogenic basis for epileptic idiocy and imbecility, and for focal epilepsy occurring in the child—namely, anomalies of growth and nutrition impressed upon the growing nerve-cell as well as the neuroglia-cell, and affecting predominantly this or that area of the brain, frequently in territories corresponding to a particular vascular distribution.

" In cases of epilepsy supervening in adult life, after the brain-cells had attained complete development, the changes found were (as regards the nerve-cells) only of the positive kind just mentioned. But, in addition, these very frequently exhibited intranuclear vacuolation of the cortical cells also, an observation of Bevan Lewis which I can fully confirm.

" In the brains of nonepileptic imbeciles, sclerosis and mycrogyria are both conspicuous by their absence. When the epileptic neurosis is present, however, this process is also present. The positive or negative changes in the nerve-elements themselves are present in varying degrees. It is in the combination of these two classes of pathologic lesions that we find the surest indication, the seal as it were, of epileptic idiocy or epileptic imbecility in the brain."

D. Telford Smith [1] calls attention to the **misshapen hands** found in the Mongol type of idiots, which he deems as significant as the cranial formation and the markings of the tongue that are described by Shuttleworth. In one of these instances he had a skiagraph made of the hand, showing defective development of the middle and terminal phalanges of the little finger, with deviation of the finger outward, giving it a convex line on the ulnar aspect of the hand. Casts and photographs from the hands of these idiots also show thickened, spade-like extremities, suggestive of those sometimes seen in cretins.

Infantile Cerebral Degeneration, with Changes of the Macula. —Kingdon and Risien Russell [2] report what they consider a peculiar disease occurring in 4 children. They look upon the disease as a family affection without reference to sex, consanguinity, syphilis, or any of the usual hereditary diseases, but common in the Jewish race. In the first stage the fully developed child, born at full term, shows symptoms toward the end of the third month in the way of muscular enfeeblement and impairment of sight. Definite changes in the macula are detected about the 4th or 5th month; the child becomes so helpless that it cannot sit up, and vision is almost or entirely lost. Muscular atrophy ensues; the deep reflexes are exaggerated; later there are rigidities. Convulsions do not usually occur, and the temperature is normal. Such children generally die within 2 years. Symmetrical degeneration of the pyramidal cells of the cortex and the fibers of the pyramidal tracts throughout their course is found upon microscopic examination. The 5th nerve and the superior cerebellar peduncle and the fillet may also show degeneration. The retina is usually much thickened and the optic nerve is atrophied. [The cases are identical with those reported by Sachs as cases of " family amaurotic idiocy," already noted in the *Year-Book* for 1897.]

[1] Pediatrics, Oct., 1896.　　　　　　　　　　　　　[2] Lancet, Jan. 16, 1897.

ORTHOPEDIC SURGERY.

By V. P. GIBNEY, M. D., and H. W. GIBNEY, M. D.,

OF NEW YORK.

Prefatory Remarks.—The advances in orthopedic surgery have kept pace with those in other departments. The correction of spinal deformities dependent upon Pott's disease promises to be a most marked advance. M. Calot, a French surgeon, has held out hope to the hunchback in some wonderful results, obtained by means which have heretofore appeared hazardous. The medical journals and daily press have been so full of Calot's work that it has been deemed unnecessary to devote space in these pages to more than a recapitulation. Management of the cold abscess is still *sub judice*. The narration of cases and the presentation of statistics and individual opinions are still as impotent as ever. The best work in orthopedic surgery is done, as a rule, by men who are fortunate enough to get cases in the early stages. The prevention of deformity is as important as the correction. Very little progress has been made in the appliances for correction. The greatest advances have been made in operative procedures. The recognition of the value of the specialty by the different medical colleges throughout the country adds fresh impetus, and it is believed that the education of students in early diagnosis will do more than anything else to enhance the value of orthopedic surgery.

DISEASES OF THE SPINE AND THORAX.

Some Apparatus for the Treatment of Pott's Disease.—J. C. Schapps[1] has devised a very convenient wheel-couch, which makes recumbent posture in the treatment of Pott's disease less distressing to the anxious mother and enables the little patient to lead an out-of-door life. The couch is so constructed that the patient can lie upon canvas, while the frame on which the canvas is stretched corresponds very closely with the Bradford frame already in use. [One chief objection to this conch is the absence of springs. So long as the patient is thus recumbent it is good to diminish jar as much as possible. For very young patients, too young for the use of plastic apparatus, or for steel braces, this seems to be an admirable device.]

Control of the Spine by a New Method.—E. A. Tracy[2] has devised apparently a very simple method of securing control of the spine, and at the same time of making traction, in efforts to *reduce deformity*. Considering the impetus given to reduction of deformity by Calot, this method of Tracy's is timely. It is illustrated in the accompanying figure, which speaks for itself. While he does not advocate the administration of an anesthetic, this can be easily done, and much more accurate traction made by means of screws at the ends of the frame. [At the International Congress in Moscow, 1897, one or two surgeons advocated mechanical means for making traction,

---

[1] N. Y. Med. Jour., Aug. 1, 1896.   [2] Boston M. and S. Jour., Oct. 1, 1896.

rather than manual force, in crowding the bosse down with the patient lying prone. The results certainly showed that this is a preferable way.]

Successful Laminectomy in Pott's Paraplegia.—J. Punton[1] records a case of great interest in a patient aged 27, who, in the spring of 1894, developed the disease. The most prominent spinous process was that of the sixth dorsal. The loss of power appeared shortly after the bosse was discovered, and within a month he was compelled to take to bed. Shortly thereafter paraplegia came on. Seven months later the bosse was larger, there was

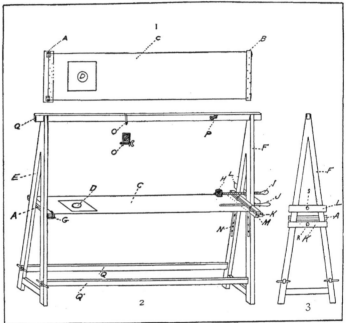

Fig. 56.—1. Cloth-stretcher for recumbent patient: *A*, clamp open; *B*, clamp closed; *C*, cloth; *D*, hole for occiput. 2. Machine in projection: *A*, clamp; *C*, cloth-stretcher; *D*, hole for occiput; *E*, left triangle; *F*, right triangle; *G*, hook holding clamp; *H*, threaded block; *I*, screw for traction upon the spine; *J*, screw for traction upon the cloth-stretcher; *K*, cross-piece for *J*; *L*, cross-piece for *I*; *M*, wooden piece for books; *N*, bracket; *O*, movable clamp; *P*, cleat; *Q*, bar. 3. End-view of right triangle: *A*, clamp; *L*, cross-piece for *I*; *K*, cross-piece for *J*; *R*, hole for screw *J*; *S*, hole for screw *I*.

general anesthesia of the limbs, deep reflexes were exaggerated, ankle-clonus present in both limbs, and motor paralysis of spastic type was complete. Bladder and rectum were never involved. Nov. 23, 1895, laminectomy of the fifth and sixth dorsal vertebræ. Ten days later there was full use of the limbs, and the paralysis seemed to have disappeared. Four weeks later there was a tendency of the deformity to return. Muscular weakness followed and the spastic paralysis returned. Jan. 28th a second operation on the seventh and eighth dorsal vertebræ, when a large abscess was discovered and its contents evacuated. A sinus remained at the date of report, but the paralysis had disappeared and the outlook was good.

[1] Jour. Nerv. and Ment. Dis., Dec., 1896.

Operative Treatment of Pott's Disease.—Diakonaft[1] reports 3 cases in which resection of the vertebral ends of the ribs was resorted to, in order to reach the seat of disease. Two of the cases died shortly after operation. In the third case, that of a child, the deformity involved the seventh cervical and first and second dorsal vertebræ, with complete paralysis of the lower extremities. The incision exposed the transverse processes of the second and third dorsal. The heads of the second and third ribs were removed, when a pus-cavity was discovered, connecting with the spinal canal. Carions bits of bone were removed by a sharp spoon, and the cavity drained; the dura was found intact. The wound was sewed up and iodoform emulsion injected through the drainage-tubes, which were removed two weeks later. Twenty-three days after operation mobility was established in the limbs, and at the end of another month the patient was walking without the use of apparatus.

Compression-paraplegia in Pott's Disease of the Spine.[2]—In December, 1896, an important discussion on this subject was held at a meeting of the New York Neurological Society. The papers for discussion were 3 in number: V. P. Gibney, 74 eases analyzed; N. M. Shaffer, 40 cases; and De Forest Willard, giving the result of operative procedures in a large number collected. In the first paper there were cured 45, improved 12, unimproved 8, died 9, in a total of 74. In the second paper there were 32 recovered, 8 still under treatment, in a total of 40. All of the cases tabulated in the first two papers were treated by mechanical appliances, and were not subjected to operation. Willard's conclusions from the operative side of the discussion were as follows: 1. Prognosis in pressure-paraplegia is hopeful unless the cord has been actually destroyed. 2. Laminectomy for Pott's paraplegia should never be undertaken until at least 1 year of persistent treatment by rest, fixation, and extension (together with alteratives, etc.) has been most patiently tested. 3. The dangers from the operation are shown by statistics to be great; 24% dying from the immediate shock, 36% within 1 month, and 46% within 1 year. At least 65% either died or were not improved by operation. 4. The dangers are hemorrhage, prolongation of the operation, and manipulation of the cord. 5. In spite of these risks the operation is justified in selected cases when persistent and carefully applied measures have failed. R. Abbe, in the discussion, was reluctant to operate because of the danger of disseminating tuberculosis by operation. Under a careful technic he believed the operation could be made without disturbing the spinal cord, and that the removal of the laminæ could be done without impairing the strength of the column. M. A. Starr, C. A. Herter, E. D. Fisher, B. Sachs, and J. Collins all expressed themselves as unwilling to advocate operative procedures, except in desperate cases.

Spinal Cord from a Case of Pott's Disease.—H. D. Boyer[3] reports on a cord taken from a case without angular deformity, but paraplegic and without control of both bladder and rectum. The laminæ of the dorsal vertebræ from the fifth down were carious. The bodies were carious and filled with cheesy matter. In the dorsal region the dura was greatly thickened, and here the cord was completely surrounded by thickened tissue, in some places to the extent of half an inch. The cord had been greatly pressed upon and nearly destroyed by both mechanical and inflammatory processes. There was no distinct line of demarcation between the cord and white matter, both being almost totally destroyed; cells were few in number; the central canal was filled by new epithelial cells. [Microscopic examination was very

[1] Centralbl. f. Kinderh., i., 309, 1896.   [2] Jour. Nerv. and Ment. Dis., Apr., 1897.
[3] Ibid., Nov., 1896.

thorough, and those interested are referred to the paper for details. The case would seem to be one of osteomyelitis of the spinal column, and emphasized the hopelessness of any operative procedures so long after the invasion of the paralysis, which was six or eight months.]

Dana and Frankel[1] have also reported a case, of which the following is a summary: the patient was a male, aged 60, of nontubercular history. He had very severe spinal pains for 6 months, followed by rapid paraplegia. There was no kyphosis. Death followed 1 year later. The autopsy showed necrosis of vertebræ, tubercular pachymeningitis, and transverse myelitis.

Posture in Diagnosis.—R. Sayre[2] has illustrated very accurately the different positions assumed in Pott's disease of the spine, and has very properly dwelt upon the assistance one gets in a diagnosis from noting carefully these different attitudes. [The paper is copiously illustrated, and while it makes no effort at presenting anything new, is certainly worthy of record in the *Year-Book*.]

Forcible Reduction of Deformity.—Perhaps the most interesting paper that has appeared in many years, and one that has elicited more discussion, is that of M. Calot, presented to the Paris Academy of Medicine.[3] He stated that he had done forcible correction of the bosse 37 times, without an accident and with the happiest results. The procedure was regarded both in this country and abroad as so radical that surgeons have been slow to adopt it. The discussion in the journals, and at foreign societies, has developed a certain distrust in the author's claims. Certain accidents have occurred. [The final results are, in some instances, not satisfactory, and the evidence furnished has not been such as to make one feel that assurance in the method that the author himself proclaims. The field is limited, but after all there are enough cases to justify a careful resort to this measure. In the more recent invasions of the column the deformity ought to be overcome and the good position maintained. In these recent cases the treatment will certainly confer a boon upon humanity. It is not a new thing to get recession of deformity. Ambroise Paré, in 1650, published a book, *De Gibborum Corrigenda Deformitatum* recommending an apparatus for forcible correction.]

Diagnosis and Treatment of Pott's Disease in the Adult.—V. P. Gibney[4] reports a variety of diseases simulating Pott's disease of the spine, and calls attention to the difficulty of diagnosis, as well as to the results obtained by appropriate treatment. The subjects are: 1st, neuroses of the spine; 2d, rheumatic spondylitis; 3d, fracture of the spine; 4th, multiple osteomyelitis, involving some portion of the vertebræ; 5th, malignant disease of the vertebræ; 6th, Pott's disease proper. All are illustrated by cases, and the protection of the spine in Pott's disease of the adult is shown to yield good results. Indeed, there is no reason why one should not get as good a result in the adult as in the child.

Lateral Curvature, Resection of the Ribs.—Hoffa[5] puts on record a case of severe scoliosis, in which he performed a section of portions of the ribs. The operation suggested by Volkmann in 1889 was carried out by Hoffa, with an improvement in the condition of the patient. He repeated the operation in a second patient, a boy of 10, presenting curvature from rhachitis. The ribs were sharply bent and made a marked projection. The incision was made from the upper border of the deformity of the ribs to the lower border downward. He made a subperiosteal resection at the ninth rib,

---

[1] Post-Graduate, July, 1896. [2] Trans N. Y. State Med. Soc., 1897.
[3] Ann. de Chir. et d'Orthopédie, Dec., 1896. [4] Med. News, Feb., 1897.
[5] Zeit. f. orthopäd. Chir., p. 401, 1896.

which was the sharpest portion of the deformity. He divided the seventh and eighth ribs the same way, while the third, fourth, fifth, and sixth were twisted out of their vertebral articulations. Although the pleura was perforated, there was no serious disturbance. After the operation the thorax was fixed by adhesive plaster. At the end of eight days the patient was allowed to go about. It is claimed that there was not only great improvement in appearance, but that considerable relief was later effected by means of gymnastic treatment supplemented by a corset. The operator recommends in scoliosis not only resection of a portion of the ribs on the convex side, but on the concave a linear osteotomy. He thinks this would enable one to correct the twist of the spine. [That this operation is radical no one will question, and it is doubtful whether any but a bold surgeon like Hoffa would attempt it. It is difficult to see how any correction of the twist can be accomplished by resection of the ribs on the convex and osteotomy on the concave side. Whether one could correct this twist if he had command of the vertebral ends of the ribs on the concave side, is a question. What should be done with the projecting ends of the ribs after correcting the twist, is a question quite as important. The damage that is likely to be done the pleura, as he himself did, must have due weight, and it is doubtful whether one would get off so well as he. The photographs published certainly show an improvement.]

Forcible Correction without Cutting.—Delore [1] advocates the forcible correction of scoliosis under an anesthetic. A cushion is placed under the axilla and under the pelvis. The patient lies upon the side, and strong force is used in pressing upon the projecting ribs. During this procedure the adhesions are broken down between the ribs and spinal column, the author claims, and a correct position is secured. In some instances the correction is easily made, while in others much force is employed. After all, no evil results have thus far been met with by the author. A fixed bandage is employed, and later, twice a day, manual force is used to secure still further correction. He follows this with the corset to maintain the good result. The patient lies upon the right, or the projecting, side at night. [While this method is radical, it is what is often done by orthopedic surgeons, viz., forcible correction in suspension. It is not uncommon, in highly deformed cases of lateral curvature, to partially suspend the patient, and have an assistant secure the pelvis while the operator presses forcibly on the ribs of the projecting side, crowding the column into a position of over-correction, so far as it is possible. The plaster bandage is immediately applied, and the parts are held in good position until the plaster sets. The idea, therefore, is not new, except in that an anesthetic is employed.]

For Lateral Curvature, the Bicycle.—O. G. Kiliani [2] recommends a modification of the seats and handle-bars, in the ordinary bicycle, in the treatment of milder cases of lateral curvature. He takes advantage of the old-fashioned chair-seat, with one side raised, and makes the seat of the bioycle correspond. The height of one or the other side of the handle-bar contributes to an elevation or depression of the shoulder, and thus one gets practically the same position of the spine as is obtained in one of Roth's movements, known as the key-note.

DISEASES OF THE HEAD AND NECK.

A Wry-necked Family.—J. H. Thompson [3] presents, in a brief com-

---

[1] Zeit. f. orthopäd. Chir., p. 416, 1896.   [2] Med. Rec., Oct. 31, 1896.
[3] Lancet, July 4, 1896.

munication, the photographs of four members of a family, all of whom have this deformity. The family history is absolutely negative. In only one case did the deformity develop in childhood, and this was the most severe of the four. The spasm was choreiform in character and the patient had great difficulty in speaking and swallowing. The limbs were likewise affected, but not to so great an extent as the head. The second patient developed wry-neck at the age of 32. There are no convulsive movements, no paralysis, and no loss of sensation. The third patient developed the deformity in adult life; the fourth when she was about 18 years of age.

Spasmodic Wry-neck.—Pattee[1] publishes a very interesting paper on the expectant treatment of 8 cases, with cure. There is no definite line of treatment carried out in any case reported, but the author seems to have studied carefully the causation, and after futile attempts at different methods succeeded in finding a method which yielded good results. The paper is well worthy of a careful study, inasmuch as this form of torticollis is usually very rebellious to treatment of any kind.

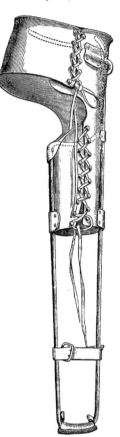

DISEASES OF THE HIP.

A Modified Splint.—Ap. M. Vance[2] presents a leather splint which he gave to the profession a few years ago, supplemented by the lower portion of the ordinary Thomas knee-splint. The foot-piece differs from the foot-piece of the knee-splint in that it has a leather splint-shoe, with means for securing traction. [There is really nothing new in principle about this apparatus, but, as the author claims, it is a simple method of fixing a hip and securing a certain amount of traction. It is shown in the accompanying figure.]

Osteotomy as a Treatment for the Disease in the Early Stage.—R. F. Tobin[3] advocates a most extraordinary method of treating the disease in its early stage: that of an osteotomy on a level with the lesser trochanter. [The case he figures in a photograph, however, is not hip-disease in the first stage. One is, to say the least, surprised that a surgeon of any standing should advocate so radical a measure in the early stage. Fortunately, however, Howard Marsh[4] writes a very just criticism.

Fig. 57.—Vance's modified hip-splint (Med. News, Aug. 29, 1896).

The orthopedic surgeon in this country who is fortunate enough to get a case in the early stage does not need to resort to operative measures, because the average splint, with attention to details, enables him to secure an excellent result. We are prepared to admit that in dispen-

[1] Jour. Am. Med. Assoc., p. 59, July 11, 1896.   [2] Med. News, Aug. 29, 1896.
[3] Brit. Med. Jour., April 24, 1897.   [4] Ibid., May 8, 1897.

49

sary practice the splint is often abused, and the disease sometimes advances to the second and third stages, but even this is exceptional. In the more advanced stages, say, where deformity has become fixed, then osteotomy is an excellent routine treatment.]

Death after Osteotomy.—W. R. Townsend,[1] at a meeting of the Orthopedic Section of the New York Academy of Medicine, presented a specimen of the hip-joint from a boy who died within 36 hours after a simple subcutaneous osteotomy. The patient reacted well from the operation, and it was not until the following day, toward the close of the first 24 hours that vomiting appeared, accompanied by a weak, rapid pulse, speedy collapse, and death. The autopsy failed to reveal any cause of death. It was the opinion of the members taking part in the discussion that an embolism had occurred, though there was no positive proof of this. [In view of the large number of patients submitted to this simple operation, the case is extraordinary.]

Muscular Atrophy; Contraction of the Arteries of the Limb as a Probable Cause.—A. G. Miller[2] claims that diminution of the blood-supply from contraction of the artery, or main arteries, is probably the cause of the atrophy which takes place so early in tuberculous disease of the hip-joint. He has frequently seen contraction of the arteries in limbs amputated for disease. He advances other arguments in favor of this theory, and closes a very interesting paper with the following conclusions: "1· Muscle-atrophy is a common symptom in tubercular joint-disease. 2. No explanation of this atrophy has been suggested hitherto, except a mysterious reflex influence. 3. Contraction of arteries has been seen and proved to exist. 4. The muscle-atrophy is likely to be caused by a diminished blood-supply rather than by nerve-influence. I assume therefore that arterial contraction and consequent diminished blood-supply are the cause of muscle-atrophy in tubercular joint-disease." [We are free to admit that the argument induced by the author is weighty, because we have always felt that there was something vague about this "mysterious reflex influence." The theory which seeks to establish reflex centers and reflex nerves has been nothing more than a suggestion accompanied by little or no proof.]

Double Excision, with Cure.—Prewit[3] reports a case in a boy whose disease developed on the left side when he was $2\frac{1}{2}$ years of age. Three years later there were indications of disease in the right hip, as an abscess had already formed. Later there were sinuses, and the disease was progressing from bad to worse, when, after unsuccessful attempts at curetting to relieve the patient, he excised the left hip, which healed without suppuration. Nearly a year later he excised the right hip, finding both head and acetabulum extensively diseased. The patient made a good recovery. When presented to a society the sinuses were healed and the boy walked without crutches. There was likewise a small range of motion. [Such instances are not new, but exceedingly rare. It not unfrequently happens in double hip-disease that a surgeon is so pleased with the result of resection on one side that he is tempted to perform it on the other. The results, are, as a rule, unsatisfactory, and the author of this report is to be congratulated.]

The Non-bloody Reduction of Congenital Dislocations.—G. R. Elliot,[4] after a visit to Lorenz, presents a very complete record of the work done by the Vienna surgeon, and demonstrates his new method with the record of a case or two. To Sept. 25, 1897, 83 cases have been operated upon by Lorenz, and the results were thought to have surpassed those obtained by the

---

[1] Am. Medico-Surg. Bull., Nov. 21, 1896.   [2] Edinb. Med. Jour., Sept., 1896.
[3] St. Louis Med. Rev., May 15, 1897.   [4] Med. Rec., May 29, 1897.

PLATE 9.

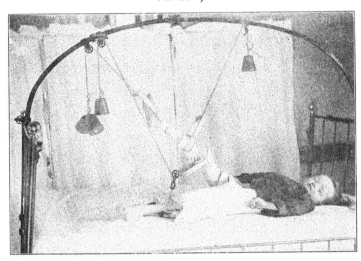

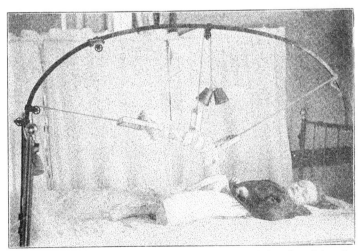

Apparatus for the gradual reduction of flexion and subluxation of the knee (from photographs furnished by E. B. Young .

open method. [Our own experience in this direction is at least satisfactory, though the results thus far secured have not been perfect. The procedure appeals to the general practitioner and to laymen with more force than ever did the bloody method—a method still on trial. As for ourselves, we believe that the cases suitable for bloody reduction are few, and that the technic of the operation, the after-treatment, and the subsequent use of splints are not fully comprehended. In Hoffa's private hospital at Würzburg great attention is given to massage and muscle-pedagogy. It may be, therefore, that the good results which the European surgeons claim to have established are largely due to the after-treatment. Lorenz has published a volume of 372 pages, with 54 figures, and the work has been translated by J. Cottet, into French, with a preface by Dr. Brun. The publishers are Geo. Carre et Acnaud.]

DISEASES OF THE KNEE.

Gradual Reduction of Deformity.—E. B. Young[1] describes and illustrates a means of gradually reducing flexion and subluxation of the knee on the principle of the genuclast. The apparatus consists of the ordinary frame for holding the patient in bed, and an arched strip of scantling supported by an upright at each end. The uprights are fastened firmly to the bed, while small galvanized iron pulleys may be fastened at any point along this arch. By means of the weights and pulleys the thigh is held in position while traction is made in the line of deformity of the leg. At the same time force is employed by means of the weights against the posterior aspect of the upper third of the leg. Indeed, the pads and straps are so applied that direct force is brought to bear against the salient points in the deformity. The author has had an opportunity of using the apparatus in the Children's Hospital, and he claims that the deformity is reduced in a remarkably short period of time—from two to three days in rather severe cases. Plate 9 represents the apparatus in use. The first step in the treatment is the reduction of the subluxation of the head of the tibia. The counterextension strap A prevents the lower end of the femur from moving forward, and the whole force of extension, B, applied to the lower limb tends to separate the tibia from the femur. The traction at C pulls forward the head of the tibia. As much weight may be applied as the patient can stand with comfort; but the amount attached to B should be sufficient to prevent the pull on C from disturbing the position of the leg while the tibia is being brought into place. After the backward displacement is fully overcome, all that is necessary is to keep the tibia in position and slowly pull out the flexion after the manner shown in the illustration. The weight at C is reduced until just sufficient to keep the head of the bone forward, while that at B is increased as much as possible. The traction at A is carried downward through a pulley attached to a frame on which the child lies, and upward over another pulley, so that the downward pull at the lower end of the femur counteracts the tendency at C to flex the knee-joint. [The method is certainly deserving of credit so far as one can judge from the study of a report, because there is nothing quite so intractable as these minor deformities of the knee, accompanied by flexion and subluxation.]

Non-calcifying Plastic Ostitis.—Pitts and Shattock,[2] at the London Pathologic Society, presented a specimen removed by amputation from a woman, aged 39, who had received an injury to her knee when she was 31. The limb was removed on account of pain and discomfort and failure to get

[1] Boston M. and S. Jour., Oct. 8, 1896.   [2] Brit. Med. Jour., Jan. 23, 1897.

relief in various hospitals. The upper half of the tibia had undergone a uniform transformation into cancellous bone-like substance so void of earthy salts that the bone itself was as pliable as India-rubber; a like tissue filled the medullary cavity. It was easy to make specimens for microscopic purposes without artificial decalcification. After appropriate staining the trabeculæ were found surrounded with osteoblasts. The spaces between the trabeculæ were everywhere occupied by highly cellular connective tissue. Quite a full description followed, and its relationship to other conditions of bone was fully discussed.

Conservative Operation in a Case of Tubercular Goneitis.—H. Lilienthal [1] reports a very rebellious case. The account given of the condition is such as to lead one to class it among the most desperate of these tubercular lesions of the bones involving the knee. The operation performed was that advised by Mayo, of Minnesota. "After applying the Esmarch constrictor, the knee was opened by a transverse incision through the ligamentum patellæ, taking in, in this case, more than two-thirds of the circumference of the limb. All the structures were divided as in resection of the knee, and so far as possible cut away. The patella was removed. The quadriceps bursa was laid open by an incision at right angles to the first one, and this last cut had to be extended nearly to the fold of the groin. All diseased surfaces were thoroughly scraped. Other extensive incisions were made longitudinally over the fibula, and also over the inner aspect of the knee. Every recess was laid open in so thorough a fashion that drainage-tubes were dispensed with, the wounds being stuffed with weak iodoformized gauze, which was, at subsequent dressings, replaced by nosophen gauze, because I feared iodoform-poisoning from the vast extent of the wounded surface. The leg was now flexed on the thigh *beyond* a right angle. The gaping knee-joint was also thoroughly packed, and the patient sent to bed with the limb in this flexed position." Under chloroform three weeks afterward the parts were flushed and an attempt made to straighten the limb. Contractures of the soft parts had resulted from this long-flexed position, and it was necessary to take a thick shaving from the femoral condyles before the limb came into a suitable position. Healing went on rapidly. Three months from the date of the first step in the Mayo operation the child was discharged cured.

Displaced Semilunar Cartilages.—Douglas Graham [2] reports several cases reduced by massage and certain movements. He makes a very fair argument for this method of treatment, and gives this rule for its replacement: "Flex the leg, then extend suddenly, rotating the leg internally if it be the internal cartilage, outwardly if it be the external cartilage, and exert pressure over the offending region." He feels that it can be held in place by a figure-of-8 bandage and a few folds of bandage as a pad. This bandage and pad, he thinks, affords a safe limit to the motion, and a dislocation is not apt to occur. [It has long been claimed by masseurs that much could be done for these displacements about the knee, but the results are not always satisfactory. Graham's paper, however, is very clear on the subject, and is worthy of record.]

DISEASES OF THE FOOT.

Metatarsalgia.—R. Jones,[3] after a lengthy discussion on the literature of the subject, recommends the following treatment: 1. Abstain from continuing any action which produces the pain; 2. Increase the depth of the inner aspect

[1] Pediatrics, May 15, 1897.   [2] Am. Jour. Med. Sci., Nov., 1896.
[3] Liverpool Med.-Chir. Jour., Jan., 1897.

of the heel in order to produce slight inversion of foot ; 3. Wear thick soles with well-fitting insteps and roomy around the heads of the metatarsals ; 4. Insist that the sole be at least one-quarter of an inch thicker behind the bases of the metatarsals. This putting of an extra heel just back of the ball of the foot is a device originating with the late Hugh Owen Thomas. The objection to it is that it makes the shoe very awkward and clumsy, and does not seem to be necessary in a large proportion of cases. Jones has not found the measures just enumerated sufficient to give relief in all cases, and he prefers exsection of the metatarsal head to incision or amputation.

W. S. Halsted,[1] of Johns Hopkins University, after a careful examination of 20 cadavers, fails to find the anatomic conditions which have been described so frequently by Morton. In no single instance did he find the head of the fifth metatarsal more than a quarter of an inch posterior to that of the fourth. As a rule, it was not more than one-eighth of an inch. He found also that the digital nerves passed below the inferior transverse ligaments, and did not appear in the normal foot between the heads of the metatarsals, or between the head of the fifth and the neck of the fourth. He found no evidence to support Morton's theory of the causation, but believed that Lorenz had given a more satisfactory explanation, which was that of the flatfoot. This giving way of the arches produces inflammatory thickening of the sheaths of the nerves, and sometimes fibroneuromata. Microscopic examination convinced him that these conditions were present, and that the nerves should be excised. Most of his cases, he believed, could be cured by the usual treatment for beginning flatfoot.

Anatomy of Congenital Clubfoot.—Nichols[2] presents a dissection of two specimens from the feet of a child stillborn. The description is supplemented by reference to other anatomic papers and goes into detail quite thoroughly. The author arrives at a conclusion which a careful study of the anatomy of clubfoot usually warrants—viz., that the deformity is due to alterations in the shape of all of the bones of the foot, and is formed by the contraction of certain tendons and ligaments. The chief deformity is at the midtarsal joint, and is due to an inequality of facets of the os calcis and astragalus. He believes that if one fails to correct this obliquity the deformity is not corrected. He also believes that in resistent cases this obliquity should be corrected by an osteotomy of the neck of the astragalus, followed by forcible reposition of the foot. [While there is nothing specially new in his work, we welcome every paper bearing upon the anatomy of clubfoot, and bespeak for it a careful study. The subject should be frequently brought before the members of the profession, and hence is referred to in these pages.]

Compression of the Front of the Foot.—E. H. Bradford[3] has made quite a study of prehistoric footprints and the foot of Art. From this study he constructs an argument against universal compression of the foot in civilized life. The article in question is a very interesting study. He concludes with the following : " It is well to remember that it is not the tail which separates man from anthropoid apes, but the shape and strength of the foot, especially of the first metatarsal and its accompanying phalanges. It is that which gives to man the erect gait, and it is a mutilation not to preserve this given strength."

Flatfoot, its Causes and Treatment.—N. M. Shaffer[4] presents in a more complete form views, which he is known to have held for many years, of the causation of flatfoot. It is due, he believes, to a shortened gastrocne-

[1] Medicine, II., No. 8, p. 631.
[2] Boston M. and S. Jour., Feb., 1897.
[3] Ibid., Oct. 29, 1896.
[4] N. Y. Med. Jour., May 29, 1897.

mius in the majority of cases. He makes this statement: "Among the hundreds of cases that I have examined during the past 8 or 10 years, I do not recall over three or four instances where I could not satisfy myself that the tendo-Achillis was tense and unyielding when flexion was attempted beyond 90°." His treatment, therefore, is to elongate this tendon, and the well-known shoe which bears his name is employed as a means of treatment.

Hallux Valgus, the Operative Treatment of.—R. F. Weir [1] has an excellent article on this subject, and recommends a curved incision, which enables one to more readily extirpate the bursa and remove any sesamoid bones.   One is further enabled to dissect out the dorsal extensor tendon, cut it near its attachment, and secure it to the periosteum at the inner side of the base of the first phalanx.   A further advantage claimed for the incision is that it leaves a cicatrix that is not rendered sensitive by shoes.   [The paper is well illustrated, and from our own experience we can heartily recommend this procedure.]

Automatic Hammer-toe Springs.—From the *Lancet*, Nov. 21, 1896, we reproduce drawings of two springs for hammer-toe (Figs. 58 and 59).

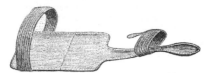

FIG. 58.—Spring for use in hammer-toe (Lancet, Nov. 21, 1896)

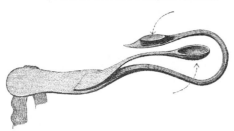

FIG. 59.—Spring for use in hammer-toe (Lancet, Nov. 21, 1896).

One of these (Fig. 58) is made to be worn within an easy-fitting boot, while the other (Fig. 59) is put on at night.   A reference to the illustration is all that is necessary, as one can easily understand how the springs should be constructed.

Achillo-bursitis, Anterior.—S. Lloyd [2] presented a paper to the Orthopedic Section of the New York Academy of Medicine, and in an abstract we find this disease is the result of traumatism from tight shoes.   It sometimes comes from bicycle-riding, or may be the result of septic, tubercular, gonorrheal, or rheumatic infection.   The most prominent symptom is pain under the tendo-Achillis when standing.   The pain is also found in the plantar region.   There are swelling on either side of the tendon and extensive inflammation of the surrounding tissues.   The paper is replete with interest, and it inclines us to classify still further the numerous affections in the

[1] Ann. of Surg., Apr., 1897.   [2] St. Louis Med. Rev., May 15, 1897.

region of the heel. The treatment naturally suggested is rest, warm baths, and in some instances counter-irritation. [We are reminded now that in many instances we have diagnosed this condition rheumatic, and without any special evidence therefor.]

Dislocation of Peronei Tendons Treated by Operation.—G. M. Smith[1] offers a cure, in suturing the tendon to the fascia behind the sheath, having excised an oblong piece of periosteum from the malleolus, and brought this over the tendon already secured to the fascia. The result was excellent, but the time elapsed had not been sufficiently great to enable him to speak with confidence of the permanency of the cure. Kousmine[2] makes a half-moon incision to the bone, behind and below the external malleolus, and a trapeze-shaped space on the periosteum is cut around so that the base of the trapeze corresponds to the lower edge of the malleolus. After doing this he cuts out a small flat piece of bone and raises it perpendicular to the malleolus. This piece of bone is not completely removed, and the tendon is placed behind it. A couple of nails are inserted to hold the bone in place and keep the tendons in position. The bone acts as a kind of trap-door. It is claimed that in 17 days the plaster-of-Paris can be removed and the nails withdrawn, when the tendons are found in normal position. It is further claimed that the operation has proved curative and brilliant.

SHOULDER.

The Treatment of Old Dislocations.—F. B. Lund[3] discusses very fully the old dislocations one encounters in the shoulder. He claims that the method of Kocher, for the reduction of old dislocations as well as recent ones, is fraught with danger. It is easy, he claims, to fracture the humerus. He quotes from Monks, who has met with this accident, and also from Morton. In recent dislocations the scapula is held by voluntary muscular spasm, while in ancient dislocations this element does not prevail; hence it is necessary to secure pretty firmly the scapula in all attempts at reduction. Failing to reduce, he advocates arthrotomy. That is, he thinks this would be an ideal operation if the glenoid cavity could be opened so as to receive the head with a fair probability of its remaining in place. As this is very improbable, he advocates resection. The literature of the subject shows that many of the arthrotomies were done with the idea of completing the operation by resection. While the mortality after resection is a little greater than that of arthrotomy, he was led to believe from his investigation that it was not less dangerous, but that even any open operation should be postponed until all reasonable attempts at reduction by the employment of manual force could be made. He cautions against misapplied force, and the danger of rupturing vessels by such procedures. In the discussion which followed his paper, presented at the Surgical Section of the Suffolk District Medical Society, it was evident that many old cases had been reduced after months had elapsed. Porter reported that he had records of a case in which reduction was accomplished 4 years after the injury. [Personally, we incline to a free resection rather than an arthrotomy. We have been led to prefer this in the management of congenital dislocations of the shoulder where the structures are more or less shortened, and where it is difficult to secure a glenoid cavity. Referring also to the good functional results obtained after resection for disease and for gunshot-injuries, we recall a number of very useful shoulders.]

[1] Brit. Med. Jour., May 15, 1897. [2] Rev. de Chir., Sept., 1896.
[3] Boston M. and S. Jour., Apr. 29, 1897.

DISEASES OF THE HAND.

Cleft Hand ; Operation for the Use of Periosteal Flaps.—C. M. Dowd[1] reports a very instructive case of cleft hand, the cleft extending down to the middle, apparently, of the palm, between the middle and ring fingers. In this case the fourth and fifth metacarpal bones were fused into one and separated from the third. The ring and little fingers were widely separated from the other fingers, and resembled the claws of a crab or lobster. The adduction was remedied by removing a wedge-shaped piece from the distal end of the fused fourth metacarpal bone, and forcibly adducting the fingers. The closure of the cleft was made by approximating the metacarpal bones, turning back the lateral flap and the periosteum from each at the place of divergence, and sewing these together with catgut. Firm apposition by a chromicized gut ligature around the shaft of the third metacarpal bone and through that of the fused fourth and fifth was made. An excellent result was obtained. In summing up, he makes the following pertinent statement : " The bones, the joints, the tendons, and the soft parts present peculiarities which must be met in each case. The device of raising the periosteal flaps, and thus joining the bones together by newly formed deposit, has been neglected, so far as I know ; but it is so manifest a thing to do, that it must have been done where suitable conditions existed." [The good result obtained we certainly commend. It has many advantages over such devices as wire, pegs, nails, etc. This union gave a most satisfactory firmness to the hand and it caused no practical inconvenience from lack of pliability. We are pleased to give place to an abstract of this case, because it is evident that much can be done by special surgery in these congenital deformities. The removal of bone to correct deformity is certainly commendable. A careful dissection is always required. Good asepsis must be secured, and the results are generally satisfactory.]

SPASTIC PARALYSIS.

S. Ketch[2] presents a very fair *résumé* of the **orthopedic treatment of spastic paralysis in children.** He very properly condemns the use of apparatus—such apparatus as is generally employed. The indications for simple mechanical procedures are usually clear enough to enable the surgeon to correct certain deformities and to maintain the foot or the knee in good position. The education of muscles by manual exercise is commended. What pleases us best is the prominence he gives tenotomy and myotomy, supplemented by overcorrection. In his experience at Randall's Island Hospital, where there are a number of idiots with spastic paralysis, he noted their mental condition before and after operative procedures. He was inclined to commend Rupperts' views. He was convinced that many of these cases after tenotomy not only showed cure of the deformities, but also a great improvement in the mental condition. We do not think he dwells with sufficient emphasis upon the importance of maintaining the position sufficiently long after tenotomy, although he makes this statement : " The danger of relapse after tenotomy is, I think, much greater in this class of cases than in either the congenital or acquired clubfoot." [What we have found in our experience is a tendency to overcorrection. For instance, if a foot is operated on for equinus, it requires a long and patient course of after-treatment to prevent calcaneus.]

H. L. Taylor[3] presented the subject in a different aspect. His treatment

---

[1] Ann. of Surg., Aug., 1896.   [2] Med. News, Mar. 27, 1897.
[3] Am. Medico-Surg. Bull., Nov. 21, 1896.

was such a management of the case as would promote coordination and self-helpfulness of the child. He insisted upon memo-muscular training by methods analogous to those of the kindergarten and manual-training school. [This treatment was successful many years ago in the hands of the elder Seguin, so that the author very properly calls attention to this method in conjunction with orthopedic measures. It is interesting to note that no orthopedic surgeon recommends electric treatment, or at least, if it is employed, it is of secondary importance.]

J. Collins[1] has a very interesting editorial on congenital spastic rigidity from a historic standpoint. [It is pleasing to note that the subject was first scientifically treated by the late Dr. Little, whose memory orthopedic surgeons love to honor. Indeed, this affection was known as Little's disease. The author of the editorial discusses likewise the clinical as well as the pathologic side of the question. It is, on a whole, a very masterly review of the subject, and well worthy of perusal.]

MISCELLANEOUS.

Sacro-iliac Disease.—F. B. Judge–Baldwin[2] gives a brief review of the literature of this disease and reports a case that is of much interest, in that it presents some unusual features, and especially a cure by operation. A woman 26 years of age, 5 months after confinement, in September, 1893, had the first train of symptoms referable to the sacrum. These were: aching at the bottom of the back, pains in the left limb as she walked, and a feeling as if she " had a broken bone." The symptoms lasted a few weeks; but 6 months later they recurred, and early in January, 1895, a swelling in the left groin appeared. The reporter saw her first in April, 1895, finding a large psoas abscess, without spinal angularity. There was no pain in the lumbar region, and no abnormality about the hip-joint. She responded to the test for sacro-iliac disease, and, although her general health was dangerously impaired, she was operated upon May 1, 1896. "The line of incision was determined by drawing a line 3 in. from the anterior superior iliac spine to the posterior inferior spine. One and a half inches from the posterior inferior spine was a point for insertion of the scalpel," and he showed a horseshoe-shaped incision about 2 in. wide downward, the muscles being divided to the periosteum and held well away. This incision gave a good view of the sacroiliac joint, which looked spotty and grayish. On introducing a chisel into this area it passed readily into the joint, and the parts immediately thereabout were scraped away, leaving a perforated pelvis. Care was taken to remove all broken-down bone. Drainage was employed; the dressing was changed 3 or 4 times during the next 18 hours, on account of impending collapse. The healing was rapid; by July 24th the patient was on a spinal carriage, and on August 13th on a Thomas splint with crutches. The sinus closed on March 17, 1896. October 1, 1896, patient was reported as "perfectly well. She has had no ill-health since the operation, and walked so well that it would be difficult to detect that she had had any disease of the joint." [The reporter is to be congratulated on this brilliant result. The difficulty of removing the bone in the neighborhood of the sacroiliac junction is recognized by all surgeons, and it is seldom that a thorough operation can be made. The details of the operation and of the subsequent history have been omitted in our abstract.]

Fragilitas Ossium in Childhood.—Griffith[3] contributes an interesting

---

[1] Med. News, Feb. 6, 1897.   [2] Brit. Med. Jour., Dec. 19, 1896.
[3] Am. Jour. Med. Sci., 1897.

paper on idiopathic osteopsathyrosis, which is supplemented by a case in a child born June, 1893, who in March, 1894, sustained a fracture of the right femur, near the hip; Sept. 11, 1894, another fracture; and up to the time of his report of the case other fractures had occurred.   The final result of the case is not given, but the presumption is that the limbs grew stronger and in time the brittleness of the bones disappeared.   This case closely corresponds with cases under our observation.   In 57 collected cases Griffith drew conclusions as to etiology, which was that of inheritance in 11 cases; in 7 there was a family predisposition without direct inheritance; in 24 cases there was no family predisposition recorded; the remaining 15 were classed as doubtful.   The disease affected males more than females, in the ratio of 47 to 19.   It began in early life—sometimes before birth; syphilis and rickets seem not to have had any direct influence in the production of the fragility.   It was noted that in this affection the union of the fractures was prompt.   The treatment which seemed to give the best results was alteratives, the maintenance of the general health, and protection of the limbs.   Muscles must not be allowed to waste for want of use, and fractures should be set as early as possible.

Congenital Defects in Long Bones.—B. E. McKenzie[1] publishes a paper detailing a number of congenital deformities of the legs, wrists, and hands, which may be found in most any large collection.   In one case a dissection was made, which gave a very clear idea of the anatomy of the parts.   After operating on some of these cases and securing results that were far from satisfactory, he concludes as follows: " All things considered, if one is to judge from the 5 cases of this kind here reported " (the kind referred to is where the tibia is absent), " I think it must be placed beyond controversy that the most convenient support to be secured for the patient is found in the artificial limb, which may be applied to a good stump."   [We agree with the author in the conclusion to which he has come.   It is seldom that a good walking limb can be secured where the tibia is absent.]

Congenital Absence of Both Patellæ.—A. T. Bristow[2] adds to the list of cases already published a case in which the radiograph showed clearly the absence of the patellæ.   The paper itself is valuable on this account, but in addition a list of cases in literature has been collected.

W. B. Hopkins[3] reports a case in which both patellæ were absent.   Fifteen cases are briefly reported in connection with this one.   [In looking over this report one finds several where the patellæ were rudimentary.   In our experience it is not so uncommon.   In a large orthopedic clinic a certain number of rudimentary patellæ are seen every year.   We find that the bones develop to a very useful size in the course of a few years, enabling the patients to walk with comparative ease.   In many instances the patellæ are reported as absent, when in reality they are simply rudimentary.   In the case reported by Bristow the radiograph confirmed the truth of his statement.]

[1] N. Y. Med. Jour., Feb. 20, 1897.   [2] Med. News, Jan. 2, 1897.
[3] Ann. of Surg., Feb., 1897.

OPHTHALMOLOGY.

HOWARD FORDE HANSELL, M. D., AND WENDELL REBER, M. D.,

General Epitome.—Advances in ophthalmology since the publication of the 1897 *Year-Book* have not been few or unimportant. The tendency seems to have been to seek the elevated standard of original research, and while many authors content themselves with the recital of a case or two and venture to draw conclusions from them as bases for universal laws, others have enriched literature with thorough investigations of disease, and, by shedding light into places hitherto dark, have helped both student and practitioner. For example, the utilization of the *x*-rays, foreshadowed in our epitome of last year, has become general, and its use in the localization of foreign bodies in the interior of the eye and orbit almost universal. No up-to-date ophthalmic surgeon would attempt to decide as to the presence of a piece of metal in a doubtful case without employing this method. Perfection in apparatus and better understanding of the properties of the rays will lead to a more intelligent use of them, and will mean much for future medicine and surgery. In the choice as to the operation—simple or compound—for cataract we are to-day in about the same position as in 1897. The caprice of the operator, rather than the peculiar indications of the case, decides the question. Americans of large operative opportunities are in favor of the simple operation. Europeans of equal authority and experience are about divided. Our own suggestion (conveyed in part in the text) is that the large majority of oculists whose cataract-extractions number perhaps 25 in a year should continue to practise the method they have pursued from the beginning. The risk of an unsuccessful termination to a single case because of nervousness or other causes originating in a novel procedure, when by following the usual method a good result would have been obtained, is not justifiable. Discission or extraction of the lens in high myopia for the retardation of pathologic changes in the choroid and the improvement of vision has proved its superiority to the correction of the optical defect by lenses, and has steadily advanced in favor, until its general adoption seems to us to be merely a question of a short time. The operation recently brought prominently before the profession by Fukala was introduced many years ago, but was abandoned later because of its risks. Asepsis and antisepsis, however, have made its revival possible. Diseases of the retina and choroid, congenital or acquired, from constitutional or local causes, are practically on their old footing. When potassium iodid fails our only resource is empiricism. Electrolysis, that promised so much when heralded as a cure for retinal detachment, has met the same fate that awaited further experience with Schöler's injections of iodin, substitution of rabbit's vitreous, and other novel procedures. Puncture, galvanocautery, rest in bed, and bandaging are still recommended and practised as the least unsatisfactory of the methods proposed. Investigation into the intimate nature of

779

interstitial keratitis has changed our old-time conception that this disease is always congenitally syphilitic in its nature. It is now frequently ascribed to other diatheses, such as acquired syphilis, influenza, rheumatism, and tuberculosis. While the general signs and symptoms are the same, irrespective of the cause, that form due to acquired syphilis has its own distinctive features. The subconjunctival treatment of this and other diseases of the cornea and of the uveal tract has been this year (as last) the subject of extended discussion. The general consensus of opinion, outside of France, relegates this form of therapy to a second or third place among the methods employed, and it seems to us is reserved for those cases in which the surgeon, having tried other means and failing to effect a cure, does not blame injections much because they fail also. The preference is given to mercuric cyanid over the sublimate or normal salt-solution. There is manifest a disposition to defer acceptance of the etiologic classification of the different forms of conjunctivitis until the responsibility of the various microorganisms can be more sharply defined. Studies of climatic environment, supposed to be an active factor in the origin and spread of granular lids and trachoma, show that altitude is a less potent factor than racial and individual peculiarities. We regret to have to record each year that, in spite of the recommendations of the value of certain medicaments, no one remedy has yet been brought forward that will replace the roller-forceps of Knapp, and subsequent treatment by copper and other astringents. Retinoscopy is slowly but surely installing itself as a reliable objective method in the daily work of many careful refractionists. The trend in refraction-methods is toward objectivity, and any objective method that offers precision of result and ease of application may be sure of just such a gracious reception as is being accorded to retinoscopy.

ANATOMY AND PHYSIOLOGY.

The Brain and Vision.—Sharkey [1] devotes the clinical and pathologic data of 3 unusually interesting cases to the solution of the problem, that, although each angular region seems to be able to subserve vision in both eyes, it cannot make up for hemianopsie defect produced by disease of the occipital lobe. To him, the only tenable explanation is that the occipital lobe is a lower center through which the visual impulses must pass on their way to the higher centers in the region of the angular gyrus, and that disease of the lower center, or of the fibers in connection with it, intercepts the visual impulses on their way to the higher centers; but each higher center being connected with the whole of both occipital lower centers, destruction of one higher center does not interfere permanently with vision in either eye. His cases would seem to indicate that the convolutions surrounding the posterior extremity of the fissure of Sylvius are especially concerned with the vision of the opposite eye, and in such a direct manner that destruction of them in one hemisphere produces transitory blindness of the opposite eye, while bilateral destruction of them causes permanent blindness in both eyes. Parinaud [2] divides vision into binocular, monocular, and simultaneous. The last is distinguished from the second by identical projection of the same object by each eye. Each form has motor, sensory, and connecting fibers. In squint, binocular vision is present, but simultaneous binocular vision is absent. The image of the squinting eye, falling on a part of the retina disassociated in function from that of the other, is suppressed. The motor apparatus is represented by convergence and the connecting fibers by a reflex established by two images that

---

[1] Lancet, May 22, 1897.　　　　　　　　　[2] Ann. d'Ocul., June, 1896.

at the first moment of vision are not on corresponding points of the retina, but when vision is established become so.

Photometry.—Snellen [1] states that, owing to the variation in illumination, reliable figures recording vision can be obtained only by the use of a photometer that shall give vision under known conditions of light. The acuity is modified according to the size of the object, the illumination, the size of the pupil, and the adaptation of the retina.

Aqueous Humor.—The labors of E. Niesmamoff [2] substantiate the conclusions formulated by Greeff two years ago (see *Year-Book*, 1896) as to the secretion of the aqueous humor and its origin. The author states that the amount of aqueous secreted is in proportion to the difference in pressure in the vessels of the ciliary body and the intraocular pressure.

Parallax Test.—A simple method of locating opacities in the cornea, lens, and vitreous is detailed by E. Jackson.[3] It is known as the "parallax test," used with the plane mirror at 10 to 12 inches. A body situated anterior to the plane of the pupil will move in the direction taken by the eye, while one posterior to the plane of the lens will move against the direction taken by the eye. Bodies lying about the same plane as the pupil will show little, if any, movement. There are many practical applications of the method.

Orbit.—L. Koenigstein [4] contributes an elaborate study of the anatomy and physiology of the orbit and its contents. It constitutes a valuable enrichment of our knowledge of this little-studied side of ophthalmology.

Color.—P. Hilbert [5] claims that abnormal color-perceptions are always subjective; that they arise centrally as conditions of irritation of the color-vision centre; and that although they cannot be originated by external conditions, they may be intensified by them. He further holds that these facts are explainable only on the hypothesis of a color-vision center distinct from the light-perceptive center. Gorty's method of color-examination,[6] priority for which is claimed by H. Adler,[7] is to lay before the candidate a number of colored pencils, the wood of each of which corresponds to that of the crayon. The pencils are taken up one by one and the candidate is to write upon a sheet of white paper the name of the color of the pencil in hand; *e. g.*, with a red pencil the word "red" is written, with a green one, "green," etc. The paper on which this writing is done is signed by the writer, and this paper filed away for future reference in case of complaint by the candidate of unfair dealing.

REFRACTION.

Accommodation.—Tscherning's theory of accommodation has been materially strengthened by the observations of Hess,[8] Stadfeldt,[9] and especially by Crzellitzer,[10] who by elaborate experimental researches have shown that during accommodation the middle portion of the lens is more highly refractive than the periphery, and that traction on the zonule produces central increase of curvature and peripheral decrease, giving a hyperbolic shape to the lens. Tscherning contends that the total change of shape which the lens will have to undergo to effect a given increase of curvature in the pupillary area would be considerably less according to his theory than according to that of Helmholtz. Hess,[11] by experiments on his own eyes, determined that

[1] Ophth. Rev., June, 1896.
[2] Arch. f. Ophth., Nov., 1896.
[3] Phila. Polyclinic, Oct. 10, 1896.
[4] Beitr. z. Augenh., Dec., 1896.
[5] Samml. Zwangloser Abhandlungen a. d. Gebieta d. augenh. Halle, 1897.
[6] Münch. med. Woch., Feb. 23, 1897.
[7] Ibid., Mar. 30, 1897.
[8] Arch. f. Ophth., vol. xlii., 1.
[9] Klin. Monatsbl. f. Augenh., Dec., 1896.
[10] Arch. f. Ophth., Nov., 1896.
[11] Ibid., May, 1897.

during accommodation the lens sinks downward about $\frac{1}{3}$ mm., and that when the head is displaced toward either shoulder there is corresponding displacement of the lens. These, he says, are passive movements, due solely to the weight of the lens.

Ocular Hygiene.—The plain truths of prophylaxis are pointed out by S. D. Risley's[1] *résumé* of the results of the examinations of many thousands of school children, truths that ought to be put into practical execution in our public-school system. Sanitary science can have no more important or fruitful field of application. W. F. Southard[2] compares the attention given by intelligent parents to their children's teeth with that bestowed upon their eyes, much to the disadvantage of the latter, and emphasizes the greater importance of good vision and ability to read without asthenopia to the development of the child's faculties. A. C. Simonton[3] objects to the glaze of the paper on which the *Jour. of the Am. Med. Assoc.* is printed. [This is a subject well worth agitating. Paper of dead finish is the only paper that should be used for literature, and if the publishers of medical journals were but properly approached in the matter, we believe that they would not be slow to make an improvement, in which they would soon be followed by publishers everywhere.] W. B. Carhart[4] submits that while the eyes of the children of the present generation are not intrinsically any weaker or more diseased than those of their forefathers, the demands of the school-life of to-day have compelled the necessity of aiding their eyes with glasses.

Statistics.—Among 53,333 pupils in the public schools of Baltimore, Harlan and Woods,[5] found vision equal to $\frac{20}{20}$ in 43%, $\frac{20}{30}$ in the better eye in an additional 39%, between $\frac{20}{30}$ and $\frac{20}{200}$ in 15%, and less than $\frac{20}{200}$ in the better eye in $\frac{1}{2}$% of the cases.

Criminology.—In an investigation of the eyes of 362 criminals, with a view to determine whether their defects might be held responsible for their criminal lives, or might be classed among hereditary characteristics of degeneracy, H. Truc, J. Gaudibett, and Rouveyroles,[6] determined that the ocular and visual defects were of no more value than other anatomico-physiologic defects in determining abnormal mental deviations.

Refraction and Body-weight.—G. M. Gould[7] suggests that increase of body-weight is attended by decrease of refraction, and that decrease of body-weight is attended by increase in refraction, owing to the influence on the form of the eyeball of the varying amount of fat in the orbit. Illustrative cases are submitted.

Eyesight and Veils.—C. A. Wood[8] voices the general sentiment of the profession when he condemns the wearing of veils. By testing the vision of an individual with normal sight while wearing the different varieties (lace, chiffon, single-thread, dotted, etc.), he found vision seriously interfered with in every case, and concludes that all veils are pernicious in their effect, the dotted kind in particular.

Visual Tests.—Brown[9] calls attention to the mistake made in prescribing plus for minus lenses by reason of the assumption that 20 feet is equal to infinity. Distances less than 20 feet would give correspondingly greater errors. J. Ramos[10] offers a new series of test-types based on a novel applica-

[1] Norris and Oliver, System of Diseases of the Eye, vol. ii., 1897.
[2] Pacific Med. Jour., Mar., 1897.   [3] Jour. Am. Med. Assoc., Apr. 24, 1897.
[4] N. Y. Med. Jour., June 12, 1897.   [5] Jour. Am. Med. Assoc., Dec. 3, 1897.
[6] Ann. d'Oculist., Apr., 1897.   [7] Med. News. June 26, 1897.
[8] Boston M. and S. Jour., Dec. 3, 1896.   [9] Jour. Am. Med. Assoc., Nov. 21, 1896.
[10] Gazetta Medica, Apr. 2, 1896.

tion of the laws of retinal perception. He favors the decimal system in expressing visual acuity. Proceeding on physiologic principles, G. M. Gould has revived the idea of a black test-card on which are lithographed white letters.[1] The great advantage to be derived from its use is the restfulness felt by the patient, to which testimony is often spontaneously given. [For 8 months we have been using one of these cards with the greatest satisfaction. Absence of retinal tire during the subjective examination has been especially noticed.]

Objective Refraction.—The principles underlying the application of this latest method in objective refraction are clearly set forth by J. Thorington,[2] in his monograph. J. W. Ellis[3] observes that one ought to test his ophthalmometer at regular intervals with a convex mirror made for the purpose, in order that the instrument may not by its faulty indications lead the worker into error. G. J. Bull[4] considers the information given by the ophthalmometer is often more trustworthy and useful than that given by skiascopy or any other objective method of refraction. [The relative merits of skiascopy and ophthalmometry are too well appreciated in this country to permit of much growth of this doctrine.]

Asthenopia.—In treating of asthenopia as a forerunner of neurasthenia St. J. Roosa says,[5] "Unless corneal astigmatism makes a dioptre with the rule, or a quarter of a dioptre against the rule, it does not of itself produce asthenopia. Given normal refraction in both eyes, there can be no such thing as want of muscular equilibrium, except in cases of paresis. When a patient comes having normal vision, a low degree of hypermetropia (1 to 3 D.), and either no astigmatism or a half dioptre with the rule, there must be something besides the eye which is at fault in the production of the asthenopia [!]." "Repeatedly I have found this condition of things to be the premonition of neurasthenia or general nervous breakdown. To give such patients" (that is, patients with 0.5 D. astigmatism or 1 to 3 D. hypermetropia) "glasses, is at best a placebo" [*sic!*]. "In my judgment, no one is ever the better for glasses unless they see better with them or are much more comfortable with them. Even when vision for distance is perfect with the glasses, I do not urge such patients to wear glasses except for the near. The point I make is that when in a case of asthenopia the refractive conditions do not justify the ordering of glasses, thorough investigation of the whole train of symptoms should be instituted." [To this last proposition we are sure every sane ophthalmologist will assent, but if 0.5 D. of astigmatism or 3 D. of hypermetropia is not a factor in neurasthenopia, what degree of ametropia does Dr. Roosa feel will "justify in ordering glasses?" This is retrogression pure and simple. It amounts to retraction of those truths which the ophthalmic world has enunciated for 20 years. Such statements proceeding from one high in authority are fraught with exceeding danger. We believe, with Dr. Roosa, that the eye is only one factor in neurasthenia, but it may easily prove the one additional factor necessary to insure nervous breakdown.] There is a much larger grain of truth in the statement of S. D. Reynolds,[6] whose study of the records of 2000 astigmatics convinced him that correction of the ametropia relieves asthenopia only in persons otherwise in good health. Recovery in all other cases is contingent upon other means of relief. P. W. Maxwell[7] traces a connection between accommodative asthenopia and nasal

[1] Ann. Ophth. and Otol., Jan., 1897.
[3] Boston M. and S. Jour., July 9, 1896.
[5] Manhattan Eye and Ear Hosp. Rep., Jan., 1897.
[6] Jour. Am. Med. Assoc., May 29, 1897.

[2] Retinoscopy, Phila., 1897.
[4] Ophth. Rev., June, 1897.

[7] Brit. Med. Jour, Sept. 22, 1896.

obstruction, claiming that many patients will lay aside their glasses after the nasal functions have been rectified. Especially did he find his idea applicable in cases presenting pharyngeal adenoids as a complication. [Maxwell's conclusions would be much more readily accepted if he had shown in the histories he cites that the refractive error had been painstakingly measured and persistently worn before proceeding to nasal treatment. Judging from his case-histories, the estimations were of the manifest refraction, or were made with the ophthalmoscope, either of which methods may lead even the most careful observer far astray.] The 4 cases of epilepsy affirmed by J. S. Kirkendall[1] to have been cured by correction of ametropia and graduated tenotomy are strikingly similar to the generality of such cases detailed by A. L. Ranney in his recent monograph.[2] [There ought to be greater reason offered for tenotomy of both interni (Kirkendall), than esophoria of 1°, even though the abduction be but 3°.] Causes for asthenopia, other than errors of refraction, are said by H. Gradle[3] to be found in inherited nervous instability, enfeebling infectious diseases, anemia, impaired digestion, faulty habits, chronic blepharitis and conjunctivitis, disturbance of the retinal pigment, muscular anomalies, nasal affections, hysteria, and insomnia. He advises absolute rest of the eyes and dark glasses. The ocular expressions of eye-strain (Clarke)[4] are blepharitis, phlyctenular keratoconjunctivitis, scleritis, recurrent iritis, and, under certain conditions, cataract and glaucoma.

Mydriatics.—Homatropin, in E. Jackson's hands,[5] has proved an efficient, reliable cycloplegic capable of producing complete ciliary paralysis, and possessing the therapeutic influences for which a mydriatic is indicated in cases of eye-strain. As compared with other drugs of the class, it is least likely to cause general poisoning or local harm by glaucoma or conjunctival irritation, and it entails upon the patient the shortest period of disability. F. Mayo[6] secures as complete cycloplegia from 6 instillations of a 2 % solution of homatropin at 5-minute intervals as from a 1 % solution of atropin used 3 times daily for 2 days. On the other hand, Hansell[7] states that homatropin is not a reliable cycloplegic in young individuals. T. E. Murrell's further trial of scopolamin hydrobromate as a cycloplegic in 150 more cases (making 200 in all) only emphasizes the commendations he bestowed on the drug last year (see *Year-Book* for 1896).[8] In his hands it has proved the ideal cycloplegic, in which opinion he is joined by C. A. Oliver.[9] An undoubted instance of poisoning following the instillation of 1 drop of a 0.2 % solution of this drug is reported by C. P. Pinckard.[10] The patient, a 48-year-old woman, had experienced no unpleasant symptoms from the use of homatropin a year previously. The case further shows that scopolamin distinctly increases the intraocular tension.

Presbyopia.—G. M. Gould[11] calls attention to a mistake that may be made by opticians of inverting the presbyopic segment frequently cemented to the distance-correction. To avoid this he recommends that the upper edge of the segment have a sharper curve than its lower edge, which is ground of the same curve as the lower edge of the distance-correction. Anent this same topic, W. F. Southard[12] claims that much comfort can be given to many presbyopes who wear bifocals, by having the reading-segments made small and

[1] N. Y. Med. Jour., Apr. 17. 1897.
[2] Eye-strain in Health and Disease, F. A. Davis & Co., Phila., 1897.
[3] Jour. Am. Med. Assoc., Mar. 6, 1897.
[4] Med. Press and Circular, 22, 1896.
[5] Jour. Am. Med. Assoc., No. 21, 1896.
[6] Med. News, June, 1896.
[7] Am. Jour. Ophth., No. 3, vol. xii.
[8] Arch. f. Ophth., July, 1897.
[9] Am. Jour. Med. Sci., Nov., 1896.
[10] Ann. Ophth. and Otol., Oct., 1896.
[11] Ophth. Rec., May, 1897.
[12] Ann. Ophth. and Otol., Oct., 1896.

almost square in shape. The inability of hyperopes and presbyopes to see clearly through their glasses at night is said by E. Jackson[1] to be due to the dilated pupil. The cornea near its periphery is less hyperopic than in the pupillary region, and therefore the glasses are too strong. He also found[2] that when the difference in the refraction of the two eyes exceeds 2 D. that the lens of the stronger eye may be decentered to save the prismatic effect and the annoyance of looking through the periphery of the lens. An examination of 300 individuals by J. Barrett[3] showed the interpupillary distance to be on an average 2 mm. greater than the distance between the visual axes.

Myopia—In a discussion before the Section on Ophthalmology of the British Medical Association (1896), Drs. J. B. Lawford, F. R. Cross, Argyll-Robertson, P. W. Maxwell, Henry Juler, and David Little were of one accord in endorsing the operative treatment of high myopia in those cases in which no contraindications presented. A. Mooren's experience with this class of cases has now reached a total of 149 without a failure [!],[4] and only serves to confirm him in his opinion of some years ago, that the procedure is markedly beneficial in the large majority of properly selected cases. Speaking elsewhere of the dangers lurking in progressive high myopia, he says: "Full myopic corrections for near-work are pernicious, as they induce exaggerated accommodative effort and ciliary spasm, and thus intensify the refractive error, causing progressive myopia. Furthermore, retinal detachment and slow inflammatory changes are much more likely to supervene." [Our own experience has been that in myopes under 25 years of age full corrections are not only tolerated, but are really welcomed for near-work after the accommodation has been temporarily assisted with pilocarpin and the convergence properly trained with prisms.] V. Fukala, in his monograph[5] and elsewhere,[6] reviews his practice of this method in high myopia for a number of years, and enunciates views that are largely held by most of the disciples of the operation. He offers as advantages after the operation: enlargement of the retinal images, better illumination of the images, simplification of the optical apparatus, and increase of the retinal functional activity. Th. Gelpke and W. Bilber,[7] basing their faith on an experience with 59 cases, are enthusiastic advocates of the surgical treatment of high myopia. Vacher's conclusions[8] are judicial and safe. He says extraction of the transparent lens is a grave operation that should only be performed with great prudence and under the most rigorous antiseptic precautions. Myopia progressing rapidly between the ages of 12 and 16 may be operated upon after the age of 12, if there be a large staphyloma and if the number of the diopters of myopia exceed the number of years of the patient. Only one eye should be operated on, and that the more seriously affected. Operation on the second eye should not be undertaken until later, and then only at the express request of the patient if the myopia continue to progress. After the 30th year myopia of more than 15 diopters, predisposing to retinal detachment, justifies extraction of the transparent lens when the visual acuity permits. Panas[9] and Ascher[10] are both advocates of discission or extraction of the lens in myopia of 16 D. or higher.

In progressive myopia of from 9 D. to 29 D., representing vision equal to $\frac{1}{3}$ or less, Drousart[11] has done iridectomy and sclerotomy 248 times, arresting

[1] Phila. Polyclinic, Aug., 1896.　　　　　[2] Am. Jour. Ophth., Oct., 1896.
[3] Intercol. Med. Jour. of Australasia, Oct. 20, 1896.
[4] Die medicinische und operativ Behandlungen kurzsichtiger Storungen, Wiesbaden, 1897.
[5] Ueber Heilung hochstgradiger Kurzsichtigkeit, etc., F. Deuticke, Leipsig und Wien, 1896.
[6] Arch. f. Ophth., Feb., 1897.　　　　　[7] Beitr. z. Augenh., Aug., 1897.
[8] Ann. d'Oculist., July, 1896.　　　　　[9] Gaz. hebdom. de Méd. et Chir., Dec. 31, 1896.
[10] Beitr. z. Augenh., July, 1896.　　　　[11] Rec. d'Ophtal., June, 1897.

the myopia, stopping fundus-changes, and greatly improving vision. There was never retinal detachment following the operation. He prefers iridectomy to sclerotomy. Along with the removal of the lens, says M. Salzmann,[1] we probably remove a source of considerable irregularity of refraction, and vision is improved for the reasons advanced by Fukala. A residual myopia of 3 D. is the ideal post-operative condition. Persons whose vocation demands continued work at the near-point will derive but little benefit from the operation, the indications for which should never be based solely on a certain degree of refraction. F. Otto's[2] conception of an ideal after-result is 4 D. of myopia. He also points out the possibility of divergent strabismus following upon the destruction of binocular vision, which, if it should happen to affect the operated eye, would vitiate the result of the operation. He believes that ancestral impress counts for more than consanguinity in the production of congenital myopia. Martin[3] says the latter condition is never axial, but depends upon the increased refraction of the ocular media. It must not be forgotten that myopia may occur in persons who have never had but one eye, as shown in Duane's[4] patient. In Philadelphia the removal of the lens for the cure of high myopia has been limited to a very few cases.[5] In the large majority of cases correction by means of a well-adapted and accurately made glass confers vision good enough to render operation unjustifiable. While Chauvel[6] grants that removal of the crystalline lens may be useful in some cases of high myopia, he maintains that our experience is still too limited to judge definitely of the modifications to which the eye may subsequently be subjected. J. Hirschberg,[7] too, thinks that reduction of progressive myopia by discission of the lens is a procedure that calls for the most judicial consideration. For high myopia F. C. Hotz[8] advocates a bifocal that is exactly the reverse of the ordinary bifocal in that the main lens constitutes the correction for near-work, while the distance-correction is secured by cementing a segment to the upper margin of the main lens. The lower edge of this segment must be at least 3 mm. above the center of the main lens.

Astigmatism.—Hess,[9] by an elaborate series of experiments on himself with cylindrical lenses, disproves the hypothesis of partial correction of corneal astigmatism by a secondary action on the part of the lens, claiming that the pupillary state and the palpebral fissure must be reckoned with in such cases. H. Gradle fails utterly in his attempt to negate the above findings of Hess as to the impossibility of unequal lenticular contraction in the correction by the patient of his own astigmatism. The 2 cases selected by Gradle[10] for the support of his hypothesis were most unfortunate in their evidence, one of them being a young astigmatic whose best corrected vision was but $\frac{1}{5}$; the other, a young woman whose best corrected vision was not only a scant $\frac{1}{4}$, but presented also congenital oculomotor palsies of some of the muscles of her left eye. Hess,[11] in responding, reaffirms his position of a year ago (see *Year-Book*, 1897, p. 325), that the whole phenomenon is explained by lid-pressure so exerted by the patient as to correct his own astigmatism. In C. Williams'[12] study (in 100 office-cases) of the discrepancy between the astigmatism indicated by Javal's ophthalmometer and the total

[1] Ann. of Ophth., July, 1897.   [2] Arch. f. Ophth., Apr. and May, 1897.
[3] Rec. d'Ophtal., Aug., 1896.   [4] Ophth. Rec., June, 1897.
[5] T. B. Schneideman and E. Jackson, Med. and Surg. Reporter, July 3, 1897.
[6] Bull. de l'Acad. de Méd., June 22, 1897.   [7] Centralbl. f. prakt. Augenh., Mar., 1897.
[8] Ophth. Rec., Jan., 1897.   [9] Arch. f. Ophth., No. 2, 1896.
[10] Ibid., Feb, 1897.   [11] Ibid.
[12] Ann. Ophth. and Otol., July, 1896.

astigmatism by trial-lenses, Javal's instruments gave the position of the axis of the cylindrical glass in about 50% of the cases, and the astigmatism to within 0.5 D. of the accepted glass in 54% of the cases. His chief use of the Javal is as a rapid approximate indicator of the axis and degree of astigmatism. [This, we think, fairly reflects the views of most careful refractionists who are skilled in the use of Javal's instrument, namely, that its best service is as an indicator in refraction.] To determine accurately the meridian in astigmatism, F. W. Coleman[1] uses a cylinder from 0.5 to 1.5 diopters stronger than the accepted cylinder, and finds the preferred axis, which will be the angle for the accepted cylinder. He resorts to this method only when the accepted cylinder is of 0.5 D. strength or less. [A useful suggestion.] It is well known that the astigmatism following cataract-operation gradually diminishes for some months, until only 1 or 2 D. remain. Lucciola[2] says that a small corneoscleral incision that does not allow the aqueous humor to escape will generally increase the corneal curvature of that meridian in which the incision is made. This is contrary to the effect of the incision for cataract, which decreases the corneal curve in that meridian, and Lucciola therefore suggests this measure as a radical cure for astigmatism. A naval officer who was the subject of acquired astigmatism, had presented 5 years before the time of report an emmetropic left eye; 5 years later F. L. Henderson[3] found a regular myopic astigmatism of 1.75 D., induced, as Henderson believes, by the pressure of the orbicularis on the left eye while using the right eye on a surveyor's sextant. H. Aschheim,[4] too, speaks of an instance of acquired astigmatism of 32 D. occurring in a young woman with scrofulous cornea. The pupil was so involved by anterior synechiæ as to assume a slit shape. In the correction of irregular astigmatism Th. Lohnstein[5] employs a hydrodiascope, his own device, fashioned on Thomas Young's theory. He has worn the apparatus himself (high M+Am.), an aggregate of 7 hours in one day, without discomfort.

Tinted Glasses.—Risley's[6] examination of a large number of coquilles showed that not one in a dozen was free from some cylindric or prismatic defect or other irregularity which could only add to any existing strain in an ametropic eye. To correct this evil and secure uniformity in smoked glasses, E. Pergens[7] proposes that a smoked glass of 1 mm. thickness should absorb $\frac{1}{10}$ of the light from a Hefner amylacetate light one meter distant.

MUSCLE-AFFECTIONS.

Paralyses.—A careful study of the oculomotor nuclear conditions secondary to long-standing isolated paralysis of some one of the ocular muscles will be of more definite value[8] to ophthalmic science than a whole array of physiologic and anatomic experiments. By combining the results obtained in a few selected and well-studied cases the relative positions of the separate nuclei can be fixed with scientific accuracy. Among the **causes** of paralyses in infants Dujardin[9] mentions traumatism from forceps during delivery. He asserts that this cause is frequently overlooked, and that when the child becomes older the squint is ascribed to hyperopia. C. A. Wood[10] observed a patient with optic-nerve atrophy accompanied by oculomotor paralysis

[1] N. Am. Pract., Aug., 1896.
[3] Ann. Ophth. and Otol., July, 1896.
[5] Ibid., Dec., 1896.
[7] Klin. Monatsbl. f. Augenh., Feb., 1897.
[9] Jour. des Sci. méd. de Lille, Nov. 28, 1896.

[2] Arch. d'Ophtal., Oct., 1896.
[4] Klin. Monatsbl. f. Augen., Apr., 1897.
[6] Am. Jour. Ophth., Nov., 1896.
[8] Th. Sachs, Arch. f. Opth., July, 1896.
[10] Med. News, May 29, 1897.

from plumbism. W. M. Leszynsky[1] refers congenital absence of outward movement of both eyes to arrested development affecting the external recti, or to a faulty insertion of those muscles. H. Spicer[2] suggests as a cause of squint the secondary contraction of the internus following paralysis of the externus in childhood from whooping-cough, fits, etc., and after recovery the squint is maintained by habit. A. Duane[3] lays particular stress on the **frequency of paralysis** of the inferior and superior recti, and asserts that it escapes attention because our visual line is ordinarily directed below the horizontal plane of the eyes. The part that these vertical paralyses play in convergence-insufficiency is worthy of consideration. C. Kunn[4] has studied 8 peculiar cases of acquired ocular palsy of some one of the ocular muscles, in which fixation was performed by the palsied eye, and that too, in several instances in spite of the fact that the **vision** of the palsied eye was much lower than that of its fellow. The 13th published case is reported by de Schweinitz[5] of **recurrent abducens paralysis** in a 6-year-old girl. M. Straub[6] adds 3 classic cases of paralysis of divergence, in all of whom lateral conjugation was perfectly performed. The patients were aged 53, 29, and 20. **The prognosis** of true nuclear traumatic paralysis of the ocular muscles, says P. Simon[7] is quite favorable. The therapy of these conditions is largely symptomatic; iodids to promote absorption and electricity to stimulate nerve-action. In a case of long-standing paralysis of the external rectus J. E. Giles[8] remedied the condition by excising a portion of the internal rectus of the paralytic eye. [This operation has been frequently performed, and is the only one that should be considered. The result, however, is improvement in appearance only, since the function of the muscle is not in the least restored.]

Nystagmus.—Nystagmus is acquired in other occupations than that of coalmining. Thus Snell[9] found it among artists and painters, compositors, metalrollers, platelayers, plankcutters, sawmakers, fitters, ironfounders, etc., in all of whom the nystagmus may be ascribed to the necessity of elevating the corneas above the horizontal line. D. Gourfein's[10] observations on 6 cases of congenital ophthalmoplegia and nystagmus, with preservation of the functions of the iris and ciliary muscles, in a father and 5 sons, convince him that the congenital variety of external ophthalmoplegia is not of nuclear origin, but is clearly a hereditary affection consisting entirely in defects of the muscles. Schwarz,[11] in speaking of Könighoefer's case of voluntary movements of one eye while the other eye was held in its primary position (Heidelberg Congress, 1896) remarks that such anomalies of ocular movements are not uncommon among hysterics, and states further that it is a faculty that is acquired with comparative ease. By finding the position of rest in nystagmus and then tenotomizing the contracted muscles so that the visual lines would be brought from deviated and abnormal directions, J. E. Coburn[12] has been able to relieve the oscillation and improve vision in nystagmic patients.

Relation of Shape of Orbits to Visual Planes.—G. T. Stevens'[13] study of the normal directions of the planes of vision in relation to certain cranial characteristics shows that in the dolichocephalic (long skull) the orbit is horizontally long and low, inducing kataphoria or restriction of upward

[1] N. Y. Med. Jour., Feb. 27, 1891.   [2] Royal London Ophth. Hosp. Rep., vol. xiv., p. 1.
[3] Arch. of Ophth., July, 1897.   [4] Beitr. z. Augenh., Oct., 1896.
[5] Phila. Polyclinic, Aug. 21, 1897.   [6] Centralbl. f. prakt. Augenh., Jan., 1897.
[7] Beitr. z. Augenh., July, 1896.   [8] Manhattan Eye and Ear Hosp. Rep., 1897.
[9] Ophth. Rev., June, 1896.   [10] Rev. méd. de la Suisse Romande, No. 12, 1896.
[11] Centralbl. f. prakt. Augenh., April, 1897.   [12] Am. Jour. Ophth., Aug., 1897.
[13] Oph Rec., July, 1897.

rotation ; in the mesocephalic (medium high head) the orbit is strongly arched above, inducing anophoria or restriction of the downward rotation ; in the brachycephalic (broad skull) the orbit is not only long and low, but is also directed down and out, inducing restriction of both upward and downward rotation. Stevens fixes the average upward rotation at 30° to 35° and the downward at 50°.

Relation of Accommodation and Convergence.—G. A. Berry[1] claims that the close theoretic relation between accommodation and convergence is maintained only in those individuals who are emmetropic, or nearly so ; that it is seldom correct to measure the meter-angles of convergence by the number of diopters of accommodation in use for certain distances, this relation depending upon the refraction and the power of fusion. In testing for operation the deviation for the far and not for the near should be the guide. It must be remembered that limitation of external rotation is not caused by structural weakness of the muscles, but is due to an increase of innervation to the interni, and limitation of internal rotation to insufficiency of convergence. Atropinization or bandaging of the good eye is seldom of benefit. The surgical treatment is tenotomy for the former and advancement for the latter. Apropos of bandaging, F. W. Martin[2] has observed that wearing a bandage a few days after tenotomy will make manifest a squint that was supposed to have been perfectly corrected. He recommends this as a means of determining heterophoria.

Center of Rotation.—E. Landolt[3] insists that the center of rotation of the eye is not a fixed point in the vitreous [as stated in his own and others' text-books], but that its location is the resultant of all the forces that hold the globe in position and which move it.

Strabismus.—C. Kuun[4] says that the existence of concomitant squint demands that the mobility of the eyes shall be normal, and that the strabismic eye shall be able to follow all movements of its neighbor fixing in any distance. In sleep and in ether-narcosis, while the squint has changed from its previous condition, it is not lost ; but the eyes present an irregular strabismus, the cortical impulse acting to produce a symmetrical displacement. This fact proves that the associated movements of the eyes are the result of experience, and not an inherent faculty. Defects of motility are always congenital, and while the eyes may be freely movable the central field of locomotion or the center governing locomotion may be defective (here locomotion differs from rotation). Factors contributing to squint are the orbit, globes, muscles, and innervation (orientation). Amblyopia is not a consequence, but often, when the mechanical conditions are not favorable to parallelism of the axes, is a cause of squint.

Malposition of the macula is held by G. M. Black[5] to be responsible for that variety of heterophoria in which there is esophoria with the phorometer in the presence of apparent divergence, or exophoria with the phorometer with apparent convergence. This condition is to be diagnosed by means of the perimeter, when the angle *a* will be found to be larger than normal in esophoria and smaller in exophoria ; while M. Sachs[6] rejects the idea of a vicarious macula (or secondary macula) in strabismus, contending that the squinter is a person who sees single with each eye, and that there can be no binocular vision because the visual fields do not overlap each other. W. B. Meany[7] assumes that binocular fixation is a faculty that

[1] Edinb. Med. Jour., Jan., Feb., Mar., 1897.   [2] Ophth. Rev., Mar., 1897.
[3] Arch. of Ophth., Jan., 1897.   [4] Rec. d'Ophth., May, 1897.
[5] Ophth. Rec., Aug., 1897.   [6] Arch. f. Ophth., May, 1897.
[7] Jour. Am. Med. Assoc., May 29, 1897.

exists from birth [this is untenable ground. As presumed evidence], he quotes an instance of convergent squint in a 19-year-old male that was completely corrected by tenotomy of the internus and advancement of the externus of the squinting eye, combined with subsequent orthoptic exercise. Savage[1] believes that the true cause of typical antipathy to binocular single vision resides in the fact that the macula of one eye is connected with the right side of the brain, while the macula of the other eye is connected with the left side of the brain [on this assumption all symmetrical motions of the limbs should be anatomical anomalies]; while C. M. Hobby[2] is convinced that accuracy of coordination when one eye is covered, as with the Maddox rod, is not essential to ease of vision, but admits the frequent coincidence of asthenopia and difficult or imperfect coordination. He further holds that a difference in size of retinal images equal to 10% is compatible with mental association.

A. Duane[3] reiterates that squint and insufficiency, or heterophoria, differ only in degree, and must be treated on the same principles based on etiology. The several causes that may induce insufficiency are each to be given proper weight in deciding treatment.

To test the degree of rotation of the cornea and, to a certain extent, the strength of the individual muscles, Wood[4] has suggested the simple method of using strips of paper on which are printed letters and numbers, to be adjusted to the perimeter. The letters that can be read nearest to the periphery indicate the degree of turning of the cornea. [The objection to this device is that patients with considerable optic defect are forced to read through the edges of their glasses, and thereby lose acuity of vision proportionately to the strength of the glasses, in addition to having the apparent position of the letters altered by the prismatic effect of the lenses.]

If in concomitant strabismus there is the slightest limitation of individual movement of either eye, says C. Kunn,[5] the case is one of congenital defect of movement of the eyes, provided other complications are absent.

G. T. Stevens[6] claims that the tropometer, his instrument designed to measure rotations of the cornea, confirms his views frequently expressed, that lateral deviations will often be found in cases in which the tension of the vertical muscles is unequal, and that the former depends upon the latter.

Heterophoria from Nasal Reflex.—H. B. Chandler[7] urges caution in approaching heterophoria from the surgical side, offering in support of his contention several histories of instances of muscular anomalies induced by enlarged turbinated bodies. [There is food for thought in his article.]

Asthenopia.—Walter[8] suggests an analogy between accommodative and muscular asthenopia and the professional neuroses, such as writer's cramp, and divides asthenopia or ocula-dyscinesia into the spastic and paretic, and believes that the best results would accrue from their treatment on this basis, rather than by surgical alterations in the tensions.

Treatment.—Marked improvement in the oculoneural reflexes resulting from paresis of the superior oblique muscle, in a youth, was afforded by division of the superior rectus of the same eye by D. Webster.[9] W. R. Parker[10] details an interesting history of a 33-year-old woman, the subject of a suppressed upward squint of 7 degrees, on whom he performed **tenotomy** of the right superior rectus, bringing the deviation down to 2 degrees, which gradu-

[1] Jour. Am. Med. Assoc., May 22, 1897. [2] Ophth. Rec., June, 1897.
[3] Va. Med. Semi-monthly, Nov. 26, 1896. [4] Jour. Am. Med. Assoc., Nov. 28, 1896.
[5] Beitr. z. Augenh., Apr., 1897. [6] Ophth. Rec., May, 1897.
[7] Ann. of Ophth., Jan., 1897. [9] Ophth. Rec., Feb., 1897.
[9] N. Y. Polyclinic, Nov. 15, 1896. [10] Physician and Surgeon, Apr., 1897.

ally increased, however, to 7 degrees, necessitating tenotomy of the inferior rectus when balance was secured. Four months later, deviation of 7 degrees was again manifested, and in a second division of the right superior rectus overcorrection occurred, which was controlled by a stitch. Several hours later the stitch gave way, and diplopia appeared, when a deeper stitch was inserted, apparently overcorrecting the new deviation. After a few weeks, however, perfect muscle-balance was found, and the patient used her eyes freely with complete relief.

In a discussion before the Section of Ophthalmology in the British Medical Association,[1] on the question of precision in squint-operations, P. W. Maxwell stated that in only about 5% of cases was perfect binocular vision obtained. His review of 179 cases, comprising his own experience, showed that **tenotomy with advancement** was equal in effect to double tenotomy. He pleaded for the angular measurement of all cases of squint. Landolt favored advancement in each eye as a measure designed to aid weak muscles, in the place of tenotomy, which at best could but weaken strong ones; moreover, the latter procedure allows the globe to come forward in the orbit and to slip partly out of the grasp of the recti muscles. Berry thought it unnecessary to attempt precise adjustment, believing it best to leave a little convergence. Bickerton resorted to advancement with great confidence, stating that personal observation of Stevens's technic had convinced him of the value of advancement, dividing the effect between the two eyes. Vignes[2] adds his testimony to the value of advancement of the externi in the treatment of internal squint. C. B. Taylor[3] expects a great deal more from advancement of the internus than from advancement of the externus. In convergent squint he believes in thorough tenotomy of the internus, with subsequent shortening of the externus if necessary. He does not hope for the establishment of binocular fixation. Repeated operations are discouraging to the patient, and he, therefore, accomplishes all he can at the primary operation. [There is a large grain of truth in this last sentence. The operator can at best but approximate the visual lines to parallelism, while the final accurate adjustment must be made by means of prisms.] After the 9th year, H. Parinaud[4] says, squint cannot be straightened without operation. The center for coordination is immature at birth, and is developed by use. Therefore, ametropic eyes in which vision is bad are infinitely more subject to strabismus than those of normal acuity. He defines concomitant strabismus as a vice of development of the apparatus of binocular vision, of which the principal symptom is the defect of convergence of the two eyes upon a fixed object. A. G. Bennett[5] is enthusiastic over the results obtained by **prism-exercise** in 46 cases of low exophoria; 30 were apparently cured, 9 were benefited, 4 showed no improvement, and in the remaining 3 the result was unknown.

Valk's operation for shortening the muscles is essentially that of Savage,[6] modified by the use of catgut instead of silk sutures. Deschamps[7] has devised a pair of strong forceps, blunt and curved, for grasping and holding the muscles before the tendon is cut in the operation for advancement (Fig. 60).

W. Rider[8] argues from 2 cases of muscular asthenopia unsuccessfully treated by **graduated tenotomies** that that operation is, as a rule, irrational and dangerous. [There is very little doubt that a reaction against operative treatment has set in, and that many cases are now treated on strictly medicinal

[1] Brit. Med. Jour., Sept. 26, 1896.
[2] Rec. d'Ophthal., Aug., 1896.
[3] Lancet, Sept. 12, 1896.
[4] Traité de Thérapeut., A. Robin, Paris, 1897.
[5] Ann. of Ophth., Jan., 1897.
[6] N. Y. Med. Jour., Nov. 7, 1896.
[7] Ann. d'Oculist., July, 1896.
[8] Buffalo Med. Jour., Mar., 1897.

principles with good result; yet it is true that speedy and certain cures have resulted from tenotomy in properly selected cases, and that operative measures cannot wholly be discarded.]

Suppurative tenonitis, with secondary perforation of the ball after a thoroughly antiseptic advancement of the externus, is reported fully by J. A.

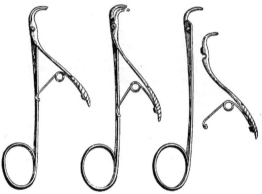

FIG. 60.—Deschamps forceps (Ann. d'Oculist., July, 1896).

White.[1] The eye finally healed, and parallel axes with good binocular vision were eventually secured.

THE EYE IN GENERAL DISEASE.

Autoinfection.—That the eye may be the seat of expression of an auto-intoxication is plainly shown by Panas.[2] The condition may be induced by germs or their toxins, brought by the circulation either from external sources or from the absorption of waste-products not eliminated by the natural emunctories (endoinfection), giving rise to disturbance of the nervous system, and thus so influencing the growth of the cells upon which the body-health depends as to produce a condition of "tendency to infection," or "latent microbism." This influence of the nervous system is seen in the bilaterality and symmetry of the infection. The sources of the intoxication are eruptive fevers, and dyscrasiæ, diabetes, albuminuria, uremia, oxaluria, phosphaturia, gout, chronic rheumatism, leukemia, scurvy, syphilis, tuberculosis, leprosy, blennorrhagia, puerperal and traumatic fevers, typhus, cerebrospinal meningitis, influenza, diphtheria, erysipelas, pernicious anemia, malarial fevers, and the nasopharyngeal tract; in women, the utero-ovarian apparatus. As chemic poisons, may be enumerated alcohol, nicotin, carbon disulphid, lead, santonin, and quinin. No ocular tissue is immune. Panas pronounces sympathetic ophthalmia an endoinfection. "The vasomotors of the sympathizing eye are influenced by reflex action, which creates in them a condition of *minoris resistentiæ.* In this case, as in others, it is a question whether the endoinfection of the sympathizing eye proceeds from toxins or from attenuated microbes charged with blood. One thing is certain—that in a traumatic eye (especially when previously irritated chemically) microbian activity is effected with the greatest facility." The necessity for local and general antisepsis in a case of traumatic

---

[1] Va. Med. Semi-monthly, Nov. 27, 1896.　　　　[2] La Clin. ophtal., May 10, 1897.

eye is obvious. Trousseau,[1] Vacher,[2] and Boucheron[3] are among Panas's supporters, while DeWecker[4] and Meyer[5] accept only in part the theory of autoinfection as the cause of many of the diseases named. D. M. Campbell[6] likewise remarks the relation between certain diathetic conditions and the correlated inflammations of the iris and ciliary body, believing that they are autoinfections, and that treatment looking to the digestive tract and all the emunctories will be vastly helpful to the local treatment of many ocular disorders. P. D. Keyser[7] also suggests regulation of the diet in all cases of subjective visual sensations. For those instances in which ocular and hepatic disorders are not simply coincident, Streminski[8] offers two hypotheses, ascribing them either to the circulation of biliary elements in the blood, or to the alteration in the blood caused by the absence of bile in the intestines. The resultant ocular disorders are sudden or gradual hemeralopia, due either to an insufficient production of visual purple or to alteration of the optic-nerve tissues, amblyopia, limitations of the fields, imperfect color-sense, xanthopsia, dilated or contracted pupils, asthenopia, moderate papillitis, altered caliber of the retinal vessels or retinal hemorrhages, and pigmentary retinal degeneration, with atrophy and proliferation of the pigment of the choroid. The anatomic changes consist in interstitial sclerosis of the retinal and choroidal elements. According to A. Wagenmann,[9] the choroid and selera are the tissues that suffer most in gout, although this diathesis also frequently underlies eczema of the lids, painful hemorrhagic iritis, migraine with visual disturbances, and especially presenile glaucoma. The effect of antiarthritic treatment upon the latter class of cases is striking—indeed, they will often yield only when general treatment is systematically resorted to. Secondary arthritis following autoinfected gonorrheal ophthalmia, in a male nurse aged 28, is reported by L. Weiss and W. Klingelhoffer.[10] The association of the gouty diathesis with cataract is clearly demonstrated by S. D. Risley.[11] "The excess of uric-acid salts in the blood-serum of gouty and rheumatic subjects may be and doubtless is sufficient to disturb the nutritive equilibrium in all the organic cells, but falls with especially disastrous results on the unstable transparent cells of the lens and vitreous body. It is a significant fact that the ectodermic structures of which the lens is one, and the avascular connective tissue in and about the joints another, are precisely the localities which suffer earliest and most constantly in the evolution of gout."

Relation to Kidney-disease.—H. F. Hansell[12] speaks of a patient exhibiting a central color-scotoma, who died 6 weeks after examination, from interstitial nephritis. Hansell says, "If this observation is confirmed in a number of cases, the discovery of central color-scotomata will afford an important indication of the speedy approach of a fatal termination." Unilateral neuroretinitis of albuminuric origin is, according to de Schweinitz,[13] not very common. It has been found by subsequent observation of some of these cases that the second eye becomes affected before death. In a nephritic, Higgins[14] notes acute edema of the conjunctiva so extensive that the cornea was covered by its folds. The choroid also showed signs of edema. This relation of deficient urinary excretion to certain obscure ocular disorders is also forcibly illustrated by E. E. Wright's array of cases.[15]

[1] La Clin. ophtal., May 10, 1897.   [2] Ibid.   [3] Ibid.   [4] Ibid.
[5] Ibid.   [6] Physician and Surgeon, Aug., 1896.
[7] Ophth. Rec. May, 1897.   [8] Rec. d'Ophtal, Feb., 1897.
[9] Arch. f. Ophth., Feb., 1897.   [10] Klin. Monatsbl. f. Augenh., Mar., 1897.
[11] Univ. Med. Mag., June, 1897.   [12] Phila. Polyclinic, Nov. 2, 1896.
[13] Med. News, Dec. 19, 1896.   [14] Jour. Am. Med. Assoc., Nov. 21, 1897.
[15] Medicine, May, 1897.

Diabetes.—Marked rapid change in the refraction of 2 glycosuries, varying with the amount of sugar in the urine, is recorded by S. D. Risley.[1] In each case, as the general condition improved, there was decided abatement in the accommodation, calling for the addition of from 1 to 4 D. spherical to the original correction; but when the sugar reappeared in the urine in any amount return to the original glasses became necessary. Risley assumes a change in the density of the tissue-fluids as the explanation of the phenomenon. [Compare with Appenzeller's case,[2] in which a transitory myopia of 1 D. disappeared along with the glycosuria.] Cataracts, in diabetics are not always dependent upon the diabetes. The age, acuity of vision before the cataract appeared, and its variation with the amount of sugar in the urine are to be considered. Sous[3] finds iritis a not infrequent complication. The lens is usually soft. In a polyuric, showing neither albumin, sugar, nor casts in the urine, H. F. Hansell[4] observed mild optic neuritis and retinitis similar in all respects to the albuminuric variety, save that the star-shaped figure, instead of affecting the foveal region, had selected the retina to the nasal side of the disk. The man died 8 months later. Contracted kidneys were found.

Tuberculosis.—A. Stiel[5] treated a patient for what he took to be iridocyclitis, and later chronic serous choroiditis, until the development of an anal fistula aroused his suspicions and led to an investigation, which revealed the tuberculous nature of the disorder. The incident teaches that tuberculosis of the uveal tract may simulate iridochoroiditis or cyclitis, chronic serous or plastic choroiditis, etc., and that exhaustive search into all the body-functions is necessary in all chronic affections of the uvea. DeWecker[6] agrees with Leber that ocular tuberculosis is not primary, and that enucleation is not advisable. He removed completely an area of tuberculous material from an iris in a 5-year-old boy whose health was good; 7 years later vision in the operated eye was normal.

Syphilis.—J. Hirschberg[7] contends that when, with a mydriatic pupil, small blood-vessels or their remains can be revealed in the cornea, careful search should be instituted for other evidences of acquired and especially hereditary syphilis.

Marasmus.—C. Koller[8] records the 18th and 19th published cases of a fatal disease of infancy, presenting symmetrical changes in the macula. The disks and retinæ atrophy, and the foveal region is occupied by a dark-red mass, circular in outline and surrounded by a clear white patch of atrophic choroid. The disease occurs often in 2 children of the same family; all die before their fourth year, of marasmus. There is no muscular paralysis, but the child is never well developed or strong enough to hold up its head or to walk. Koller attributes the malady to progressive degeneration in the cortex of the brain and the retina.

Malaria.—Guarnieri[9] enumerates the following retinal lesions found in the graver forms of malarial poisoning: swollen arteries and veins, perivascular edema, sometimes swelling of the papilla itself. In the blood of the retinal vessels were found the well-known changes in the red blood-corpuscles characteristic of malaria, thus explaining most of the visual disturbances complained of by victims of malarial fever. Basseres[10] considers retinal hemorrhage a

[1] Phila. Polyclinic, May 29, 1897.
[2] Year-Book, p. 945, 1897.
[3] Rec. d'Opthal., Aug., 1896.
[4] Phila. Polyclinic, Jan. 30, 1897.
[5] Centralbl. f. prakt. Augenh., May, 1897.
[6] La Clin. ophtal., May, 1896.
[7] Deutsch. med. Woch, Oct. 7, 14, 28, 1896.
[8] Med. Rec., Aug. 22, 1896.
[9] Arch. per la Sci. Med., No. 1, 1897.
[10] Arch. d'Ophtal., July, 1896.

more frequent complication of malaria than is generally supposed. The lesion is due to thrombi of parasitic origin, alterations in the blood, or weakening in the coats of the vessels through the irritating action of the malarial germs. Litten's [1] case of leukemia presented a peculiar affection of the eyelids, which at first had the aspect of edema, but on closer examination proved to be small lymphatic tumors which were not adherent to the skin. Köbner [2] looked upon the case as remarkable because of the rarity of skin-lesions in leukemia.

Goiter.—The course of exophthalmic goiter is pretty well illustrated by R. T. Williamson's study of 24 cases that were followed for some years; most of the cases were very little influenced by treatment.[3] Six terminated fatally, 7 recovered completely, 7 others were much benefited, and 4 remained unchanged by treatment. The above therapy did not include any of the animal extracts. [It would be interesting to have contrasted 3 series of cases: the first dealing with cases treated according to the usual therapy, the second being an animal-extract series, and the third a surgical series.]

In a discussion on the pathogeny of exophthalmic goiter Murray [4] stated that the cause of the disease must be sought in the thyroid gland. He knew of no case in which it was found normal after death. Edmunds and Robert Hutchinson,[5] dissenting from Murray, were of like mind in considering Graves' disease essentially a specific change in tissue-metabolism, due probably to a functional alteration in the central nervous system. The cardinal symptoms of Graves' disease are put down by W. C. Krauss [6] as tachycardia, exophthalmos, tremor, and goiter. Sänger [7] inveighs against meddlesome surgery in exophthalmic goiter, and challenges surgeons to show lasting benefit following extirpation of the gland. [The results in such cases reported from thyroid-feeding in the last year relegate surgery (at least temporarily) to a secondary place in the treatment of this disorder.] Grocco [8] refers to certain atypical instances of Graves' disease described in literature that were accompanied by paresis of the extrinsic ocular muscles, weakness of the extremities, and variable ability to speak, masticate, and swallow. These, he suspects, are really examples of Erb-Goldflam disease, and he suggests that when there is associated with a transient or variable ophthalmoplegia easily induced fatigue of other muscles of the body and exophthalmos, with no decided evidences of organic lesion, a suspicion of the presence of the Erb-Goldflam symptom-complex is justifiable.

Diphtheria.—Schirmer [9] states positively that postdiphtheric ocular palsies are not directly due to the presence of virulent microbes. The fact that these paralyses have been so frequently noted since the application of serum-therapy to diphtheria would rather indicate that the antitoxic serum does not destroy the toxins. In summarizing the results of serum-treatment in 16 cases of conjunctival diphtheria, R. Greeff [10] observes that the severe forms of the disorder prove a test for the value of serum-treatment, as formerly the most careful treatment was unavailing. Serum-treatment is without effect in pseudodiphtheria of the conjunctiva, nor is it prophylactic against postdiphtheric ocular paralyses. H. Bruns saw 3 cases presenting so little membrane on the conjunctiva and such slight symptoms in the first case that diphtheria was not suspected until a bacteriologist verified the diagnosis of

[1] Med. Bull., Mar., 1897.   [2] Ibid.
[3] Brit. Med. Jour., Nov. 7, 1896.   [4] Ibid., Oct. 3, 1896.
[5] Ibid.   [6] Alienist and Neurol., Jan., 1897.
[7] Neurol. Centralbl., Apr. 15, 1897.
[8] Ann. of Ophth., Jan., 1897, from Arch. di Ottalmol., Sept. and Oct., 1896.
[9] Ann. d'Oculist., Aug., 1896.   [10] Deutsch. med. Woch., Sept. 10, 1896.

diphtheria of the conjunctiva. The author [1] comments fittingly on how such mild cases of so deadly a disease may become particularly dangerous as sources of infection, remarking that they have probably caused many cases the etiology of which was shrouded in mystery. The conclusion is obvious that during the prevalence of diphtheria-epidemics or -endemics children with sore eyes are to be viewed with wholesome suspicion, and should be quarantined until the exact nature of their malady shall have been shown by bacteriologic examination. In the case observed by C. D. Westcott [2] membranous conjunctivitis occurring in a 3-year-old boy was traced postmortem to the streptococcus pyogenes in the blood and the eye, although the antemortem conditions led to the diagnosis of diphtheric conjunctivitis. [All of which goes to prove that we are yet far from possessing all the truth about membranous conjunctivitis.]

Chlorosis.—As a complication of chlorosis, Dieballo [3] mentions optic neuritis and aggravated headaches, suggesting brain-tumor. When treatment had restored the hemoglobin and corpuscular elements of the blood the optic neuritis faded away.

Typhoid.—Spontaneous orbital and intraocular hemorrhages, one of the rarest complications of typhoid fever, were seen by C. E. Finlay [4] in a 10-year-old boy, presenting also subcutaneous ecchymoses and epistaxis. Vision in both eyes was completely abolished, secondary metastatic choroiditis supervening in the left one.

Menstruation.—A young woman who applied to A. E. Davis [5] because of sudden blindness in her left eye was found to be the subject of vicarious hemorrhage from the choroidal vessels into that eye. Friedenwald [6] also speaks of cases of punctate keratitis, recurrent conjunctivitis, iritis, and hemorrhages into the vitreous that appeared during the menstrual periods only, although that function was normally performed.

Hysteria.—F. S. Millbury cured 3 cases of confirmed hysteric amblyopia by suggestion.

Puerperium.—Puerperal infection of both eyes was observed in 2 instances by Janerskierwicz.[8] The first woman became blind 10 days after parturition; in the other, aged 36, both eyes became swollen and blind a few weeks after her 7th normal pregnancy.

Epilepsy.—After correction of the refraction, a neurotic patient of Marlow's [9] gained 20 pounds, and at the end of 5 years continued free from an intense nervousness and occasional epilepsy that had baffled many physicians for some years prior to the correction of the refraction.

Whooping-cough and Tonsillitis.—G. Futterer [10] speaks of paresis of the muscles of both eyes associated with tonsillitis, and Craig [11] of palsy of the 6th and 7th nerves occurring during whooping-cough, probably induced by a small venous hemorrhage into the 4th ventricle.

Vaccination.—A. F. Rutherford [12] reports an instance of accidental vaccination of both eyelids and the conjunctiva of the left eye, in a 28-year-old woman who had inoculated herself from her child's arm.

The Eye as a Help in Diagnosis.—Ocular symptoms are often found

[1] New Orl. M. and S. Jour., July, 1897.　　　[2] Medicine, June, 1897.
[3] Deutsch. med. Woch., July 9, 1896.　　　[4] Arch. of Ophth., Jan., 1897.
[5] Manhattan Eye and Ear Hosp. Rep., 1897.
[6] Jour. of Eye, Ear, Throat, and Nose Dis., Oct., 1896.
[7] Med. Rec., Mar. 20, 1897.　　　[8] Centralbl. f. prakt. Augenh., No. 20, 1896.
[9] Med. News, July 4, 1897.　　　[10] Ann. Ophth and Otol., July, 1896.
[11] Brit. Med. Jour., June 13, 1897.　　　[12] Quart. Med. Jour., July, 1896.

helpful by H. Gradle [1] in establishing a diagnosis, for instance : edema of the lids suggests arsenic-poisoning or Bright's disease ; blood in the lids, scurvy ; pallid conjunctiva is associated with anemia ; a suspicion of accident, whooping-cough, or general vascular disease is aroused by hemorrhages under the conjunctiva ; deep infiltration of the cornea may mean inherited syphilis, while superficial streaks of opacity are sometimes found in malaria ; plastic iritis points to syphilis or rheumatism ; the Argyll-Robertson pupil is an early indication of tabes ; contracted pupil is associated with the acute stage of cerebrospinal diseases, and with opium- or chloroform-narcosis, while a dilated pupil may mean any one of several cerebrospinal affections, asphyxia, diphtherio paralysis of accommodation, intraocular hemorrhages, leukocythemia, hysteria, muscular paralyses, and cerebral syphilis.

Miscellaneous.—K. Goh [2] says that septic retinitis and metastatic chorioretinitis are not inflammatory processes in the sense that they are the only parts affected by the microorganisms, but that they are secondary to somatic changes in the blood which induce degeneration of the tunica intima, and thus predispose to hemorrhage.

C. S. Bull [3] refers to panophthalmitis and orbital cellulitis, with subsequent diaphragmatic abscess, the latter probably metastatic. Among miners Bourguet [4] found nystagmus, and choroidal and optic atrophy to be the prevailing ocular lesions, and attributes them principally to the poison-laden atmosphere, for in well-ventilated mines the men were found to be comparatively free from ocular lesions. A case of chloroma is fully described by S. C. Ayres and A. Alt.[5]

Cerebrospinal Diseases.—H. de Gouvea [6] reports a case of transitory blindness, followed by loss of the lower field of vision of one eye that continned four weeks, in an epileptic. The ophthalmoscope showed marked edema of the upper halves of the retinæ. The ocular manifestations of epilepsy, in the order of their frequency, are : affections (spasm) of the ciliary muscle, of the muscular tunics of the retinal arteries, and of the extrinsic muscles. As the literature of tumors of the pons increases, it is becoming evident that the ocular symptoms play no little part in making up the symptom-complex. Disturbances of function of the 3d, 4th, and 6th nerves seem to be the most frequent symptoms (Hoffman [7] and Bischoff[8]). To the above symptom-complex H. Upson [9] adds orbicular paralysis and bilateral optic neuritis. H. F. Hansell's [10] case illustrates how closely all the symptoms of brain-tumor may be simulated by cyst of the brain. The cyst involved the right frontal lobe, producing high-grade bilateral choked disk, concentric narrowing of the visual field terminating in blindness, and intense headaches, with general convulsions shortly before death. Syphilitic growths at the sphenoidal window involving the optic foramen also simulate brain-tumors ; e. g., Rochon-Duvignead [11] reports several such cases, with a characteristic array of ocular palsies and amblyopia, always of grave prognosis. Some cases recover under mixed treatment. The symptoms referable to tumor of the pituitary body noted by Stirling [12] were bilateral optic atrophy, giddiness, iris-paralysis, frequent flushings and perspiration of the head and neck, sleepiness, increase of body-fat, and photopsiæ. In 2 cases of polyencephalitis

[1] Medicine, Mar., 1897.
[3] Ann. Ophth. and Otol., July, 1896.
[5] Am. Jour. Ophth., xiv., No. 3.
[7] Virchow's Archiv, vol. cxxxxvii., 1896.
[9] Ann. of Ophth., Jan., 1897.
[11] Arch. d'Ophtal., Dec., 1896.

[2] Arch. f. Ophth., Feb., 1897.
[4] Gaz. des Hôpitaux, Nos. 139 and 140.
[6] Ann. d'Oculist., Aug., 1897.
[8] Jahrb. f. Psych. u. Neurol., Bd. xv., 1896.
[10] Ann. Ophth. and Otol., Oct., 1896.
[12] Ann. of Ophth., Jan., 1897.

superior acuta[1] the main symptoms were extra- and intraocular palsies. G. Hinsdale,[2] in his monograph on syringomyelia, classifies the ocular symptoms of this recently much-studied disorder into symptoms referable to the pupil, the oculomuscular apparatus, the fundus, and the visual field. Franke[3] saw akromegaly unfold its features in a 31-year-old woman previously healthy, producing in time typical bilateral temporal hemianopsia. There was some improvement in her condition following the use of powdered extract of hypophysis taken from an ox. There is much added to the knowledge of this subject by Streminski's[4] study.

J. Soury[5] investigates comprehensively the relations of the retina, the optic path, and the occipital lobe to the completed visual act, and confirms Munk in his view that the region of the calcarine fissure is especially concerned in central visual acuity. A 74-year-old patient of B. Schirmer's[6] experienced fiery photopsiæ at the time of rupture of the deep cerebral artery into the occipital lobes in the region of both calcarine fissures. Schirmer claims that this is the first instance of well-proved subjective sensation excited by the pressure-stimulus communicated to the occipital cortex. A wonderfully interesting instance of word-blindness is recorded by W. P. Morgan,[7] occurring in a bright, well-grown 14-year-old son of intelligent parents. The only words he read at all were "the," "and," "that," "of," while other words meant absolutely nothing to him. He conversed well, read figures quickly and correctly, and was fond of arithmetic and algebra. The case is unique in that it was congenital and secondary to some lack of development in the region of the left angular gyrus. J. M. Rattray,[8] alludes to an instance of word-blindness accompanying degeneration of the cerebral blood-vessels in a 75-year-old man who had been a teacher of no little ability up to within a few months of his illness. P. Steffan[9] says sensory anopsia (soul-blindness) may be subcortical, cortical, or transcortical, in which latter case the association-fibres are involved. Sensory anopsia may be either physiologic or pathologic, and mixed forms may also appear. According to F. Peterson,[10] between 7% and 8% of idiots are congenitally blind. Many present certain visual and ocular defects, such as hyperopia, defective color-sense, strabismus, nystagmus, congenital cataract, inequality of the pupils, and microphthalmos, and good binocular vision is uncommon. He states that the normal child takes pleasure in the sight of objects as early as the 11th day; the eyes are coordinated by the end of the second month, and he begins to distinguish colors correctly about the age of 2 years. In a child 12 years old there appeared myosis, retraction of the globe, narrowing of the palpebral fissure, and paralysis of the vasa motores of the same side secondary to caries of the first dorsal vertebra, which Cousoy[11] adduces as additional evidence that nerve-filaments to the iris proceed from the ciliospinal center in the cord between the 7th cervical and 1st dorsal. The most frequent eye-symptom in Friedreich's ataxia is nystagmus of the ataxie variety, says C. W. Burr.[12] Marked optic atrophy never occurs, while strabismus, diplopia, and ptosis are met with as complications rather than a part of the disease. To the eye-symptoms of a kindred disease to the foregoing (multiple sclerosis), C. Kunn[13]

[1] Neurol. Centralbl., Feb. 1, 1897.
[2] Syringomyelia, International Medical Magazine Co., 1897.
[3] Klin. Monatslbl. f. Augenh., Aug., 1897.   [4] Arch. d'Ophtal., Feb., 1897.
[5] Rev. Philosophique, Feb. and Mar., 1896.   [6] Klin. Monatsbl. f. Augenh., Sept., 1896.
[7] Brit. Med. Jour., Nov. 7, 1896.   [8] Ibid., Dec. 5, 1896.
[9] Arch. f. Ophthal., May, 1897.   [10] Am. Jour. Insan., July, 1896.
[11] Sem. méd., No. 63, 1897.   [12] Ann. of Ophth., Jan., 1897.
[13] Beitr. z. Augenh., July, 1896.

adds 3 that he claims are new, namely—nystagmus when a near object is fixed upon, dissociation of the normal ocular movements (developed strabismus), and a sort of nystagmus of the ciliary muscle evidenced by rapid variation in the accommodation.

CONGENITAL AFFECTIONS.

Of the Cornea.—Congenital opacities of the cornea in an infant the subject of purulent conjunctivitis were observed by Barbacheff.[1] Their origin has been demonstrated by Kölliker to be a retardation or cessation in the process of the mesoderm that differentiates the cornea from the sclera. In W. Reber's ease[2] the opacity was central, 5x5½ mm., and unilateral, and within 2 years shrank fully 2 mm. without treatment. He does not commit himself either to the inflammatory or the arrest-of-development theory, but says that "when embryologists tell us whether the cornea clears from periphery to center, or from center to periphery, we will have taken a long step toward a better understanding of the etiology of this affection." Peltesohn[3] describes a defect in the stroma of the anterior layer of the iris, situated in the outer lower quadrant, that at first produced the impression of an iridodialysis. Patient was a 52-year-old laborer.

Of the Anterior Chamber.—Hartridge[4] speaks of an instance of a cyst moving freely in the anterior chamber both in a mother and her son. It was dark in color and about the size of a large shot.

Of the Vitreous.—J. A. White[5] refers to bilateral persistent hyaloid artery, which he discovered in a highly myopic woman whose refraction he was estimating.

Of the Choroid.—Dunn[6] says that in coloboma of the choroid the scotoma is not necessarily the size of the coloboma, and indeed it may be absent. Its presence and size depend upon the amount of damage done to the overlying retinal tissue by the processes, whatever they may be, that determine the choroidal coloboma.

In treating of the pathology of this affection Ginsberg[7] says it has no relation to the ocular fissure, and that it is probably due to some disturbance in the mesodermic layer.

Of the Optic Nerve.—Fournier and Sauvineau[8] attribute the cause of congenital optic-nerve atrophy, absorption of choroidal and degeneration of retinal pigment, paralysis of external rectus, and immobile pupil coexisting in the left eye, while the right eye was normal, to inherited syphilis, in spite of a nonsyphilitic history. Two cases of coloboma of the optic nerve and one of medullated nerve-fibers associated with myopia are reported by Moll.[9]

Anophthalmos.—Complete anophthalmos in a 7-year-old Chinese girl was observed by L. Steiner.[10]

DISEASES OF THE LIDS.

Association-movements.—[Association of lid-movements with jaw-movements is not uncommon, but association of movements of the upper lid with the movements of the external ocular muscles other than the superior

[1] La Clin. ophtal., Oct., 1896.
[2] Ophth. Rec., July, 1897.
[3] Centralbl. f. prakt. Augenh., Apr., 1897.
[4] Lancet, Sept. 22, 1896.
[5] Ann. Ophth. and Otol., July, 1896.
[6] Va. Med. Semi-monthly, June 12, 1896.
[7] Centralbl. f. prakt. Augenh., Sept., 1896.
[8] Rec. d'Ophtal., Jan., 1897.
[9] Centralbl. f. prakt. Augenh., Nov., 1896.
[10] Ibid., Sept. 26, 1896.

rectus is rare.]   J. Brixa[1] details fully 2 such cases in which, in addition to
Graefe's sign, there was elevation of the upper lid associated with action on
the part of the internal recti, while any attempt at abduction brought the upper
lid down quickly. H. Friedenwald[2] saw 2 cases of this kind, one peculiar
by its late appearance (at the 14th year), the other unique in showing association of the levator with the pterygoid of the opposite side.

Itching of the lids, as a result of nasal stenosis, and cured by opening of
the nasal passages, is recorded by Prince.[3]

Molluscum Contagiosum.—The 3 cases detailed by H. Muetze[4] indicate that molluscum of the lids or lid-margins is frequently the cause of conjunctival catarrh, and that it is undoubtedly contagious.

Tuberculosis.—Bacteriologic examination was required to determine to
Armignac's[5] satisfaction the tuberculous nature of a lid-affection that was followed some weeks later by involvement of the larynx and lungs, leading to
death.

Vaccine-pustule.—J. H. Egbert[6] tells of a 11-year-old girl who, while
sleeping with her sister, who had been recently vaccinated on the arm, acquired
a vaccine-pustule on her eyelid.

S. Reiner[7] puts on record the 17th case of syphilitic tarsitis in medical
literature, classic in all its features except that the conjunctiva bulbi was
rather extensively involved. Gallaemarts[8] considers extragenital chancre
not more predisposed to produce constitutional syphilis than chancre on the
genitals. He reports an instance of lid-chancre caused by the application o
the tongue of a syphilitic. Chancre of unknown origin, found on the eyelid
of a 5-year-old negro boy is recorded by J. H. Egbert.[9]

Ptosis.—Ed. Pergens[10] refers recurrent unilateral ptosis, after operation
for its relief, to astigmatism, because the patient is inclined to close partially
the palpebral fissure in his efforts to see. Advancement of the levator palpe-
bra superior for traumatic ptosis occurring in a child was done by C. A.
Oliver[11] with marked success. In view of the failure of many operations
practised for the cure of ptosis, Motais[12] proposes to remove a tongue of muscle
and tendon, 3 mm. wide and 10 mm. long, from the middle of the superior
rectus and suture this into the cartilage of the lid. Parinaud[13] suggests suturing the entire superior rectus to the lid by passing the thread under the muscle
through the adjoining conjunctiva into the posterior extremity of the lid,
bringing the two ends of the suture out from the lid at its ciliary margin and
tying them. Both writers claim good results and no interference with the movements of the ball. Harold Wilson[14] prefers pedicellate flaps for the repair of
lid-malposition, except in those cases in which the cicatrix, involving not only
the lids but also the surrounding parts, has not the necessary qualities for
plastic purposes. In this class of cases Thiersch's method promises the best
results.

C. H. Beard claims that the chief ends to be gained in operations for
ectropion and trichiasis following conjunctival cicatrization are to replace the
atrophied tissues and to relieve the lid-tension. For the first he transplants
mucous membrane from the mouth, and for the second he does a free cantho-

[1] Beitr. z. Augenh., Apr., 1897.   [2] Johns Hopkins Hosp. Bull., July, 1896.
[3] Eye, Ear, Nose, and Throat Clinic, Apr., 1897.   [4] Arch. of Ophth., Jan., 1897.
[5] Rec. d'Ophtal., June, 1897.   [6] Phila. Polyclinic, Mar. 13, 1897.
[7] Beitr. z. Augenh., July, 1896.   [8] Rec. d'Ophtal., Aug., 1896.
[9] Phila. Polyclinic, Mar. 13, 1897.   [10] Rec. d'Ophtal., May, 1897.
[11] Ann. of Ophth., Apr., 1897.   [12] Ann d' Oculist., July, 1997.
[13] Ibid.   [14] Arch. of Ophth., Jan., 1897.

plasty, including a division of the external canthal ligament. F. C. Hotz[1] splits the margin of the lid back of the hair-bulbs in correcting the deformities after trachoma, and speaks highly of the efficiency of Thiersch's skin-transplantations in repairing the disfigurements of ectropion. Argyll-Robertson[2] employs the device of cutting out of a piece of paper an exact pattern of the surface that has been bared and placing this pattern upon the skin at the part whence the graft is to be taken, allowing about a fifth or sixth of the width of the flap all around the pattern for shrinkage. He also employs what he terms the "tether"-stitch to keep the transplanted flap in position (Fig. 61).

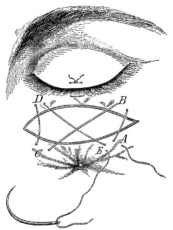

FIG. 61.—Argyll-Robertson's "tether"-stitch for holding the skin-graft in position by lacing the thread over it (Practitioner, Aug., 1896).

Tumors.—An unusual form of growth proceeding from the inner canthal portion of the lower lid is reported by A. A. Hubbell.[3] The tumor, globular in form and about 1 in. in diameter, was successfully removed. A young Egyptian woman, under the observation of Kenneth Scott,[4] submitted to operation for a tumor of the upper lid that displaced the globe 24 mm. downward. Microscopic examination of the tumor revealed small-celled sarcoma, although 10 months after operation there was no indication of recurrence. Trousseau[5] finds that epithelioma of the lids and conjunctiva, after removal, is less frequent and longer in recurring than epithelioma in other parts of the body, and Fage[6] states that sarcoma of the lids, having its origin in the conjunctiva or neighboring parts, is frequently observed, but that only 7 or 8 authentic cases of true primary sarcoma of the lids have been reported.

DISEASES OF THE CONJUNCTIVA.

Bacteriology of the Normal Conjunctiva.—R. Randolph's bacteriologic investigations of 100 perfectly healthy eyes[7] demonstrate that the normal conjunctiva always contains bacteria, among which the staphylococcus epidermis albus is found with such frequency that it must be regarded as a regular inhabitant of the conjunctival cul-de-sac. This coccus, though but slightly pathogenic ordinarily, may under certain conditions become harmful. Neither irrigation with distilled water nor instillation of a 1 : 5000 solution produces sterility of the conjunctiva, all of which facts induce Randolph to conclude that in operating upon the normal conjunctiva or cornea, as in cataract-operations, the surgeon would do well, in the present state of our knowledge, to direct his asepsis and antisepsis chiefly, if not solely, to the hands, instruments, cocain, and atropin. Our knowledge of the microorganisms of the normal and abnormal conjunctiva and lacrimal sac is also much enriched

[1] Ann. Ophth. and Otol., July, 1896. [2] Practitioner, Aug., 1896.
[3] Ann. Ophth. and Otol., Oct., 1896. [4] Ann. of Ophth., July, 1897.
[5] Arch. d'Ophtal., Oct., 1896. [6] Rec. d'Ophtal., Dec., 1896.
[7] Arch. of Ophth., July, 1897.

by the contribution of J. McFarland and S. S. Kneass.[1] The form of muco-purulent conjunctivitis, described by Morax [2] and T. Axenfeld,[3] is another addition to the comparatively small list of microbic eye-diseases in which there seems little doubt that the microorganism has been identified.

Epidemic Conjunctivitis.—S. Stephenson [4] believes, with Morax, Weeks, and Beech, in a specific microorganism which is accountable for epidemic acute catarrhal conjunctivitis, and he considers the diagnosis in such cases incomplete without a microscopic examination of the secretion. The bacilli are to be found at some stage in every instance of the disorder, and their numbers stand in direct relation to the severity of the inflammation. They are readily killed by antiseptics or by drying. 2% silver solution is his main reliance in the treatment of this affection. He further details [5] the incidents of an epidemic of catarrhal ophthalmia affecting 23 out of 25 male infants in one of the wards of the London Central District School, although, by rigorous prophylaxis and quarantine, the epidemic was confined to this one ward. All the affected cases made a good recovery. In an epidemic of acute conjunctivitis that swept through 2 schools near Karlsruhe Gelpke [6] saw 22% of the children fall victims to it, although within 8 weeks all had recovered. Fränkel's pneumococcus is held responsible by H. Clifford [7] for most cases of catarrhal conjunctivitis. To all these contagion-theories of catarrhal ophthalmia A. H. Jacob [8] demurs, holding overcrowding, dark and ill-ventilated rooms, damp soil, and insufficient diet accountable for the affection. He bases his contention on many years' experience with the disorder among the paupers of Ireland.

Purulent Conjunctivitis.—L. Howe [9] draws a striking picture of the results that would follow compulsory observation of Credé's method in the prophylaxis of conjunctivitis of the newborn. He says there is a direct proportion between case of transportation and a low rate of blindness, while a higher ratio is to be expected where travel is poor and inconvenient. He pleads for renewed activity in promoting legal measures looking to the prevention of ophthalmia neonatorum, in which plea he is joined by Zimmerman [10] and Ferguson.[11]

The latter writer urges the Canadian government to pass laws regulating its treatment, as has been done in many of the United States, mainly through the instrumentality of Howe, of Buffalo. Kuies [12] holds that subsequent infection is as often responsible for purulent conjunctivitis as immediate infection occurring during delivery, while A. E. Adams [13] condemns the obstetrician who neglects to adopt Credé's method when there is the least suspicion that the conjunctiva may be infected. Walter, on the other hand, lays stress [14] on attention to general nutrition and the necessity of promoting active circulation in the subjects of this condition. K. Hoor [15] does not favor Kalt's irrigation-method for purulent conjunctivitis, although he himself has employed a somewhat similar method for 12 years. He objects to Kalt's tube or any other hard instrument that may abrade the cornea. In pediatrics A. Pukalow [16] is

[1] System of Diseases of the Eye, Norris and Oliver, vol. ii., 1897.
[2] Ann. d'Inst. Pasteur, June, 1896.
[3] Centralbl. f. Bakteriol., Parasitenk. u. Infektionskrank., No. 1, 1897.
[4] Lancet, June 5, 1897.　　　　　[5] Brit. Med. Jour., July 11, 1896.
[6] Twenty-fifth Ophthal. Congress, Heidelberg, 1896.　　[7] Arch. of Ophth., No. 3, 1896.
[8] Lancet, June 5, 1897.　　　　　[9] N. Y. Med. Jour., June 26, 1897.
[10] Medicine, Oct., 1896.　　　　　[11] Am. Medico-Surg. Bull., Sept. 26, 1896.
[12] Samml. zwangloser Abhandl. a. d. geb. d. Augenh., 1896.
[13] N. Y. Med. Jour., Apr. 3, 1897.　　　　[14] Ibid., June 16, 1897.
[15] Centralbl. f. prakt. Augenh., Aug., 1896.　　[16] Dietskaj. Medicin., p. 184, 1897.

credited with having made use of calomel in 57 cases of purulent conjunctivitis, with results superior to those secured from any other remedy.

Gonorrheal Conjunctivitis.—Chartres[1] asserts that the serious ophthalmias are those produced by streptococci or by an association of streptococci and gonococci, or by the combination of these 2 with others. The gonococci when alone are comparatively harmless [?] and yield to treatment, which should be prompt and vigorous, consisting of copious irrigations with potassium permanganate, boric acid, and cauterization with silver nitrate. This combination acts on all the various species of microbes which may be producing the ophthalmia. He concludes by insisting on the necessity of bacteriologic investigation. Hansell[2] has seen gonorrheal conjunctivitis secondary to a gonorrhea induced by intercourse during menstruation. Formalin has proved effective in his hands in this affection. Aqueous extract of suprarenal capsule produces great bleaching of the conjunctiva, but after the astringent action has passed away the inflammation returns in greater force than before. Hansell favors exclusion of the sound eye, providing that the dressing is changed and the eye sealed often enough. [In a case of postoperative congestion of the anterior ocular segment, occurring in our own experience, the extract of suprarenal capsules induced marked ischemia of the eye in 10 minutes, but the patient returned the following day suffering excruciating pain from the terrific engorgement of the anterior ocular circulation. It will require some study to determine just what may be the most effective sphere of action of the aqueous extract of suprarenal capsules.] In the gonorrheal conjunctivitis of adults, Knies[3] uses fluorescin to map out for cauterization any denuded or desquamating corneal areas. Wandless,[4] from an experience of 1 case, advocates the application of 8 % silver solution in gonorrhea of the conjunctiva.

Phlyctenular Conjunctivitis.—The treatment of phlyctenular conjunctivitis by subconjunctival injections of sublimate 1 : 3000, advocated by Evans,[5] is mentioned only that it may be condemned. [The well-known simple and effective remedies, attention to the nares and intestinal tract, and alteratives are greatly to be preferred.]

Membranous Conjunctivitis.—Until the etiologic classification of the different forms of conjunctivitis assumes more definite outlines, H. Coppez,[6] prefers to retain the old anatomic classification, though he looks forward to the day when treatment will have reference to etiology rather than to symptoms only. A. Pilcher is convinced that the Löffler bacillus bears a causative relation to ordinary membranous conjunctivitis, and argues for the retention of the generic term "membranous conjunctivitis" for all of the varieties until the etiology of the different forms can be sharply defined. Ewetzky[7] and H. Woods[8] associate themselves with the above views, while C. H. Sproneck[9] contends that Behring's serum can be used to differentiate between nonmalignant and true diphtheria of the conjunctiva. In a false membrane removed from the neighborhood of the caruncle in a case of membranous conjunctivitis J. Ehre[10] found numerous bacilli of Friedländer. Cultures were injected into the tail of a mouse, and 48 hours later the heart-blood of the mouse was filled with encapsulated Friedländer bacilli.

Granular Conjunctivitis.—In granular conjunctivitis, Kalt[11] recom-

[1] Arch. Clin. de Bordeaux, Dec., 1896.   [2] Editorial, Phila. Polyclinic, 1897.
[3] Samml. zwangloser. Abhandl. a. d. geb. d. Augenh., 1896.
[4] Jour. Am. Med. Assoc., Jan. 23, 1897.   [5] Med. News, Nov. 7, 1896.
[6] Centralbl. f. prakt. Augenh. Apr., 1897.   [7] Berlin. klin. Woch., Aug. 3, 1896.
[8] Ann. of Ophth., Jan., 1897.   [9] Deut. med. Woch., No. 36, 1896.
[10] Lancet, Mar. 20, 1897.   [11] Arch. d'Ophtal., Aug., 1896.

mends free application of 1 : 5000 to 1 : 300 potassium permanganate in addition to the usual remedies, and Dubat[1] speaks well of the effect of raw petroleum applied twice daily with a brush.

Vernal Catarrh.—Darier[2] differentiates graphically between trachoma and the palpebral form of vernal catarrh. Trachoma attacks by preference the fornix of the conjunctiva, while vernal catarrh limits its invasion to the tarsal portion of that membrane ; again, the semicartilaginous character of the papillæ in spring catarrh is almost pathognomonic. For the latter condition, Wechsler[3] finds antipyrin and sulfate of quinin quite effective. In some cases the disposition is to become chronic, in which case the disease persists without regard to season. Infectious conjunctivitis originating in animals is characterized by two main symptoms,[4] distinct voluminous granulations resembling trachoma-cells and a subacute adenitis attacking the preauricular and cervical glands. The affection is benign and usually monocular. It has also been studied by Despagnet[5] among workmen in slaughter-houses, and the main symptoms put down by him as glandular swelling of the conjunctiva with pus containing granulations on the lid. M. Villard,[6] during his studies of the normal conjunctiva of rabbits, found granulations much resembling trachoma in man, and he demonstrated lymphatic vessels directly connected with the granulations. The verification of these findings is important, as it brings into close relation the granulations and the lymphatic glandular tissues. Villard infers by analogy that the same condition exists in man.

Trachoma.—According to T. Federow,[7] there is no anatomic identity between trachoma foci and granules of the conjunctiva. The greatest evils following in the wake of trachoma, says M. Kirsch,[8] are the limitation to education, susceptibility to inheritance, influence upon the capability of armies, the latter in itself a calamity to the home and a danger to the monarchy. J. W. Heustis[9] points out the danger that lurks in the slightest corneal abrasion when complicated with granular lids. The dissemination of trachoma can be diminished, it is claimed by Probsting,[10] by state supervision of school hygiene. Chibret,[11] reporting on the geographic distribution of trachoma, says : " In Cuba the three great branches of the human family are represented by the negroes, the whites, and the Chinese. The Chinese are affected twice as often as the whites and 8 times as often as the negroes. Santos Fernandez (quoted by Chibret) found 16 cases of trachoma among the negroes to 67 among the whites and 111 among the Chinese. The freedom from trachoma of the eye of the negro is shown by J. M. Ray.[12] Chibret further states that occupation plays an insignificant part in immunity from trachoma, while hygienic conditions are of great importance Lymphatic temperament and malarial infection favor its inroads. Irritation from dust is considered by S. M. Burnett[13] an important causative factor in trachoma, especially in those predisposed to conjunctival irritation. An altitude of 3000 meters furnishes the ideal climate. It is in part due to this latter advantage that Ole Bull[14] ascribes the immunity of the Norwegians from trachoma. G. Hirsch,[15] however, opposes Bull's view that trachoma is largely a matter of race, disposition, and approach

[1] Münch. med. Woch., Dec. 29, 1896.   [2] Ann. of Ophth., July, 1897.
[3] Beitr. z. Angenh., Apr., 1897.   [4] J. Dominique, Rec. d'Ophtal., May, 1897.
[5] Bull. Med , No. 89 ; Med. News, May 29. 1897.   [6] Thése de Montpelier, 1896.
[7] Zur Anatomie d. follikularentzundung d. Bindehaut in Zuzammenhang mit ihrem physiologischen Bau, Moscow, 1896.
[8] Berlin. klin. Woch., Mar. 1-8, 1897.   [9] Ophth. Rec., Aug., 1897.
[10] Centralbl. ; Ann. Ophth. and Otol., July, 1896   [11] Méd. mod., May 16, 1896.
[12] N. Y. Med. Jour., July 18, 1896.   [13] Am. Jour. Ophth., July, 1897.
[14] Centralbl. f. prakt. Augenh., Nov., 1896.   [15] Arch. f. Ophth., May, 1897.

to the sea-level, claiming that trachoma has been brought into his district (eastern Germany) by miners and artisans, who poured into the region spreading trachoma through the province notwithstanding that the altitude was fair and trachoma had been previously quite rare in that locality. D. Reynolds[1] is satisfied that trachoma is, *per se*, the local manifestation of a constitutional infection just as urgently demanding mercury and quinin as though it were some other form of that miasmatic infection which begets remittent and intermittent fevers. [The facts do not lend probability to this theory.]

E. Nesnamoff[2] finds unusually rapid good results wait on the treatment of trachoma with the following: pure iodin, 1 to 2 pts.; liquid white vaselin, 100 pts.; sulphuric ether q. s. to make thorough solution. To be applied once daily, taking care to protect the cornea from contact with the solution. Burchardt's[3] treatment consists in touching all the granules (even to 400) with the point of a narrow galvanocautery. In the intervals between the cauterizations he uses tannate of quinin, which has proved quite effective. Unusual results in the handling of trachoma are spoken of by T. Proskauer[4] from the application of a 1% solution of formalin, which must necessarily be preceded by 8% cocain solution. If the application is quickly and lightly made, there will be little or no reaction. The large gray granules will be the first to disappear, then the follicles, while the smaller whitish follicular bodies will often resist treatment for a long time. J. S. Fernandez[5] claims the credit of introducing jequirity in the treatment of trachoma. For small discrete trachomatous granules R. H. Elliott[6] prefers the actual cautery, because of its painlessness, even in children. For trachoma with pannus, Trousseau[7] considers iodized glycerin (equal parts of glycerin and tinct. iodin) the best treatment. J. W. Bullard, on the other hand, relies on silver and copper; surgery is his last resort. J. H. Claiborne[8] discountenances the continued use of atropin in granular conjunctivitis, as it may cause the formation of granulations, which cannot be distinguished from true trachoma.

H. Armaignac[9] reports a case of undoubted primitive tuberculosis of the palpebral conjunctiva, verified by the finding of a few Koch's bacilli. The eye in other respects remained uninvolved. The palpebral ulceration was treated and cured by frequent application of silver nitrate, bathing with saturated solution of potassium chlorate, and curettage. The patient died, 2 years later, from laryngeal and pulmonary phthisis. E. Valude[10] describes another case similar in all respects to that of de Wecker.

Syphilis.—Another instance of primary lesion occurring on the conjunctiva is reported by R. Hitchman.[11]

Urticaria.—Urticaria of the conjunctiva following the ingestion of veal and strawberries is noted by S. M. Stocker.[12] The analogy between the conjunctival condition and the cutaneous lesion which coexisted was complete.

Ophthalmia Nodosa.—G. Knapp[13] believes that many cases of so-called ophthalmia nodosa, in which the history is vague and uncertain, are caused by the confinement in the conjunctiva of caterpillar hairs that have escaped casual examination, and can be found only by the use of a strong magnifying lens.

Phlebolith.—A perfectly smooth oval body, 4 by 6 mm., which S. Bur-

[1] Jour. Am. Med. Assoc., Dec. 19, 1896. [2] Centralbl. f. prakt. Augenh., Aug., 1897.
[3] Centralbl. f. prakt. Augenh., Feb., 1897. [4] Ibid., May, 1897.
[5] Cronica Medici de Habana, Dec., 1896. [6] Indian Med. Gazette, Jan., 1897.
[7] Ann. d'Oculist., June, 1896. [8] N. Y. Polyclinic, Jan. 15, 1897.
[9] Ann. d'Oculist., Aug., 1897. [10] Ann. d'Oculist., Aug., 1897.
[11] Wien. klin. Woch., Dec. 24, 1896. [12] Ann. Ophth. and Otol., July, 1896.
[13] Am. Jour. Ophth., Aug., 1897.

ιett[1] removed from one of the conjunctival veins of a 30-year-old woman proved to be a, typical phlebolith.

Pterygium and Plastic Operations.—In 3 different instances C. H. Baker[2] repaired large denudations of the bulbar conjunctiva with Thiersch's skin-grafts, with the most gratifying results. K. Hoor[3] employed with equally good results the membrana testæ from boiled eggs in restoring 2 conjunctivæ buttonholed during the operation for symblepharon. In dealing with large pterygia, F. C. Hotz[4] dissects the growth, allows it to retract toward the inner canthus, and then places parallel with the cornea a narrow Thiersch skin-graft, about 2 by 10 mm., which, when it becomes attached, forms a smooth white barrier, over which the pterygium never advances. Trousseau[5] removes the head of the pterygium, and cauterizes the union of the head and body a little behind the limbus.

Tumors.—True papilloma of the conjunctiva occurring in a 47-year-old healthy man came under O. Stuelp's[6] observation. The microscope fixed the diagnosis. S. Bomboletti[7] refers serous cysts of the conjunctiva to an enlargement of an emissary duct of one of Krause's glands of the lower fornix of the conjunctiva. Injury may originate the condition.

An unusual sequel to exenteration is mentioned by W. A. Wagemann,[8] who saw carcinoma develop in the conjunctival cicatrix left by the operation. The patient was 70 years old. Small-celled sarcoma of the upper lid, probably the result of inoculation during an operation for removal of a melanosarcoma at the limbus, is reported by A. Szulislawski.[9] The patient was a 55-year-old farmer.

AFFECTIONS OF THE LACRIMAL APPARATUS.

Physiology.—The part that the facial nerve plays in lacrimal secretion is well shown by Tribondeau's experiment on a dog[10] that developed a perfectly dry eye 3 weeks after deep section of the facial nerve, thus confirming Goldschneider's and refuting Tepliaschin's theory.

Congenital Anomalies.—In a patient showing double harelip and coloboma of both eyelids van Duyse and Rutten[11] traced the tear-duct from the coloboma of the lower lid all the way down to the left half of the upper lip. J. H. Eyre[12] observed a case of congenital supernumerary caruncle in a 38-year-old man that was strikingly similar to the one described by Stephenson last year (see *Year-Book*, 1897).

Sarcoma.—C. A. Veasey[13] and S. Snell[14] add two more to the few reported cases of sarcoma of the lacrimal carunele. Both were nonpigmented and contained large and small round cells.

Inflammation.—R. Randolph[15] has met with an instance of bilateral nonsuppurative inflammation of the lacrimal gland, the so-called "mumps of the lacrimal gland."

Obliteration of the Duct.—For impassable bony stricture Scott[16] passes an ordinary small pointed drill attached to a dental machine along the pre-

[1] Arch. of Ophth., Jan., 1897.
[2] Ann. Ophth. and Otol., July, 1896.
[3] Wien. klin. Woch., Aug. 15, 1896.
[4] Ann. of Ophth., Jan., 1897.
[5] Ann. d'Oculist., June, 1896.
[6] Centralbl. f. prakt. Augenh., Feb., 1897.
[7] Arch. of Ophth., July, 1897.
[8] Klin. Monatsbl. f. Augenh., Aug., 1896.
[9] Centralbl. f. prakt. Augenh., Oct., 1896.
[10] Jour de Méd. de Bordeaux, No. 44, 1895; Centralbl. f. prakt. Augenh., Mar., 1897.
[11] Centralbl. f. prakt. Augenh., Apr., 1897.
[12] Arch. of Ophth., July, 1897.
[13] Ibid., Apr., 1897.
[14] Ibid., July, 1897.
[15] Ibid., Jan., 1897.
[16] Ann. of Ophth., July, 1897.

viously slit lower canaliculus, directing it exactly in the way in which a lacrimal probe is introduced, tilting it and then drilling through the bony tissue into the unobstructed portion of the duct. Three other burrs, respectively 2, 3 and 4.5 mm. in diameter, are made to pass through the opening, and the advantage thus gained is maintained by the introduction of a leaden style. He claims uniformly good results from this method. R. S. Miller[1] finds styles much the most satisfactory way of treating lacrimal obstructions, especially those following abscess.

Anesthesia.—A. E. Davis[2] has used hypnotism in a number of cases to pass lacrimal probes, and even for slitting up the canaliculus without pain. Its quieting influence was a source of much comfort to nervous patients, for by suggestion alone he prevented these patients from worrying about their eyes and from dreading the next visit, with its attendant pain. [It is a matter of surprise that hypnotism, highly extolled by some writers as the most desirable means of preventing pain, has not had more general application.]

AFFECTIONS OF THE CORNEA.

Ulceration.—Evidence collected by J. E. Weeks[3] is sufficient to establish the fact that the pneumococcus of Friedländer is capable of producing grave ulcerative conditions in the eye, and that the pneumococcus of Fränkel has been observed as the pathogenic microorganism in case of tenonitis, panophthalmitis, hypopion keratitis, conjunctivitis, and probably in some cases of dacryocystitis. Nuel[4] says that punctate keratitis and analogous forms that are characterized by the presence of spiral microbes, of which he found many in a case studied, are diseases of special microbes that are absolutely typical. Antonelli and Giglio[5] have shown that many of the asthenic ulcers are really tuberculous lesions. Cultures of the detritus from the floor of the ulcer should be made in every instance to determine its character.

Burnett,[6] de Schweinitz,[7] and O. Belt[8] endorse formol as an efficient remedy in 1% solution in arresting ulceration and in lessening opacities. C. Mayet[9] has tried with success, in chronic indolent ulcers that refused to be cured by other means, transplantation of a flap of conjunctiva to the ulcer. H. Sureau[10] substitutes for hot compresses and hot bathing (universally recommended and of the greatest service in relieving pain and stimulating healing) "cataplasms of linseed meal" [a dangerous substitution.] W. Bruner[11] recommends the actual cautery when simpler methods have been tried unsuccessfully or "occasionally in severe cases in which it is evident from the first that something radical will be necessary." The remedies found most useful by Kalt[12] are the galvanocautery, tinct. iodin, iodin-glycerol, phenique and methylblue, preferably the first named. The proneness of the eye of the negro to diseases of the cornea and uveal tract is pointed out by J. M. Ray.[13]

Interstitial Keratitis.—The **causes** mentioned by different writers are: hemorrhagic urticaria, E. Stern;[14] the menstrual epoch, König and Meyer;[15] in the order of their frequency, hereditary syphilis, tuberculosis, acquired syphilis, influenza, malaria, rheumatism, R. Greef,[16] and

[1] Brit. Med. Jour, Mar. 13, 1897.
[3] Ophth. Rec., June, 1897.
[5] Rec. d'Ophtal., Jan., 1896,
[7] Phila. Polyclinic, Aug. 21, 1897.
[9] Rec. d'Ophtal., July, 1897.
[11] Med. Rec., Feb. 27, 1897.
[13] N. Y. Med. Jour., July 18, 1896.
[15] Rec. d'Ophtal., June, 1897.

[2] Post-Graduate, Nov., 1896.
[4] Arch. d'Ophtal., Dec, 1896
[6] Therap. Gaz., Nov. 16, 1896.
[8] Med. News, Sept. 5, 1897.
[10] Ibid.
[12] Traité de Thérapeut. A. Robin, Paris, 1897.
[14] Klin. Monatsbl. f. Augenh., Jan., 1897.
[16] Ophth. Rev., June, 1897.

Achenbach;[1] beginning phthisis, O. Schirmer.[2] E. Valude[3] says that the interstitial keratitis of syphilis is characterized by its unilateral character, slight tendency to vascularization, and beneficent results of treatment. The prognosis is more favorable than in the hereditary form. C. D. Marshall[4] differentiates the two forms thus: the anterior part of the eye is most commonly affected in tertiary or congenital, while the choroid is peculiarly susceptible to inflammation during the course of acquired syphilis. K. Moulton[5] observed in a man, 67 years old, a true nonsyphilitic **annular interstitial keratitis** that surrounded the central two-thirds of the cornea; recovery ensued. W. Reber[6] and H. Moulton[7] report cases of **congenital corneal clouding,** in neither of which were there any signs of inflammatory or syphilitic origin. Reber inclines to the arrested-development theory as a cause for the phenomenon.

Treatment.—Greef's theory[8] of this disorder is German in its adherence to inunction as the elect method in specific cases. This, in connection with a "sweat cure," accomplished by the liberal use internally of sodium salicylate, has proved highly efficient in his hands. He utterly discountenances the subconjunctival injections of "homeopathic" amounts of mercury to hasten the absorption of post-inflammatory cloudings of the cornea. During the recent epidemic of small-pox in Havana C. E. Finlay[9] saw 24 cases of **variolous pustule of the cornea,** although for some unknown reason the lesions appear at a later period than in other tissues. A translucent facet, eccentrically situated, slow in progress, and interminable in healing, developed in the third week. Treatment has little or no influence on the duration of the affection.

The Electric Light.—J. Ogneff,[10] after exposing the eyes of rabbits, frogs, and pigeons to a powerful arc light, found that the cornea and conjunctiva were the parts to suffer most, while the retina (contrary to the usual findings) was least affected.

Neuroparalytic Keratitis.—I. Luseh[11] saw this condition in a married woman 42 years of age, who was otherwise perfectly healthy.

Lead-deposits.—H. Derby[12] describes a peculiar incrustation of the cornea secondary to ulcer that presented all the characteristics of deposit after using a lead collyrium, although chemical examination of the scale failed to reveal lead.

Herpes.—The treatment advised by Galezowski[13] consists in weak duboisin and eserin, insufflation of powdered iodoform and cocain, and the same in ointment once daily, occlusion, galvanocautery if necessary, and in infecting progressive ulcer, injections under the conjunctiva of antitoxin.

Blood-staining.—De Schweinitz[14] refers to a case of this kind in a 4-year-old girl, in whose right eye there occurred several hemorrhages secondary to abscission of a prolapsed iris.

Tumors.—Thomas[15] reports the removal of a dermoid cyst attached to a linear base extending from the cornea to the inner canthus. The major part of the tumor was covered with skin and hung out between the lids. C. D. Westcott[16] describes keloid of the cornea encountered by him in a 3-year-old

[1] Berlin. klin. Woch., Jan. 4, 1897.　　[2] Arch. f. Ophth., July, 1896.
[3] Ann. d'Oculist., Jan., 1897.　　[4] Ann. of Ophth., July, 1897.
[5] Ann. Ophth. and Otol., July, 1896.　　[6] Ophth. Rec., July, 1897.
[7] Ibid.　　[8] Loc. cit.
[9] Arch. of Ophth., July, 1897.　　[10] Arch. f. d. Ges. Physiol., Pts. 5 and 6, 1896.
[11] Wien. med. Woch., Feb. 13, 1897.　　[12] Boston M. and S. Jour., Apr. 22, 1897.
[13] Rec. d'Ophtal., June, 1896.　　[14] Phila. Polyclinic, Sept. 5, 1896.
[15] Pacific Med. Jour., Dec., 1896.　　[16] Ann. of Ophth., July, 1897.

child as secondary to ophthalmia neonatorum. The microscope confirmed the diagnosis.

Congenital defects of the cornea are classified by Barabacheff[1] thus: glaucomatous, adherent leucoma, sclerosis—all of which are the result of intrauterine inflammation. He cites a case of undoubted interstitial keratitis of syphilitic origin occurring in the second generation. C. A. Woodruff's[2] case of binocular and monocular diplopia is unusual and interesting, as presenting varying vision and refraction dependent upon the relation of the pupil to the corneal cicatrices [and unless carefully studied would suggest intracranial complications]. A. Tepljaschin[3] enjoyed the unusual opportunity of examining microscopically the eyes of a child born with opacity of both corneæ. There were no other congenital anomalies, and the infant died on the third day. Tepljaschin concludes that the opacities originated in an intrauterine inflammation.

Leukoma.—Associated with conjunctivitis of the newborn J. S. Fernandez[4] saw 2 instances of complète corneal clouding that slowly disappeared without treatment. In 3 cases of nebulous cornea in which iridectomy had improved vision, Stern[5] added to the vision in each case by tattooing the cloudy corneal area.

E. Stephenson[6] lauds **electrolysis** for the dissipation of corneal opacities. He employs a current of from $\frac{1}{4}$ to $\frac{1}{2}$ ma. under a pressure of $1\frac{1}{2}$ to 3 volts. Any excess of these amounts will defeat the purpose of the treatment by its over-effect. The current should be accurately controlled by a rheostat and milliampèremeter, the galvanometer being placed near the patient's head, so that variations of the current may be closely followed. The indifferent electrode is held in the patient's hand, while the active pole is attached to a bulb-pointed silver probe, which is gently, but rather rapidly, passed over the opacity. The cornea must be kept moist. Slight frothing will be noticed during the manipulations, which ought to be continued for about a minute. In the list of cases published the average improvement in vision was from 50% to 66%. After 15 to 20 daily applications it is well to suspend treatment for a month. [We are glad to note that Stephenson insists upon the use of a milliampèremeter in the work To our minds, no intelligent and accurate electrolysis can be applied without one which graduates the amount administered as accurately as does a medicine-glass the dose of a remedy at the bedside.]

ANOMALIES AND DISEASES OF THE LENS.

Congenital displacement of the lens occurring in 7 members of a family of 10 is recorded by E. S. Miles.[7] Cramer[8] speaks of meeting with an instance of lenticonus posterior in a 9-year-old girl. The refraction of the peripheral portions of the lens was plus 4 D., while the central portion was minus 11 D. A well-authenticated case of retention of transparency of a lens in which a foreign body had lain quiescent for 16 years is reported by T. B. Archer.[9] At the expiration of that time, when the man was 30 years old, the lens became opaque without assignable cause.

Moon-blindness.—Ole Bull[10] believes that moon-blindness is due to a

[1] La Clin. ophtal.,.Oct., 1896.
[2] Ophth. Rec., June, 1897.
[3] Arch. of Ophth., Jan., 1897.
[4] Ann. of Ophth., Apr., 1897.
[5] Berlin. klin. Woch., May 3, 1897.
[6] Brit. Med. Jour., Sept. 26, 1896.
[7] Ann. Ophth. and Otol., July, 1896.
[8] Klin. Montasbl. f. prakt. Augehn., Aug., 1897.
[9] Lancet, Mar. 20, 1897.
[10] Ann. d'Oculist., July, 1896.

partial change in the lens, leading to a collection of opaque spots on the surface and radiating opaque fibers in the center of the lens.

"**Second Sight.**"—St. J. Roosa [1] attributes so-called second sight to lenticular myopia—a swelling of the lens-nucleus that may or may not be the forerunner of cataract. [This opinion is recorded, not because of its novelty, but because the explanation of the condition is not generally known.]

A. Dnane [2] corroborates E. Jackson's [3] explanation of the method of determining the **position of an opacity** in the lens by means of the corneal reflex of the ophthalmoscopic mirror, namely, the real corneal reflex is always seen in the direction of the center of curvature of the cornea, but as the eye is rotated the reflex appears to move across the pupil exactly as would an opacity situated just behind the posterior pole of the lens. The comparison of the relative rate of movement of opacities with the movement of the reflex across the pupil determines the depth of such opacities.

The claim made by Wolff that **regeneration of the lens** is possible, is substantiated by Erick Müller. [4] The lens was removed from larvæ 3 to 6 cm. in length. Within one day changes were noted in the posterior layer of cells of the iris that in 2 months resulted in the formation of a new lens that had every appearance of a normal one [!].

Causes of Cataract.—The presence of a cilium in the anterior chamber produced capsular cataract in a patient of E. Schwartz. [5] Hennecke [6] ascribed unilateral cataract, observed in a 14-year-old boy, to intestinal worms. That cataract may follow a blow that in no wise compromises the other ocular structures is demonstrated by the case reported by Lenz, [7] which occurred in a young farmer. Wettendorfer [8] includes attacks of epilepsy among the causes.

Diabetes.—Boucheron, in speaking of the proneness of diabetics to suppuration, referred incidentally to the prophylactic use of the antistreptococcic serum previous to operation, and related the ease of a 66-year-old diabetic, in whom, about the time that the injections of the streptococci had become most attenuated, cataract-extraction was done, followed by normal healing and perfect ultimate result. [9] The author claims this to be the first case of its kind published.

At what Age should Cataract-extraction be Performed?—A. Elschnig [10] says "those cataracts which show intensely white nuclei and transparent, bluish-white anterior cortices are least suitable for operation. All other cataracts in persons over 50 years of age may be safely extracted as soon as the vision is so reduced that the patient cannot perform his usual duties." De Schweinitz [11] prefers to wait for maturity, or for that time of life when the lens, even though immature in the ordinary sense of the term, will cleanly leave its capsule. According to C. B. Taylor, [12] there is no limit to the age for cataract-extraction, even if the patient's physical condition is only fair. In his experience he has operated on a number of people over 80 and 3 over 90, one of these being 96 years of age.

Artificial Ripening.—D. Little [13] gives his adherence to Förster's method, basing his conclusions on his experience with 40 cases. The final extraction then resolves itself into a normal operation for thoroughly mature

[1] Med. Rec., Jan. 2, 1897.   [2] Ophth. Rec., June, 1897.
[3] Phila. Polyclinic, Oct. 10, 1896.   [4] Med. Age, Jan. 25, 1897.
[5] Beitr. z. Augenh., July, 1896.   [6] Klin. Monatsbl. f. Augenh., Dec., 1896.
[7] Centralbl. f. prakt. Augenh., Jan., 1896.   [8] Wien. med. Woch., Mar. 13, 1897.
[9] Ann. d'Oculist., Aug., 1896.   [10] Wien. med. Woch., Dec. 13, 1896.
[11] Ophth. Rec., Jan., 1897.   [12] Lancet, Nov. 7, 1896.
                    [13] Brit. Med. Jour., Aug. 8, 1896.

cataract. De Schweinitz[1] prefers extraction of immature cataract by the combined method to the performance of an operation for ripening. Del Toro[2] prefers early extraction to artificial ripening. On the other hand, W. F. Coleman,[3] B. F. Fryer,[4] and Stevenson[5] argue for preliminary iridectomy, especially in the practice of young ophthalmic surgeons, as conferring the greatest safety to the patient. [While much is to be said in favor of preliminary iridectomy, and while Coleman has enumerated the advantages and disadvantages attending two operations instead of one, he has not reckoned with the nervous shock incident to every ophthalmic operation, no matter how slight, a factor that demands recognition in all surgery.] The point is well made by J. Widmark[6] that surgeons who will operate only upon naturally ripe cataracts will at times be beset with many difficulties. From 1882 to 1892 he has dealt with 79 immature cataracts; those occurring after 55 years of age were extracted as immature cataracts; those between 40 and 55 were subjected to Förster's operation, and those under 40 were treated by discission. In 89 % the visual result was good, and in 9 % relatively good, and in 2 % unfavorable. He would operate on any unripe, slowly progressing cataract in a person over 55 as soon as the vision sinks below $\frac{1}{16}$. He has performed Förster's operation 10 times in private practice, and 16 times in his hospital work, without a failure.

Simple or Combined Operation?—A review of the facts deducible from the statistics[7] of 11,250 cataract-extractions reported by F. M. Wilson[8] (see *Year-Book*, 1897), J. B. Story,[9] D. Webster,[10] J. E. Weeks,[11] O. Hallauer,[12] W. Albrand,[13] W. Berger,[14] indicates what we have before stated (see epitome, *Year-Book*, 1898), that the choice as to simple or combined operation will be largely according to the caprice of the operator, each surgeon offering statistics that support his own method. Two of the Germans adhere to Graefe's operation, while Story and the Americans are all advocates of simple extraction. G. A. Berry[15] will find many supporters of his claim that no fixed rule can be observed in determining whether the simple or combined operation shall be done in a given case. The utmost discrimination is called for. His experience would indicate that vision is perhaps better after combined than after simple extraction.

Plettinick-Bauchau[16] extracts cataract according to Galezowski's method as follows: with the Graefe knife the puncture is made exactly at the junction of the opaque border of the cornea 3 mm. below the horizontal diameter. If the pupil is large enough (atropin is used if necessary), the point of the knife divides the capsule in all directions. Counterpuncture is made directly opposite, and the cutting edge of the knife is so directed that it emerges in the cornea 2 mm. from its superior border. Iridectomy he seldom practises on account of its immediate disadvantages, namely, hemorrhage from the iris and choroid, prolapse of vitreous, and escape of the lens into the anterior chamber instead of out through the cut. He considers its antiphlogistic effect exaggerated. The author says, "In the interest of suffering humanity and of ophthalmic science we hope that the better procedure of simple extraction

[1] Ophth. Rec., p. 810, Jan., 1897.   [2] Ann. of Ophth., Jan., 1897.
[3] Ibid., Apr., 1897.   [4] Am. Jour. Ophth., July, 1897.
[5] Trans. Indiana State Med. Soc., 1896.
[6] Jahrb. ueber d. Augenk. des Serafimerlazereths, Stockholm, 1896.
[7] Klin. Monatsbl. f. Augenh., Nov., 1896.   [8] Trans. Am. Ophth. Soc., 1896.
[9] Trans. Royal Acad. of Med., Ireland.   [10] Manhattan Eye and Ear Hosp. Rep., 1895.
[11] N. Y. Med. Jour., No. 5, vol. lxii.   [12] Jahrsb. der Augenanstalt, Basel, 1896.
[13] Bericht ueber 295 Staaroperationen in der Schoeler's chen Klin., Arch f. Augenh., xxxii.
[14] Verhandlungen der Physik.-med. Gesell. zu Würzburg.
[15] Brit. Med. Jour., Sept. 26, 1896.   [16] Rec. d'Ophtal., Aug., 1896.

812   *OPHTHALMOLOGY.*

made by the elliptical incision of Galezowski will be adopted throughout the entire world."

Complications.—Infiltration of the cornea near the cut and slow recovery after extraction are explained by Abadie.[1] He found that because of the slanting incision the cut edge of the iris becomes adherent to the posterior surface of the corneal wound. This hitherto unsuspected accident can be avoided by making the puncture as normally and as peripherally as possible, so as to penetrate into the anterior chamber through the minimum corneal thickness, and the same maneuver and precaution should be observed for the counterpuncture. The section must be continued and finished exactly in the periphery.

Bourgeois[2] calls attention to a cause for retardation of the cicatrization of the wound after cataract-extraction, namely, entropion of the lower lid, caused and maintained by the dressings applied to the eye.

Darier,[3] in a case of cataract with obliteration of the anterior chamber, introduced two lance-shaped knives inversely to each other in the corneoscleral border, one at the right, the other at the left, a little above the horizontal diameter of the cornea. As soon as the points had perforated the cornea they were withdrawn and a cataract-knife, curved and sharp on its convex edge, *with a button at its end,* was entered through one of the incisions, brought out through the other, and the cornea incised, the incision measuring about one-third the circumference of the cornea.

Sanford's[4] experience in extraction of cataracts **in albinoes** has taught him to avoid iridectomy because of prolonged hemorrhage from the cut edge of the iris.

Complete atrophy of the iris followed the third discission of a cataract in a 24-year-old man in a case of F. H. Edsall.[5]

Dislocation of the Lens.—Slight partial dislocation of the lens, Dunn[6] asserts, can be cured by the continued use of atropin, which gives the zonula a chance to repair, or by eserin if vision is improved by its instillation and where the tests show atropin produces a still further tilting of the lens. Higgins[7] removed a lens dislocated into the vitreous without iridectomy while the patient was lying prone on an operating-table. K. Hoor[8] saw a case in which a lens dislocated into the vitreous during a cataract-operation set up so much sympathetic disturbance 6 months later that enucleation was necessary. [This is not an infrequent eventuality. Since the cortical portion of the lens becomes absorbed while lying in the vitreous extraction of the nucleus is not always a difficult feat.]

Discission in Secondary Cataract.—Da Gama Pinto[9] is enthusiastic over the operation for secondary cataract, and feels that even Knapp does not speak highly enough of the blessings of a successful secondary operation. Pinto performed discission in 61% of 529 cases, giving the preference to what he terms posterior discission, in which the narrow Graefe knife is introduced 7 mm. back of the limbus and the capsule divided from behind; 70% of such discissions were successful. A modified cataract-knife is preferred by A. Elschnig[10] to the needle for discission of either primary or secondary cataract.

Jocqs[11] believes that in cases of occlusion of the pupil following iritis and in circumscribed and stationary lenticular opacities, discission and extraction

[1] Ann. d'Oculist., July, 1896.   [2] Rec. d'Ophtal., Mar., 1897.
[3] Ann. d'Oculist., June, 1896.   [4] Rec. d'Ophtal., Dec., 1896.
[5] Med. News, Jan. 23, 1897.   [6] Va. Med. Semi-monthly, Jan. 2, 1897.
[7] Lancet. Dec. 26, 1896.   [8] Wien. med. Woch., Aug. 22, 1896.
[9] Klin. Monatsbl. f. Augenh., Sept., 1896.   [10] Wien. klin. Woch., No. 53, Dec 13, 1896.
[11] Rec. d'Ophtal., Dec., 1896.

will give far more acute, hence useful, vision than the traditional optical iridectomy.

DISEASES OF THE IRIS.

Congenital Anomalies.—In recording instances of partial aniridia and corectopia (slit-shaped pupil), W. C. Posey [1] assumes that these anomalies represent non-development of the arteries which, springing out into the anterior chamber from the major circle of the iris, collect about them the tissue that makes up the iris-stroma. He believes that this theory is applicable to all congenital malformations of the iris. In K. Hook's case the aniridia was bilateral.[2] W. Goldzieher [3] found glaucoma and ectopia lentis associated with bilateral congenital absence of the iris in a 14-year-old girl, and congenital eversion of the posterior pigment-surface of the iris (ectropium uveæ congenitum) is recorded by G. Spiro.[4]

Functional Diseases.—A strong, healthy young lady whose hair, previously dark, turned gray when she was 18 years old, was observed by J. C. Clemensha [5] to have irides that varied in color, ranging from black to bluish-gray through the various shades of brown, brownish-yellow, and yellowish-green. Mental emotion seemed to be a factor in the causation of the changes. A case of voluntary dilatation of the pupil in a woman is held by Bechterew [6] to be due to the existence of an established relation between the upper psychical center (center for voluntary impulse) and the center which innervates the dilator muscle of the pupil. Two facts argue for this hypothesis: 1. At the same moment when the pupil became dilated the patient felt a sensation of protrusion of the eyeball; 2. When the pupil became dilated it remained in this condition for some time, and the dilatation did not disappear until after repeated closure of the lids. The faculty of voluntary dilatation had been acquired 5 years before Bechterew saw the patient.

Paralyses of the Iris.—F. W. Marlowe [7] holds a hemorrhage into the 3d nerve-centers responsible for incomplete sudden paralysis of both 3d nerves observed in a young man. Complete recovery ensued without treatment. T. K. Monro [8] asserts that the Argyll-Robertson pupil has for its cause a lesion of the center in the 4th ventricle, is not due to a degeneration of the spinal center in the lower cervical region, and therefore ought to be grouped with the other varieties of ophthalmoplegia. Speaking of unilateral iris-paralysis occurring in connection with an affection of the sympathetic in a 37-year-old syphilitic, W. H. Wilder [9] says: "this condition is supposed to depend on a nuclear lesion, but here we have the rare example of a one-sided reflex iridoplegia with involvement of the sympathetic. I am, therefore, strongly inclined to locate the lesion in or about the ciliary or ophthalmic ganglion which lies in the orbit about $\frac{3}{4}$ of an inch behind the globe." [This is in accord with the theory of Mendel (see *Year-Book*, 1897).] Recurrent oculomotor paralysis with anesthesia of any or all of the branches of the 5th nerve is attributed by W. H. Haynes [10] to a vascular change, excitation, or edema affecting the root of the 3d nerve and spreading to the 5th.

Myotics.—H. Snellen, Jr.,[11] pronounces pilocarpin the best myotic known

[1] Arch. of Ophth., July, 1897.   [2] Wien. med. Woch., Aug. 15, 1896.
[3] Centralbl. f. prakt. Augenh., Apr., 1897.   [4] Ibid., Oct., 1896.
[5] St. Louis Med. and Surg. Jour., Apr., 1897.
[6] Gaz. hebdom. de Méd. et de Chir., May 9, 1897.
[7] Ann. of Ophth., Apr., 1897.   [8] Am. Jour. Med. Sci., July, 1896.
[9] Chicago Med. Recorder, July, 1896.   [10] N. Y. Med. Jour., Feb. 13, 1897.
[11] System of Diseases of the Eye, Norris and Oliver, vol. ii., 1897.

because of the permanence of its solution and the absence of conjunctival irritation and other complications or general disturbances following its use.

Iritis.—Iritis giving rise to deposits on the posterior surface of the cornea in the manner described by Friedenwald (see *Year-Book*, 1897) is alluded to by J. Dunn.[1] Two full histories of **gonorrheal iritis** occurring in young men are given by R. del Castillo.[2] While anointing the upper lid with the milky juice of a plant belonging to the euphorbia family, for the removal of warts from the eyelid, some of the juice got into the eye, and when R. Hilbert[3] saw the case there was violent iritis with hypopyon, which, however, yielded quickly to treatment. W. Cheatham[4] is persuaded that **serous iritis** never exists without coincident cyclitis and choroiditis, and sometimes hyalitis, and he therefore argues for the use of Noyes' term, "serous uveitis," as a better description of the true pathologic condition. Gertrude Walker[5] well says that painless iritis, easily mistaken for less serious diseases, and readily diagnosed by the instillation of a mydriatic, is an insidious and dangerous affection, because not brought to the notice of the oculist until late in the disease, when synechiæ have formed. Under the title "uveitis iridis," Grandclement[6] describes an inflammation of the posterior wall of the iris which he claims is a continuation of the ciliary part of the retina. It is distinct from iritis, is essentially chronic, and attacks women, occurring preeminently during menstruation and recurring during the menstrual periods for many years. It is not caused by syphilis, rheumatism, or gout, and, although of unknown origin, is favorably affected by iridectomy.

A nice point in the pathogeny of **rheumatic iritis** comes out in the report of the Calcutta Ophthalmic Hospital[7] of the work done from 1890 to 1895. Of the 670 cases of iritis seen, but one was rheumatic in nature, which fact Col. Sanders (the reporter) ascribes to the almost exclusively vegetable diet of the East Indians.[8]

Tuberculosis.—Tubercle of the iris was studied by E. Ammann[9] in a 3-year-old boy and also in a 50-year-old man. In both cases enucleation became necessary.

Gumma of the Iris and Ciliary Body.—True gumma of the ciliary body that finally yielded to specific treatment was seen by H. C. Highet[10] in a 31-year-old Malay, 2½ years after the primary infection. He says that, in addition to the signs of syphilitic iritis, there was bulging forward of the iris adjacent to the tumor, producing different depths in the anterior chamber, gummatous growths in the iris, circumscribed discoloration and distention of the sclera (ciliary staphyloma), and almost total loss of vision from exudation into the vitreous and the pupillary area. [This is described as a rare disease by the author. It is, we believe, very common, but escapes notice because attention is usually confined to the iris, which by its great similarity to the tissue of the ciliary body is seldom affected without coincident involvement of the ciliary body.

Uveal Cysts.—M. W. Zimmermann[11] advised iridectomy for 2 brownish tumors protruding from behind the outer lower quadrant of both irides. Operative interference was declined, and now these melanotic tumors, probably benign, are very little larger than they were 4 years ago. Zimmermann ven-

[1] Ann. of Ophth., Jan., 1897.
[2] Revista de Medicine y. Cirurgia Practicos, Feb. 15, 1897.
[3] Centralbl. f. prakt. Augenh., Feb., 1897.　　[4] Ophth. Rec., Aug., 1897.
[5] Phila. Polyclinic, Jan. 9, 1897.　　[6] Arch. d'Ophtal., Oct., 1896.
[7] Centralbl. f. prakt. Augenh., Apr., 1896.　　[8] Ibid., Apr., 1897.
[9] Klin. Monatsh. f. Augenh., May, 1897.　　[10] Brit. Med. Jour., Nov. 7, 1896.
[11] Ann. of Ophth., July, 1897.

tures the opinion that these are uveal cysts, not secondary to malignant neoplasms, and perhaps arising from the anterior border of the ciliary body. A. L. Whitehead[1] has also seen an instance of cyst of the iris, the result of the introduction into the anterior chamber of a 29-year-old man of a particle of corneal tissue during the performance of an iridectomy for rheumatic iritis 2 years before. **Tumors.**—J. Hirschberg and A. Birnbacher[2] claim to have found a carcinoma spongiosum proceeding from the posterior surface of the iris in a 26-year-old man, and in a young woman of about the same age F. H. Edsall[3] discovered primary sarcoma of the iris.

AFFECTIONS OF THE CHOROID.

Inflammation.—C. A. Oliver[4] records the changes in the field, and the daily alterations in the form, of the scotomata in 2 cases of acute double retinochoroiditis following a flash of lightning and a flash from burning lycopodium. Galezowski[5] protests against the common supposition that such diseases as atrophic choroiditis, interstitial disseminated choroiditis, with either pigmented or white patches, and herpetic choroiditis, are scrofulous, and declares that they should be regarded as syphilitic and treated with mercury.

R. S. Randolph[6] met with metastatic iridochoroiditis ending in panophthalmitis in a 9-months-old infant. Rupture of the globe finally ensued. No rational origin could be made out.

Detachment.—A case of spontaneous detachment of large sections of the choroid, the space intervening between the sclera and choroid filled with greenish exudation that was partly purulent, but without special microbes, and probably originating from a small malignant tumor of the ciliary body, is recorded by Dor.[7] Contrary to the experience of previous writers, Dor's patient had severe pain and increased intraocular tension.

Sarcoma.—J. Hirschberg[8] speaks of sarcoma of the choroid with retinal detachment, in which he punctured the globe far back with a cataract-knife, and the next day the outlines of the tumor were plainly visible. Enucleation became necessary later. Neese[9] does not agree with Fuchs that carcinomatous sarcoma or mixed sarcoma of the choroid occurs twice as frequently in the posterior half as in the anterior half of the eyeball, contending that an analysis of the literature shows the liability to invasion of either half is about the same.

SYMPATHETIC OPHTHALMIA.

Under the title of "A New Form of Sympathetic Ophthalmia," Nuel[10] describes what are only the manifestations of a tardy sympathetic ophthalmia leading to secondary optic atrophy. Donaldson[11] enucleated the right eye of a young woman for cyclitis following traumatic rupture of the sclerotic. Four weeks later there developed sympathetic inflammation in the left eye, relapsing with more or less irregularity for 5 years. At the end of this time the eye became injected and painful during an attack of acute catarrhal conjunctivitis, and eventually vision was almost entirely lost. K. Hoor[12] relates an

[1] Brit. Med. Jour., Mar. 20, 1897.
[3] Med. News, Jan. 23, 1897.
[5] Rec. d'Ophtal., Mar., 1897.
[7] Arch. d'Ophtal., Dec., 1896.
[9] Arch. f. Ophth., Apr., 1897.
[11] Ophth. Rev., Feb., 1897.
[2] Centralbl. f. prakt. Augenh., Oct., 1896.
[4] Internat Med. Mag., Oct, 1896.
[6] Ann. Ophth. and Otol., Oct., 1896.
[8] Centralbl. f. prakt. Augenh., Sept., 1896.
[10] Ann. Soc. Méd.-Chir. de Liege, Jan., 1897.
[12] Wien. med. Woch., Aug. 15, 1896.

instance in which a bit of copper entered the ciliary region of one eye, and was finally discharged from a small abscess 3 months later, when the sympathetic signs in the other eye immediately disappeared. In 2 cases of sympathetic ophthalmia L. Dor[1] saw great improvement in the condition of the remaining eye a long time after enucleation of the primarily diseased one, brought about by the instillation of the extract of the ciliary body of an ox into the conjunctival sac every 2 hours. In one case withdrawal of the treatment caused immediate return of the inflammation. This case had been previously treated by all the usual remedies without success. In the management of this disorder A. Trousseau[2] does not approve of the application of the galvanocautery to an inflamed eye that is causing sympathetic inflammation.

GLAUCOMA.

Classification.—L. Connor[3] believes that the foundation of glaucoma is a constitutional dyscrasia which should be sought out in every case and removed as far as possible. S. O. Richey[4] reaffirms his position of two years ago (see *Year-Book* for 1896) that glaucoma is nothing more than a chronic interstitial ophthalmitis or gout of the eye. He believes[5] more in the causative possibilities of the vortex veins in glaucoma than in a vicious anterior filtration angle. Schoen[6] asserts that it is caused by accommodative strain, and that it can be prevented by early correction of errors of refraction. Of 140 cases 48% were hyperopic and 33% astigmatic, and none of these patients possessed a lens correcting the refraction for distance. Schoen does not speak of glaucoma in myopia, but R. Randolph[7] had a case in a high myope 61 years old that presented typical attacks daily, with complete subsidence of the symptoms in the intervals. Sulzer[8] draws the following conclusions from his researches: 1. Glaucoma may be divided into 3 classes—the circulatory, vascular, and nervous; 2. They have in common vascular degeneration, primary in the second class, secondary in the first, and tertiary when it depends on a disturbance of arterial circulation produced in the first class by an inequality between the intraocular and arterial tension, and in the third by direct nervous influence; 3. The degenerative and nervous circulatory troubles are mutually interdependent and reinforce each other; 4. Circulatory disturbances play the principal role in all glaucomas; 5. The excavation of the optic disk is not a mechanical effect of plus tension, but is dependent upon degeneration of peripheral fibers of the retina and nerve and loss of nutrition from insufficient circulation.

Malignant glaucoma is defined by H. Friedenwald[9] as an intense acute increase of tension of an eye on which iridectomy for simple glaucoma has been recently performed and the anterior chamber has failed to become reestablished. It is followed in nearly all cases by incurable blindness. He considers that it arises from structural alterations in the lymph-vessels of the posterior portion of the eye rather than dislocation forward of the edge of the lens into the angle of the anterior chamber, or to irritation of the ciliary body, or to sudden exudation after iridectomy from the choroidal veins into the vitreous, altering the character of the latter. Recovery followed in one case after the hourly exhibition of strong solutions of eserin, and in another from internal

[1] Gaz. hebdom. de Méd. et de Chir., June 24, 1897.
[2] Rec. d'Ophtal., May, 1897.
[3] Jour. Am. Med. Assoc., Aug. 29, 1896.
[4] Ann. of Ophth., Oct., 1896.
[5] Jour. Am. Med. Assoc., May 29, 1897.
[6] Wien. med. klin. Rundschau, Nos. 26 and 31, 1896.
[7] Ann. of Ophth., Oct., 1896.
[8] Rec. d'Ophtal., Jan. and Feb., 1897.
[9] Ann. of Ophth., Oct., 1896.

administration of sodium salcylate. Where malignant glaucoma has developed after iridectomy in one eye, that operation should not be employed as a means of cure of glaucoma in the second.

Valois[1] warns against accepting the **diagnosis** of glaucoma in cases that seem to have all the symptoms, including cupping of the nerve-head, without careful examination to determine whether other causes are not acting, and whether the excavation is a true cupping, the vessels bent on the edge, and their continuity lost, or a shallow depression that may be only physiologic. He calls such cases " pseudoglaucoma." Randall[2] emphasizes the importance of testing for knee-jerk and other reflexes, and of carefully measuring the field for white and colors in the differential diagnosis between simple glaucoma and atrophy of the optic nerve. Reisse[3] diagnosed by exclusion an absolute glaucoma occurring in an eye injured 18 years previously by a blow from a ball.

Treatment.—In the irritative or prodromic stage myotics may ward off active disease for 4 or 5 years. Rochon-Duvignaud[4] and Trousseau[5] find no benefit from iridectomy in simple glaucoma, and Hansell[6] opposes iridectomy because it may precipitate an acute attack and produce astigmatism of the cornea and irregular refraction through the enlarged pupil, perhaps malignant glaucoma following nonclosure of the wound (see above), and finally because eserin will retard for some years the progress of the disease. Chavellereau[7] relies upon medical treatment alone. After total loss of vision, including light-perception, had existed for 3 weeks after an acute onset of glaucoma, Taylor[8] iridectomized and restored useful vision. The curative action of iridectomy is believed by Abadie[9] to be due to the section of vasodilator veins which course circularly in the diaphragm of the iris and which incision interrupts. Chavellereau[10] speaks highly of De Vincenti's operation of incision of the tissue of the iris in the angle of the anterior chamber. Pflüger[11] proposes to exsect the iris, leaving the pupillary border intact, thus permitting contraction of the pupil to myotics, which may subsequently be employed. Connor[12] advises that such attention should be given to the bowels, skin, and kidneys as will secure the most prompt elimination of effete tissue. The diet should be regulated to such articles and in such quantities as can be perfectly digested. The liberal use of water internally and externally greatly assists in restoring the fluids of the body to a state of reasonable purity. To all this S. O. Richey[13] agrees, and suggests therapeutically a mixture of sodium salicylate, ammonia, and taraxacum, taxis, and weak eserin solution. He says that cases under his observation for 10 years with persistent halo-symptom, increasing refraction, and progressive excavation of the disk, have shown but little, if any, loss of vision and no persistent contraction of the field.

Glaucoma with Ocular Tumors.—A. S. Martin's comments[14] on C. D. Marshall's paper on "Tension in Intraocular Tumors"[15] are important. He says: "There is nearly a constant relation between closure of the angle of the anterior chamber and increased tension; many eyes with normal tension have been known to contain tumors. Tension is more often raised in the presence of a choroidal than a ciliary tumor. The plus tension is due to the glaucoma and only secondarily to the tumor." For the differentiation of primary and secondary glaucoma he offers the following working rule: "When

[1] Rec. d'Ophtal., Dec., 1896.
[2] Jour. Am. Med. Assoc., Nov. 7, 1896.
[3] New Orl. M. and S. Jour., June, 1897.
[4] Rec. d'Ophtal., June, 1897.
[5] Ann. d'Oculist., June, 1896.
[6] Phila. Polyclinic, Jan. 2, 1897.
[7] Traité d'Thérapeut. A. Robin, Paris, 1897.
[8] Lancet, Dec. 5, 1896.
[9] Rec. d'Ophtal., June, 1897.
[10] Traité d'Thérapeut. A. Robin, Paris, 1897.
[11] Ann. d'Oculist., July, 1896.
[12] Loc. cit.
[13] Loc. cit.
[14] Practitioner, Feb., 1897.
[15] Trans. Oph. Soc. Unit. Kingdom, 1896.

an eye has gradually become blind, and develops an attack of acute glaucoma without involving the second eye, a tumor is probably present in the affected eye ; if, however, the eye has lost its sight, and glaucomatous signs appear in the fellow eye, tumor will hardly be found in the offending eye."

The subject of glaucoma is thoroughly reviewed by A. W. Stirling[1] in a series of articles.

AFFECTIONS OF THE RETINA.

Congenital Anomalies.—We note records of the following anatomic curiosities : coloboma of the retina without fissure of the choroid, by Fr. Hosch[2]—the 19th published case ; unusual tortuosities of the retinal arteries, by S. E. Cook ;[3] angioid striæ in the fundus, by J. Dunn ;[4] medullated nerve-fibers continued far out onto the retina along some of the vessels, associated with posterior polar cataract and fine vitreous opacities, by de Schweinitz ;[5] anomalous oval bodies in the retina, by Tiffany.[6] [These were probably choroidal and not retinal. Such opaque ganglionic cells in the vesicular layer would certainly interfere with the acuity of vision, which in this case was normal. Congenital anomalies are for clinicians merely curiosities. Few opportunities present themselves for examination after death from which the study of embryology and the origin of disease might be enriched.]

The restoration of vision to an eye that had been blind as the result of traumatism, iritis, and cataract for 17 years, by D. Webster,[7] is another instance of the **retention of function of the retina** after having been for a long time in abeyance.

Glioma.—S. E. Cook[8] says that if the tumor be not too far advanced and is still intraocular, and the vessels be not too numerous, the living cells are arranged in a cylinder or zone around each vessel. A proper regard for the embryonic origin of the tissues from which it springs and the character it assumes would, he thinks, place this tumor in closer relationship with the carcinomata than with the sarcomata.

E. Wintersteiner[9] has found glioma to be binocular in 24% of all cases reported, and he states plainly that the seed of the trouble is sown in utero, no matter how late in life it may make its appearance, and that it is curable in its earliest stages. Nieden[10] used cancer-serum unsuccessfully on a child. Six weeks later he injected a 2% formol solution, which caused sloughing of the parts and seemed to limit the progress of the tumor. He thinks that the formol treatment may prolong the life of such patients. Grand,[11] on the contrary, thinks that the contraction in size and improvement in appearance claimed by Nieden are to be attributed to the lowered vitality of the patient, since death followed in some of the patients 2 months after use of formol.

Embolism.—Nuel[12] is convinced from anatomic investigation that the cherry spot seen in the macula in embolism of the central artery is due to engorgement of the macular arteries. All other vessels in his case, excepting those around the papilla which anastomose with the vessels of the nerve-entrance, were atrophic. C. F. Clark[13] considers from a review of the litera-

[1] Ann. of Ophth., Jan., 1897.   [2] Arch. f. Augenh., Dec., 1896.
[3] Ann. of Ophth., Apr., 1897.   [4] Ibid., July, 1897.
[5] Phila. Polyclinic, July 18, 1896.   [6] Eye, Ear, Nose, and Throat Clinic, Apr., 1897.
[7] Arch. of Ophth., Oct., 1896.   [8] Ophth. Rev., Aug., 1897.
[9] Das Neuro-Epithelioma Retinæ, F. Deutche, Leipsic, 1897.
[10] Twenty-fifth Ophthal. Congress, Heidelberg, 1896.
[11] Ann. d'Oculist., July, 1897.   [12] Arch. d'Ophtal., Mar. and Aug., 1896.
                      [13] Arch. of Ophth., July, 1897.

ture and a study of his own cases that the time-honored theory that in "embolism of the central artery" a so-called "cilioretinal" vessel serves to preserve the integrity of the papillomacular area," is not proved; but Wadsworth [1] reports his second case, in which central vision was preserved and the foveal region nourished by large cilioretinal vessels (Fig. 62). Embolism of a

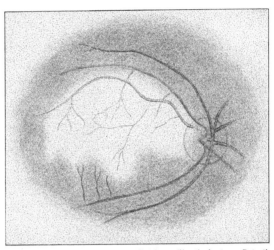

FIG. 62.—Embolism of central artery; macula supplied by a cilioretinal artery. Retention of central vision (Boston M. and S. Jour., Dec. 24, 1896).

branch of the central artery occurring 8 weeks after a normal childbirth in a perfectly sound woman is fully described by O. Stuelp.[2]

Thrombosis.—T. A. Woodruff [3] encountered a thrombosis of the central retinal vein with tremendous choked disk. The patient was 48 years old, and presented no especial lesion that could be held to account for the condition. A full histologic description of the pathologic changes is recorded by S. Tuerk [4] as seen in a 67-year-old tavern-keeper, the subject of emphysema.

Hemorrhage.—De Schweinitz [5] describes an unusual form of macular change after iritis, consisting in an oval reddish area at the macula, giving the impression of a disintegrating hemorrhage and containing in its center 2 white dots. This spot was surrounded by a greenish ring somewhat raised, so that the reddish ring portion appeared as if at the bottom of a small pit, the sides of which were composed of the greenish border described. The macular reflex was unusually distinct and the nerve-head and the retinal vessels were normal. In explanation of the greenish ring he thought it was likely that in such instances of macular lesion, in addition to the change visible to the ophthalmoscope in the center, there must occur some thickening of the extra layer of ganglionic elements in the circummacular region. As a symptom of vascular degeneration in a 60-year-old woman, the subject of aortic stenosis and asthma, F. Pincus observed hemorrhages between the

---

[1] Boston M. and S. Jour., Dec. 24, 1896. [2] Centralbl. f. prakt. Augenh., Feb., 1897.
[3] Ann. Ophth. and Otol., July, 1896. [4] Beitr. z. Augenh., Oct., 1896.
[5] Phila. Polyclinic, July 18, 1896.

vitreous and retina produced by a coughing-fit.[1] Postmortem examination of a case of retinal hemorrhage by J. H. Fisher[2] showed that the blood was effused between the hyaloid membrane of the vitreous and the internal limiting membrane of the retina, and was contained between these membranes. It had not perforated the latter, nor was it found in the true retinal tissue. R. Simon[3] reports another instance of retinal hemorrhage secondary to retinal vascular changes similar to the cases mentioned by Friedenwald (see *Year-Book* for 1897, p. 926). C. A. Oliver[4] observed rupture of the inferior retinal vein in the eye of a young man who was struck in that eye by a flying missile, not otherwise compromising the structure of the globe.

Central Retinitis.—C. S. Bull[5] calls attention to the patches of yellowish exudation in the retina near its center and inflammation of the optic nerves consecutive to angiosclerosis of the walls of the vessels, dependent upon gouty conditions of the blood. Marked impairment of vision from excessive use of the eyes in close and very fine work, followed by perfect recovery, is reported by S. M. Theobald.[6] The defect consisted of an exudative central retinitis with corresponding scotoma for white.

Commotio retinæ with retinal odema, as the result of contrecoup, was seen by M. Linde[7] in 17 cases.

Retinitis Pigmentosa.—A 30-year-old woman applied to W. Goldzieher[8] for failing vision, which he found to be due to glaucoma complicating retinitis pigmentosa. Though the patient's parents were not blood-relations, 6 of her 8 brothers and sisters were the victims of nyctalopia that had incapacitated 3 of them for work. Gould[9] reports 2 cases, a brother and sister, whose only subjective symptoms of retinitis pigmentosa were a partial night-blindness, shown by stumbling, etc. The fields showed considerable limitation for white and colors, and in 1 case extreme irregularity with limitation. There was not a particle of abnormal pigmentation, except at the extreme periphery a minute brown stipling. The patients' paternal grandfather was night-blind all his life, and became wholly blind at 70, but his eyes were never examined by an oculist. In a review of the literature there are found only 5 cases that may be relied on as similar to Gould's cases. In the French reports no fields are given, and records of the refraction and other details are omitted. For the closer study of this subject Gould suggests interrogation of every office-patient as to his vision after dark, and as to whether they bow their heads at night (to see the floor or ground in darkness); that careful account be taken of the form- and color-fields and of the refraction. The important facts to determine are: (*a*) Is the disease progressive? (*b*) If so, is it the incipient stage of what later becomes typical retinitis pigmentosa? (*c*) What is the pathology of the abnormal color-fields? and What is the etiology of the disease?

A decidedly unique pigment-anomaly of the retina, occurring in both eyes and supposed to be congenital, was studied and is pictured by H. Pretori.[10] (See Plate 10, Fig. 1.) The patient was a glassblower 52 years old, with normal vision in right eye and $\frac{1}{10}$ of normal in left eye. The changes were practically identical in both eye-grounds.

"Hemeralopia."—Krienes[11] ascribes this symptom to a disturbance or

[1] Beitr. z. Augenh., Oct., 1896.   [2] Royal London Hosp. Rep., Dec., 1896.
[3] Centralbl. f. prakt. Augenh , Nov., 1896.   [4] Ann. Ophth. and Otol., Jan., 1897.
[5] Med. News, May 8, 1897.   [6] Am. Jour. Ophth., July, 1897.
[7] Centralbl. f. prakt. Augenh., Apr., 1897.   [8] Ibid.
[9] Ann. of Ophth., Oct., 1897.   [10] Beitr. z. Augenh., Oct., 1896.
[11] Ueber Hemeralopia, speziel Akute Idioptische Hemeralopia, Wiesbaden, 1896.

PLATE 10.

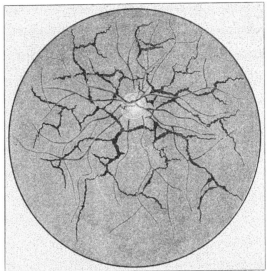

FIG. 1.—Anomalous pigmentation of an eye-ground (Beit. z. Augenh., Oct., 1896).

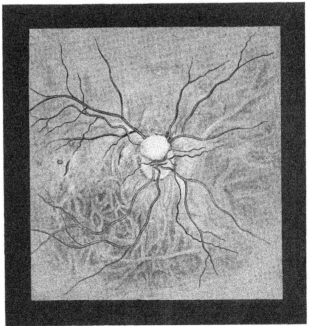

FIG. 2.—Cyst of the optic nerve (Ann. of Oph. and Otol., Oct., 1896).

destruction of the relation between waste and repair of the visual substance. He claims that it is not a functional disease, for it always originates in some form of chorioretinitis. [The term hemeralopia, from the doubtfulness of its meaning, should not be used.] Wilbrand[1] concludes that in the neurotic eye there is relatively slower restoration of the visual purple after light-stimulation than that which occurs in the normal eye. While fundus-changes in hemeralopia are sometimes not visible with the ophthalmoscope, there must be some lesion in the nerve, retina, or choroid following chorioretinitis syphilitica, choroiditis disseminata, or retinitis pigmentosa. The association of night-blindness with xerosis of the conjunctiva and cornea was noted by C. Kollock[2] in negro children of tuberculous, scrofulous, or syphilitic diathesis living on the South Carolina coast. The ocular media, other than the cornea, are clear, and the nerve-head is slightly swollen and of a dirty white color.

Retinitis proliferans was the final outcome of two instances of laceration of the optic nerve and central blood-vessels recorded by C. Zimmerman.[3]

Albuminuric Retinitis.—J. Hinshelwood[4] contributes a notable exception to the ordinary gloomy prognosis of albuminuric retinitis in the case of a 62-year-old woman, who was alive and in good health 3 years after an attack that had reduced her vision to $\frac{1}{60}$ in each eye.

Detachment.—As causes H. O. Reik[5] mentions granular kidney, albuminuria of pregnancy, diabetic retinitis, tumors, and pregnancy, in addition to the most frequent factor—namely, high myopia. Nuel[6] adds disease of the macula and exudation into the posterior layers of the retina of albuminous material, as in albuminuric retinitis; disease of the walls of the retinal vessels, which leads to changes in their level and length; retraction of the vitreous and alterations in the rods and cones, producing a relaxation of their adherence to the choroid.

R. L. Randolph[7] found the microscopic changes in the vitreous body of eyes exhibiting detached retina to consist in fibrillary alterations in the vitreous, sustaining the position of Nordenson and Nuel. I. Casper's 4 cases of striæ in the fundus showed the course of development so plainly that he does not hesitate to assert that all retinal striations represent the residue of cured detachments.[8]

B. L. Millikin[9] comments on the finding of progressive retinal detachment in 3 brothers, none of whom had suffered from any marked constitutional disorders. They were of a large family, characterized in an unusual degree by long life and general good health.

Detachment of the superior temporal vein, occurring as the terminal stage of a previous hemorrhage, is fully detailed by J. Dunn.[10]

Indications of Choroidal Disease.—Elschning's[11] theory that idiopathic detachment is primarily caused by localized retinochoroidal disease received confirmation from two cases studied by T. Collins. A circumscribed, extending detachment is one of the earliest symptoms, and may be for a long time the only one, of choroidal tumor, according to Rockliffe.[12]

Treatment of Detachment.—Electrolysis, according to the method of Terson (see *Year-Book*, 1897), was employed by Montgomery[13] in 4 cases un-

[1] Die Erholungsausdehnung unter Normalen und Pathologischen Bedingungen, Wiesbaden, 1896.
[2] Ophth. Rec., Feb., 1897.
[3] Arch. of Ophth., Jan., 1897.
[4] Brit. Med. Jour., May 8, 1897.
[5] Jour. Am. Med. Assoc., Oct. 3, 1896.
[6] Arch. of Ophth., Oct., 1896.
[7] Jour. Am Med. Assoc., Oct. 3. 1896.
[8] Arch. of Ophth., Jan., 1897.
[9] Ann. Ophth. and Otol., Oct., 1896.
[10] Ann. of Ophth., July, 1897.
[11] Ophth. Rev., June, 1896.
[12] Ibid.
[13] Jour. Am. Med. Assoc., Sept. 26, 1896.

successfully. In one of them it undoubtedly caused glaucoma. It is painful, valueless as a curative agent, and may excite glaucoma. Chavellereau,[1] Fromaget, and Lagrange[2] have rejected it because, they say, it increases the area of separation. Eve[3] evacuated the fluid by means of a cannula, through which he introduced a small bundle of horsehairs. This was removed in a few days on account of conjunctival inflammation. After recovery the field was normal. [We think Eve's surprise was as great as it was agreeable.]

C. A. Wood[4] sums up the whole subject when he says "that we have as yet discovered no better device than that reported by some of the older ophthalmologists with occasional success—namely, rest in bed, bandages, atropin, and the internal use of some absorbent." He reminds the profession that spontaneous cure often occurs, in which case the measures employed are wrongly given the credit.

DISEASES OF THE OPTIC NERVE.

Anatomy.—Partial crossing of the optic nerves at the chiasm is now reaffirmed by Gruetzner.[5] This theory was temporarily abandoned when Kölliker, as a result of the study of microscopic sections, reported at the Anatomic Congress in Berlin that the nerves crossed entirely. [There is little reason to believe that Kölliker's position can be maintained.] E. Berger[6] proposes a division of the fibers of the distal portion of the optic nerve into 3 groups—namely, central, supplying the anterior retina; intermediate, supplying the equatorial region; and peripheric or subpial, supplying the peripapillary zone. Lesions of the central group are characterized by peripheral contractions of the visual field, lesions of the intermediate group produce a zone of amblyopia around the blind-spot, and lesions of the peripheral group increase the size of the blind-spot.

Functional Diseases of the Nerve.—As the result of an application of a 5% solution of cocain to the posterior nares, J. H. Shastid[7] witnessed complete amblyopia lasting 4 days. Beauvais[8] speaks of a patient who, after watching vivid lightning, claimed to be blind. The man directed his gaze downward and held the lids closed, the exact reverse of the usual position of the sightless globes of an amblyopic. The pupils reacted normally and the fundi were healthy, showing plainly that the blindness was simulated.

Perimetry.—Willetts[9] continues to insist that our present method of perimetry is faulty, inasmuch as it fails to take account of the fact that the retina is histologically the same throughout its whole expanse. He offers as the practical corollary of this fact his own demonstration that the true visual field is round, extending 70° in all directions from the fixation-point, and contends that any method that shows the usual nasal limitation of the normal field of vision for form or color is wrong, for no such contraction exists. [This is an advanced position which will require abundant anatomic and clinical evidence to render it tenable.] H. Wilbrand[10] emphasizes the point that perimetry can only be of diagnostic value when considered in connection with the central visual acuity and the fundus conditions. [The real clinical worth of perimetry, as set forth in the publication mentioned, can be

[1] Traité de Thérapeut. A. Robin, Paris, 1897.
[2] Soc. Méd. et Chir. de Bordeaux, May 28, 1897.
[3] Ann. d'Oculist., June, 1896.
[4] Jour. Am. Med. Assoc., Oct. 3, 1896.
[5] Deut. med. Woch., Nos. 1 and 2, 1897.
[6] Arch. d'Ophtal., Nov., 1896.
[7] Jour. Am. Med. Assoc., Feb. 13, 1897.
[8] Rec. d'Ophtal., Aug., 1896.
[9] Ann. Ophth. and Otol., July, 1896.
[10] Norris and Oliver, System of Diseases of the Eye, vol. ii., 1897.

unhesitatingly pronounced the most comprehensive and authoritative work on this subject that has appeared in the English language.] Wilbrand[1] shows elsewhere that the absolute extent of the visual field can be determined only by the smallest and least luminous object which can be perceived by the most peripheral cones of the retina. To meet this proposition he has devised what he calls his " Dunkel-perimeter," of the usual hemispheric form, to be used in a thoroughly darkened room, in connection with pin-head-sized test-objects made of phosphorescent material. The normal retina will recover itself in the dark room, and show a normal field a few minutes after entering the room, and each half-hour in excess of this time will be the measure of the pathologic condition. He claims for the method an exactness not obtainable by ordinary perimetry.

Hemianopsia.—In the case of binasal hemianopsia reported by C. A. Veasey,[2] there were associated nausea and vomiting, tremor, numbness, and heaviness of the left leg, vertigo terminating in coma, which after 20 hours ushered in death. Coggin's 7 cases of homonymous hemianopsia,[3] loosely and inaccurately described and without report of autopsies, are of no particular interest. W. A. Holden[4] says that hemiachromatopsia, accompanied by a hemiopic light-sense disturbance, must be due to an affection of the fibers of the visual path, and not of the ganglion-cells of the cortex.

Optic Neuritis.—G. E. de Schweinitz[5] reports 5 cases of unilateral optic neuritis assigned severally to rheumatism, syphilis, chlorosis, albuminuria of pregnancy, and degenerative changes in the vessels of the optic nerve, or endovasculitis. In the optic neuritis or amblyopia accompanying purulent disease of the sphenoidal cavities Holmes[6] urges immediate and effective drainage by drilling through the anterior wall, removing if necessary the middle turbinated bone. Partial retention of the placental membranes and menorrhagia following miscarriage were found by Minor[7] to give rise to acute optic neuritis and considerable loss of vision, a condition of things which was soon righted when the uterine functions had been restored. In specific neuritis P. Webster[8] found contracted fields and scotoma for red. When optic neuritis coexists with otitis media purulenta Ostman[9] thinks that the ocular condition is the expression of a meningitis secondary to the otitic process.

"Choked Disk."—The origin of choked disk is still unsettled. In a discussion at the March meeting of the Berlin Neurologic and Psychiatric Society,[10] Jacobson, in reporting a case, committed himself to the mechanico-inflammatory theory, stating that the primary agent was the irritant toxins, the stagnation being a secondary, yet powerful, factor. Bruns,[11] attacking the inflammatory theory, observed that the toxins would never find their way down the optic-nerve sheaths to the nerve-head were it not for the increased intracranial pressure ; and that even if the cerebral fluid were rich in toxins, it could avail nothing save in the presence of increased intracranial pressure. Jacobson[12] replied that as yet no one has succeeded in producing choked disk experimentally, and that therefore Bruns' position, along with that of Schmidt and Manz (see *Year-Book* for 1897, p. 933), is untenable. E. von Grosz's division of choked disk into inflammatory and edematous[13] is based on the microscopic examination of the optic nerves of 3 sufferers from brain-tumor, and a consid-

[1] Monatschr. f. Psychiat. u. Neurol., Jan., 1897.
[2] Ophth. Rec., Feb., 1897.   [3] Boston M. and S. Jour., Dec. 24, 1896.
[4] Med. Rec., Oct. 31, 1896.   [5] Phila. Polyclinic, Dec. 12, 1896.
[6] Arch. of Ophth., Oct., 1896.   [7] Ophth. Rec., Feb., 1897.
[8] Intercol. Med. Jour. of Australasia, June 20, 1897.
[9] Arch. f. Ophth., Feb., 1897.   [10] Neurolog. Centralbl., Apr. and May, 1897.
[11] Ibid.   [12] Ibid.   [13] Centralbl. f. prakt. Augenh., May, 1897.

eration of the literature of the subject. To his mind, edematous choked disk is the accompaniment of true brain-tumor, while tubercle and gumma give rise to the inflammatory form, although these differences can be made out only in the early stages of the disorder. Vision will obviously be better with the first form. Unfortunately, we are not yet able to localize the cerebral process by means of any special characteristics on the part of the neuritis. He thinks that, even if the tumor cannot be removed, the effect of trephining is not injurious to the patient, and is markedly beneficial to the optic nerves. Epe- ron [1] is an adherent of the mechanical hypothesis.

Optic Atrophy.—Treacher Collins' [2] report of permanent scotoma with partial atrophy of the optic nerve, due to 5 minutes' exposure of the retina to direct sunlight, by a young man, clinically illustrates the result arrived at experimentally by Usher and Dean,[3] that wounds of the retina in animals can set up nerve-degeneration corresponding to the part of the retina that has been injured. O. J. Short [4] says that mercurial inunctions in conjunction with hot baths are always beneficial in partial optic atrophy; that unless the origin is specific or from some blood or mineral poison, potassium iodid is oftener harm- ful than helpful. When vision is $\frac{20}{200}$ or more, benefit may be expected; when it is less we can only hope to arrest the progress of the disease; while in those cases showing light-perception only, treatment is unavailing. Strychnin is serviceable only in spinal atrophies. Rapid acute atrophy associated with tabes dorsalis in a 40-year-old farm laborer was ascribed by W. Reber [5] to syphilis. M. Benedikt [6] inveighs against too heroic treatment in the optic- nerve degenerations of tabes [but just why, we cannot imagine]. L. R. Cul- bertson's suggestion,[7] that ovariotomy in women and castration in animals are a cause of optic atrophy, cannot be viewed as more than a coincidence in the 2 cases he reports—a woman and a colt. [A deduction from 2 cases when hun- dreds of such operations are done daily is absurd.] C. W. Kollook [8] records permanent improvement in a patient with optic-nerve atrophy from $\frac{20}{200}$ to $\frac{20}{30}$, following systematic inhalations of amyl nitrite, after persistent medication with potassium iodid and strychnin had failed.

Toxic Amblyopia.—Nüel [9] controverts the accepted idea that the cen- tral scotoma of toxic amblyopia is due to interstitial neuritis of the macular fibers of the optic nerve, and finds that the earliest changes take place in the macular cells themselves, and that the atrophy of the macular bundle is sec- ondary and consecutive to the atrophy of the retinal cells from which they arise. C. A. Wood [10] believes that secondary alterations in the nerve in chronic plumbism are the result of fatty metamorphosis consequent upon peri- and endarteritis, and that the ocular lesions are peripheral and distinct from those changes which coincidently occur as results of renal or cerebral complications arising in the course of long-standing intoxication. Higgins agrees with other writers,[11] that tobacco-amblyopia is more common among the poor, because they smoke the cheaper tobaccos, which are richer in nicotin. In Belt's ease,[12] al- cohol-tobacco amblyopia and multiple neuritis were encountered in the same patient. F. van Fleet [13] speaks of what may be a true amblyopia potatorum occurring in an artist addicted to rum. The blindness followed a debauch, and despite strychnin carried to $\frac{2}{3}$ gr. hypodermically per day, the amblyopia

[1] Albany Med. Ann., May, 1897.   [2] Royal London Ophth. Hosp. Rep., Dec., 1896.
[3] Trans. Ophth. Soc., vol. xvi., p. 248.   [4] Jour. Am. Med. Assoc., Dec. 5, 1896.
[5] Phila. Polyclinic, Aug. 21, 1897.   [6] Arch. f. Ophth., May, 1897.
[7] Am. Jour. Ophth., Aug., 1897.   [8] Ophth. Rec., May, 1897.
[9] Arch. d'Ophtal., Aug., 1896.   [10] Med. News, May 29, 1897.
[11] Jour. Am. Med. Assoc., Jan. 9, 1897.   [12] Ann. Ophth. and Otol., Oct., 1896.
[13] Manhattan Eye and Ear Hosp. Rep., 1897.

became permanent and the nerves thoroughly atrophic. Ellis'[1] patient, a
tobacco-, alcohol-, and morphin-slave, was given 120 gr. of quinin in 24 hours
for an acute malaria. He became perfectly blind, but in 2 weeks recovered
a part of his former vision. · Ellis queries whether this was toxic amblyopia,
and, if so, was it from the tobacco, alcohol, morphin, or quinin? [It was
plainly induced by the quinin in a subject whose optic nerves had long since
been prepared for the easy engrafting of such a condition.] Toxic amblyopia
following the prolonged internal use of iodoform has been twice seen by J. W.
Russell,[2] who treats his cases of phthisis systematically with iodoform, sometimes working the dose up to 10 gr. 3 times a day. Both of his cases were
pronounced upon by Wood White, who said of them, "this amblyopia differs
from that of tobacco in that there is no color-scotoma." [This is a strange
assertion on the part of White. Priestly Smith[3] distinctly states in the history of his case that there was not only central color-scotoma, but that it was
absolute at a point below the fixation-point.] A. G. Thomson[4] ascribes the
amblyopia in a case observed by him to drinking large quantities of Jamaica
ginger. The ophthalmoscope showed the classic changes of alcohol- and
tobacco-amblyopia. In the treatment of toxic amblyopia de Wecker[5] advocates the injection of artificial serum, 60 to 100 gm. (Cberon's serum). Pari-
nand, Darier, and others,[6] consider the method inferior to milk-diet, purgatives, and pilocarpin.

Cyst of the Optic Nerve.—S. D. Risley[7] furnishes a beautiful drawing
of a cyst of the optic nerve accompanying bilateral chorioretinitis, which he
observed in a 38-year-old Polish woman (see Plate 10, Fig. 2).

INJURIES TO THE GLOBE.

The first two recorded instances of the **diagnosis of the presence of
pieces of metal in the eyeball by means of the Röntgen process**
were that of C. F. Clark and that of C. H. Williams.[8] Both were eminently
successful. Since then G. O. Ring,[9] H. F. Hansell,[10] and G. E. de Schweinitz[11]
have published details of cases confirmatory of the value of this means of
diagnosis. Experiments and the practical application of the methods found
most useful in determining the location of the foreign body have been successfully made by Lewkowitch,[12] who claims that his calculations, based on
double images, have never been more than 1 mm. wrong; by Sweet,[13] who
has had equally successful results by the use of an especially devised apparatus (see Figs. 63, 64), and by Oliver and Leonard.[14] J. Hirschberg[15] holds
that skiagraphy can be of no use in assisting the determination of the location
and the extraction of bits of copper that have entered the eye. [Copper cannot be extracted by the magnet, but can be diagnosed and located by the
x-rays.] He related 2 histories of copper-injuries to the eye, both successfully
operated.

Ardoin[16] substantiates Leber's observations on the extreme danger to the
eye and the susceptibility to sympathetic inflammation from wounds made by
copper, and advises immediate removal if possible, and, when impracticable,

[1] Jour. Am. Med. Assoc., Nov. 7, 1896.
[2] Lancet, June 12, 1897.
[3] Ophth. Rec., Apr., 1893.
[4] Phila. Polyclinic, Sept. 11, 1897.
[5] Rec. d'Ophtal., May, 1897.
[6] Ibid.
[7] Ann. Ophth. and Otol., Oct., 1896.
[8] Trans. Am. Ophth. Soc., 1896.
[9] Trans. Sec. Ophth., College of Physicians of Phila.
[10] Ibid.
[11] Amer. Jour. Med. Sci., May, 1897.
[12] Lancet, Aug. 15, 1896.
[13] Ophth. Sect., Am. Med. Assoc., June, 1897.
[14] Trans. Am. Ophth. Soc., May, 1897.
[15] Berlin. klin. Woch., Apr. 12, 1897.
[16] Rec. d'Ophtal., Dec., 1896.

the enucleation of the ball. Another instrument, less practical than the
Röntgen apparatus, is the "siderescope," invented by Asmus. It consists
essentially of two magnetic needles so suspended in appropriate tubes that
their slightest turnings can be observed and registered. A. Barkau[1] used it
in connection with either Haab's or Hirschberg's magnets with success.

Instances of **extraction of pieces of steel and iron** from the vitreous,
with preservation of the globe, and in some cases of the sight, are recorded

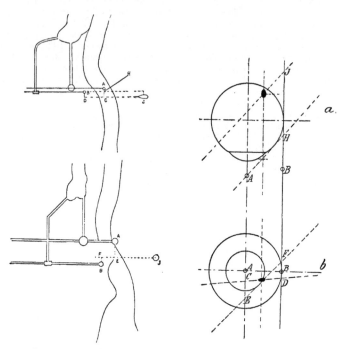

FIG. 63.—Outlines of negative taken by Sweet's method.

FIG. 64—Sweet's projection-lines for locating foreign bodies in the eye: *a*, transverse section; *b*, vertical section.

by F. Buller[2] [6 cases, 1 unsuccessful], H. F. Hansell,[3] J. E. Weeks,[4] who
used Haab's magnet, and G. O. Ring,[5] and in some of the cases in which the
x-rays were used, mentioned above.

Traumatism.—Buckner[6] reports a case of rupture of the choroid from
traumatism to the forehead, and de Wecker[7] mentions instances of emptying
the orbit, paralysis of an external rectus, ptosis and keratitis, in each instance
produced by compression on the parts of the mother or by the forceps in
instrumental delivery. He calls attention to the fact that the eyes of the

[1] Occidental Med. News, Mar., 1897.
[2] Ann. Ophth. and Otol., Oct., 1896.
[3] Am. Jour. Ophth., Dec., 1896.
[4] Arch. of Ophth., Jan., 1897.
[5] Univ. Med. Mag., Feb., 1897.
[6] Charlotte Med. Jour., Nov., 1896.
[7] Ann. d'Oculist., July, 1896.

infant in the process of birth are exposed to other dangers than infection. Penetration of all the tunics of the eyeball by a piece of window-glass is reported by Marie Haydon.[1] The conjunctiva was drawn over the wound and sutured ; recovery was uninterrupted. C. A. Oliver[2] does not recommend suturing the edges of the rupture in the sclera made by the escape of the lens when dislocated by traumatism, or of the cut in the conjunctiva through which the lens has been removed.

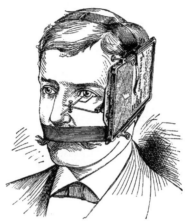

FIG. 65.—W. M. Sweet's *x*-ray apparatus for locating foreign bodies in the eye, applied.

Meningitis after Operation.—G. E. de Schweinitz[3] prefers evisceration to enucleation when acute panophthalmitis is present, feeling that the chances of secondary infectious meningitis are thus lessened. Lapersonne[4] enucleated an eye on account of an injury received. Ten days later fatal meningitis developed. Pneumococci were abundant in the pus found at the base of the brain. The most active antiseptic, he says, is hypochlorite of calcium purified in sterile water.

DISEASES OF THE ORBIT.

Functional Diseases.—J. Terson[5] affirms the existence of an orbital affection of spontaneous or traumatic origin, which is characterized by alternation of the two opposite conditions, enophthalmos and exophthalmos, the former succeeding transient attacks of the latter until the exophthalmos becomes permanent. The exophthalmos originates in voluntary and involuntary efforts, and in compression of the jugular veins. The connective tissue and fat of the orbit are absorbed, the veins become dilated and varicose from atrophy of their muscular fibers, and there is atrophy of the muscular fibers of Müller. The disease is a trophic neurosis depending on lesions of the sympathetic nervous system. Treatment consists in electrization, tonics, and the local application of hamamelis virginica. This disease should not be confounded with the stabile exophthalmos due to orbital tumors or goiter.

[1] Phila. Polyclinic, Oct. 24, 1896.   [2] Ophth. Rev., June, 1897.
[3] Phila. Polyclinic, Sept. 6, 1896.   [4] Rec. d'Ophtal., June, 1897.
[5] De l'Enophthalmie et de l'Exophthalmie Alterans, 1897.

A. B. Kibbe's[1] ease of pulsating exophthalmos, exhibiting an unusually complete picture of cavernous sinus thrombosis, belongs to that rare class of cases (*e. g.*, Churchman's, *Year-Book*, 1897, p. 912) in which all the symptoms are dissipated by ligation of the common carotid.

Periostitis.—W. Reber[2] refers to an instance of bilateral tertiary orbital periostitis and cellulitis encountered in a married woman aged 41. Despite the most active treatment from the start, one optic nerve atrophied completely as the result of long-continued stretching attending the accompanying exophthalmos, while the other nerve escaped injury.

Pseudoplasmes.—S. Snell[3] counsels caution in approaching surgically certain apparently organic tumors of the orbit. His 3 case-histories, showing disappearance of the tumor in each case under potassium iodid, teach plainly that medical treatment should be resorted to before operation. Snell concurs with Panas in believing that there is a class of orbital tumors amenable to drugs, and that they are neither specific nor malignant. [These tumors would likely fall into the class " pseudoplasmes " proposed by Panas (see *Year-Book* for 1897, p. 911).] Ayres[4] met with an orbital condition in a 7-year-old boy that might also be styled a " pseudoplasm " because of its indeterminate character. The exophthalmos became so great as finally to usher in death from conjunctival hemorrhage [a rare occurrence]. The patient was the subject of leukocytosis, or " chloroma," as Ayres prefers to style it.

Tumors.—An orbital tumor, ill defined in character, affecting a 2-year-old child, was removed because of threatened destruction of the left eye. Fifteen months later, when the growth had recurred, the patient's parents refused F. H. Knagge[5] permission to operate again, and the child died soon afterward. C. S. Bull[6] concludes, from a study of 36 cases, that the prognosis of malignant tumors of the orbit is highly unfavorable; that surgical interference is almost invariably followed by a return of the tumor; and that repeated operations shorten the life of the patient, in which opinion he is joined by R. Sattle,[7] who feels that in such cases surgery ought only to be exploratory. The same author says elsewhere[8] that epithelioma of the soft tissues of the orbit is more amenable to surgery than the other forms of malign neoplasms. Of 3 cases detailed, one was alive 2 years and another 5 years after operation. The third one died a week after removal of the tumor. The ocular disturbances observed in epithelioma of the sphenoidal sinus by Morax[9] were continuous headache, progressive failure of vision, with sudden blindness later, although there was no lesion of either fundus; finally, optic atrophy, oculomotor palsy, exophthalmos, and death from intercurrent bronchopneumonia. H. Knapp[10] removed a congenital cavernous angioma, 27 by 24 mm., from an orbit, restoring the displaced eye to the normal position and to the full exercise of its functions.

Hydatid Cyst.—Two cases of hydatid cyst of the orbit have been reported during the year. one by P. Varese,[11] who saw the condition in a 15-year-old girl, in whom the disease induced optic neuritis, and the other by L. von Issekutz,[12] who successfully removed the parasite.

[1] Arch. of Ophth., Jan., 1897.
[2] Ann. of Ophth., Apr., 1897.
[3] Lancet, Jan. 23, 1897.
[4] Jour. Am. Med. Assoc., Nov. 7, 1896.
[5] Lancet, Sept. 19, 1896.
[6] Trans. Am. Ophth. Soc., 1896.
[7] Ophth. Rec., June, 1897.
[8] Cleveland Med. Gaz., July, 1897.
[9] Ann. d'Oculist., June, 1896.
[10] Arch. f. Augenh., No. 4, 1896.
[11] Arch. di Ottalmo logia, Feb., 1897.
[12] Centralbl. f. prakt. Augenh., Apr., 1897.

OPERATIONS.

P. Fridenberg[1] employs 2 radiographs in **locating foreign bodies with the x-rays.** He cuts a plate so that it will fit into the anterior orbital margin, protects the cornea with cotton, and bandages the plate against the eye. The Crookes tube is held 14 in. back of the head, and the rays are passed through the opposite temple. In this way he located 5 bird-shot that had gone entirely through an eye and lodged in the orbit. [Fridenberg's method is practically that employed by Dahlefeld and Pohrt[2] and in the laboratories of Philadelphia.]

Asepsis and Antisepsis.—Absolute alcohol, while a valuable disinfectant for instruments infected under the conditions which ordinarily surround us in everyday life, has been proved by R. Randolph[3] to be unreliable for the sterilization of instruments infected with a pure culture of septic micrococci. His contention is supported by an extensive array of bacteriologic experiments. A sterile conjunctival sac will most likely be secured by combining asepsis and antisepsis, and E. Franke,[4] therefore, cleanses the sac thoroughly by simple irrigation, and then instils the antiseptic, preferably sublimate in 1:5000 to 1:10,000 solution. In this way, although all the bacteria may not be destroyed, they will at least be rendered inert. Bach[5] considers that asepsis is all that is necessary in ophthalmic surgery. Antiseptic treatment not only does not destroy all the germs, but it also irritates the conjunctiva, inducing a catarrhal condition highly unfavorable to operations. The open-wound treatment of all operations on the eye is lauded by J. Hjort,[6] who supports his contention with statistics covering 112 operations, including 52 cataracts and numerous iridectomies, discissions, and sclerotomies. His preparation of the eye is essentially aseptic, while the after-treatment practically resolves itself into the use of cold compresses and the injunction of quiet. Viewing the cilia as the most likely source of infection, he frequently epilates both lid-margins before operation. He does not hesitate to apply the open method to cataract-extraction in the presence of dacryocystitis. His series of 112 cases treated after this method does not include one failure.

For Epithelioma.—F. T. Smith[7] tells of a case in which he proposed to remove the inner half of an upper lid for epithelioma. While preparing for operation the patient fell into the hands of an empiric, who cauterized the growth thoroughly, and, to Smith's surprise, there was perfect healing. [By means of glacial acetic acid we have succeeded in removing repeatedly just such growths, but they have invariably recurred, until there was no remedy other than the knife.]

For Ectropion.—Terson[8] excises redundant conjunctiva and sutures the edges; he then removes a triangular piece of skin and the underlying orbicularis muscle from the neighborhood of the external canthus. He has operated 4 times, with excellent result.

Pterygium.—Boeckman[9] dissects the apex from the cornea and the body from the underlying connective tissue, cleaning up the sclera from all connective tissue to which the pterygium had been attached and replacing the pterygium in the space thus cleared. It adheres to the sclera and remains fixed for all time.

Iridectomy.—Lawford[10] prefers Schöler's method of performing iridot-

---

[1] Med. Rec., May 15, 1897.
[2] Deutsch. med. Woch., Apr. 29, 1897.
[3] Johns Hopkins Hosp. Bull., Oct., 1896.
[4] Arch. f. Ophth., Feb., 1897.
[5] Arch. f. Augenh., 1 and 2, 1896.
[6] Centralbl. f. prakt. Augenh., May, 1897.
[7] Jour. Am. Med. Assoc., Oct. 3, 1896.
[8] Arch. d'Ophtal., Dec., 1896.
[9] Jour. Am. Med. Assoc., Jan. 14, 1897.
[10] Ophth. Rev., Aug., 1896.

omy—so-called extraocular—to iridectomy for artificial pupil made for optical purposes. A small incision is made through the cornea near, but not at, the limbus; the iris is carefully withdrawn and divided perpendicular to its pupillary margin. He claims that this method avoids the disturbing refraction of the lens-periphery. Prolapse of the retina through the corneal wound made during iridectomy for glaucoma, and occurring the day of the operation, is recorded by D. Webster,[1] who ascribes the unusual complication to choroidal hemorrhage.

Hemorrhage after Enucleation.—Sattler's experience[2] teaches that removal of the eye in bleeders sometimes involves serious consequences. Once in a young hereditary hemophilic, and once in an elderly arteriosclerotic, he rescued his patient from fatal syncope only after the most vigorous treatment continued 24 to 36 hours. G. F. Suker[3] employs a spray of hot sterilized water in arresting hemorrhage after enucleation.

Enucleation, or Mules' Operation.—The question of the choice of these 2 operations has been freely discussed. The weight of authority seems to be in favor of the latter if care is exercised in the selection of the case, but most writers agree with Kalt[4] that it is not preventative of sympathetic inflammation. In panophthalmitis it is said to be the safer procedure, and Hughes[5] claims it does not provoke postocular inflammation or meningitis; but Stocker and Pflüger[6] have both enucleated and eviscerated in many cases of panophthalmitis without ill-results. James Barrett's case[7] of death following excision of an eye would indicate that the excision had determined the fatal result, had not the autopsy shown the existence of previous meningitis. F. Allport,[8] H. Schmidt,[9] F. W. Coleman,[10] and H. Bickerton[11] are strongly in favor of evisceration. The last is enthusiastic over the results obtained in 40 cases. Communications from Brudenell Carter and H. Juler, warmly commending the method, appear in his article. R. del Costello[12] states that the operation is preferable only in leucomatous eyes, and surgeons should be slow to abandon the safer and oftener indicated enucleation. H. Claiborne,[13] has substituted glass-wool and asbestos for the glass ball of Mules, without success. Where removal of the ball and its contents is indicated he considers enucleation to be the better operation, although Belt[14] has had fair success with the substitution of a fine, soft sponge, which, he says, fills with new tissue, the sponge-fibers being apparently absorbed. A. Bourgeois[15] condemns Mules' operation because of the danger of sympathetic inflammation from the resistless glass ball, and has substituted for it with success in 2 cases the employment, after a modified enucleation, of a ball of black silk. The center or nucleus of the ball is made from a wad of catgut. Finally, E. Pflüger[16] believes that enucleation is the only operation that will insure against sympathetic ophthalmia.

Tattooing.—L. de Wecker[17] performs the operation of tattooing for 2 purposes—optical and cosmetic. Improvement of vision has been decidedly greater after iridectomy and tattooing than after iridectomy alone, because the total exclusion of the rays of light by a dense black patch prevents the irreg-

[1] Manhattan Eye and Ear Hosp. Rep., Jan , 1897.
[2] Jour. Am. Med. Assoc., Nov. 21, 1896.   [3] Medicine, May, 1897.
[4] Traité de Thérapeut. A. Robin, Paris. 1897.   [5] Thesis of Montpelier, 1896.
[6] Medicine, Jan., 1897.
[7] Internat. Med. Jour. of Australasia, Nov., 1896.
[8] Ann. of Ophth., July, 1897.   [9] Klin. Monatsbl. f. Augenh., Nov., 1896.
[10] N. Am. Pract, Aug., 1896.   [11] Brit. Med. Jour., Sept. 26, 1896.
[12] El Sigla Medico, Madrid, Dec. 13, 1896.   [13] Jour. Am. Med. Assoc., No. 21, 1896.
[14] Ibid., Nov. 7, 1896.   [15] Rec. d'Ophtal., June, 1897.
[16] Wien. klin. Woch., Feb. 18, 1897.   [17] Ann. d'Oculist., Aug., 1897.

PLATE 11.

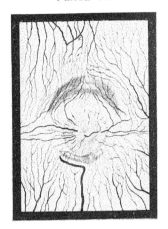

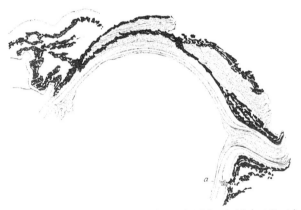

Subconjunctival injections : showing penetration of injected material about the globe
(Knapp's Arch. of Oph., July, 1897).

ular and imperfect refraction through a semitransparent spot. Care must be taken to accurately outline the spot and thoroughly saturate it with the ink.

THERAPEUTICS.

Subconjunctival injections of mercuric cyanid have been employed in checking panophthalmitis by Lagrange and Fromaget,[1] in vitreous opacities as well as in many diseases of the choroid and retina by Chavellereau,[2] and in hypopyon keratitis by J. Dunn.[3] Healing was wonderfully rapid in Dunn's case. [In one instance of ulcer cornea serpens one of the editors of this department had an absolutely parallel experience.] In a case of paralysis of the superior oblique followed by interstitial keratitis S. M. Payne[4] records the development of corneal inflammation while the patient was taking 75 gr. of potassium iodid daily for the muscular paralysis. After 4 injections of sublimate, aimed at the keratitis, the muscle completely regained its power. In those affections amenable to mercury internally, namely, iritis, iridocyclitis, iridochoroiditis, specific hyalitis, and optic neuritis, W. Wilder claims the subconjunctival treatment is particularly serviceable. The case of a 9-year-old boy with optic atrophy, whose vision Wilder improved from $\frac{20}{120}$ to $\frac{20}{40}$, is interesting. In the discussion before the Section on Ophthalmology of the American Medical Association of the value of subconjunctival injections of mercury E. H. Bernstein advocated the use of mercuric cyanid rather than bichlorid,[6] claiming for it quicker and more complete absorption. He finds this treatment to be of considerable use in infectious diseases of the anterior ocular segment and in specific iritis. DeSchweinitz, Baker, and Roy join him in this opinion, while Stirling, Savage, and Reynolds have had unfavorable experiences with this method. Impelled by the controversy over the rationale of subconjunctival injections C. Mellinger and D. Bossalino[7] introduced sterilized India ink beneath the conjunctivæ of rabbits, and demonstrated beyond cavil that fluids so introduced follow the greater lymph-spaces and surround the entire globe, the amount of ink actually entering the eyeball (see Plate 11) being small in comparison with the total amount injected. They believe that the fluids not only surround the eye and the optic nerve, but also communicate with the suprachoroidal and intravaginal spaces of the optic nerve. After having produced an ulcer in the center of the cornea in rabbits by injecting cultures of staphylococci, von Sicherer[8] treated one eye with subconjunctival injections of the various medicaments used for the purpose, leaving the other eye untouched. He found that the injections produced in fact a slight salutary effect, by causing a considerable leukocytosis around the infected focus. The simple 2% salt-solution is as effective as the more irritating salts, and deserves preference over these injections; but there is no necessity for the injections at all, as the same effect is produced by the simple application of a salve of the yellow oxid of mercury, followed by an occlusive dressing. The leukocytosis thus produced is equal in extent to that caused by any other method, and the ulcer heals as promptly. Wilder[9] says it is impossible to obtain as good results from salt as from bichlorid solutions. Abadie[10] repeats his injunctions against bichlorid solutions, and especially when iodoform is used

[1] Soc. anat. et Physiol. de Bordeaux, June 14, 1897.
[2] Traité de Thérapeut. A. Robin, Paris, 1897.
[3] Va. Med. Semi-monthly, Nov. 13, 1896.
[4] Manhattan Eye and Ear Hosp. Rep., 1897.   [5] Medicine, Dec., 1896.
[6] Jour. Am. Med. Assoc., Sept. 12, 1896.   [7] Arch. of Ophth., July, 1897.
[8] Rev. gén. d'Ophtal., Nov., 1896.   [9] N. Y. Med. Jour., Nov. 28, 1896.
[10] Eye, Ear, Nose, and Throat Clinic, Apr., 1897.

contemporaneously in purulent ophthalmia, on account of their evil effects on the cornea. He insists that boric acid and potassium permanganate 1 : 1000 are equally useful and not injurious. Galezowski[1] has abandoned mercurial injections in the treatment of syphilitic eye-affections, because he believes them inefficacious, dangerous, and likely to cause thrombi and erysipelas. D. Roy[2] feels that we cannot depend exclusively upon this treatment in ulcerative or interstitial keratitis, iritis, and lesions of the uvea, but as an adjuvant it is most useful.

Intravenous Injections.—Notwithstanding the urgent claims of Bacelli, who introduced the method of treatment of grave ocular syphilitic lesions by intravenous injections of mercury, that it is absolutely free from danger, Galezowski[3] urges against its adoption. He reasons that the insertion of the needle into the vein will cause erysipelas, the incorporation into the blood thrombi and embolism, and the absorption of mercury ptyalism of serious nature.

Yellow Oxid.—W. D. Babcock[4] has yellow ointment made according to the following formula: English graphite, 10 gr.; yellow oxid, 20 to 40 gr.; theobroma oil, $\frac{1}{2}$ oz.; antimony butter, 2 gtt. This prevents precipitation of the mercury and its decomposition by light. W. M. Sweet[5] finds that Jamieson's salve, consisting of 3 parts of lanolin, $\frac{1}{2}$ part of oil of sweet almond, $\frac{1}{2}$ part of distilled water, is not only a bland and soothing application in itself, but is a useful base for other eye-ointments. Coleman[6] prefers the red to the yellow oxid. While chemically the same, the latter commonly contains free sublimate. He states that experiments upon animals show that the yellow is more irritating than the red oxide.

Formol.—Compresses soaked in formol in increasing strength from 2% to 10% were effective in reducing the volume and cicatrizing the ulceration in an inoperable tumor of the face after failure of the cancer-serum of Emmerich-Scholl in a patient of Nieden.[7]

Serum.—The same writer has essayed the cure of recurring melanosarcoma of the eye and recurring glioma by injections of the cancer-serum, with negative results. Despagnet[8] treated 10 cases of diphtheric ophthalmia by means of serotherapy. He reports cure in 9 and loss of the cornea in 1.

Electrotherapy.—D. A. von Reuss'[9] method of electrotherapy is novel enough to merit description. In using the constant current he employs a small platinum disk slightly concave on one side, isolated entirely, except on the concave surface, with a coat of varnish. This plate is applied directly to the eyeball after it has been thoroughly cocainized. The positive or negative pole is used according as it is desired to obtain a greater or less degree of irritation. Treatment should be from 60 to 80 seconds of 1 to 1$\frac{1}{2}$ ma. every other day. This method has proved in his hands very beneficial to episcleritis. His use of the faradic current is also unique in that he has the patient take one of the electrodes in his hand while the operator takes the other, and then with the free hand gently presses upon or strokes the closed lids. In this manner great relief from pain was afforded in recent iritis and in iridocyclitis. In a case of inflammatory glaucoma two applications dispelled all the symptoms. In a case of episcleritis periodica fugax (Fuchs) that had resisted all recognized treatment less than a dozen faradizations were necessary to dissipate the symptoms. These results are unusual, and ought

[1] Rec. d'Ophtal., Dec., 1896.   [2] Va. Med. Semi-monthly, Oct. 9, 1896.
[3] Rec. d'Ophtal., Dec., 1896.   [4] Ophth. Rec., Aug., 1897.
[5] Phila. Polyclinic, Feb. 14, 1897.   [6] N. Am. Pract., Aug., 1896.
[7] Arch. d'Ophtal., Oct., 1896.   [8] Ibid., Dec., 1896.   [9] Beitr. z. Augenh., July, 1896.

to prompt investigators to renew their efforts in the electrotherapy of the eye.

Heat and Cold.—W. C. Posey[1] lays down the following rules for the application of cold and heat in ocular disorders : cold in the form of compresses in hyperemia of the conjunctiva, in the early stage of purulent ophthalmia (unless there is corneal involvement), after penetrating wounds of the eye, especially when the iris and lens have been injured. Moist heat is to be used in the later stages of purulent ophthalmia and pannus, in all forms of keratitis, in suppurative ophthalmitis, in muscular asthenopia, and in secondary iritis ; while the primary form of iritis will be found more amenable to dry heat. Hot applications are to be avoided when there is any tendency to disease of the deeper structures, for fear of adding to the congestion of these delicate membranes. With healthy eyes it matters little whether cold or warm water be used to bathe the eyes.

Curettage.—T. H. Pleasants[2] endorses Santarnecchi's method[3] of hydraulio curettage in the treatment of corneal ulcers.

Antipyrin.—A. Sallard[4] does not agree with Valude as to the good results of hypodermic injections of antipyrin in optic-nerve atrophy, and prefers injections of strychnin sulfate.

Homatropin.—The use of homatropin, 2–5 %, as a cycloplegic is preferred to that of the other mydriatics by Jackson,[5] when instilled by the surgeon himself, by dropping 1 to 2 drops on the upper corneal border every 5 minutes until 6 applications are made. He finds it entirely reliable, and its brevity of action is a great advantage. On the other hand, H. F. Hansell[6] says that it cannot be relied upon to paralyze accommodation completely in young persons.

Scopolamin.—For quick pupillary dilatation in incipient iritis C. A. Oliver[7] prefers scopolamin hydrobromate to atropin. Where prolonged use of such drugs is necessary the alternate use of scopolamin and atropin seems the best method. The duration of the healing and soothing powers is not so lasting with the former as with the latter.

Ichthyol.—In 3 % solution or ointment ichthyol has been found serviceable in Panas' clinic in catarrhal conjunctivitis, phlyctenular and follicular conjunctivitis, and in blepharitis. Its action is astringent and antiseptic.[8] G. D. Jacovides[9] recommends it in 50 % solution or in ointment, 2.5 to 5 gr. in 100 gr. vaselin, in the treatment of the various forms of conjunctivitis.

NEW REMEDIES.

Holocain.—This new aspirant for anesthetic honors is, like phenacetin and lactophenin, a synthetic derivative of phenetedin. According to Tauber,[10] it is feebly soluble in water, is neutral in reaction, and should be warmed in porcelain vessels. 1 % solutions remain clear for 2 months. R. Kuthe[11] has used it in 45 eyes for removal of foreign bodies, and Gutmann,[12] in tenotomies, discissions, tattooing of the cornea, and galvanocautery work, with great satisfaction. R. Heinz[13] pronounces it a protoplasmic poison, stating that it arrests ameboid movements, and that it is also inimical to bacterial growth in the

[1] Univ. Med. Mag., Aug., 1896.
[2] Cleveland Med. Gaz., July, 1897.
[3] Ann. d'Oculist, Sept., 1895.
[4] Rev. de Thér., Sept. 15, 1896.
[5] Jour. Am. Med. Assoc., Nov. 21, 1896.
[6] Am. Jour. Ophth., xiii., 8, 1896.
[7] Am. Jour. Med. Sci., Nov., 1896.
[8] Munch. med. Woch., Feb. 23, 1897.
[9] Thèse de Paris, 1896.
[10] Centralbl. f. prakt. Augenh., Jan. 1, 1897.
[11] Ibid., Feb., 1897.
[12] Deut. med. Woch., Mar. 11, 1897.
[13] Centralbl. f. prakt. Augenh., Mar., 1897.

strength of $\frac{1}{10}\%$ solution. 1% solution will arrest putrefaction or fermentation completely, thus rendering unnecessary any preliminary sterilization in operations. [If these last two statements are verified, we have been presented with an ideal local anesthetic.] A large number of experiments with 5% solution caused no intoxicating symptoms. Anesthesia supervenes 1 to 3 minutes after the use of a 1% solution, and lasts 10 minutes. Gutmann[1] remarks that the pupil, ocular tension, and accommodation are unchanged. The advantages over cocain are its inherent antiseptic qualities, its rapid action, the preservation of the corneal epithelium, and no after-effects. These statements are substantiated by the labors of Hirschfeld[2] and Lowenstamm.[3] It must not be forgotten that subcutaneously the drug is an active poison, though this does not lessen its efficiency and safety in ocular practice. Brudenell Carter[4] used holocain once for cataract-extraction and once for slitting the canaliculus, securing complete anesthesia in each instance in 4 minutes. There was no particular effect on the conjunctival blood-vessels, the pupil, or the accommodation.

Eucain.—This other claimant for the position now occupied by cocain is endorsed by J. E. Jennings[5] as superior to the latter because it does not decompose when kept in solution, is rendered aseptic by boiling, is less poisonous, dilates the pupil but slightly, and does not paralyze the accommodation or denude the cornea of its epithelium. The only point in which it is inferior is that it causes smarting and conjunctival injection. Vollert,[6] on the other hand, tested eucain in Leber's clinic, and found that it produces a considerable mydriasis, is similar to cocain in its action, and affects the corneal epithelium much more than cocain. He thinks that eucain will hardly find a place in ophthalmology, and quotes Hirschberg, who for a while used it for removing foreign bodies, but has discarded it. These views of Vollert and Hirschberg are shared by J. E. Willetts,[7] F. Wustfeld,[8] and Best.[9]

Mydrol.—Mydrol, or iodothylate of phenylpyrazolin, is offered as a new mydriatic by Cattaneo.[10] It dilates the pupil slightly, anesthetizes the conjunctiva but not the cornea, partially paralyzes the ciliary muscle, diminishes tension in strong solution, and enlarges the palpebral fissure, the effects disappearing entirely in 20 to 36 hours. He recommends it for ophthalmoscopy.

Scopolamin.—C. A. Oliver[11] recommends scopolamin hydrobromate in 1% solution as the best mydriatic in plastic iritis and the best cycloplegic for refraction. C. S. Hawkes[12] noticed sleepiness and delirium with hallucinations of sight and hearing in a young person after the absorption by the conjunctiva of 2 tablets of scopolamin hydrobromate, each containing $\frac{1}{100}$ gr.

Argentamin.—According to K. Hoor,[13] argentamin, in 3% to 5% watery solution once or twice a day, or oftener if required, seems, by reason of its alkalinity, to possess all the advantages of silver nitrate without any of its disadvantages.

Formalin.—E. O. Belt[14] and S. Burnett[15] both add their testimony to the efficiency of formalin in from 1 : 1500 to 1 : 3000 solution in arresting corneal ulceration.

[1] Loc. cit.
[2] Klin. Monatsbl. f. Augenh., May, 1897.
[3] Therap. Monatsh., May, 1897.
[4] Lancet, May 22, 1897.
[5] Am. Jour. Ophth., Dec., 1896.
[6] Münch. med. Woch., No. 22, 1896.
[7] Am. Jour. Ophth., July, 1897.
[8] Münch. med. Woch., Dec., 1896.
[9] Deutsch. med. Woch., Sept., 1896.
[10] Ophth. Rev., Sept., 1896.
[11] Am. Jour. Med. Sci., Nov., 1896.
[12] Ann. d'Oculist., July, 1897.
[13] Klin. Monatsbl. f. Augenh., July, 1896.
[14] Med. News, Sept. 5, 1896.
[15] Therap. Gaz., Nov. 16, 1896.

NEW INSTRUMENTS.

Colored Glasses.—S. B. Allen's studies[1] lead him to believe that not the light- but the heat-rays do most harm to the eye. Redness of the disk and of the retina to the nasal side of the disk are the resulting changes. He hopes to compass the difficulty by having constructed 2 thin surfaces of lightly smoked glass containing a solution of alum between them, as he has found that this solution has the property of cutting off the heat-rays. [If alum has this effect, it occurs to us that lenses ground from glass into which ammonioferric alum enters as a constituent would fulfil the purpose.]

Axonometer.—Williams[2] has devised an apparatus for the rapid and accurate determination of the axis of a cylinder worn in glasses or spectacles. [The objection to the instrument is that since a large proportion of corrections are compound, and since the spherical must be determined in the usual way with lenses from the test-case, it has little value.]

Bifocals.—Bourgeois[3] commends superimposed double spectacles for patients requiring two corrections, in which the near correction shall be a single lens and the distance-correction equal to the combined strength of both lenses. Thus, in a cataract-patient who accepts + 10 D. for distance and + 16 D. for near work, he places the near correction in a permanent frame and − 6 D. in the movable portion that is joined by a pair of hinges to the upper rim of the frame and can be raised and lowered at will. [This cannot compare with the lenticular bifocal (cemented bifocal) in any of its features.]

Binocular Lens.—E. Jackson[4] offers a binocular lens, to be used with oblique illumination, which consists of 2 segments of planoconvex lenses of from 20 D. to 40 D. joined at an angle of 20 to 30 degrees. It gives a magnification of from 8 to 15 diameters, but its chief advantage is the impression it conveys of the depth of the object surveyed. [In furnishing the third dimension, this instrument adds not a little to the accuracy ordinarily obtainable in inspection of the anterior section of the eye.

Ophthalmoscopic Mirror.—The same author also suggests that to obviate the annoying reflex from the sight-hole of the ophthalmoscopic mirror a thin piece of glass should be cemented to the glass of the sight-hole, and that its edges should extend beyond the margin of the opening in the silvering.[5]

Skiascopy.—Instruments to facilitate skiascopy are offered by Mitchell[6] and by J. E. Jennings.[7] The former is light and cheap, the latter cumbersome and expensive.

Accommodation-stick.—A. E. Prince[8] adds to our armamentarium a combined age- and refraction-scale for the rapid determination of accommodation (see Fig. 66).

Combination Spectacle and Hand Reading-glass.—C. Koller[9] describes a combination of a spectacle and hand reading-glass, which he devised to facilitate reading with defective vision. It is based on the observation that vision of at least $\frac{6}{24}$ is necessary to the discernment of ordinary type. He accomplished his object by mounting a very strong convex lens, 15 to 30 D., in a 2-inch tube fitted into the eye of an ordinary spectacle-frame (see Fig. 67).

Clinoscope.—The clinoscope recently devised by G. T. Stevens[10] meas-

[1] N. Y. Med. Jour., Oct. 10, 1896.　　[2] Boston M. and S. Jour., Jan. 14, 1897.
[3] Rec. d'Ophtal., Aug., 1896.　　[4] Ann. Ophth. and Otol., Oct., 1896.
[5] Ophth. Rec., June, 1897.　　[6] Ibid., Feb., 1897.
[7] Ann. of Ophth., Jan., 1897.　　[8] Arch. f. Ophth., Jan., 1897.
[9] Ann. Ophth. and Otol., Oct., 1896.　　[10] Arch. of Ophth., Apr., 1897.

ures the torsion of the eyes when gazing at a fixed object with the axes of vision presumably parallel. The instrument is practically useful in examining for functional anomalies, or for paralysis or paresis of one or more of the ocular muscles.

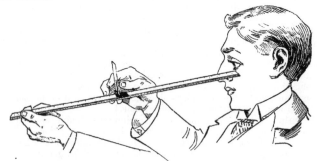

FIG. 66.—Prince's combined age- and refraction-scale (Arch. of Ophth., Jan., 1897).

Advancement.—Valk[1] likes a double hook for elevating and stretching the muscle to be advanced. He uses catgut instead of silk sutures, and one needle in taking the tuck in the muscle.

Speculum.—R. Murdoch[2] adds to his speculum a small fixation-forceps, which he can attach to the speculum for steadying the eyeball during iridectomy for cataract.

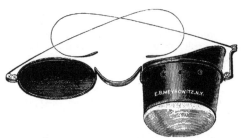

FIG. 67.—Koller's combination spectacle and hand-glass (Ann. Ophth. and Otol., Oct., 1896).

Photography.—Th. Guilloz[3] has completed an apparatus for instantaneous photography of the fundus oculi. The photographs show a reversed image, from which the author has succeeded in eliminating the reflection from the cornea and the optic disk.

[1] Med. Rec., Nov. 7, 1896. [2] Ann. Ophth. and Otol., July, 1896.
[3] Am. Jour. Med. Sci., Nov., 1896.

OTOLOGY.

By CHARLES H. BURNETT, M. D.,

OF PHILADELPHIA.

During the past year many valuable articles have been written upon diseases of the external ear, the most important of them pertaining to foreign bodies in the auditory canal, malignant diseases of all parts of the external ear, and myringodermatitis. The last-named disease may be easily overlooked. It is likely to occur in measles, and in this disease, therefore, myringodermatitis should be looked for. The most important of all diseases, acute otitis media, has received widespread attention. Since upon the prevention, or upon the proper treatment, of this disease depend the hearing, and in some instances the life of the patient, the importance of this malady cannot be overestimated. The secondary results in many of the cases reported do not seem to have been necessary. They tend to show that too much caution cannot be observed in the avoidance of all forms of irritant treatment, nor too close an adherence to conservative, aseptic measures in acute otitis media. It is a regrettable fact that much of the secondary infection of an acutely inflamed ear is due to the domestic treatment, always septic, the patient receives before the physician is called in. The latter must bear in mind, therefore, that usually in such cases he has to combat at the outset of his services artificial lesions of an inflamed organ.

The great advantages of intratympanic surgery in chronic purulent and in some forms of chronic catarrhal otitis media continue to be shown by numerous reports of the results obtained by reliable operators, to which reference is made in the following pages. The brilliant results of surgical interference in otitic lesions of the cranial cavity are also demonstrated by a review of the writings of both general and special surgeons in Europe and America. In fact, the literature of otology for the past year shows that important advances have been made in every department of this specialty.

DISEASES OF THE EXTERNAL EAR.

Malformation of the Auricle.—J. F. Binnie[1] has reported a case of microtia on both sides in an adult man, without much evidence of the presence of an osseous auditory canal on either side; also a case of malposed auricle (below the normal position) associated with harelip. Max[2] reports rectification of malformation of the auricle by operation, under cocain-anesthesia. An **acquired circular defect** in the auricle near the bifurcation of the antihelix, the consequence of an ulcer, is reported by the same writer.[3]

Othematoma, cured by incision of the sac and packing, is reported by G. A. Webster.[4] A. D. McConachie[5] reports the occurrence of 3 cases of

---

[1] Ann. of Surg., Aug., 1896.
[2] Aust. Otol. Soc. ; Jour. Laryn., Rhinol. and Otol., 1896.
[3] Wien. med. Woch., Nov. 7, 1896.   [4] Boston M. and S. Jour., Oct. 8, 1896.
[5] Jour. Eye, Ear, and Throat Dis., vol. i., No. 3.

hematoma auris in the sane. In the first case the blood-tumor was considered to be an idiopathic one. The sac was opened 3 times, refilling twice; but the third time injections of carbolic acid solution (strength not given) were followed by agglutination of the perichondrium to the cartilage, and healing with considerable deformity. No history of traumatism could be found in this case. In the second case, traumatism being the cause of the formation of the blood-tumor, prompt incision without injections was not followed by healing. Finally, after several incisions, recovery followed an injection of a carbolic acid solution and tight bandaging. There was considerable deformity of the auricle subsequently. In the third case, also caused by violence, prompt incision, evacuation, and firm bandaging were followed by quick recovery with the usual puckering of the auricle. L. P. Clark [1] regards the occurrence of hematoma arising in the insane as justifying a very grave prognosis. W. F. Robertson [2] has demonstrated that degenerative areas in the cartilage of the auricles occur in the insane, and that hematoma may occur easily without the aid of anything that could be fairly termed traumatism. An ordinary slight touch on the auricle of the insane may produce traumatism.

Degenerate Auricle.—Scientists and neurologists, however, are forced to lay little stress upon the occurrence of any one or two stigmata. It is only the combination of several that is indicative of a corresponding degeneration of the cerebral tract.[3]

Angioma of the Auricle.—J. Gruber [4] reports the occurrence of an angioma, mistaken at first for a sebaceous tumor, in the concha of a man. The growth was attacked by incisions through the skin as for removal of a sebaceous cyst, the profuse hemorrhage revealing its true nature. The contents were scraped away, little blood was lost, and under iodoform-compresses recovery took place quickly.

Keloids of the Auricle.—W. Scheppegrell [5] reports 2 cases of keloid tumor of the auricle, the result of piercing the lobule for earrings. The tumors were removed after local injections of a 4% solution of cocain muriate. There were no recurrences after 6 and 14 months respectively.

Lupus of the Auricle.—Ciarrocchi [6] reports a case of lupus pernio of the left auricle in a man of 35. It was relieved by the use of ignipuncture with the thermocautery of Paquelin and cataplasms of rice-water.

Hemorrhagic Ecthyma of the Auricle.—Two cases of partial necrosis of the auricle, the so-called "ecthyma térébrant" of infancy, are reported by O. Barnick [7] as occurring in the clinic of Habermann, in Gratz. The patients were 3 and 4 years old respectively, and died shortly after the aural condition was noted, of chronic tuberculosis of the glands and bones. In each instance the disease began on the front surface of the helix, and extended from this point, gradually spreading until it reached and implicated the hairy scalp above and the skin below the auricle. In the pus from these latter ulcers tubercle-bacilli were found.

Epithelioma of the Auricle.—Compaired [8] reports 2 cases of epithelioma of the auricle and auditory canal, cured by amputation, followed by treatment with potassium chlorate. Roncali [9] reports a case of melanotic sarcoma

[1] Am. Medico-Surg. Bull., Aug. 22, 1896.   [2] Brit. Med. Jour., Sept. 26, 1896.
[3] Editorial in Am. Med. Rev.; see Laryngoscope, vol. i., No. 4.
[4] Aust. Otol. Soc.; Jour. Laryn., Rhinol. and Otol., 1896.
[5] N. Y. Med. Jour., Oct. 17, 1896.   [6] Arch. Ital. di Otol., Jan., 1897.
[7] Arch. f. Ohrenh., Apr. 9, 1897.
[8] First Spanish Oto-rhinol. Cong., Nov., 1896; Ann. des Mal. de l'Oreille, May, 1897.
[9] Arch. Ital. di Otol., Jan., 1897.

of the auricle, which spread from the zygomatic region to this part of the ear, and thence to the middle ear, notwithstanding an operation on the auricle early in the disease.

Artificial Diseases of the Lobule.—According to Vior-Travieso,[1] gangrene, noma, septic phlegmons, chronic exudative erysipelas, and eczema, both humid and impetiginous, are caused by the ordinary septic method of piercing the lobule of the ear.

Congenital Aural Fistula.—A case of congenital aural fistula or sinus, with recurring inflammation, is reported by A. H. Cheatle.[2] Under a general anesthetic this sinus was laid open, all suspicious-looking membrane cut away, the cavity thoroughly mopped with pure carbolic acid, and the whole wound packed with double cyanid gauze and allowed to heal from the bottom. In 1 month recovery had taken place.

Reflex Effect of Cerumen Plugs.—R. W. Merrick[3] reports the occurrence of ear-cough, deafness, vertigo, and nausea from the presence of hard cerumen in the ear. He thinks that in nervous patients a melancholic form of dysthymia may be produced by mechanical irritation in the external ear.

Epidermis-plugs in the Ear.—H. Hessler[4] reports 35 cases of epidermis-plugs in the external ear observed in his own practice within the last 17 years. These foreign bodies of endogenous origin are best removed with a hooked instrument; not by syringing, as fluids cause them to swell. Their instrumental removal, however, should not be attempted by any one but an expert, as improper force in such an operation may cause fatal irritation.

Herpes of the Meatus.—Herpes at the orifice of the external auditory canal is reported by L. S. Somers.[5] This was cured by tonics and the local application of yellow oxid of mercury.

Foreign Bodies in the Ear.—Preobraschensky[6] presents safe conclusions regarding extraction of foreign bodies from the ear that can be summed up by saying that no inexpert hand should attempt instrumental extraction, and that syringing will usually remove a foreign body if it has not been previously impacted by unskilful efforts at removal with instruments. Letting alone foreign substances in the ear is far better than inexperienced efforts to get them out. Yearsley[7] observed severe ear-pain resulting from the entrance of a pellet of wool through a perforation in the membrana tympani in a case of chronic purulent otitis media. The wool had been inserted into the meatus for protection, but slipped into the canal and thence into the drum-cavity. Upon removal of the foreign substance all acute inflammation disappeared. Lalatta,[8] in an article on foreign bodies, demonstrates by 3 cases how innocuous an inanimate foreign body in the ear is, so long as it is not touched by an unskilful hand. No endeavor at removal is better than rough and unskilful ones.

Hummel,[9] in a lecture on foreign bodies in the ear, delivered to military surgeons, formulates these conclusions: 1. There is no reaction between the normal auditory canal and the foreign body placed in it; as such, the foreign substance is unattended with danger. 2. Therefore, every hasty endeavor at removal is not only unnecessary, but may be injurious. 3. In all cases in which no rough endeavors at removal are made, syringing with warm water is

---

[1] First Spanish Oto-rhinol. Cong., Nov., 1896.   [2] Arch. of Otol., Apr., 1897.
[3] Brit. Med. Jour., Oct. 10, 1896.   [4] Arch. f. Ohrenh., Dec., 1896, and Feb., 1897.
[5] Am. Medico-Surg. Bull., Oct. 31, 1896.
[6] Wien. klin. Rundschau, 33–36, 1896; Times and Register, Mar. 20, 1897.
[7] Brit. Med. Jour., Sept. 26, 1896.   [8] Arch. Ital. di Otol., Jan., 1897.
[9] Münch. med. Woch., Apr. 27, 1897.

sufficient to remove the foreign body. 4. The general physician should never employ anything but the syringe to remove foreign bodies from the ear. 5. An instrumental removal should never be attempted by any one but a specialist skilled in the use of ear-specula and the technic necessary in such cases.

Fracture of the External Auditory Canal.—Galetti[1] has contributed an account of 5 cases of indirect fracture of the external auditory canal. The prognosis is generally favorable; there is, however, danger in some instances, of injury to the cerebral meninges. Denker[2] observed a fracture of the anterior lower wall of the auditory canal, caused by the force of a fall upon the lower jaw. The blood was removed by syringing with an antiseptic solution (bichlorid 1 : 1000), and the ear gently tamponed with iodoform-gauze. Recovery soon took place. [This is a rare form of accident to the ear.] Ostmann[3] has treated successfully connective-tissue **strictures of the auditory canal** by means of electrolysis with a current of 4–5 ma. in four or five sittings at intervals of 8–10 days.

Hyperostosis of the external auditory meatus, according to A. Hartmann,[4] is simply an anomaly of development, and has nothing to do with inflammatory or morbid processes. J. Dunn[5] has operated successfully by way of the mastoid upon hyperostosis of the auditory canal, caused by chronic purulency of the middle ear.

Respiratory Movements in the Membrana Tympani.—V. Hammerschlag[6] has demonstrated that there are normally motions in the membrana tympani synchronous with the respirations and pulsations of the heart. E. Donaldson[7] describes a flaccid cicatrix in the membrana tympani, movable with respiration, observed by him in a woman of 25. This condition was a variable one, and whenever observed was attended with autophony. B. Gomperz[8] draws attention to the fact that subjects of valvular occlusion of the Eustachian tubes suffer at times from modified tensions (bulging) of the upper posterior quadrant of the membrana, accompanied by sensations of tension or compression in the ears and tinnitus. Masini[9] reports the occurrence of **aural myoclonus** in 3 men, all the subjects of marked dyspepsia and neurasthenia. L. S. Somers[10] reports a case of autotraumatic **rupture of the membrana tympani.** The deafness was finally relieved some weeks after the accident by drawing the impacted membrana into proper isolation by the pneumatic speculum. [No secondary infection had occurred in this case, as nothing was dropped or put into the ear after the traumatic perforation ensued.] C. J. Colles[11] reports 2 cases of traumatic rupture of the drum-head from the concussion caused by a discharge of artillery. [Both of these cases would have done much better if the ears had not been syringed immediately after the rupture of the membrane before they were seen by Colles. Simple stopping the meatus with antiseptic cotton or gauze is sufficient in such cases.]

Syphilitic Exudation in the Membrana.—J. Dunn[12] reports the occurrence of syphilitic exudation into the folds of mucous membrane about the head of the malleus. The patient was a man with syphilitic history and chronic catarrhal deafness in the affected ear. The exudation was confined to the region of the membrana flaccida and malleus. It was attended with pain in the ear and mastoid tenderness. Pricking the exudation-sac and the ad-

[1] Arch. Ital. di Otol., Jan., 1897.   [2] Arch. f. Ohrenh., Feb., 1897.
[3] Berlin. klin. Woch., Aug. 24, 1896.   [4] Arch. of Otol., Jan., 1897.
[5] Va. Med. Semi-monthly, Feb. 26, 1897.   [6] Wien. med. Woch., Sept. 19, 1896.
[7] Lancet, Oct. 10, 1896.
[8] Aust. Otol. Soc., June, 1896; Ann. des Mal. de l'Oreille, Jan., 1897.
[9] Arch. Ital. di Otol., Jan., 1897.   [10] Phila. Polyclinic, Mar. 6, 1897.
[11] Am. Medico-Surg. Bull., Dec. 5, 1896.   [12] Va. Med. Semi-monthly, Aug. 7, 1896.

ministration of potassium iodid were followed by recovery. Courtade[1] has observed in hereditary syphilis, in a woman of 21, intense injection in Shrapnell's membrane and of the handle of the malleus.

B. Gomperz[2] succeeded in bringing about the **closure of chronic perforations** in the membrana in 4 cases out of 10 in which the effort was made by touching their edges with trichloracetic acid preceded by local anesthesia with 10 % solution of cocain. [As no advantage is to be gained by the closure of such perforations, we wonder at the time wasted on such experiments.]

Myringodermatitis.—J. E. Sheppard[3] calls attention to the important fact that a form of inflammation in the outer layer of the drum-membrane may exist with the formation of blebs either behind or below the malleus. [We have found such conditions of not uncommon occurrence, and suggest for them the name of myringodermatitis. They occur in measles and from exposure to cold winds or cold-water baths. In cases we have treated, dry heat has controlled the pain, while spontaneous rupture of the blebs has been awaited. Paracentesis has not been found necessary in our cases. If, in performing paracentesis of the blebs, the perforation should be carried into the drum-cavity, a secondary inflammation of this cavity would certainly follow. Spontaneous rupture of the blebs is likely to occur within 24 hours.]

DISEASES OF THE MIDDLE EAR.

Etiology of Acute Otitis Media.—J. Holinger[4] claims that in all cases acute otitis media is largely due to adenoids in the nasopharynx. These are primarily the seat of acute inflammation in coryza, and even in the infectious diseases of childhood, the sepsis spreading from them to the middle ear. In all instances treatment and cure of the ear-disease must therefore be preceded by treatment and cure of the nasopharyngeal adenoid inflammation. [This is true to some extent, but we often see perfectly healthy ears, with normal functions, become the seat of acute inflammation as the result of the treatment of nasopharyngeal catarrh, adenoids, etc.] Lannois[5] has shown we cannot establish any pathologic differences between acute catarrhal and acute purulent otitis; the same microbes determine both conditions, and it is merely a question of resistance of the organism. A case of acute otitis media caused by the nasal douche, with distinct secondary infection of the middle ear and mastoid cavities by improper treatment of the inflamed ear, necessitating mastoid trepanation finally after 4 months of pain, is reported by C. H. Burnett.[6] Acute otitis media followed by mastoiditis and an epidural abscess, entirely relieved by operation, is reported by J. E. H. Nichols.[7] A case of acute purulent otitis media complicated by a retropharyngeal abscess, which apparently had formed by burrowing along the tract of the tensor tympani muscle, was observed by F. L. Stillman.[8] The abscess was discharged into the pharynx, and entire recovery of the patient in all particulars ensued in the course of 2 months after the initial inflammation in the ear.

Acute otitis media, followed by mastoiditis in the course of 2 months, unrelieved by operation, is reported by Grunert and Leutert.[9] Ten days after the mastoid-operation the patient died with symptoms of meningitis. The autopsy revealed chronic leptomeningitis, with edema of the pia mater. [It

---

[1] Jour. de Méd. de Paris, Dec. 6, 1896.   [2] Wien. klin. Woch., Sept., 1896.
[3] Am. Medico-Surg. Bull., Feb. 25, 1897.   [4] Chicago Med. Rec., Aug., 1896.
[5] Ann. des Mal. de l'Oreille, June, 1896; Jour. Laryn., Rhinol. and Otol., Dec., 1896.
[6] Phila. Polyclinic, July 11, 1896.   [7] Manhattan Eye and Ear Hosp. Rep., Jan., 1897.
[8] N. Y. Med. Jour., Feb. 6, 1897.   [9] Arch. f. Ohrenh., June, 1897.

would be interesting to know what treatment was applied to the ear in the acute stage of inflammation. We have never observed mastoiditis succeed acute otitis, except as the artificial result of improper treatment of the primary otitis.]

Middle Ear in Diphtheria.—In 25 autopsies upon children who had died of true diphtheria E. Lommel[1] found only 1 case in which the middle ear was unaffected. He concluded, therefore, that otitis forms part of the clinical picture of diphtheritic inflammation of the respiratory tract.

Diagnosis of Acute Otitis Media.—The importance of early diagnosis and treatment of inflammation of the middle ear, especially in children, is pointed out by J. H. Fruitnight.[2]

Richard Frothingham[3] shows that "on account of the anatomic relations of the middle ear and the gravity of some of the results of middle-ear disease, as regards not only permanent loss of hearing, but also danger to life, no part of the body is of more importance to all practitioners; and still there is no branch of medicine about which the majority of physicians know so little." He then gives a most significant list of incorrect diagnoses of ear-diseases he has known to be made within a short time, viz., "unrecognized acute middle-ear suppuration followed by meningitis;" acute mastoid disease diagnosed as "cellulitis;" furuncle of the canal diagnosed as "mastoid-disease;" "acute middle-ear suppuration" diagnosed and treated as "neuralgia;" otolgia dentalis diagnosed as "a gathering in the ear;" acute middle-ear suppuration diagnosed on the right, but the same disease on the left overlooked; polypus from Shrapnell's membrane the unrecognized cause of head-symptoms; polypus of the ear diagnosed as "chronic catarrhal disease;" acute middle-ear disease with a bulla of the membrane diagnosed as a "malignant growth;" and dried white desquamated epithelium in the canal diagnosed as "the ossicles coming out."

Treatment of Acute Otitis Media.—N. H. Pierce,[4] in an article on the modern pathology and treatment of acute otitis media, presents a valuable reiteration of the rational treatment of acute otitis media as set forth by Gradenigo and Pes and Lermoyez and Helme (see *Year-Book* for 1896, pp. 836–841), by which secondary infection and chronicity are avoided. Briefly, this means apply no local anodyne-treatment to the ear, as it is useless and harmful: employ dry heat. If pain continues without spontaneous rupture in 12 hours, puncture the drum-membrane at the lower posterior border; then do nothing but place a thin strip of antiseptic gauze in the canal, a tuft of the same in the concha, and let the ear alone till the dressings are moist with secretions; then remove and renew them. Avoid all forms of inflation of the tympana, as well as all forms of aspiration, swabbings, etc. Timely remarks in the same direction upon the modern and rational (nonirritative) treatment of acute otitis media are also made by R. Otto.[5] Karminski[6] enjoins upon aurists the greatest care in avoiding infection of the acutely inflamed ear. He shows that the staphylococcus is often conveyed to the ear by the finger of the surgeon, by instruments, and by medications. R. W. Seiss[7] makes an earnest plea for conservative treatment in acute otitis media, maintaining justly that lavage of and syringing the inflamed ear can be done properly only by the aurist. D. M. Campbell[8] demonstrates the value of cautious aseptic treatment in acute and chronic catarrhal diseases of the nose and ear in children.

[1] Arch. of Otol., Apr., 1897.   [2] Med. News, Sept. 12, 1896.
[3] Med. Rec., Aug. 8, 1896.   [4] Jour. Am. Med. Assoc, Dec. 19, 1896.
[5] St. Petersburg. med. Woch., Sept. 21, 1896.
[6] First Spanish Oto-Rhinol, Cong., Nov., 1896.   [7] Univ. Med. Mag., Apr., 1897.
[8] Physician and Surgeon, Feb., 1897.

Acute Otitis Media in Acute Polyarthritic Rheumatism.—O. Wolf[1] claims that acute otitis media is often a prodrome of acute articular rheumatism, and suggests that the bacteriologist in searching for the microbe of polyarthritis should examine the secretions taken from the drum-cavity immediately after paracentesis of the membrane has been performed in a case of acute rheumatic otitis media.

Complications of Acute Otitis Media.—J. E. Sheppard[2] has given an instructive "analysis of 114 cases of mastoid involvement complicating acute middle-ear suppuration . . . . of less than 6 weeks' duration;" 51 were operated upon by Sheppard, 3 were operated upon by others, 1 died without operation, 34 recovered without operation, while the result in 25 is unknown. Sheppard makes the following summary based on the above very large number of cases of what may be termed acute mastoiditis: 1. For opening the mastoid the gouge or the chisel has invariably been used, excepting when the cortex was so much softened as to make the sharp curet more applicable; 2. For clearing out the mastoid sharp curets were used for the outer, the blunt curet for the deep portions; 3. Grippe, outside of the acute affections of the nose and nasopharynx due to cold, etc., has played the most important role in the etiology. Of those operated upon, 4 died; 2 from meningitis about 3 days after operation, 1 from erysipelas and then meningitis 2–3 weeks after operation, and 1 from erysipelas 2 weeks after operation. 4. The symptoms are important in about the following order: (*a*) pain in the mastoid, or in some part of the affected half of the head; (*b*) tenderness, either of the whole or of some part of the mastoid (oftenest of the apex); (*c*) drooping or bulging of the posterior superior canal wall, especially if close to the membrane; (*d*) posterior superior perforation of the membrane, especially if pointing or teat-like; (*e*) pulsating tinnitus, when it continues as a marked symptom after the time it should have ceased were the case a simple middle-ear suppuration; (*f*) the external symptoms are redness and edema of the mastoid, and pushing outward of the auricle; 5. Abortive measures should be employed in a majority of cases for from 2 to 5 days, and will be successful in curing a fair proportion of all cases. If these fail, then the conclusions are that " we must time and again operate on the strength of one or two symptoms, and often with these only slightly marked. If a patient is seen before the external manifestations of mastoiditis have developed, we should not wait for their appearance (symptoms of empyema being present), because by so doing we give the pus the same opportunity to break through the internal as through the external mastoid cortex, and while awaiting the latter event we leave the patient exposed to the former danger. The operation, if performed with due care, is relatively free from danger. Danger to the patient arises, not from the operation, but from delay in performing it."

Pyemia in Acute Otitis Media.—Röpke[3] reports a case of well-marked pyemia fully established in the third week of the aural disease. The secondary infection in this case was evidently due to the improper treatment of the ear in the acute stage of inflammation by syringing with chamomile-tea and poulticing, as ordered by the family physician. The local mastoid symptoms were largely negative. There was nearly constant pain in the left temple. The eye-ground was not examined. Chills, rapid rise and fall of temperature, the permanently rapid pulse, even in intervals of normal temperature, tumor of the spleen, and the dry, cracked, thickly coated tongue, were relied upon in establishing the diagnosis of otic pyemia from osteophle-

[1] Arch. f. Ohrenh., Dec., 1896.　　　　[2] Trans. Am. Otol. Soc., July, 1896.
[3] Arch. of Otol., Oct., 1896.

844   *OTOLOGY.*

bitis. Suppuration of the mastoid cells and probably acute necrosis of the
bone-tissue of this cavity were evidenced by the profuse discharge from the
ear and the tenderness of the mastoid to pressure. No external symptoms of
sinus-phlebitis were present. There was no edema, neither at the region of the
temple nor at the posterior boundary of the mastoid. The mastoid cavity and
antrum, when opened, were found filled with pus and granulations, and were
completely cleared out. The vertical portion of the lateral sinus was then
found to be exposed from necrosis of its bony covering. The sinus-wall was
free from disease, but it did not pulsate. It was punctured, but neither blood
nor pus was aspirated. It was evident that the thrombus thus shown to be
present was solid, and *further interference with it was deemed unadvisable.* The
wound was tamponed and bandaged. The temperature fell immediately, but
rose the next day to 39.8° C. after a chill. The spleen could not be felt.
From the 5th day after the operation the temperature remained normal. On
the 10th day the patient left her bed, and in one month she was dismissed
from the hospital entirely well, with very good hearing in the previously diseased ear. [But the secondary infection of the middle ear, from the improper
treatment of the ear in the acute stage of inflammation jeopardized the life of ·
the patient.]

Cerebral Abscess from Acute Otitis Media.—Gorham Bacon [1]
reports the occurrence of abscess in the temporosphenoidal lobe, in connection
with acute otitis media. The first symptom, loss of memory, occurred in
about the fifth week of the disease, and in the eighth week there ensued sensory but no motor aphasia, severe headache, and subnormal pulse. The temperature and pulse remained normal, but the mastoid was somewhat swollen
and tender. The latter was chiselled open with difficulty, as eburnation had
taken place, and the antrum freed from granulations and pus. In 10 days
the patient complained of general headache and became delirious at times.
Slight optic neuritis with faint edema was detected. An abscess was sought
for, found, and emptied, but the patient died, apparently from shock, about
10 hours after the operation. A communication was found to have formed
between the suppurating attic and the cranial cavity. W. Milligan [2] reports
a case of abscess of the same region of the brain, following acute otitis media.
The symptoms were similar to those in the case reported by Bacon, having,
however, motor, in addition to sensory aphasia. There was dilatation of the
left pupil—*i. e.*, on the affected side—a symptom frequently noted of late, viz.,
the wider pupil on the side corresponding to that of the brain affected with
abscess. The cerebral abscess was evacuated by operation. The patient did
well for nearly two months after the operation, when hernia cerebri occurred
and the patient died with symptoms of basal meningitis. The postmortem
examination revealed no erosion of the roof of the parietes of the middle ear
and no symptoms in the mastoid cells. "Apparently the pathogenic organisms had been carried directly from the middle ear to the interior of the
temporosphenoidal lobe by way of the lymphatics or small venous arteries,
no bone-lesion intervening." [In reflecting upon the notes of this case we feel
that the secondary infection of the ear, which passed to the brain at last, was
due to the three months of "various forms of local treatment which were
tried" before Milligan was consulted. Three months' trial of "various forms
of local treatment of an acutely inflamed ear could not fail to convey sepsis
to the ear and result in secondary infection, chronicity, and final infection of
the cranial cavity.]

¹ Trans. Am. Otol. Soc., July, 1896; Arch. of Otol., July, 1896.
² Arch. of Otol., July, 1896.

Meningitis in Acute Otitis Media.—H. Knapp[1] reports "a case of acute purulent otitis media in which marked symptoms of meningitis developed," and in which the opening of the mastoid and cranial cavities was followed by prompt improvement and subsequent recovery. No pus was found in this case, but the extensive area of "destructive osteitis in which suppuration might occur any day," discovered in the mastoid, antral, and sigmoid regions, seems to have justified the operation.

Meningismus in Acute Otitis Media.—Cozzolino[2] calls attention to the fact that very frequently pseudomeningeal symptoms, or meningismus, in young children are due to acute inflammation of the middle ear. In many of these cases perforation of the membrana tympani and discharge from the ear are wanting. It is claimed that this is due to the fact that the disease is produced by the Talamon-Fränkel microbe, which, possessing very feeble destructive power, the membrana is left intact, but the disease is perhaps all the more likely to travel to the internal ear and brain. [A paracentesis of the membrana in such cases would save the ear and the life of the patient.]

Facial Paralysis in Acute Otitis Media.—In a case of acute suppuration of the middle ear, followed by caries of the Fallopian tube and paralysis in five weeks, in which there had been most of that time intense pain but no fever, F. L. Jack[3] opened the mastoid cells, but found no pus, nor carious bone in the thick outer walls. Continuing the chiselling a quarter of an inch farther inward and forward a small pus-cavity was discovered in the Fallopian region. Under antiseptic irrigations and dressings the pain was entirely and promptly relieved, the temperature became normal, and the paralysis disappeared.

Cozzolino,[4] in an article on the "surgery of the Fallopian canal in cases of otitic facial paralysis," shows that in removing septic and phlogistic matter from the tympanic and mastoid zones of this canal the paralysis may be relieved. His method he terms "radical mastoidotomy," by which he frees the nerve from diseased bone surrounding it. It is worthy of note that Politzer[5] records two instances in which facial palsy due to chronic purulency in the middle ear was entirely cured by surgical exposure and thorough curetting of the suppurating ear-cavities. Geronzi[6] reports a case of facial paralysis of otitic origin followed in three years by labio-glosso-laryngeal paralysis from ascending degeneration of the seventh nerve on the same side, in a man of 45, of intemperate habits. O. Barnick[7] observed facial paralysis supervene after curetting the drum-cavity in a man of 40, in whose case the mastoid cavity was found to be the seat of a cholesteatoma metamorphosed into a blood-cyst. This case was finally cured after operation upon the middle-ear cavities and the mastoid process, clearing the spaces of a sanious fluid, and the formation of a permanent opening behind the ear. Eitelberg[8] reports the occurrence of facial paralysis, without aural suppuration, associated with Ménière-symptoms. These phenomena appeared in a man of 35, after a fall from a horse, but recovery ensued after months of treatment. It was thought that the facial paralysis might have been rheumatic, as it appeared shortly after a painful swelling of the cheek from a carious tooth.

Simulated Deafness.—Ostmann[9] demonstrates that minute acquaintance with otologic diagnosis ranks above all other means for the detection of aural malingering.

[1] Trans. Am. Otol. Soc., July, 1896.   [2] Med. Bull., Dec., 1896.
[3] Trans. Am. Otol. Soc., July, 1896.   [4] Arch. Ital. di Otol., Jan., 1897.
[5] Austr. Otol. Soc., June, 1896; Ann. des Mal. de l'Oreille, Jan., 1897.
[6] Arch. Ital. di Otol., Jan., 1897.   [7] Arch. f. Ohrenh., Apr., 1897.
[8] Ibid., Feb., 1897.   [9] Monats. f. Ohrenh., Sept., 1896.

Impaired Auditory Center.—Functional impairment of the auditory center as the result of catarrhal deafness is pointed out by J. A. Mullen.[1] [This is analogous to atrophy of the auditory center, supposed by some to occur in deaf-mutes.] F. Alt[2] reports **deafness from mumps** cured by potassium iodid, pilocarpin injections, and acoustic exercises. Gruber claims that bilateral deafness after mumps is incurable. J. L. Minor[3] has reported 8 cases of deafness following mumps. The left ear was affected in 5 of these; when the middle ear alone is attacked there is some hope of recovery of hearing. but there is none when the internal ear is the seat of the lesion. Trifiletti[4] describes a case of **deafness due to atheroma** of the arteries, and ascribes to the same cause the pathogenesis of senile deafness.

The Ear in Bright's Disease.—Haug[5] has reported a case of nasal and aural hemorrhage in Bright's disease from alcoholism. There first occurred very severe pain in both ears, together with tinnitus and some deafness, and then hemorrhages as above stated, especially in the drum-cavities.

A. H. Buck[6] in an elaborate paper presents the relations of goutiness to diseases of the ear, showing that this diathesis may induce disease in different portions of the organ of hearing.

Middle Ear in Malignant Disease of the Nasopharynx.—A case of fibrosarcoma of the nasopharynx and middle cerebral fossa, with associated ethmoiditis, empyema of the sphenoid cells, otitis media, and pachymeningitis, is reported by T. Hubbard.[7]

Gellé[8] claims that **ankylosis of the stapes** enfeebles but does not abolish hearing. Therefore, when deafness has become chronic, the stapes being ankylosed, the aurist is confronted with a lesion of the labyrinth or even of the brain causative of deafness. In his opinion this should call for hesitation before mobilization or removal of the stapes is effected, with a view to relieve the deafness. [Retraction and impaction of the stapes in the oval window are more important considerations than simple ankylosis of this bonelet.]

Treatment of Catarrhal and Sclerotic Diseases of the Middle Ear.—R. H. Fridenberg[9] suggests some hygienic principles in the prevention of ear-disease, consisting in maintaining an aseptic condition of the nasopharynx by treatment with gargles and sprays and the removal of any possible nidus for pathogenic germs, such as diseased tonsils, decayed teeth, etc. H. Jackson[10] calls attention to the great importance of carefully examining the nose, throat, and ear during the course of **scarlet fever**. There are pseudomembranous lesions of the palate, and these processes may spread to the postpharyngeal wall and, after invasion of the pharyngeal vault, to the nose. Such a process is usually found on the third or fourth day of the disease, and is the direct cause of the most alarming and fatal complications of scarlet fever, namely, septicemia, purulent otitis media, and infection of the cervical glands, besides serious kidney-lesions. He advises sprays of Dobell's solution for the mouth and nose. The nasal douche is condemned. In order to prevent infection of the mucous membrane of the middle ear, by forcing nasal mucus through the Eustachian catheter, A. Lucae[11] proposes to pass a

[1] Med. Age, Jan. 25, 1897.　　　　　　[2] Aust. Soc. of Otol., Oct. 27, 1896.
[3] N. Y. Med. Jour., Mar. 27, 1897.　　[4] Arch. Ital. di Otol., Jan., 1897.
[5] Deutsch. med. Woch., Nov. 5, 1896.　[6] N. Y. Med. Rec., May 22, 1897.
[7] Arch. of Otol., Apr., 1897. [This resembles a case observed by C. H. Burnett and Harrison Allen, and reported in the Transactions of the American Otological Society, 1881.]
[8] Soc. de Biol., Dec. 4, 1896; Ann. des Mal. de l'Oreille, Jan., 1897.
[9] Med. News, Aug. 6, 1896.　　　　　[10] Arch. of Otol., Apr., 1897.
[11] Arch. f. Ohrenh., June, 1897.

constant stream of air through the catheter during the introduction of the latter through the nose, thus keeping nasal secretions from the beak. [This current of air ceases, of course, as soon as the beak of the catheter reaches the nasopharynx and is about to be inserted into the mouth of the Eustachian tube, when a renewed air-current is demanded.] E. Morpurgo,[1] as a result of careful observation of cases in the Marine Hospital at Trieste, concludes that sea-baths exercise a beneficial effect upon ear-diseases in the **scrofulous.** B. A. Randall[2] deems it of the first importance in the treatment of chronic catarrhal deafness to place the nasopharynx in the best possible condition before treatment of the Eustachian tube and middle ear can relieve the hardness of hearing. "Only a small proportion of cases will present deformities or hypertrophies which compel operative intervention to free the air-passages."

Massage of the membrana and ossicula by means of the pneumatic speculum is also advocated, while the Politzer form of inflation of the tympana is not employed in such cases. The foregoing form of treatment may have to be carried out a year before any improvement is seen, though usually good results have been obtained sooner. Even pneumomassage must be applied to the ear with caution, or pain and permanent injury to the already weakened ear may occur. A. Lucae[3] therefore places a small slit in the air-conducting tube near the ear-piece, thus forming a "safety valve," for the escape of excessive inward pressure upon the membrana tympani. Unusual dryness of the nose and throat, with increased deafness, in chronic aural catarrh is said by T. H. Shastid[4] to follow doses of **belladonna.**

W. Vulpius[5] draws attention to the fact that Kinnicut and M. A. Starr, while employing **thyroid extracts** in cases of myxedema with which hardness of hearing was associated, observed that with improvement of other symptoms the hearing was also greatly improved.

Gradenigo,[6] recognizing the infective origin of ozena, probably from a diphtheritic bacillus (Belfanti), has found that ozena and concomitant chronic otitis in some cases are greatly benefited, at least for a long time, by hypodermic injections of **diphtheritic serum.** Bayer[7] regards ozena as a trophoneurosis, and proposes to treat it with **interstitial cupric electrolysis;** but this treatment is always painful, and in 7 cases thus treated by Bayer 2 suffered from acute otitis media, 1 of which succumbed apparently from an intracranial abscess. [The method is highly censurable.] Nonfetid ozena, first described by Abel,[8] has been observed in two cases, and reported by C. H. Burnett[9] in connection with chronic aural catarrh, which it had produced. The nasal and aural lesions were improved by the use of sprays of Dobell's solution and Boulton's solution of iodin and carbolic acid.

Botey[10] claims that **puncture of the membrane of the round window** and aspiration of the endolymph will relieve vertigo, tinnitus, and some of the affections of the labyrinth, due to excessive intralabyrinthine pressure. Cozzolino[11] claims to have suggested puncture of the round window for the relief of tinnitus and vertigo, in 1888, at the International Congress of Otology held at Brussels. A similar suggestion, puncture of the outer labyrinth wall, to relieve increased labyrinth tension, is made by A. H.

[1] Arch. Ital. di Otol., Jan., 1897.   [2] Univ. Med. Mag., July, 1896.
[3] Arch. f. Ohrenh., June, 1897.   [4] Jour. Am. Med. Assoc., Sept. 19, 1896.
[5] Arch. f. Ohrenh., July, 1896.   [6] Ann. des Mal. de l'Oreille, Aug., 1896.
[7] Rev. de Laryn., d'Otol., etc., No. 22, 1896.   [8] Ann. des Mal. de l'Oreille, Aug., 1896.
[9] Phila. Polyclinic, Oct. 5, 1896.   [10] Ibid., Dec., 1896.
[11] Ibid., Feb., 1897.

Cheatle.[1] Forns[2] has demonstrated that the operation of puncture of the round window, as suggested by Botey, is almost impracticable in any case, but especially so when the plane of the round window is turned backward, instead of outward toward the membrana tympani. In any case Forns justly claims that puncture of this window is very likely to permanently injure the soft tissues of the labyrinth.

Cohen-Kysper[3] makes the general statement that deafness due to the sequels of catarrhal and suppurative inflammations of the tympanum may be successfully treated by injections of **digestive ferments,** especially of dog's pepsin, into the drum-cavity, so as to bathe the stapes and oval window, allowing the injected fluid to lie in such position one hour. Such treatment, however, he does not employ in sclerosis of the drum-cavity. [No statistics are given.]

Vibration or massage of the nasal mucous membrane is highly recommended by T. H. Shastid[4] for improving the hearing in chronic aural catarrh. The same writer[5] has found that Lucae's vibrating sound applied to the membrana tympani in chronic catarrhal deafness has better effect after tenotomy of the tensor tympani than before it. Wegener[6] claims to have produced good results in sclerosis of the mucous membrane of the drum-cavity by means of gentle pneumatic massage, the tinnitus especially being relieved. [This instrument acts like the well-known Siegle pneumatic speculum.]

A. Iljisch[7] draws attention to a form of **" double massage "** for the treatment of chronic catarrhal otitis media, consisting of inflation of air into the drum-cavity, by a catheter, at the same moment that the membrana tympani is drawn outward by rarefaction of the air in the external auditory canal, by means of a simple arrangement of rubber ball and tubing worked by the hand. Instead of the hand, an electric motor may be arranged to effect the pumping for the rarefaction. [Pneumomassage may be of the greatest value in the treatment of chronic catarrhal otitis media, but phonomassage, or massage with a pressure-sound, is not only irrational, but usually injurious.]

Stapedectomy.—C. De Rossi[8] reports his observation of stapedectomy in 4 four cases of hyperplastic catarrh of the middle ear with ankylosis of the ossicula. [While no good results seem to have been obtained by the operation in the above-named cases, no harm occurred to the patients.]   The operations were performed in the ear clinic of the University of Rome. According to the observations and data accumulated by C. Grunert,[9] there is little to hope for the betterment of the hearing in the removal of the stapes in cases of ankylosis between the stapes-foot-plate and the vestibule (oval window). E. B. Gleason[10] reports benefits to hearing from tenotomy of the stapedius, section of the incudostapedial joint, and mobilization of the stapes. The operations are performed under local anesthesia of the membrana by cocain.

Removal of the Incus.—Chronic tympanic vertigo (Ménière's symptoms), a paroxysmal condition of impaction of the stapes in the oval niche and compression of the labyrinth-fluid, the compensatory yielding of the round window membrane being inhibited by its rigidity, induced by the catarrhal state of the mucous lining of the tympanic cavity, can be entirely re-

---

[1] Arch. of Otol., Apr., 1897.
[2] First Spanish Oto-rhinol. Cong., Nov. 18 and 24, 1896; Ann. des Mal. de l'Oreille, Mar., 1897.
[3] Arch. of Otol., Apr., 1897.
[5] Ibid., Sept. 19, 1896.
[7] Ibid., June, 1897.
[9] Arch. f. Ohrenh., Dec., 1896.
[4] Jour. Am. Med. Assoc., Sept. 9, 1896.
[6] Arch. f. Ohrenh., Dec., 1896.
[8] Arch. Ital. di Otol., Jan., 1897.
[10] Med. Bull., Mar., 1897.

lieved by the surgical removal of the incus, and the consequent liberation of the stapes, as shown by C. H. Burnett[1] in a report of 26 cases operated upon by him.

CHRONIC PURULENT OTITIS MEDIA.

Tuberculous otitis media is said by H. Monscourt[2] to occur in 3 different forms: 1, the subacute; 2, the chronic; and, 3, the acute form. The latter is rare. Heuss[3] recommends **xeroform** as an insufflation-powder in otorrhea. W. Cheatham[4] has found the instillation of 10 drops, 2 to 3 times daily, of a mixture of dilute **hydrochloric acid**, 10 drops, with 1 fluidounce of **pyrozone,** to effect a cure of chronic suppuration of the middle ear, even in attic complication, in a short time. **Camphorated salol** is employed with advantage in purulent otorrhea of children, by Campo and Compaired.[5] W. H. Fritts[6] reports a case of chronic otitis media with great tissue-destruction in both ears, in which excellent results were finally obtained by a careful, judicious **local antiseptic method** combined with tonics, after the removal of the malleus and sequestra from the right ear. Zeroni[7] discovered in a polypus which he removed from the chronically suppurating ear of a girl of 16, true **cholesteatoma.** He says that though such an occurrence has been observed before, it is a rarity. After the removal of the polypus and treatment of the ear the suppuration soon ceased. R. E. Moss[8] demonstrates by notes of 3 cases the advantages of free exposure of the middle-ear cavities in chronic purulent otitis media, and in 1 case the advantage of simpler methods, like instillations of strong solutions of nitrate of silver.

Rueda,[9] in an article on the conservative treatment of **attic suppuration,** admits that after months of unsuccessful conservative treatment by means of the curet, injections with the tympanic syringe, etc., surgical removal of diseased bonelets is the only hopeful method of cure. He also thinks prompt operation by removal of diseased bonelets will obviate the necessity of the more heroic operations of Stacke, Zaufal, and others upon the attic by way of the mastoid. [This corresponds entirely with our experience in attic suppuration.]

Excision of Necrotic Ossicula.—J. H. McCassy[10] demonstrates the importance and advantages of treatment in both acute and chronic suppuration of the middle ear. In 1 case he reports prompt and entire cure of chronic purulency by excision of the remnants of the chronically inflamed membrana, malleus, and incus. Bing[11] reports cure of chronic suppuration after removal of the malleus in a case which defied all other treatment. The hearing became very good. C. Grunert and E. Leutert,[12] in a report on excision of the diseased ossicula in chronic purulency of the ear, as observed in the clinic of Halle, state that such operation, if it did not result in a cure in a few months, was succeeded by the Stacke operation for exposure and evacuation of the attic and antrum. [This is very surprising to us, as we have waited patiently as long as a year before rewarded by seeing entire cure of the purulency by excision of necrotic tissue in the drum, by way of the auditory canal.]

[1] Am. Jour. Med. Sci.. Oct., 1896.   [2] Gaz. hebdom. de Méd. et de Chir., Sept. 6, 1896.
[3] Arch. f. Ohrenh., Feb., 1897.   [4] Med. Rec., Sept. 12, 1896.
[5] First Spanish Oto-rhinol. Cong., Nov., 1896.   [6] Phila. Polyclinic, .Dec. 12, 1896.
[7] Arch. f. Ohrenh., June, 1897.   [8] Med. Rec., Feb. 27, 1897.
[9] First Spanish Oto-rhinol. Cong., Nov., 1896; Ann. des Mal. de l'Oreille, May, 1897.
[10] Med. Rec., Aug. 29, 1896.
[11] Aust. Otol. Soc.; Jour. Laryn., Rhin. and Otol., Oct., 1896.
[12] Arch. f. Ohrenh., June, 1897.

J. A. Stuckey[1] reports the good effect of excision of the diseased ossicles and membrana in chronic suppuration of the middle ear.   E. J. Moure[2] demonstrates the advantages of generous surgical exposure of the middle-ear cavities and removal of ossicles in 59 cases of chronic suppurative otitis media.

H. Schwartze[3] presents the following conclusions respecting caries of the ossicula and the operations indicated : 1. When isolated caries of the ossicula is diagnosed, extraction of the diseased ossicula by the external auditory canal is indicated ; 2. When the existence of isolated caries of the ossicula is doubtful, extraction of the diseased ossicula through the external meatus should be performed, as it is a minor and less destructive operation than that through the mastoid, and in any event, even if it does not effect a cure, the removal of the diseased ossicles lessens the danger of retention of pus in the epitympanic cavity ; 3. When caries in the antrum or cholesteatoma is present in addition to caries of the ossicles, the extraction of the ossicles through the external meatus should not be relied upon, but a radical operation for the exposure of all middle-ear cavities should be performed immediately.

Ferreri[4] has contributed an excellent article on the extraction of the malleus and incus in chronic suppuration of the middle ear, and in lesions the result of chronic suppuration of the middle ear ; 45 cases were operated upon with the following results : chronic suppuration : 24 cured ; 5 improved ; 1 unchanged.   In the lesions following chronic suppuration, 15 cured.

Urbantschitsch[5] has demonstrated that in 8 cases of the radical or Stacke operation on chronically suppurating middle-ear cavities good results were obtained notwithstanding the closing of the retroauricular opening.   Again, Urbantschitsch[6] reports his results and experiences based on the surgical exposure of the middle-ear cavities in 12 cases.   " Operative exposure of the middle-ear cavities—the so-called radical operation of the middle ear—consists in the formation of a wide communication between the auditory canal and the drum-cavity on the one side, and the mastoid antrum and varying areas of the mastoid process on the other, so that all these parts are thrown into a common cavity.   At the same time the malleus, incus, and the remnant of the membrana tympani are removed and the posterior wall of the cartilaginous auditory canal is split and thrown back, so that from the entrance to the ear the tegmen tympani and mastoid antrum are brought into view and rendered easily accessible to necessary treatment."

This author observed among his cases 6 in which necrotic disease had exposed the dura mater of the cerebellum, and 3 in which it had exposed the dura mater of the temporal lobe over the tegmen tympani.   In all of the latter cases the disease penetrated the dura, and portions of the brain-tissue escaped into the middle ear and were syringed out at the meatus in one case.   This case got entirely well after surgical exposure of all diseased parts.   In another case the cerebellar dura was penetrated by the necrotic disease and portions of cerebellar tissue escaped through the middle ear.   In this case, too, entire recovery ensued after surgical exposure and cleansing of the diseased middle ear and cranial tissues.

" Operative exposure of the middle-ear spaces affords us the important information that frequent grave and far-reaching destruction induced by various middle-ear affections may penetrate to the brain and the sinus, not only with-

[1] Jour. Eye, Ear, and Throat Dis., Oct., 1896.
[2] De l'Ouverture large de la Caisse, etc., Bordeaux et Paris, 1897.
[3] Arch. f. Ohrenh., Dec., 1896.   [4] Arch. Ital. di Otol., Jan., 1897.
[5] Aust. Otol. Soc., June, 1896 ; Jour. Laryn , Rhin. and Otol., Oct., 1896.
          [6] Wien. klin. Woch., July 16, 1896.

out striking symptoms, but even in the midst of those of perfect health, so that it is only when the diseased nidus is exposed by operation that the real danger in which the patient stands is fully shown. The more cases of chronic purulent inflammation of the middle ear, and also cholesteatoma of the middle ear, that are subjected to this radical operation, the more plainly is the great worth of the operation shown. Furthermore, as experience teaches that the operation is usually well borne and is followed by the best effects in the most varied conditions, we may conclude that the operative exposure of the middle-ear cavities is one of the most valuable of otiatic interferences."

A. Politzer,[1] in 53 cases of chronic suppuration of the middle ear, has exposed the middle-ear cavities by surgical operation. In 17 instances the suppuration stopped at once; 6 patients died, 3 from pyemia existing before the operation, 2 from chronic tuberculosis, and 1 from cerebral abscess existing before the operation on the ear. The rest of the 53 cases remained under observation. [To say the least, these measures in cases of chronic otitic suppuration are plainly indicated as prophylaxis of deeper cranio-otic lesions.] Mongardi[2] reports the good effects of exposure of the middle-ear cavities by the Stacke-Küster method. The chronic purulency was cured and the hearing restored. A case of chronic purulency of the middle ear of $3\frac{1}{2}$ years' duration after scarlatina, in a child 7 years old, which yielded only to complete surgical exposure of the middle-ear cavities, is reported by Gomperz.[3] The tympanic antrum was found full of cholesteatomatous material, granulations, and pus.

A. Politzer[4] reports a reduction of otorrhea, existing from birth, in a woman of 30, after surgical exposure of the middle-ear cavities, and the removal of granulations, pus, and sequestra, one of which was the modiolus and the lamina spiralis ossea of the cochlea. O. Barnick[5] reports 20 cases of surgical exposure of the middle-ear cavities in Habermann's clinic, in Gratz. In one-half of these cases simple caries of the bone was present, while in the rest of the cases cholesteatomatous masses were found in addition to the carious process. The retroauricular opening is maintained only when the bone has been largely destroyed by the cholesteatoma, and the opening shows no marked tendency to close by granulations. As a rule, these operators endeavor to bring about a closure of the tympanic mouth of the Eustachian tube by cauterizations during the after-treatment in order to prevent the subsequent passage of septic matter from the nasopharynx to the middle ear. Max Toeplitz[6] reports 5 Stacke operations in 2 years for the relief of chronic purulency of the middle ear; 2 have recovered entirely and 3 are greatly improved and bid fair to be soon entirely cured. E. J. Moure[7] admits the advantages of intratympanic surgery in chronic purulent otitis media, but cannot admit that ossiculectomy is of benefit in the progressive deafness of sclerosis or dry chronic otitis with arthritis or anchylosis of the stapes. H. A. Alderton[8] has devised an antrotome for the accurate performance of mastoid antrotomy in chronic purulent otitis media. [An ingenious instrument, but only to be used with safety in an antrum and mastoid cavity in which the lateral sinus lies far behind. The position of the latter cannot be positively known until the mastoid is opened by a chisel or a hand drill carefully managed.] J. Habermann[9] points out the important fact and illustrates it by 5 cases,

[1] Aust. Otol. Soc., June, 1896; Ann. des Mal. de l'Oreille, Jan., 1897.
[2] Arch. Ital. di Otol., Jan., 1897.
[3] Aust. Otol. Soc.; Ann. des Mal. de l'Oreille, Feb., 1897.
[4] Ibid. [5] Arch. f. Ohrenh., Apr., 1897.
[6] Post-Graduate, Nov., 1896. [7] Med. Age. Nov. 25, 1896.
[8] Arch. of Otol., July, 1896. [9] Arch. f. Ohrenh., Apr., 1897.

that purulent disease of the middle ear may pass directly from the tympanic cavity by a carious process directly into the labyrinth and the petrous pyramid. 4 of the cases referred to proved fatal, 1 from meningitis and thrombophlebitis, and 3 from pyemia; the fifth was successfully operated upon for an abscess 1 cm. in diameter which lay in the *petrous part of the temporal bone,* over the bulb of the jugular.

MASTOIDITIS.

Acute Mastoiditis.[1]—A. H. Cheatle[2] claims that "on examining the formation of the 'mastoid' antrum in fetal life it can be clearly seen that it is a definite and regular part of the middle ear." A. Broca[3] draws attention to the fact that furuncle near the ear, accompanied by lymphangitis, may be mistaken for mastoiditis. Primary inflammation and abscess of the mastoid are reported by Dunbar Roy.[4]

Chronic Mastoiditis.—Latent otitic mastoiditis presenting the appearance of trigeminal neuralgia has been reported by R. Spira,[5] and "latent" mastoid disease in which the external symptoms are slight in comparison to the deep underlying mastoid lesions, is described and illustrated by 3 cases by E. Fridenberg.[6] Chincini[7] regards the wholesale condemnation of the so-called Wilde's incision, as expressed by Duplay, and later by Chipault and Demoulin (see *Year-Book* for 1896), as unjustifiable, since it is not sustained by facts, and is too theoretical. [Wilde's incision is useless unless there is periostitis of the outer mastoid table or pus beneath the soft tissues over the mastoid.] "When the symptomatology of mastoid disease is obscure the indication is to operate, not to delay. The mastoid operation is harmless; delay may be fatal."[8]

A. Bronner[9] delineates the indications for **surgical treatment** of diseases of attic and mastoid as set forth by Schwartze: 1. In acute primary or secondary inflammation of the mastoid process, if under antiphlogistic treatment the symptoms of pain, tenderness, and fever do not improve in a few days; 2. Chronic inflammation of the mastoid process, with recurrent attacks of swelling; 3. Fistula over or near the mastoid process; 4. Chronic inflammation (purulent) of the middle ear without apparent affection of the mastoid process if there are any symptoms of retention of pus, or of diseased bone (pain, fever, etc.), or if there is a cholesteatoma; 5. Persistent pain over the mastoid process; 6. Chronic otorrhea without any symptoms of retention of pus or swelling of the mastoid process, as soon as we have reason to think that the inflammation has spread beyond the middle ear.

Purulent inflammation of the middle ear with surgical perforation of the mastoid cells, followed by erysipelas and recovery, has been reported by Kipp.[10] O. Barnick[11] reports 18 cases of simple perforation (Schwartze's method) of the mastoid in Habermann's clinic, in Gratz, 14 of which recovered. One of the cases died of intercurrent pneumonia and one died of scarlatinous nephritis. Barnick[12] also reports a case of extensive destruction of the temporal bones after scarlatina, in a child. The mastoid cavities were opened freely on both sides, and granulations, sequestra, and the diseased tissues, extending even into the

[1] See also mastoiditis in acute otitis media (p. 843).
[2] Arch. of Otol., July, 1896. [3] Presse méd., Aug. 12, 1896.
[4] Jour. Am. Med. Assoc., Sept. 12, 1896. [5] Arch. f. Ohrenh., Nov., 1896.
[6] Med. News, Oct. 24, 1896. [7] Arch. Ital. di Otol., Jan., 1897.
[8] Felix Cohn, N. Y. Med. Jour., Aug. 8, 1896. [9] Brit. Med. Jour., Oct. 17, 1896.
[10] Trans. Am. Otol. Soc., July, 1896. [11] Arch. f. Ohrenh., Apr. 9, 1897. [12] Ibid.

internal ears, removed. The patient recovered her health, but the hearing was irrevocably destroyed by the extensive necrosis.

M. D. Lederman[1] reports extensive necrosis of the petromastoid bone following chronic suppurative otitis media on the right side in a deaf-mute woman of 62. After the disease had lasted 9 months facial paralysis occurred suddenly on the right side. A mastoid operation was indicated, and performed at the end of a year of chronic aural suppuration. At this operation, in "clearing out the upper and posterior portion of the antrum and cells, the finger encountered the dura mater." After the operation exposing the middle-ear cavities there was improvement for a month, when sudden hemorrhages from the ear, nose, and mouth, preceded by paralysis of the left leg and arm, ended the patient's life. It seemed plain in this case that long and extensive disease had existed within the ear and cranium without much external manifestation. Softening of the lower portion of the right temporosphenoidal lobe of the brain was found postmortem, accounting for the paralysis in the leg and arm of the left side.

Lake[2] proposes in Stacke operations on the mastoid to pave the floor of the artificial opening between the external ear and the antrum with skin of the meatus only, the cartilage being dissected off at the time of the operation. A. C. Smith[3] reports uniform success in 13 mastoid operations, and Dunbar Roy[4] reports a case of primary inflammation and abscess of the mastoid, occurring in a negro girl 10 months old. B. Gomperz[5] reports a successful radical operation with Koerner's autoplasty, upon a case of mastoid caries in a young girl. Grunert and Leutert[6] report 87 cases of mastoid operation in Schwartze's clinic, in Halle, for the year ending April, 1897. Of these, 46 recovered, in 21 the result is unknown, 7 were still under treatment, 8 were not cured, and 5 died of intracranial complications. H. L. Swain[7] reports two instances of purulent inflammation of the mastoid cells, followed by epidural abscess and relieved by trepanation. Stern[8] opened the mastoid in a case presenting nervous phenomena. The sinus appeared healthy, but later the jugular vein became painful and the region infiltrated. Finally an incision into this tumefaction liberated pus, and recovery ensued without further operation. Hemorrhage from the carotid sinus during an operation on the mastoid was observed by Bloch.[9] This patient died 14 months later of hemorrhage from the carotid.

Sheibe[10] has operated successfully on the mastoid under local anesthesia by chlorid of ethyl. The antrum and an extradural abscess in the posterior cerebral fossa were exposed without causing any pain. In 6 other cases of mastoid disease chlorid of ethyl was used successfully as a local anesthetic in 5, general anesthesia being necessary in 1. Abscess of the mastoid extending along the course of the lateral sinus, with pus resting on the dura, but without any local or general symptoms beyond fulness in the head, and entirely relieved by operative exposure of the mastoid cells and sinus region, is reported by W. G. E. Flanders.[11] C. J. Blake[12] obviates the objections to a drill in mastoid operations by the "use of a long, broad-bladed drill, cutting at an obtuse and not at an acute angle, rotated with one hand and held firmly with the other at a point so near the blade that a very slight deviation of the operative end is represented by a wide and easily appreciable movement of the

[1] Laryngoscope, July, 1896.   [2] Arch. of Otol., July, 1896.
[3] Med Sentinel, Mar., 1897.   [4] Jour. Am. Med. Assoc, Sept. 12, 1896.
[5] Aust. Otol. Soc., June, 1896; Ann. des Mal. de l'Oreille, Jan., 1897.
[6] Arch. f. Ohrenh., June, 1897.   [7] Arch. of Otol., Jan., 1897.
[8] Ibid., Apr., 1897.   [9] Ibid.   [10] Ibid.
[11] Med. Rec., Apr. 17, 1897.   [12] Trans. Am. Otol. Soc., July, 1897.

handle." The preliminary opening in the cortex made with this drill is to be enlarged with a chisel.

Lichtwitz[1] reports a case of **Bezold's mastoiditis** (burrowing of pus from the mastoid into the neck) successfully operated upon. The cervical abscess was opened first, then the antrum and mastoid cells. H. du Fougeray[2] has observed that abscesses of the neck, consecutive   acute and chronic inflammations in the middle ear, form in 3 ways: 1.to.Abscess by direct irruption of pus into the tissues of the neck; 2. Abscess by way of the veins; 3. Abscess by way of the lymphatics. Luc[3] reports a case of Bezold's mastoiditis (perforation of the medial plate into the cervical region) terminating fatally with symptoms of encephalic abscess. An operation was not permitted and there was no postmortem. H. L. Swain[4] observed a trapezius abscess the result of spontaneous perforation of the inner and posterior wall of the tip of the mastoid, that had become diseased from chronic purulent otitis media. Entire recovery followed complete trepanation of the mastoid and drainage of the abscess by counter-openings.

CHOLESTEATOMA OF THE TEMPORAL BONE.

H. Schwartze[5] discovered at a postmortem a true **cholesteatoma of the squama** in a man of 41, who had died of pulmonary phthisis. There was no trace of cholesteatoma in any portion of the middle ear. The origin of the growth in this case was probably from an embryonal offshoot of laminated epithelium. During an operation by A. Kuhn[6] on the mastoid for the removal of a cholesteatoma death occurred by the entrance of air into the injured sigmoid sinus, as shown by finding air in the right ventricle at the autopsy. He suggests that keeping fluid over the opening in the sinus would tend to prevent the entrance of air into the circulation. R. Sattler[7] observed a case of secondary cholesteatoma of the mastoid in a girl of 17, relieved by trepanation and evacuation of the growth. The opening behind the auricle was maintained.

Spontaneous recovery of true cholesteatoma and cholesteatomatous retention-cysts, without retroauricular openings, is pointed out by K. Redmer.[8] Four illustrative cases are given, and the author concludes that all such masses of whatsoever nature ought to be removed by Zaufal's method, if operation is resorted to, without a permanent retroauricular orifice. He also thinks that surgical closure of the Eustachian tubes, according to Hang's suggestion, is not necessary for the permanent cure of cholesteatomatous cavities, as shown by one of Redmer's cases, in which a cure had persisted for 10 years, with entirely patulous Eustachian tubes. Koerner,[9] too, reports spontaneous recovery of cholesteatoma without permanent opening, as after Zaufal's operation. A. Politzer[10] reports a case of cholesteatoma of the middle ear, with pyemic symptoms, cured by operative opening of the cavities of the middle ear. He is in favor of maintaining a permanent opening behind the auricle, in order to be able to remove any recurrent cholesteatomatous flakes which may form. J. Gruber,[11] however, is of the opinion that in the case of small cholesteatomatous collections in the tympanum, and even in the antrum, all desired

[1] Arch. Internat. de Laryn., Otol., etc., Sept., 1896.
[2] Tenth Congress of Surgery, Paris, Oct. 10, 1896.
[3] Arch. Internat. de Laryn., Otol., etc., Oct., 1896.
[4] Arch. of Otol., Jan., 1897.
[5] Arch. f. Ohrenh., Dec., 1896.
[6] Arch. of Otol., Jan., 1897.
[7] Ibid.
[8] Ibid., Oct., 1896.
[9] Ibid., Apr., 1897.
[10] Aust. Otol. Soc., Apr., 1897.
[11] Ibid., Jan. 26, 1897.

results can be obtained in the majority of cases by removal of the pars epitympanica. In the case of large ones in the mastoid there would be absolute necessity for free opening of the mastoid process and the maintenance of the aperture.

Guranowski[1] observed, in a man who had suffered from childhood with chronic purulency of the ear, cholesteatoma filling the drum-cavity, the attic, and the antrum, which were found to have been converted into one cavity by natural processes. This circumstance had acted as a prophylactic against encroachment of disease upon the cranial cavity. P. Bolewski[2] detected cholesteatoma in the middle-ear cavities of a child of 7. Thorough surgical exposure of these cavities and evacuation of the nonsuppurating cholesteatomatous masses were followed by entire recovery, without a permanent opening behind the ear.

INTRACRANIAL COMPLICATIONS OF OTITIS.

A quotation from A. Broca[3] will form a proper introduction to this subject: "When an otitis improperly treated passes into a chronic state it frequently leads to the death of the patient by an intracranial complication. This complication will be, according to the nature of the ear-disease, an acute meningitis, a thrombosis of the dural sinuses, an abscess situate between the petrous bone and the dura, or an abscess in the cerebrum or in the cerebellum. Frequently several of these lesions are associated, constituting a malady beyond the reach of art. At the onset this complexity is not present, and the diagnosis of the solitary or predominant lesion is often possible and some of the lesions are surgically curable."

T. R. Pooley[4] claims that the condition of the fundus of the eye often confirms a diagnosis of otic intracranial disease arrived at from other symptoms, and sometimes is the only symptom. If optic neuritis is found, the diagnosis of extension of ear-disease to the brain is certain, no matter whether other evidence exists or not. Unfortunately, optic neuritis does not explain the nature of the intracranial lesion. Marked optic neuritis alone occurring in chronic otorrhea is sufficient indication for opening the mastoid, even when only a slight optic edema exists. Optic neuritis as an indication for exploratory opening into the cranium, in otitic lesions, can be considered only in connection with other symptoms. It seems, however, to make the presence of other intracranial disease more certain.

Lumbar Puncture in Otic Intracranial Lesions.—E. Leutert[5] contributes a most interesting article on the "Importance of Puncture of the Lumbar Spinal Cavity in the Diagnosis of Intracranial Complications of Otitis," based on 11 cases in which the method was employed in the differential diagnosis between diffuse meningitis and abscess of the brain, apparently with considerable advantage. [The operation of puncturing the lumbar rhachitic space seems to be attended with no disadvantage.]

Sinus-thrombosis.—Fever extending over several days in an acute otitis media, after cessation of the first acute stage, free discharge of pus from the drum-cavity continuing, and also especially in the course of a chronic purulent otitis media without an acute process and without great retention of pus in the drum-cavity, continuous high fever is practically an unmistakable evidence of the existence of a sinus-affection, according to the observations of

---

[1] Arch. f. Ohrenh., June, 1897.   [2] Ibid.
[3] Ann. des Mal. d'Oreille, Nov., 1896.   [4] Med. Rec., Aug. 15, 1896.
[5] Münch. med. Woch., Feb. 23, 1897.

Leutert.[1] The same eminent observer has formulated the following conclusions :[2] " 1. An otogenous pyemia without sinus-thrombosis has never yet been
observed.   2. The occurrence of such a disease is so improbable as not to
enter into diagnostic consideration.   3. The variety of metastases occurring
in sinus-thrombosis, both in acute and in chronic aural suppuration, is explained by the different quality of the thromboses, especially whether tubular
or solid.   4. Therefore, immediate surgical exposure of the sinus is advised
in every case of empyema of the mastoid process occurring after acute otitis
media, if, after the acute stage has passed and the escape of pus from the
drum-cavity is ample, fever of 30° C. (102.3° F.) and over sets in.   5. In
recent cases the result of this must be awaited.   If the fever does not abate by
the 3d day, or if after abatement of the fever for a short time the temperature
again goes up, either with or without a chill, the sinus should be immediately
opened.   6. If the case has become subacute and high fever has been present
for some time, especially, however, if to a chronic suppuration without marked
mastoid implication continued high fever for several days occurs, and diffuse
meningitis can be excluded by lumbar puncture, then too must the sinus already
exposed by operation be laid open.   (Exception : When there is perisinuous
suppuration confined under high pressure, which condition can sometimes cause
fever, even if not as high as that caused by thrombosis.)   7. In young children
the diagnostic value of high fever is not so great, but the possible presence of
sinus-thrombosis must be kept in view.   8. Isolated thrombosis of the bulb of the
jugular vein generally occurs indirectly through the agency of microorganisms
which have passed from the diseased sinus-wall and have found in the jugular
bulb favorable conditions for lodgement and the formation of a thrombus on
the intima.   9. Exploratory puncture of the sinus is of value only when the
result is positive."

E. B. Dench[3] reports a successful exposure and removal of a thrombosis
of the lateral sinus, on the fifth day after the acute inflammation in the
middle ear.   A. Broca[4] observed an acute otitis followed by mastoiditis and a
collection of pus surrounding the lateral sinus in a child of eight.   Evacuation
of the pus-cavity, by surgical exposure, through the mastoid, and packing with
iodoform-gauze were followed by prompt recovery.   J. L. Adams[5] reports a
successful operation in a similar affection of the lateral sinus, the result of
septic treatment of an acutely inflamed ear.   Prompt recognition of the
disease and operative relief of the thrombosis resulted in entire recovery.
Wall[6] reports a case of lateral sinus-thrombosis, with operation and recovery.   The patient was diabetic.   A case of septic otitic sinus-thrombosis
cured by operation is reported by Zaufal.[7]   Ligation of the jugular was performed in this case.   Denker[8] reports a case of otitic sinus-phlebitis and
metastatic purulent pleurisy cured by operation first on the mastoid and
the sinus, though the firm, cheesy clot found in the latter was let alone,
and then in three days on the chest by resection of the sixth rib in the
anterior axillary line, with the evacuation of a liter of fetid pus.   A. J.
Horsey[9] reports a case of chronic suppuration of the middle ear, mastoid
infection, sigmoid sinus-thrombosis, septic pneumonia, and death.   A mastoid operation, and five days later trepanation over the temporosphenoidal
lobe, failed to save life.   [It seems to us, from perusal of the notes of this

[1] Arch. f. Ohrenh., Dec., 1896.   [2] Loc. cit.
[3] Trans. Am. Otol. Soc., July, 1896.   [4] Ann. des Mal. de l'Oreille, Nov., 1896.
[5] Trans. Am. Otol. Soc., July, 1896.   [6] Ann. of Ophth. and Otol., July, 1896.
[7] Prag. med. Woch., Dec. 3, 1896.   [8] Monatschr. f. Ohren., Sept., 1896.
                       [9] Canada Lancet, Apr., 1897.

case; that the only hope of success in operation lay in prompt and thorough exposure of the lateral sinus at the time of the mastoid operation, or perhaps before that time.]

A. Broca[1] observed thrombosis of the lateral sinus without cervical swelling as the result of chronic otorrhea in a boy of 12. An operation upon the apophysis and sinus failed to relieve, as general pyemia induced a fatal gangrenous pneumothorax, surgical intervention having been delayed too long. The same observer[2] successfully operated in a case of lateral sinus-thrombosis, with phlebitis of the jugular, by simple disinfection of the sinus and vein, the latter being ligated. The sinus-disease was the result of chronic purulent otitis media. Necrosis of the petromastoid portion of the temporal bone, producing perforation into the middle and posterior cranial fossæ, with softening of the temporosphenoidal lobe of the brain and ulceration of the sinus, with fatal hemorrhage, is reported by M. D. Lederman.[3] Mayo Robson and Herbert Keighley[4] report a case of mastoid suppuration followed by lateral sinus pyemia, successfully treated by partial excision of the sinus and ligation of the internal jugular vein in the neck.

Extensive, noninfected thrombosis of the several sinuses of the brain, and of the jugular vein, due to operative injury of the lateral sinus, followed by recovery, is reported by R. Hoffman.[5] There was also in this case crossed facial paralysis supposed to be due to cerebral congestion, as there were on the right side opposite the affected ear and sinus optic papillitis and edema of the lids. [We venture to suggest that the optic and facial symptoms on the right side may have been due to stasis induced by the thrombosis of the left lateral sinus and extending through the torcular around to the right lateral and ophthalmic sinuses.] K. Weissgerber[6] reports a case of sinus-thrombosis, following acute otitis media, cured by exposure of the diseased sigmoid sinus, and then four days later by ligation of the nonthrombotic internal jugular vein. Two cases of sinus-thrombosis with marked involvement of the internal jugular vein, the result of chronic suppuration of the middle ear, are reported by the same writer as unrelieved by operation, death occurring from embolic abscesses in the lungs. [These cases show that in the acute form prompt surgical interference offers great hope of saving the patient, while delay in operating in any case, permitting the disease to extend beyond the diseased sinus, is fatal to the patient.]

In a boy of 14 chronic purulency of both ears resulted fatally, notwithstanding free surgical exposure of the middle-ear cavities on both sides and of the sinus on the right side. The autopsy revealed cholesteatoma of the left antrum, inflammatory thrombosis of the right transverse, the right inferior petrosal, and basilar sinuses, and of the jugular vein. There were also purulent infiltration of the muscles of the neck, lung abscesses, and purulent infarction of the lungs. Grunert and Leutert,[7] who report this case, say that the diagnosis of sinus-thrombosis was made very late in this case, as the fever was not very high at first. They also claim that meningitis could have been excluded, and the diagnosis of sinus-thrombosis differentiated by lumbar puncture. Chronic purulent otitis media in a tuberculous child of 7, resulting in fatal thrombosis of the right transverse sinus, is reported by Grunert and Leutert.[8] In this case both ears and mastoids were affected, and the middle-

[1] Ann. des Mal. de l'Oreille, Nov.; 1896. [2] Loc. cit.
[3] Jour. Am. Med. Assoc., Sept. 12, 1896. [4] Lancet, Feb. 6, 1897.
[5] Arch. of Otol·, Apr., 1897. [6] Deutsch. med. Woch., June 3, 1897.
[7] Arch. f. Ohrenh., June, 1897. [8] Ibid.

ear cavities on both sides were exposed by a Stacke-operation. A cysticercus was found in the pia mater at the base of the brain.

Otogenous Pyemia.—O. Brieger[1] has contributed a most valuable article on otogenous pyemia. He shows that this disease may occur under three different forms: 1. Without sinus-phlebitis; 2. With thrombophlebitis of the lateral sinus; 3. With thrombosis of the cavernous sinus. The first-named form is rare, and usually appears as a dermatomyositis, without muscle-abscesses. It may also appear as an osteophlebitis without involvement of the lateral sinus (Körner). In the latter form the metastases are rarely located in the lung, while arterial emboli are observed much more frequently than in sinus-phlebitis. H. Hessler's[2] recent article substantiates Körner's statement that a large group of cases of otogenous pyemia, which differ clinically by the absence of all local symptoms of sinus-thrombosis, by the greater benignity of the entire disease-picture, by the unity of pulmonary metastases and relatively frequent metastatic joint- and muscle-involvement, indicate a special classification.

This classification is not impaired by the occasional occurrence of pulmonary abscesses, as is shown by a case reported by Brieger, and also by one reported by C. H. Burnett.[3] Brieger states that "in operation on the mastoid undertaken during the early days of the disease the subjective mastoid symptoms were lessened, but the general condition was not only repeatedly uninfluenced, but increased fever and chills were observed. The local course was also more unfavorable and more tedious than usual in cases operated upon before the inflammation had reached its height and pus was demonstrable."

In speaking of pyemia with thrombophlebitis of the lateral sinus, the second class named above, Brieger says that while the treatment of sinus-phlebitis has improved, no great advance has been made in its diagnosis. "The most weighty indication of its existence, according to our present knowledge, has been the general evidence of pyemia." The temperature-curve, however, in sinus-phlebitis does not always follow the pyemic type. This form of pyemia is often confounded with typhoid fever, malaria, and tuberculosis. Peptone has been found in the urine in this form of pyemia, disappearing after successful operation on the sinus. "Among the most important symptoms of sinus-phlebitis are changes in the background of the eye." Griesinger's symptom—circumscribed, hard infiltration extending backward from the posterior border of the mastoid—is not considered by Brieger pathognomonic of sinus-thrombosis. Extension of the thrombosis to the jugular vein is occasionally directly perceptible, but swelling and sensitiveness along this jugular tract must be taken with caution, as Schwartze has observed these symptoms without coexisting inflammatory change in the vein, the sensitiveness in this region being due to changes in the lymph-plexus near it. The diagnosis of sinus-thrombosis is still obscure. Brieger, in common with H. Hessler, J. O. Green, E. A. Crockett, and others, deem prompt exploratory exposure of the sinus in suspected sinus-phlebitis as entirely justifiable and much more advantageous to the patient than waiting for positive symptoms of the presence of sinus-thrombosis, when it is generally too late to operate with any hope of relief. An exploratory incision may be more advantageous than an exploratory puncture and aspiration of the sinus. Sinus-thrombosis may be cured by clearing out the primary pus-collection and evacuating the pus which bathes the sinus. Mere pulsation of the exposed sinus does not preclude the presence of a thrombus within, as this pulsation

---

[1] Arch. of Otol., Oct., 1896.   [2] Arch. f. Ohrenh., Bd. xxxviii.
[3] Trans. Am. Otol. Soc., 1883.

is due to the impression made upon its walls by the general pulsation of the cranial sinuses.

Ligation of the jugular is unquestionably justified only when it is locally indicated. . . . The systematic application of ligation as an integral part of the operative therapy of sinus-phlebitis is not justified. It is an error in pyemia without sinus-phlebitis. . . . The principal point, in Brieger's opinion, in deciding as to whether or not the vein should be ligated, is dependent upon the local findings in the vein itself, or at least at the cranial end of the thrombus. The sole contraindication for the operation, aside from the conditions of the heart, Brieger believes to be purulent leptomeningitis, the presence of which is to be demonstrated not only by diffuse meningeal symptoms, which under certain circumstances accompany sinus-thrombosis, but most certainly by spinal (lumbar) puncture.

The third form of otitic pyemia characterized by thrombosis of the cavernous sinus requires, according to Brieger, a special classification in contradistinction to lesions of other cranial sinuses. Körner has shown that this form of thrombosis is due frequently to the passage of infection from the middle ear, by way of the carotid canal, to the cavernous sinus. While no one symptom may be considered positively pathognomonic of its existence, the occurrence of edema about the brow and orbit, exophthalmos, paralysis of the ocular muscles, immobility of the eyeball, edema of the lids, chemosis of the conjunctiva, and often choked disk on the side of the chronic aural suppuration, justify the surgeon in concluding that he is confronted with thrombosis of the cavernous sinus.

The only treatment so far successful is prompt exposure of the middle-ear cavities, opening freely the *lateral* sinus, and permitting judicious hemorrhage in the hope that the normally forcible blood-current in the sinuses will eject the thrombus either at the artificial opening in the lateral sinus or throw it into the general circulation, when, if not infectious, it may be dissolved without metastases. Brieger reports one case, a man of 22, in which recovery ensued rapidly after generous opening of the *lateral* sinus, though all the above-named serious symptoms were present before the operation. Isolated otitic thrombophlebitis of the cavernous sinus has not been successfully treated by the Krause method of exposing it as for intracranial resection of the trigeminus. The sinus has been repeatedly reached and injured by Krause, Finney, and Czerny in trigeminus resection.

E. Rimini[1] observed a case of pyohemia consecutive to an acute purulent otitis media, following diphtheria, in a child of 3. One injection of serum No. 1, of Behring, had caused the disappearance of the false membranes in the fauces, in 3 days. Ten days later, symptoms of scarlatina ensued, with aural pains and suppuration, and in six days later death supervened after general pyemic symptoms. A. Politzer[2] reports recovery after otitic pyemia. First, there was an operative exposure of the mastoid cavity and the lateral sinus; later, there was thrombosis of the jugular vein, with phlegmonous inflammation about it. On the 22d day purulent metastasis occurred in the elbow-joint, when all rigors ceased and recovery set it. J. H. Clayton[3] reports a ease of peripetrous suppuration resulting from chronic purulent otitis, mastoid caries, and involvement of the lateral sinus on the left side. A small abscess in the temporal lobe near the sinus was found after death, and pus had found its way from the mastoid over both surfaces of the petrous

[1] Berlin. klin. Woch., July 6, 1896.
[2] Aust. Otol. Soc., 1896 ; Jour. Laryn., Rhin. and Otol., Oct., 1896.
[3] Birmingham Med. Rev., Aug., 1896.

bone and into the left orbit. F. W. Mackenzie[1] reports a fatal case of otitic pyemia in a man of 39. An operation on the mastoid and lateral sinus was suggested promptly, but rejected by the patient, who succumbed in three weeks after the initial pyemic symptoms. Well-marked otitic pyemia, terminating apparently in embolic abscess of the liver, is reported by M. D. Lederman.[2]

A case of otitic pyemia cured by excision of the thrombosed internal jugular vein is reported by H. Eulenstein.[3] This operation was performed 3 days after surgical exposure of the middle-ear cavities, the lateral sinus, the posterior cerebral fossa, and the evacuation of a large pus-cavity near the jugular bulb. Chills and fever continuing after this operation, the ligation was considered as the last resort, though there were no external symptoms pointing to its thrombosed condition. F. P. Hover[4] reports the case of a man of 47, who suffered with great pain and tumefaction of the left side of the head. Incision into this region gave vent to a quantity of pus, and finally dead bone and granulations were removed ; but the temperature of the patient rose to 105° F., coma supervened, and the man died 10 days after the above operation. The autopsy revealed a purulent thrombus in the left lateral sinus extending back as far as the torcular and forward into the superior petrosal sinus, the inferior petrosal being normal. E. Rimini[5] reports a case of pyemia following acute otitis media of a benign form. The patient was a child of 7. The mastoid was opened, but showed no disease. The sinus was then opened and pus escaped. Thrombi were found and removed, but the sinus was free from pus. Recovery finally took place in three months. A case of septic otitic thrombosis of the sigmoid sinus cured by ligation of the jugular and laying bare the sinus is described by Zaufal.[6] Notwithstanding metastatic abscesses in the glutei muscles of the left side and purulent pleurisy entire recovery ensued in six weeks. W. Ridley[7] has reported "middle-ear" pyemia cured by ligation of the internal jugular vein, and removal of a fetid clot from it. An epidural abscess was also opened, and the lateral sinus, blocked only in its mastoid portion, was cleaned out, and recovery ensued. W. R. H. Stewart[8] reports a case of pyemia following middle-ear suppuration in a boy of 11. With vomiting, rigors, and a temperature of 97°, the antrum was laid open, with temporary relief. The lateral sinus was then explored and found to contain a healthy clot. The dura was incised, letting out a large quantity of serous fluid. Rigors still continuing, the lateral sinus was slit, the healthy clot removed, and then recovery took place.

Otitic Meningitis.—E. B. Dench[9] reports a case of otitic meningitis occurring as a result of chronic suppuration in the left ear of a man of 60. For 3 weeks the patient suffered from dizziness and pain in the left ear and corresponding side of the head, without elevation of temperature. Suddenly at the end of this time the temperature rose, the other symptoms continuing. Dench then etherized the patient and opened the cranial cavity so as to expose that part of it immediately above the drum-cavity. The tympanic roof was found roughened and bloody serum escaped from the epidural space ; a dural flap was turned down, and the aspirator thrust into the brain-substance, but no pus was found. The dural flap was then replaced and the lateral sinus was explored in both directions, but was found to contain fluid blood. The evacuation of the bloody serum from the epidural space and the antiseptic

[1] New Zealand Med. Jour., July 1, 1896.   [2] Jour. Am. Med. Assoc., Sept. 12, 1896.
[3] Arch. of Otol., Apr., 1897.   [4] Med. Herald, Aug., 1896.
[5] Arch. of Otol., Apr., 1897.
[6] Prag. med. Woch, No. 49, 1896 ; Arch. of Otol., Apr., 1897.
[7] Lancet, Nov. 28, 1896.   [8] Ibid., Nov. 7, 1896.
[9] Trans. Am. Otol. Soc., July, 1896.

treatment of this region and of the entire wound-cavity were followed by rapid recovery. The case was regarded as one of infective meningitis. [The latter was due probably to osteitis of infectious origin from the suppurating drum-cavity.]

Acute, diffuse, suppurative meningitis of otitic origin A. Broca[1] regards as beyond the reach of surgical art, but as often in the presence of meningitic symptoms the chief lesion is really a cerebral (epidural) abscess, he believes that an exploratory operation is demanded. He reports[2] 2 cases of acute otitic meningitis unsuccessfully operated upon, in one of which diffuse osteitis of the temporal bone was marked. Both patients were children of 5.

Riehl[3] observed an otogenous meningitis with thrombosis of the sigmoid sinus, the tympanic cavity, antrum, and mastoid cells being filled with a dark-red jelly-like mass, but the membrana atrophic and imperforate. The origin of the disease was considered hematogenous after influenza.

Otitic Cerebral Abscess.—Luc[4] presents an excellent review of the generally accepted laws of diagnosis and treatment of cerebral abscess consecutive to cranial suppurations—*i. e.*, in the frontal sinuses and middle ear. Lannois and Jaboulay[5] observed in a man who had been affected with chronic otorrhea for 25 years sudden symptoms of cerebral abscess: vertigo, staggering, nausea, dysphasia, violent headaches, and hemiparesis of the right side, without rise of temperature. Sensory aphasia and homonymous hemianopsia, with preservation of pupillary reaction, pointed to the temporal lobe as the seat of the abscess. Amnesic aphasia, a symptom suggesting an abscess in the left temporal lobe, and leading to an operation, is reported by A. Kuhn.[6] But the autopsy revealed diffuse suppurative meningitis and the sac of the spinal dura filled with pus. [Lumbar puncture would have aided in a differential diagnosis in this case.] T. R. Pooley[7] observed a case of chronic purulent otitis media in a boy of 12, followed by mastoid periostitis, mastoiditis interna, abscess of the cerebrum, thrombosis of the lateral sinus, meningitis, optic neuritis, and death. Mastoid chiselling, removal of pus, and curetting of the cells and the antrum revealed carious destruction of the lateral sinus and exposure of the dura at that point. [As within three days of that time the choked disk in the eye on the side of the affected ear was marked and the headache increased for a month until the patient died, it seems that a deeper penetration into the cranial cavity in the tract of the sinus at the time of the mastoid operation might have been attended with the happiest results.] C. Grunert[8] reports the occurrence of an otitic abscess of the temporal lobe, the result of chronic purulency of the ear, relieved by thorough exposure of the middle-ear cavities first, and then, a month later, by trepanation of the cranium through the squama. G. Bacon[9] reports the successful operative treatment of an abscess in the temporosphenoid lobe on the left side, the result of chronic otitic suppuration. [The case presented an instance of the exceptional occurrence of chills, high temperature, rapid pulse, and convulsions—symptoms of thrombosis of the lateral sinus rather than brain-abscess, in which we expect subnormal pulse and temperature. There were, however, aphasic symptoms in Bacon's case, which led to the suspicion of the presence of a temporosphenoidal abscess, in spite of the apparently contradictory ones of chills, fever, and convulsions.] R. C. Myles[10] reports a

[1] Ann. des Mal. de l'Oreille, Nov., 1896.   [2] Loc. cit.
[3] Wien. klin. Rundschau, No. 49, 1896; Arch. of Otol., Apr., 1897.
[4] Méd. moderne, Nov., 1896.   [5] Arch. of Otol., Apr., 1897.
[6] Ibid., Jan., 1897.   [7] Trans. Am. Otol. Soc., July, 1896.
[8] Berlin. klin. Woch., Dec. 28, 1896. [9] Trans. Am. Otol. Soc., July, 1896.
                    [10] Ibid.

case of brain-abscess, the result of chronic suppuration in the middle ear of a child 7 years old. After removal of the mastoid cortex a flexible curet was passed into the attic, and while curetting the tegmen the instrument passed without force and resistance, into the cranial cavity. This was followed by a gush of pus—more than a wineglassful. After two abscesses in the connective tissue about the mastoid, in the course of 3 months after relief of the brain-abscess, entire recovery ensued. D. Kaufmann[1] reports a case of chronic suppurative otitis media in which pyemic symptoms led to radical operative exposure of the middle-ear cavities and opening of an extradural abscess. 15 days later symptoms of cerebral compression led to opening of an abscess in the right temporal lobe, but this was followed by thrombophlebitis, meningitis, and death. Gilbert Barling[2] reports the occurrence of an abscess in the temporal lobe, resulting from purulent otitis, successfully operated upon, with speedy recovery of the patient. Before the operation there were unconsciousness, and paralysis of the left arm, opposite the diseased ear, as guiding symptoms of abscess in the temporal lobe. These phenomena disappeared immediately after the evacuation of pus from the brain by operation. [We are not informed that the middle-ear cavities, from which the infection of the brain originates in such cases, were cleansed and the infectious nidus destroyed. Unless this is done, if the patient survives the first attack of otitic brain-disease, he still remains exposed to the liability of further infection from the diseased ear.]

Gradenigo,[3] in an article on the operative treatment of otitic cerebral abscess, shows, first, that local treatment of the ear in chronic purulency, if not based on rational surgical laws, will lead to the development of endocranial complications; whereas a rational local treatment of purulent inflammation of the middle ear will be a benefit to the patient, both in preventing the formation of endocranial complications, or leading to their spontaneous resolution if only in their initial stage, " as, for example, circumscribed foci of pachymeningitis above the tegmen tympani." In doubtful cases it is more of a risk to wait for decided symptoms of intracranial complications than to perform an exploratory operation on the cranium. The best way of approach to exposure and evacuation of an otitic abscess of the temporosphenoidal lobe is through the mastoid and then the tegmen of the antrum and tegmen tympani. If the condition of the patient makes the operation directly upon the brain imperative, the mastoid and tympanic openings may be deferred to a second intervention. When the symptoms of the patient are equally grave, but when the diagnosis of meningitis has the greater probability, the suspected region of the brain must be approached through an opening just above and in front of the osseous auditory canal.

As to whether the aural surgeon or the general surgeon should operate in cases of otitic endocranial lesions, Gradenigo says "the operator ought to possess, by frequent operations on the temporal bone, the best anatomic and pathologic knowledge of these parts, and that we cannot conceive of a modern otologist who would not be a surgeon before he became an otologist." Two cases of otitic cerebral abscess are reported by Gradenigo.[4] In the first, a child of 6, the subject of chronic otorrhea, was attacked with symptoms of pyemia and cerebritis. Though in a comatose state, the child was etherized, the mastoid and middle-ear cavities opened, and relief given to coma and some other symptoms. Two days later an epidural abscess was opened into the middle ear by puncture of the denuded dura over the tegmen tympani. In the

[1] Aust. Otol. Soc., Oct. 27, 1896. [2] Brit. Med. Jour., June 12, 1897.
[3] Arch. Ital. di Otol., Jan., 1897. [4] Ann. des Mal. de l'Oreille, Apr., 1897.

second case, a man of 20, surgical exposure of the middle-ear cavities revealed a cerebral abscess directly over the tegmen tympani. This was punctured and evacuated through the drum-cavity. Trepanation of the squama was also performed, but no further abscess was found in the brain, and the man recovered. Urbantschitsch[1] reports what might be termed a spontaneous evacuation of an epidural abscess through the tympanic cavity after surgical exposure of the middle-ear cavities. The pus-cavity was entirely healed under the instillation of a 10% emulsion of glycerin and iodoform every other day for 3 weeks. B. A. Randall[2] reports the occurrence of an extradural (epidural) abscess from mastoid empyema, and states that in ten instances within a year after trephining a suppurating mastoid the caries of its inner plate was so great as to necessitate exposure of the dura and liberation of pus between it and the bone. P. Avoledo[3] reports his results with craniotomy in 4 cases of otitic purulent processes within the cranium. Recovery ensued after operative relief in 1 case of cerebral abscess and 2 instances of circumscribed purulent inflammations of the dura. The operation failed to relieve in a case of diffuse purulent meningitis.

A temporosphenoid abscess, the result of chronic purulent otitis of 28 years' duration, was successfully operated upon by J. M. Cotterell.[4] The pulse and temperature became subnormal in this case, and the cerebration very dull, symptoms indicating the operation on the brain, three days after the mastoid had been opened. N. S. Roberts[5] reports 4 successful operations on the mastoid in children : one in a child of a year and a half, involving the middle cerebral fossa, in the form of an epidural collection of pus. An otitic brain-abscess, the sequel of chronic purulent otitis media, in a boy of 13, entirely relieved by trephining the squama, and, after the escape of an epidural collection of pus, freely incising through the healthy dura into the anterior convolutions of the temporosphenoidal lobe, is reported by J. E. H. Nichols.[6] In this case, before entire recovery ensued, erysipelas occurred, which was greatly benefited by the local application of a saturated solution of aceto-tartrate of aluminum.

Cerebellar Abscess.—H. Schwartze[7] observed a case of otogenous cerebellar abscess, from chronic purulent otitis, in a woman of 22. The prominent symptoms for seven weeks were intense, though intermittent, pain in the occiput, nausea and vomiting, subnormal temperature, but very rapid pulse, 100–150 (accounted for postmortem by the discovery of chronic endocarditis deformans), and varying width of pupils, the *right* being generally the wider. After death an abscess the size of a walnut was found in the *right* cerebellar hemisphere, with circumscribed lepto- and pachymeningitis interna. The rapid pulse was considered incompatible with the presence of brainabscess, and an operation therefore contraindicated.

Macewen[8] says "when you have a cerebellar abscess caused by a focus in the middle ear, we find that that abscess is in immediate contiguity with the lateral sinus ; we do not find it occurring in other parts. If, therefore, after opening the middle ear, we find that the erosive process has taken a backward direction, and that it comes in contact with this sinus, and if the symptoms of an abscess have already been noted, you may be assured that you can get at that abscess by going around this large blood-channel to its posterior surface : . . . in every case of cerebellar abscess which I have had, arising from middleear disease, this has been the course that it has taken."

[1] Aust. Otol. Soc., Apr., 1897.

[2] Jour. Am. Med. Assoc., Sept. 12, 1896.

[3] Arch. Ital. di Otol., Jan., 1897.

[4] Scot. M. and S. Jour., Apr., 1897.

[5] N. Y. Med. Jour., May 23, 1897.

[6] Manhattan Eye and Ear Hosp. Rep., Jan., 1897.

[7] Arch. f. Ohrenh., Dec., 1896.

[8] Occidental Med. Times, Nov., 1896.

A cerebellar abscess following otitis media of four months' duration, successfully treated by operation, is reported by H. S. Walker.[1] The only symptom which may be called characteristic of cerebellar abscess was increased knee-jerk on the side of the diseased ear and abscess in the cerebellum. Acland and Ballance call attention to this symptom, as well as muscular weakness, chiefly of the arm, and conjugate deviation toward the unaffected side from weakness of the ocular muscles, as characteristic of the presence of a cerebellar abscess. Gilbert Barling[2] reports two cerebellar abscesses the result of purulent otitis media. In one instance there was also an extradural suppuration and in the other a second abscess in the cerebellum not reached by the operation. Both cases proved fatal. There were horizontal nystagmus in both of these cases, and paralysis of the sixth nerve in one, on the side of the diseased ear. T. Heiman[3] has observed his 7th case of cerebellar abscess of otitic origin. The patient was 21 years old, had fever with morning remissions and marked cerebral symptoms. When first seen by Heiman the temperature was 37° C. and the pulse 54–48, with intense headache, especially in the region of the right occiput, the side of the more diseased ear, increased by percussion. The right pupil was the wider, there was choked disk, and the right eyelid could not be closed. There was also inconsiderable paresis of the lower facial branches. The tongue turned toward the left, there were thirst and apathy, and the speech was slow and indistinct. In a sitting posture the head fell forward, then turned toward the left and continued to move with pendulum-like oscillations. The vertigo was intense in the sitting posture and with the least movement of the head. There were paresis of the upper and weakness of the lower extremity on the left side. Foot- and patellar-reflex were increased. Vomiting was frequent and persistent. The temporal bone was trephined in three places, the dura did not pulsate, and at two points the temporal lobe was punctured, but no pus was found. After this operation the headache and paresis were lessened and the speech improved. Two weeks later all the symptoms grew worse, and there was added twitching of the left arm and of the right side of the face. The middle-ear cavities and the dura over the tegmen were exposed by operation, and pus escaped, but relief did not ensue, and two weeks later the right occiput was trephined and the right cerebellar lobe explored, but no pus was found. Slight improvement for a few days, and then all the symptoms of central pressure returned, and the patient died with symptoms of general tubercular marasmus. The autopsy revealed an abscess of the right lobe of the cerebellum and the processus vermicularis, superficial cysts in the right cerebral hemisphere, caries of the right tympanum, and chronic purulency of both ears. There were also cavities in the lungs, pyopneumothorax, and general marasmus.

Carcinoma of the Temporal Bone.—Danziger[4] reports 2 cases of this rare malady. One occurred in an unmarried woman of 54, who suffered from chronic otorrhea, the result of scarlatina in her 10th year. The ear-disease had never received any treatment. The second case was that of a man of 53, syphilitic, but not before affected with ear-disease. Both cases proved fatal.

Alveolar sarcoma of the cerebellum, giving rise to disturbances in gait, hearing, and vision, is reported by H. M. Thomas.[5] W. Milligan[6] reports 2 cases of malignant growth—one angiosarcoma, the other myxosarcoma—in

[1] Brit. Med. Jour., Mar. 6, 1897.   [2] Ibid., June 12, 1897.
[3] Medycyna, Sept. 8, 1896; Arch. f. Ohrenh., June, 1897.
[4] Arch. f. Ohrenh., Aug., 1896.   [5] Bull. Johns Hopkins Hosp., Sept., 1896.
            [6] Arch. of Otol., July, 1896.

ears for a long time the seat of chronic suppuration. The first-named growth occurred in a woman of 63 ; the other in a woman of 18. In the latter a very radical removal of diseased tissue was effected, but repullulation of the morbid growth soon ensued. Hogg[1] observed a case of sarcoma of the base of the skull involving the middle ear.

Tuberculous Disease of the Temporal Bone.—O. Barnick[2] reports 3 cases of tuberculous inflammation of the temporal bone, 1 terminating in extensive destruction of the mastoid, the lower part of the squama, the petrous pyramid, and partial thrombosis of the superior petrosal and sigmoid sinuses, with tuberculous disease of the sphenoid and occipital bones. Manasse[3] discovered a solitary tubercle on the eighth nerve, in a consumptive. The growth was situated to the left of the pons. The facial and auditory nerves were imbedded in the cheesy mass and could not be isolated. Tubercular caries of the middle ear, perforating the fenestræ, and invading the internal ear, in a child 3 months old, is reported by W. Haenel.[4] The pathologic process, as shown by section of the decalcified bone, had begun near the tympanic mouth of the Eustachian tube and passed backward as far as the autrum. The infection apparently had reached the middle ear through the Eustachian tube. The infection of the dura mater, which had taken place through the petrosquamous suture, had remained localized. Poli[5] reports a case of purulent otitis media in a child 18 months old. Endocranial symptoms led to exploratory craniotomy and the discovery of tubercle of the left cerebral peduncle. Death occurred 3 months after the operation. H. L. Swain[6] observed a purulent collection in the lateral ventricle as a result of chronic purulent otitis media, with caries of the roof of the tympanum. Death occurred with a temperature of 107° F.

The relation of the aurist to the surgery rendered necessary by chronic purulent otitis media is well summed up by C. J. Blake.[7] "The surgery of a suppurative process within the temporal bone which, beginning in the middle ear, has implicated the mastoid process and threatens contiguous structures, has to take into consideration, not merely the effort to save life, but also to conserve, as far as possible, the hearing power, and to leave undisturbed the equilibrating function of the ear ; it has also to take into consideration the possibility of injury to important structures lying in minutely close relationship to the necessary operative field. Under these circumstances it is a tenable proposition that no aural surgeon should undertake an operation upon the mastoid in a case of suppurative implication of that cavity without being prepared by his mental and material equipment to enlarge his operative field to any extent demanded, or without having, if he does not possess it himself, the necessary surgical assistance and counsel at hand.

"The fact that it is easier for the aurist to learn to open the cranial cavity and to operate upon the lateral sinus in the brain, than for the general surgeon to acquaint himself with the technical procedures of operation within the temporal bone and middle ear, is an argument in favor of leaving the subject of the intracranial complications of suppurative middle-ear disease where it now largely stands—in the hands of the special practitioner."

[1] Austral. Med. Gaz. ; Laryngoscope, Oct., 1896. [2] Arch. f. Ohrenh., Apr., 1897.
[3] Arch. of Otol., Apr., 1897.   [4] Ibid.   [5] Arch. Ital. di Otol., Jan., 1897.
[6] Arch. of Otol., Jan., 1897.   [7] Am. Jour. Med. Sci., June, 1897.

DISEASES OF THE INTERNAL EAR.

Syphilis of the Internal Ear.—E. A. Crockett[1] describes a form of acute syphilitic affection of the ear, probably due to an effusion into the labyrinth in a previously normal ear, characterized by sudden deafness, tinnitus, and vertigo, coming on in the late secondary or early tertiary stage of systemic syphilis. The difference between this form of sudden deafness, tinnitus, and vertigo, and that due to nonsyphilitic causes, is that the deafness is not so profound in the specific form. The syphilitic aural affection yields promptly to a few doses given hypodermically of pilorcarpin ($\frac{1}{6}$ gr.), whereas nonsyphilitic labyrinth-diseases are entirely unaffected by pilocarpin. According to an article on disease of the internal ear, by Thomas J. Harris,[2] pilocarpin gives the best results in syphilitic diseases of the internal ear.

Caries of the Internal Ear.—Extensive caries of the petrous bone, the result of purulent otitis media after scarlet fever in a child $2\frac{1}{2}$ years old, terminating in sequestration of the osseous semicircular canals and the posterior part of the vestibule, has been reported by Guranowski.[3] H. S. Walker[4] removed a sequestrum consisting of the cochlea, semicircular canals, the internal auditory meatus, and parts of the mastoid cells, following scarlet fever. A large cavity was left, the posterior and upper walls of which were formed by the dura mater of the middle and posterior fossæ.

Internal Ear in Submarine Workers.—F. Alt[5] reports apoplectiform affections of the labyrinth in 3 men employed in submerged caissons. When the Eustachian tube is permeable the ear endures the increased atmospheric pressure in submarine caissons; when it is not permeable, the inward pressure of the membrana produces congestion of the drum-cavity and finally of the internal ear, as Alt has shown by experiments on animals.

Anemia of the Labyrinth.—Lermoyez[6] claims that deafness, tinnitus, and vertigo may be caused by either congestion or anemia of the labyrinth. The inhalation of a few drops of nitrite of amyl will temporarily relieve these symptoms if they be due to ischemia, but will increase them if they be due to congestion. This differentation in etiology will enable the physician to properly treat the disease. In a case of anemia of the labyrinth Lermoyez found that trinitrin in doses of $\frac{1}{100}$ gr. three times daily permanently relieved the deafness, tinnitus, and vertigo. In cases of congestion of the labyrinth an alterative or absorbent treatment would be indicated.

Internal Ear in Leukemia.—A case of so-called Ménière's disease, caused by leukemic disease of the auditory nerve, in a man of 66, is reported by F. Alt and F. Pineles.[7]

Internal Ear in Diphtheria.—Sudden, bilateral, total deafness in true diphtheria in a woman of 33, with previous good hearing and no history of syphilis, is reported by J. C. Wilson.[8] The middle ears seemed in no way affected. The tinnitus and vertigo were marked at first, but gradually in six months the tinnitus greatly diminished and the vertigo ceased. [The onset of the ear-disease in this case resembled that of the internal ear affection occurring in syphilis and mumps.]

Traumatism of the Internal Ear.—Ménière's group of symptoms

---

[1] Boston M. and S. Jour., Feb. 11. 1897.
[2] Manhattan Eye and Ear Hosp. Rep., Jan., 1897.
[3] Monats. f. Ohrenh., No. 12, 1896 ; Arch. of Otol., Apr., 1897.
[4] Brit. Med. Jour., Oct. 31, 1896.
[5] Aust. Otol. Soc., June, 1896 ; Ann. des Mal. de l'Oreille, Jan., 1897.
[6] Ann. des Mal. de l'Oreille, July, 1896.   [7] Wien. klin. Woch., Sept. 17, 1896.
            [8] Trans. Cong. Am. Phys. and Surg., May, 1897.

following traumatic lesion of the labyrinth have been noted by Politzer,[1] in a case of fracture of both temporal bones (from a blow on the head) involving the labyrinth. Death occurred in about six weeks from meningitis; the day before death albuminuria appeared. New growth of connective tissue in both labyrinths was detected by microscope after death. Politzer draws attention to this rapidity of formation of connective tissue, and believes that the rapid and incurable deafness which occurs in various kinds of panotitis can be explained by the development of new growth of connective tissue in the labyrinth. It also shows why prompt and energetic absorptive treatment fails entirely in such cases. Whether the fatal meningitis resulted from the fracture, or from purulency of the sphenoid sinus or the middle ear, could not be determined, as there was no demonstrable connection between these foci of suppuration and the cranial cavity. D. Kaufman[2] reports a case of complete ambilateral deafness three days after a fall upon the occiput. This result was supposed to be due to traumatic apoplexy in the labyrinth terminating in degeneration, necrosis, and secondary hemorrhages in the internal ear. J. Gruber[3] observed a fracture of the temporal bone, caused by a fall upon the head. The case proved fatal in four days from widely diffused meningitis. T. A. Kenefick[4] reports a case of the apoplectic form of Ménière's disease, in which, as the author thinks, spontaneous recovery of the tinnitus, dizziness, and deafness, ensued in about two weeks from the time of sudden onset at night. [So far as we know, the deafness resulting from an intense extravasation within the labyrinth, such as occurs in Ménière's disease, never disappears and is usually bilateral. Therefore, we think this was a case of vertigo, nausea, etc., of tympanic origin.]

Thos. Barr[5] points out that many cases of drowning from "sudden cramps" are in reality cases of fatal ear-giddiness, induced by the sudden entrance of cold water into the drum-cavity in persons with perforated membranæ.

Psychic Deafness.—Psychic deafness is often confounded with deaf-muteness. The former is rather an inability to learn to talk in one who can hear, rather than muteness in one who cannot hear, and has therefore never learned to talk, as in cases reported by S. Heller[6] and V. Urbantschitsch. In Heller's[7] case, a boy of 3½ years, there was great nervous excitability, evinced as paroxysms of rage. The hearing was good, but the power to speak remained latent. By combating this excitability and awakening and cultivating the faculty of concentration and perception, the power of speech was gained. In Urbantschitsch's case[8] a teacher, a woman of 22, grew dull of hearing without apparent cause, and, as a result of the impaired function, became melancholic and subject to delusions with suicidal intentions. Under careful acoustic exercises—words spoken slowly and near the ear, fair hearing was slowly regained. [Many cases of psychic deafness seem to possess what is termed "latent hearing," by some observers.]

Deaf-mutes.—Ottolenghi[9] advises education of deaf-mutes with the idea of giving them full use of what powers they have, and to restore them to civil and penal responsibility if possible. V. Pendred[10] reports two cases of associated goiter and deaf-mutism in the same family. Mingazzini[11] offers a clinical observation of a case of so-called hysteric deaf-muteness in a man with a neurotic history. Recovery took place after both intra- and extra-

[1] Arch. f. Ohrenh., Dec., 1896.   [2] Aust. Otol. Soc., Ann. des Mal. de l'Oreille, Feb., 1897.
[3] Aust. Otol. Soc., Apr., 1897.   [4] Med. Rec., July 25, 1896.
[5] Brit. Med. Jour., May 1, 1897.
[6] Aust. Otol. Soc., June, 1896; Jour. Laryn., Rhin. and Otol., Oct., 1896.
[7] Loc. cit.   [8] Loc. cit.   [9] Jour. of Laryngol., No. 1; Arch. of Pediatrics, Aug., 1896.
[10] Lancet, Aug. 22, 1896.   [11] Arch. Ital. di Otol., Jan., 1897.

laryngeal application of faradic and galvanic currents. G. Alvarez[1] claims to have cured deaf-muteness in a girl of 15, by treatment of the nasopharynx and the removal of the nonabsorbed gelatinous matter of infancy which had remained in the drum-cavity. Barbera[2] maintains that deaf-muteness is a stigma of degeneration, while Verdos[3] claims that many cases can be cured, especially those resulting from rhinitides that have passed into the middle ears. Forns[4] claims that this is the only class of curable mutes, while those resulting from nonabsorption of the connective-tissue jelly present in the middle ears at birth, and those caused by disease of the internal ear and auditory nerve-center, are incurable. J. Sendziak[5] maintains that an early operation on adenoid vegetations, even in infancy, will prevent the development of deaf-dumbness.

Hallucinations of Hearing.—Kaufman[6] claims that the ear in those affected with hallucinations of hearing generally presents organic changes, and also that a vicious interpretation of subjective noises in the ear causes hallucinations. Séglas,[7] too, states that all hallucinations of hearing are not due to purely neuro- or psychopathic causes, but that alterations in the peripheral sensorial apparatus will be found to have a large share in their production.

Tinnitus.—G. W. McCaskey[8] writes on the diagnostic significance of subjective head- and ear-sounds, chiefly in neurotic cases without ear-disease. In all cases coming before the neurologist the ear should be examined at the outset, in order to find out whether or not local ear-disease is present. The diagnosis of tinnitus can be made in obscure cases (those not caused or aggravated by local ear-disease) only "after the broadest and most searching clinical investigation that rational, scientific medicine can give." Auditory allochiria and extracranial noises were observed by Verdos[9] in a man of 50. At the time of writing no remedy had given any relief, and no explanation of the causes of the disease was offered. Tinnitus, when a warning of epileptic fits must be regarded according to W. R. Gowers[10] as originating in the auditory center in the cortex, not in the nerve.

Fibrosarcoma of the Acoustic Nerve.—W. Anton[11] reports the occurrence of fibrosarcoma of the acoustic nerve in a man of 55. The man was seized with headache and blindness of the right eye, and three days later with blindness of the left eye. At times he vomited, and he suffered from roaring and hissing-sounds in the ears, and hardness of hearing. Optic neuritis occurred on both sides and facial paralysis on the right. Death occurred 8 months after the first symptoms. The autopsy revealed a tumor the size of a hen's-egg, rather soft, with rough surface, situated between the pons and the cerebellum. The origin of the nerves on the left was normal; on the right side the 5th, 7th, and 8th nerves ran on the under surface of the tumor, and then over the latter. The 7th and 8th nerves were imbedded in the tumor, and were accompanied by the morbid tissue as far as the internal porus acusticus.

The same author reports the accidental discovery of a similar kind of tumor at the autopsy of an old man. The growth was the size of a nut, and rough, connected with the left acoustic nerve and extending as far as the internal porus acusticus. The acoustic and the facial nerves were separated by the tumor, but connected by a bridge of partly degenerated medullary fiber. In both these cases the fibrosarcoma originated from the sheath of the acoustic and partly from that of the facial nerve.

[1] First Spanish Oto-rhinol. Cong., Nov., 1896.   [2] Ibid.   [3] Ibid.   [4] Ibid.
[5] Jour. Laryn., Rhin. and Otol., Apr., 1897.   [6] Ann. des Mal. de l'Oreille, Jan., 1897.
[7] Ibid.   [8] Fort Wayne Med. Mag., Sept., 1896.
[9] First Spanish Oto-rhinol. Cong., Nov., 1896; Ann. des Mal. de l'Oreille, May, 1897.
[10] Jour. Laryn., Rhin. and Otol., May, 1897.   [11] Arch. f. Ohrenh., Nov., 1896.

DISEASES OF THE NOSE AND LARYNX.

BY E. FLETCHER INGALS, M. D., AND H. G. OHLS, M. D.,

OF CHICAGO.

Review of the Year's Work.—While no brilliant discoveries have illumined the field, a vast amount of faithful clinical work has led to improved methods and apparatus in various lines. Hypertrophic rhinitis, as usual in late years, has been a fruitful subject for study. Turbinotomy, as practised by Carmalt Jones, has its enthusiastic supporters; but equally competent operators raise a note of warning which will doubtless be generally heeded by the profession. D. Bryson Delavan suggests a plan of incision that is certainly simple. John Edwin Rhodes outlines a plan of treatment of atrophic rhinitis for which he does not make extravagant claims, but which certainly enables patients to live in comfort. E. B. Gleason and Arthur W. Watson offer operations for the relief of deflection of the septum. Thomas Fillebrown made a study of the anatomy of the frontal sinus and the antrum, throwing new light upon the relation of suppuration in these cavities. Much study has been devoted to the subject of laryngeal tuberculosis, and the experience of Solomon Solis-Cohen with formic aldehyd and that of W. Scheppegrell with cataphoresis with copper electrodes promise relief of much suffering. Electrolysis has been applied by Arthur B. Duel to the dilatation of the Eustachian tubes for the relief of throat-deafness.

Anesthesia.—Barclay J. Baron[1] reports a case of severe strangulation following an operation on adenoids under nitrous oxid gas, according to the method advocated by W. G. Holloway.[2] As a local anesthetic, J. E. Newcomb[3] recommends guaiacol as a substitute when cocain is contraindicated. [We have been disappointed in the results in attempting to get local anesthesia by the application of guaiacol. After cocain has been applied guaiacol has appeared to cause more smarting than when no cocain had been used, and it has frequently utterly failed to secure anesthesia.] He has used it 36 times in the nose, pharynx, and larynx, and on the average obtains anesthesia in 10 minutes. He proposes a solution as follows: to olive oil add 10% of dry zinc sulfate; heat over a water-bath one hour and add 12½% absolute alcohol; shake several times during 24 hours; decant and add 5% guaiacol. M. Broeckhaert[4] had a patient, an army officer, whose skin was blistered by solutions of cocain. C. W. Ingraham[5] believes that a 2% solution of cocain applied thoroughly to the olfactory region will immediately relieve nausea in 9 out of 10 cases.

Eucain.—The earlier reports of eucain indicated that it caused hyperemia of the mucous membrane, and Lewis A. Somers[6] said that property militates greatly against the use of the drug in active inflammatory conditions. A 4% solution applied on a cotton swab caused anesthesia in from 8 to 10 minutes,

[1] Bristol Med.-Chir. Jour., Dec., 1896.   [2] Med. Mag., June, 1896.
[3] Laryngoscope, June, 1897.   [4] Jour. Laryn., Rhinol. and Otol., Dec., 1896.
[5] Am. Medico-Surg. Bull., Aug. 15, 1896.   [6] Therap. Gaz., Jan. 15, 1897.

lasting about 20 minutes. A 10% solution in sterilized water will keep indefinitely, and may be boiled without impairing its efficiency. W. Jobson Horne and Macleod Yeardsley[1] found that eucain causes no hyperemia, but, on the contrary, slight ischemia, not to be compared to that caused by cocain. The only ill effect noted was the unpleasant taste, lasting half an hour. One patient in whom cocain had previously caused alarming syncope was, later, under the influence of eucain 3 times without ill effect. Joseph Gibb[2] concludes: 1. Eucain is equal to cocain in its anesthetic effects; 2. Eucain is nearly as effective as cocain in reducing engorged turbinates; 3. Eucain is superior to cocain in being less likely to produce toxic symptoms; 4. Eucain is superior to cocain in producing far less unpleasant subjective symptoms, especially in the larynx. Vinci[3] finds that the toxic dose of eucain for the rabbit is 15 to 20 cgm.; of cocain, 10 to 20 cgm. The only alarming report on eucain available is that by T. H. Shastid.[4] In his patient, a man of 32, the application of a 5% solution to the turbinate caused slight intoxication, with amblyopia lasting several hours.

Bacteria in the Nares.—W. H. Park and Jonathan Wright[5] have recently examined the mucus of 36 healthy nares, and conclude, contrary to their investigations of 10 years ago, that the bactericidal properties of the mucus are poor or absent, though it does not form a good culture-medium. E. L. Vansant[6] examined the mucus from 100 cases of chronic nasal disease. Although none of the cases were febrile or showed other clinical signs of diphtheria, 30 cultures from 26 cases showed diphtheria-bacilli. The diseases in which they were found included: 11 of 25 cases of atrophic rhinitis; 3 of 16 cases of chronic purulent rhinitis; 5 of 14 cases of rhinitis; 3 of 7 cases of nasal syphilis; 3 of 31 cases of hypertrophic rhinitis; none in 2 cases of diseased accessory sinuses; none in 1 case of fibrinous rhinitis; in 58 cultures staphylococci were found. He emphasizes the importance of disinfection of the nares. The patients with diphtheria-bacilli were pale and listless, showing apparently a slow chronic toxemia.

Nasal Malformation.—W. R. H. Stewart[7] operated on a man with a bifid nose, due probably to imperfect fetal development, caused by a dermoid cyst that was removed in infancy. The removal of excessive bone and cartilage from the septum and a flap-operation restored the normal shape. Robt. C. Myles[8] notes the liability to stenosis following operations involving the vestibule. To relieve the contracted band he passes a trephine along the floor and inserts a long tube, to be worn several months. Later the bridge may be removed by a Graefe knife and a Berens' cork or Asch's tube worn for a week. In that form of nasal occlusion caused by enlargement of the anterior edge of the triangular cartilage the excess of cartilage is removed by subperichondrial dissection. Geo. C. Stout[9] reports a case of atresia in an infant of 3 months, whose respirations were habitually 105 per minute. Dilatation of the nares by bougies reduced the respirations in a few weeks to 45, and stopped the attacks of laryngismus stridulus to which it had been subject.

Physiology of the Nose.—J. L. Goodale[10] studied experimentally the action of the nasal mucous membrane upon the air inhaled; the normal alterations in intranasal air-pressure, and the route taken by respired air within the nose. He finds the relative humidity of the air after passing the nasal

[1] Brit. Med. Jour., Jan. 16, 1897.   [2] Jour. Laryn., Rhinol. and Otol., Apr., 1897.
[3] Ibid , May, 1897.   [4] Ibid., Apr., 1897.
[5] Laryngoscope, June, 1897.   [6] Phila. Polyclinic, Mar. 13, 1897.
[7] Lancet, Mar. 27, 1897.   [8] Jour. Am. Med. Assoc., Sept. 16, 1896.
[9] Ibid., May 22, 1897.   [10] Boston M. and S. Jour., Nov. 5 and 12, 1896.

chambers is near the saturation-point with reference to its own temperature, but falls considerably below the saturation-point for the temperature which it subsequently attains. The nose is also, in an atmosphere not excessively dust-laden, a nearly complete filter for the inspired air.

Acute Rhinitis.—H. J. Mulford[1] offers a protest against the classic treatment. He attributes acute rhinitis to the accumulation within the blood of the products of tissue-waste, urea, uric acid, etc. The indication is to restore the activity of the emunctories and to neutralize the foreign matter in the blood. Calomel or podophyllin stimulates the liver; lithia or soda overcomes the condition of the blood, and a free supply of water opens the kidneys. Pilocarpin would seem an ideal remedy, but it is unreliable. By this method the cold is cured in from 24 to 48 hours. M. Courtade[2] recommends saline douches at 122° F. to abort coryza. The heat is the important factor, and either sodium chlorid or bicarbonate may be used with good effect.

Phenacetin in Nasal Catarrh.—J. S. Woodruff[3] found that phenacetin applied locally gives satisfactory results in nasal catarrh. He mentions two cases, one in which a profuse nasal discharge following scarlet fever had lasted four years, and another in which there were itching and dryness of the nasal passages, with frontal headache. In the first, phenacetin was administered in the form of snuff; in the second, dissolved in glycerin, with success. The author does not mention to what the above symptoms were due.

Nasal Hydrorrhea.—D. Braden Kyle[4] relates a case and reviews the literature of 26 others. The profuse discharge of clear alkaline, irritating fluid was preceded by headache and sneezing. The mucous membrane presented the appearance of chronic congestion, as if the venous return were obstructed. Examination of the blood showed the plasmodium malariæ, and the patient improved on quinin ·bromid and arsenic sulphid.

Fibrinous Rhinitis.—Lewis S. Somers[5] describes a case of membranous rhinitis, in which repeated bacteriologic examinations were made before the Klebs-Löffler bacillus was discovered. The disease pursued a mild course. Of two children infected by exposure to this case one developed a laryngeal diphtheria and died; the other had a membrane on both tonsils without severe constitutional disturbance. He thinks the first was originally a case of fibrinous rhinitis, becoming infected later with Klebs-Löffler bacillus. Glover[6] gives the autopsy of a woman of 67, in whom a false membrane extended throughout the respiratory tract, serum-cultures from which developed only pure staphylococci.

Turbinotomy for Hypertrophic Rhinitis.—Peter Abercrombie[7] gives an analysis of 66 cases of turbinotomy by Carmalt Jones with his spokeshave. Relief from obstruction was obtained in 62. Patients varied in age from 6 to 71 years. In 49 cases both sides were operated on. As to anesthetics, nitrous oxid gas was given to 5 patients, who felt no pain at all. In 31 cases in which a 10 % solution of cocain was applied more or less pain was felt, in some cases severe. Hemorrhage, free at first, was controlled by cotton-wool plugs. In no cases has atrophic rhinitis resulted. On the contrary, a reproduction of normal mucous membrane takes place, becoming in a few cases excessive. Finally, he recommends the operation as both successful and highly desirable in many instances. Henry B. Hitz,[8] from an experience in many cases, in-

[1] Am. Medico-Surg. Bull., Nov. 21, 1896.
[2] Bull. gén. de Thérap.; Am. Jour. Med. Sci., May, 1897.
[3] Jour. Laryn., Rhinol. and Otol., June, 1897.
[4] Jour. Am. Med. Assoc., Sept. 26, 1896.   [5] Univ. Med. Mag., Aug., 1896.
[6] Ann. des Mal. de l'Oreille, May, 1896; Jour. Laryn., Rhinol. and Otol., Dec., 1896.
[7] Ibid., Oct., 1896.   [8] Laryngoscope, Nov., 1896.

dorses the spokeshave, and meets the objection that the function of the turbinate is thereby destroyed, with the question whether the function is not already destroyed when hypertrophy is sufficient to cause obstruction. Fayette C. Ewing,[1] although formerly an assistant in Mr. Jones' clinic, voices the sentiment felt by all those whose motto is to "restore as nearly as possible the relationship of the parts," when he says, "reason knows no rationalism that will justify the spokeshave." The Laryngologic Society of London[2] discussed turbinotomy, Dundas Grant exhibiting 18 cases out of 35 operated on by himself. Half of this number remained completely free from their primary symptoms, and the rest were relieved. Notable regeneration of the turbinate took place in 6. Hemorrhage was serious in 1, free in 5, moderate in 7. In 8 cases of anterior partial turbinotomy the nasal symptoms were cured in 5 and relieved in 2. He considers the partial resection advisable if only as a preliminary to posterior operation. Cresswell Baber recommended the operation, especially when the removal of septal obstruction does not give free breathing-space. Lambert Lack maintained that the cases must be very exceptional in which complete relief could not be obtained by other and milder measures. [We agree with Lack, but have seen a few cases in which turbinotomy became necessary. In most of these a nasal scissors was the only instrument needed; bleeding was checked by packing with a long strip of antiseptic surgeons' lint.] Semon reported the case of a theologic student in whom turbinotomy was followed by typical atrophic rhinitis, and an increase of the laryngitis to which he had been subject. Scanes Spicer never noticed pharyngitis sicca following the operation, but, on the contrary, found that the temporary dryness of the throat that sometimes followed was far less annoying than the dry mouth and throat before. Watson Williams condemned the operation as unnecessary, dangerous, not under perfect control, and liable to be followed by unfortunate complication.

Transfixion.—Blondian[3] passes a lance-shaped cautery at dull-red heat beneath the mucous membrane of the inferior internal angle of the turbinate for a distance of 7 or 8 cm. A single operation is usually sufficient; the mucous surface is uninjured and synechiæ are never produced. [We have tried this frequently, but have been disappointed in the results.] Marked polypoid degeneration of the posterior end usually shrivels up after one transfixion. The Eustachian tube should be avoided. D. Bryson Delavan,[4] noting the inefficiency of snare and caustics, though they are not conservative, for the reduction of hypertrophies, described a method of incision with a small ophthalmic knife. The point of the knife is carried obliquely as far as possible into the turbinate, and with a slight sweeping motion is brought out of the same opening. The parts are kept contracted with cocain for some hours after the operation, which causes little irritation. Arthur W. Watson,[5] after trying the cautery to reduce the granulation-tissue following removal of the spur of the septum without permanent relief, obtained rapid reduction of the mass by friction, as advocated by C. C. Rice.

Nasal Reflexes.—Chas. N. Cox[6] reports a case of redness of the tip and alæ of the nose due to swelling of the turbinate, and relieved by cauterization of the latter. Touching the inferior turbinate with a probe caused swelling, and at the same time the tip and alæ suddenly became red. Max Thorner[7] had a case of amaurosis of the right eye following the

[1] Laryngoscope, Mar., 1897.　　[2] Brit. Med. Jour., June 12, 1897.
[3] Jour. Laryn., Rhinol. and Otol., Dec., 1896.　　[4] Laryngoscope, Aug., 1897.
[6] Phila. Polyclinic, Nov. 7, 1896.　　[5] Brooklyn Med. Jour., Oct., 1896.
[7] Jour. Am. Med. Assoc., Sept. 26, 1896.

removal of polypi on that side with the cautery. Rethi[1] relates 2 cases of chlorosis due to hyperesthesia of the olfactory nerve, and relieved by light cauterization of the olfactory area. Horace Clark[2] thinks that hyperesthesia of the pharynx is the most common reflex disturbance of intranasal disease, and that the nasal disease most often causing a reflex is posterior polypoid degeneration. Arthur J. Hobbs[3] inadvertently relieved 2 cases of priapism by a spray of cocain applied to the nares to relieve the congestion of the erectile tissue there. He also mentions several cases of sneezing due to erotic emotions accompanied by the same turgescence of the turbinate.

Rhinitis Sicca.—U. Ribary[4] says rhinitis sicca anterior may be regarded as atrophic rhinitis confined to the septum. In this condition the ciliated is converted into pavement epithelium. It precedes erosions and exposes the subject to various infections. Acute cases are susceptible to treatment by ointments containing zinc oxid and bismuth subnitrate. When chronic, a return to the normal is not to be expected [but ointments to prevent drying of the mucus upon the surface give much relief, and mild cauterizations with nitrate of silver sometimes give permanent benefit].

Atrophic Rhinitis.—W. Peyre Porcher[5] says atrophic rhinitis is not a disease *per se*, but is the result of any inflammation, acute or chronic, specific or nonspecific, which ends in a purulent discharge sufficiently prolonged to wash away the epithelia and destroy the nasal mucosa, turbinates, etc. [The belief that atrophic rhinitis is the result of varying degrees of inflammation excited by various causes appears to be strengthened by the reports of many observers; but the etiologic relation of the purulent discharge cannot be accepted by most pathologists.] Ralph W. Seiss[6] extols massage with a cotton swab for 3 to 6 minutes at a sitting. The swab may be dipped in ointment with 5% or 10% of europhen to advantage, or in solution of thymol in albolene. The europhen is less painful than thymol, and may be used as a dusting-powder with stearate of zinc. He claims arrest of the disease and great comfort from treatment extending over several months. The need is for an agent to control fibrosis. W. Peyre Porcher[7] gets the best results by packing the vault of the nares daily with cotton tampons carrying a strong solution of iodin, glycerin, and potassium iodid. Capart and Cheval[8] still use the bipolar method of electrolysis, and claim cures in 90% of cases so treated. [This claim is so remarkable that we are led to suspect that their cases were not all fully developed, or else that the word "cures" was used in the Latin sense.] John Edwin Rhodes[9] gives a thorough review of the literature, and notes cases in which hypertrophy preceded the atrophic process and others which presented atrophy in one part of the nares and hypertrophy in another. As a cleansing douche he recommends the following tablet, dissolved in 4 ounces of tepid water: potassii chloratis, gr. iiss; sodii bicarbonatis, gr. x; sodii chloridi, C. P., gr. x; sodii salicylatis, gr. v; sodii biboratis, gr. v; thymol., gr. $\frac{1}{8}$; eucalyptol., $\mathfrak{m}\frac{1}{4}$. After cleansing the nares with the douche $1\frac{1}{2}$ gr. of the following powder should be blown into the nares two or three times a day: sodii biborat., gr. ij; hydrarg. oxid. flav., gr. ij–v; iodol., gr. j; cocain. hydrochlorat., gr. iiss; magnes. carb., gr. ij; sacch. lactis, q. s. ad gr. 100.

Animal Parasites in the Nares.—H. M. Folkes[10] removed from the

---

[1] Rev. Internat. de Rhinol., in Am. Medico-Surg. Bull., Aug. 1, 1896.
[2] Buffalo Med. Jour., Jan., 1897.   [3] Jour. Am. Med. Assoc, Apr. 12, 1897.
[4] Arch. f Laryn. u. Rhinol. in Jour. Laryn., Rhinol. and Otol., May, 1897.
[5] N. Y. Med. Jour., Aug. 29, 1896.   [6] Med. News, Nov. 28, 1896.
[7] N. Y. Med. Jour., Aug. 29, 1896.   [8] Jour. of Laryn., Rhinol. and Otol., Jan., 1897.
[9] Jour. Am. Med. Assoc., June 26, 1897.   [10] Med. Rec., May 8, 1897.

nares of a negro in Guatemala 131 screw-worms, none of which were under 10 mm. in length. A spray of an alcoholic solution of chloroform followed by irrigation assisted in the process of removal.

Rhinolith.—P. McBride[1] removed from the naris of a woman of 32 a rhinolith measuring $1\frac{1}{2}$ by 1 by 1 in., but found no ulceration and no evident loss of substance or cicatrization.

Etiology of Hay-fever.—Chas. P. Grayson[2] thinks that the digestive system rather than the nervous system is at fault in the development of hay-fever. [We have observed pronounced and peculiar symptoms referable to the digestive system in this disorder, but they have appeared to us rather a result than a cause, and could not be taken as an evidence that the nervous system was not primarily at fault.]

Deflection of the Septum.—John O. Roe[3] concludes: 1. That devia-

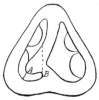

FIG. 68.—Vertical, transverse section through the anterior portion of the nose; angular deviation of the septum, with hypertrophy of the tissues at the angle of the deviation. The dotted line indicates the direction of the saw-cut for the removal of the obstruction (Gleason).

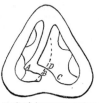

FIG. 69.—Vertical, transverse section through the anterior part of the nose; angular deviation of the septum without hypertrophy of the tissues at the angle of the deviation. The dotted line indicates the direction of the saw-cut for forming the tongue-shaped flap covering the button-hole in the septum; *A B* and *D C,* portions of the septum to be denuded (Gleason).

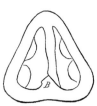

FIG. 70.—Vertical, transverse section through the anterior portion of the nose, showing position of the septum after the tongue-shaped flap has been thrust through the button-hole in the septum. After healing has occurred, the parts at *B* are sometimes abnormally thick; but redundant tissue can readily be removed with the saw (Gleason).

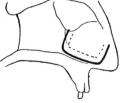

FIG. 71.—Sagittal section through the nose to the right of the septum. Convex surface of deviated area of the septum. The dark line shows position of U-shaped saw-cut through the septum about the deviated area on the convex side, and the dotted line the position of the same saw-cut on the side of the septum. In some instances the mucous membrane on the concave side of the septum apparently rides over the saw teeth and is not cut to the extent shown in the diagram (Gleason).

tions of the septum are produced by a variety of causes operating upon different persons; and that upon the same person several different influences may be operating at the same time. 2. That heredity plays a very important part as a predisposing cause, not only by the dyscrasias which may be transmitted, but by the blending of different races in the composite type, which brings

[1] Jour. Laryn., Rhinol. and Otol., Feb., 1897.   [2] Univ. Med. Mag., July, 1896.
[3] N. Y. Med. Jour., Oct. 10, 1896.

about an infinite variation in the conformation of the osseous and cartilaginous structures. 3. That the three local causes most frequently producing deviation, spurs, and ridges of the septum are trauma, nasal obstruction, and unequal growth of the different component parts of the vomer. The last-mentioned cause is itself produced mainly by local malnutrition or diseased conditions of the structures of the nasal passages, inducing an unequal development of the two sides of the septum, which causes a bulging or bending to the side of greatest development. The fact that the vomer is composed of two laminæ, separated by a plate of fibrocartilage, which is continued forward to form the triangular cartilage of the nose, readily explains how the unequal development takes place. E. B. Gleason,[1] instead of overcoming the resiliency of the deflected septum, makes it a factor in holding it in the proper position (see Figs. 68–71). He saws a U-shaped incision through the base of the septum so as to surround, except above, the whole deflected area. After paring the convex edge of the flap and the concave edge of the base of the septum he forces the flap through the incision and lets the resiliency "do the rest." Arthur W. Watson[2] takes advantage of resiliency by a similar operation, but uses a knife and makes the incision along the crest of the deviation.

E. J. Moure[3] says these are due to luxations of the cartilaginous septum from the shallow groove in the superior maxilla, complicated by thickening. The septum may be forcibly replaced or gradually brought into position by the redresseurs of Delstanche.

Abscess of Septum.—W. E. Casselberry's[4] patient, a boy of 16, was supposed to have asthma owing to dyspnea caused by the abscess. Early incision at the lower edge of the abscess and daily opening with a probe until the cavity is effaced are essential to prevent the destruction of the cartilage and deformity. H. G. Ohls had an unreported case in which moderate depression of the bridge of the nose had already occurred. Suppuration had ceased, leaving a separation of the plates of cartilage. Tubes of dental rubber with a packing of gauze above the tubes, worn for about 5 weeks, restored the patency of the nares and corrected the deformity. Gouguenheim[5] believes that the cause of abscess is always trauma, though traumatic hematoma does not always lead to abscess.

Acute Purulent Perichondritis.—Gottleib Kicer[6] describes a rare affection of the septum as primary acute perichondritis, with phlegmonous symptoms occurring in otherwise healthy persons. Tumors form on both sides of the quadrangular cartilage, often communicating by a necrosis or perforation of the septum.

Tubercular Ulceration of Septum.—Hill,[7] in the discussion of Symonds' case of rapid ulceration of the septum in spite of scraping and applications of lactic acid, suggested trichloracetic acid, 25 %, in these cases, as lactic acid is not strong enough.

Nasal Syphilis.—Albert Kohn[8] removed a large granulating mass which developed in connection with a chancre of the nares. This was twice reproduced at intervals of 2 days, following removal. The disease was checked by inunctions, but the naris was occluded except a small passage through the lower meatus. J. Dionisio[9] describes 31 cases of tertiary syphilis charac-

---

[1] Laryngoscope, Nov., 1896. [2] N. Y. Med. Journ., Oct. 13, 1896.
[3] New Orl. M. and S. Jour., July, 1896; Jour. Laryn., Rhinol. and Otol., Mar., 1897.
[4] Jour. Am. Med. Assoc., Feb. 20, 1897.
[5] Jour. Laryn., Rhinol. and Otol., Apr., 1897; from Ann. des Mal. de l'Oreille, Jan., 1897.
[6] Laryngoscope, Mar., 1897. [7] Jour. Laryn., Rhinol. and Otol., Apr., 1897.
[8] N. Y. Med. Jour., Mar. 27, 1897.
[9] Gaz. Med. di Torino, June 11, 1896; Jour. Laryn., Rhinol. and Otol., Mar., 1897.

terized by simple tumefaction of the mucous membrane, running its course without any signs of ulceration or purulent secretion. Chas. H. Knight[1] cautions against the use of destructive agents in treating syphilitic disease of the nose, but says that necrosed bone may be removed before it is completely detached after the active symptoms have been controlled by treatment. This is especially important before inserting the Martin bridge (Fig. 72) to correct the deformity. If the disease is active, the pressure of a bridge is very liable to cause extensive ulceration. At least 3 years should have elapsed after active symptoms cease before the bridge is inserted. [Two years more should elapse before the case is reported as improved or cured.]

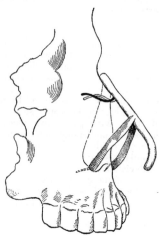

FIG. 72.—The Martin bridge (N. Y. Med. Jour., Sept. 19, 1896).

Sarcoma of the Nares.—Wm. Thomson[2] saw a round-celled sarcoma of the antrum extending into the nose and recurring after two operations. Within a month following the last operation the tumor protruded through the incision in the cheek. It was blue, tense, lobulated, and had almost closed the eye. Further operation was declared useless. Three months later the tumor had disappeared, with unbroken covering and with no other treatment than poultices of comfrey root. G. Melville Black[3] reports removing with the cold snare and curetting the attachment of an alveolar sarcoma involving the middle turbinated region, in a woman aged 38 years, in April, 1894. In 2 years it had not recurred. H. Lambert Lack[4] exhibited before the Laryngologic Society of London a man aged 65, from whom in Feb., 1895, he had removed with polypus-forceps a sarcoma of the middle turbinate, and r d away a large portion of the lateral mass of the ethmoid with Meyer's ring-knife. No recurrence has taken place.

Anosmia.—M. Joal[5] recommends inhalations of carbonic acid gas, from an inverted siphon-bottle with a nasal tip, both to restore the sense of smell and to arrest acute coryza and vasomotor attacks.

Nasal Dermoid Cyst.—Albert Kohn[6] removed from a woman 65 years old several dermoid cysts attached to the middle turbinate. The cysts contained cheesy material. They had not recurred within 6 months.

Epistaxis.—C. G. Cowie[7] plugged the anterior naris of a woman aged 65, to control a moderate epistaxis. A few hours later blood escaped from the lacrymal canal and filled the conjunctival sac. He then made 2 attempts to plug the posterior nares, but on both occasions the patient retched so violently when the plug touched the enlarged tonsils that she sustained a double dislocation of the jaw. Swoboda[8] quotes 4 cases of death from epistaxis. One was a case of hemophilia due to septicemia in an infant with gonorrheal

[1] N. Y. Med. Jour., Sept. 19, 1896.   [2] Brit. Med. Jour., Nov. 28, 1896.
[3] N. Y. Med. Jour., Aug. 15, 1896.   [4] Jour. Laryn., Rhinol. and Otol., May, 1897.
[5] Am. Med. Compend., Nov., 1896.   [6] N. Y. Med. Jour., Mar. 27, 1897.
[7] Brit. Med. Jour., Sept. 19, 1896.
[8] Wien. klin. Woch., in Jour. Laryn., Rhinol. and Otol., Dec., 1896.

conjunctivitis and rhinitis. In another case purulent rhinitis was accompanied by epistaxis. In 2 other deaths from epistaxis the patients had diphtheria.

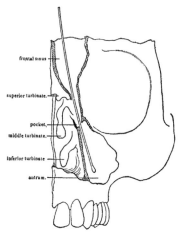

FIG. 73.—Infundibulum terminating in foramen of maxillary sinus (Dental Cosmos, Nov., 1896.)

Anatomy of Frontal Sinus and Antrum.—Thomas Fillebrown[1] found that in 8 specimens the infundibulum, instead of terminating in the middle meatus, continued as a half tube, terminating directly in the foramen

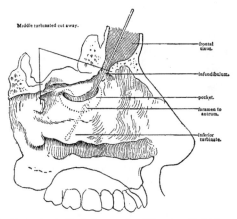

FIG. 74.—Infundibulum terminating in foramen of maxillary sinus (Dental Cosmos, Nov., 1896.)

of the maxillary sinus (see Figs. 73, 74). In 7 of these there was a fold of mucous membrane covering the foramen and forming a pocket, which pre-

[1] Dental Cosmos, Nov., 1896.

vented any secretion from the frontal sinus getting into the meatus until the antrum and pocket were full.

Sinusitis.—W. E. Casselberry[1] thinks that 9 out of 10 cases of acute empyema recover spontaneously. Henry L. Wagner[2] described a case of seropurulent sinusitis of 3 years' duration, with severe neuralgic pains, in a painter. All the upper teeth had been removed, and the supraorbital nerve had been resected, without relief of the neuralgia. The writer opened the antrum freely and noted a bluish-gray hypertrophy of the mucous membrane, which gave the lead-reaction with sodium sulphid. Iodids internally relieved the pain in a few days and caused the discharge to cease. Frank C. Todd[3] had a case of frontal sinus disease in which paroxysms of pain in the frontal region were followed by epileptic convulsions. Reducing the swelling of the ethmoid by cocain solution allowed pus to escape from the sinus, and as the inflammation subsided the convulsions ceased.

The Accessory Sinuses in Zymotics.—M. Wolff[4] examined the accessory sinuses in 22 cases of diphtheria, in 12 of which the diphtheria-bacillus was found in the antra, with inflammatory edema. Various cocci were also present. One frontal sinus and 6 out of 7 sphenoidal sinuses examined contained diphtheria-bacilli. The sphenoidal sinuses were not developed in 15 cases. Five cases of measles and 2 of scarlatina showed various bacteria, with severe inflammatory changes.

Transillumination.—F. E. Sampson[5] says of the indications obtained

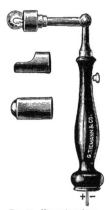

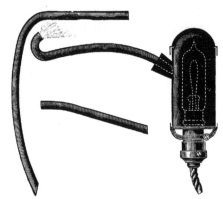

FIG. 75.—Heryng's antrum-illuminator.

FIG. 76.—Chevalier Jackson's lamp for transillumination.

by transillumination: "Ordinarily, when the sinus shows dark, we will find pus, or at least a greatly thickened mucosa; but let us run briefly over the possibilities: if the sinus shows clear, it means one of two things—it is either healthy or contains a mucocele; if clearer than its fellow, it does contain a mucocele, unless the other sinus be diseased, absent, or contains a solid neoplasm. If it shows dark, the sinus contains pus or has a thickened mucosa—unless it be a solid neoplasm or the sinus is absent." W. Scheppegrell[6] reviews

[1] Medicine, Oct., 1896. [2] N. Y. Med. Jour., Aug. 15, 1896.
[3] Laryngoscope, Oct., 1896. [4] Medicine, Sept., 1896; Zeit. f. Hyg. u. Infectionskrank.
[5] Laryngoscope, Aug., 1897. [6] Ann. Otol., Rhinol. and Laryn., May, 1897.

the various methods of transillumination and gives a comprehensive analysis of the indications obtained by this method of diagnosis. He recommends Heryng's lamp (Fig. 75) as the most useful. He has adapted a more powerful light to it, and removed the interrupter from the handle, and uses a foot-switch for completing the circuit. He commends also the ingenious lamp of Chevalier Jackson (Fig. 76). The glass rods, *A, B, C,* are silvered on the sides and covered with enamel, so that the light of the 50-candle-power lamp issues from the end of the rod with undiminished intensity. The different shapes of the rods facilitate their use in every procedure to which the method is adapted. He classifies the different methods of examination of the antrum as follows: 1. Opacity of the cheek of the affected sides, or the method of Voltolini-Heryng. 2. Opacity of the pupil of the affected side, or the method of Davidsohn. 3. Absence of the luminous sensation of the diseased side, or the method of Garel. 4. A modification of the above methods by placing the lamp directly under the maxillary sinus, not under the nasal fossæ, or the method of Ruault. 5. Opacity of the nasal wall of the sinus observed by rhinoscopy, or the method of Robertson. In conclusion, he finds transillumination a valuable addition to our means of diagnosis, but believes that it must be corroborated by other signs.

Congenital Stenosis of the Nasopharynx.—St. Clair Thomson [1] quotes Escat on stenosis of the nasopharynx simulating adenoids. Fig. 77 shows the average anteroposterior section of the healthy nasopharynx of a child of 10. Fig. 78 represents the same space of a child of 11½ years with congenital stenosis. Fig. 79 represents a man of 45 who had congenital sten-

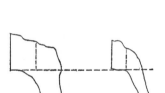

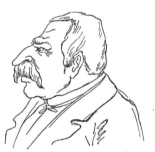

Fig. 77.—Average anteroposterior section of the healthy nasopharynx of a child of 10 years (Practitioner, Jan., 1897).
Fig. 78.—Average anteroposterior section of the nasopharynx of a child of 11½ years wi h congenital stenosis (Practitioner, Jan., 1897).

Fig. 79.—Man of 45 years who had congenital stenosis and emphysema for 10 years, necessitating constant mouth-breathing (Practitioner, Jan., 1897).

osis and emphysema for 10 years, necessitating constant mouth-breathing. This individual was not insane, but was a marked degenerate.

Etiology of Acute Nasopharyngitis.—J. Lewis Smith [2] states that a large proportion of cases are due to microbic infection, especially to influenza in this country. He recommends having the air of the nursery moist and impregnated with the vapor of eucalyptus, carbolic acid, and turpentine.

Medication of the Nasopharynx.—John H. Hollister [3] describes Liebreich's method of medicating the nasopharynx as follows: 30 to 40 drops

---

[1] Practitioner, Jan., 1897.   [2] Med. News, Aug. 12, 1896.
[3] N. Am. Pract., Feb., 1897.

of the medicament are dropped upon a cotton-wool tampon large enough to fill the nasal vestibule. With the mouth open the ala nasi is compressed and the fluid passes into the nasopharynx.

Ultimate Prognosis of Adenoids.—D. Bryson Delavan[1] notes a variety of pathologie conditions in the adult following adenoids in youth, and concludes that adenoid hypertrophy does not tend to spontaneous cure; that when present in any marked degree it demands thorough treatment; and, finally, that if left to itself the prognosis is far from satisfactory.

Adenoids in Adults.—Edward F. Parker[2] notes the frequency with which spurs of the septum are found in adults with adenoids persisting, and he believes that the spurs are an important factor in preventing the atrophy of the hypertrophied lymph-tissue at puberty, by keeping up the irritation and vascularity which were the original causes of the growth.

Unusual Symptoms of Adenoids.—John A. James[3] was asked to tracheotomize a 3-year-old child for croup, with respiration 45 per minute and extreme dyspnea. Learning that the child was a mouth-breather and had enlarged tonsils and adenoids, he removed them, with immediate relief of the dyspnea. Boulay[4] noted the case of a boy of 12 who had adenoids and enlarged tonsils, and who for two years suffered with epileptiform crisis between 4 and 6 A. M. The attacks ceased after removal of the adenoids and tonsils. Grondech[5] noted enuresis in 13% of children with adenoids, operation giving relief in half the cases and improvement in a third more. Upon recurrence in 4 cases, enuresis followed in all. John Sendziak[6] operated on a congenital deaf-mute, 5 years old, removing adenoids, and thereby restoring the hearing so that the child soon began to talk and made rapid intellectual advancement.

Lymphotome.—Jacob E. Schadle[7] has devised an instrument on the

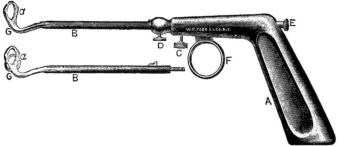

FIG. 80.—Schadle's lymphotome: *A*, aluminum handle; *a*, cutting blade; *B*, cannula; *C* and *D*, thumb-screws; *E*, push-button; *F*, ring trigger; *G*, Gottstein's curve.

principle of the tonsillotome, with a flexible cutting-blade for the removal of adenoids (Fig. 80).

Forceps for Adenoid Operation.—James J. Concanon[8] recommends the removal of adenoids without anesthesia by means of a cutting-forceps (Fig. 81) of his design, with a guard that acts as a palate-retractor and pro-

[1] N. Y. Polyclinic, Dec. 15, 1896.   [2] N. Y. Med. Jour., June 5, 1897.
[3] Med. Rec., Apr. 17, 1897.
[4] Rev. hebdom. de Laryn., in Am. Medico-Surg. Bull., Oct. 24, 1896.
[5] Arch. of Pediatrics, Oct. 1, 1896, from Arch. f. Kinderh.   [6] Laryngoscope, Apr., 1897.
[7] Ibid., Apr., 1897.   [8] N. Y. Med. Jour., June 12, 1897.

teets the septum. When the adenoids extend low in the pharynx he supplements the use of the forceps by one sweep with the Gottstein curet.

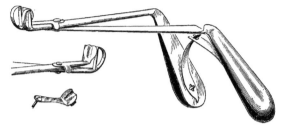

Primary Tuberculosis of the Pharyngeal Tonsil.—F. Pluder and W. Fischer[1] found latent tubercles in the mucosa of 5 out of 32 hypertrophied pharyngeal tonsils examined; bacilli were only scantily present in the diseased part, never in the epithelium or healthy lymph-follicles. The disease was sometimes confined to a small part of the tonsil, but distinct caseation was found in half the cases. The following list includes the microscopic observations recorded:

Lermoyez	in 32 cases found tuberculosis			2	times
Gottstein	in 33 "	"	"	4	"
Brindel	in 64 "	"	"	8	"
Pluder and Fischer	in 32 "	"	"	5	"

Nasopharyngeal Fibromata.—E. Fletcher Ingals[2] reported a large fibroma removed by electrocautery snare in 1894, and the base cauterized several times until the growth in the nares and nasopharynx was destroyed. Part of the tumor passing behind the palate-bone and beneath the zygomatic arch caused a swelling in the cheek. After injecting a 4% solution of cocain, 15 minims of an aqueous solution containing 25% of lactic acid and 15% of carbolic acid were injected into the mass through the mucous membrane of the cheek. This caused severe pain and reaction. Several subsequent injections of lactic acid, 25%, and carbolic acid, 5%, with glycerin, 12%, preceded by the cocain solution, produced little pain or reaction, and caused the growth to almost entirely disappear. [A year after this report the growth had not recurred. He recommends the lactic acid especially in all inoperable tumors, the carbolic acid and cocain being used to minimize pain.]

Alcohol Injections for Cancer.—Edwin J. Kuh[3] reports that he removed from a man of 36, with atrophic rhinitis, a tumor that appeared to be an enlarged pharyngeal tonsil, in July, 1896. Sections of the tumor showed it to be epithelial cancer, and it recurred so rapidly that the nasopharynx was nearly filled by a soft bleeding mass within a month. The diagnosis of carcinoma being confirmed by Nicholas Senn and operation being considered hopeless, Kuh made daily injections of erysipelas prodigiosus toxins. After 10 injections two-thirds of the growth disappeared, but growth began in spite of subsequent injections. In October injections of alcohol, after the method of C. Schwalbe and O. Hasse, were begun with 3 minims, and increased to 30 minims. After the seventh injection reduction in the size

[1] Arch. f. Laryn. u. Rhinol., in Jour. Laryn., Rhinol. and Otol., June, 1897.
[2] N. Y. Med. Jour., Sept. 18, 1896.   [3] Chicago Med. Recorder, Apr., 1897.

began, and after the eleventh little of the growth remained. At the time of writing the nasopharynx was free from growth. The principle of treatment is to surround the periphery of the neoplasm with the alcohol to induce seir-rhous contraction in the connective tissue, and thus reduce the blood-supply. The tumor itself is supposed to undergo sclerotic contraction in its interstices and a fatty regressive metamorphosis in its parenchyma. [If it is true that a few injections of alcohol will produce sclerosis of any tissue, it would seem to resemble the effects on the liver of chronic alcoholic irritation. Many obser-vations will be necessary before such an assumption can be considered proved.]

Electrolysis for Stricture of the Eustachian Tube.—Arthur B. Duel [1] reports brilliant results in the rapid dilatation of the Eustachian tube by electrolysis. After a few treatments patients have remained free from tin-nitus and vertigo, and the hearing has been greatly improved for several months or until the report was made. He uses copper bougies from No. 3 to No. 6, French, mounted on No. 5 piano-wire. These are carried through insulated silver catheters (Fig. 82). The bougie is connected with the negative

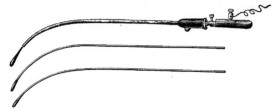

FIG. 82.—Duel's electrodes.

pole of the galvanic battery, the positive pole being applied to the patient's hand by the ordinary sponge electrode. The current should be accurately regulated and never exceed 5 ma.

Epithelioma of the Soft Palate.—Thomas Hubbard [2] injected liquor potassæ into an epithelioma developing in the soft palate and anterior pillar of the fauces, causing the growth to slough. There was no return of the tumor, and the patient gained 40 pounds within a few months. The growth was due to irritation by a tooth-plate. The patient had previously acquired the cocain-habit from Birney's catarrh-snuff.

Glossitis.—J. L. Goodale [3] reviews the literature of "wandering rash of the tongue" and "Moeller's superficial glossitis," and cites cases to show the probable identity of these affections, for which he proposes the name glossitis superficalis migrans.

Foreign Body in the Tongue.—A. V. Anderson [4] removed from a man's tongue an amber mouth-piece of a pipe one inch long which had been forced into the tongue a month before from contact with a hawser when jump-ing off a pier to rescue a man from drowning. In the excitement the man forgot his pipe.

Actinomycosis of the Tongue.—Claissé [5] describes a case in which aspiration of a gumma-like tumor of the tongue revealed the ray-fungus and potassium iodid effected a cure.

[1] Laryngoscope, July, 1897.   [2] N. Y. Med. Jour., Sept. 12, 1896.
[3] Am. Jour. Med. Sci., Nov., 1896.
[4] Laryngoscope, Nov. 18, 1896; Australian Med. Gaz., Sept. 21.
[5] Jour. of Laryn., May, 1897; Presse méd., Mar. 31, 1897.

Lingual Tonsil.—J. F. Barnhill[1] accounts for the great difference in the disturbance caused in different people by the presence of lingual tonsils or other growths in the glosso-epiglottic spaces in two ways: first, in persons of highly sensitive nervous systems the slightest touch of a foreign body against the hypersensitive epiglottis will excite the reflex centers of the air-tract in a degree that would not be possible in one whose nervous tone is normal; second, the conformation of the epiglottis in many cases is such that, instead of standing up and away from the base of the tongue, as it normally should, it curls unduly forward, projecting its crest directly against the base of the tongue and over the glosso-epiglottic spaces, thus unduly infringing upon the smallest nodule of lymphoid tissue, and giving rise to symptoms equal in severity to those found in cases in which the spaces are filled with tumors many times larger, but with normal epiglottis. Functional heart-disease is often much aggravated, and he believes sometimes wholly caused, by disease of these spaces. Globus hystericus usually accompanied such cases, together with other symptoms commonly classed hysteric. He believes some of these cases are cured by proper attention to the upper air-tract, and particularly the spaces under consideration. Other symptoms are sore throat, the nature of which can only be determined by laryngoscopic examination, when there may be found to exist any one of the varieties of tonsillar affections which are better known in connection with the diseases of the faucial tonsil, such as acute lingual tonsillitis, acute follicular lingual tonsillitis, etc.

Malignant Disease of the Tonsil.—David Newman[2] quotes five cases in which cancerous growths of the tonsil were completely removed by five different surgeons through the month without external incision, and reports two cases of his own operated on in 1890 and 1891. He then describes fully two cases requiring external operation. In one the tumor was small and strictly limited to the tonsil. After splitting the cheek to the ramus of the

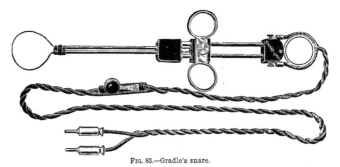

Fig. 83.—Gradle's snare.

jaw, he dissected out the tonsil with blunt scissors. In the other case the growth involved the tonsil and edge of the posterior pillar, without affecting the lymphatics. He removed it by lateral pharyngotomy, with division of the jaw at the angle. These cases were reported 5 and 8 months respectively after operation. The diagnosis must be made early by microscopic examination of the new tissue, not the glandular tissue surrounding it. He prefers the knife to the cautery, on account of the greater ease in distinguishing healthy from diseased tissue.

[1] Laryngoscope, Aug., 1897.   [2] Brit. Med. Jour., Jan. 2, 1897.

Hypertrophy of the Tonsils.—Lacoanet[1] noted a case of great enlargement of the tonsils following diphtheria, which was treated by serum. Under astringents, diet, and sulphur baths the tonsil atrophied. He ascribes the enlargement to either the poison of Löffler's bacillus or the serum, and advises against surgical intervention.

Tonsil-punch.—W. Hill[2] recommends the punch devised by Kretschman for the removal of tonsils, when the guillotine is not practicable.

The Hot Snare.—Henry Gradle[3] devised a hot snare (Fig. 83) for using either platinum, or preferably steel wire. The current-closer is placed in the cable a foot from the handle and is operated by the hand that holds the tenaculum. [The galvanocautery is especially valuable in removing tonsils when there is danger of hemorrhage, but it is followed by much greater reaction than the tonsillotome, and in some cases by a large amount of cicatricial tissue; therefore, usually it is an unsatisfactory instrument in tonsillotomy.]

Bone-growths in the Tonsil.—Alex. W. Sterling[4] exhibited 3 patients with bony growths projecting into the tonsillar region. The first case was a young lady of good personal history. Her tonsils had been cauterized, and when tired she often complained of pain originating in the right tonsil and radiating through the right side of head and right shoulder. On palpation an immovable hard mass was detected below the tonsil and projecting to the level of its anterior surface. By exclusion, he determined that it was the styloid process of the temporal bone. The two other cases were a brother and sister, aged 65 and 64. In each both styloids could be detected, but neither patient had suffered in any way from the anomaly. Deichert,[5] in tonsils removed from 3 persons, found connective tissue with cartilage and bone-cells, which he attributed to aberration of foetal cartilage.

Calcium Sulphid in Tonsillitis.—W. Bayard Shields[6] recommends calcium sulphid in 1 gr. doses to abort tonsillar inflammation and prevent abscess-formation (quinsy). He gives 4 doses at hourly intervals, 6 doses at intervals of 2 hours, and then every 3 hours till inflammation subsides. In 150 cases this treatment gave relief in from 2 to 6 days. If this dose causes depression, heart-stimulants are given. [This does not appear a very rapid result of treatment; indeed, there may be some question whether many of the cases would not have recovered in the same time if left entirely to themselves. The application of a spray of guaiacol, 50%, in oil of sweet almonds, in most cases cuts short the inflammation in from 12 to 36 hours.]

Scarlatinal Sore Throat.—Lape[7] recommends **resorcin,** 5% to 10% in glycerin, applied on a brush or swab two to four times a day, after gargling with boric acid solution.

Reflex Cough.—Furet[8] says reflex cough may be due to any pathologic alteration of the tonsil owing to the involvement of the tonsillar plexus of nerves. Emil Mayer[9] says cough is reflex in its origin: 1. When it is spasmodic, practically constant, without expectoration and temperature; 2. When the physical signs of pulmonary disease are absent; 3. When it persistently resists all medication; 4. When the general health remains comparatively undisturbed; and, 5. When upon removal of the cause it promptly ceases.

---

[1] Rev. hebdom. de Laryn., in Am. Medico-Surg. Bull., Aug. 15, 1896.
[2] Brit. Med. Jour., Sept. 26, 1896.   [3] Jour. Am. Med. Assoc., Sept. 26, 1896.
[4] Ibid., Oct. 3, 1896.   [5] Virchow's Archiv, in Am. Medico-Surg. Bull., Oct. 24, 1896.
[6] Jour. Am. Med. Assoc., Jan. 16, 1897.
[7] Rev. internat. de Méd. et de Chir., Mar. 25, 1896.
[8] Presse méd., in Med. Rec., July 25, 1896.   [9] Laryngoscope, Mar., 1897.

Enlarged Pharyngeal Arteries.—P. McBride[1] traced a pulsating artery across the pharynx of a woman of 67. In a second case a pulsating tumor in the region of the tonsil simulated an aneurism, but proved to be a cyst. In a woman of 61, not only the pharyngeal, but a number of arteries in different parts of the body pulsated visibly. E. Harrison Griffin[2] noted a pulsating tumor with old syphilitic scars in the pharynx of a woman of 49,; the swelling was about the size and shape of a lead-pencil. In another woman of 45 he saw a similar artery traversing the visible length of the pharyngeal wall.

The Bucco-pharyngeal Zona.—Lermoyez and Barozzi[3] described a case of bilateral zona of the mouth and pharynx occurring in a man of 78. The vesicles were arranged with geometric symmetry over the palate, uvula, and inner surface of the lips, the successive crops of vesicles lasting several weeks. The differential diagnosis follows:

HERPETIFORM ANGINA.	PHARYNGEAL ZONA.	RECURRENT PHARYNGEAL HERPES.
Sudden onset, with headache, rigor, and intense general disturbance.	Insidious onset; very little general disturbance.	General disturbance often absent.
Pain in the throat increases. It is slight at first, but becomes intense at the time of eruption, and lasts to the end of the attack.	Less pain in the throat. It is most marked at the onset, and then decreases. It has disappeared almost as soon as the eruption appears.	Very little pain. Burning sensation often unnoticeable.
Eruption bilateral.	Eruption unilateral.	Eruption very intense. Often localized to the same area during each relapse.
Attacks the tonsil particularly; but also affects simultaneously the pharynx, larynx, and lips.	Limited to the area supplied by a nerve, usually the second division of the 5th. It affects the palate, uvula, gums, and cheeks, leaving the tonsils and pharynx intact.	A particular spot; often in the neighborhood of the anterior pillar.
Short duration—four to six days.	Longer duration—fifteen to twenty days.	Eight to ten days' duration.
Acute course.	Subacute course.	
Frequently recurs.	Never recurs.	Always, recurs, often with periodicity.

Primary Tuberculosis of the Pharynx.—Walter. F. Chappell[4] noted tubercular infection following the removal of the pharyngeal tonsil from a girl of 19. The cervical glands soon become enlarged and tender, and the lateral pharyngeal folds resembled collections of granules—hard, tender, and blue. Frequent examination of the lungs revealed no pulmonary involvement for 4 months. Then rapid development of miliary tuberculosis caused her death in 3 months.

Thyroid Extract in Myxedema.—J. Woodman[5] reports the case of a woman of 38, who had developed myxedema 8 years before. Her weight had increased from 120 to 240 pounds; sweating ceased with the onset of the disease, and the skin became hard, dry, and deeply pigmented; the hair was coarse and brittle. Nothing was lacking of the typical symptoms of a severe case. Four months' treatment with thyroids reduced her weight 60 pounds, and in all

---

[1] Edinb. Med. Jour., Dec., 1896. [2] Med. Rec., Aug. 15, 1896.
[3] Ann. des Mal. d'Oreille, in Jour. of Laryn., Rhinol. and Otol., May, 1897.
[4] N. Y. Med. Jour., Sept. 19, 1896. [5] Med. Rec., Oct. 31, 1896.

other respects the patient returned to her normal condition. John W. Farlow [1] reports a localized myxedema lasting 2 years, in a woman of 46. The face was slightly involved, but general symptoms were not marked. Under thyroid extract the patient made slight gain.

Iodin in the Thyroid Extract.—Baumann and Goldmann [2] found that thyro-iodin, 3 to 6 gr. a day, prevents tetanic symptoms in thyroidless dogs. The same remedy cures the tetany, but is all excreted by the kidneys. Hennig [3] says iodin is combined in the gland with albumin and globulin. The physiologic effect of thyro-iodin is to increase the excretion of phosphoric acid, nitrogen, chlorin, and sodium chlorid.

Pharyngeal Teratoma.—A. W. de Roaldes [4] removed from a male infant of 6 weeks a sessile dermoid tumor attached to the posterior pillar of the fauces, and large enough to cause dyspnea when falling into the larynx. It had much the shape of an auricle. Section showed fibrocartilage, fat, loose connective tissue, and skin. Achard classifies it as a simple form of the very rare epignath monsters.

Apomorphin in Acute Laryngitis.—Thos. Hubbard [5] recommends apomorphin, gr. $\frac{1}{30}$, in freshly compounded acidulated mixture, as a most efficient relaxing expectorant. Given every 2 or 3 hours, it causes a free seromucous flow in from 12 to 36 hours.

Edema of the Larynx.—W. P. Meyjes [6] reports a case of acute idiopathic edema of the epiglottis in a man of 41. A spray of ichthyol, $\frac{1}{3}\%$ in ice-water every 15 minutes, with ice externally, gave rapid relief. Dunbar Roy [7] describes a case of suddenly appearing and disappearing swelling of all the tissues of the neck in a man of 36. By measurement the neck was found to be actually greater in circumference during the attacks, which occurred about 10 A. M. at frequent intervals, lasting only a short time. The swelling of the neck was firm, and did not pit on pressure. The attacks were accompanied by palpitation of the heart and some dizziness. The thyroid was not enlarged. The interarytenoid space was obliterated by swelling without congestion. The vocal cords were normal. No organic disease except myopia was discoverable. Max Thorner [8] intubated a man of 18 who had suffered with dyspnea for 8 years, from a stenosis of the larynx of unknown origin; 15 hours later the tube was removed at the request of the patient. A few moments of comfortable breathing were followed by a rapid edema of the larynx and death. This case emphasizes the necessity of watching carefully, and for some time after removing the tube, cases of chronic stenosis.

Varicella of the Larynx.—M. Marfan and J. Halle [9] describe 2 cases of varicella in which dyspnea necessitated intubation. Antitoxin was given in both cases before the vesicular eruption, on the supposition that it was diphtheria. One of these cases is said to be the only recovery on record.

Urticaria of the Larynx.—Delbril [10] says the symptoms may simulate edema of the larynx when the respiratory trouble precedes the skin eruption. On examination red, raised erythematous patches may be seen in the pharynx, even when a view of the larynx and trachea is impossible. For acute cases with severe pulmonary symptoms and no cutaneous eruption, he recommends brisk friction to induce its appearance.

[1] N. Y. Med. Jour., Sept. 26, 1896.
[2] Münch. med. Woch., in Jour. Laryn., Rhinol. and Otol., Mar., 1897.   [3] Ibid.
[4] N. Y. Med. Jour., Feb. 6, 1897.   [5] N. Y. Med. Jour., July 18, 1896.
[6] Jour. Laryn., Rhinol. and Otol., Mar., 1897.   [7] N. Y. Polyclinic, Nov. 15, 1896.
[8] Jour. Am. Med. Assoc., Sept. 26, 1896.   [9] Rev. mens. des Mal. d'Enfance, Jan., 1896.
[10] Jour. de Méd., July 25, 1896 ; Brit. Med. Jour., Oct. 3, 1896.

Fracture of the Larynx.—A. W. de Roaldes[1] describes a fracture of the left cornu of the thyroid cartilage caused by forcible manipulation of the larynx by a man who was partly suffocated by an olive-pit. The sensation of a foreign body persisted several months.

Foreign Bodies in the Larynx.—Guy Hinsdale[2] made an autopsy on a boy 4 years and 9 months old who died suddenly, and found a pencil $2\frac{1}{4}$ in. long impacted in the larynx and trachea (Fig. 84). Cyanosis just before death was supposed to indicate heart-disease.

E. W. Davis[3] describes the case of a child of 15 months, who choked on a piece of peanut-shell. A man introduced his finger forcibly into the larynx, which relieved the dyspnea partly. The following day tracheotomy was performed, and 52 days later the child expectorated the shell, the tube being worn for 75 days. He thinks that the injury done by introducing the finger violently caused an edema that prevented the shell being discovered. Max Thorner,[4] by means of Kirstein's autoscope and Krause's straight tube-forceps, removed a chicken-rib, $1\frac{1}{2}$ in. long, lodged in the right ventricle, extending across the cavity. N. Palazzolo[5] removed a large leech that had been in one of the ventricles for 10 days. J. Walker Downie[6] located a pin in the larynx by means of **x-ray** photographs, and removed it by median thyrotomy. Ten days after using the x-ray prickling and heat were felt over the back of the head and neck; vesication and sloughing of the skin followed, and the hair over a large area came out.

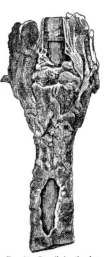

Fig. 84.—Pencil in the larynx (Internat. Med. Mag., Feb., 1897).

Papillomata in the Larynx.—G. Hunter Mackenzie[7] shows the success that may follow simple **tracheotomy** for papillomata. A child with congenital papillomata wore a tracheotomy-tube for 7 months, during which time a number of papillomatous particles were detached and expectorated. The dyspnea following final removal gradually improved, and the voice became normal for the first time. He believes that the rest from coughing and phonation causes atrophy of the growth. F. Lohrstorfer[8] intubated a child three times for papillomata, with relief of dyspnea each time. Later a tracheotomy preparatory to a radical removal of the growth was followed by death, owing to some obstruction in the cannula. H. Heryng[9] recommends sulphoricinate of phenol, 30%, applied thoroughly, to cause absorption of papillomata. On the aryepiglottic folds and cartilages of Santorini the application will cause them to disappear. In other parts they should be operated on before applying the remedy. [There is reason to believe that the neglected *thuya occidentalis*, applied in the form of fluid extract or tincture, and at the same time administered internally, will cause the destruction of papillomata.]

Acute Perichondritis of the Thyroid Cartilage.—C. W. Richardson[10] reported a case of acute suppurative perichondritis in a man of 24 with-

[1] N. Y. Med. Jour., Feb. 6, 1897.
[2] Internat. Med. Mag., Feb., 1897.
[3] Physician and Surgeon, Sept., 1896.
[4] Jour. Laryn., Rhinol. and Otol., Jan., 1897.
[5] Ibid., Mar., 1897.
[6] Glasgow Med. Jour., Nov., 1896.
[7] Lancet, Feb. 13, 1897.
[8] Med. Rec., Oct. 10, 1896.
[9] Therap. Monats., Mar., 1897.
[10] Ann. of Otol., Rhinol. and Laryn., May, 1897.

out discoverable cause. Swallowing became extremely painful, and edema of the larynx caused such dyspnea that incisions into the edematous tissues became necessary. Finally, evacuation of a large abscess just above the sternal notch gave relief to the acute symptoms, and was followed by rapid gain of strength and weight, though the voice gained strength very slowly, and after 9 months was easily fatigued.

Gonorrheal Perichondritis.—H. S. Birkett[1] relates an interesting case of inflammation of the left crico-arytenoid joint, with edema of the mucous membrane covering it and tenderness on external pressure, occurring during an attack of gonorrheal rheumatism. Application of Leiter's ice-coil gave marked relief. Within a week the swelling disappeared and the voice became normal.

Feeding in Paralysis of the Larynx.—Frank Savery[2] had a case of malignant stricture of the esophagus, involving and causing paralysis of both recurrent laryngeal nerves, with aphonia, dyspnea, and dysphagia. To avoid the latter symptom, he recommends giving liquid food from a feeding-cup introduced into the lower angle of the mouth, the patient lying on his side with the head well over the side of the bed. In this position the fluid passes not over, but by the side of the larynx, through the hyoid fossa, and enters the esophagus without coming in contact with the posterior commissure of the larynx.

Laryngeal Vertigo.—Albert C. Getchell,[3] from a study of 77 cases, including 2 of his own, concludes that laryngeal vertigo occurs in persons in whom there is evidence of unstable equilibrium of the central nervous system. There is some abnormal condition of the air-passages, likely to produce laryngeal irritation, with cough and glottic spasm. The spasmodic closing of the glottis may, and in many cases does, act directly and immediately upon the inhibitory centers of the brain and cause syncope. A severe paroxysm of coughing, which produces congestion of the cerebral vessels, may also cause syncope; but it will not cause it unless there be an existing disorder of the central nervous organ.

Laryngeal Tuberculosis.—S. Oakley Vander Poel[4] calls attention to the appearance of the larynx in early tubercular disease. In the case described there was no evidence of ulceration or of tumefaction of the posterior laryngeal wall, but merely a slight thickening of the mucous membrane, with a white, milky, somewhat purulent mucus containing no tubercle-bacilli, but which he considers almost pathognomonic. In his case this condition occurred in a patient with a healed tubercular cavity of long standing, and it was followed by a rapid development of typical ulceration and death in a few months. F. Brannsfeld[5] finds that inhalations of from 10% to 30% solutions of **lignosulphite** cause increased expectoration, with easier respiration and improved appetite. In laryngeal cases cough becomes easier, dysphagia diminishes, and ulcers clean up to a certain extent. However, no specific influence on the bacilli or on the tubercular process is claimed for this inhalation. J. Lardner Green[6] strongly recommends the inhalation of 1 or 2 drops of **formalin** from a Jeffery's respirator in the early stage of phthisis. Both the micrococcus pneumoniæ and the bacillus tuberculosis rapidly decrease in number under the treatment. For acute cases the formalin should be diluted with water. Solomon Solis Cohen[7] has had good results in infiltrative, ulcerative, and vegetative cases from the use of **formic aldehyd** in $\frac{1}{2}$% to 4% solutions.

---

[1] N. Y. Med. Jour., Sept 19. 1896.   [2] Lancet, Sept. 18, 1896.
[3] Boston M. and S. Jour., Nov. 5. 1896.   [4] N. Y. Med. Jour., July 18, 1896.
[5] Deutsch. med. Woch., Apr. 1, 1897.   [6] Brit. Med. Jour., Jan. 23, 1897.
[7] N. Y. Med. Jour., Oct. 24, 1896.

The intense burning and strangling sensation can be prevented to a large extent by the previous application of cocain solution of proportionate strength, from 4% to 20%. He begins with $\frac{1}{2}$% solution of formic aldehyd and gradually increases to 4%, equivalent to 10% of the commercial preparation, rubbing the remedy into the tissues thoroughly twice a week. He attributes to the formic compounds iodoform, chloroform, bromoform, and formaldehyd, a specific antitubercular influence. **Bromoform** is recommended as a local analgesic for painful tubercular ulceration. In several early lesions the application of bromoform followed by insufflations of iodoform has been followed by healing. W. Scheppegrell[1] recommends **cataphoresis with a copper laryngeal electrode,** as preferable to curetting or the cautery in laryngeal tuberculosis. With the Kirstein autoscope a slightly curved electrode may be used to better advantage. The advantages which he found in the method of applying cupric electrolysis in the treatment of laryngeal tuberculosis are as follows: 1. There is no real destruction of the tissues, and there are no lacerations of the surfaces which might form a point of entrance for new pathogenic germs for reinfection, as in the case with the method of curettage, and, to a certain extent, also with the galvanocautery and simple electrolysis. The cure is effected by the healthy reaction of the tissues in the same manner in which we often see specifie lesions heal when the system is under the influence of mercurials. 2. In the cases which he treated by this method there was absolutely no reaction or hemorrhage following the application—a point of great importance with tuberculous patients. 3. This method does not demand the high degree of manipulative skill required for curettage, or for the manipulation of the electrocautery in the larynx, and is especially simple when direct laryngoscopy can be used. 4. This method is applicable in all cases of laryngeal tuberculosis.

Tuberculosis and Syphilis of the Larynx.—E. Harrison Griffin[2] claims that a constitution that is prone to tuberculosis renders the patient more susceptible to its development if the syphilis is not quickly and properly treated. He quotes cases to prove: 1. Tubercular and syphilitic ulcerations are found side by side in the larynx. 2. That the presence of a syphilitic ulcer by the side of a tubercular ulcer in the anatomy exercises a moderating influence upon the tubercular deposit, if the syphilis be treated, and prolongs the life of the patient. 3. Do not rely upon the report of the microscope in all these cases, as the tubercle-bacilli will be found if there be phthisis, but the syphilitic element, if present, is overlooked. 4. In the case of a mixed sore the syphilitic ulcer will generally progress quicker than the tubercular, but can be easily controlled if the right diagnosis is rendered. [The diagnosis of mixed infection of this kind is extremely difficult, and cases bearing out this position are very rare in the practice of the most experienced laryngologists.] Leopold Glück[3] treated a series of 30 cases of syphilis of the larynx with intermuscular injections of **corrosive sublimate.** Mucous patches were present in many cases. Of 14 ulcers, 10 were located on the vocal cords. None of them left a cicatrix, thus indicating that they all belonged to the secondary stage. The strength of the solutions used varied from 3% to 5%, beginning with the weakest. The treatment averaged from 15 to 18 days, and the total amount injected in each case varied from 9 cgm. to 2.53 gm. The results obtained were gratifying, and the author recommends the method as best adapted for lesions in the larynx. Irsai,[4] from 4 years' ex-

---

[1] Med. Rec., May 29, 1897. [2] Laryngoscope, Apr., 1897.
[3] Wien. med. Woch., Jan. 9, 1897.
[4] Rev. hebdom. de Laryn., in Am. Medico-Surg. Bull., Aug. 15, 1896.

perience with the injections, recommends them highly for speedy relief when the lesions cause dyspnea. He injects a 5% solution once a week into the gluteal muscles.

Chorditis Tuberosa.—Johnson Elliott[1] notes that improper or excessive use of the voice is the cause of chorditis tuberosa in adults subject to chronic nasal catarrh. Sopranos are not subject to it, though the Italian method of singing is said to induce it in some cases. [We have not found sopranos exempt.]

Changes in the Voice.—Cartex[2] found only 1 case of injury to the voice in 6 oöphorectomies. In some cases the voice gained both in tone and compass. C. Biaggi[3] describes the voice due to arrest of development of the larynx during puberty. In 2 cases complete cure followed removal of nasal obstructions. [This defect in the voice is seldom, if ever, due to want of development of the larynx. It may be speedily cured in most, if not in all, cases by the method recommended by Mulhall, of St. Louis, in the *Transactions of the American Laryngological Association.* In a number of cases that have come under our observation the cure has been effected in from 2 to 10 days.] Felix Semon[4] applied the galvanocautery to a singer's nodule, and thereby changed the high falsetto voice of a clergyman to a deep basso.

Stammering and Stuttering.—Geo. A. Lewis[5] defines stammering as the inability, under certain conditions, to articulate or control the organs of speech, which are usually, under such circumstances, tightly held together, accompanied in many cases by the substitution of one sound for another. Stuttering is a defect in respiration and vocalization, oftentimes causing spasmodic action or the rapid repetition of one word or syllable before the following can be uttered. He indicates by a graphic representation the relative influence of the physical and mental types of defective speech. Stammerers of the former class are troubled continually about the same. Mental emotions and impaired health do not much increase the severity of their affliction. When the mental type predominates they can speak well when free from excitement, but stammer violently under a variety of emotions when tired or ill.

Stammering and Hypnotism.—Thos. B. Keyes[6] reports 2 cures of stammering by hypnotic suggestion. One patient, a man of 22, had stammered 16 years, and was cured by 3 treatments. The other case required 11 treatments. From these cases he believes that hypnotic suggestion offers a reliable method of treatment.

Surgical Treatment of Stammering.—G. Hudson Makuen,[7] in the case of a youth of 19, who had never been able to speak intelligibly, found that the tip of the tongue was too short. Dividing the genio-hyo-glossi muscles freely, following by tractions on the tongue and vocal exercises, gave him almost perfect articulation, and was followed by rapid mental development. Another boy of 8 years was cured of stammering within 2 months by the removal of adenoids and the amputation of the tip of the uvula.

Intubator.—Louis Fischer[8] describes a new aseptic intubator which grasps the head of the tube without obstructing the lumen, thus allowing more time for the operation. He also devised a corrugated rubber tube, which is not as easily coughed up as the smooth tubes, nor do secretions adhere to it as to the metal tubes.

[1] Va. Med. Semi-monthly, July 10, 1896.
[2] Bull. de la Soc. Franc. d'Otol., in Practitioner, Jan., 1897.
[3] Bull. del. Mal. del. Orec. in Jour. Laryn., Rhinol. and Otol., Mar., 1897.
[4] Jour. of Laryn., Rhinol. and Otol., Mar., 1897.   [5] Physician and Surgeon, Sept., 1896.
[6] Columbus Med. Jour., Sept. 1, 1896.   [7] Therap. Gaz., Dec. 15, 1896.
[8] Med Rec., June 19, 1897.

CUTANEOUS DISEASES AND SYPHILIS.

By LOUIS A. DUHRING, M. D.,

OF PHILADELPHIA.

INFLAMMATIONS.

Two Cases of Urticaria Treated by the Administration of Calcium Chlorid.—According to A. E. Wright,[1] "serous hemorrhage" (an increased transudation of the fluids of the blood into the tissues) may be due to a diminished blood-coagulability, and, therefore, we may hope to control the transudation by correcting this defect. To this end he recommends that large doses of calcium chlorid (30 gr. t. i. d.) be administered at the outset to supply the deficiency of lime and to bring the patient rapidly under the influence of the drug; afterward reducing the dose (to 5 gr. t. i. d.), so that excessive quantities of lime shall not accumulate in the system. One of the cases, reported had followed the injection of 25 c.c. of antitoxin.

Urticaria following an Enema.—J. E. Moorhouse[2] reports the case of a woman of 38, who suffered from an attack of dysenteric diarrhea followed by constipation. An enema of soap and water was followed by urticaria, which lasted 4 days. The itching and discomfort were slight. The author believes that the eruption was the direct result of a toxemia due to the absorption of fecal matter liquefied by the warm water. All other causes were excluded in considering the case. [The case bears points of resemblance to that reported by Hale in the *Brit. Med. Jour.*, vol. i., p. 474, 1895.]

Case of Ritter's Dermatitis Exfoliativa Neonatorum.—W. A. Newman Dorland[3] describes a case of this rare disease (termed by Ballantyne keratolysis neonatorum), which is characterized by an acute cutaneous hyperemia, followed by an excessive exfoliation of the epidermis, and accompanied at times by a vesicular or bullous formation and by a high mortality. It is more common in male than in female infants, and generally appears in the second week, and rarely after the fourth or fifth week. At first apparently healthy, an erythematous hyperemia or superficial dermatitis appears on the face or the buttocks, which soon becomes generalized. There is no elevation of temperature nor gastric disturbance. Exfoliation of the epidermis soon sets in, large flakes coming off. The entire process occupies a week or two, and may be unaccompanied by systemic disturbances; but in many cases there will develop complications, as diarrhea, pneumonia, or marasmus, the infant ultimately dying from exhaustion or from loss of body-heat due to the extensive exfoliation. The author's case was of a mild type, and recovered.

Notes on Dermatitis Venenata.—James C. White[4] calls attention to some cases of dermatitis due to poisons not commonly recognized. One was that of a young woman with hands and wrists greatly swollen, and the dorsal

[1] Brit. Jour. Dermatol., viii., No. 3, 1896.   [2] Brit. Med. Jour., May 29, 1897.
[3] Phila. Polyclinic, Sept. 26, 1896.   [4] Boston M. and S. Jour., Jan. 28, 1897.

surfaces of her hands thickly occupied by a papulo-vesicular efflorescence in process of development, with much heat and itching. Two days previously she had washed five bushels of recently dug parsnips (*pastinaca sativa*). Another case was that of an inflammation of the skin of the hands excited by oil of cassia, the girl having been engaged in dipping wooden tooth-picks in oil of cassia for the purpose of giving them an agreeable perfume. Reference is also made to the stinging properties of the hairs which grow at the base of the point of the hop hornbeam, and a case is mentioned in which an irritation was caused which did not disappear for several hours. A case of a fireman is given whose skin was poisoned by wearing a shirt dyed in anilin-black. It caused an infiltrated erythema of a brilliant red color, decidedly elevated above the general surface, occurring either in uniform areas of considerable extent or in smaller, discrete, circular patches, varying in size from a pea to a dime. [Dr. White is an authority on this subject, having published valuable articles and a book on dermatitis venenata. The cases referred to are new in the literature of affections of this kind.]

The Relation of Dermatitis Herpetiformis to Erythema Multiforme and to Pemphigus.—Louis A. Duhring[1] discusses this subject, stating that some cases of dermatitis herpetiformis possess similar features to those characteristic of erythema multiforme, especially to the erythematous and bullous varieties of that disease. In dermatitis herpetiformis, however, the cutaneous manifestations are in most instances more intense, more persistent, and more chronic. The formation of pustules, especially miliary and acuminate, so common in dermatitis herpetiformis, is a symptom that is lacking in erythema multiforme. The other well-known disease to which dermatitis herpetiformis bullosa bears likeness is pemphigus, but from which it differs in important particulars. As characteristic of dermatitis herpetiformis may be mentioned irregularity or even capriciousness in the production of the lesions; polymorphism, more notable even than in erythema multiforme or eczema; the tendency to relapses and to recurrences; the irregularity in the evolution of the lesions, especially a tendency to radical and abrupt changes in the kind of lesions; and, finally, the presence of herpetiformity, without which dermatitis herpetiformis cannot exist. All these features are peculiar to the disease and are wanting in pemphigus. The conclusions reached are: 1. That dermatitis herpetiformis is in most instances a disease with well-defined, tolerably constant clinical features; 2. That it is more closely allied to erythema multiforme than to any other generally recognized disease; 3. That the bullous variety resembles pemphigus, but differs from it in the peculiar inflammatory and herpetiform character of the lesions, as well as in the tendency to polymorphism, the irregular and peculiar evolution of the lesions, and in its cause.

Case of Dermatitis Herpetiformis involving the Alimentary Canal and Ending Fatally.—J. Kenneth Watson[2] reports the case of a woman of 52, who was admitted into the hospital with the following history: after family bereavement, which had brought about serious mental depression, she began to complain of an eruption which commenced at the back of the shoulders, and had continued to spread rapidly up to the time of admission. The skin was covered with an eruption consisting chiefly of large bullæ, irregular in shape and size, situated on an erythematous base. In addition to the bullæ there were scales and pustules. The temperature was not raised, nor were there any signs of acute illness. There was a general feeling of "soreness" rather than of great irritation, accompanied by constitutional depression.

<hr/>

[1] Am. Jour. Med. Sci., Feb., 1897.   [2] Lancet, July 11, 1896.

PRESS NOTICES

Pepper's New "American Text=Book of Practice."

"We reviewed the first volume of this work and said : 'It is undoubtedly one of the best text-books the practice of medicine which we possess.' A consideration of the second and last volume leads us odify that verdict and to say that the completed work is, in our opinion, the BEST of its kind it has ever n our fortune to see. It is complete, thorough, accurate, and clear. It is well written, well arranged l printed, well illustrated, and well bound. It is a model of what the modern text-book should be."

"An American Text=Book of Gynecology."

"As a text-book it is well up to the most advanced views of the day, and embodies all the essentia nts of advanced American gynecology. It is destined to make and to hold a place in gynecologica rature which will be peculiarly its own."

"An American Text=Book of Surgery."

"If this text-book is a fair reflex of the present position of American Surgery, we must admit it is very high order of merit, and that English surgeons will have to look very carefully to their laurels hey are to preserve a position in the van of surgical practice."

"An American Text=Book of Diseases of Children."

"This is far and away the best text-book of children's diseases ever published in the English lan ge, and is certainly the one which is best adapted to American readers. We congratulate the editor h the result of his work, and heartily commend it to the attention of every student and practitioner."

"An American Text=Book of Obstetrics."

"We can truly say of this magnificent work that it marks a distinct advance in the literature o stetrics, and we hope, for the sake of womankind, that it may find a place in the library of every prac ng obstetrician. It is almost encyclopedic in its scope."

"An American Text=Book of Physiology."

"The names of the authors alone would command respect, and this feeling is considerably anced after a perusal of their productions. The book is certainly the best thing in the way of physio- cal text-books that America has produced."

"An American Text=Book of Applied Therapeutics."

"The whole field of medicine has been well covered. The work is thoroughly practical, and while intended for practitioners and students, it is a better book for the general practitioner than for the dent. The young practitioner especially will find it extremely suggestive and helpful."

surfaces of her hands thickly occupied by a papulo-vesicular efflorescence in process of development, with much heat and itching. Two days previously she had washed five bushels of recently dug parsnips (*pastinaca sativa*). Another case was that of an inflammation of the skin of the hands excited by oil of cassia, the girl having been engaged in dipping wooden tooth-picks in oil of cassia for the purpose of giving them an agreeable perfume. Reference is also made to the stinging properties of the hairs which grow at the base of the point of the hop hornbeam, and a case is mentioned in which an irritation was caused which did not disappear for several hours. A case of a fireman is given whose skin was poisoned by wearing a shirt dyed in anilin-black. It caused an infiltrated erythema of a brilliant red color, decidedly elevated above the general surface, occurring either in uniform areas of considerable extent or in smaller, discrete, circular patches, varying in size from a pea to a dime. [Dr. White is an authority on this subject, having published valuable articles and a book on dermatitis venenata. The cases referred to are new in the literature of affections of this kind.]

The Relation of Dermatitis Herpetiformis to Erythema Multiforme and to Pemphigus.—Louis A. Duhring [1] discusses this subject, stating that some cases of dermatitis herpetiformis possess similar features to those characteristic of erythema multiforme, especially to the erythematous and bullous varieties of that disease. In dermatitis herpetiformis, however, the cutaneous manifestations are in most instances more intense, more persistent, and more chronic. The formation of pustules, especially miliary and acuminate, so common in dermatitis herpetiformis, is a symptom that is lacking in erythema multiforme. The other well-known disease to which dermatitis herpetiformis bullosa bears likeness is pemphigus, but from which it differs in important particulars. As characteristic of dermatitis herpetiformis may be mentioned irregularity or even capriciousness in the production of the lesions; polymorphism, more notable even than in erythema multiforme or eczema; the tendency to relapses and to recurrences; the irregularity in the evolution of the lesions, especially a tendency to radical and abrupt changes in the kind of lesions; and, finally, the presence of herpetiformity, without which dermatitis herpetiformis cannot exist. All these features are peculiar to the disease and are wanting in pemphigus. The conclusions reached are: 1. That dermatitis herpetiformis is in most instances a disease with well-defined, tolerably constant clinical features; 2. That it is more closely allied to erythema multiforme than to any other generally recognized disease; 3. That the bullous variety resembles pemphigus, but differs from it in the peculiar inflammatory and herpetiform character of the lesions, as well as in the tendency to polymorphism, the irregular and peculiar evolution of the lesions, and in its cause.

Case of Dermatitis Herpetiformis involving the Alimentary Canal and Ending Fatally.—J. Kenneth Watson [2] reports the case of a woman of 52, who was admitted into the hospital with the following history: after family bereavement, which had brought about serious mental depression, she began to complain of an eruption which commenced at the back of the shoulders, and had continued to spread rapidly up to the time of admission. The skin was covered with an eruption consisting chiefly of large bullæ, irregular in shape and size, situated on an erythematous base. In addition to the bullæ there were scales and pustules. The temperature was not raised, nor were there any signs of acute illness. There was a general feeling of "soreness" rather than of great irritation, accompanied by constitutional depression.

[1] Am. Jour. Med. Sci., Feb., 1897.   [2] Lancet, July 11, 1896.

She was a year past the menopause. A mixture containing potassium iodid, perchlorid of mercury, and liquor arsenicalis, was ordered, and an ointment containing zinc oxid and ammoniated mercury. Under this treatment the skin improved very rapidly, the contents of the bullæ drying up and the lesions being replaced by raised pigmented and discolored patches. On the fourth day two bullæ were noticed, one on each side of the hard palate posteriorly, and at this time diarrhea set in, which became very intractable, although it was partially held in check by copper sulphate and opium in pillform. Mercurial treatment was now stopped, and on the eleventh day opium in larger quantities had to be administered. From this time the patient rapidly became weaker, and for two days before death the diarrhea was accompanied by vomiting, which could only be partially controlled. She died on the fourteenth day. The points of interest in this case are: 1. The universal distribution, almost no part of the trunk or limbs being free; 2. The apparent lack of any cause beyond the mental condition; 3. The coincidence of the rapid healing of the skin-lesions with the commencement of the diarrhea, indicating the involvement of the alimentary canal by the disease; 4. The rarity of death from this disease.

Herpes Zoster following Extraction of Teeth.—George Pernet [1] reports the case of a woman aged 25, from whom six teeth were extracted under gas (four lower incisors, right lower canine, and a left molar). Six days afterward a marked herpes zoster appeared in the right axillary region and over the right mamma. A year before, twelve teeth were removed under ether, when she suffered much from shock, loss of blood, and from the anesthetic.

Counterirritation in the Treatment of Herpes.—Theodore Wilkins [2] states that in nearly all cases of herpes zoster a tender spot may be found higher up over the nerve-trunk. At this point he recommends the application of a counterirritant in the form usually of fly-blisters or turpentine. The pain in most cases is speedily relieved, and the eruption dries up much sooner than would be the case in the natural evolution of the disease.

Case of Duhring's Impetigo Simplex.—N. J. Kaufman [3] reports an example of the impetigo simplex of Duhring, some authors inclining to doubt the existence of the disease. The subject was a child 4 days old. There was no history of impetigo contagiosa in the family or neighborhood. There existed about 12 straw-yellow, firm, discrete, elevated, thick-walled, semiglobular pustules, about the size of a finger-nail, surrounded by a pronounced dark-red areola, disseminated over the chest, abdomen, and legs. There was no depression nor umbilication, nor did the lesions coalesce. After 7 or 8 days some of the pustules became slightly bloody, and then dried to yellowish or brownish crusts, fell off, and left no scar, but a slightly reddish spot which faded in a few days. The disease lasted four weeks. The general health was good. The microscopic examination showed many agglutinated pus-corpuscles, a few red corpuscles, pus-cocci, and broken-down epithelial cells.

Blood-erythema.—Harrison [4] calls attention to a peculiar state of the skin in which arterial blood sprinkled upon it causes irritation and sets up an erythema (first described by Shield). The case of a surgeon, who for a great many years was annoyed by the irritation resulting from arterial blood coming in contact with his skin, making him uncomfortable, is cited. It was not

---

[1] Brit. Med. Jour., Jan. 30, 1897.   [2] Med. Rec., Sept. 26, 1896.
[3] Jour. Cutan. and Genito-Urin. Dis., June, 1897.
[4] Brit Jour. Dermatol., p. 42, June, 1897.

altogether a subjective sensation, for after washing off the blood a pink stain was left on the skin, which lasted for 15 minutes or longer. He was also very susceptible to the smell of blood. Mr. Chappell Fowler was acquainted with a surgeon who suffered from the same irritation. He was asthmatic and of very neurotic temperament, and the smell of blood was loathsome to him. After a case of postpartum hemorrhage he had seen an erythematous rash on the arm where the blood had been projected some hours after carefully washing the part, and there was irritation.

A Puzzling Eruption following Sunburn.—Erythema—edema—purpura—ulceration.—What was it?—The patient-physician [1] reports the case as follows: in apparently perfect health the physician drove in an open-case carriage, bare-handed, starting, on a very hot summer day, at 7 A. M. At 10 A. M. the neck, backs of hands, and thumbs began to burn. At 11 A. M. the burning was so intolerable that he stopped at a druggist's and applied watery extract of hamamelis. By noon, when he returned home, the burning was unbearable, lead-and-opium wash affording no relief. At 4 P. M. he left by train for Boston. About midnight the parts began to swell, and by the next morning edema was very pronounced, the face and hands resembling erysipelas. Next day petechial spots appeared, the burning and itching continuing. On the third day extravasation of blood began, and after the ninth day ulceration and sloughing set in. Though in good health, the patient had been addicted for fifteen years to the daily use of morphin, but had been cured of this habit two years before. For two months before the attack he had used 3 or 4 ounces daily of fluid extract of coca. During the first five weeks of the cutaneous disease a condition of nervous erethism existed constantly. Appetite was "extra good" until the end of the third week, then fair. The bowels were regular until the fourth week, then constipated for ten days; afterward they were all right. The temperature was normal throughout attack.

Dermatitis, etc., due to the X-rays.—T. C. Gilchrist [2] records the case of a man of 32, who, after he had exposed his right hand, wrist, and lower portion of the forearm for three weeks for four hours daily to the x-rays, noticed that the skin turned red and swollen, without pain. The swelling first occurred on the back of the hand, then active inflammation set in. Three weeks later there were aching, darting pain up the forearm, and throbbing pain, preventing sleep. Under the use of hot-water applications and the internal administration of bromids the swelling and the other signs of acute inflammation subsided. Three weeks from the beginning the dorsal aspect of the hand was pigmented a dark-brown color, and the epidermis was exfoliating, the skin beneath being dry and of a dull reddish color. Ten days later the skin was stretched and glossy, and there was a distinctly thickened state of the first and second phalanges of all the fingers. All movements of the hand were painful. Sensation was much impaired before exfoliation of epidermis took place. An excised portion of the skin examined histologically showed the vessels of the corium to be dilated, and the pigment-cells of the papillæ to be almost as numerous as are usually found in a section of negro skin. Photographs were at this stage taken of the sound as well as of the affected hand, and revealed a distinct osteoplastic periostitis and probably an osteitis.

E. E. King [3] reports a case in which, after six weeks' exposure of from two to six hours daily of the right side, the right hand began to swell, the feet became stiff, and large blisters appeared on the dorsal aspect, which produced great pain. The demonstrations were discontinued, and the hand recovered. Two

[1] Phila. Polyclinic, July 11, 1896.   [2] Johns Hopkins Hosp. Bull., Feb., 1897.
[3] Canad. Pract., Nov., 1896.

PLATE 12.

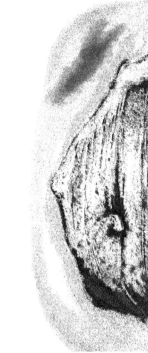

H. R. Crocker's case of dermatitis from Röntgen rays (Brit. Med. Jour., Jan. 2, 1897).

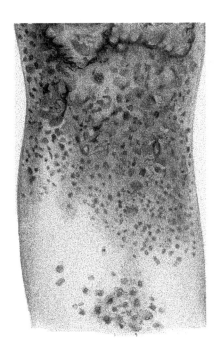

J. A. Fordyce's case of hypertrophic lichen planus (Jour. of Cut. and G.-U. Dis., Feb., 1897).

months later the patient was again exposed to the rays, this time the left side being placed toward the instrument. In about six weeks swelling of the lips and left cheek occurred, and a few days later the left hand swelled with blebs, ached like a severe sunburn, and the skin was discolored. The finger-nails showed signs of shedding ; the eyelids were edematous and there was conjunctivitis on both sides. About two-thirds of the side of the face exposed to the rays was affected. Subsequent notes state that the skin of the hands was congested, infiltrated, and unusually smooth, the left being almost entirely devoid of hair. All the nails were in a state of exfoliation. The hair on the left side of the face was to a great extent lost, the eyebrows, moustache, and whiskers being almost gone, the skin in these regions being very smooth and different from that of the other side.

H. R. Crocker[1] reports (with portrait in color, Plate 13) the case of a boy aged 16, upon whom the experiment of radiographing the spine was made. A Crookes tube was placed about 5 inches from the epigastrium, a flannel shirt intervening between the tube and the skin. The next day the skin felt irritated, and was of a deep red color in the area subjected to the rays from the tube. Six days after the experiment the skin felt stiff when he bent his body, and a few days later vesicles formed. Subsequently the patch was the size of a hand, very sharply defined, and raised. The lower border was sharply outlined ; the upper much less so. The color was a dark or purplish red. Numerous flat vesicles occupied the surface of the skin. The skin felt sore, but was not very tender. There was only moderate itching. A week later the epidermis became detached, leaving a raw surface which healed very slowly.

Hypertrophic Lichen Planus.—J. A. Fordyce[2] records the following case : the subject was a man, aged 54, the skin-disease having appeared two and a half years before. The anterior surface of the right leg was the seat of numerous, closely aggregated, flat-topped, warty elevations, of a purplish-red to a brownish-red color, and of irregular outlines. These lesions were moderately firm, and covered by a thickened stratum corneum, which could be seen as minute horny plugs dipping below the cutaneous surface. Surrounding the warty lesions were a great number of brownish-red papules situated around and independent of the hair-follicles. These papules corresponded in their main features with lichen planus papules, having flat, shiny tops, angular outlines, and some showing the central dell. The lesions varied in size from a pin's head to a pea, or even larger. Intermingled with and about the smaller papules were individual and grouped sepia-brown to black pigment-spots, which evidently represented the involution-stage of the papules that had not developed into the larger tumors. This pigmented area extended upward and outward over the leg until it became continuous with a similar group of lesions in the right popliteal space. Here the same general condition existed of warty growths, small papules, and pigmented spots, as seen on the anterior surface of the leg. The warty growths in this locality were softer, pinkish to bluish-red in color, and formed the most prominent feature of the clinical picture (see Plate 12). They were elevated from a quarter to half an inch above the skin-level, and formed a band-like group extending across the popliteal space for a distance of three inches or more. At right angles to this band another group of lesions extended upward. The left popliteal space and the sacral region on either side of the gluteal fold were affected in a similar, though less pronounced, manner. The genital region was implicated in a most curious and striking manner by the new growths, which occurred as isolated, dome-shaped, hard, purplish-red papules in the hair over the pubes. The skin of the penis, with

---

[1] Brit. Med. Jour., Jan. 2, 1897.   [2] Jour. Cutan. and Genito-Urin. Dis., Feb., 1897.

the exception of a narrow ring about the prepuce, was almost completely surrounded by the papillomata, which had coalesced in a diffuse infiltration made up of elevations and depressions. The growth here was distinctly pinkish in color, quite firm, painless to pressure, perfectly dry, and not marked by evident desquamation. The skin which was not attacked was the seat of a deep patchy pigmentation, and spots of leukoderma. On elevating the organ its under surface was seen to be the seat of similar warty tumors, which were arranged in the form of bands on either side of the raphe, and extended in a continuous, beadlike line of nodules along the raphe of the scrotum, suggesting an autoinoculation from contact with the apposed surface. The scrotum was deeply pigmented; the inguinal nodes somewhat enlarged, but painless. The posterior surfaces of the forearms were a trifle pigmented, rough, and showed a papular development not unlike that seen in prurigo mitis.

Prurigo.—James C. White[1] gives a critical review of our knowledge of this disease, and finds that the views of dermatologists in all countries are discordant. He says: "We find wide differences of opinion held by accomplished dermatologists concerning the primary manifestations and their mutual relations upon the anatomic character of the so-called characteristic lesion or lesions and upon their pathologic significance; deviations from the Hebra standard in point of the parts affected and course of the disease; marked variations in type and prevalence in different countries and nationalities." He sums up his views of the situation by stating that he can go no farther than to "accept the existence of a condition of early childhood allied to pruritus and urticaria in its visible manifestations, and not to be positively distinguished from them in its first stages, often becoming in certain parts of the world a chronic affection due to some inexplicable national cutaneous traits, or inherent customs of living—a condition which certainly lacks many of the essential elements of individuality."

E. Besnier,[2] of Paris, discusses this disease in its totality, but especially its position among other allied diseases of the skin, and concludes that it begins in early childhood as a cutaneous disturbance manifesting symptoms closely related to pruritus and to urticaria, from which disease it is indistinguishable in the beginning; that it occurs in certain parts of the world in consequence of inexplicable national peculiarities of the skin or of heredity, taking on a chronic form characterized by certain well-defined clinical features. [The paper thus succinctly abstracted is an elaborate, lengthy, and valuable contribution to the pathology of this much-discussed disease, which in some large centers of population in the United States is practically unknown (as in Philadelphia), and in others (as Chicago) is only rarely met with. It occurs in its most pronounced form in Austria.]

On the Restriction of Meat in the Treatment of Psoriasis.— L. Duncan Bulkley[3] states that there are few who will contend that this disease is wholly local in its origin, either in the line of idiopathic cell-derangement or external causation. All who are familiar with the disease know only too well how temporary and relatively unsatisfactory local treatment proves to be. Observation and study, with a large amount of material, extending over many years have led the author to the conclusion that the disease is dependent upon a blood-state closely allied to that belonging to gout and rheumatism, which is perhaps best expressed by the term "uricacidemia." The chief point in the article is that free indulgence in meat is very likely greatly to aggravate the eruption of psoriasis, whereas its restriction (especially

---

[1] Jour. Cutan. and Genito-Urin. Dis., Jan , 1897.
[2] Monatsh. f. prakt. Dermatol., Sept. 15, 1896.   [3] Med. Rec., Jan. 9, 1897.

the avoidance of beef and mutton, including meat-extracts and strong soups) will materially aid in its removal. The author does not wish to be understood as saying that the eating of strong meat alone will produce the eruption, or that its avoidance will surely cure the eruption, but that the element under consideration is of great importance in the management of psoriasis.

Local Treatment of Variola.—F. S. Purman,[1] stimulated by Bryan's success, treated 2 cases of variola antiseptically by a somewhat different method. As soon as the papules developed into vesicles the surface was scrubbed with soap and water, followed by solution of hydrogen dioxid. The vesicles were then opened, the fluid permitted to escape, and the cavity touched with pure carbolic acid, and the surface again washed with solution of hydrogen dioxid, oiled to relieve the smarting, and finally covered with cloths wrung out of carbolized water. No pitting of the skin resulted in either case.

Arrest of Variola in its Vesicular Stage.—Alonzo Bryan[2] thinks that the eruption can be arrested in its vesicular stage, and that the pustular stage is due to infection of the vesicles by pyogenic organisms. A case is narrated in which the hands and forearms, the seat of a papular eruption, were disinfected by means of soap and water, alcohol and corrosive sublimate (1 : 500), and a solution of hydrogen dioxid. The parts were then wrapped in borated cotton. On the parts thus treated most of the vesicles dried up into adherent dry scales, without any suppuration, only a small number forming pustules. When vesicles only had formed there was no scarring or pitting. On the rest of the body the disease ran its usual course.

Treatment of Acne.—G. T. Elliot,[3] after discussing the general treatment of the disease, says : There are innumerable local remedies employed in the treatment of acne, but all those which are of any benefit are to a certain degree antiseptic in action. They are in the forms of lotions, salves, and powders. When the process is acute, and the inflammatory symptoms are active, then soothing applications are at first preferable, such as a 2 % salicylic acid ointment, or a lotion of magnesiæ carbonat., zinc. oxid., $\bar{a}\bar{a}$ $\mathfrak{z}$j ; hydrarg. bichlorid., gr. j to ij; aq. rosæ, $\mathfrak{z}$iv. M. In place of this, a dilute lead wash, or the lotion of lead water and opium can be used, or any other mild application. The remedy used should be kept as long as possible in contact with the surface, and not simply dabbed on once or twice daily.

When the acute symptoms have subsided, or when the inflammatory reaction is more of a chronic type, and this is the rule, then more stimulating applications are necessary. The majority of those which offer good results contain sulphur, either in powder form, or in an ointment or a lotion. The sulphur mixed with starch in the proportion of 1 to 8 or 1 to 4 may be used, or it may be incorporated in Bassorin paste. When used as an ointment, its strength should be at least 10 %, and even 20 % or more. ℞. Sulph. sublim., $\mathfrak{z}$ij ; ætheris, spts. vini, glycerin., $\bar{a}\bar{a}$ $\mathfrak{z}$ij ; aq. calcis, aq. rosæ, $\bar{a}\bar{a}$ $\mathfrak{z}$iv. M. or, ℞. Sulph. lactis, $\mathfrak{z}$iv ; tinct. saponis viridis, $\mathfrak{z}$x ; glycerin., $\mathfrak{z}$vj ; spts. vini, $\mathfrak{z}$j. M. Both are good lotions in chronic cases. One of the most useful is potass. sulphuret., zinc. sulphat., $\bar{a}\bar{a}$ $\mathfrak{z}$j ; aq. rosæ, $\mathfrak{z}$iv. M. All of these are applied at night after a preliminary soap-and-water washing, and allowed to remain over night. They produce a certain amount of reaction, a more or less marked temporary shrivelling and scaling of the skin, but are not to be dispensed with for that reason. If their effects are severe, they can be weakened in strength or used less frequently. Vleminckx's solution is also at times of benefit, as is also a paste : ℞. Sulph. sublim., $\mathfrak{z}$iss ; glycerin., $\mathfrak{z}$j ; spts. vini camphorat., $\mathfrak{z}$x ; aq. rosæ, q.s. M. (Besnier).

[1] Med. Rec., Sept. 5, 1896. [2] Ibid., July 10, 1896. [3] Post-Graduate, Oct., 1896.

The mercurial preparations are much esteemed, but care should be taken not to use them when any sulphur preparation is being or has been applied. A favorite lotion is : ℞. Hydrarg. bichlor., gr. xv ; ammon. chlor., gr. 30–70 ; spts. vini, ʒiv ; aq. rosæ, ad Oj. M. or, the corrosive sublimate can be used in any other combination desired.

Ointments are extensively prescribed, though in Elliot's experience they are of value only in particular cases, when uncomplicated by a seborrhœa oleosa, and when there is a natural dryness of the skin. The ointment may be a sulphur one, or of beta-naphthol, 5 % to 15 % ; or of ichthyol, 10 % to 25 %, or more ; or of resorcin, 5 % to 20 % ; or of some of the mercurials—the white precipitate, the ungt. hyd. oxid. rub., 5 %, or the ungt. hyd. nitratis, ʒj to ʒiij, ad. ʒj. A very useful combination when much pustulation exists is : ℞. Ungt. hyd. oxid. rub., ʒiij ; ungt. sulphuris, ʒvj ; ungt. zinc. oxid. ad. ʒij. M.

Care in the local treatment of acne should be taken that too severe measures are not employed, so as to avoid secondary injuries to the tissues, which may be of more moment than the skin-disease itself, and in consequence the effects of the remedies should always be carefully watched, and the amount of reaction should be controlled. Success in the treatment of acne depends particularly upon the proper conception of both the etiologic factors existing in each case presenting itself, and also in a knowledge of the pathology of the disease. Every example of acne should be regarded as distinct and whatever remedy or mode of treatment is instituted should be prescribed after careful investigation into the indications furnished by the patient's history. Routine treatment cannot but furnish more failures than successes.

Etiology of Acne.—Lomry,[1] from a bacteriologic examination of comedo and pustular acne, concludes that the staphylococcus pyogenes albus is constantly present in the pustule of acne, but that it possesses a very weak virulence. By passing it through the animal body it can be made as virulent as the yellow staphylococcus, becoming at the same time yellow and acquiring the faculty of liquefying gelatin. Besides the staphylococcus albus, there are present also occasionally a yeast-fungus and a bacillus, always in small numbers. In noninflamed comedo there is an abundant development of microbes, the staphylococcus albus always being present, but not in such numbers as in the acne-pustules. In comedo one observes at the beginning of the inflammatory process a microbic development intermediate between that of the pustule and that of the noninflamed comedo. When inflammation sets in in comedo there occurs a considerable diminution in the number of kinds of microbes. The skin of those not affected by acne is as rich in microbes as that of the acne-subject. In the comedones and pustules which sometimes occur on those not affected by acne the same microbes are found as in those who have acne. The presence of certain microbes is not sufficient to explain the occurrence of the malady. There must be a peculiar soil. We cannot accept the theory of a specific cause in acne. The staphylococcus albus is seen in many other diseases of the skin. The clinical features which Unna brings forward to contrast acne with other staphylococcic infections of the skin may be explained by the difference in the virulence of the microbes. The special bacillus of Unna is only a variety of the bacterium coli with attenuated virulence.

Case of Folliculitis Decalvans.—George Thomas Jackson[2] reports, with photographs, a case of this rare disease. The subject was a woman 35 years old, nervous and worried over family matters. Her appearance showed that she was harassed. She was very thin and her face was drawn. The hair turned gray prematurely. She suffered with intense headache. The disease had

[1] Dermatol. Zeit., Bd. iii., H. 4.   [2] Jour. Cutan. and Genito-Urin. Dis., July, 1896.

begun 6 years before, on the vertex. Since then new patches had formed from time to time, especially since she was injured in a railroad accident one year ago. None of the old patches have got well, but, on the contrary, have spread slowly into the surrounding parts. There are now some ten patches scattered over the scalp. They are irregular in shape, cicatrized in their centers, and push out into the surrounding parts, so that the full extent of the ravages of the disease can be seen only by raising the hair about them. They vary in size from a marrowfat pea up to a patch 2 in. or more in diameter. They seem to begin by the appearance of a small red spot with stumps of hair in it. This slowly invades the surrounding parts, the oldest part becomes crusted, and when the crust falls the scalp is found to be cicatrized and reddened. The disease is attended by no discomfort. Ever since the beginning the patient has been treated by various physicians, but without any benefit. In the diagnosis tinea tonsurans was excluded. Alopecia areata is another possible diagnosis, and one that probably would have been made before we knew of the existence of folliculitis decalvans. It differs from alopecia areata in the chronicity of the patches, in the redness of the scalp, in the crusting that is seen in one part of their course, in the irregular shape of the patches, in their peculiar invasion of the surrounding parts, and in the cicatrization of the center of the patches. The course of the disease is inflammatory, and it spreads as if from local infection. We are ignorant as to its cause. The cases observed have been refractory to treatment.

Chronic Equinia of the Skin.—Buschke,[1] as the result of his study of the literature of the subject and the examination of a case of his own, concludes that there is a form of chronic equinia localized upon the extremities, the ulcers of which have nothing characteristic in their appearance, being almost the same as syphilitic ulcers. The diagnosis is to be made by bacteriologic examination and intraperitoneal inoculation according to the method of Straus, supplemented by the identification of the bacilli by staining and culture. Mallein is possibly available for diagnostic purposes in human equinia. The treatment is extirpation when possible, or cauterization with the Paquelin.

Case of Bucco-facial Actinomycosis Cured.—M. Duguet[2] reports a case (with portraits taken before and after treatment) of this rare disease which was radically cured. The subject was a young man, and the disease recent, the fungus having very probably penetrated a carious tooth. Cure was obtained after 4 months by treatment with potassium iodid taken internally and injections of tincture of iodin into the fistules and diseased structures. The lesions bore more resemblance to syphilis than to either cancer or lupus.

Some Glycosuric Dermatoses.—C. W. Allen[3] observes that if there were sufficient marked characteristics to distinguish the diabetic eruptions from those of similar nature, but of distinct non-diabetic causation, we might be warranted in making of them a class apart, as the syphilides, leprides, etc. The writer's objection to this is that many of the cutaneous manifestations due to the presence of sugar in the system occur in glycosuria (which is not to be confounded with the disease diabetes). Instances of dermatoses disappearing with a transient glycosuria are quoted, and the possibility of glycosuria following furuncular and suppurative processes is referred to. Both symptoms might depend upon a common cause. An instance of true diabetes following carbuncle, or at least not being detected until some time afterward, was mentioned. A series of eruptions which the writer had not found mentioned in the literature of *dermatoses diabeticæ* are recorded. The first of these is an eruption involving

---

[1] Arch. f. Dermatol. u. Syph., Bd. xxxvi., H. 3.   [2] Presse méd., No. 39, 1897.
[3] Jour. Cutan. and Genito-Urin. Dis., Dec., 1896.

the scalp, extensor surfaces of the arms, backs of the hands, thighs, legs, and backs of the feet. It consists of rounded lesions, either with a "scooped-out" center or covered with crusts which had a central depression somewhat like those seen in acne varioliformis of Hebra. Other lesions have the appearance of superficial erosions, rather oblong than rounded, presenting a glazed surface. They are irritable rather than itchy. The picture as a whole is more suggestive of acne cachecticorum than of the acne necrotica above mentioned, which is usually limited to the forehead and a few hairy regions, and has smaller lesions with a crust "mortised-in" at the summit. The lesions, too, are much more obstinate than those of acne varioliformis.

A nother form of lesions which occurred in the presence of a high percentage of sugar is described as acute multiple gangrene of the skin, of very superficial nature, the ulcerations extending at the periphery until some reach the size of a quarter-dollar ; the base grayish-yellow, with the red points of papillæ showing through. [The patient was confined to bed for a fortnight.] Pigmented areas remained where many of the lesions had existed, and some of them became covered with a strong growth of hair. Bronzing of the skin as a condition *per se* is spoken of, and the fact that Mossé demonstrated pigmentations on mucous membranes in diabetics, contrary to the generally accepted view. Erysipelas in diabetics is then taken up, and an instance of death related in which the patient was syphilitic, very obese, and affected with extensive sloughing and undermining of the skin about the trunk. Erythema, dermatitis, and eczema about the genitals, possibly leading to gangrene, receive passing notice, and xanthoma diabeticorum, which some observers maintain is not a xanthoma at all, but more properly called lichen diabeticus, is touched upon. The latter is not thought by the author to bear a close clinical relationship to the xanthoma usually seen about the eyelids. The peculiar vulnerability of the skin in diabetics is referred to, and the slight tendency to heal which lesions from injury or disease manifest. [The article is interesting and instructive.]

Balsam of Peru in Scabies.—Jullien[1] states that he has used balsam of Peru, according to the method of Peters and Tanturri, in about 300 cases of this disease. Balsam of Peru contains an essential oil, the vapor of which is extremely toxic to the itch-mite. The patient is rubbed in the evening for fifteen or twenty minutes with the balsam. The vapor itself is sufficient to kill the parasite. The patient sleeps afterward in a night-shirt impregnated with balsam of Peru, and the next morning he is well soaped and has a bath. This treatment is particularly useful in patients affected with secondary eczematoid and other inflammatory lesions, and in weakly persons, in the subjects of heart-disease, in pregnant women, and in nurslings.

Tinea Versicolor on the Soles of the Feet.—E. D. Smith[2] reports the case of a man addicted to drink the soles of whose feet gave him much uneasiness. The soles of both feet were the seat of patches of a considerable size and of pale-red color, their peripheries being darker than their centers, which were nearly of the color of the normal skin. There was slight itching especially annoying after going to bed. The patches were easily distinguishable by daylight, but with difficulty by lamplight. The microscope revealed the fungus peculiar to tinea versicolor. A few applications of tincture of iodin effected a cure. [Such cases are very rare, and the importance of employing the microscope as an aid to diagnosis in cutaneous diseases is admirably illustrated.]

Bald Ringworm.—Dubreuilh and Frèche[3] call attention to a form of

---

[1] Sem. méd., Apr. 15, 1896.   [2] N. Y. Med. Jour., Oct. 31, 1896.
[3] Brit. Jour. of Dermatol., Nov., 1896.

ringworm, under this title, which resembles alopecia areata so closely as to be distinguished from it with difficulty. They report two cases, one certainly, the other probably, of animal origin, due to the ectothrix variety of the trichophyton. The transformation from the ordinary form of ringworm to that resembling alopecia areata was sudden. These cases, the authors think, give a positive foundation for the belief in a relationship between ringworm and alopecia areata.

A Study of the Trichophyton Fungi.—As the result of his investigations Krösing [1] concludes in part that Sabouraud's division of the trichophyton fungi into large-spored and small-spored (megalosporon and microsporon) is unwarranted. The size of the spores varies in the same fungus and in the same culture. Classification of the human trichophytoses therefore, according to their localization (trichophytosis of the scalp, of the heard, of the non-hairy parts), based upon the size of the fungus, cannot prove satisfactory.

Deep and superficial affections (sycosis and trichophytia circinata) may be caused by the same fungus. There are forms of suppuration produced by the trichophyton alone. It is thus far impossible to draw conclusions concerning the fungus at the bottom of it from the clinical picture presented by any trichophytosis.

The Anatomy of Trichophytosis.—Waelsch [2] finds that the trichophyton tonsurans grows through the cortex of the hair, upward and downward, for a variable distance, but spares the hair-bulb. It develops in the lower corneous layers, as well as in the cells of the hair-follicle in process of cornification. By its growth in the skin the fungus produces inflammation of the skin, causing exudation on the surface, proliferative processes in the epithelial layers, folliculitis, perifolliculitis, and ultimately destruction of the follicle.

The degree of the inflammation, and especially the depth to which it penetrates, are dependent upon the anatomic structure of the parts affected. When the follicles are superficial the inflammation will be less than when they are deep-seated. The presence of the fungus alone is sufficient to cause severe inflammation. To ascribe severe inflammation to a mixed infection with staphylococci, the author thinks, is not justifiable. From a pathologico-anatomic point of view all the morbid processes in the various forms of trichophytosis are the same, varying only according to the anatomic structure of the affected parts, the susceptibility of the individual, and the virulence of the fungus.

Tinea Tonsurans in an Adult.—J. Abbott Cantrell [3] reports the following rare case: the subject was a man aged 25, who was employed as salesman in a hat-store, it being his custom to place on his head every hat that had been handled by him, and in doing so it was supposed he contracted the disease. Immediately upon its being discovered by him he presented himself for diagnosis. The scales examined microscopically showed that the trichophyton tonsurans was present. The lesion was situated upon the vertex; it was circular, with the edges sharply defined, the center being somewhat scurfy or nutmeg-grater-like, the hairs being dry, brittle, and broken off. After 4 months' treatment the condition resolved itself into a kerion and got well in a short time. [Tinea tonsurans is a rare condition in adults, being very seldom met with in countries where dermatology is cultivated.]

Formic Aldehyd in the Treatment of Ringworm of the Scalp. —Alfred Salter [4] treated 40 cases of ringworm of the scalp in the outpatient

[1] Arch. f. Dermat. u. Syph., Bd. xxxv., H. 1 u. 2.   [2] Ibid., Bd. xxxv., H. 1.
[3] Phila. Polyclinic, Aug. 22, 1896.   [4] Brit. Med. Jour., Sept. 12, 1896.

department at Guy's Hospital with this remedy. The preparation most used was Schering's "formalin" in full (40%) strength. The fluid was rubbed in with a brush or mop for ten minutes, the hair having been shaved round the margin of the patches. The application was repeated every other day on four occasions and then discontinued. In some patients the head was painted every day for four successive days. Of the 40 cases only 5 required repainting from noneradication of the disease, and in these the fault lay not with the remedy, but in the fact that, owing to the struggles of the children, no proper application could be made. The ages of the children treated ranged from 4 to 12, and the extent of the disease varied from a small, strictly localized patch to areas which were practically coextensive with the whole scalp. Microscopic examination was always made before commencing the treatment, and the actual presence of the trichophyton verified, whilst before pronouncing any case cured microscopic examination was again made. In 38 of the cases the fungus presented the characters of trichophyton microsporon. Formalin thus applied induces discomfort and irritation of very brief duration rather than actual pain, and does not vesicate the scalp as it does the skin elsewhere. Only 3 cases showed any suppuration after its use, and in these the process was slight and did not destroy any of the follicles. It produces, however, a thick crust, and the subsequent application of some emollient is advisable. Growth of healthy hair commences immediately, and in three or four weeks the denuded patch is covered with hairs $\frac{1}{8}$ in. long Allusion must be made to a remarkable occasional complication of the treatment. In 6 cases edema of the face was noted some hours after the painting. In one case this was so extensive as to completely prevent vision from swelling of the eyelids, and the forehead pitted $\frac{1}{2}$ in. on pressure. The skin, however, was neither hot nor red, and there was no pain nor constitutional disturbance. The edema only occurred when the area treated was very large, and the condition is probably analogous to that produced by a nettle-sting. It is interesting in this connection to remember that the active toxic agent in the nettle is formic acid, and that it is thus closely related to the substance now under discussion. The occurrence of this edema renders it advisable to deal with limited areas at a time.

Treatment of Chronic Tinea Tonsurans.—Herman B. Sheffield[1] treated in an institution 369 cases of tinea tonsurans, most of which had previously resisted varied forms of treatment. The diagnosis in all cases was confirmed by the microscope. Chrysarobin had been freely used during a period of four months, with the result of setting up a suppurative inflammation of the scalp and face in about 20% of the cases, and acute conjunctivitis in more than half of them. After some experimentation the following combination of drugs was found to constitute "the most reliable formula, curing all cases in about four weeks:" R. Acidi carbolici, ol. petrolei crudi, āā ʒij; tinct. iodini, ol. ricini, āā ʒiiiss; ol. rusci, q. s. ad Oj. M. Sig. Apply over entire scalp once a day for four successive days; wash off thoroughly with green soap on the sixth day; then clip the hair close and wash again as before. Repeat this course of treatment regularly for three successive weeks. After this plan had been followed for the period stated the microscope failed to reveal the trichophyton fungus in the majority of the cases. To relieve the slight eczematous eruption which was still present the following was ordered: R. Resorcin., acid. salicylic., āā ʒiv; alcoholis, ʒiv; ol. ricini, q. s. ad Oj. This was well rubbed into the scalp. After about two weeks the hair in the bald spots began to grow, and no relapse of the disease has since occurred. The advantages are that the cure is speedy, and attended with but little inflammation. It can be

[1] Am. Medico-Surg. Bull., Sept. 5, 1896.

easily and rapidly applied. The mixture being thickly applied excludes the air, thus retarding the growth of the fungus, while by keeping the scales and broken-down hair closely adherent to the primarily affected spots the liability of autoinfection is lessened.

The author also praises highly glacial acetic acid as a destroyer of the trichophyton fungus. In 8 acute sporadic cases of tinea tonsurans it was tested with excellent results. It was applied in the following manner: after clipping the hair close to the scalp the affected areas were touched with the acid by means of a cotton swab once every third day, making in all three applications. Care was exercised to prevent the acid reaching the healthy scalp. Two days after the third application the scalp was washed with soft soap and covered with a sulphur ointment ($\mathfrak{z}$j ad $\mathfrak{z}$j), after the hair had been clipped again. The resorcin-salicylic oil referred to is useful as a preventive, and should be used toward the end of the treatment with stronger remedies.

Henry A. Pulsford[1] gives his **experience in the treatment of ringworm of the scalp in the New York Skin and Cancer Hospital,** the material upon which his paper was based being the clinical records of 75 cases treated during the ten years ending in 1892. All the cases were inmates of this hospital during the entire course of their treatment. All the circumstances were favorable, not only for the cure of the cases, but for the accumulation of data as to the value of the various methods of treatment employed. From the author's analysis we may conclude that, of all the remedies used upon these 75 cases, the preparations of mercury proved the most efficient. Of the others, iodin, naphthalin, salicylic acid, and chrysophanic acid seem worthy of further trial, while croton oil, properly used, was as valuable as electrolysis in eradicating the last traces of the disease. The results obtained in the treatment of ringworm of the scalp, finally, give full corroboration to the recent dictum of Wickham, of Paris, that "No matter what methods are employed, the duration of treatment necessary to the thorough cure of ringworm of the scalp cannot practically be reduced to less than eight months."

ATROPHIES AND HYPERTROPHIES.

Alopecia Areata as a Result of Exposure to the Röntgen Rays.—Frederick S. Kolle[2] reports the following case (with photograph): the subject was a boy, 12 to 13 years of age, who had sat for some pictures before. A radiogram of his skull was made. The exposure was one of forty minutes, made in the usual way, with a Thompson double-focus or standard vacuum-tube. The distance between the tube and skull was a little over eighteen inches. As the time of sitting was long for him, he was advised to close his eyes and so overcome the monotony of watching the minutes pass by on a clock hanging directly in front of him. He did so, fell asleep, and slept throughout the sitting. This was the only radiogram made that day. Radiograms of his body were subsequently completed in the four sections necessary, and the boy disappeared until three weeks later, when he reappeared, showing a large area of hair missing upon that side of the head exposed to the vacuum-tube, as shown by the photograph. There had been no premonitory symptoms of itching or inflammation; all the patient knew was that on the night previous the hair had suddenly fallen out. The integument, or scalp, appeared bald and somewhat elevated, and slightly edematous. There was no redness, sensibility was not impaired, the patch was regular, and scaling was absent. The area was perfectly bald, not even lanugo-hairs being present.

---

[1] Jour. Am. Med. Assoc., Jan. 9, 1897.   [2] Brooklyn Med. Jour., Dec., 1896.

Common Alopecia: its Nature, Cause, and Mechanism.—R. Sabouraud,[1] who has studied ringworm so thoroughly, summarizes his conclusions on common alopecia as follows: I. The specific microbacillus of oily seborrhea introduced into the pilosebaceous follicle causes there four constant results—namely, (*a*) sebaceous hypersecretion; (*b*) hypertrophy of the sebaceous glands; (*c*) progressive papillary atrophy; (*d*) death of the hair. II. On the scalp, this infection has the vertex for its usual site, oily seborrhea giving rise to the baldness. *Common alopecia is only oily seborrhea of the vertex in a chronic state.* The follicular seborrheic infection is indispensable to the baldness. The infection remains intense, pure, and permanent until the alopecia is fully constituted and the ultimate sclerosis of the follicles occurs. III. Common alopecia is then a microbic, specific, well-characterized disease. A remarkable statement of the author in this paper relates to the action of the seborrheic toxin on the hair-papilla. The cocoon (described elsewhere) remains circumscribed in the upper third of the hair-follicle, consequently the bacilli themselves do not reach the papilla. Death must then be produced by toxins generated in the neighborhood of the cocoon of the hair. Cultures of the microbe on artificial media furnished a toxin which, when injected into sheep, rabbits, and guinea-pigs, produced loss of hair without any other symptom. These inoculations, done under all conditions, would seem to preclude errors in the results obtained. The author points out certain errors of observation as to these facts, which have led such observers as Unna and others astray. They are: (1) examination of seborrhea by surface-scraping, instead of section through the integument; (2) the misconception that the pathology and physiology of the follicle are the same as those of the epidermis, than which nothing is more erroneous; (3) the presence of pityriasis accompanying alopecia. When the two occur coincidently the baldness is due to a subjacent seborrheic infection, but they may be commingled. [This work by the distinguished dermatologist, microscopist, and pathologist, is experimental and novel. The conclusions should be received cautiously. They require to be verified by other observers before being accepted as final.]

Pitting about the Hair-cups.—Browning[2] describes a trophic change of the skin in certain nervous disorders of central origin. It consists in a faint depression, frequently oval, in the direction of the lines of the skin, about the exit of each hair. It is slightly paler than the surrounding skin, like a minute cicatrix, but soft to the touch, and is usually found upon the extremities, most markedly upon the lower. On the upper it is seen best on the outer side of the forearms; on the lower, chiefly on the front and outer side of the leg below the knee. In chronic anterior myelitis associated with progressive muscular atrophy the author has never found this pitting absent. It has been noted also in paralysis due to lead-poisoning, spastic tabes of syphilitic origin, and grave hysteria. It would seem that this pitting is indicative of disease of the spinal cord, especially of the anterior horns, and is useful in differentiating central from peripheral disease. Its occurrence indicates a grave disorder.

Too Much and Too Little Hair.—G. T. Jackson[3] concludes, from a study of the first hundred cases of hirsuties in his case-book, that hypertrichosis in women is very largely a matter of heredity, especially on the maternal side. It has comparatively little to do with disorders of the reproductive organs. Brunets are more prone to it than blondes. A woman with hirsuties is a little less apt to bear children than one without hirsuties. The

[1] Ann. de Dermatol. et de Syph., t. viii., No. 3, 1897.
[2] Jour. Nerv. and Ment. Dis., Sept., 1896.   [3] Med. News, July 11, 1896.

most frequent age for the appearance of the affection is between the sixteenth and thirtieth years. There is but one treatment—by electrolysis, which the author recommends under certain conditions. With regard to premature alopecia, he states that in men seborrhea and heredity are the main causes. In women anemia, chlorosis, and neurasthenia are contributory factors. The chances of improvement and restoration are much greater in women than in men. Massage is highly esteemed in the treatment. [The operation of electrolysis for the removal of superfluous hair from the face of women in marked cases should never be undertaken without due consideration of the ability of the subject to carry out the treatment to the end. A face operated on here and there, and left "half-finished," is more disfigured than if nothing had been done. The operation is tedious and expensive, and is generally followed by obvious, often disfiguring, scarring.]

A Rare Case of Acquired Hypertrichosis.—Valentine Zarubin, of Charkoff, Russia,[1] gives the notes of this case: the subject was a woman of 38. She married at 23, and bore a child after a year. Two years later a pregnancy was interrupted at the eighth month, the child dying. She was in bed for 6 weeks, and had much pain in the sexual region. She first remarked an abundant growth of hair on the breast. A little later the whole body was covered, and finally, after 3 months, the face. From this time, her head began to grow bald ; 6 weeks after childbed her abdomen began to enlarge enormously, but pregnancy was not recognized by the accoucheurs consulted. For three years the patient consulted physician after physician, and tried every means to rid herself of beard and moustache (shaving, pulling the hair out, epilation by electrolysis), but without avail ; 6 months after, the abdominal swelling was reduced, but the pain continued. Having exhausted her money, she exhibited herself to the public. The family history showed no such anomaly. The woman was tall, strong, and well nourished ; a brunet. The whole surface was abundantly covered with hair, especially the face, where it was nut-brown in color. The hair of the beard was soft and fine. The same was true of the body, except that the growth was shorter. The head was so bald that a wig was worn to cover it. The genital and axillary hair was normal. No peculiarities were remarked in the teeth. The breasts were well developed, the carriage was masculine, and the voice coarse. Menstruation appeared at 16. After the first year the periods were abundant, regular, and lasted 7 days. After the premature labor the menses did not appear for 11 years. Sexual sense was normal. Gynecologic examination showed hypertrophy of the clitoris, with a well-developed glans and prepuce. The other organs were normally feminine. There was a left-sided salpingo-oöphoritis. As to the etiology of the case, one sees that heredity has no place. The anomalies in the sexual sphere pointed out by various authors were present in this instance (amenorrhea). In the cases of De Creccio,[2] E. Hoffmann,[3] Durval,[4] and others, beard and moustache existed in pseudohermaphrodites of feminine sex. In this case a false feminine external hermaphroditism (*pseudo-hermaphroditismus ¡femininus externus*) existed. The etiologic factor was, very possibly, a severe psychic disturbance.

Lesser[5] has reported a similar case in a girl of 6, in whom the growth began at the age of 4. Besides the hair on face, pubes, axillæ, and the body in general, the child exhibited signs of precocious development, menstruating first when 3 years of age.

[1] Jour. of Cutan. and Genito-Urin. Dis., Feb., 1897.   [2] Il Morgagni, 1865.
[3] Wien. med. Jahrb., iii., S. 293, 1877.   [4] Virchow's Jahrbucher, S. 81, 1877.
[5] Correspondenzbl. f. Schweizer Aerzte, xxvi., p. 355.

Ichthyol in Ichthyosis.—Max Klonk [1] reports a severe case of ichthyosis treated by him in a boy 15 years of age. The disease first manifested itself in infancy, and had resisted all previous treatment. The patient first received a warm bath of 20 minutes' duration, containing 10 oz. of pure ichthyol, and was then rubbed down with a bland soap and water, a rough towel being used for drying. The skin was now rubbed with pure ichthyol, the patient wrapped in woollen blankets, and given repeated doses of extract of jaborandi to stimulate diaphoresis. The next day the patient was rubbed down with soap and water, and in the evening a warm bath containing sea-salt was given. On the third day the treatment of the first day was repeated. Thus, the patient received, in the course of 1 week, 3 ichthyol baths and inunctions, 3 warm soap-baths (in the morning), and 3 sea-salt baths (in the evening). Three 2-gr. capsules of ichthyol were taken daily for the first week, 6 daily the second week, and 8 daily the sixth week, this latter quantity being continued for some time. Under this treatment the patient gained rapidly in weight, and the horny masses were cast off. After 4 weeks' treatment the greater portion of the surface was free from disease, the skin being smooth, soft, and moist. During the day the body was kept moist with glycerin and water (1 : 3); occasionally an ointment of sulphur, resorcin, zinc, and benzoinated lard was substituted. Another case is cited in which the most remarkable results were obtained in the short period of 18 days. The unusually favorable results achieved by this treatment have convinced the author that ichthyol is a remedy possessing specific virtue in ichthyosis. [It is not stated how long the cases remained free from disease.]

Streaked Skin Affections of the Lower Extremity.—Julius Heller [2] believes that the striated distribution of the disease over a part or the whole of the lower extremity is dependent upon anatomic conditions, and is common to the whole class of such affections. The cases depicted and described were observed by Unna, Shearer, Philippson-Unna, and Neumann. Some were of an inflammatory nature, others possessed the general characters of nevi, for the most part unilateral. Heller concludes that all attempts to explain by any one system the streaked or striated affections of the lower extremity fail. In one case involvement of the larger lymphatics can without doubt be considered the cause of the streaked character of the eruption, but in other cases this factor can be with certainty excluded. The anatomic basis of every case must be separately determined.

Case of Symmetric Morphea attended with the Formation of Bullæ and Extensive Ulceration.—Prince A. Morrow,[3] after referring to the statistic frequency of morphea and scleroderma in this country, reports a case of morphea which was remarkable for the number and size of the plaques, their symmetric distribution, the occurrence of bullæ, and the extensive breaking down and ulceration of some of the patches. The patient was a man 66 years of age, who had always enjoyed excellent health with the exception of attacks of inflammatory rheumatism. One year before, the first patch appeared upon the anterior surface of the right thigh. Similar patches were soon observed upon both right and left thighs and over the tibial regions. Three months later, broad, bandlike patches appeared upon the lower abdomen, the sides of the trunk, on the back between the shoulders, and along the spine. These patches were symmetric in form and disposition. Over the right thigh they had become confluent and formed a continuous sheet, completely investing the limb in its upper and middle thirds. On the left limb they were for the

---

[1] Ohio Med. Jour., vii., 1896.   [2] Internat. Atlas of Rare Skin Diseases, part xii., 1895.
[3] Jour. Cutan. and Genito-Urin. Dis., Nov , 1896.

most part discrete. They presented a white, lardaceous appearance, were slightly elevated and surrounded by a well-defined lilac border. To the feel they were hard, rigid, and unyielding. The integument could not be pinched up. The white surfaces were stippled over with numerous punctiform indentations corresponding to the follicles of the skin. There was complete absence of hairs on the affected surfaces, with suppression of the sudoral and sebaceous secretions. Sensation was but slightly impaired. The affected surfaces below the knees soon became ulcerated. Cicatrization of those surfaces did not take place until six months later. A noticeable feature was the formation of numerous bullæ of the size of a marrowfat pea or larger, which upon rupturing later discharged an amber-colored fluid, leaving superficial excoriations which healed in a few days. These blebs occurred here and there upon the cicatricial area without assignable cause. Their occurrence was a constant feature for 2 or 3 months. Under large doses of potassium iodid and the thyroid extract there occurred a notable and steady improvement. Later sodium salicylate was substituted for the iodid. The skin lost its boardlike hardness and many of the patches underwent involution.

Porokeratosis.—M. B. Hutchins[1] describes a case of this new and rare disease of the skin, to which Mibelli, of Italy, first directed attention in the *International Atlas of Rare Skin Diseases*, in 1893. The case occurred in a man of 32, the disease having first appeared in early childhood on the border of the left palm as a "seedwart"-like growth, spreading gradually until the age of 15 years. The patch involved the palm and dorsum of the hand, the boundary of the described area being irregular, wavy, about one line in width and height, and formed of horny epidermis. "The border is like the outside of a seam, with a longitudinal thread-like line dividing its lateral halves. Here and there in this line are round, millet-seed-sized or smaller, blackish epidermic concretions, which can be picked out." The "seam" can be snipped off without causing pain or injury to the papillæ. On the dorsum of the first phalanx, external to this "seam," the hairs are broken in their follicles, and the latter show dirty, horny plugs. There existed several other similar areas of disease on the palm, fingers, and dorsum of the hand, and one on the face, the size of small coins. Some of the "seams" or ridges were tortuous in outline, like a burrow. The area of the patch included in the border showed the skin to be smoother than normal (slightly atrophic). All the epithelial structures were involved in the process. A photograph is given. [Mibelli called the disease, based on its histology, "porokeratosis," or keratosis of the sudoriparous ducts. Respighi designated it "hyperkeratosis eccentrica." It is allied to ichthyosis hystrix linearis.]

Nævus Acneiformis Unilateralis.—S. B. Selhorst[2] reports a case of this rare disease, to which he thinks the name given is suitable. The subject was a woman of 24, in good health. The condition existed from birth; it was limited to the left side of the body, occupying the thorax, neck, abdomen, and arm to the second phalanges, the point at which the sebaceous glands cease. It followed the course of the cutaneous nerves. The lesions consisted of oval spots, which coalesced to form one large patch, on which were numerous flat scars bounded by raised patches of skin. The diseased area was dotted over with large, single and double comedones. Occasional small ulcers were met with, resulting from the destruction of tissue following folliculitis and perifolliculitis round the comedones. The microscope verified the clinical picture, so that the term nævus acneiformis of this strange disease is not inappropriate. Photographs accompany the description.

[1] Jour. Cutan. and Genito-Urin. Dis., Oct., 1896.   [2] Brit. Jour. Dermatol., Nov., 1896.

Hypertrophic Rosacea (Pachydermatosis).—Isadore Dyer [1] reports the case of a man, aged 60, a native of Germany, and a farmer by occupation. The disease of the skin of the face had been gradually developing for many years. The skin was thickened in rugæ, running chiefly in parallel lines, crossed at many points, thus giving the skin a tessellated appearance. There was extensive sealing, with excoriations here and there, due to scratching, itching being almost constant. The color of the skin was a dull red, but in nowise brownish, bronzed, or dusky, as one would expect to note in leprosy. There were no tubercles nor telangiectases. The backs of the hands were similarly affected. The condition seemed to warrant designating the disease pachydermatosis. After one month's use of thyroid extract great amelioration of all the symptoms occurred, and later the case was regarded as cured. [The case is interesting because of the resemblance of the lesions to those of lepra. A similar case is reported with the title " Hypertrophic Rosacea " in the *Pictorial Atlas of Skin Diseases* of the models of the Hôpital St. Louis, Paris.]

NEW FORMATIONS.

Treatment of Keloid with Thiosinamine.—R. C. Newton,[2] from his experience in 2 cases, thinks favorably of this mode of treatment. It has a distinct action on sear-tissue [as H. Hebra pointed out in connection with lupus vulgaris and corneal opacities in *Internat. klin. Rundschau*, 1892]. Tousey [3] first called attention to its value in keloid. Newton used a 10% solution in absolute alcohol, 18 minims being injected into the deltoid muscle, and subsequently every 4 or 5 days. There were nausea and vomiting, and the injections were painful. The cicatricial tissue (in one case) and keloid (in the other case) became softer and smaller under the treatment. One case received 29 injections in all. [The treatment seems to have been followed by moderately satisfactory results; but it cannot be regarded as of great value.]

Myoma Multiplex of the Skin.—H. R. Crocker [4] reports a case of this rare skin disease. Babes divides it into 4 varieties, namely: 1. Myomata springing from the vessel-walls; 2. Hyperplasias of the arrectores pili; 3. Neoplasms from the deep muscular layer of the skin; 4. Myomata from embryonic "remnants." Crocker's case was in a man aged 43. Eighteen years before, there appeared on the left side of the lower jaw a small tumor, which was at first regarded as a fibroma. Slowly a number of similar tumors formed around the primary one, until a patch of closely aggregated, painless, brownish-red tumors formed, each tumor occupying a space $1\frac{1}{2}$ by 1 in. in area. The tumors were excised. A short account of 12 cases observed in various countries is given.

Xanthoma Diabeticorum.—A. R. Robinson [5] describes the case of a woman who had never been jaundiced herself and had never had a relative thus affected. During the past 10 years, however, she had suffered from gall-stones. The eruption first showed itself in 1891, especially upon the anterior surfaces of the forearms and about the elbows, with a few scattered spots upon the knees. With the exception of those about the elbows, they all disappeared. In the second attack about 150 lesions made their appearance upon the right arm, and about the same number upon the left; but in the latter there was none over the fingers or joints. About 50 lesions were present upon each leg, from the calf to the middle-thigh region. The face and eyelids were free. The

---

[1] New Orl. M. and S. Jour., Jan., 1897.   [2] N. Y. Med. Jour., Mar. 20, 1897.
[3] Ibid., May 2, 1896.   [4] Brit. Jour. Dermatol., Jan., 1897.
[5] Jour. Cutan. and Genito-Urin. Dis., Dec., 1896.

size ranged from that of a pin's point to a pin's head. The color was yellowish, with a tinge of red. On pressure the yellowish color was intensified. The urine showed no sugar, but the report of the examiner was that it appeared "glycosuric." It contained 20 % by bulk of albumin and a few granular casts. The interesting features of the case were the absence of sugar in a person who had the physical appearances of a diabetic, the presence of a parenchymatous nephritis, the desquamative hidradenitis, and the condition of the gall-bladder.

The Treatment of Lupus Vulgaris with Salicylic Acid and Creosote Plaster.—W. Dubreuilh and Bernard[1] observe that Unna's salicylic-acid-and-creosote plaster has the advantage of attacking the diseased parts alone, the tubercles being thoroughly destroyed by the salicylic acid, and the healthy tissue remaining unaffected ; the creosote subdues the pain of the application. The plaster contains equal parts of salicylic acid and creosote, or a larger quantity of creosote. It should be large enough to include some of the healthy skin, and should be renewed once daily. The application is painless at first ; burning pain is experienced when the lupus begins to ulcerate. According to Unna, the pain lasts from 5 to 15 minutes, but the authors say it seldom exceeded 1 minute in their experience. After the plaster is removed the surface is cleansed with moist cotton, and the application renewed. After 3 or 4 applications the lupus-nodules begin to ulcerate separately, and after 8 to 10 applications the entire diseased area is either ulcerated evenly or is covered with deep, cup-like ulcerations. The healthy skin and cicatrices are never attacked by the salicylic acid. The authors have treated 10 cases according to this method. They prefer the stronger plasters for the treatment of the deeper foci of disease, and use about 20 plasters on an average in every case. In the treatment of sclerosed lupus the plaster did not answer well ; the authors are of the opinion that in this form of lupus surgical treatment, especially scarification, is more useful.

Like other methods of treatment, the plaster does not bring about a complete cure. Relapses may occur. Patients who object to surgical treatment may be treated advantageously with the salicylic-acid-and-creosote plaster. It is less severe than by mercuric chlorid and caustic potassa, and less painful and dangerous than arsenical paste. The treatment of lupus superficialis with the plaster promises the best results. Suspicious points can be cauterized with silver nitrate, or destroyed with galvanocautery or with other local remedies, like pyrogallic acid, during cicatrization.

Treatment of Lupus Vulgaris by Means of Electrolysis.—A. Ravogli[2] states that electrolysis acts very gently, destroying the tubercle by the combination of scarification with its histochemic action. In cases of lupus in which small tubercles are scattered, especially on the face, it is a good method. It leaves a small and scarcely perceptible scar. A salve consisting of salicylic acid, 20 gr., creosote, 30 drops in 1 oz. of vaselin, is first employed ; with this application the crusts fall off and the tubercles show plainly as whitish points. Each of the tubercles is then treated with electrolysis, the application of the salve being continued. When the necrosed tissue has sloughed off and granulation commences, the sites of the tubercles are touched every alternate day with a 5 % solution of nitrate of silver, covering the surface with a salve of zinc or boric acid until recovery. With this method perfect success was obtained in 5 weeks in 1 case. Two more cases are at present under treatment with similar results, showing that electrolysis is to be considered as a valuable agent in the treatment of this disease.

[1] Monatsh. f. prakt. Dermatol., xxii., Feb., 1896.   [2] Jour. Am. Med. Assoc., Dec. 5, 1896.

Thyroid Extract in Lupus.—J. Barclay[1] reviews the use of this drug in lupus vulgaris, quoting the favorable experience with it of P. Abraham, B. Bramwell, and Lake. He records three cases with favorable results after the drug had been administered for a long period. The reaction in one case was very severe, the burning pain being very distressing, and similar (though less violent, both locally and constitutionally) to that observed after the use of tuberculin injections. Two of the cases he believes to have been permanently cured in one year. The dose of the drug required is larger than for myxedema.

F. G. Proudfoot[2] has also had good results with the same drug in two cases of lupus. By degrees one case took as much as 75 gr., the other 90 gr. daily, but later about 15 gr. daily was the dose administered. The treatment was continued over a period of eight months, both cases, it is said, having departed from the hospital absolutely well.

An Oidium in the Skin of a Case of Pseudo-lupus Vulgaris.— T. C. Gilchrist and W. R. Stokes[3] report the results of microscopic investigation in a case of disease of the skin which resembled lupus vulgaris more than any other well-known disease. Miliary abscesses were found in the epidermis and in the upper portion of the corium, in all of which were numbers of doubly contoured, refractive, round, and ovoid bodies, many of them with buds, others with vacuoles. They were arranged singly or in groups, contained granular protoplasm, and resembled closely blastomycetes. No tubercle-bacilli could be found in any of the sections. The writers were of opinion that this extensive cutaneous disease was caused by the species of oïdium described, and that this is the only example in literature of a pure disease of the skin which has been shown to be caused by a species of oïdium, and the third example in which lesions of the human skin have been produced by organisms allied to the yeast-fungi, Busse's case and Gilchrist's case being the other two. [The case is of much interest, especially in connection with Wernicke's, Busse's, and Gilchrist's investigations in other similar cases recently reported.]

Case of Erythematous Lupus Cured by Injections of Lamb-serum.—Legrain[4] reports a case of erythematous lupus of the face cured by injections of serum obtained from a lamb. The disease had been treated for more than a year with the local applications and internal remedies usually employed in such cases, without success. Linear scarifications, while producing a slight improvement, had not been of more than transient benefit. Two months after cessation of all treatment two injections of lamb-serum, of 10 c.c. each, were given at intervals of five days. Three days after the first injection the patches were paler, and ten days after the second they had disappeared without leaving any signs of disease.

Importance of Early Treatment in Cutaneous Malignant Epitheliomata.—A. R. Robinson[5] states that in all cases of malignant epitheliomata there are : 1. An abnormal and excessive proliferation of epithelium ; 2. The proliferation is atypical, and is associated with the production of a poison which injures the surrounding tissues ; 3. Changes, usually of an inflammatory character, occur in the surrounding connective tissue, lessening the resisting power of the skin ; 4. Invasion of the connective tissues by the new epithelial elements by way of the lymph-channels, tending to secondary infection of lymphatic structures. The author further says that "it seems that carcinomata contain a poison, a toxin—as shown by experimental injections

[1] Brit. Med. Jour., Oct. 24, 1896.   [2] Ibid., Jan. 2, 1897.
[3] Bull. Johns Hopkins Hosp., July, 1896.   [4] Ann. de Dermatol. et de Syph., No. 1, 1896.
                [5] Med. News, Apr. 10, 1897.

and implantations of cancerous material—which injures connective tissues, differing in this respect from the benign epitheliomata." Injury to the connective tissue of the part favors a more rapid extension of the disease, and should always be borne in mind in locating a case of this kind. Thus mild caustics, which can only destroy the growth to a limited extent, act injuriously on the surrounding connective tissue, and thus favor the extension of the epithelial proliferation. Nothing is worse than meddlesome treatment in epithelial cancers. Whatever the method employed for their removal or cure, it should be effective. [The article contains much that is of value to the practitioner and is replete with sound teaching.]

Dermatitis Papillaris Maligna (or Paget's Disease).—A. M. Sheild[1] reports a case in which the lesion, occupying the breast of a woman aged 47, measured 11 in. vertically and 10½ in. from before backward. It was dusky-red, glazed, and possessed a slightly thickened, quite definite margin. The nipple was destroyed by ulceration. The gland was not enlarged. The disease began six years before, after an abscess of the breast. [The case is interesting on account of the large size of the lesion.]

Lymphendothelioma Cutis Multiplex.—Gustav Riehl[2] reports the case of a rare disease occurring in a woman aged 75, a native of Hungary, characterized by numerous, circumscribed, firm and hard, uneven, nodular, symmetrically distributed tumors, varying in size from a pea to a small hen's egg, occupying the skin and subcutaneous tissue, and also the mucous membrane of the mouth. They had begun to form on the face three years before. The clinical diagnosis was that of a peculiar form of sarcoma cutis. Later the lymph-glands began to swell; fever set in; a few of the tumors ulcerated, especially on the face, followed by erysipelas; and the woman died from bronchitis six days after the erysipelas began. The principal structure of the tumors was alveolar. Microscopic sections showed in numerous places that the lymph-vessels were enlarged and in direct relation to the neoplasm, and that the tumors began to form in the endothelium of the lymph-spaces. The diseased lymph-glands showed the same alveolar structure as the cutaneous tumors, the same arrangement and order of cells, and an absence of any relation with the blood-vessels.

Concerning differential diagnosis, it may be said that carcinoma, except in the case of the lenticular variety, never occurs so markedly multiple and over so large a surface. Sarcomata, with or without pigment, as a rule are less hard and ulcerate more rapidly. For the same reasons granuloma fungoides would be excluded. The clinical picture of the case was regarded as unique.

A Case of Sarcoma of the Skin successfully Treated by Arsenic. —Pospelow[3] reports a case of sarcoma in which the use of arsenic in increasing doses was followed by the complete disappearance of the tumor, which was situated upon the nose, and had been excised, but returned after six weeks. New lesions beginning to appear upon other parts of the face, further surgical treatment was deemed useless, and recourse was had to the internal use of arsenic. The drug was prescribed in the form of Asiatic pills, each containing one-twelfth grain, and of these at first one, finally nine, were taken daily. One month after beginning this treatment the tumor was decidedly smaller, the secondary lesions much flatter and apparently undergoing retrogression. These large doses of arsenic were well borne, and occasioned no disturbance of the digestive tract. At the end of ten months the cure was apparently complete.

[1] Brit. Jour. Dermatol., p. 443, Nov., 1896.   [2] Wien. klin. Woch., Nov. 12, 1896.
[3] Arch. f. Dermatol. u. Syph., Bd. xxxiv., H. 2.

The author emphasizes the necessity for perseverance in the treatment, since the good effects of the arsenic only appear slowly.

An Unnamed Granuloma.—Tenneson, Leredde, and Martinet[1] endeavor to show that the affection which has been described by Brocq, Barthélemy, and others, under the names "symmetrical disseminated folliculitis of smooth parts," "acnitis," "folliclis," "acne varioliformis, hidradenitis destruens suppurativa," "disseminated suppurative idrosadenitis," "disseminated suppurative spiradenitis," does not originate in the hair-follicles, the sebaceous nor the sweat-glands, but that it is a granuloma which can invade the glands secondarily, but does not begin in them. The authors believe that the discrete form is more common than is supposed; that it develops upon a scrofulous soil; and that it is of microbic origin.

Congenital Sarcomatosis of the Skin.—Neuhaus[2] states that of all the neoplasms of childhood sarcoma is the most frequent; of congenital sarcomata the commonest occur in the kidneys. Metastasis of internal sarcomata to the skin is not rare, but primary sarcoma of the skin is extremely rare. The case of a child two months old, of healthy parents free from syphilis and tuberculosis, is cited. The infant appeared normal at birth, but when bathed on the fifth day by the mother the left leg was noticed to be thicker than the right. At the age of five weeks an incision was made into the leg and a gelatinous mass as large as a hen's egg was removed. The bones were apparently healthy and not connected with the growth. At about this time the mother noticed on the external aspect of the right ankle a bluish nodule as large as a pea. Similar nodules appeared upon other portions of the body, some undergoing ulceration. The child was large and apparently well nourished. The nodules varied in size from a lentil to a small apple, were elastic, and presented pseudofluctuation. They were sharply circumscribed and movable upon the subjacent tissues. They were seated in the skin and in the subcutaneous connective tissue. The lymphatic glands were slightly enlarged. There was no evidence of involvement of any internal organ. Examination of the growths disclosed round-cell sarcoma. The child died in ten days. Postmortem examination disclosed widespread metastasis, the evidence pointing to the cutaneous covering of the left leg as the seat of the original growth, which must have been congenital.

Nonidentity of Yaws and Syphilis.—C. W. Daniels,[3] of British Guiana, concludes that yaws has no resemblance to primary or to secondary syphilis, and shows none of the associated lesions, and that if it be considered as a tertiary manifestation there are neither primary nor secondary stages.

THERAPEUTICS.

Gelanthum in Skin-diseases.—P. G. Unna,[4] of Hamburg, after two years' experience with this vehicle, recommends it very strongly. The difficulty with the soluble varnishes used heretofore has been that insoluble substances like zinc oxid, sulphur, and chrysarobin, cannot be suspended in them, but collect in lumps or fall to the bottom, but in gelanthum they are evenly divided and remain suspended. Hygroscopic substances, like ichthyol, easily form a dry coating in this vehicle, and large quantities of the necessary mediaments can be added, as of ichthyol 30%; of salicylic acid, resorcin, and pyrogallol 4%; and of carbolic acid 5%, without destroying its varnish-like properties. Two incompatible bodies, such as salicylic acid and zinc oxid,

[1] Ann. de Dermatol. et de Syph., No. 7, 1896.   [2] Arch. f. Kinderh., Bd. xxi., H. v., vi.
[3] Brit. Jour. Dermatol., Nov., 1896.   [4] Therap. Woch., Sept. 13, 1896.

which in watery solutions undergo chemical reaction, can be used together in gelanthum. Fats can be fixed with it to the amount of 10 %, and glycerin 20 %, to prevent its drying too quickly.

Gelanthum—named from its principal constituents—consists of equal parts of gelatin and tragacanth (about $2\frac{1}{2}$ % of each). Each substance is macerated slowly in cold water, then subjected to steam and filtered. By this means the gelatin is deprived of a part of its gelatinous property. The two substances are then mixed and subjected to steam for two days, and then pressed through gauze. Glycerin 5 %, some rose-water, and 2 % of thymol are added. The medicament to be added, if not soluble in water, must be rubbed into a soft paste with water, and fats must first be emulsified by gums and water. As compared with the old soluble varnishes, it presents the following advantages : it spreads easier, dries more quickly, and with a smoother surface ; it holds the solid substances evenly suspended and finely divided upon the skin ; it tolerates all substances singly and together ; hygroscopic substances are made to dry ; it bears an addition of fat to prevent drying too quickly. Finally, it is a cheap vehicle. [The preparation is difficult to make on account of the apparatus required. It may be obtained from New York importing-houses.]

Use and Abuse of Arsenic in Dermatologic Affections.—Albert E. Carrier,[1] a number of years ago, read a paper before a society, in which he took the ground that arsenic was too freely used in the treatment of cutaneous diseases. A larger experience convinced him more fully of the truths of the statements made in that paper, and he does not prescribe arsenic now in one-quarter of the cases that he then thought demanded it. In getting the previous history of patients that have been referred to him for treatment he usually finds that arsenic has been used, and he concludes from this that the remedy is still very freely used by the general practitioner in the treatment of skin diseases.

The diseases in which arsenic has been used with benefit are : pemphigus, herpes zoster, lichen ruber, lichen planus, psoriasis, chronic urticaria, dermatitis herpetiformis, and some forms of erythema multiforme ; yet even in these cases, prescribed by those skilled in its use, it often fails to benefit. To illustrate some of its unfavorable effects, a case of psoriasis was cited, in which arsenic in small doses had been given for some time, when without any apparent cause the whole body became pigmented. Previous to this the palms and soles became the seat of small, warty growths, which completely covered their surfaces and required frequent paring in order to make walking possible, or to enable the patient to follow his occupation of a carpenter.

The abuse of the remedy consists, first, in its administration indiscriminately, in giving it for acne, or for eczema, or even for scabies, etc. Another abuse consists in the lack of care in the selection of the preparation to be used. The aqueous solutions of pure arsenious acid are the most convenient to give, and if freshly prepared are the best for use ; but these solutions deteriorate with age, losing some of the arsenic, and no case should be held as not yielding to arsenic until arsenious acid has been given. Good results are slow in following its use, and we should be content to wait even months for a cure ; in order to prevent relapses it should be continued for a considerable length of time after all evidences of the disease have disappeared.

In conclusion, arsenic is useful in only a very limited number of skin-diseases. Second, its use in apparently selected cases is often disappointing. Third, it must be given for a long time before deciding that no good will result from its use. Fourth, we should be careful in the selection of the prep-

[1] Physician and Surgeon, July, 1896.

58

aration to be used, and a verdict should not be rendered against the value of the drug unless arsenious acid has been used. Fifth, its use in cases that are liable to return must be continued for some months after apparent cure is obtained; lastly, it must be borne in mind that when it is given in properly selected cases it may be followed by untoward effects that are not amenable to treatment.

[This subject is one of great importance to the profession, and the sooner physicians unfamiliar with the treatment of cutaneous diseases become impressed with the observation that arsenic may be harmful as well as beneficial, the better for all concerned. There is a vast amount of mischief made by the indiscriminate and reckless administration of this potent drug.]

Uses of Resorcin in Dermatology.—M. B. Hartzell[1] states that this drug in many of the milder forms of eczema often proves extremely serviceable in allaying itching and diminishing hyperemia; and even in the oozing stage, when the inflammation is not too acute, it often acts most happily in diminishing the discharge and favoring the speedy formation of cornified epithelium. Many cases of erythematous eczema will recover under the judicious use of this remedy alone. It is best used in aqueous solutions, 10 to 15 gr. to the ounce; ointments are more likely to prove irritating. The addition of $\frac{1}{2}\%$ sodium chlorid to aqueous solutions has seemed to increase the sedative action, possibly by favoring the absorption of the drug. The following formulæ are given: ℞. Resorcin., gr. x–xv; glycerin., ℳx; liq. calcis, ℥j. When there is oozing a half dram of bismuth subgallate to the ounce may be added. In other cases the following paste is useful: ℞. Resorcin., gr. xv; amyli, zinc. oxidi, āā ℥ij; petrolati, ℥iv. The drug is also useful in painful ulcers of the leg, which so frequently complicate varicose veins and eczema. In these cases it is especially useful in ointment-form, 5 to 20 gr. to the ounce. In seborrhea of the scalp it is one of the most valuable remedies, in the strength of about 20 gr. to the ounce. In blondes it causes a slight brownish tinge of the hair. Resorcin is also valuable in epithelial cancer, acting in a remarkable way in promoting cicatrization. In this disease it is best used as a plaster, about 70 gr. to 3 drams of the plaster-mass. It is also useful as a parasiticide, especially in ringworm in its several forms.

Filmogen (liquor adhæsivus).—E. Schiff,[2] of Vienna, recommends this as a vehicle for the application of drugs upon the skin. It is "a solution of nitrated (*nitrirter*) cellulose in aceton," which is painted on the epidermis in the form of a thin film. It resembles elastic collodion mixed with a corresponding amount of oil, such as castor oil. It forms an adhesive, impermeable coating on the skin, and on account of the oil it contains follows the movements of the skin without breaking or cracking. The solution is clear, of a pale yellow color, and through the evaporation of the aceton is cooling, but burns on abraded epidermis or on wounds. Most of the drugs in everyday use in dermatology may be applied successfully with it, either in solution or suspension. It is insoluble in water. The preparation is highly recommended by the author as an elegant method of applying drugs to the skin, possessing fewer objectionable features than most similar varnishes before the profession.

Notes on Some of the Newer Remedies used in Diseases of the Skin.—L. Duncan Bulkley[3] calls special attention to the value of resorcin in seborrheic eczema, used in the strength of about 6 % in zinc ointment or as a lotion with a little alcohol and glycerin. The solution is particularly applicable to the scalp. The same remedy used stronger, even up to 25 %,

[1] Therap. Gaz , June, 1896.   [2] Wien. med. Woch., No. 46, 1896.
[3] Jour. Am. Med. Assoc., Nov. 28, 1896.

will sometimes give excellent results in acne rosacea. The application is kept on for several days, and causes some little inflammation, after which the previous redness and pustular condition will be found to have largely disappeared. Resorcin is also valuable in certain ulcerative conditions, notably those of a tuberculous nature, used as a 10 % ointment. The author speaks highly of the value of ichthyol. As an antipruritic remedy it is often of great service. As an ointment, 6 % to 10 % strength, it is often very valuable in eczema, and may be used in quite acute conditions. In dermatitis herpetiformis a watery solution, 5 %, 10 %, or even 20 %, will often give more relief than any other local remedy. Taken internally, it is useful in hemorrhoids, 5 to 15 drops after each meal. It relieves the congested vessels of the rectum and anus.

A New Traumaticin.—Ducommun's [1] method of preparation consists of mixing an aqueous solution of soap with a solution of alum. A magma is formed, from which the excess of water is squeezed out with the hands, and the residue, while still moist, is dissolved in ether. It is much used in the clinic in Berne.

Nitrate of Silver in Diseases of the Skin.—R. Abrahams [2] speaks of the value of this drug in warts, every variety of " wart " being amenable to it. The silver stick should be worked down to the bottom of the wart and around its interior. In some cases the lesion should first be scraped. In corns, after maceration, a 30 % solution is valuable. The solid stick is useful in lupus vulgaris ; the nodules should be bored into, as F. Hebra first pointed out many years ago. The author also refers to its use in suitable cases of epithelioma, to be used as in lupus. Reference is also made to its value in leg-ulcers and in chancroids and phagedenic ulcers. The application of a saturated solution in neglected or maltreated venereal ulcers will quickly change their aspect and bring about healthy granulating tissue. In erysipelas, as well as in eczema, it is useful. It is especially useful in eczema intertrigo, the result of friction and sweating. It abates the itching and the discharge, and cures the disease of the skin. It should be used in solution, from 3 % to 10 % or even 20 %. In marginate eczema complicated with a fungus it is particularly useful in 20 % or 50 % strength.

Absorption of Methyl Salicylate by the Healthy Skin.—Linossier and Lannois [3] find that the healthy skin is capable of absorbing certain substances in larger amounts than are generally used therapeutically. In persons upon whose skin guaiacol had been applied, upward of 3 gm. were recovered in the urine passed in twenty-four hours. Methyl salicylate is readily absorbed by the skin ; after an application of 4 gm. to the thigh as much as 1.3 gm. of salicylic acid may be found in the urine passed during the following twenty-four hours, and at the same time an analysis of the evacuations from the bowel shows that a large quantity is eliminated in this way. The method of applying methyl salicylate to the skin is the same as that employed for guaiacol. The liquid is spread out on the skin (usually on the thigh) by means of a dropper or brush ; the part is then covered with waterproof and cotton-wool (to keep the temperature up), the whole being left in place for twenty-four hours ; 4 gm. of methyl salicylate are usually employed each time. Mixing the drug with lard or other oils interferes with its absorption.

Local Treatment of Seborrhœa Capitis.—Herbert Skinner [4] advocates the following formula for cleansing the scalp in seborrhea : sapo cast.

[1] Rev. internat. de Méd. et de Chir., Sept. 25, 1896.
[2] Jour. Am. Med. Assoc., Jan. 30, 1897.   [3] Med. Weekly, Mar., 1896.
[4] Brit. Jour. Dermatol., p. 70, 1897.

alb., ʒj ; alcohol., ʒj ; æther. methyl., ʒij ; aq., ʒij. Dissolve the soap in the water, add the spirit, clarify by filtration through kaolin, and then add the ether. Various ingredients can be added to this, even mercuric chlorid. One of the best methods to cleanse the scalp is with the following shampoo-liquid : ammonii carbonat., ʒss ; boracis, ʒj ; aq. Oj. Dissolve and add glycerin, ʒiv ; bay rum, Oj.

Quillaia-washes, consisting, for example, of two parts of a perfumed spirit or lavender-water and one part of fluid extract of quillaia, are soothing, but possess doubtful cleansing properties. The following is a new formula made with saponin, and is an improvement on most of the preparations of this kind : saponin., ʒj ; tinct. benzoin. simpl., ʒj ; aq., ʒss ; glycerini, ʒj ; acid. carbolici, ʒj ; aq. cologniensis, ad ʒj. Dissolve the saponin in the water and add the other ingredients. An antiseptic and stimulating "hair-tonic," containing no alkali, and therefore having no tendency to bleach the hair, may be compounded as follows : acid. salicylic., gr. xv ; resorcinol, ʒss ; tinct. cantharidis, ʒss ; tinct. capsici, ʒj ; saponin., ʒj ; lanolin., ʒj ; aq. rosæ, ad ʒx. Melt the lanolin, dissolve the saponin in the same quantity of water, and incorporate the two. Dissolve the acid and resorcinol in the tinctures and rose-water respectively. It should be brushed into the scalp once daily.

The following "tonic for the hair" is recommended, having several points to commend it, not the least being the combination of a small percentage of oil with alcohol : tinct. cantharidis, ʒxiv ; tinct. cinchonæ, ʒij ; tinct. benzoin. simpl., ʒvj ; spirit. lavandulæ, ʒiss ; ol. ricini, ʒij ; alcohol, ad ʒx. Dissolve the castor oil in the alcohol, mix with the tinctures and spirit, and filter through kaolin. For a natural grease for the scalp the following, the liquid lanolin preparation, will be found useful : lanolin., ʒss ; saponin., gr. iv ; aq., ʒss ; alcohol., ʒj. Dissolve the saponin in the water, stir in with the lanolin, which has been previously melted, and when cooling add the spirit. This makes a thick cream, devoid of stickiness or greasiness, which can be poured out of a bottle.

The Pathology of Itching, and Its Treatment by Large Doses of Calcium Chlorid, with Illustrative Cases.—Thomas D. Savill[1] states that he has had success in the use of calcium chlorid in the treatment of this affection. It has been shown that this drug has a marked effect on the blood—namely, increasing its coagulability. The author believes that the irritated state of the nerve-endings and fibrils which exists in this complaint, manifested by itching and tingling, is due to some change in the quality and composition of the blood. The paper is accompanied by an elaborate table of cases thus successfully treated, with the remedies previously used without effect. In each case either a cure was made or great benefit obtained. The doses must be not less than 20 gr. three times a day, and should be gradually increased ; 30 or even 40 gr. have often succeeded where less have failed. As thirst frequently follows the administration of the drug, it is best to cover the salt taste with a dram of tincture of orange-peel and one ounce of chloroform-water, in which form it is an acceptable medicine. The diet during its use should be restricted, especially as to sugar. The bowels should be kept freely active. Improvement may be noted after the first dose, but recovery sometimes does not take place until the blood has become saturated with the drug. Upon recovery the dose should be gradually, not suddenly, reduced.

Picric, or Carbazotic, Acid as a Therapeutic Agent, especially in the Treatment of Certain Inflammatory Skin-affections.— William Maclennan[2] states that picric, or carbazotic, acid, in watery and alco-

[1] Lancet, Aug. 1, 1896.   [2] Brit. Med. Jour., Dec. 26, 1896.

holic solutions, has for long been recognized, especially in France, as a useful application for superficial burns. The admirable results which the author has seen follow the free application of picric acid in solution to painful and extensive burns led him to try its effect in the treatment of certain skin-affections. In 1877 L. L. Grangé drew attention to the healing-power of this remedy in some varieties of eczematous eruption. Acute eczema, associated as it usually is with burning, severe itching, and profuse discharge, is rapidly relieved and cured under the influence of picric acid. Owing to the powerful astringent properties which this chemical possesses, it forms, when applied over a discharging or denuded surface, a protective layer of coagulated albumin and epithelial debris, under which healing rapidly proceeds; and as a potent antiseptic, by inhibiting the action of, or destroying, the microbes on which the formation of pus depends, it completely prevents suppuration.

Applied as a pigment with a brush or piece of absorbent wool, even to an extensive surface, it is quite free from danger, and causes not the slightest pain, however vascular the surface may be. Almost immediately itching and smarting abate, and in a few days, when the protective crust is removed or separates, the underlying skin is found to be comparatively dry, free from redness, and covered with a new epidermis.

In acute eczema occurring in children (eczema capitis et faciale), which is usually so intractable to the ordinary methods of treatment, the author has had most encouraging results from its use. If the hair on the child's head happens to be long, it should be cropped short and all adherent crusts removed by means of poulticing. The raw surface should then be freely painted over, morning and evening, for three or four days in succession with a saturated watery solution. During this treatment the scalp, and the face when it is involved, should be protected by means of a calico mask. After the lapse of a few days the pellicle which has been formed by the action of the picric acid can be removed by some emollient if it has not previously separated, and if any undue redness or moisture remain a fresh application may be made. The cessation of irritation permits the child to sleep, and its general health soon improves.

Although picric acid is so specially valuable in acute discharging eczemas, it will be found an efficient remedy in almost any superficial inflammatory affection. Thus in 3 cases of erysipelas the author found a saturated solution of picric acid superior to any local remedy he had hitherto tried. It arrested the inflammation and prevented the disease from spreading, and much more rapidly diminished local discomfort than carbolic acid, dusting-powder, or ichthyol. Carbazotic acid is a harmless topical agent. Although so nearly akin to carbolic acid, no apprehension need be entertained as to its absorption, even when applied to extensive surfaces. Like nitric acid it limits its own action by coagulating the albumin of the tissues to which it is applied. As heat readily decomposes the acid, accidental stains may be removed from the underclothing by boiling.

The Action of Salicylic Acid on the Sound Skin.—Menahem Hodara[1] has studied its action histologically, in order to better understand its effects clinically. The action of the acid is confined to the horny layer; an oozing surface is never seen. The experiments were made by applying salicylic acid in varying strengths, and in the form of ointments and collodion, to the skin of man and of rabbits. When applied to the human skin for 2 or 3 days in the form of plaster it produced a swelling of the horny layer and moderate intercellular edema of the prickle and granular layers. When the

[1] Monatsh. f. prakt. Dermatol., Aug. 1, 1896.

salicylic plaster was allowed to remain for from 8 to 10 days the prickle layer was found necrotic to various depths. After the skin has become necrotic the process of casting off and of new formation begins at once. Active proliferation begins in the deeper layers and in the adjacent epithelium, a new prickle-cell layer appears beneath the necrotic mass, and a new granular and horny layer is produced. Salicylic acid (30%) in collodion acts more energetically. Salicylic acid in man causes no emigration of polynuclear leukocytes. Its action is rather that of causing in the corium a slight inflammation. In the rabbit a concentrated salicylic acid plaster causes a complete necrosis of the whole epidermis, with suppuration. Briefly, it may be stated, salicylic acid in small amount on the healthy skin causes an exfoliation of the horny layer. Employed in larger quantity and for a longer time, it produces a desquamation, derived partly from the corneous layer, partly from the mucous layer, which has become necrotic in places.

SYPHILIS.

Treatment of Syphilis by Intravenous Injections of Mercury.

—According to J. Ernest Lane,[1] the plan of treating syphilis by intravenous injections of mercurial solutions was originally suggested by Baccelli in 1893, and has since been carried out by many Continental surgeons : in Italy by Jemma, Colombini, Nieddu, Campana, and Bruni ; in Germany by Görl, Neumann, and Lewin ; in France by Abadie ; and in Russia by Stoukovenkoff and Kusel. Lane, having charge of all the male wards in the London Lock Hospital, had unusual opportunities of giving a fair and impartial trial to this novel method of treatment. He systematically adopted it in every case of syphilis that came under his care in the hospital during 9 months, and states with conviction that he has formed a very favorable opinion as to its merits, and believes that, with certain reservations,, it compares favorably with other methods of treatment, whether it be by inunction, by intramuscular injection, or by internal medication, its special feature being the rapidity with which patients can be brought under the influence of mercury.

The preparation he has utilized throughout has been cyanid of mercury in 1% solution, and the amount used at each injection was usually 20 minims, or about $1\frac{1}{4}$ gm., though in some of the more severe cases he commenced with double this dose for the first 1 or 2 injections. At first the injections were employed every other day, but after a short time he introduced them daily. A loop of bandage was first tightly applied round the upper arm, and selection was made of the most prominent vein in the neighborhood of the elbow-joint ; the skin in that region was rendered aseptic in the customary manner, and the needle was thrust into the vein, the syringe filled with the solution being attached to it ; the bandage was then removed, and the syringe was emptied into the vein and then rapidly withdrawn ; the finger was placed on the puncture for a few seconds, and the operation was complete.

The advantages may be summarized as follows : the injections are absolutely painless, in which respect they are in direct contrast with intramuscular injections ; the functions of the digestive tract are not interfered with ; the doses of the mercurial salt are small, are certain of absorption, and can be easily regulated to the varying susceptibilities of different individuals ; with ordinary precautions the treatment is perfectly safe, and, even if the vein is missed, little or no inconvenience is caused thereby ; the resulting improvement is certain and rapid, and consequently it would seem to be indicated in .cases of cerebral

[1] Brit. Med. Jour., Dec. 12, 1896.

syphilis; the author's experience does not warrant him in offering an opinion as to whether this treatment is followed by relapses, but so far he has not met with any. The only real objection he can see to the method is the difficulty experienced in some instances of bringing the veins into sufficient prominence, and in a certain proportion of cases, especially amongst women, this is an insuperable obstacle. In conclusion, he is of opinion that in intravenous injections we have a valuable addition to our antisyphilitic theraputic agents, though the plan is one which obviously cannot be recommended as a routine practice.

Injections of Calomel for Syphilis.—Louis Jullien [1] remarks that the subcutaneous method possesses the two advantages that the liver and the alimentary mucous membranes are spared. The vehicle used is liquid vaselin. The dose varies from 1 to 2 gr., according to the size of the individual. The locality is preferably the supra- and infraspinous fossæ of the scapular region. Strict asepsis must be enforced. The interval between the injections varies according to circumstances; it may be from 8 to 20 or more days. Among the advantages can be cited the promptitude of its effects, the intensity of its action, and the persistence and positive character of its cures.

Sixteen Years' Experience in the Treatment of Syphilis by the Hypodermic Injection of Mercuric Chlorid.—T. S. Dabney [2] states that the hypodermic method of treating syphilis possesses many advantages over other methods when used by physicians bold enough to disregard the dosage recommended by most writers on therapeutics. The only test in giving medicines is the effect, and the dose should be increased until that is obtained. The author reports seven cases taken from his case-book in which the treatment advocated was employed successfully. The following objections raised against the treatment by subcutaneous injections are considered. They are (1) unnecessary pain; (2) subcutaneous infiltration; (3) large indurated and painful swelling; (4) inflammation; (5) abscesses; (6) stomatitis; (7) ptyalism; (8) disturbances of circulation and respiration. Pain does occur in some cases. In hyperesthetic cases the treatment is hardly admissible and cannot be recommended. The injection of morphin with the mercury is condemned. The author sees no objection to subcutaneous infiltration. When the needle is not thrust in deep enough an area of inflammation may in some instances be set up. Ptyalism and stomatitis have never been observed by the author in cases treated in this way, whereas he has rarely seen a case treated by other methods without them.

The advantages claimed for this method are (1) accuracy of dose; (2) exactness in intervals between doses; (3) rapidity of action of the medicine; (4) small amount of mercury and the short time needed to effect a cure; (5) the constant effect of the drug, day and night, and the personal supervision of the physician; (6) the certainty of the patient getting the right medicine, and of its being properly administered at regular, stated intervals; (7) absence of gastrointestinal disturbance; (8) quick diagnosis in questionable cases.

The needle should be plunged quickly through the skin and well into the subcutaneous tissue, care being taken to avoid adipose or muscular tissue. The injection should be made very slowly. As soon as the bichlorid solution comes in contact with the albuminous serum, the soluble mercuric chlorid immediately becomes the albuminate, which is not very soluble, and herein lie the efficacy and safety of these large doses of this highly corrosive poison. The solution usually employed is 8 grains to the ounce, from 5 to 15 minims being used for each injection, every second, third, or fifth day, until, say, ten or more injections have been given. The dosage should be gradually increased.

---

[1] Arch. gén. de Méd., No. 5, 1896.   [2] New Orl. M. and S. Jour., Apr., 1897.

Serum-therapy in Syphilis.—Mueller-Kannberg[1] reports 12 cases treated with serum. He calls attention to Kollmann's negative results obtained in 1890; and to the favorable results of Tommasoli's six experiments with serum taken from lambs, in which all the symptoms rapidly disappeared after the injection of from 2 to 8 c.c. In seven other cases the symptoms disappeared so rapidly that it was not found necessary to use more than 50 c.c. in each case, and none of these showed any recurrent symptoms. Fournier and Feulard, however, after using this serum, were unable to corroborate the above results. Lewin used serum obtained from horses prepared by Aronsohn. The first two cases treated were girls, aged 17 years, neither of whom had received any previous antisyphilitic treatment; they received 5 c.c. of the serum by injection in the gluteal region; after the fifth injection one was attacked by persistent urticaria, when corrosive sublimate treatment had to be substituted. There had been no change in the syphilitic symptoms. The third case was an 18-year-old girl, with initial chancre on the upper lip and enlargement of the glands; after the first injection her general condition became so serious that it was necessary to discontinue the treatment. The fifth patient showed urticaria eleven days after the first injection. The sixth patient was treated for five consecutive days with 5 c.c. of the serum, with some rise of temperature after the last injection. This case was also followed by erythema and urticaria.

In all other subsequent cases the treatment, for like reasons, has to be discontinued. As a result of these experiments, Mueller-Kannberg says he cannot see that the treatment with serum has any decided influence upon the course of syphilis.

Treatment of Malignant Syphilis.—Albert Neisser[2] defines "malignant syphilis" to be a severe form of the disease characterized by certain symptoms differing rather in their nature than in mere severity from the usual forms of the malady. Every case of severe syphilis must not be included under the designation of "malignant." For example, when syphilis is rendered a dangerous disease on account of the relation of the organs invaded the term "malignant" is inappropriate, the term "grave" being more suitable. Subjects suffering from malignant syphilis do not bear mercurial treatment well. No successful result is to be looked for from "forced cures." In former times the rule was laid down that mercury should never be prescribed in malignant forms of the disease; but Neisser thinks this is an extreme view. The insoluble salts, in the form of subcutaneous injections (valuable as they are in Neisser's opinion), should never be employed in malignant syphilis. A certain degree of success follows the use of potassium iodid, especially if it is administered when fever is present. In cases in which antisyphilitic treatment, even when persevered in, is ineffective, the only possibility of benefiting the patient is by the use of tonics (arsenic, strychnin, iron, quinin, baths, especially sea-baths) and the external use of sulphur in the form of sulphur ointment or the sulphur-bath. The latter often proves successful. The early employment of mercury and its administration in large doses have nothing to do with the development of the malignant form of the disease. Neisser agrees with Fournier in insisting that the individuality of each case must be borne in mind, and that the pauses between the courses of treatment should be properly observed. "Antisyphilitic serum" is not regarded as a valuable remedy, either in malignant or in any other form of syphilis.

Value of Potassium Iodid in the Hypertrophic Lesions of Syphilis.—T. Baer[3] calls attention to this subject, especially as such lesions

[1] Arch. f. Dermatol. u. Syph., vol. xxxv., H. 2.
[2] Brit. Jour. Dermatol., Jan., 1897.   [3] Med. Week., 1896.

are met with in women. Granulating papules, tubercles, etc., do not improve readily under mercury; but they yield rapidly to the iodin salts. The doses should begin with 15 and increase to 300 gr. daily.

How Long is Syphilis Contagious?—C. T. Drennen [1] would assert dogmatically that treatment does remove, not only the manifestations of this disease, but the disease itself, and with it its contagiousness. Syphilis loses its virulence as time progresses, and by the end of the sixth year it has practically lost its contagiousness, with here and there an exception. Patients who have been well treated may marry in three or four years after the primary lesion.

Syphilitic Reinfection.—H. Fitzgibbon [2] gives a valuable article on this subject, with some personal cases, and also discusses the nature of syphilis and its place in classification. The conclusions of the lengthy and interesting paper may be given as follows : 1. Syphilis is a specific fever of the same class as the other major exanthemata. 2. That if uncomplicated by pre-existing constitutional cachexia or coexisting septic influence, it runs a definite course, by which it exhausts in the system of its recipient the elements upon which its virus can feed. Thus, like variola, vaccinia, etc., the first attack is followed by a period during which the same individual is insusceptible of reinfection. 3. That the effects of syphilitic infection are no more necessarily lifelong than the effect of any other zymotic eruptive fever, although slower in its course. 4. Too much importance has been attached to the question of the possibility of second infection with syphilis as the only reliable proof of complete recovery from the disease. 5. From reported cases it would appear that when second infection with syphilis occurs the disease is more likely to be of an aggravated type than in first attacks. This the author is inclined to regard as due to contact with septic infection rather than to pure syphilitic virus. [The large experience of the author with syphilis entitles his views to respect.]

H. P. Collings [3] also reports a case of syphilitic reinfection. The second chancre occurred 9 years after the first chancre and 28 days after exposure. [The history is clear, and there seems every reason to accept this case as an authentic instance of reinfection.]

J. D. Thomas [4] likewise reports a case of syphilitic reinfection, in this instance the second chancre occurring five years after the first chancre. The first lesion was a characteristic Hunterian chancre ; the second manifested itself 2 weeks after exposure as an indurated and characteristic abraded sore in the right sulcus. There was no question as to the disease on both occasions.

The Pigmentary Syphiloderm and its Diagnostic Value.—G. Lewin [5] regards this manifestation as of importance, but states that it is not an absolutely certain diagnostic sign of syphilis, for he has observed it upon a large number of men who never had syphilis. Since it may exist upon nonsyphilitics, its presence is no indication for syphilitic treatment. Antisyphilitic remedies possess no influence over the disease. Syphilitic women who become pregnant do not show the leukoderma more pronouncedly than those who are not pregnant. It may appear upon parts of the skin that before had been the seat of some syphiloderm. It is not established that there exists any connection between the two affections. It is necessary, perhaps, to seek the cause of the leukoderma in a paralysis of certain centers which govern the movements of pigment—paralyses which have been caused by a toxin of syphilis.

[1] Cleveland Med. Gaz., Jan., 1897.   [2] Canad. Pract., Oct., 1896.
[3] Jour. Cutan. and Genito-Urin. Dis., Aug., 1896.
[4] Am. Jour. Dermatol. and Genito-Urin. Dis., Apr., 1897.
[5] Charité-Annalen, xviii., Berlin.

MATERIA MEDICA, EXPERIMENTAL THERAPEUTICS, AND PHARMACOLOGY.

By HENRY A. GRIFFIN, M. D., and J. R. TILLINGHAST, JR., M. D.,

OF NEW YORK.

The progress of the past year in pharmacology has been marked rather by that development of former knowledge which is of lasting value than by brilliant achievements which so often are ultimately but disappointments. Animal therapy has received considerable attention, and much good work has been done in its study, notably by Oliver, Mairet, and Bose. It must be confessed, however, that little of therapeutic value has been added to our knowledge of this subject, although it is equally clear that its limitations are as yet unreached. The usual number of pharmacologic novelties has been forthcoming, and of them the most important, so far as can now be judged, are considered in the body of this report. Among all these it is presumable that some may demonstrate a practical value, although the experience of previous years would prognosticate for the majority a brief tenure of life. In dulcin a distinct advantage would seem to have been attained as compared with saccharin, and the combined actions of disinfection and astringency represented in tannoform, especially in its internal employment, would suggest for this remedy a future of considerable usefulness. In view of the hopes placed upon antistreptococcic serum and the urgent necessity for a remedy which may be relied upon in septic infection, it is unfortunate that the later reports of its use are far from encouraging. Recalling the successes obtained by other protectant and curative serums, it would appear reasonable to hope that streptococcic infection might be similarly combated. Certainly the results so far obtained are not to be considered as final, since faulty technic may be the explanation of present disappointment. The mescal button has attracted considerable attention during the last twelve months, and a further understanding of its activities has been gained. From this it would appear that the drug, though interesting in no small degree, and useful no doubt in some of the conditions it is expected to combat, is scarcely to be rated of greater therapeutic reliance than cannabis indica, whose activities indeed its own in many respects resemble. Formaldehyd has received abundant attention, and much testimony is forthcoming as to its value. Indeed, so unanimous is the opinion as to its usefulness that it seems quite within the bounds of reason to hope that we have at last found an ideal disinfectant.

Acetanilid continues to be largely used both in its topical application and in the popular " headache powders," of which there are so many. That its reckless administration is by no means without danger, however, is indicated by the frequent reports of toxic effects produced (see *Year-Book* for 1897, p. 1101). A. E. Brindley,[1] of Manchester, England, reports the case of a woman who had

[1] Brit. Med. Jour., Sept. 12, 1896.

taken "kaputine" powders for neuralgic pain without the advice of a physician. The number of powders taken is not stated, but the patient had taken one just before her admission to the hospital, where she came under Brindley's observation. One of these powders, on chemie examination, proved to consist mainly of acetanilid. On admission the skin of the entire body was of a bluish-gray color, and the same appearance extended to the lips and tongue. The skin was warm and moist, and the patient complained of no distress. There was no dyspnea even on movement, and examination of the heart and lungs gave a negative result. There was no sensory disturbance, and the reflexes were normal. The conjunctivæ were yellowish and the urine contained a good deal of bile. There was bile also in the feces. Spectroscopic examination of both blood and urine was made, and was negative, as was the microscopic examination of the blood. From these symptoms it was believed that the acetanilid had caused a sufficient destruction of the coloring-matter of the blood to give rise to the symptoms of a nonobstructive jaundice. The patient was put on a milk-diet and salines were administered. Under this treatment the skin regained its normal appearance and the symptoms gradually disappeared.

Acetylene.—Considerable interest has recently been taken in the poisonous effects of acetylene. Experiments have been conducted by Grehant, Berthelot, and Moissan,[1] upon dogs, with a view to determining its poisonous properties as compared with carbonic oxid. The acetylene used was prepared carefully from calcium carbid, as Moissan found that the gas thus made, and purified subsequently by being liquefied, had a very pleasant ethereal odor, and when inhaled in not too large quantity produced no ill effects. If, however, it contained calcium sulphid and phosphid, as may be the case when the calcium carbid is made from coal and impure lime, the odor is most unpleasant. From the experiments of these observers it would appear that, while acetylene in proportions as high as 40% by volume may be fatally poisonous, yet it is much less poisonous than ordinary coal-gas. The toxic effects of acetylene, therefore, as it was formerly prepared, were, it is now thought, due to the presence of carbonic oxid or hydrogen cyanid. The researches of Mosso and Ottolenghi,[2] working with dogs, guinea-pigs, and other animals, seem to lead to similar conclusions. They found that if the gas was rapidly administered the animals were much more apt to recover when placed in the air than when it was given more slowly. Large doses seemed to cause death chiefly by respiratory paralysis, and, indeed, the paralytic phenomena seemed to preponderate throughout.

Ammonol, also called ammoniated phenyl-acetamid, is a substance whose formula and preparation have not been made public. R. G. Eccles,[3] however, has examined the substance chemically, and reports great variation in its composition, even to the degree that "no two samples were alike." He states that ammonol is composed of acetanilid, sodium bicarbonate, and ammonium bicarbonate. The drug is said to be antipyretic and analgesic, but recent publication upon the subject are few in number.

Analgene is the name given to a new antipyretic and analgesic remedy derived from coal-tar. The drug is soluble in slightly acidulated water, and, having no taste, is especially applicable to the treatment of children's disorders. Mongorvo[4] has employed it in 59 cases of children sick with various ailments, of whom 33 were suffering from malarial poisoning. The 33 cases ranged

[1] Boston M. and S. Jour., July 30, 1896.
[2] Brit. Med. Jour., Apr. 17, 1897, from Riforma Med., Jan. 23, 1897.
[3] N. Y. Polyclinic, Aug. 15, 1896, from Charlotte Med. Jour., vol. viii., No. 8.
[4] Univ. Med. Mag., May, 1897, from Bull. de l'Acad. de Méd. de Paris, Nov. 10, 1896.

MATERIA MEDICA, EXPERIM:'

AND PHARMA:

By HENRY A. GRIFFIN, M. D., AND

The progress of the past year i
rather by that development of former kno
by brilliant achievements which so often
Animal therapy has received considerabl
been done in its study, notably by Olive
fessed, however, that little of therapeut
edge of this subject, although it is equ:
unreached. The usual number of pha:
ing, and of them the most important, ;
ered in the body of this report. Am·
may demonstrate a practical value, alt
would prognosticate for the majority
advantage would seem to have been
the combined actions of disinfection
especially in its internal employmer
of considerable usefulness. In view
serum and the urgent necessity for
tic infection, it is unfortunate th:
encouraging. Recalling the suc
tive serums, it would appear re
might be similarly combated.
be considered as final, since fa
disappointment. The mescal |
ing the last twelve months, a
been gained. From this it v
no small degree, and useful n
combat, is scarcely to be ra
indica, whose activities indee
dehyd has received abunda
as to its value. Indeed, so
it seems quite within the b
an ideal disinfectant.

Acetanilid continues
in the popular "beadache
reckless administration i
by the frequent reports of
A. E. Brindley, of Man

eturns to the normal during the
·ffect upon the stomach seems to
-ional fulness and uneasiness to
rsisting for a number of hours,

Lewin, in 1888, separated a sub-
alkaloid, which has since been
ibed as " a white, strongly alkaline
utiou in prismatic, sometimes tabu-
oluble in a large quantity of water,
loroform, benzin, and petroleum-
it can be sublimed without decom-
acids." Anhalonin hydrochlorate,
-like crystals, has also been obtained.
nich solution it is very bitter, and to
with decomposition, at 254°–255° C.,
to the left. A sulfate of somewhat
cribed by Lewin. It is almost insol-
r which the name " mescalin " is pro-
It forms a salt with hydrochloric acid
d in alcohol than is the similar salt of
ı separated by Ewell from the mother-
alonin and mescalin. It also forms a
ghtly yellow color, neutral in reaction,
·ohol· The taste is acid and slightly
)eriments upon animals with these three
materially in their effects. The results
justify a detailed account at the present
nous substance, apparently of complex

anhalonin are said by Prentiss to be
nervous headache, nervous irritative
iping of the intestines, hysteric mani-
s in which an antispasmodic is indi-
henia and in depressed conditions of
and allied conditions ; as a substitute
eat nervous irritability or restlessness,
somnia caused by pain. In the last
hypnotic, but by relieving the cause
s it produces insomnia, but in thera-
Several cases of its use in neuralgia
already on record, but its use as a
experimental.
· value of extracts of the various so-
e of the attention of investigators (see
ontradictory results that are common
period. George Oliver [1] gives the
)ecially as regards their effect on the
ould appear that the blood is sup-
s which powerfully affect the ciren-
omotor muscles. This effect seems
njected so that it reaches the blood
ct. 16, 1896.

from 20 days to 13 years in age, and the dose of the remedy varied from 25 cgm. to 3 gm. in 24 hours. No injurious influence was observed upon the respiration or circulation, and though large and long-continued doses produced a more deeply colored urine, neither albumin nor sugar was ever found in it. In all malarial cases the action was favorable and rapid, the temperature being lowered and the duration of the disease apparently being made shorter. The other cases treated (26) by Mongorvo included " tuberculosis, lymphangitis, arthrosynovitis, parotiditis, Pott's disease, hip-disease, epilepsy, hysteria, chorea, otalgia, herpes zoster, urticaria, and painful tumor of the liver." In these, too, the action of the remedy was excellent, fever being reduced and pain made less. In hysteria, chorea, and epilepsy the nervous symptoms were benefited.

Anhalonium Lewinii, mescal button, has been made the subject of considerable study of late, and, if we may judge by the reports, we are in a fair way to have another "habit" on our hands in mescal intoxication. The very complete review of our present knowledge of the subject by Prentiss and Morgan[1] has led to personal experiments by S. Weir Mitchell[2] and Havelock Ellis.[3] We have, therefore, a very complete picture of the phenomena of mescal-poisoning, for the drug interferes but little with clear mental action.

Anhalonium Lewinii is a plant belonging to the genus Anhalonium, of the natural order Cactaceæ or Cacti (see Pellotin, p. 947). The exact place of this species in the genus is as yet a matter of discussion among botanists. It grows in rocky and barren soil, often in places almost inaccessible, in the valleys of the Rio Grande and Pecos Rivers in Texas and New Mexico. The mescal buttons, the commercial form of Anhalonium Lewinii, consist of the dried tops of the plant, and are of brown color, $\frac{1}{2}$–$1\frac{1}{2}$ in. in diameter by about $\frac{1}{4}$ in. thick, with curled-up edges. The average weight is about 4 gm. They are rather hard, but brittle, and can with difficulty be pulverized in a mortar. In the mouth the button swells, becoming soft under the influence of the saliva, and has a persistent, nauseous, and very bitter taste, with a marked sensation of tingling in the fauces. The powdered drug acquires a nauseous odor when moistened.

Physiologic Action.—Prentiss and Morgan[4] reported the results of some experiments upon man to determine the physiologic action of this drug (see *Year-Book* for 1897, p. 1103). The most remarkable effect was in the production of visions of color in rapidly changing and very varied forms. These could, as a rule, be seen only when the eyes were closed, and were distinctly heightened by rhythmic noise. The sensation accompanying these visions was one of pleasure, and the memory was also agreeable. They were rarely under the control of the will, and were about as often subject to the suggestion of others. At times there was occipital headache, as in the case of Mitchell, which persisted for some days, but that this is not an invariable sequel is shown by the experience of Ellis. The effect upon the mind seems to be comparatively slight. In some cases the reason and will are said to be entirely unaffected; in some, slowness of thought and loss of the power of expression or of attention are mentioned. All observers seem to agree that a dilatation of the pupil, which is well marked and persists for from 12 to 24 hours, is one of the phenomena following the administration of the drug. Accommodation seems to be but little affected, however. Depression of the muscular system in greater or less degree is apparently always present, and in some cases partial anesthesia of the skin was noticed as the effects of the drug began to pass away. The respiration was rarely affected, and the heart-action,

[1] Med. Rec., Aug. 22, 1896.   [2] Brit. Med. Jour., Dec. 5, 1896.
[3] Lancet, June 5, 1897.   [4] Therap. Gaz., Sept., 1895.

which at first becomes slower and stronger, returns to the normal during the period of greatest activity of the drug. The effect upon the stomach seems to vary with the individual, from a sense of occasional fulness and uneasiness to actual nausea and vomiting. Insomnia, persisting for a number of hours, appears to be a uniform effect.

Several alkaloids have been obtained. Lewin, in 1888, separated a substance which he called anhalonin. This alkaloid, which has since been obtained in a pure state by Ewell, is described as "a white, strongly alkaline substance. It crystallizes from aqueous solution in prismatic, sometimes tabular crystals of the rhombic system. It is soluble in a large quantity of water, and is very soluble in alcohol, ether, chloroform, benzin, and petroleum-ether. Its melting-point is 77.5° C., and it can be sublimed without decomposition. It forms salts with the ordinary acids." Anhalonin hydrochlorate, a white, odorless substance forming needle-like crystals, has also been obtained. It is soluble in 50 parts of water, in which solution it is very bitter, and to some extent also in alcohol. It melts, with decomposition, at 254°–255° C., and rotates the plane of polarized light to the left. A sulfate of somewhat similar appearance and properties is described by Lewin. It is almost insoluble in alcohol. A second alkaloid, for which the name "mescalin" is proposed, is now being studied by Ewell. It forms a salt with hydrochloric acid which is much more soluble in water and in alcohol than is the similar salt of anhalonin. A third alkaloid has been separated by Ewell from the mother-liquor left after the separation of anhalonin and mescalin. It also forms a hydrochlorate, crystalline and of a slightly yellow color, neutral in reaction, and readily soluble in water and alcohol. The taste is acid and slightly bitter, with persistent after-taste. Experiments upon animals with these three alkaloids seem to show that they differ materially in their effects. The results are not sufficiently definite, however, to justify a detailed account at the present time. The buttons also contain a resinous substance, apparently of complex nature, one or more wax-like bodies, etc.

The probable **therapeutic uses** of anhalonin are said by Prentiss to be as follows: "In general 'nervousness,' nervous headache, nervous irritative cough, abdominal pain due to colic or griping of the intestines, hysteric manifestations, and in other similar affections in which an antispasmodic is indicated; as a cerebral stimulant in neurasthenia and in depressed conditions of the mind—hypochondriasis, melancholia, and allied conditions; as a substitute for opium and chloral in conditions of great nervous irritability or restlessness, in active delirium and mania, and in insomnia caused by pain. In the last condition it acts to produce sleep not as a hypnotic, but by relieving the cause of the insomnia. In full physiologic doses it produces insomnia, but in therapeutic doses it does not have this effect." Several cases of its use in neuralgia and general neurasthenic conditions are already on record, but its use as a therapeutic agent must still be considered experimental.

Animal-extracts.—The therapeutic value of extracts of the various so-called ductless glands has received its share of the attention of investigators (see *Year-Book* for 1897, p. 1104), with the contradictory results that are common to all remedies during the experimental period. George Oliver [1] gives the result of his work with these extracts, especially as regards their effect on the circulatory system. From his report it would appear that the blood is supplied by the ductless glands with materials which powerfully affect the circulation, especially by their action on the vasomotor muscles. This effect seems to be produced both when the extract is injected so that it reaches the blood

[1] Indian Med. Rec., Oct. 16, 1896.

directly and when it is exhibited by the mouth. These are both important facts if further research shall establish them.

In detail: the **thyroid extract** seemed to cause a fall in blood-pressure. Apparently this action was due to the effect on the vasomotor system, causing an increase in the caliber of the arteries, as the force and frequency of the heart appeared to be unaffected. An extract of the spleen also produced a fall in blood-pressure, but this was followed later by a rise, the meaning of which has not been explained. On the other hand, the extracts prepared from the **pituitary body** (see p. 949) and from the **suprarenal capsules** (see p. 954) seemed to exert a contrary effect. A powerful contraction of the arteries was noted, with a corresponding rise in blood-pressure. At the same time the force of the heart's action was increased, but these extracts appeared to affect the frequency of the beats in different ways. The extract obtained from the pituitary body, while it did not inhibit the heart's action, diminished the frequency of the beats. That from the suprarenal capsules, however, increased the number of beats until the contractions were almost continuous, dilatation being incomplete, and the heart eventually stopped in systole.

The activity of both these extracts is destroyed by long boiling. The active principle of the suprarenal capsule is said to be found in the medullary portion. It is a dialyzable, organic principle soluble in water, and its activity is destroyed by alkalies as well as by boiling. It is unaffected, however, by acids, and its action is not interfered with by stomach-digestion. It is active in very minute doses, and the maximal effect may be produced when not more than fourteen millionths of a gram of active adrenal material to the kilogram of body-weight is given. Muret[1] reports some clinical results from the use of an **ovarian extract.** He was led to try this remedy from a consideration of these facts: 1. Without ovaries there is no uterine development of menstruation; 2. Ablation of ovaries in young children causes them to grow up without any feminine attributes; 3. After puberty loss of ovaries entails cessation of menstruation and atrophy of the genital organs; 4. Osteomalacia is believed to have been cured by oöphorectomy. He argues from these facts ' that there exists an internal ovarian secretion the absence of which would explain the first, second, and third conditions, while if it were excessive or altered osteomalacia might occur. He publishes 21 cases treated since 1893. A glycerin-extract of the ovaries of young cows, known as "liquid ovarin," which contained 1 gm. of ovarian tissue in 0.5 gm. of glycerin, was used at first. This was injected into the buttocks daily in doses of 0.5 to 1. gm. Later it was found that compressed tabloids, each containing 25 to 30 gm. of dried gland, were quite as efficacious as the injections, and this method of administration was therefore adopted. Two or three tabloids were given daily, and were well borne, even when the treatment was continued for a month or more.

The cases on which the report is based were: 9 patients who sought relief from nervous disorders accompanying the physiologic menopause, 3 whose symptoms were due to premature menopause following removal of the ovaries, and 4 cases of chlorosis. In the remainder menstruation was irregular from various local causes. In all these cases it is claimed that improvement followed the use of the ovarian extract, and that in some a cure was effected. The chlorotic patients were treated for two weeks by rest in bed alone, and then ovarin was given for two weeks. A more marked improvement is said to have occurred during the second than during the first fortnight.

Antipyrin.—That antipyrin still has an extended use is shown by the very

---

[1] N. Am. Pract., Dec., 1896, from Rev. méd. de la Suisse Romande, July 20, 1896.

considerable number of articles which have appeared in regard to it during the past year. These articles are very largely in reference to the toxicology of the drug.

Edwin Webster [1] reports a case of poisoning (see also p. 931) in a girl of 19, in which the recovery was rapid and complete, but which presents interesting features. The patient was anemic, and was being treated with Blaud's pills. One morning, as she complained of headache, the following draught was prescribed : antipyrin, gr. v ; potass. bromid., gr. vij ; spts. ammon. camp., ʒj ; aq., q.s. ad. ʒj. About 10 minutes later the physician was hurriedly summoned and found the following condition : there were " cold shivers, severe and gasping dyspnea ; the face was swollen, especially about the eyes, and so much so as to prevent any possibility of opening them or of seeing, except with great difficulty, the pupil ; and the body was covered with a bright-red rash like scarlet fever and resembling that of urticaria, in that it presented wheals which were of different sizes, from that of a small papule to some as large as a five-shilling piece. The temperature in the axilla was 97° F., and the pulse, which was very intermittent, was only 50. She complained of no pain. The tongue was very dry. The lips and general aspect were decidedly cyanotic." The patient was immediately put to bed and external heat applied. Whiskey, strychnin, and digitalis were administered, and at the end of 3 hours the shivering ceased. The other symptoms, however, continued, and the breathing was at one time so bad that artificial respiration was considered. At the end of 8 hours, however, the breathing began to improve, and after 4 hours more the only symptoms remaining were a faint rash and slight puffiness about the eyes. The rash did not completely disappear for 30 hours, but on the next evening, though suffering somewhat from weakness, she was up and on the following day went about her work as usual.

Of the reports on *idiosyncrasy,* among the most interesting are that of Steinhardt [2] regarding the effects of the drug on himself, and that of Briquet [3] of a case of acquired idiosyncrasy. Steinhardt suffered from migraine and habitually took 15 gr. of antipyrin during the attacks. He was greatly annoyed by the occurrence of small aphthous ulcers on the mucous membrane of the lips, cheeks, and tongue, which were slow to heal, but which he did not think of connecting with the antipyrin. In April, 1888, however, he noticed that the under lip became swollen and edematous immediately after taking a dose of the usual size, and 2 hours later an ulcer appeared on the tongue, followed shortly by several on the cheeks and lips. These healed only after a fortnight. He then stopped taking the drug for 2 years. On repeating the dose at the expiration of this time the same symptoms again occurred, and were not only more severe, but were accompanied by a dermatitis of the genital region. Four years later another dose of the drug brought about a repetition of the symptoms. A similar intolerance developed in him to all drugs of this kind which he used for the headache, but in the case of antipyrin alone was it so pronounced. He reports a similar idiosyncrasy in one of his patients.

Briquet's case was that of a young man who, previous to an attack of typhoid fever, from which he fully recovered, had no intolerance of antipyrin. Since his recovery, however, the most minute doses have caused an erythematous eruption, accompanied by bullæ, about the genital organs and on the mucous membrane of the mouth. A somewhat larger dose (1½ gr.) caused ulceration

[1] Lancet, Jan. 30, 1897.
[2] Edinb. Med. Jour., Jan., 1897, from Therap. Monatsh., Nov., 1896.
[3] Am. Medico-Surg. Bull., Apr. 10, 1897, from Méd. moderne.

directly and when it is exhibited by the mouth. These are both important facts if further research shall establish that.

In detail: the **thyroid extract** seems to cause a fall in blood-pressure. Apparently this action was due to the effect on the vasomotor system, causing an increase in the caliber of the arteries; the force and frequency of the heart appeared to be unaffected. An extract of the spleen also produced a fall in blood-pressure, but this was followed later by a rise, the meaning of which has not been explained. On the other hand, the extracts prepared from the **pituitary body** (see p. 949) and from the **suprarenal capsules** (see p. 954) seemed to exert a contrary effect. A powerful contraction of the arteries was noted, with a corresponding rise in blood-pressure. At the same time the force of the heart's action was increased, but these extracts appeared to affect the frequency of the beats in different ways. The extract obtained from the pituitary body, while it did not inhibit the heart's action, diminished the frequency of the beats. That from the suprarenal capsules, however, increased the number of beats until the contractions were almost continuous, dilatation being incomplete, and the heart eventually stopped in systole.

The activity of both these extracts is destroyed by long boiling. The active principle of the suprarenal capsule is said to be found in the medullary portion. It is a dialyzable, organic principle soluble in water, and its activity is destroyed by alkalies as well as by boiling. It is, unaffected, however, by acids, and its action is not interfered with by stomach-digestion. It is active in very minute doses, and the maximal effect may be produced when not more than fourteen millionths of a gram of active animal material to the kilogram of body-weight is given. Muret[1] reports some clinical results from the use of an **ovarian extract.** He was led to try this remedy from a consideration of these facts: 1. Without ovaries here is no uterine development or menstruation; 2. Ablation of ovaries in young children causes them to grow up without any feminine attributes; 3. After puberty loss of ovaries entails cessation of menstruation and atrophy of the genital organs; 4. Osteomalacia is believed to have been cured by oöphorecton. He argues from these facts that there exists an internal ovarian secretion the absence of which would explain the first, second, and third condition, while if it were excessive or altered osteomalacia might occur. He publishes 21 cases treated since 1893. A glycerin-extract of the ovaries of young cows, known as "liquid ovarin," which contained 1 gm. of ovarian tissue in 0.5 gm. of glycerin, was used at first. This was injected into the buttock daily in doses of 0.5 to 1. gm. Later it was found that compressed tabloids each containing 25 to 30 gm. of dried gland, were quite as efficacious as the injections, and this method of administration was therefore adopted. Two other tabloids were given daily, and were well borne, even when the treatment was continued for a month or more.

The cases on which the report is based were: 9 patients who sought relief from nervous disorders accompanying the physiologic menopause, 3 whose symptoms were due to premature menopause following removal of the ovaries, and 4 cases of chlorosis. In the remainder menstruation was irregular from various local causes. In all these cases it is claimed that improvement followed the use of the ovarian extract, and that in some a cure was effected. The chlorotic patients were treated for two weeks by rest in bed alone, and then ovarin was given for two weeks. A more marked improvement is said to have occurred during the second than during the first fortnight.

Antipyrin.—That antipyrin still has an extended use is shown by the very

[1] N. Am. Pract., Dec., 1896, from Rev. méd. de la tisse Romande, July 20, 1896.

considerable number of articles which have appeared in ... past year. These articles ar very largely in ... ... drug.

Edwin Webster¹ reports case of poisoning ... ... 19, in which the recovery was rapid and complete, but ... ing features. The patient was anemic, and was ... pills. One ... orning, as s! complained of headache, th... ... was prescribed: antipyrin, c. v; potass. bromid, gr. v; ... ... ℥j : ᴢj., q.s. ... ℥. About 0 minutes later the physician was ... ... moned and ... und the following condition: there were ... ... and gasping dyspnœa; the ce was swollen, especially about th... ... much so as to prevent an possibility of opening the... ... ... with great difficulty, the poil; and the body was covered with a ... ... rash like scarlet fever and resembling that of urticaria, in that ... ... wheals which were of different sizes, from that of a small papule to a size large as a five-shilling piece The temperature in the axilla was 97° F., an the pulse, which was very intermittent, was only 50. She complained of ... pain. The tongue was ver dry. The lips and general aspect were decidedly cyanotic." The patient was immediately put to bed and external heat applied. Whiskey, strychnin, and igitalis were administered, and at the end of 3 hours the shivering ceased The other symptoms, however, continued, and the breathing was at one tine so bad that artificial respiration was considered. At the end of 8 hours, hovver, the breathing began to improve, and after 4 hours more the only symptms remaining were a faint rash and slight puffiness about the eyes. The rash id not completely disappear for 30 hours, but on the next evening, though suffering somewhat from weakness, she was up and on the following day went bout her work as usual.

Of the reports on *idiosyncrasy*, among the most interesting are that of Steinhardt² regarding the effects of the drug on himself, and that of Briquet³ of a case of acquired idiosyncrasy. Steinhardt suffered from migraine and habitually took 15 gr. of antipyrin during the attacks. He was greatly annoyed by the occurrence f small aphthous ulcers on the mucous membrane of the lips, cheeks, and torue, which were slow to heal, but which he did not think of connecting with te antipyrin. In April, 1888, however, he noticed that the under lip became swollen and edematous immediately after taking a dose of the usual size, and 2 hours later an ulcer appeared on the tongue, followed shortly by several o the cheeks and lips. These healed only after a fortnight. He then stoppl taking the drug for 2 years. On repeating the dose at the expiration of his time the same symptoms again occurred, and were not only more severe but were accompanied by a dermatitis of the genital region. Four years later another dose of the drug brought about a repetition of the symptoms. A similar intolerance developed in him to all drugs of this kind which he use for the headache, but in the case of antipyrin alone was it so pronounced. He reports a similar idiosyncrasy in one of his patients.

Briqnet's case was the of a young man who, previous to an attack of typhoid fever, from whiche fully recovered, had no intolerance of antipyrin. Since his recovery, howeve, the most minute doses have caused an erythematous eruption, accompanied by ullæ, about the genital organs and on the mucous membrane of the mouth. A somewhat larger dose ($1\frac{1}{2}$ gr.) caused ulceration

---

¹ Lancet, Jan. 30, 897.
² Edinb. Med. Jou., Jan., 1897, from Therap. Monatsh., Nov., 1896.
³ Am. Medico-Sur Bull., Apr. 10, 1897, from Méd. moderne.

of the bullæ, the ulcers healing with difficulty after about 2 weeks.   He was steadily becoming more susceptible to the drug.   [The similarity between these cases is noteworthy and interesting.]

Incompatibility with Calomel.—H. Werner[1] has made a study of the reaction that occurs on mixing antipyrin with calomel outside the body, testing both qualitatively for the presence of mercuric chlorid, and quantitatively to ascertain the relative amount of this poison produced.   The results of his investigation lead us to think that the utmost care should be taken to prevent these two drugs from coming together in the human stomach.   Should they be thus combined the reaction, which, according to Werner, may be roughly expressed thus :

$$6HgCl + H_2O + 2 \text{ antipyrin} = 2Hg + Hg_2O + 2 HgCl_2 + 2 \text{ antipyrin hydro-chlorate,}$$

would probably give rise to a sufficient amount of mercuric chlorid to seriously endanger the patient's life.   A table is given in which the results of Werner's experiments are compared with the maximum doses of mercuric chlorid at a given age, according to Biedert, as follows :

Age.	Calomel and Antipyrin given	Mercuric Chlorid formed.	Max. Doses acct. to BIEDERT.
2 years	0.2 gm.	0.00468 gm.	0.002 gm.
4 "	0.3 "	0.00696 "	0.004 "
8 "	0.4 "	0.00928 "	0.008 "
20 "	1.0 "	0.0232 "	0.020 "

The experimenter did not acidify his solutions ; but if we accept the theory that the action of calomel is due to the formation, in the presence of the acid gastric juice, of corrosive sublimate, it will be readily seen that the quantity of the latter would be even greater than that shown by the tests.

New Compounds.—G. Patein and E. Dufau[2] have given us a description of two new compounds of antipyrin.   Antipyrin para-oxybenzoate is a crystalline solid, which may be recrystallized from its solution in boiling water or alcohol. With ferric chlorid it gives the antipyrin reaction.   It melts between 78° and 82° C. ; is soluble in 130 parts of cold and much more freely in boiling water ; is very readily soluble in alcohol, and but slightly so in ether.   It is obtained as follows : to an aqueous solution of 8 gm. of antipyrin is added a concentrated alcoholic solution of 5.5 gm. of para-oxybenzoic acid.   There ensues a union of a molecule of each of these substances without the elimination of water, and the result is an oily liquid which slowly crystallizes.   Antipyrin meta-oxybenzoate is obtained in a similar way and by a similar molecular union, but remains a liquid under ordinary conditions.

The reports on the *therapeutics* of antipyrin show that its use by itself is relatively decreasing.   It is being employed rather as a corrective and adjuvant to other preparations, and as such is largely used.   By such combinations the toxic effects appear to be diminished, while the antipyretic, analgesic, and hypnotic effects remain.   Leprevost[3] reports from France 47 cases of measles in which antipyrin was used to reduce the temperature.   He sums up his conclusions thus : " 1· Antipyrin is well tolerated by children. 2. It pro-

[1] Am. Medico-Surg. Bull., Aug. 29, 1896, from Pharm. Zeit., xli., p. 395, 1896.
[2] Am. Medico-Surg. Bull., July 25, 1897, from Journ. Soc. Chem. Indust., xv.
[3] N. Y. Med. Journ., vol. lxiii., p. 192.

duces prompt lowering of the temperature, not always to a very great extent, but with certainty in the immense majority of cases. 3. The maximum of the fall of temperature is obtained at the end of two hours in most cases. 4. Antipyrin seems to act in cases in which simple baths, or those to which mustard has been added, and moist applications have failed ; in all cases, if the immediate antithermic effects were not more intense, they were more lasting. 5. It has no action on the classic thermic cycle of measles, or on any of its complications. 6. The most varied complications have no influence at all on the results obtained with antipyrin, and the failure of the drug should not be imputed to them. 7. No antithermic reaction, or a very feeble one, is often an unfavorable element in the prognosis ; this rule is not absolute, and, as recovery may supervene in a case in which there has been no reaction, so may death occur with an abnormally high or an abnormally low temperature in patients who previously showed a notable lowering of the temperature. 8. Antipyrin has no action at all on the rapidity of the pulse. 9. It seems to ameliorate dyspnea in a slight degree. This action does not often begin until two hours after the ingestion of the drug."

Rousseau,[1] of Bordeaux, reports most favorably upon 500 of his hospital cases in which he used antipyrin in very small doses in infantile diarrheas and colic, especially when they occurred during teething.

Frederick Graves,[2] of Birmingham, England, reports the successful use of antipyrin in a case of diabetes mellitus with sudden onset, fever, epileptoid attacks of a nature resembling those of uremia, maniacal raving, and the presence of acetone ; 10 gr. were given t. i. d. for three days, and from this time the improvement was steady and rapid under appropriate diet and treatment.

Several reports[3] have appeared regarding the use of antipyrin as an anesthetic locally applied in the surgery of the genito-urinary tract and in obstetrics. Much is claimed for its efficiency, and no toxic effects are noted, but a more extended observation of clinical data is desirable.

Antistreptococcic Serum.—As is often the case, the later reports of experiments with this remedy are less promising than were those first published. Petruschky[4] reports his experiments with cultures of streptococci and an antistreptococcic serum which he obtained from Marmorek. He found, on giving a dose which Marmorek had stated to be absolutely fatal, that his rabbits were killed only in exceptional instances. He then used two of his own cultures of streptococci which he had grown for two years, and found them to be much more virulent. The action of these cultures was not checked by the antistreptococcic serum even when the latter was injected during the first twenty-four hours after infection. In consideration of these facts Petruschky thinks the following conclusions are justifiable : " That the therapeutic action of the serum is not yet to be recommended in man ; and that up to the present time there is no certain proof of the possibility of serum-therapy in streptococcic infection."

Calomel and Potassium Bromid Incompatible.—In an article by W. J. Robinson[5] on the incompatibility of antipyrin and calomel the assertion was made that potassium bromid formed a very poisonous compound with calomel. This having caused some surprise and comment, the author has further set forth this subject in a letter[6] to the editor of the *New York Medical Journal*, which, because of the importance of the subject, we quote all but entire :

[1] Ephemeris. p. 1786, Jan., 1897.   [2] Ibid., from Brit. Med. Journ., vol. i., p. 970, 1896.
[3] Ibid., p. 1787.   [4] Med. News, Jan. 9, 1897, from Presse méd., Nov. 11, 1896.
[5] N. Y. Med. Jour., Feb. 13, 1897.   [6] Ibid., Apr. 17, 1897.

"In many minds there seems to be the impression that when a mercurial salt is combined with another salt there is only a liability of the acid radical being changed, but not of the base—*i. e.*, mercurous chlorid, for instance, may become converted into a mercurous bromid, but not into mercuric bromid. This is, of course, wrong. Any mercurous salt may, by some of the mercury being precipitated in the metallic state, become converted into a mercuric salt. This is exactly what takes place when calomel and potassium bromid are triturated together; mercury is separated, and mercuric bromid—a highly poisonous compound—is formed.

"The reaction is plainly expressed by the following equation :

$$Hg_2Cl_2 + 4KBr = Hg + HgBr_2 + 2KBr + 2KCl.$$

Calomel. Potassium   Mercury.   Mercuric   Potassium   Potassium
          bromid.   bromid.   bromid.   chlorid.

"The presence of water or moisture seems to be necessary for the reaction to take place, because if the potassium bromid is dried, so that all interstitial moisture is driven off, no change occurs in the mixture; but the reaction occurs immediately on the addition of water.

"The bromid and calomel should therefore never be prescribed together, whether in powder-form or in a mixture; and when they are administered separately the interval should not be too short—say, one or two hours."

Chloralose appears to have given considerable satisfaction as a hypnotic, but reports are not wanting as to unfortunate manifestations produced by it, generally, however, as a result of doses unnecessarily large. James Tyson [1] gives us a valuable contribution upon the subject, reporting his experiences with the drug. In one case of obstinate insomnia 10 gr. of chloralose were given at bedtime each night. For three nights nothing but sound and refreshing sleep was the result. During the fourth and fifth nights, however, the patient arose and entirely disrobed himself, remaining naked until morning, but awakening quite unconscious of what had taken place in the night. In the second case, one of habitual insomnia, 5-gr. doses of chloralose had for two nights afforded refreshing sleep. On the third night, the usual dose failing to cause sleep, a part of another 5-gr. cachet was taken after several hours, and later the remaining part. In the morning the patient was found sleeping heavily and breathing stertorously, and could not be aroused. Later, however, he awoke feeling well and unconscious of anything unusual. In a third case a 10-gr. dose of the drug having failed to affect an habitual insomniac, the dose was repeated in an hour, with the result of causing at first restlessness with sleep, but later excessive violence, which required forcible restraint. At the same time there was involuntary evacuation of the bladder and bowels. A quiet sleep finally occurred, from which the patient awoke in his usual state. Tyson believes that in these cases the untoward results were caused by doses too large, and recommends that the dose employed should be between 3 and 5 gr. for adults. He thinks highly of the remedy when thus used, but insists upon certain precautions of administration. It should always be given in solution, in either hot water or hot milk. If its bitterness is objected to, then it may be given in cachet, but the objection to giving in cachet or powder is the danger of its being unabsorbed in the stomach and so causing failure, while if repetition is practised the conjoint action of these doses may cause unfortunate results. The cases most benefited by chloralose appear to be the simple insomnias, for it is little if at all analgesic. It may also be used in insanity, in cardiac disease, and in Bright's disease. In tuberculosis,

[1] Univ. Med. Mag., Dec., 1896.

however, the dangerous effects of the drug seem most likely to occur, and therefore, especially if debility is present, it should be withheld. The advantages of chloralose as properly given are its rapidity of action and freedom from dulness, sleepiness, and other ill results on the following day (see *Year-Book* for 1896, p. 1032).

Coal-tar Antipyretics.—J. A. Martin[1] gives a brief review of the results of his study of the coal-tar derivatives—antipyrin, acetanilid, phenacetin, and lactophenin. He undertakes to show the relation existing between these drugs from a chemic, physiologic, and therapeutic standpoint. *Chemically*, all these preparations are obtained from carbolic acid through some of its derivatives, and contain also the radical of some organic acid. Thus antipyrin is obtained by the action of heat on phenyl-hydrazin and diacetic ether; acetanilid, by boiling pure aniline (phenyl-anim) with glacial acetic acid, equal parts by weight, for a day or two, when acetanilid and water result. Phenacetin again is para-phenetidin in which an atom of hydrogen has been replaced by the acetic acid radical, acetyl; and similarly in lactophenin an atom of hydrogen in para-phenetidin is replaced by lactyl, the lactic acid radical. It will be noticed that in the first three compounds the hydrogen is replaced by acetyl, while in lactophenin lactyl is substituted. This fact is said to have an important bearing on the relative action of the drugs.

As to the *physiologic action*, it must be borne in mind that the aim has been to retain the antipyretic effect of carbolic acid, while doing away with its caustic and poisonous properties. Carbolic acid diminishes heat-production while at the same time it increases the dissipation of heat. But, unfortunately, aside from its caustic action, which was readily got rid of in its derivatives, it reduces arterial pressure by paralysis of the vasomotor centers and by markedly depressing the heart. Furthermore, death is generally due to respiratory paralysis.

Antipyrin meets the requirements only to a limited degree. It is, to be sure, noncaustic and freely soluble in water, and it reduces febrile temperature to a marked degree. But it is decomposed in the body, the products of its decomposition acting on the hemoglobin of the blood to form methemoglobin. Thus, it is said, it gives rise to the symptoms of poisoning—ataxia, paraplegia, convulsions with general rigidity, stupor and coma, with dilated pupils, sweating, cyanosis, and marked depression of both heart and respiration. In addition, there often exists a personal idiosyncrasy against antipyrin which makes its promiscuous administration very dangerous. A most alarming condition of the patient has more than once been produced by a very small dose (see p. 927).

Acetanilid has a similar action when given in large doses or to patients having an idiosyncrasy against it. The action on the blood is the same, and while the sweating, when it occurs, is less severe, the cyanosis is said to be more marked than that which follows the administration of antipyrin (see p. 927; also *Year-Book* for 1897, p. 1101). The pulse-rate falls markedly, and its character becomes thready. The fall in temperature seems to be due to a diminished heat-production.

Phenacetin, on the other hand, while it lessens heat-production, does so by an influence on the nervous system, while the blood-pressure, according to Martin, remains unaltered. But, again, we find among the unpleasant symptoms the profuse sweating and the cyanosis. This cyanosis, Martin believes, is due to the action of the acetic acid on the hemoglobin, as in the case of antipyrin and acetanilid (see *Year-Book* for 1897, p. 1131).

[1] Atlanta M. and S. Jour., July, 1896.

Lactophenin, like phenacetin, lessens the production of heat by an action on the nervous system, without affecting the blood-pressure. It is said that this antipyretic action, though rapid, is not abrupt, and lasts from four to six hours. Martin has not found that the subsequent rise of temperature was accompanied by shivering or other unpleasant effects, and he has never known cyanosis to follow its administration. The reason for this he believes to be that none of its decomposition-products affects the hemoglobin. He considers the analgesic and hypnotic effects to be decidedly more pronounced than those that are produced by either of its three predecessors, while the heart and respiration seem to be entirely unaffected (see *Year-Book* for 1896, p. 1064; also see p. 942).

In regard to the *therapeutics* Martin makes the following statement: " In my opinion, the day is not far off when antipyrin will be almost wholly discarded on account of the uncertainty of the degree of its action, and on account of its incompatibility with a large number of drugs in common use; acetanilid will find a home with the surgeon as an antiseptic dressing; and phenacetin, which has done a noble work as a forerunner, will give way to its younger and more worthy brother, *lactophenin*."

Codein.—Although we much doubt how widespread is the failure to appreciate this valuable remedy, for our observation has led us to believe that it is in very general employment, still it may be that some have failed to realize its advantages. For this reason the attention called to codein by a recent writer[1] is a matter which should be widely published, for the facts he points out are true beyond question and valuable to the utmost. Although codein suffers from its relationship with morphin, and is overshadowed by a comparison with it, in many respects it has the advantage of the comparison, for it seldom disturbs digestion and is less likely than morphin to constipate. Furthermore, it is not so dangerous a remedy as is morphin used habitually, for it has not the enslaving and therefore dangerous tendencies of that drug. Among the conditions most benefited by codein are irritating coughs. In these, especially that of pulmonary tuberculosis, from ½ to 1 gr., in pill, taken at bedtime will do much to promote quiet and rest. In pneumonia ¼ gr. is an excellent sedative addition to a cough-mixture when cough is causing suffering and exhaustion. In pelvic discomfort and pains of varying kind the remedy is remarkable in its power to relieve. In nausea due to nervous causes its action is often good. In the abdominal distress and post-prandial diarrhea of some varieties of dyspepsia codein has unique power to benefit, the method of administration recommended in such cases as these being ½ gr. in pill taken 10 minutes before meals. In the cure of the opium-habit, too, codein may be employed as a sedative substitute for temporary and diminishing employment. The writer emphasizes what is a matter of vast importance, namely, that if good results are expected, a reliable drug should be employed. [This is of rather more importance in the case of codein than in the case of most drugs.] He furthermore thinks that codein pills should be gelatin-coated, made as ordered, and compounded with the addition of a sufficient quantity of aromatic sulphuric acid. Codein sulfate is preferable to the alkaloid itself. [As supplementary to what is here said of the usefulness of codein in irritating and exhausting cough, the formula of a cough-mixture much employed in the hospitals of New York is given: ℞. Codeinæ, gr. ¼; ac. hydrocyanic. dil., ♏iij; ammon. chlorid., gr. iij; syp. prun. virg., ad ℥j. Sig.: Dose ℥j.][2]

Commelina (*Yerba del Pollo*) is the name under which several plants

---

[1] Therap. Gaz., Aug. 15, 1896, from Maryland Med. Jour., Apr. 18, 1896.
[2] Formulary of the Roosevelt Hospital, New York City.

of the family *Commelinaceæ* are known in Mexico. Alfonso Herrera[1] has recently contributed a very interesting article upon this subject. Although the chief activity of commelina is as a hemostatic, of old the remedy had extensive employment by the Aztecs in the treatment of fevers, headaches, neoplasms, and hemorrhages, as well as in certain conditions associated with parturition. The remedy was neglected for a long time, and in fact, until the experiments conducted with it in 1863 by Hernandez and Alzate, it was little esteemed. Since that time, however, it has been largely employed as a hemostatic. What may be the active principles of yerba del pollo it is difficult to say, though acetic acid may be found in the juice, and in the extract obtained from the plants ammonium acetate, potassium chlorid, albuminoids, vegetable albumin, chlorophyll, extractive, and cellulose.

It would appear that the most frequent hemostatic use of commelina in Mexico is in metrorrhagia and hemoptysis, the extract being employed in injections for the former condition and in pills in the latter. The pills may contain 1 or 2 gr. of the extract, and from 24 to 48 pills even may be given in a day. For injection from a dram to an ounce of the extract may be added to a pint of water. Commelina, in the form of the extract, has also some employment in leucorrhea and as a hemostatic in capillary hemorrhage. For wounds a strong solution of the extract may be applied upon lint, or a poultice made from the powdered plant. [Although commelina cannot but interest us, and while no doubt it may be in many cases a remedy of value, it is unnecessary to more than call attention to the very limited employment which styptic drugs now have and the very manifest dangers associated with their local application.]

Condurango, it will no doubt be remembered, enjoyed a brief notoriety some few years ago as a remedy for gastric cancer. That its curative power against this condition does not exist is generally conceded, but many observers have called attention to its undoubted stomachic influence, an action which has, no doubt, made the remedy at times productive of relief from many of the dyspeptic symptoms of gastric carcinoma, and has even led to the error crediting it with curative power. In this connection the report of G. Bardet[2] is of interest. He regards condurango as sedative, and valuable therefore in nerve-irritability. The sedative influence, he thinks, is especially manifested in gastric pain, and at the same time stomach digestion is improved. Not only is condurango a stimulant to gastric digestion, but, according to Tcheisow, it promotes biliary and pancreatic digestion as well. Bardet suggests that when prescribing condurango it is wise to specify the bark of the white variety, this being the variety which has received most study. Of a 20% tincture the dose is from 2 to 4 teaspoonfuls; and of the extract 7 to 15 gr. may be given.

Creolin.—Results are not wanting to show that this substance is not as innocuous as has been believed, and in this connection the investigations of Hobday,[3] of the Royal Veterinary College, are both interesting and instructive. A solution containing about two ounces of creolin to the quart of water was applied to a couple of valuable ferrets to eradicate lice and mange, with the result that within half an hour both animals were dead. This called the attention of Hobday to the possible toxic effects of the preparation, and he undertook a series of experiments upon dogs and cats, the results of which he thus states: "That creolin is an irritant and narcotic poison to the dog and cat; that it is especially toxic when spread in emulsions of a certain strength

[1] N. Y. Med. Jour., June 19, 1897, from Am. Jour. Pharm., June, 1897.
[2] Am. Jour. Med. Sci., May, 1897, from Nouveaux Remèdes, No. 3, p. 65, 1897.
[3] Ephemeris, p. 1817, Jan., 1897, from Lancet, vol. i., p. 1733, 1896.

over a large area of the body; that its effect is more rapid and violent when mixed with water than when applied pure or in an ointment; that applied externally in certain proportions it will act as a violent irritant; that the pure creolin is more toxic than the less refined preparations; and that it is less readily absorbed from the stomach, from small wounds, and from the subcutaneous tissue than from a large area of skin-surface."

Digitoxin.—The confusion which has long existed in connection with the digitalis glucosids is a matter of as much practical importance as theoretic, and all efforts made to solve the problems which pertain to foxglove are to be encouraged. Actuated by a desire to bring order out of the present chaos M. L. Adrian[1] advances several propositions which we quote entire: "1· The digitoxin studied in 1888 by Lafont and Bardet is not identical with the more active commercial article of 1893–'94. 2. This difference leads us to believe that digitalis, besides the digitalin already isolated in purity, contains a very active glucosid of the strophanthin type. 3. This digitoxin is not in every case a pure drug, for its variations have been demonstrated, and for this reason it should be omitted from the pharmacopeia for fear of accidents. 4. The digitalin of Nativelle is a pure, crystallized product of constant composition and of constant pharmacologic action, and for these reasons should be the only one admitted to the pharmacopeias. Recently Kiliani[2] has presented a glucosidal body of the chemical formula $C_{36}H_{50}O_{6}$, or exactly that established by Arnaud for crystallized digitalin. This substance, designated as digitoxin, is none other than the crystallized digitalin of Nativelle." [It need not be said that such statements, if confirmed, are important; but until pharmacy shall provide us with more reliable and constant digitalis principles, and ones which, however pure, are not variable with their manufacture, we must confess a preference for the preparations of digitalis itself, howsoever objectionable these may be as compared with idealized glucosids.]

A New Disinfectant Derived from Petroleum.—Although the substance described is not as yet obtainable commercially, and therefore its medical importance is rather more theoretical than real, yet the researches of Bartochewitch,[3] of Kharkow, with a substance he obtained from petroleum are full of interest. To petroleum-refuse he added 20 parts by volume of strong sulphuric acid, and, mixing thoroughly, he allowed a precipitate to form during 24 hours and in the cold. This precipitate was a mass resembling tar, and above it was an opalescent black fluid. This fluid having been decanted, there was added a 10% solution of caustic potash somewhat less in amount than the original volume. By shaking there was developed a smooth, soapy, yellowish-brown mass, from which emulsions could be prepared. The emulsion which Bartochewitch employed in his experiments contained 200 parts of the disinfecting substance shaken for 15 or 20 minutes with 800 parts of water at 75° C., and subsequently filtered through cotton-wool. The result of this treatment was a dirty, milky liquid containing fatty particles and an aqueous solution of the disinfectant, free from every sort of microorganism. Separation took place in this emulsion after standing for 2 or 3 days, but slight shaking restored its former condition. Investigation showed that the alkalinity of the fluid was equivalent to 1% of caustic potash. For purposes of investigation he employed spores of bacillus anthracis on silk threads, cultivations of the same organism in broth, and similar cultivations of bacillus prodigiosus, bacillus typhi abdominalis, bacillus choleræ asiaticæ, staphylococcus pyogenes, and

---

[1] Am. Jour. Med. Sci., May, 1897, from Nouveaux Remèdes, No. 3, p. 78, 1897.
[2] Compare Year-Book for 1896, p. 1035, and for 1897, p. 1116.
[3] Medicine, Sept., 1896, from Med. Week., Feb. 14, 1896.

streptococcus erysipelatis. He also applied his testing to the disinfection of fecal matter. As an index of the strength and power which the disinfectant showed, it may be said that the anthrax bacillus was killed by it in 24 minutes, and the same bacillus with its spores in 48 minutes.

The conclusions which Bartochewitch[1] reached from these experiments are : 1. Being without any odor of its own, the disinfectant destroys evil smells, developing only at the beginning of its action a slight ammoniacal smell; 2. Its oily particles, resulting from the decomposition of the soapy, disinfecting mass, gradually rising to the surface of the liquid to be disinfected, prevent the access of oxygen from the air to the putrefying products, and thus hinder their further decomposition ; 3. The liquid being disinfected gradually separates out of the disinfectant the active constituents, whereby the continuance of its action is insured ; 4. The disinfectant need only be added to the contents of cesspools, etc., in the proportion of 1 % or 2 % of the refuse, feces, etc. ; thus, calculating the normal amount for each person at 1500 c.c. of urine and 400 gm. of feces, it is necessary to pour into a privy or cesspool from 20 to 40 gm. of the disinfecting substance, an average of 30 gm., instead of about 2000 gm.; 5. The cheapness of this mode of disinfection is beyond doubt, for to render innocuous the excretions of one man costs from $\frac{3}{4}$ to 1 kopek—*i. e.*, one farthing—a day. Thus, with the exception of tar and its products, this is the cheapest disinfecting-substance known.

Dulcin[2] is the name given to a substance obtainable from Berlin-blue, and said to be 250 times sweeter than cane-sugar. It is a white, crystalline powder, which is soluble in 800 parts of water at 15° C., in 50 parts of boiling water, and in 15 parts of 90% alcohol. The long-continued use of dulcin by diabetics is said to be unproductive of injury or disagreeable effect, and as compared with saccharin it is advantageous from having a taste more nearly resembling that of sugar. Dulcin has been employed in pastils, which contain 25 mgm., the equivalent of 5 gm. of sugar. [See *Year-Book* for 1896, p. 1037.]

Eosote is a commercial name given to the valerianate of creosote, a fluid distilling at 240° C. It is to be had in gelatine capsules, each of which, it is said, contains about 3 gr. The drug is said by E. Grawitz[3] not to be caustic or poisonous. Its therapeutic applications are those of creosote. The beginning dose is a capsule 3 times a day, given with milk in plenty; later 2 or even 3 capsules may be given at a dose.

Grawitz[4] has employed eosote in 35 cases of tuberculosis, and as an intestinal antiseptic, in many cases of gastrointestinal disturbance. In most of these the treatment was very successful, and it was rarely necessary to withhold the drug because of digestive disturbance, even after administration for many weeks. Grawitz is warm in his recommendation of eosote because of its cheapness, its palatability, the comfort with which large doses are taken, and the freedom from toxic effect.

Euchinin is a recently introduced preparation of quinin which is asserted to have the curative power of the latter without to the same degree its property of causing noises in the ears, heaviness, and gastric disorder, and also without its disagreeable taste. The drug is produced by the action of ethyl-chlorocarbonate upon quinin, and occurs in needle-shaped crystals which are soluble in alcohol, chloroform, and ether, but little soluble in water. We owe our infor-

[1] N. Am. Pract., Aug., 1896, from Med. Week., Feb. 14, 1896.
[2] Med. Rec., June 19, 1897, from Jour. de Méd. de Paris, Feb. 7, 1897.
[3] N. Y. Med. Jour., Aug., 15, 1896, from *T*herap. Monatsh., 1896, No. 7 ; *T*herap. Woch., July 19, 1896.   [4] Brit. Med. Jour., Oct., 1896, from *T*herap. Monatsh., July, 1896.

mation upon this subject mainly to O. Van Noorden.[1] Euchinin has basic properties, and uniting with certain acids it forms crystallizable salts. Of these the chlorid is freely soluble in water, the sulfate is somewhat soluble, and the tannate is less soluble. This euchinin tannate is highly to be recommended, and is advantageous in that it is without taste. The chlorid or hydrochlorid, on the other hand, has an exceedingly disagreeable taste, while euchinin itself is without taste unless left long upon the tongue, in which case it is somewhat bitter, but if given in milk or sherry or cocoa no unpleasant taste is noticed. The usual dose of euchinin is between 1 and 2 gm., and it is said that this dose may be given daily for a considerable time without ill effect. A single large dose (2 gm.) in one case produced sensations of heaviness in the head. The drug is advantageously administered in tablet or enclosed in cachet, and to children it may be given in milk, soup, or cocoa, its tastelessness rendering it peculiarly fitted for pediatric practice.

It is to be regretted that Van Noorden was unable, owing to the absence of cases, to test the action of euchinin upon malarial disease. He has reported upon the action of the drug in whooping-cough (15 cases), hectic fever in tuberculosis (14 cases), sepsis from various causes (5 cases), as well as in pneumonia, typhoid fever, and neuralgia. In pertussis and in febrile states Van Noorden states that from 1½ to 2 gm. of euchinin are required to accomplish the work of 1 gm. of quinin. As to the result accomplished, it is stated that 12 cases of whooping-cough were rapidly benefited, and in the febrile cases the temperature was lower within a few days. In neuralgia the effect was also good, and especially brilliant in one case in which the pain was supraorbital, a dose of 0.6 gm. of quinin or 1 gm. of euchinin acting when other remedies had failed, the favorable influence being witnessed in several later attacks.

Ferrostyptin is a substance of recent introduction, said to be antiseptic and styptic and valuable as a substitute for ferric chlorid. Its composition[2] is unpublished as yet, but it is thought to contain about 20% of iron together with ammonium chlorid and, perhaps, acetanilid. It occurs as a yellow, crystalline powder of sharp and saline taste and an odor which resembles that of carbolic acid. It is freely soluble in water, but is insoluble in alcohol and ether. The watery solution if heated to boiling undergoes coagulation, and a gelatinous precipitate is formed in it by the addition of acids. This, however, is dissolved if the acid is added in excess. If alkalies are added, ferric hydroxid is precipitated. Ferrostyptin melts at 112° C. The clinical value of ferrostyptin is undetermined, but it has been regarded as likely to be of value in dentistry and gynecology. Among the advantages[3] claimed for it are freedom from caustic properties, the pulverulent condition, and its action as an antiseptic. The remedy was introduced by Eichengrun.

Formaldehyd, formyl or formol (see *Year-Book* for 1896, p. 1039, and for 1897, p. 1120), is a colorless gas of pungent odor, very irritating to the mucous membrane of the nose and throat if inhaled for more than a few seconds. Chemically it is formic aldehyd, and has the formula CH_2O. It combines with hydrogen sulphid and with volatile compounds derived from ammonia, acting thus as a deodorant. With water it forms a stable, colorless solution, somewhat volatile and having the odor of the gas, not inflammable and practically nontoxic. The 40% (saturated) solution is the commercial formaldehyd, or formalin. It also forms an effective combination with gelatin, known as glutol (see p. 939).

---

[1] Jour. Am. Med. Assoc., Mar. 10, 1897, from Centralbl. f. innere Med., Nov. 28, 1896.
[2] Ephemeris, p. 1838, 1897.
[3] Am. Medico-Surg. Bull., Sept. 5, 1896, from Apoth. Ztg., xi., p. 440, 1896.

Preparation.—Formaldehyd is usually prepared by incomplete combustion of methyl alcohol. Thus far, the most effective and economical method has seemed to be to pass a current of air saturated with methyl alcohol over a heated spiral coil of platinum. On condensation the product is a solution of formaldehyd in methyl alcohol. A. Brochet[1] points out an element of danger in this method, for he has found that the gas when made in this way is mixed with not inconsiderable amounts of carbon monoxid. He recommends a method by which hot air is made to pass over finely divided para-formaldehyd. The gas thus prepared is so dilute that no polymerization takes place on cooling.

Uses.—As an antiseptic, germicide, and disinfectant, formaldehyd has been the subject of many reports, and while we must not lose sight of the tendancy to favorable reports on new preparations, the fact that it has some value in this direction would seem to be pretty well established so far. Nearly all observers appear to unite in emphasizing its freedom from taste and odor in weak solutions, together with its ready volatility and the absence of poisonous effects. F. C. J. Bird[2] thus summarizes the effects produced by the various solutions: "1 : 125,000 kills anthrax-bacilli ; 1 : 50,000 prevents the development of typhus-bacillus ; 1 : 25,000 forms a useful injection in leucorrhea ; 1 : 2500 destroys the more resistant microorganisms in one hour ; 1 : 500 is useful for the irrigation of catheters and as a mouth-wash ; 1 : 200 or 1 : 250 is a general disinfectant solution for washing hands and instruments, spraying in sick-rooms, and as a deodorant ; 1 : 100 is used for lupus, psoriasis, and other diseases of the skin." Aronsohn and Burkhardt, as quoted by H. C. Wood,[3] conclude from their experiments that formaldehyd is not only germicidal, but that it also deprives the toxins of diphtheria and of tetanus at least of their poisonous power. Should further observation confirm this belief its importance is evident. The general opinion seems to have been that as a germicide formaldehyd is as powerful as the bichlorid of mercury. Later reports do not appear to establish this fact altogether. Walter,[4] after an exhaustive series of experiments, states his conclusions thus: "1. Formalin in the strength of 1 : 10,000 arrests the growth of the germs of anthrax, cholera, typhoid fever, diphtheria, and staphylococcus pyogenes aureus. 2. In the gaseous form it arrests growth, even when greatly diluted. 3. In 1% solutions it kills pure cultures of pathogenic germs in an hour. In diluted alcoholic solutions the effect is more intense. 4. In 3% solutions, especially with the addition of alcohol, the hands may be freed from all germs. More extended investigations are necessary to show the degree to which the skin is affected. 5. By spraying artificially infected matter with formalin solution, and afterward enclosing it in air-tight vessels, such matter may be sterilized. 6. By means of formalin (or, in other words, formaldehyd) leather articles, uniforms, etc., may be thoroughly disinfected in large quantities, and without in any way injuring these articles ; 24 hours' exposure is requisite for such disinfection. The possibility of disinfecting rooms may be considered as demonstrated by other experts. 7. Feces are almost instantly deodorized by a 1% solution, and are disinfected (germ-free) in 10 minutes by a 10% solution. 8. Formalin acts well as a caustic. 9. It is an excellent preservative."

To the surgeon this substance presents many possible improvements in methods of sterilization. It is said not to affect instruments, leaving the edges of knives undulled, while the hands may be rendered aseptic by a 3% solu-

[1] Quart. Med. Jour., July, 1896, from Compt. rend. de la Soc. de Biol., 122, 201-203.
[2] Am. Jour. Med. Sci., Jan., 1897, from Am. Jour. Pharm., No. 11, 1897.
[3] Univ. Med. Mag., June, 1897.
[4] Ibid., May, 1897, from Zeit. f. Hyg., vol. xxi., 1896.

tion, especially if subsequently rinsed in alcohol. It is also said to be a very efficient aid in sterilizing catgut, and several methods have been recommended. It acts by so hardening the gut that it is not damaged by subsequent boiling. As a local application, also, it is said to offer many advantages, though in too concentrated solution it is irritating to the sound tissues. No case of poisoning is reported. H. C. Wood[1] refers to its use in Philadelphia, both in hospital and private practice, for all sorts of wounds, carbuncles, and infected sores. For cleansing infected wounds a 2% solution was used, and for continuous application $\frac{1}{4}$%. In strong solution a mild caustic action results. Von Winckel, in Berlin, found that irrigation with a solution containing 1 part in 10,000 was effective in diseases of an infectious nature in the female genital organs. O. Hasencamp,[2] of Toledo, Ohio, also reports favorably on the use of a 5% solution in gonorrhea in the male.

Much is said in favor of formaldehyd in ophthalmologic practice. Its value in this connection was noted by Valude in 1893, but recently it has come into more extended use. J. M. Davidson,[3] of Aberdeen, Scotland, gives a very conservative and, therefore, valuable account of his use of this agent. He finds the most serviceable solution to be 1 part of formalin to 2000 or 3000 of water. This he has found to be of very great value when used freely in infected abrasions of the cornea and in hypopyon ulcers. Hasencamp[4] also finds it of use in conjunctivitis.

Salter[5] reports good results from the use of the 40% solution painted on in ringworm of the scalp; 40 cases were thus treated, and microscopic examinations made both before and after the application showed the trichophyton to have disappeared in each case. A temporary irritation and the production of a thick crust rendered the subsequent application of an emollient advisable. Edema of the face, unaccompanied by pain or constitutional disturbance, was a remarkable complication in 6 of the cases, but was only noticed when the area painted was large.

By far the most important fact in regard to this substance appears to be that it will act as a germicide in the gaseous state, owing to its power to permeate almost all organic substances. In this way, by the use of one of the many formaldehyd-generators now for sale in this country, it seems possible to completely disinfect a room with the contained furniture in about six hours. The experiments of Roux, Trillat, and Bose[6] gave remarkable results in this connection. The only resistant germs that were found were bacillus subtilis (of hay) and bacillus mesentericus, neither of which is of pathologic importance. The process was found to be more certainly effective the more perfect the contact of the infected materal with the gas, although many remarkable instances of its power of penetration are reported by these and other authors. At the conclusion of the process of disinfection the windows were opened and allowed to remain so for two days, when the room was found to be odorless and habitable. No injury to any object in the rooms followed the use of this method. F. C. Robinson,[7] of Bowdoin College, has devised a lamp, which is automatic, to produce the vapor of formaldehyd.

E. G. Horton[8] has conducted experiments at the University of Pennsylvania to test the value of this agent in disinfecting books. He finds that:

[1] Loc. cit.   [2] Columbus Med. Jour., Mar. 2, 1897.
[3] Ephemeris, p. 1843, Jan., 1897.   [4] Loc. cit.
[5] Ephemeris, Jan., 1897, from Brit. Med. Jour., vol. ii., p. 650, 1896.
[6] Ephemeris, Jan., 1897, from Lancet, vol. i., p. 1678, 1896.
[7] Jour. Am. Med. Assoc., vol. xxvii., p. 675.
[8] Ephemeris, Jan., 1897, from Med. News, vol. lxix., p. 152.

" 1. Books can be disinfected in a closed space simply by vapor of commercial formalin, by using 1 c.c. of formalin to 300 c.c., or less, of air. 2. The effect produced in the first 15 minutes is practically equivalent to that observed after 24 hours. 3. An increase in the amount of air to each c.c. of formalin is not counterbalanced by an increase in the length of time of exposure. 4. In case the disinfection has been incomplete, the vitality of the organisms has been so weakened that they survive only if transferred in a few hours to media suitable for their development. 5. The use of the vapor of formalin is not detrimental, as far as observed, in any manner to the books, nor is it objectionable to the operator beyond a temporary irritation of the nose and eyes."

H. C. Wood [1] states that the action of the drug upon the higher animals is comparatively feeble. In sufficient doses it acts as a violent irritant. It is worthy of note that the poisonous effects are much more marked after exhibition by the stomach than after hypodermic injection. Free inhalation, as noted by Mosso and Paoletti, is liable to cause a pulmonary inflammation which may be severe enough to cause death.

The purely medicinal uses of formaldehyd have so far been few, though Rosenberg [2] has given it internally in a solution of milk-sugar, which he calls sterisol. Examination of the urine, shows that it is eliminated very slowly by the kidneys. Hamaide [3] describes an inhaler devised for the treatment of pulmonary tuberculosis by this agent, which produces a vapor of 2% to 10% strength. The odor may be disguised by Austrian Pine. The coughing-spells are said to become less troublesome and the quantity of fetid expectoration is diminished.

In preserving and hardening pathologic and anatomic specimens formaldehyd is most useful. The specimens are rendered hard without shrinking, and retain the original colors to a much greater degree than when other agents are used. The penetrating and preservative powers are also said to be good. Lester [4] has found it very efficient as a preservative for ointments in proportion of about 2 drams to the pound. He found it useful also in mucilages and pastes.[5]

Formopyrin is the name which Marcourt [6] has given to a combination of antipyrin and formaldehyd. It is prepared by dissolving equal molecular weights of the two components in water and mixing the solutions. The mixture having stood for eight or ten days, there is formed a crystalline substance, which is formopyrin. The next step in the process is the drying of the precipitate upon a porous slab, by which the excess of formaldehyd is absorbed, and its purification by recrystallization from alcohol. Formopyrin is insoluble in cold water, somewhat soluble in boiling water, insoluble in ether and benzine, but freely soluble in alcohol and chloroform. It melts at 142° C., and is decomposed at a temperature higher than this. At the present time the value of formopyrin is purely one of inference, for it has had no reported clinical use to justify the supposition that it will act as an anodyne, antipyretic, and antiseptic.

Glutol is a combination of formalin (see page 936) with gelatin which promises to be of considerable value, if we may judge from the early reports.[7]

[1] Loc. cit. [2] Med. News, Feb. 27, 1897, from Deutsch. med. Woch., Nos. 39 and 40, 1896.
[3] Bull. Acad. de Méd. [4] Ephemeris, p. 1839, Jan., 1897.
[5] Those who wish to look up the literature of this agent will find a very complete bibliography in a "Résumé of the Uses of Formalin," by Geo. C. Freeborn in N. Y. Med. Journ., vol. lxiii., p. 770.
[6] Am. Medico-Surg. Bull., July 25, 1896, from Report de Pharm., vii., p. 214, 1896.
[7] Ephemeris, p. 1848, Jan., 1897.

To make it, 2% of formalin is added to a warm aqueous solution of gelatin. On stirring there results a combination in the form of a clear, transparent mass having a glassy lustre. This may be powdered, and is usually presented in this form. The advantage claimed is that in contact with animal tissues the compound is decomposed, setting free the formalin, which acts as a continuous antiseptic. The many uses to which such a compound might be put will be readily seen.

Grindelia Robusta.—The following is an abstract[1] representing the result of laboratory investigation which Dott. Luigi d'Amore has conducted with this drug: " He finds that in frogs it produces first a paralysis of the higher nerve-centers, then of the lower. The nerves and muscles preserve their excitability only through direct action upon them, so they at last lose their irritability. With dogs it is found that large doses depress and weaken the nerve-centers after having markedly excited them. With frogs, when the drug is applied to the heart, there is a slow and progressive diminution of the beat and a lengthening of the systole; sometimes the action is so energetic that there is a rapid diminution of the number of beats and arrest of the heart in systole and with an inexcitable myocardium. With warm-blooded animals the phenomena which it produces may be ascribed to an exciting action upon the bulbar center of the pneumogastric, which, when a large dose is introduced at one time into the circulation, appears to be paralyzant. The effects upon blood-pressure are that with small doses there is a slight raising, which is more evident with medium doses; but as the amount is increased the pressure gradually and continually falls during the same time that the oscillations are shorter. In its action upon the respiratory system we have the most interest, for here we find the most extensive use of the drug. Experiments show that when its effects on the pneumogastric are considered, and also its power of contracting bronchial muscles and its action on the heart, that it is likely, in proper doses, to be of value as a remedy for the symptoms of asthma. When in addition we bear in mind that the drug contains an active principle, likely a terpene, which benefits the associated catarrh, the clinical use of the drug has a scientific foundation. So far as its effect on bodily temperature exists, it apparently possesses a paralyzing action on the thermogenic center. The secretions are changed as follows: the urine is increased by small, and diminished by large doses, partly from changes in blood-pressure and partly from direct action on the renal epithelium. The saliva and bile are increased. Both urine and saliva are of greenish tinge."

Hemol.—From the application of this remedy in 30 instances J. Bartelt[2] has reached the following conclusions: " 1. There is no doubt that this remedy is capable of absorption, and in very debilitated individuals is useful for the building up anew of the red blood-corpuscles. 2. The relatively small content of iron frequently, even after three weeks' use, does not present any clinical results; therefore the favorable action of hemol must be due to the entire constitution of the remedy, which may be designated as a blood-corpuscle extract. 3. Its administration is very simple, for, with the exception of gastric ulcer, which it may irritate, there are no untoward symptoms arising from its use. It does not give rise to constipation, the appetite remains unchanged or improved, and the teeth do not become blackened nor carious. 4. There is especially to be commended for the use of neurologists and dermatologists a combination with as much arsenous acid as may be necessary, of a hundred times as much of the

[1] Am. Jour. Med. Sci., Apr., 1897, from Giornale della Associazone Napoletana di Medici e Naturalisti, Puntata 5a e 6a, p. 331, 1896.
[2] Am. Jour. Med. Sci , Jan., 1897, from Therap. Monatsh., H. 10, S. 533., 1896.

drug, which should then be given in pill-form. In this way the unpleasant gastric symptoms to which arsenic may give rise are obviated. Doubtless the arsenous acid combines with the drug, forming an arseno-hemol analogous to the copper-, zinc-, or mercury-hemol, and it is probable that there is a rapid absorption."

Holzinol.—Oppermann has used formaldehyd (see p. 936) in a 60% solution in methyl alcohol, which he called *holzin.* Rosenberg,[1] in order to do away with the irritating effects of this solution, combined it with a small quantity of menthol, giving to the combination the name of *holzinol.* He says that by allowing this fluid to evaporate slowly in a room, from a small apparatus, the room and its contents, even including food, may be rendered sterile without injury. He used it also in whooping-cough, and found its influence favorable in all stages. In solution of a strength of only 1 part in 100,000 he states that the development of bacteria is prevented, and 1 part in 75,000 is germicidal.

Improved Mercurial Ointment.—L. A. Harding[2] has devised a new method for making mercurial ointment, the advantages claimed for it being rapidity of making and a.product which keeps well. The ingredients and proportions are as follows: mercury, 12 oz.; expressed oil of almond, 1 oz.; ether, 2 dr.; gum benzoin, 2 dr.; lard and suet, mixed in the proportions of the U. S. P., $10\frac{1}{2}$ oz. The benzoin is powdered, placed in a bottle, and shaken with the ether. The mercury and the oil of almond are then added, and the mixture is shaken with a rotary motion until it gathers into a mass. This is placed in a mortar and rubbed up with a part of the mixed lard and suet; the remainder is finally added, and trituration is continued until the mercury disappears and a perfect mixture is obtained.

Intestinal Capsules and Pills.—The use of keratin and of shellac for coating pills designed for intestinal action only is well known. Several new methods of coating pills intended for this purpose have been devised, and Weyland[3] cites that of C. F. Hausmann among others. This process consists of placing gelatin capsules, which have been filled with the medicament, in an 0.8% solution of formaldehyd and allowing them to remain for 18 minutes. They are then removed, washed with water, and dried at 50° C. By this treatment the capsules are rendered insoluble in the stomach, but are dissolved with ease by the pancreatic juice. According to Weyland, the essentials in the process are the strength of the formaldehyd solution and the duration of maceration. Properly treated these capsules are insoluble in water at 38° C., though soluble if long exposed to the action of boiling water. If placed in artificial gastric juice, they are soluble, it is true, but only after an exposure of 10 or 12 hours, a duration of exposure which will seldom be encountered therapeutically. The action of artificial pancreatic juice is quite the opposite, for, whether the capsules have previously been exposed to the action of gastric juice or not, a solution is effected in one or two hours. [It is much to be hoped that this process may demonstrate its value clinically, for in many instances the keratin process has been a disappointment, apart from the very tedious and troublesome manipulations which it involves. We have had, however, no personal experience with the new coating.] (See Glutol, p. 939.)

Iodol continues to be extensively employed, though recent literature upon the subject is not rich. From its use in 558 cases, of which 187 were chancre

[1] Med. News, Feb. 27, 1897, from Deutsch. med. Woch., Nos. 39 and 40, 1896.
[2] Am. Medico-Surg. Bull., Aug. 15, 1896, from Am. Druggist, xxviii., p. 297, 1896.
[3] Am. Medico-Surg. Bull., Sept. 5, 1896, from Pharm. Rev., iv., p. 164, 1896.

or chancroid, Dominico Majacchi[1] finds reason to praise it most highly.   It is advantageous for several reasons : 1. Its freedom from odor renders it more acceptable to patients than iodoform ; 2. It is nontoxic even when used very freely ; 3. It hastens healing ; 4. The preparations employed are stable and nonirritant.   A number of formulæ for preparations of iodol have recently been published and are here presented :[2]

"*Iodol-ether*.—A 10-to-20% ethereal solution for injection into fistulous tracts and for sprays. By spraying it upon the gauze with which a wound has been bandaged an excellent iodol gauze is had.

"*Iodol-ether-collodion :* iodol, 1 part ; ether, 5 parts ; collodion, 10 parts. For applying to open or sewed wounds.

"*Iodol-alcohol-glycerin :* iodol, 1 part ; alcohol, 16 parts ; glycerin, 14 to 34 parts.

"*Iodol-lanolin*, containing 5% to 10%, for inunction in glandular tumors.

"*Iodol-vaselin :* iodol, 1 to 2 parts ; vaselin, 10 to 15 parts.   For internal as well as external abscesses.

"*Iodol Paste*.—Iodol triturated with a few drops of alcohol and sufficient glycerin to yield the desired consistency, for vaginal tampons.

"*Iodol gauze and cotton*.

"Iodol is also used in powder in ophthalmic practice, and as a substitute for potassium iodid internally (up to 1 gm. per day).   In the last case its action is said to be of greater persistence than that of potassium iodid, for its presence in the urine can be shown even after six days, whereas potassium iodid disappears in 1½ to 2 days."

Lactophenin.—Hermann Strauss, of Giessen, Germany, and F. Kolbl,[3] of Vienna, after using lactophenin for considerable periods of time in large doses in the treatment of neuralgia and muscular pains, have concluded that it is far from harmless. Strauss reports three cases in which jaundice and dyspeptic disturbances were produced, owing to retention of bile, as was shown by the colorless condition of the feces. Kolbl reports two cases of a similar character.

Loretin, though still in use, it would seem, has not been the subject of much report during the past year.   E. Wyllys Andrews,[4] however, has pursued its study, and speaks highly of it.   According to him, the substance is somewhat irritant to new wounds, and, therefore, is not desirable save in cases of sepsis.   The mixture of loretin in the proportion of about 1 to 10 of boric acid, magnesia, or starch, is also recommended as an application to ulcerated surfaces, and the effect produced upon sluggish and varicose ulcers is said to be stimulant and beneficial, while even phagedenic ulceration is favorably influenced.   To small chancroids it may be applied pure, with the result of stimulating their rapid cicatrization.   Andrews is emphatic in his preference for loretin over iodoform, so far as its freedom from toxic properties is concerned, for in several hundred cases of its employment he failed to discover any evidence of poisonous effect.   In the disinfection of old fistulæ this writer thinks that loretin is of unusual value, and was favorably impressed with its influence upon carbuncle.   To the report of Andrews is appended a bacteriologic report upon loretin by S. P. Black, which leads to the conclusion that the real antiseptic power of the drug is slight.

Herbert Snow,[5] surgeon to the Cancer Hospital, London, in the course of a

[1] Ephemeris, p. 1866, Jan., 1897.
[2] Am. Medico-Surg. Bull., Dec. 19, 1896, from Pharm. Centralbl., xxxvii., p. 475, 1896.
[3] Ephemeris, p. 1867, Jan., 1897.   [4] Chicago Med Rec., July, 1896.
[5] Ephemeris, Jan., 1897, from Brit. Med. Jour., vol. ii., pp. 1549 and 1637, 1895.

report upon loretin, says: "My own experience is confined to the powder, which I have never found occasion to mix with any other substance. Dashed on the skin, or over a granulated wound, this causes not the slightest irritation or unpleasant sensation. It immediately destroys the malodor of the most fetid cancerous sore, controlling this in a manner which no other agent I have yet tried will do. Copiously puffed with an insufflator into the deep cavity formed by evacuating the axilla of carcinomatous glands, it efficiently precludes suppuration, even when free hemorrhage has taken place after closing the wound, an occurrence almost inseparable from anesthetic vomiting when the patient has been removed from the operating-table. Not the slightest bad symptom from its employment in this way has so far been detected. When there is no deep cavity a wound dusted with loretin heals rapidly by first intention. I have had recourse to loretin in some 60 cases, mainly operations on the breast and axilla, notoriously a test-region for antiseptics. In my hands it has proved an ideal antiseptic and deodorant, with no single drawback ; and I am sure that no surgeon who has once tried it will ever again resort to the noisome and toxic iodoform, from the free use of which I have seen more than one death. Though whenever old-established agents answer sufficiently the purpose I have a strong prejudice against novelties, yet this substance—nonpoisonous, devoid of smell, and absolutely preventative of suppuration—seemed to me so marked an advance upon anything previously brought forward, that I felt constrained to direct thereto the notice of the section." Somewhat later Snow adds to the above : " by pointing out a peculiar quality which the 6 months' experience gained since the July meeting has shown me it possesses. While taking first rank as a nonpoisonous, nonirritating, odorless antiseptic and deodorant, I find that when dusted on a raw surface it relaxes the blood-vessels. Hence the wound is prone to become subsequently filled by a clot, which, however, does not suppurate, as would be the case under almost any other circumstance, but is eventually reabsorbed. The incident is not desirable, and I now apply loretin only to the skin-surface, never dusting it into a cavity unless there be special risk of suppuration, and then only very sparingly. I would take leave to add that long experience has shown me the ideal condition in which to leave any operation-wound to be the utmost attainable maximum of dryness, avoiding all swabbing with fluids, however antiseptic. It is probably that the efficacy of iodoform, loretin, and the like is very largely due to their capacity for absorbing microbe moisture, without which microbe proliferation does not occur." [The value of a report such as this is necessarily very great, but of all its wisdom the wisest is contained in the concluding sentences, a truth which too many are unaccountably apt to disregard.]

Magnesium Sulfate.—Few cases of poisoning by Epsom salts have been noted, but the importance of knowing that such symptoms may occur is evident. J. H. Neale,[1] of Leicester, England, observed such a case in a boy of 15. The day before he was seen by the physician he had taken an ounce of magnesium sulfate, proved by subsequent analysis to be pure, and which caused only three slight movements from the bowels. Soon after he began to feel sick, and continued growing worse until the following evening. When seen then he was conscious, but apathetic, markedly cyanosed, the trunk covered with a roseolous eruption, pulse too feeble to be counted, and temperature 105°. The stomach and bladder were dilated and there was an occasional tetanie spasm of the right side of the face and of the right arm. There was some vomiting of greenish fluid. The only treatment employed was directed to the relief of symptoms and stimulation. The patient made a good recovery. [Although of exceed-

---

[1] Lancet, Aug. 15, 1896.

ingly uncommon occurrence, poisoning by magnesium sulfate is not unknown. A case reported by Christison in some respects resembles that reported by Neale. In Christison's case a fatal result in a boy of 10 was attributed to 2 oz. of the salt, and that without purgation. Absorption sufficient to cause poisoning is, in truth, very rare, but the experiments of Recke, Hay, and Curci show that the injection of magnesium sulfate within the veins is productive of circulatory disturbance and death from respiratory or circulatory failure.[1]]

Malarin is the name given to a new patented compound said to be [2] " the citrate of a condensation-product of aceto-phenon and para-phenetidin " or [3] "acetophenonphenetidin." The name " malarin " is copyrighted. The preparation of the substance is by heating acetophenone and paraphenetidin in molecular proportions, alone or with dehydrating substances, in a vessel having a return-condenser. The drug occurs in needle-shaped crystals, which are lemon-yellow in color and of slightly acid taste. It is insoluble in water, but is readily soluble in hot alcohol and in ether. It is said that malarin is free from injurious properties to man, and that doses of 30 gm. for every 75 kilos of body-weight cause neither sugar nor acetone to appear in the urine. Furthermore, no injurious effect is noted upon the urinary apparatus. The application of the compound medicinally is as an antipyretic and antineuralgic, and thus employed in doses of 0.5 gm. is said to be prompt in action and harmless. Thus have been treated fevers, toothache, neuralgic headache, and nervous excitement. [Although the reports which have reached us of " malarin " are in its favor, it is far too early to express opinions as to its worth, for as yet it has had little employment other than in Germany, and, so far as we are aware, no observations have been made upon it in this country. It is possible that we shall find it a preparation of value, but it is difficult to see how it can be superior to others of its class which are now in general use, apart from the very decided prejudice which prevails in this country against drugs of the patented order.]

Mercuro-iodo-hemol (see *Year-Book* for 1897, p. 1127), according to Kobert,[4] contains mercury, 13 % ; iodin, 28 % ; and hemoglobin. It has received commendation from a number of sources, and is held advantageous not only for its antisyphilitic powers, but because of its freedom from irritant properties and its action as a bloodmaker. It is especially of value, therefore, in the presence of debility and anemia, and may be administered for a long period without ill result. The preparation is ordinarily given in pills, for whose preparation the following formula is employed : mercuro-iodo-hemol, 10.0 gm. ; opium, 1.0 gm.; glycerin ointment, enough to make 100 pills. To be given three times a day ; at first one, then two, three, and later four pills.

Metallic Mercury for Hypodermic Injection.—The following formulæ are given in a recent publication [5] as the most important ones in which mercury and fatty substances are combined, constituting the so-called gray oil (huile grise), for the purpose of subcutaneous introduction. The dose is not more than $\frac{3}{4}$ gr., and should be given not oftener than once a week.

1. (Lang.) ℞ : mercury, lanolin, each 3 parts ; olive oil, 4 parts.—M.
2. (Gay.) ℞ : mercury, 20 parts ; lanolin, 5 parts ; liquid vaselin, 35 parts. —M.

[1] U. S. Dispensatory, p. 846, 1894.   [2] Ephemeris, p. 1872, Jan., 1897.
[3] Am. Medico-Surg. Bull., Dec. 19, 1896.
[4] Am. Medico-Surg. Bull., Aug. 15, 1896, from Centralbl. f. Nervenh. u. Psychiat., xix, p. 233, 1896.
[5] N. Y. Med. Jour , June 19, 1897, from Gaz. hebdom. de Méd, et de Chir., May 16, 1897.

3. (P. Vigier.) ℞ : purified mercury, 3 parts; mercurial ointment, 2 parts; soft white vaselin, 19 parts; liquid vaselin, 40 parts.—M.

4. (P. Vigier.) ℞ : solid white vaselin, 5 parts; mercurial ointment, 2 parts; mercury, 39 parts. Triturate, and add : solid white vaselin, 14 parts; liquid vaselin, 40 parts.

5. (Neisser, Balzer.) ℞ : metallic mercury, 20 parts; tincture of benzoin, 5 parts; vaselin oil, 40 parts.—M.

6. (Thibierge, Balzer.) ℞ : purified mercury, 20 parts; ethereal tincture of benzoin, 5 parts; liquid vaselin, 30 parts; solid vaselin, 10 parts.—M.

Nitroglycerin.—It has been the experience of all observers that the dose of nitroglycerin is a very variable matter, and latterly there has been a growing tendency to disregard all arbitrary measurements in its continued use, and to grade the doses employed solely with regard to the physiologic effects produced. Acting under this plan many have succeeded in giving doses of nitroglycerin far in excess of the text-books—$\frac{1}{100}$ or $\frac{1}{50}$ gr.—and with most beneficial results. W. L. Armstrong,[1] writing upon this subject, speaks of the variability in response to nitroglycerin, and quotes the cases reported by H. C. Wood, in one of which one drop of a 1 % alcoholic solution caused insensibility, and in two of which two drops caused abolition of consciousness and the radial pulse ; these as examples of smallness of active dose. As showing the other extreme of therapeutic doses there is cited the case of Whittaker, in which $1\frac{1}{10}$ gr. was given every 3 hours, a matter of $8\frac{4}{5}$ gr. in 24 hours. The writer goes on to say that he is unable to find in literature a suggestion that arterial contraction affords a toleration of the drug, as compared with arteries in their normal condition, and argues that toxic symptoms from nitroglycerin are present only after "the drug has relaxed the arterial walls beyond their normal tonicity."

The experiments reported by Armstrong, as tending to prove his belief, are full of interest. In six cases with normal circulation nitroglycerin was given in doses of $\frac{1}{100}$ gr. every hour. In all of these headache was the result observed within 24 hours—*i. e.*, a dose of $\frac{1}{5}$ gr. in 24 hours caused poisoning. In the next instance it was observed that a patient with atheromatous arteries, but no increase of tension, and who previously had taken none of the drug, upon taking $2\frac{1}{2}$ gr. of nitroglycerin at a single dose, suffered no inconvenience whatever. From this it is argued that the atheroma prevented the relaxation of the arteries supposedly necessary for toxic manifestations. In the third set of cases patients were employed whose arterial tensions were high, but whose arterial walls were free from atheroma. Of these cases there were two. The first patient received gradually increasing doses of nitroglycerin during a period of 25 days, at the end of which time the daily amount taken was 76 gr. The clinical result of this was the loss of arterial tension and the disappearance of the symptoms previously experienced, but at no time was headache complained of or other manifestation of toxicity. The abrupt cessation of the remedy then resulted in a rapid return of the arterial tension as well as of the subjective symptoms. In the second case the nitroglycerin was given in increasing amounts during a period of four weeks, at the end of which time the dose amounted to 125 gr. in 24 hours, the only result of this enormous dose being beneficial, the arterial tension having disappeared.. The dose of 8 gr. every hour while awake was finally increased to 9 gr., when slight headache resulted and no further increase was made. In both these cases it is emphasized that the relaxation of the radial arteries was observed some time before the largest doses were reached, and increase was practised farther simply that the limit

[1] Med. News, Oct. 31, 1896.

of toleration might be observed. The author's conclusions seem well warranted, and indeed the study which he reports is one of much interest and importance. He sums up as follows: " 1. It is only when dealing with arteries in which there is no more than the normal tonicity of the walls that the drug is liable to produce disagreeable effects. Under this condition it should be administered with caution and in small doses. 2. In cases of arterial tension the drug can be used more freely than has been customary among practitioners, the dose being proportioned to the 'degree of tension. 3. In cases of arterial tension tolerance of the drug is rapidly acquired, and by a slight increase day by day very large doses can soon be taken with safety, the constant guide being the degree of tension in the arterial wall."

Orphol is the name employed to designate betanaphtol-bismuth, a substance partaking of the actions of betanaphtol and bismuth, and therefore employed as an intestinal antiseptic and astringent. It is said to contain about 20 % of betanaphtol and about 80 % of bismuth oxide chemically combined. The doses recommended are from 2 to 5 gm. for children and from 5 to 10 gm. for adults.[1] Orphol occurs as a powder light brown in color, of agreeable odor and aromatic taste. Golnier,[2] of Erfurt, speaks highly of this remedy in diarrhea due to tuberculous inflammation of the intestinal canal. This observer calls attention to what is already well known, namely, the disadvantages which tannin and opium have in such cases, and declares that the remedy needed in these diarrheas is a reliable intestinal antiseptic which at the same time is astringent. This combination he finds ably represented in orphol. Among the cases which Golnier reports there is one whose record is most interesting and instructive. The patient was 52 years of age and phthisical, suffering much from thin, watery movements, flatus, and abdominal pain. He received opium with no benefit, and then orphol was given in doses of 15 gr. every two hours and continued for several days. As a result of this, diarrhea ceased and the movements lost their previously foul odor. The appetite at the same time improved, together with the general appearance. The remedy was continued in the same doses and with the same frequency, with the result, however, of producing constipation. Upon lessening the amount given, however, and increasing the length of the intervals this over-astringent effect disappeared, the bowels moving daily and the feces being of a gruel-like consistency. Golnier believes that the action of orphol depends upon its being decomposed in the intestines into its components the naphtol manifesting antiseptic effect and the bismuth astringency. It is said that a little naphtol may be found in the urine. (See *Year-Book* for 1896, p. 1027.)

Parthenium Hysterophorus is a plant growing in some of the Southern States, as well as in Cuba and Jamaica. Its medical introduction is due to José R. Tovar, who in 1885 proclaimed its advantages in neuralgia and in certain fevers. H. V. Arny,[3] writing upon this subject, calls attention to the confusion which has surrounded the discussion of its active principles, some speaking of an alkaloid called partheninin and others of a parthenicin. From a thorough and prolonged study of the subject Arny has isolated, besides the usual plant-constituents, a volatile oil which has the heavy odor of the plant, and yields a stearopten of camphoraceous taste; as well as a principle to whose presence is due the intense bitterness of the plant. This principle appears to be neither an alkaloid nor a glucoside, and the author places it as a proximate principle similar to santonin. The name given to this sub-

---

[1] Ephemeris, p. 882, Jan., 1897.
[2] Am. Medico-Surg. Bull., Feb. 25, 1897, from Allg. Med. Central-zeit., No. 96, 1896.
[3] New Orl. M. and S. Jour., May, 1897.

stance is parthenin, and since Arny obtained no other principles from the plant he is disposed to regard the so-called partheninin and parthenicin as impure forms of parthenin.

As to the therapeutics of parthenin there has been some discussion, and Arny reports that in Jamaica the drug is thought remedial in certain skin-diseases, especially those which are herpetic and pustular, as well as in ulcers. Tovar speaks of his parthenin as beneficial in facial neuralgia, as well as in a case of fever and anorexia in which quinin had failed. Its antineuralgic character was confirmed by Guyet, though he failed to obtain antipyretic action from it. The dose of either partheninin or parthenicin is placed at 0.05 gm. every hour in neuralgia and at 1 gm. in intermittent fever, and parthenin can, therefore, be given on this basis, according to Arny. This investigator proposes to prepare a sufficient amount of parthenin to enable thorough clinical trial to be made, and we may therefore expect further reports upon this subject, which at present has reached no very practical status.

Pellotin, a hypnotic of recent introduction, is a crystalline substance of bitter taste. Its solubility in water is slight, but alcohol, ether, and chloroform readily dissolve it. Crystalline salts are produced by the combination of pellotin with acids, and of these the hydrochlorid has had some therapeutic employment, being exceedingly soluble in water. The medical introduction of pellotin is due to F. Jolly, of Berlin. The chemical formula of the substance is said to be $C_{13}H_{19}NO_3$.

From experiments which A. Heftner[1] has conducted with pellotin we gather the following information : injected into frogs it produces slight narcosis in 10 or 15 minutes, the reflexes being diminished and responsive only to strong irritation. Later, however (after 20 or 30 minutes), reflex irritability becomes much accentuated, even to the production of tetanic movements. It is noted, too, that the condition of great nerve irritability may remain pronounced for a considerable time, even for several days. Finally, however, and after prolonged tetanus, the motor irritability is lost. The channel by which pellotin is eliminated is renal, at least in part, the drug having been recovered in the urine. The action of the drug upon man in many respects resembles that of morphin, for following its administration by mouth there occur drowsiness and lassitude, followed presumably by sleep. It is noticeable that during the sleep so caused the pulse-rate may be lowered. Headache and nausea have been attributed to the use of pellotin. [Pellotin is as yet little known in this country, and our information upon the subject is therefore obtained chiefly from European sources. The following, though doubly a quotation, has appeared to us the best brief which we have encountered in our search of the literature of the subject and worthy of verbatim repetition.]

From this source[2] we learn that pellotin "is an alkaloid discovered in a species of Mexican cactus called anhalonium." (See Anhalonium Lewinii, p. 924. See also *Year-Book* for 1897, p. 1103.) "The natives of Mexico are reported to swallow slices of this plant, to which they give the name of 'pellote,' and Heftner, of Leipsig, has now succeeded in isolating its soporific alkaloid. Pellotin itself is not soluble in water, but its hydrochlorate is extremely soluble. Its physiologic action was first tried on frogs, and then on mammals, which very soon became unable to stand or perform spontaneous movements, and shortly afterward an increase of the reflexes was observed, followed by tetanic convulsions. This action of the drug on animals was not identical with that which Heftner observed in himself, for after taking 5 cgm.

[1] Am. Jour. Med. Sci., Nov., 1896, from Therap. Monatsh., H. 6, S. 327, 1896.
[2] Ephemeris, Jan., 1897, from Lancet, vol. i., p. 1760, 1896.

($\frac{3}{4}$ gr.) he became very drowsy and ultimately fell asleep. The drug was then given by Jolly to a number of patients in the neurologic wards of the Charité Hospital in Berlin. The first case was that of a man suffering from alcoholic neuritis who, after an injection of 4 cgm. became very drowsy, and one hour afterward he fell into a sleep which lasted for four hours. Heftner had observed in himself a diminished pulse-rate, and the same symptom was perceptible in this patient, during the first hour of whose sleep the pulse fell to 56 per minute, rising again to 76 before the man awoke. Another patient with multiple sclerosis took 5 cgm. during the afternoon, and after half an hour he also slept soundly for several hours. Similar results were obtained in a series of other cases. In patients suffering from tabes the soporific action was equally satisfactory, but the pains returned after they woke. In delirium tremens the effect was less prompt; in one instance 12 cgm. (equal to 1$\frac{3}{4}$ gr.) were needed only to tranquillize an excited patient, and no sleep ensued. In 20 cases of different kinds the remedy was given as a hypnotic in the evening; 2 cgm. had no effect, but from 4 to 6 cgm. were efficacious in producing sleep, and no injurious consequences of any kind were observed. Some patients complained of giddiness, and declined to take the medicine, but the greater number did not suffer in this way. Jolly says that 6 cgm. (equal to about 1 gr.) of pellotin are equal to 1 gm. (equal to 15$\frac{1}{2}$ gr.) of trional, or 2 gm. (equal to 31 gr.) of hydrate of chloral. The number of cases is yet too small to justify the formation of a definite opinion as to the new remedy, but it undoubtedly deserves further trial."

Although it is true that 58 cases are too few to afford the drawing of conclusive deductions as to the value of a remedy, yet in reporting his experience with pellotin in the treatment of insomnia Pilcz[1] has given us much valuable information. His patients were inmates of insane asylums in Vienna. Of the entire number (58) treated with pellotin there was produced a most excellent result in 29 cases, sleep appearing within an hour and a half and continuing through the night. In 17 cases the result was less pronounced, but still beneficial, while absolute failure of hypnotic effect was experienced in but 12 cases, and of these Pilez regards 4 as inappropriate subjects for the test. The smallest dose which Pilcz employed was $\frac{1}{3}$ gr., given subcutaneously, and 19 of the cases treated responded to this amount. In no case was more than 1 gr. administered, and though Jolly has taught that 2 gr. of pellotin hydrochlorid may be given hypodermically without ill-effect, Pilcz places the range of dose between $\frac{1}{3}$ and $\frac{2}{3}$ gr., repeated 3 times if required. In one of the cases reported by this writer $\frac{1}{3}$ gr. of pellotin was productive of sleep in a patient in whom 60 gr. of paraldehyd had failed to affect, and in another to whom 75 gr. of the same drug had been given without success. In none of his cases did Pilcz observed the slowing of the pulse already mentioned, but in 2 cases there occurred coma and dizziness, although one of these patients was suffering from paronoia with sensory hallucinations. The author thinks highly of pellotin, and rates it as often successful where other drugs have failed.

Picrocarmine solution, of a stability sufficient to remain good for 5 years, is said to be prepared as follows:[2] a solution is made of pure carmine in a mixture of 1 part (by volume) of ammonia-water and 4 of water, the carmine being in slight excess. The solution is allowed to stand for 2 days, and is then filtered. Following this it is exposed (though protected from dust) until a precipitate commences to form, when it is filtered again, and to it is added a concentrated solution of picric acid. The mixture is then stirred

---

[1] Brit. Med. Jour., June 5, 1897, from Wien. klin. Woch., No. 48, 1896.
[2] Am. Medico-Surg. Bull., Sept. 12, 1896, from Pharm. Jour., No. 1357, p. 505, 1896.

and allowed to stand for a day, when it is filtered, and to it is added 1 part of chloral hydrate for each 1000 parts. After standing for one week a final filtration is done and the product is bottled in small glass-stoppered vials.

The pituitary gland remains an enigma in spite of attempts to solve its function. The recent investigation of the subject by Mairet[1] and Bosc[2] is interesting, although the result of their experimentation is negative. As subjects of experimentation they have employed rabbits, dogs, healthy men, and epileptics. The pituitary gland of the ox repeatedly fed to dogs apparently produced no effect whatever. A solution of the gland made by pounding it up in water was administered to dogs hypodermically, but no sequelæ were observed, save for the slight and temporary elevation of temperature and slight wasting. The intravenous introduction of this solution caused death from thrombosis, a result not unnatural, and certainly not peculiar to the substance employed.

The internal administration of the gland to man in health was productive of no result whatever, and its subcutaneous introduction caused slight fever with malaise, which continued for about one day. The administration of the gland, both by mouth and by hypodermic injection, was practised upon 21 patients the subjects of epilepsy. So far as the convulsive attacks are concerned, their number was certainly not diminished by the treatment, but rather they seemed to be made more frequent. In many of these cases the ingestion of the gland seemed to be the cause of mental exaltation or delirium, which appeared 3 or 4 days after the administration of the gland. These delirious attacks in some cases resembled those sometimes seen in epileptics, and, therefore, the element of coincidence must be entertained. In other cases, however, the attacks were of an aberration different from that which had previously been observed in these cases.

Poisonous Honey.—Lyman F. Kebler[3] has made an exhaustive study of this subject from a historic standpoint in connection with a case which came under his observation. He is of the opinion that the toxic properties of the honey are determined by the character of the flowers on which the bees feed. At times examination reveals poisonous alkaloids, but this is by no means always the case. At times also the poisonous character can be detected by the color and taste of the honey.

Purity of Drugs.—Several articles bearing on this question have appeared during the past year, and all show a desire on the part of both physicians and pharmacists for some means by which drugs and galenical preparations of a definite and uniform strength may be obtained.

G. F. Hanson,[4] of San Francisco, gives many examples of the adulteration of drugs. Among the gums, gum arabic and gum tragacanth have long been subject to substitution by cheaper gums. In America apple and mesquite gums are used. The gummy exudate of the almond and palm is added to the inferior grades of tragacanth, and even the dark caramania or mosul gum is said to be similarly used after being brought to the proper color with white lead, while the untaught native of Nubia or Abyssinia, scorning such scientific mendacity, simply adds anything he can get in the way of sticks, dirt, pebbles, and bark, and thus makes up the additional weight.

An investigation of some specimens of powdered licorice of late has shown that the drug had been exhausted for the preparation of the solid extract and

[1] Brit. Med. Jour., Oct. 3, 1896, from Arch. de Physiol., No. 3, p. 600, 1896.
[2] Am. Jour. Med. Sci., Nov., 1896, from Arch. de Physiol., No. 3, p. 600, 1896.
[3] Medicine, Jan., 1897, from Med. and Surg. Reporter, Sept. 12, 1896.
[4] Pacific Med. Journ., Sept., 1896.

ammoniated glycyrrhizin, the residue being the "powder." Digitalis-leaf is said to be often adulterated by the addition of the leaves of mullein and elecampane. Ergot also often contains substitutes, such as the fungus of wheat. These, however, as a rule do no harm, and some are said to be even more active than the pharmacopeial preparation. At the worst, we shall get only a less active drug.

A mixture of resin with oil of turpentine is very frequently substituted for Venice turpentine; and one of resin and fat, with a little water to make it turbid, often takes the place of Burgundy pitch.

It is an interesting fact that the consumption of copaiba balsam yearly exceeds the importation by something like 40,000 pounds, if the figures for 1893 and 1894 can be taken as a criterion. The most frequent addition is of Gurgin balsam, or East India wood-oil. It may be easily recognized by the greenish-violet tinge that it gives when examined in strong sunlight to a specimen of copaiba to which it has been added. Paraffin or vaselin oil is also used. Once in a while some Para copaiba is said to be found on the market from which the oil has been distilled.

The fact that aconite root often lacks proper alkaloidal strength is rather due to ignorance on the part of those who gather it regarding its condition, the season in which it should be taken, and the proper method of preservation. Gamboge is sometimes found in the market filled with sand, powdered bark, and rice-flour.

Flaxseed-meal is an article that suffers frequently from adulteration. It contains at times traces of rape or mustard seed; but as these have a higher commercial value than the flaxseed itself, it is only fair to suppose that the addition is accidental. For intentional adulteration the simplest material is ground "oil-cake," the residue left after the linseed oil has been pressed out from the seeds. But crushed wheat, bran, cornmeal, middling, etc., are also often used for this purpose.

Of the various wood-chips imported for use both as drugs and as dyes, there is often an adulteration by mixing in the chips of inert woods. Thus to the resinous heartwood of guaiacum is added not infrequently the useless sap-wood; quassia-chips are adulterated with other bitter woods or simply with oak; and logwood with Brazil-wood chips.

The leaves of buchu are occasionally mixed with those of an inferior species of Barosma or with the leaves of altogether different plants. Senna often contains a large amount of argel leaves, which considerably increase the griping without adding at all to the purgative power of the drug. Hyoscyamus alba, which grows along the northern coast of the Mediterranean Sea, is sometimes sold for hyoscyamus niger. The leaves of the bearberry are sometimes mixed with those of the red whortleberry, probably through ignorance on the part of those by whom they are gathered.

The oils, especially the more expensive of the essential oils, are largely adulterated, for the temptation is great. For instance, in the oil of rose there is often a goodly quantity of Indian grass or of geranium oil. Attar of rose crystallizes at 12.5° C., and to the resulting stearopten spermaceti or some form of paraffin is added to increase the bulk. The ingenuity displayed in the adulteration of the oils of peppermint, spearmint, cajuput, lemon, etc., is almost beyond belief. Olive and cod-liver oils bear the greatest part of the attacks upon the fixed oils, both because the price is high and because the consumption is large. To olive oil are added generally the cheaper nut- and seed-oils, such as cottonseed, walnut, peanut, poppy, rape, and benne oils. Cod-liver oil often contains a large proportion of porpoise and other fish-oils, the favorite being that obtained from shark liver, as this gives the tests for cod-liver oil. It is, however, of less specific gravity.

As a rule, the adulterants used, as may be seen from the foregoing examples, are not actively harmful. They are used rather to increase the bulk with a cheaper article and thereby to add to the profits.

Pyramidon, a drug proposed as a substitute for antipyrin, is of an introduction so recent that little is known either of its properties or of its usefulness. Huchard[1] has prescribed it in maximum daily doses of 15 gr., and has never observed from it any influence upon arterial tension, though the opposite has been asserted by German observers. He reports that Deguy, as a result of his experimentation with it, rates it as exceedingly poisonous, and warns that its use must be attended with much care. [We are not aware of any other than meager reports upon pyramidon, and, in fact, the statements of Huchard were made verbally at a meeting of the Société de Thérapeutique.]

Pyrantin, or para-eth-oxyl-phenyl-succinamic acid, the recently introduced antipyretic, is derived from the reaction taking place between succinic acid (obtained by the distillation of amber) and phenacetin. These are melted together and boiled with alcohol, when pyrantin will crystallize out in prismatic, colorless needles. These crystals are but slightly soluble in cold water (1 in 1317), though more soluble in boiling water (1 in 86.6).[2] The action of pyrantin is said to resemble that of phenacetin, but A. Piretti, its introducer, claims that it is devoid of the objectionable features of phenacetin's action as well as superior to other similar antipyretics. It is said that the drug is without injurious effect upon the digestion, circulation, and respiration, and Renzi and Di Giovanni have reported it as a remedy of value in acute rheumatism, having administered it in doses of 1 to 3 gm. per diem.[3] Caution should be observed that pyrantin is not confused with the antipyretic and analgesic mixture known as "pyretine." [It is too early as yet to assign to pyrantin its proper pharmacologic place, for reports as to its clinical employment are scanty.] (See *Year-Book* for 1897, p. 1135.)

Quinin sulphovinate has been highly recommended by Alex. K. Finlay[4] as suitable for hypodermic administration, since it possesses marked solubility in water (1 in 3) and freedom from irritant after-effects. Its quinin-value is about equal to that of quinin sulfate. The use of the remedy in the form of tablets for the preparation of solutions is objectionable, it is said, because in tablet-form it is but slowly dissolved. The preparation of a solution from the crystals, however, is easily accomplished, and is rendered possible within a few seconds if gentle heat be employed. The solution of quinin sulphovinate is said to keep for a long time, and especially is preservation secured by the addition of a little alcohol. [It is much to be hoped that further use will establish the value of this salt for subcutaneous administration, for though the need for thus giving quinin is often urgent, it cannot be said that the salts previously used thus are always free from objection.]

Salacetol is a compound of salicylic acid and acetol. In some respects it resembles salol in action, though far more rapid in effect. Unlike salol, however, its separation into its component parts is not productive of poisonous substances. According to Ricchetti, salacetol is superior to other salicylates as an intestinal antiseptic, and is non-poisonous even in large doses. It is said to be inactive against the soluble ferments, and to antagonize the bacillus coli

---

[1] N. Y. Med. Jour., June 5, 1897, from Indépendance méd., May 12, 1897.
[2] Med. Bull., Dec., 1896.   [3] Ephemeris, Jan., 1897.
[4] Am. Medico-Surg. Bull., June 10, 1897, from Med. and Surg. Jour., xlix., p. 200, 1896.

communis and the organisms of cholera and typhoid fever. Mosso[1] reports his results from its external application in powder or salve and with glycerin. He says that in external use the body-heat and the presence of a liquid somewhat alkaline promote its decomposition, and its antiseptic action follows without irritation. (See *Year-Book* for 1896, p. 1067.)

Sanoform is still another substitute for iodoform, though as yet we know it only by report from abroad, and we cannot arouse ourselves to great enthusiasm over a remedy thus described when we remember the many drugs which have claimed the same substitution, and recall the fact that iodoform survives and thrives, while the larger number of its substitutes are forgotten. Perhaps we have at last found the ideal substitute for iodoform; certainly the reports upon sanoform thus far received are in its favor. The name sanoform has been applied to what is, chemically speaking, di-iodo-methyl salicylate, a substance brought forward by A. Arnheim, of Berlin. It is prepared by the action of iodin upon oil of gaultheria (methyl salicylate). It appears as a colorless, crystalline powder which has neither odor nor taste. It is unaffected by light and air, and may be heated to 200° C. without undergoing decomposition. It is insoluble in water and in glycerin, but is readily soluble in ether, chloroform, and benzol, and soluble in 200 parts of cold alcohol and in 10 parts of hot alcohol. It contains 62.7 % of iodin.

As to the clinical value of sanoform, Schlesinger[2] is convinced of its superiority over iodoform, quoting Arnheim's report. According to these observers, healing would appear more rapid and certain from the application of sanoform than from iodoform; irritation, too, was unnoticed, and not the least of its valuable qualities are nontoxicity and freedom from odor. Of the cases which Arnheim reported, 22 were chancroid, 20 chanere, 6 bubo, 16 phimosis, and 3 surgical wounds. From his experience with these he concludes that the application of sanoform in powder produces dryness in a secreting ulcer practically within two days, the powder and the secretion uniting to form a protective beneath which suppuration soon stops. The iodin of sanoform seems in strong combination, and not to be released by cell-action, for after the hypodermic injection of a fine emulsion of sanoform potassium iodid was not discoverable in the urine, and iodin only by careful search. It would seem, too, that absorption of sanoform is exceedingly slow, and after injection it is discoverable in the urine only after 24 hours, and being eliminated with much slowness may be found in the urine for about two weeks. As to the method of applying the drug, Schlesinger commends a 10 % gauze, and it is certainly advantageous that this can be sterilized without the decomposition of the sanoform. In addition to this gauze a 10 % ointment of sanoform may be employed, a 1 % collodion solution, or the substance may be applied in powder. It is to be noted as an additional advantage of sanoform that it is free from staining-properties (see *Year-Book* for 1897, p. 1137).

Sodium Chlorid as an Iodin Solvent.—As regards the employment of sodium chlorid to effect the solution of iodin in water, Müller[3] thinks it more desirable when the solution is intended for internal employment. For example, to produce a local effect on the pharynx he adds to the water used ½ % to 1 % of sodium chlorid. The following is suggested as a suitable prescription : tincture of iodin, 1 to 2 gm.; sodium chlorid, 2 gm.; distilled water, 200 gm. The tincture of iodin is that of the " Codex Medicamentarius," and is made by dissolving 10 gm. of iodin in 120 gm. of alcohol.

[1] N. Y. Polyclinic, Aug. 15, 1896, from Gazetta degli Ospedali e delle Clin., Apr. 14, 1896.　　　[2] Univ. Med. Mag., Jan., 1897, from Therap. Monatsh., Sept., 1896.
[3] Am. Medico-Surg. Bull., Aug. 29, 1896, from Pharm. Jour., No. 1357, p. 505, 1896.

Soluble bismuth phosphate is said to be prepared by the fusion of bismuthic oxid, soda, and phosphoric acid. Of the first-named ingredient it contains about 20 %. The chief value of the salt lies in its ready solubility in water, a solubility so great that a 33 % solution may be prepared. To solutions so strong, however, there is the objection that they soon become clouded ; a 5 % solution will, on the other hand, remain unaffected for a day or more. If bases or acids be added to a solution of this salt, it rapidly becomes cloudy, and boiling is said to produce a similar result. The reaction of these solutions is almost neutral and their taste saline and bitter. Dörffler[1] has employed the preparation with success in the acute intestinal catarrhs of early years. Gastric sedation is said to be a prompt result of this treatment, and so soon as the presence of bismuth in the stools is indicated by their black color their disagreeable character also disappears and the movements become fewer in number. A persistence in the treatment is usually productive of recovery within a few days, and it is recommended that the remedy be not discontinued until the diarrhea has been absent for some days. The dose of the remedy employed is, unfortunately, not stated.

Sphygmogenin is the name given to the substance which Fränkel[2] has obtained from the suprarenal body (see p. 954). The substance has not as yet been isolated in a pure state, though sufficiently for obtaining characteristic reactions. Among the various substances which have been found in the adrenals sphygmogenin is thought to be the one which increases arterial tension.

Strophanthus was first brought to the notice of the French Academy of Medicine in 1865, but the practical demonstration of its use as a valuable remedy in cardiac disease did not occur until 20 years later, when the result of the careful and patient researches of Frazer was reported. Of late, there has been an endeavor on the part of clinicians and therapeutists to discover the exact therapeutic value of this remedy, and to obtain reliable and uniform preparations of it. With this end in view H. C. Wood and W. S. Carter[3] have directed their studies to the effects of strophanthin, in order to determine whether the action of this active principle represents that of the crude drug. A series of experiments on mammals was made, and seemed to show that the strophanthin put upon the market by first-class manufacturers is exceedingly active. The arterial pressure was found to be somewhat increased, but rather by an action on the heart and vessel-walls than by any effect upon the vasomotor centres. Experiments were also made with an extract of strophanthus, from which it would appear that this preparation is also active. Its effect upon the blood-pressure is, however, less marked than that of strophanthin.

A series of clinical experiments is also being conducted by Reynold W. Wilcox with preparations of strophanthus from various sources, by which he hopes to establish a practical working-basis for the tincture from a particular drug-source. The first report on these researches, giving the results of the use of strophanthus in 12 cases, has already appeared.[4] The preparation employed was a tincture made especially for the purpose from the *strophanthus hispidus* (variety *Kombé*) of the U. S. Pharmacopeia. It was, therefore, a uniform preparation from a reliable source. Its use led Wilcox to the conclusion that this so-called variety (*Kombé*) of strophanthus was rather one of several absolutely distinct species of strophanthus. Should this opinion prove to be correct, it will doubtless have an important bearing on the therapeutic

[1] Am. Medico-Surg. Bull., Aug. 29, 1896, from Wien. med. Presse, xxxvii., p. 712, 1896.
[2] Am. Medico-Surg. Bull., June 6, 1896, from Pharm. Ztg., xli., p. 195, 1896.
[3] Therap. Gaz., Oct. 15, 1896, from Am. Jour. Pharm., July, 1896.
[4] Am. Jour. Med. Sci., May, 1897.

value of preparations of the drug. To record the effect of the remedy upon the circulatory system Dudgeon's sphygmograph was used. The object of the study was to ascertain the dose more exactly, to find out the real effects of the administration of the remedy, and what, if any, were its advantages over other drugs when properly employed. The 12 patients who were the subject of this report all showed marked cardiac symptoms. In some there were evidences of a valvular lesion; in some there was dilatation of one of the chambers of the heart, and in some the heart-action was enfeebled by a weak heart-muscle. In most, two or more of these conditions were combined. In all, the blood-pressure was low, as shown by the tracings of the sphygmograph. In all there is said to have been. an improvement both in symptoms and physical signs. The author concludes that the proper dose of the preparation used is about 5 drops in water, three or four times a day. He considers that the advantages that have heretofore been claimed for strophanthus over digitalis are borne out by this series of experiments. These advantages he sums up as follows: 1. Greater rapidity of action; 2. Absence of vasoconstrictor effects; 3. Greater diuretic power; 4. The absence of digestive disturbance following its use; 5. No cumulative action; 6. Its greater value in childhood and safety in old age. The contraindications to the use of strophanthus are also summar-ized, namely: when compensating hypertrophy is sufficient or excessive, and when the heart presents an advanced state of muscular degeneration or a high degree of mechanical defect. With these limitations, and provided a reliable preparation is used in doses not too large nor too frequently repeated, Wilcox prefers strophanthus in: 1. All cases in which we wish to establish compensa-tion; 2. All cases of arterial degeneration in which a remedy that causes more energetic cardiac contractions is required; 3. All cases of cardiac disease in which diuresis is necessary; 4. All cases of weak or irritable heart; 5. All cases of cardiac disease in childhood or old age.

The observations of Balfour[1] have led him to a rather different conclusion, for he decidedly prefers digitalis to strophanthus. He believes that the unfor-tunate symptoms which at times follow the administration of digitalis are due to a misconception of the true action of the remedy, and a consequent abuse of it. Digitalis acts, he says, by improving the general nutrition of the organism and by improving the metabolism of all the tissues, this action being particu-larly marked in the case of the cardiac muscular fiber. Thus the cardiac muscle is strengthened and its elasticity increased, the irritability of the heart being thereby relieved. The good results obtained are, therefore, permanent. Strophanthus, on the other hand, has proved in his hands an uncertain and dangerous drug. It acts as a heart-poison rather than as a heart-tonic. It stimulates the heart to increased action, it is true, but in so doing it calls upon the reserve of cardiac energy without improving the metabolism. Thus the more feeble the heart, the greater is the danger attending the use of this rem-edy. It acts only by helping the patient through an emergency until rest, warmth, and nutritious food shall have accomplished what the drug has failed to do.

Suprarenal capsules, it would appear from the report of Gourfein,[2] are by no means altogether benign in their influence. He tells us that in the glycerin extract of these bodies there are proteid substances which are precipi-tated by alcohol and are devoid of poisonous influence, but that the extract also contains materials which are not precipitated by alcohol and are exceed-

[1] Boston M. and S. Jour., Oct. 8, 1896.

[2] Buffalo Med. Jour., Aug., 1896, from Compt. rend. de la Soc. de Biol., 1895; Jour. Chem. Soc., 1896.

ingly toxic in action. These poisonous substances, being uninfluenced by heat, may be obtained by extracting the adrenals with hot water, precipitating with alcohol, and evaporating the remaining clear liquid over a water-bath. The substance thus obtained, if injected hypodermically, appears to violently attack the central nervous system and promptly causes death. The amount of this poison which the suprarenal bodies contain is said to vary considerably, and it is asserted that extracts of muscle and spleen obtained in precisely the same manner manifest no such influences.

Tannoform is a condensation-product of nutgall tannin and formic aldehyd. It is an odorless and tasteless powder of light, yellowish-gray color. It is insoluble in water, but is soluble in alcohol. It is also soluble in dilute alkaline solutions, but is precipitated from this solution if an acid is added. Although formaldehyd uncombined has a pronounced action upon the tissues, its combination with tannin is devoid of injurious properties, though the antiseptic and drying powers of the formaldehyd are said to remain. The remedy, in addition to its antiseptic power, is useful as an astringent, and has the great advantages of tastelessness, absence of irritant effect upon the stomach, and finally, since it is not dissolved by the gastric secretions, a power to reach the intestine unchanged. Zuntz[1] thus reports the results of his experimentation with this agent. A small quantity placed upon the healthy skin much diminishes the secretion of sweat; moreover, it deodorizes this and indirectly prevents the cutaneous irritation which may follow excessive sweating. For chafing and certain cases of eczema thus caused he rates tannoform as superior to any agent now employed. In such ailments the combined properties of the remedy render it unique, and it is as pleasant in action as it is effective. Zuntz has also used the remedy upon wounds, a crust forming from it which serves as a protectant; he is as yet, however, undetermined as to its value in such cases as compared with other applications. The field of usefulness of tannoform, according to D. de Buck and L. de Moor,[2] is a little more extended, and they value it as an application to wounds, ulcers, and bedsores, and in bromidrosis as well as in inflammations of mucous membranes, such as ozena, balanitis, and vaginitis. They report upon 2 cases so treated, and regard it as an efficient remedy in both acute and chronic intestinal catarrhs. A dose so large as 15 gr. may be given without causing irritation, and since it is both astringent and antiseptic its action is explained, for we have already said that the drug is not dissolved in the stomach, and therefore cannot exhaust its astringent properties upon the stomach and its contents. The same observers[3] have employed tannoform in combination with starch or talc in the proportion of 1 to 5, and have applied it pure as well. They have also used it in ointment with vaselin or lanolin in a variety of skin-diseases in which astringent and antiseptic action is required, and in the cases both of children and adults.

Traumatol (iodokresin) is described by W. Schatlenmann[4] as a fine, amorphous powder, which is without odor and in color is violet-red. It is a compound of cresylic acid and iodin, and is said to contain 54% of the latter. It is not soluble in water or alcohol, and it is not dissolved by acids. It is readily soluble, however, in chloroform and alkaline solutions, if strong. Clinically the drug may be applied for antiseptic effect, the form of application being in powder, gauze, collodion, vaselin, glycerin, or plaster. Crayons of

[1] Am. Medico-Surg. Bull., Sept. 5, 1896.
[2] Am. Jour. Med. Sci., Jan., 1897, from Rev. de Thérap. Medico-Chir.. No. 19, p. 579, 1896.
[3] Am. Medico-Surg. Bull., No. 7, 1896, from Belg. méd., ii., No. 33, 1896.
[4] Am. Jour. Med. Sci., May, 1897, from Thérap. Monatsh., H. 2, S. 89, 1897.

value of preparations of the drug.
the circulatory system Dudgeo s
study was to ascertain the dose ˥
administration of the remedy, a ˩
drugs when properly employed
report all showed marked card a
a valvular lesion; in some ther ᴌ
heart, and in some the heart-actio
most, two or more of these con
pressure was low, as shown by h
there is said to have been. an imp
signs. The author concludes that
about 5 drops in water, three or
advantages that have heretofore bee
are borne out by this series of exper
follows: 1. Greater rapidity of actio.
3. Greater diuretic power ; 4. The al)
its use; 5. No cumulative action ; 6.
in old age. The contraindications to ti ⸲
ized, namely : when compensating hyɪ ⸱
when the heart presents an advanced ˢta
degree of mechanical defect. With the·
preparation is used in doses not too larg
prefers strophanthus in : 1. All cases in
tion ; 2. All cases of arterial degenera
more energetic cardiac contractions is req
in which diuresis is necessary ; 4. All ca⸜
cases of cardiac disease in childhood oɪ ⟩

The observations of Balfour[1] have le h
for he decidedly prefers digitalis to stroph
tunate symptoms which at times follow t̩
to a misconception of the true action of tʰ r
it. Digitalis acts, he says, by improving ɪe
and by improving the metabolism of all ɪe t ˢ
larly marked in the case of the cardia mu˰
muscle is strengthened and its elasticity ɪcrea˲
being thereby relieved. The good result obtaiɪ
Strophanthus, on the other hand, has pɪved iɪ
dangerous drug. It acts as a heart-poiɪn rather
stimulates the heart to increased action, it˴ true, l
the reserve of cardiac energy without inɪroving t
more feeble the heart, the greater is the dɒger att n ˙
edy. It acts only by helping the patieɪ through an
warmth, and nutritious food shall have aᴄomplished w
to do.

Suprarenal capsules, it would aɪear from the
are by no means altogether benign in the influence. H
glycerin extract of these bodies there are ⸱ᴄreid ˢubsta⸵˲
tated by alcohol and are devoid of poisᴄoua influence,
also contains materials which are not precpitated by alcᴄ

[1] Boston M. and S. Jour., Oct. 8, 1896.
[2] Buffalo Med. Jour., Aug., 1896, from Cont. rend. de la Soᴄ
Chem. Soc., 1896.

e rece:ly studied the subject and reported upon the
ın.¹ Ie belittles its harmful properties, it is true,
poiɔ.ing as rare.   He has given the remedy with
ca: indeed he gave almost 3500 gr. within 6
.ɔ hiɐly of trional as a hypnotic for children, and
ɔn : to the appropriate doses : for infɒnts of ·from
·. ; to 2 years, 6 to 12 gr. ; 2 to 6 years, 12 to
ɔ5 r.   These doses will doubtless impress those
ɟe.   They certainly are excessive, and to us
Ruhemann is in conflict with many observers
··iews of trional as well.   The adult maxi-
30 gr., but in the presence of dyspepsia
· in milk, and says that the action of
leep appearing in from a quarter
Às to the cumulative action of
issue with some who think
ɞ in which he finds trional
childhood, but he denies
with favorable influ-
that of phthisical
mnia due to pain
fɑ contrast with
·hile praising
er nervous
ɔases as
This
cir-
the
in-

traumatol are also employed. Among the preparations whose appropriate strength is mentioned are a 5% to 10% traumatol-zinc paste, a 10% traumatol lanolin vaselin, and a 10% to 50% chloroformic solution. The powder is advantageously applied in many conditions of genito-urinary surgery as in bubo, phimosis, and the removal of papillomata, and it is recommended that collodion be afterward applied as a covering. In powder, too, as well as in solution in chloroform, its action upon syphilitic disease of mucous membranes is said to be good, and the crayons are valuable as stimulants to the healing of fistulæ. In addition to the antiseptic action of the drug it is thought to have a drying effect; and since it is not irritant, a number of cutaneous disorders are appropriately treated with it. Schatlenmann thinks highly of this substance, and cites in its favor the very excellent action which it manifested in 75 cases in which it was employed to the exclusion of other agents.

Traumatol appears to have certain advantages over iodoform, especially as a surgical application; but when we recall the many drugs which have appeared as contestants for iodoform's field of usefulness, and note how few have survived, a certain amount of skepticism in the ease of each new aspirant would seem not without justification. Traumatol has been thoroughly tested by Ladevie,[1] however, and his report of cases treated by himself and others is highly in favor of the drug. Its employment was in essentially the same cases as are so often treated with iodoform, and much benefit has followed the application. The antiseptic power of traumatol has been demonstrated bacteriologically, and it is said that the drug is neither irritating nor poisonous. It is claimed, also, that by internal administration traumatol is productive of antiseptic action upon the bronchi, and that its effect upon tuberculous diarrhea is most excellent.

Trional must be held to have established itself firmly as an excellent and reliable hypnotic. Indeed, many go so far as to pronounce it ideal, and call special attention to its value in childhood and its harmlessness. That serious results seldom follow its use is true, but that it is harmless is an error which cannot be too promptly corrected. It is in its prolonged employment that trional is likely to cause toxic symptoms, and, therefore, during such a course there should occur intervals of several days in which no trional is given; the possible necessity for hypnotic action during these periods being met by the administration of another drug. In this way the cumulative tendency of trional may be avoided, for the danger of toxic action from occasional or interrupted use is slight. This poisoning from the long-continued use of trional is well illustrated by a case reported by Gierlich.[2] The patient was addicted to the use of morphin, and in order to produce sleep (presumably because insomnia resulted when morphin was withdrawn) took about 45 gr. of trional per diem for a period of two months. As a result there occurred pronounced ataxia, tremor throughout the body, and great mental depression, together with weakening of memory and some disturbances of speech. The withdrawal of trional was followed by the improvement of the patient (the morphin being given in the customary amount), but the nerve-disorders did not altogether disappear until five weeks later.

Another element of danger in the prolonged employment of trional is the necessity for increase of dose. We think that this is a matter which is too little appreciated; necessarily, however, as the power of the drug appears rapidly to diminish with habit, there is demanded the use of larger amounts, and from this the danger of accumulation is apparent.

[1] Brit. Med Jour, Oct. 17, 1896, from Allg. Wien. med. zeit., Sept. 1 and 8, 1896.
[2] Univ. Med. Mag., Apr., 1897, from Centralbl. f. innere Med., No. 51, 1896.

Among those who have recently studied the subject and reported upon the uses of trional is Ruhemann.[1] He belittles its harmful properties, it is true, and rates the occurrence of poisoning as rare. He has given the remedy with much freedom, and in one case indeed he gave almost 3500 gr. within 6 months. Ruhemann thinks highly of trional as a hypnotic for children, and gives the following information as to the appropriate doses: for infants of from 1 month to 1 year, 3 to 5 gr.; 1 to 2 years, 6 to 12 gr.; 2 to 6 years, 12 to 20 gr.; 6 to 10 years, 20 to 25 gr. These doses will doubtless impress those familiar with the subject as large. They certainly are excessive, and to us would seem scarcely prudent; but Ruhemann is in conflict with many observers not only upon this, but upon other views of trional as well. The adult maximum dose of the remedy be places at 30 gr., but in the presence of dyspepsia he recommends the rectal injection of 20 gr. in milk, and says that the action of trional when so given is remarkably prompt, sleep appearing in from a quarter to a half hour, and lasting from 6 to 9 hours. As to the cumulative action of trional, Ruhemann is more than skeptical, and takes issue with some who think that cardiac disease is a contraindication. The cases in which he finds trional of value are severe chorea and cerebral excitement in childhood, but he denies that it is a specific against insomnia, though crediting it with favorable influence in the sleeplessness of neuroses and neurasthenia, in that of phthisical night-sweats, and that which follows acute disease. In insomnia due to pain or to cough he thinks little of it, save when in combination. In contrast with these views in many respects are those of Scognamiglio,[2] who, while praising the remedy highly for its influence in mania, melancholia, and other nervous disorders, is also of the opinion that it is valuable in pulmonary diseases as well as in pain from various causes, neuralgia, and even pains of tabes. This observer is of the opinion that trional has no ill effect upon the digestion, circulation, or respiration, but his observation upon the real influence of the drug, in view of the opinion of many that it is the cause of hematoporphyrinuria, is full of interest. In the urine of men taking this drug he failed in every case to detect hematoporphyrin, and similarly in the urine of dogs and of rabbits to which moderate doses (7 to 15 gr. a day to dogs, 1 to 7 gr. to rabbits) were given. It was only when the dose was much increased (45 gr. a day) that hematoporphyrin was detected in the urine upon the third day. As a result, therefore, of his observations, both clinical and experimental, Scognamiglio rates trional as powerfully hypnotic, and safe as well, providing its daily dose is from 15 to 30 gr. He ranks it the superior of sulphonal, morphin, and chloral hydrate, and thinks that the danger of hematoporphyrinuria is very remote. Another report upon the use and action of trional is that of von Mering,[3] and, representing as it does the deductions afforded by almost a thousand cases, it is of great value. In view of the doses prescribed by others it is interesting to note that von Mering found it rarely necessary to give more than 15 gr. of the remedy, or at most 20 gr. in cases of insomnia pure and simple, and that he regards drowsiness occurring upon the following day as indicative that the dose was excessive. What we have already said as regards the continued use of trional is corroborated by von Mering, who advises, if a daily hypnotic is required for a long time, that the trional be occasionally substituted by another remedy, such as chloralamid, chloral hydrate, or amyl hydrate. In this connection, too, it may be said that although in a number of von Mering's cases the remedy was continued for 3 or 4 months, and with no ill effect, the

[1] Therap. Gaz., Dec. 15, 1896, from Jour. des Praticiens, July 25, 1896.
[2] Therap. Gaz., Aug. 15, 1896; Rivista clinica e Terapeutica, No. 11, 1895.
[3] Med. News, Nov. 7, 1896, from Therap. Monatsh., Aug., 1896.

administration was on every second or third day only, and the doses from 15 to 25 gr. As to the power of trional, von Mering, in common with most observers, rates it as superior to sulfonal, and less likely than that remedy to cause disagreeable results. He evidently does not value the remedy as a reliable anodyne or analgesic, as does Scognamiglio, for in cases of insominia caused by pain he recommends its combination with $\frac{1}{16}$ gr. of morphin. Much that is recommended by von Mering is also advised by a writer in the *Journal de Neurologie*,[1] who places the maximum adult dose at 15 or 20 gr., amounts in excess of this being permitted only in the insane, and for children of 10 about 12 gr. He, too, regards the drng as harmless even if given for long periods of time, but wisely recommends that it be given on alternate days and in a large quantity of hot water. (Compare *Year-Book* for 1897, p. 1144.)

Unguentum durum is a recently introduced ointment-base which has the following composition : paraffin (solid), 4 parts ; wool-fat, 1 part ; liquid paraffin, 5 parts. F. Miehle[2] says that it resembles white-wax ointment, and therefore that it is a desirable substance for protectant applications, while at the same time it has a considerable power of penetration. It will absorb over 10 % of water, and is useful in the preparation of lead ointment, carbolic ointment, and ointments which contain liquid antiseptics.

Unguentum molle is a new ointment-base which has the following composition : paraffin (solid), 11 parts ; wool-fat, 5 parts ; liquid paraffin, 34 parts. This resembles white vaselin. It is easy to make, is not expensive, and is said to be absolutely permanent. It is superior to petroleum in some respects, being more active in penetrating ability and of superior consistence. The ointment is said to absorb a weight of water equal to its own, and with an equal weight of glycerin to make an exceedingly smooth ointment. The subject has been fully presented by F. Michle.[3]

Urea, according to Klemperer and Friedreich, is actively diuretic. The cause of this action, according to Friedreich,[4] is a stimulation of the renal epithelium similar to that brought about by caffein. In support of his belief, Friedreich has conducted experiments upon the subject, and has also employed the agent clinically with success. Among the cases which he treated thus in 1892–93 was one of hepatic cirrhosis without renal lesion, and to this patient urea was given and gradually increased in amount until 12 gm. were taken in a day. By this the amount of urine voided was increased sevenfold. A second and similar case showed a like result, and in a third the urine was increased from 400 c.c. to 750 c.c. Of these patients the first took in all 157 gm. of urea without untoward effect, and the second 200 gm. In the third, treatment by urea was suspended because of the occurrence of pneumonia. Had the doses in the first two cases been larger from the beginning (in Klemperer's case 10 gm. were given from the outset), it is possible that the resultant diuresis would have been even more pronounced (see *Year-Book* for 1897, p. 1144). [Although the results of this experimentation are both interesting and valuable, the excrementitious nature of urea and practically complete ignorance as to its toxic possibilities would suggest great caution in its use. In the absence of renal lesion its use would seem permissible in view of the report of Klemperer, but renal impairment would seem to considerably curtail its field of usefulness.]

Viburnum Prunifolium.—A very thorough experimental research has recently been conducted by Theodore Sherman[5] upon the action of black haw,

---

[1] Am. Medico-Surg. Bull., Dec. 26, 1896, from Jour. de Neurol., No. 14, 1896.
[2] Am. Medico-Surg. Bull., Sept. 5, 1896, from Pharm. Ztg., xli, p. 403, 1896.
[3] Ibid.   [4] Am. Medico-Surg. Bull., Oct. 10, 1896, from Brit. Med. Jour.
[5] Edinb. Med. Jour., Nov., 1896.

and forms the basis of an admirable report. The subject, as obtainable from medical literature, is graphically presented, and botanic and clinical matters discussed. The chief part of the report, however, concerns the experiments which the author conducted upon both warm-blooded and cold-blooded animals, and his conclusions thus based are as follows : " In mammals, warm-blooded animals, owing to the difficulty of giving a large enough dose hypodermically, there is no marked effect except drowsiness and some lessening of motor power. If the substance be introduced into the heart directly, there is rapid lowering of blood-pressure to about one-half the normal, with slow return to near the normal as the drug is eliminated. Although too much reliance must not be placed on experimental results in cold-blooded animals as applicable to warm-blooded animals, including man, we may be allowed to take something from these results and use them as *probably* applicable. Thus, there is *probably* some diminution of reflex irritability, a quieting effect on involuntary muscle, possibly some lowering of blood-pressure, which, even though small, might afford relief in congested conditions. Then, and very important, there is the effect of the valerianic or viburnic acid in neurotic and hysteric conditions. In the pharmacopeia there are many drugs capable of bringing about all these desired effects. Why, then, use Viburnum prunifolium ? Opium is one of our sheet-anchors, but then there are dangers and inconveniences attending its use. The patient may acquire the opium-habit ; the constipation caused by it is very troublesome, and it is very toxic. Viburnum has similar good effects, though not so strong. It is a good form in which to administer valerianic acid. Its effect upon unstriped muscle, though not so strong as that of opium, gives the relief necessary. It has scarcely any effect in causing constipation. Toxic effects have only been noticed with very considerable doses. Herrick has seen disturbance of vision, dryness of mouth, and headaches ; and Wilson has observed similar conditions, but these were with doses larger than are usually administered to man." The article is concluded by a list of viburnum preparations which, though varied, includes little that requires submitting to the American reader.

Since viburnum is a drug of American medical introduction, and furthermore is extensively employed among us, the familiarity of readers of the *Year-Book* with the subject may to a certain extent be assumed, but the indications for its employment as set down by Sherman are none the less useful. They are : In *habitual abortion*, where this is not caused by syphilitic infection or by fatty placenta, there seem, undoubtedly, good results to follow the use of Viburnum prunifolium. In *threatening abortion*, however caused, and at any period of gestation, if the case is seen soon enough, it seems to be very successful. In *dysmenorrhea*, if functional, spasmodic, or ovarian, or attended with menorrhagia, it often cures. If there is flexion or stenosis, it gives great relief, though, of course, it cannot cure. In the menorrhagias and metrorrhagia of the *menopause* and in the nervous disorders of that time it is very beneficial. *After-pains* are so readily relieved by it that some (*e. g.*, Auvard) consider that its use is dangerous unless all clots are cleared out of the uterus previously. It may be used in the diagnosis of *false pains*, speedily relieving them. It is also used with success in *colicky diarrhea* and in *dysentery*. Some even claim that it has a curative effect on cramps of voluntary muscles.

Wine of Iron and Quassia.—The following is a recently published [1] formula : ℞ : tincture of quassia, 30 parts ; pyrophosphate of iron and sodium, 5 parts ; Malaga wine, 1000 parts. M. S. : a tablespoonful before each of the two principal meals.

[1] N. Y. Med. Jour., June 19, 1897, from Gaz. hebdom. de Méd. et de Chir., May 20, 1897.

ANATOMY.

By C. A. HAMANN, M. D.,

OF CLEVELAND, OHIO.

OSTEOLOGY.

Sesamoid Bones of the Hand.—Edward Fawcett[1] has studied these bones in 38 persons by means of skiagraphy. His results confirm Pfitzner's observations, which were made on a very large number of hands. The two metacarpophalangeal sesamoids of the thumb were found in every case examined; considerable variation in size was noted. A single sesamoid was present in $68\frac{1}{2}\%$ of the cases in the interphalangeal joint of the thumb. A single radial sesamoid was found in the metacarpophalangeal joint of the index finger in 55.2% of the cases; it is oval in shape and its long axis is placed in the long axis of the finger. In the metacarpophalangeal joint of the little finger a sesamoid bone was present in 71% of the cases. In the middle and ring fingers no sesamoids were met with. Fawcett did not find that the age or the muscular development of the individuals had any bearing on the number or *size of these bones.*

Ossification of the Third Trochanter in Man.—A. F. Dixon[2] found in the femur of a young subject a small epiphysis for the gluteal ridge of the third trochanter; it was 25 mm. in length and 12 mm. in width. In examining a large number of human femora this epiphysis was found in two other bones, and a number of mammals, among them the rabbit, tapir, and horse, also show it. "The fact that the third trochanter of man thus closely resembles in its mode of development that of lower mammals adds to it an interest, especially as the presence of this trochanter is stated to be a characteristic of the femora of higher rather than of lower races, and of man rather than of apes."

Metopic Suture.—G. Papillault,[3] in an investigation on this suture carried on in the Anthropologic Laboratory in Paris, arrived at the conclusion that metopism is due to a greater development of the brain, the pressure of the cranial contents being greater in such cases than in others. The cause of a persistent frontal suture is thus to be sought for in the brain itself. Of 807 male crania, 9.91% were metopic; of 329 female crania, 11.85%.

Asymmetry of the Sternum.—A. Birmingham,[4] upon examining 54 sterna, found that 87% were asymmetrical and 13% were approximately symmetrical. He found that the most marked irregularity was a depression of the clavicular facet, which was associated with a corresponding diminution of the vertical depth of the sternum on the same side; this was found on the right side in 50% of the specimens, and on the left side in 37%. The line of

---

[1] Jour. Anat. and Physiol., vol. xi., part i, p. 157.   [2] Ibid., vol. x., part iv., p. 502.
[3] Mém. de la Soc. d'Anthropol. de Paris, t. ii. (iii e serie) 1er Fasc., and Jour. Anat. and Physiol., vol. x., part iv., p. 584.
[4] Dublin Jour. Med. Sci., Jan., 1897.

junction between the manubrium and gladiolus is oblique, and slopes down-ward on the right side oftener than on the left. In about 59 % of sterna there is a longitudinal curve occupying the entire bone; this curve is more often directed to the right than to the left.

Congenital Absence of both Patellæ.—A. T. Bristow[1] describes a case in which both patellæ were absent, the fifth on record. The patient, a child of 2½ years, was the subject of pes varus on both sides. In all the recorded cases there were additional developmental errors. [The writer has the limbs of a peromelic monster in which both patellæ are absent; there is also absence of both tibiæ and of certain of the tarsal bones. In connection with Bristow's case, it is to be remembered that at the age of 2½ years the patella is still cartilaginous, and would therefore give no indication of its presence in a Röntgen photograph.]

THE HEART AND BLOODVESSELS.

Moderator Band in Left Ventricle.—Sir William Turner[2] describes a second case in which he found the so-called moderator band in the left ven-tricle. It was 38 mm. in length, 9 mm. in its greatest diameter, and ½ mm. in its narrowest part. It consisted of muscular fibers covered with endocar-dium, and passed from the anterior to the posterior wall of the ventricle, thus enabling it to exert a moderating influence on the dilatation of the cavity. The septal wall presented a large smooth surface—*i. e.*, the columnæ carneæ were absent over it. [Though such bands in the left ventricle are but rarely met with, still it would seem that their occurrence would be nothing very strange or inexplicable when we consider the mode of development of the musculature of the heart; the columnæ carneæ, as is well known, represent the enlarged and thickened remains of the trabeculæ which in early embryonic life unite the endothelial heart-tube with the outer fibromuscular tube. Such trabeculæ might remain attached to opposite walls of the ventricle by their extremities, and being free in the rest of their extent, just as certain of the columnæ are normally, would appear as moderator bands.] Such moderator bands have also been seen in the left auricle.[3]

Structure of the Larger Arteries at different Times of Life.—N. Grünstein[4] has made some investigations on the structure of the arterial wall which are of practical interest. The intima and media increase in thickness as age advances; in the carotid, subclavian, and aorta the intima increases rela-tively more in thickness than the media, whereas in the common iliac the media increases more than the intima. In the larger vessels, as Unna has shown, part of the elastic tissue becomes changed into elacin, and thus the elasticity of the vessel-walls is diminished. Upon staining with methyl-blue Grünstein found localized patches in the aorta, and in the carotid and subclavian vessels, which stained more deeply than the rest of the arterial wall; this would indicate a change in the tissue the nature of which is not known.

Elastic Tissue in the Walls of the Cerebral Arteries.—Triepel[5] has studied the structure of the internal carotid, anterior, middle, and posterior cerebral, basilar, and vertebral arteries, with reference to the amount and arrangement of the elastic tissue. The sections were stained with orexin. It was found that the coats of these arteries contain but little elastic tissue. The elastica interna is present; a few circular fibers are found in the middle coat, and

---

[1] Med. News, p. 15, Jan. 2, 1897.   [2] Jour. Anat and Physiol., vol. x., part iv., p. 569.
[3] Ibid., Apr. and July, 1896.   [4] Arch. f. mikroskop. Anat., xlvii., p. 583, 1896.
[5] Deutsch. med. Woch., Feb. 4, 1897; Vereins Beil., No. 5, p. 31.

rather more circular fibers in the external coat, together with a few longitudinal fibers. The elastica externa and marked longitudinal elastic fibers in the outer coat are thus practically absent. Where the vertebral artery passes through the foramen magnum it contains numerous and well-marked longitudinal and circular fibers in the outer coat, and also elastic fibers among the circular muscular fibers. The changes in the structure of the vessel here are to be attributed to the elongation to which it is subjected in the movements of the head. In the neck the media of the vertebral contains elastic plates; this vessel shows distinctly how mechanical influences modify the structure and arrangement of the elastic tissue in the arterial coats.

Vasa Vasorum and Lymph-paths of the Vessel-walls.—Schiefferdecker[1] gives a summary of the main facts concerning the mode of distribution of the vasa vasorum. The main deductions that can be made from the work of previous investigators are as follows: 1. The muscular coat of the vessels is the chief tissue requiring nutrition; the muscular tissue is nourished either by capillary vessels in the adjacent adventitia, or by capillaries which enter the muscularis itself. 2. It seems that the presence of capillaries in the muscularis is dependent upon the thickness of the intima and upon whether the vessel is an artery or a vein. 3. The vessel-wall is nourished both from without (*i. e.*, by the vasa vasorum) and from within (*i. e.*, by the blood traversing the interior of the vessel). 4. When thickening of the intima occurs the blood contained in the lumen of the vessel can no longer nourish properly the tissues of the wall that it formerly did; then the vasa vasorum multiply and enter the muscularis and even the intima, which are ordinarily devoid of vasa vasorum. Thus the thickening of the intima is primary and the proliferation of the vasa vasorum is secondary. Schiefferdecker then describes subendothelial lymphplexuses which he found in the pig's aorta by means of staining with lactate of silver; stomata were not present. These subendothelial lymph-spaces have been described by Hoggan in the veins.

THE DIGESTIVE SYSTEM.

Secretion of Saliva.—Erik Müller[2] has examined the salivary glands of man, the cat, dog, and rabbit, and the results of his works agree in the main with the views of Altmann, that the saliva is formed from typical intracellular granules; these granules undergo changes in size as assimilative processes go on. Some of the results of the investigation are as follows: 1. The saliva is a product of granules which undergo characteristic transformations. 2. The secretion is present in the gland-cells in the form of small round vacuoles, which are separated from the surrounding protoplasm by a wall which can be stained. These vacuoles were first demonstrated by Retzius in Golgi preparations and by the author in ordinary preparations. 3. These vacuoles are formed in granules in the cells. 4. The cells have a different appearance, depending upon their richness in granules; some of them have large clear granules, separated from one another by a reticulum containing very small granules that take the stain; other cells have large granules that can be stained. 5. During very active secretion the granules which can be stained become changed into secretory vacuoles. 6. The secretory capillaries of albuminous glands are all intercellular.

Topographic Anatomy of the Spleen, Pancreas, Duodenum, Kidneys, etc.—A. Birmingham[3] gives the results of his examination of the

[1] Deutsch. med. Woch., Sept. 16, 1897; Vereins Beil., p. 185.
[2] Arch. f. Anat. u. Entwickelungsgesch., H. 5 u. 6, p. 305, 1896.
[3] Jour. Anat. and Physiol., vol. xi., p. 95.

viscera in three subjects hardened with chromic acid solution. Among them are the following: " 1. The lobus Spigelii of the liver has an anterior free surface as well as a posterior, and it lies in a special 'recessus Spigelii' on the posterior abdominal wall. 2. The empty stomach is in shape that of an attenuated and modified pear, with its wide end directed backward and to the left; the greater part of the long axis runs forward and a little inward in the horizontal plane, and turns to the right and downward a few inches from the pylorus. Its great curvature looks forward and to the left, its lesser to the right and backward. Special attention is called to the 'stomach-bed,' which forms the floor of a chamber in which the stomach lies. [The "stomach-bed" is a shelf-like arrangement supporting that organ. It is formed by that portion of the pancreas situated to the left of the median line; this part of the pancreas is quite thick anteroposteriorly, and its upper surface (anterior surface of His) forms a large part of the shelf. The pancreas is in such relation with the left kidney that the top of that organ forms part of the shelf. The tail of the pancreas extends to the spleen, so that the plane of its superior surface runs upward and backward into the gastric surface of the spleen, and thus the bed is completed behind and to the left. The transverse mesocolon, supported by coils of the small intestine, extends the bed anteriorly.] 3. The duodenum does not lie in the coronal plane, as usually represented; the first half of the first stage and all beyond the middle of the transverse stage lie approximately in the coronal plane; the intermediate part is moulded backward by the side of the cava, and lies almost in the sagittal plane. The cava does not lie behind the descending duodenum, but to its left. The duodenum is also connected behind to the right ureter and psoas. 4. The body of the pancreas projects forward as a distinct ridge into the abdominal cavity and is not flattened against the posterior wall. It is prismatic, but the three sides of the prism are nearly equal. Two forms of tail are described—one, which is long and slender and curves back beneath the basal surface of the spleen, the other, short and stout, which abuts against the lower part of the gastric surface of the spleen. 5. The suprarenal bodies lie not very far from the sagittal plane, and the right is nearly posterior to the vena cava. 6. The names 'anterior' and 'posterior' are suggested, instead of superior and inferior pancreaticoduodenal, as probably being more correct."

Innervation of the Dentine.—Michael Morgenstern [1] has investigated the nerves of the dentine by means of the modified Golgi method. He finds that there are nerve-fibrillæ, between the elementary cells of which the odontoblasts are formed. The nerves of the dentine are found in the dentinal canals (intratubular fibers) and also outside of the canals (intertubular fibers), the latter being more numerous. In the crown of the tooth most of the nerve-fibers are parallel with the dentinal tubules, whereas in the neck of the tooth and in the fang they in part follow the tubules and in part lie in the long axis of the tooth. By the formation of anastomoses a plexus is formed. The nerve-fibers of the dentine pursue a wavy course, divide dichotomously, and give off numerous branches. Most of the ramifications end free. Intertubular fibers frequently enter the tubules. At the border of the dentine and enamel is a more or less separate system of nerve-fibrillæ, which, however, anastomose in many places with the intradentinal fibers.

The Duodenum and Pylorus.—Thomas Dwight,[2] in the examination of 70 adult bodies, finds that the V-shaped duodenum is more frequently met with in women than in men; the irregular forms of the duodenum preponder-

[1] Arch. f. Anat. u. Physiol. (Anat. Abth.), p. 378, 1896.
[2] Jour. Anat. and Physiol., vol. xi., part iv., p. 516.

ate in males. In the majority of adults of both sexes the lowest point of the duodenum is opposite the fourth lumbar vertebra, or the disks above and below it; in about one-fourth of 54 bodies examined it was opposite the third, and in about half a dozen opposite the fifth lumbar vertebra. "In the 54 cases already mentioned, the duodenum was on the right of the aorta till just before the terminal flexure 26 times; it was wholly on the right 6 times. The fourth part lay in front of the aorta 11 times, and the third part actually crossed the aorta 11 times." In many of the cases a fold of peritoneum intervened between the aorta and the gut. The fourth part of the duodenum is prerenal in exceptional cases only. The pyloric opening in 30 cases was found to be practically always oval, though the long axis of the opening may lie in any direction. The average size of the orifice was 14 × 11 mm., the extremes being 7 × 4 mm. and 20 × 18 mm.

THE NERVOUS SYSTEM.

Course of the Taste-fibers.—A. F. Dixon[1] discusses the unsettled question of the course taken by the taste-fibers. He opposes the belief of Gowers and others, "that the path of taste from all parts in which this sense exists reaches the brain by the root of the fifth nerve," which belief is chiefly based on clinic and pathologic evidence. Dixon refers to the fact that both the facial and glossopharyngeal nerves, "which are denied the possibility of carrying taste-impulses," are anatomically, in part at least, nerves of sensation, for the facial possesses a ganglion (geniculate) which is as much a homologue of the spinal ganglia as the Gasserian ganglion is; the chorda tympani, the nerve of taste for the anterior portion of the tongue, is connected with the seventh. Furthermore, the pars intermedia of Wrisberg is in part continuous with the chorda tympani, and seems to "represent the continuation of the chorda tympani fibers, through the ganglion-cells to the brain;" if we do not regard the chorda tympani as a nerve of sensation, then it is difficult to see what are the sensory branches of the geniculate ganglion that correspond to the fibers passing from the ganglion to the brain in the pars intermedia. The ganglia of the glossopharyngeal resemble the ganglia of the posterior spinal nerve-roots structurally, and in all likelihood "as many fibers leave the ganglion as enter it." When we consider this, it is difficult to see how the small nerve of Jacobson can contain all the fibers of the glossopharyngeal nerve which convey taste-impulses, as the adherents of the view of Gowers would have us believe. The point is also made that if "the taste-impulses passing in the facial and glossopharyngeal nerves leave them by the great superficial petrosal and Jacobson's nerve to join the trigeminal, as has been maintained, then these impulses in their course to the brain pass not only through ganglionic nerve-cells of spinal ganglion type twice in each case (namely, of the seventh and fifth nerves and of the ninth and fifth nerves), but they also pass through the otic or Meckel's ganglion. If they have this complicated course, they are the only special sense-impulses which pass through multipolar sympathetic nerve-cells on their way to the brain." He then brings evidence that seems to show that the chorda tympani and the great superficial petrosal are to be regarded as afferent branches of the seventh nerve, and that Jacobson's nerve is a branch of the ninth.

Change of Brain-weight after Preservation in Formalin Solutions.—Edw. F. Latan[2] finds that the weight of the human brain when preserved in 10% formalin solutions increases during 1 month from 2% to 3%;

---

[1] Edinb. Med. Jour., p. 395, Apr., 1897.   [2] Antom. Anz., vol. xiii., p. 323.

after conservation for 5 months and over the increase amounts to 1%. In 5% solution the weight increases 9% in the first 4 days; after 1 month, 10%; after 5 months, 7%; and after immersion for 1¼ years the increase is 6%. In 1% solution the weight increases during the first 2 days 14%; after 1 month, 23%; and after 1¼ years, 19%. The spinal cord placed in a 10% solution increases 10% during the first 3 days; after 50 days, 14%. In 1% solutions the cord during the first 3 days increases 11%; after 50 days, 13%. Thus it appears that the lower the percentage of formalin in the solution the greater is the increase in weight of the brain; the spinal cord increases in weight considerably more than the brain.

Position and Dimensions of the Optic Chiasm.—Zander[1] has studied the gross relations of the chiasma opticum in connection with the subject of acromegaly and enlargements of the pituitary body. He found in the examination of 23 specimens that the pituitary body had a sagittal diameter of 8 mm. on the average, the extremes being 6 mm. and 10.5 mm. The average transverse diameter was 11.9 mm., the extremes being 10 mm. and 14.5 mm. The average vertical diameter was found to be 6.55 mm. Enlargement of the pituitary body has been found to cause certain visual disturbances, and these have usually been ascribed to pressure upon the posterior surface of the chiasm and upon the optic tracts. Zander states that this is not the case, for the position of the chiasm is such that the enlarged hypophysis would not press in that direction. He examined 55 preparations in which the optic tracts, chiasm, and nerves were exposed from above. In none of the preparations did he find the chiasm occupying the optic groove, as is stated in most anatomic text-books; in fact, the optic groove was found to be present in only 34 out of 100 skulls, while in 44 this surface was plane and in 22 it was convex. The anterior border of the chiasm never reaches the optic groove, being distant from it 10.34 mm. on the average, the extremes being 4.75 mm. and 17 mm. The intracranial portion of the optic nerve was found to vary in length from 6 mm. to 21 mm. This portion of the nerve would necessarily be very short if the chiasm lay in the groove; furthermore, the angle of divergence is less than a right angle, whereas if the chiasm had the position it is usually said to occupy the angle would have to be very much larger. Again, the groove is too small for the chiasm. The posterior border of the commissure extended behind the upper edge of the dorsum sellæ for a distance of 1.58 mm. on the average, and only in a few cases was it found in front of it, so that the hypophysis cannot lie behind the chiasm; it lies in front of it and when the diaphragma sellæ is removed the chiasm can be seen to lie in the angle of divergence of the two optic nerves. The sagittal diameter of the chiasm was found to vary from 4 mm. to 13 mm.; the transverse from 9.75 mm. to 19.75 mm.; the vertical diameter is greatest at its anterior border, where it averages 3.1 mm. It is interesting to note that in 60% of the cases the commissure was placed to one or other side, so that it did not lie symmetrically; this would cause variations in the length of the intracranial portion of the optic nerves. Tumors of the hypophysis would not be likely to grow upward, behind the chiasm, but would bulge between the two optic nerves into the cisterna chiasmatis, a small recess of the subarachnoid space situated between the chiasm, olivary eminence, and diaphragma sellæ; in some cases the inferior surface of the commissure would be subjected to pressure. The enlargement in a vertical direction would have to amount to at least 0.5 cm. before the optic paths could be compressed by the tumor.

The Eye of the Newborn.—E. v. Hippel[2] finds that hardening in

[1] Deutsch. med. Woch., Jahrg. xxiii., No. 3; Vereins Beil., No. 3, p. 13, 1897.
[2] Deutsch. med. Woch., Aug. 26, 1897; Vereins Beil., p. 162.

Müller's fluid changes most markedly the lens; less markedly the cornea. The retinal fold at the ora serrata, described by Lange, he considers an artefact. v. Hippel found the thickness of the fresh lens to be 3.76 mm.; its posterior surface is more curved than the anterior. He finds that the ora serrata are well developed, contrary to the opinion of Schoen (see *Year-Book* for 1896, p. 1086), and distinguished ora serrata of the pigment-epithelium and of the retina proper. The physiologic cup is present, and has the same appearances as in the adult. The optic-nerve fibers are nonmedullated. The fovea centralis is quite flat, and the bodies of the cones in its deepest portions are but imperfectly developed. Retinal hemorrhages are frequently encountered.

The Glands of the Ciliary Body.—Leslie Buchanan [1] finds that the pigmented cubical cells of the pars ciliaris retinæ have small processes or outgrowths, which lie adjacent to the hyaloid membrane and are structurally to be regarded as glands. They are always deeply pigmented. In cases of increased intraocular pressure these processes are in a condition of increased activity, whereas when the intraocular pressure is diminished they are less active. He therefore believes that they have to do with the secretion of intraocular fluids. The structures were first described by Treacher Collins.

Histology of the Ciliary Nerves.—G. Gutmann [2] finds that a transverse section of the ciliary nerves is elliptical in man as well as in animals. The fibers are small and medullated, though nonmedullated fibers also occur; a fine endoneurium is present. The sheath contains a small amount of pigment. The interfibrillar tissue is small in amount and finely granular. In a transverse section of the ciliary nerve 10μ in diameter 314 medullated fibers were counted.

On the Presence of Ganglion-cells in the Iris.—Authors differ in regard to the question as to whether ganglion-cells are found in the iris. N. Andogsky [3] finds bipolar and multipolar cells only in the superficial nerve-networks of the ciliary processes, and none in the iris.

THE GENITO-URINARY ORGANS.

Elastic Tissue in the Fallopian Tubes.—A. Buchstap [4] has made an examination of the oviducts of 102 individuals of different ages to determine the amount and arrangement of the elastic tissue. Some of his results are as follows: up to the end of the first year elastic fibers are found only in the peritoneum and subserous tissue, especially about the bloodvessels. From the age of 3 to 7 years the elastic tissue increases in amount, the previously existing fibers becoming larger. Fine fibers are also met with in the deep circular muscular layer. In the tubes of girls of 14 to 17 years elastic fibers are met with in the mucous membrane. In women of 21 to 45 years the elastic network is fully developed. Climacteric changes begin at about the 45th year; the elastic tissue has entirely disappeared from the mucosa by the 55th year, and to a large extent from the other layers of the tube. In senile tubes elastic tissue is found only in the serosa. Apparently the amount of elastic tissue is the same in the uterine, outer, and intermediate portions of the tube.

Anatomy of the Ureters.—Schwalbe [5] describes the ureter as consisting of an abdominal and a pelvic portion. In the abdominal portion there is always a spindle-shaped dilatation, situated just above the brim of the pelvis,

[1] Jour. Anat. and Physiol., vol. xi., N. S., part ii., p. 262, 1897.
[2] Arch. f. Anat. u. Entwickelungsgesch., xlix., 1, p. 1, 1897.
[3] Arch. f. Augenh., p. 86, Feb., 1897.   [4] Centralbl. f. Gynäk., xxi., 28, 1897.
[5] Centralbl. f. die med. Wissensch., Nov. 21, 1896.

and known as the greater dilatation; this is more marked on the right side. The narrowest part of the ureter is about 70 mm. from the kidney; this is the "superior isthmus." The "inferior isthmus" is the junction of the pelvic and abdominal portions. The pelvic portion of the tube also has fusiform enlargements. These characteristics are more marked in the female. As the above-mentioned dilatations are not present in quadruplets, the conclusion is drawn that the upper dilatation is to be looked upon as caused by the obstruction to the flow of the urine by the angle at the brim of the pelvis. Schwabel and Solger,[1] as well, found these dilatations in the fetus. They had been described previously by Luschka and others.

Pyramids of Malpighi.—Rudolph Maresch[2] reaches the following conclusions concerning the number and arrangement of the renal pyramids: 1. The kidney of man is made up of many more renculi than has previously been believed. In addition to the complete and distinct furrows seen in lobulated kidneys, there are numerous incomplete ones, so that there are in reality two or three times as many as the number (8–18) usually given. 2. For every incompletely circumscribed renculus of a lobulated kidney there is a single pyramid. 3. For each completely circumscribed renculus there are usually at least two or more pyramids. 4. The Malpighian pyramids coalesce extensively as the papillæ are approached, so that scarcely ever one papilla corresponds to one pyramid; usually two to four pyramids combine to form one papilla, and sometimes as many as nine. 5. A papilla which corresponds to several pyramids need not necessarily be unusually wide or show traces of subdivision.

Intraepithelial Glands in the Urethral Mucosa.—G. Klein and K. Groschuff[3] describe intraepithelial "glands" in the mucous membrane of female infants from 1 to 3 years of age. They exist in the form of cup-shaped cavities within the epithelium, looking very much like a single alveolus of a gland; they are quite numerous, sometimes 30 to 40 being found in a single section. Many of them resemble the taste-buds in that they have a narrow, tapering porus, and are apparently devoid of a distinct lumen; others are in wide, open communication with the surface, and their cavities are filled with a secretion. Their diameter varies from 20μ to 50μ. That they are not pathologic formations is evident from the fact of their being found within the intact epithelium, and from the regular arrangement of their cells. Whether they are to be looked upon as glandular in character or as nervous organs cannot be positively stated as yet. These structures were not found in adult females or in children under one year of age.

Lymphatic Vessels of the Urinary Bladder.—D. Gerota[4] corrects a previous assertion made by himself, that lymphatic vessels are to be found in the mucous membrane of the bladder. In the examination of more than 60 bladders he could not demonstrate, either macroscopically or microscopically, the presence of lymphatic vessels belonging to the mucous membrane. None are found in the trigonum. The few vessels found in the submucosa of the vesical neck are lymphatics of the urethra, which extend for a short distance into the neck of the bladder, but soon enter the muscular coat.

Membrana Propria of the Uriniferous Tubules.—It was shown in 1891 by Mall that the membrana propria of the uriniferous tubules consists of fine fibers of reticulated tissue. George Rühle[5] has also investigated the subject, and his results confirm in the main those of Mall. He finds that the membrana propria consists of fine, circular and longitudinal fibers, which are

---

[1] Anatom. Anz., Bd. xii., p. 347.   [2] Ibid., p. 299.
[3] Ibid., p. 197.   [4] Ibid., Bd. xiii., Nos. 21 and 22, p. 605.
[5] Arch. Anat., p. 153, 1897.

only a somewhat thicker and more regularly arranged layer of the interstitial reticulated tissue of the kidney. The layers of fibers vary in thickness in the different portions of the tubules; they are very thin around Bowman's capsule and around the tubuli contorti; around the excretory ducts they form thick, concentric layers. The fibers are not connected with the spindle-shaped cells of the connective tissue, no processes of the cells being continued into the fibers. The cells lie in more or less intimate contact with the fibers. In the kidney of the newly born infant there is no organic connection between the connective-tissue cells and the fibers of the reticulated tissue. By boiling the reticulated tissue gelatin can be obtained.

THE MUSCULAR SYSTEM.

Innervation of Muscles.—K. V. Bardeleben,[1] with Dr. Frohse, has made some important observations on the innervation of muscles, the description of the details of which are to be published in the *Handbuch* edited by Bardeleben. The authors find that the point of entrance and the branching of the nerve do not have a definite relation to the form of the muscle. Every nerve divides dichotomously, or the main trunk gives off but a single branch at any one place. Every motor nerve, prior to entering the muscle, gives off one or more nerves to vessels (vasomotor nerves). The nerve either enters with the vessels, thus forming a sort of hilus, or it enters the muscle independently of the vessels. As soon as the nerve approaches the muscle it gives off at least one recurrent branch to the proximal portion of the muscle. The points of entrance may be upon the deep surface of the muscle, at the margin, or on the surface. The nerve may enter the proximal portion of the muscle, as, for instance, in the semitendinosus—this is rare; at the junction of the upper and middle thirds; or at the middle of the muscle. It never enters the extreme distal portion. The point of entrance is assumed by the authors to be where a nerve-fiber about 0.03 mm. in thickness (just visible macroscopically) enters a muscle-bundle about 1 mm. in diameter. Intramuscular plexuses, which have not previously been described in higher vertebrates, were found in all the muscles examined, as the deltoid, biceps brachii, brachialis anticus, supinator longus, long muscles of forearm, sartorius, gracilis, etc. Frohse has found an anastomosis of the deep branch of the ulnar nerve and the branch of the median nerve supplying the flexor brevis pollicis.

Variations of the Facial Muscles and their Relation to Expression.—That a number of the muscles of expression are derived from the platysma myoïdes was first pointed out by Gegenbaur and Ruge; the platysma itself is to be regarded as an unused portion of the common muscular mass, which in its facial portion has become divided and differentiated into the muscles of expression. The occasional connection of the platysma with the orbicularis palpebrarum, zygomaticus minor, and other muscles of the face, is one of the evidences of the common origin of these muscles. The facial muscles in the lower mammals and in the anthropoids do not present the complexity and degree of development that they do in man, nor are they so independent of the platysma; the greater development of the cerebral functions of man, and the consequently more marked expression of the emotions, have led to the specialization of the facial muscles. These muscles, phylogenetically speaking, are younger than others, and are to be regarded as "progressive muscles" in the sense of Wiedersheim. They are, furthermore, quite variable,

[1] Deutsch. med. Woch , No. 23, p. 115, June 3, 1897.

and often are not alike on the two sides. In the lower races the more primitive condition of these muscles is apparent.

J. Popowsky [1] describes the facial muscles in a native of Ashantee. The platysma, besides being continuous with the zygomaticus minor, was also united to the retrahens airem ; an orbito-auricularis was also present. The levator labii superioris, zygomaticus major and miìor, and levator labii superioris alæque nasi were united to one another ; this reminds one of the condition found in the anthropoids. It can readily be surmised that the facial expressions in such an individual would be modified considerably from the lack of differentiation of these muscles. Popowsky concludes from the examination of numerous dissections that the muscles first appearing in man, viz., the zygomaticus minor, corrugator supercilii, and transversus glabellæ, are the most variable. Particularly is this the case with the first-named, and this muscle may be looked upon as passing through an intermediate phase of its development, and as not yet having reached its highest degree of specialization. The corrugator supercilii is a derivative of the orbicularis palpebrarum, and in the adult presents varying degrees of union with that muscle ; in the fetus these two muscles cannot be separated from each other. Vertical fibers of the corrugator are met with, sometimes well developed and independent ; at other times existing rather as parts of the frontalis. The existence of these vertical fibers is to be regarded as a higher degree of development of the muscle ; when they contract they produce short transverse wrinkles above the root of the nose, as seen in the expression of grief and sorrow. In some works of art these transverse furrows, which are intended to express the emotion of grief, are represented as extending entirely across the forehead ; such furrows are, of course, produced by the contraction of the frontalis, and are not correct anatomically. The occasional occurrence of the transversus glabellæ indicates a progressive development of the muscles of the forehead, these muscles being the ones concerned in the expression of some of the higher intellectual functions. When this muscle is present the upper portion of the orbicularis palpebrarum is more highly developed ; the orbicularis is, according to Duchenne, the muscle of reflection (" le muscle orbiculaire palpébral supérieur est le muscle de la réflexion, de la méditation)." [2] It is to be assumed that the appearance of the transversus glabellæ in man as a variation is due to the greater development of the upper part of the orbicularis, and that this in turn is due to the higher development of the psychical functions. It is possible that the two vertical furrows between the eyebrows seen in the portraits of some gifted persons, as Hippocrates, Blumenbach, Franklin, Beethoven, Johannes Müller, Gladstone, v. Bismarck, and others, are due to the contraction of the transversus glabellæ. In the future, it is possible that this small muscle, now occurring only as an anomaly, may be constantly present, just as the other muscles of expression now are.

A Method of Injecting the Bony Labyrinth.—Gustav Brühl [3] suggests the following method for preparing the labyrinth : macerated temporal bones are washed for several days in running water, and then decalcified, using for this purpose 2 % to 5 % hydrochloric acid solutions for the bones of the newborn, and 5 % to 10 % solutions for those of adults. After washing the decalcified bone for 24 hours in running water it is dehydrated with alcohol in gradually increasing strength ; to the alcohol is later added cupric sulfate. The fenestra rotunda and internal auditory meatus are closed with collodion,

---

[1] Internat. Monatsh. f. Anat. u. Physiol., Bd. xiv., p 149, 1897.
[2] Duchenne : Mecanisme de la physiognomie humaine, etc., pp. 19-25, Paris, 1896.
[3] Anatom. Anz., Bd. xiii., p. 93.

celloidin, cork, or, best of all, sponge ; then the needle of a hypodermic syringe, surrounded by a piece of sponge, is inserted into the oval window, and mercury to which has been added a small quantity of glycerin is injected under low pressure. The injection is continued until the mercury flows out of the aqueducts; the aqueducts are then occluded with sponge or cement. The preparation is then placed in carbol-xylol to remove any remaining water, and is then suspended in xylol. In this way preparations are secured which show plainly the topography of the internal ear ; the variations in the structure of the cochlea and semicircular canals in different animals can be shown. If the bones are weighed before and after injection, the volume of the bony labyrinth can be determined. Brühl found this to be about 120 c.mm. in the newborn and 210 c.mm. in the adult.

Method for Studying Macroscopically the Development of the Bones in the Fetus.—O. Schultze [1] describes a simple and effective method for clearing the soft tissues so that the bones can be plainly seen through them. [Th. Kölliker made use of an analogous procedure in his studies on the intermaxillary bone some years ago.] The fetus, which has been preserved in alcohol, is placed in an aqueous solution of caustic potash (3 % to 5 %), where it remains until the bones become plainly visible ; the length of time varies with the size of the fetus, the time that it has previously been in alcohol, and the degree of concentration of the potash solution. In large fetuses it is necessary to remove the brain and viscera. The preparations can be preserved in a 2 % solution of formalin, to which 30 % of glycerin is added.

MISCELLANEOUS.

Development of the Mammary Gland.—E. Kallius [2] has described a human embryo about 15 mm. in length, in which the "milk-line," first observed in pig embryos by O. Schultze, was present. Extending from just below the upper extremity, along each side of the trunk in the midaxillary line, for a distance of 1.5 mm., was a ridge-like elevation of the epidermis ; it was about $\frac{1}{3}$ mm. in width and $\frac{1}{4}$ mm. in height. No local enlargement of the ridge was present. Microscopically it is seen that the entire ridge is due to a thickening of the epithelium ; this thickening of the epithelium is most marked in the situation of the future mammary gland, and here the cells extend downward into the mesodermic tissue. As the caudal extremity of the embryo is approached the ridge gradually becomes less conspicuous. Kallius regards this ridge as the earliest, or, at any rate, a very early stage, of the developing mammary gland. Whether it is present in all embryos will have to be determined by future observations. The subject is an interesting one in connection with supernumerary mammæ and nipples. Hugo Schmidt [3] has observed similar elevations in two embryos of about the same age as those of Kallius ; the ridges were asymmetrical. It is probable that the "Milchleiste" of man is a suddenly appearing and rapidly disappearing structure, as Kallius expresses it.

Placenta.—Th. W. Eden,[4] from his studies of the placenta in the early and in the late stages of pregnancy, concludes that this organ toward the end of pregnancy shows degenerative and senile changes, just as the organs present in old age. Degenerative changes in the vessels—*i. e.*, endarteritis—and infarcts are met with. Atrophy and degeneration of epithelial structures occur.

[1] Grundriss d. Entwickelungsgesch. d. Menschen.
[2] Merkel u. Bonnet's Anatom. Hefte, Bd. viii., H. i , p. 155, 1897.
[3] Anatom. Anz., Bd. xi., p. 702.   [4] Jour. Pathol. and Bacteriol., p. 265, 1896.

These changes in the "senile" placenta are responsible for intrauterine death of the fetus in some cases.

Histology of Adenoid Tissue.—Erwin Hoehl[1] reaches the following conclusions in his investigations of the adenoid tissue in various organs: 1. The connective-tissue framework of the organs belonging to the lymphatic apparatus consists, after it has reached complete development, partly of collagen-containing fibers and partly of a reticulum destitute of cells. 2. The trabeculæ of this reticulum are composed of very many fine fibers of equal size; some of these are united into bundles, others spread out like a fan; they are imbedded in a homogeneous ground-substance. 3. The finer trabeculæ are surrounded by elastic fibers which wind spirally about them, while in the larger trabeculæ the bundles of elastic fibers can be seen in the interior. 4. In many places, for instance in the lymph-sinuses, the trabeculæ are covered with cells which are morphologically and physiologically related to endothelium; in other places the trabeculæ are not covered with cells. The trabeculæ form the supporting framework of the organ. 5. Essential differences in different species of animals (man, ox, dog, cat) are not found. The author concludes that the artificial digestion of histologic specimens with trypsin does not produce artefacts if the process is carefully carried out.

The Mammary Gland in its Active and in its Resting Condition.—Josef Szabo[2] distinguishes three states of the secreting cells of the mamma: 1st, that of absolute inactivity or rest; 2d, that of activity; and, 3d, that of relative inactivity, in which the gland is prepared for secretion. The active gland-cells can be distinguished from those in a state of relative inactivity by a characteristic peripheral grouping of the chromatin. He finds that the epithelium of the gland is always in a single layer, and believes that the cells in the exercise of their function do not perish, but remain capable of secreting during the entire period of lactation. Mitotic changes were found only in the glands of pregnant animals and in those examined in the first few days of secretory activity; no mitoses were seen after the gland had been active for several days.

Form of the Follicles of the Thyroid Gland.—J. J. Streif[3] finds that along with the rounded, oval, and polyhedral follicles of the gland there are also forms which closely resemble the tubules of a tubular gland, though the tubules are closed at each end. Some of the vesicles have secondary outgrowths, and at times two vesicles of equal size are in open communication with each other. A system of canals or ducts, however, is not found. The author conceives that the gland originates as a branched tubular gland. The secreting parts are not connected by ducts as in a gland, however, for the secretion has to escape through the walls of the vesicles, and thus finds its way into the lymph-spaces of the connective-tissue septa.

Prepatellar Bursæ.—Bize[4] describes the bursæ and connective-tissue spaces in front of the patella He states that the connective-tissue spaces are subcutaneous, subaponeurotic, and subtendinous. A superficial mucous bursa, lying in the superficial fascia over the lower extremity of the patella, is found in 88 % of cases; it is usually single. A subaponeurotic bursa lying between the fascia lata and the tendon of the quadriceps is found in 95 % of cases; it lies most often over the lower and inner portions of the patella. A subtendinous bursa, lying between the two portions of the tendon of the quadriceps,

[1] Arch. f. Anat. u. Entwickelungsgesch., H. 1 u. 2, p. 133, 1897.
[2] Arch. f. Anat. u. physiol. Anat., Abth. 5 u. 6, p. 352, 1896.
[3] Arch. f. Mikroskop. Anat., vol. xlviii., p. 579, 1897.
[4] Jour. de l'Anat. et de la Physiol., xxxii., p. 85, 1896.

over the inner portion of the patella, is found in 80 % of cases. These bursæ, or the spaces from which they originate, are formed in the latter half of intrauterine life. Hygromata of these 'bursæ are due to an accumulation of fluid in them. [Gruber, Linhart, and Luschka long ago described multilocular and superimposed prepatellar bursæ; their presence would account for the recurrence of bursal swellings after excision.]

Congenital Anonychia.—Paul Jacob[1] records a case of this kind, which, on account of its great rarity, is deserving of being mentioned. The patient, a boy, 14 years of age, had no nails on either the fingers or the toes. In place of them there was delicate skin. No other congenital anomalies existed, though the teeth were defective. Two sisters of the boy had the same defect of the nails, but the parents had normally formed nails. Anatomically and embryologically it was impossible to explain satisfactorily the anomaly.

[1] Deutsch. med. Woch., Dec. 10, 1896; Vereins Beil., No. 32.

PHYSIOLOGY.

By G. N. STEWART, M. D.,

OF CLEVELAND, OHIO.

THE BLOOD, THE LYMPH, AND THE CIRCULATION.

Coagulation of the Blood.—[This subject has been further illuminated by a vast amount of painstaking research during the past year.] The mechanism of the anticoagulant action of albumose has been to a certain extent elucidated by C. Delezenne,[1] who finds that when a solution of this substance is caused to circulate through the liver a body is formed which is capable of suspending the coagulation of the blood *in vitro*, a property which [as is well known] albumose itself does not possess. A similar, or perhaps identical, body is produced when the serum of the snake is made to pass through the liver.[2] He accordingly supposes that this anticoagulant substance is the product of a secretive reaction of the organism, and particularly of the hepatic cells [a view originally brought forward by Gley and Pachon]. Incidentally he confirms the result of Starling (*Year-Book* for 1897, p. 1162), that ligation of the lymphatics of the liver does not prevent the anticoagulant action of "peptone," and rejects the counterstatement of Gley and Pachon,[3] who, however, reaffirm their view [but without bringing forward anything materially new]. On the other hand, Athanasiu and Carvallo[4] lay stress on the fact that "peptone blood" will always ultimately coagulate if time enough be given, and interpret this [too hastily, we think] as a proof that it is not the presence of an anticoagulant substance which hinders coagulation, but something else. This "something else" they find in the lack of fibrin-ferment, due to the profound modification in the formed elements of the blood, and particularly in the increased mobility of the leukocytes, in virtue of which they wander out of the vessels into the tissue-spaces. They deny that the leukocytes are destroyed [as Löwit, Wright, and others had stated]. Fano,[5] however, defends his position that there is no want of fibrin-ferment in "peptone blood," and Dastre and Floresco[6] bring forward evidence to the same effect, and assert that it is the over-alkalinity of the "peptone plasma" which prevents it from coagulating. Athanasiu and Carvallo[7] reply that peptone plasma is certainly not more alkaline than normal plasma, and accuse Dastre and Floresco of inaccuracy in comparing the alkalinity of peptone *plasma* with that of normal *serum*, which is less alkaline than normal *plasma ;* and they clinch the matter by showing that no fibrin-ferment can be obtained by Schmidt's method from peptone plasma [thus bringing us round once more, after so much work and so much controversy, to the already ancient view of Wooldridge. It is evident that much remains to be cleared up before the last word shall have been spoken on this question. In the meantime, it seems

---

[1] Arch. de Physiol., p. 655, July, 1896.
[3] Ibid., p. 715, July, 1896.   [4] Ibid., p. 866, Oct., 1896.
[6] Ibid., p. 216.

[2] Ibid., p. 646, July, 1897.
[5] Ibid., p. 239, Jan., 1897.
[7] Ibid., p. 375, Apr., 1897.

to us that no theory can be complete which does not take account of the facts, that injection of albumose may under certain conditions, some of which are known and others as yet undiscovered, produce not retardation, but hastening of coagulation, and that if a first injection fails to be followed by the ordinary anticoagulant effect, a second, repeated under conditions which would usually insure success, is equally ineffective. It might be plausibly suggested that if the immediate and most common effect of the presence of albumose in the blood be to stimulate the hepatic, or other, cells to the secretion of a substance that hinders coagulation, the organism in its turn reacts against the presence of this substance, and makes an effort to protect itself by the production of a second body with fibrinoplastic powers. In this case the final result of an injection of albumose would be determined, in any given case, by the relative intensity of two antagonistic processes.]

[The old statement of Claude Bernard and others that the blood of the hepatic vein coagulates more slowly than the venous blood in general, which might seem to indicate that even under normal circumstances, and in the absence of any artificial stimulus, the liver produces an anticoagulant substance, is put in doubt] by the experiments of N. Paulesco,[1] who failed to detect any such difference in the blood of fasting dogs.

· Arthus and Huber[2] show that the primary cleavage-products of the digestion of gelatin and casein have the same effect as the fibrin proteoses in preventing coagulation.

Pickering,[3] working with Norway hares, some specimens of which are albino in summer and pigmented in winter, has found that intravascular clotting is caused by the injection of nucleoproteids or certain synthesized colloids during the pigmented, but not during the albino condition. [This is an observation of great interest, because it brings the previously observed difference between albino and pigmented rabbits in regard to intravascular coagulation into relation with a periodically recurring metabolic change. Not less curious, although strangely overlooked till this late day] are the facts reported by C. Delezenne,[4] that the blood of birds, when drawn without coming into contact with the tissues, coagulates with marked slowness, and that coagulation is greatly hastened by the addition of extracts of the muscles or other organs.

Blood-pigment.—A. Gamgee[5] has reinvestigated, by the aid of photography, and greatly extended Soret's discovery of the absorption-band in the extreme violet, which, according to him, is much more characteristic of hemoglobin and several of its derivatives than any of the bands in the less refrangible portions of the spectrum. [It is of considerable theoretic interest that] turacin, the copper-containing pigment first investigated by Church, shows a precisely similar band (Gamgee);[6] while of some practical importance is the announcement by A. Jolles[7] of a method adapted both to the scientific and the clinical estimation of the iron in small quantities of blood. The method depends on a comparison of the color of a solution of ammonium sulphocyanid, to which a known amount of iron has been added, with that of a similar solution after addition of the ash of a known quantity of blood.

Hemopoiesis.—To the vexed question of the part played by the spleen in the formation of the blood, J. Laudenbach[8] makes an elaborate series of contributions. He supports the orthodox conclusion that the spleen takes a

---

[1] Arch. de Physiol., p. 21, Jan., 1897. [2] Ibid., p. 857, Apr., 1897.
[3] Jour. of Physiol., vol. xx., p. 310. [4] Arch. de Physiol., p. 333, Apr., 1897.
[5] Lancet, Aug. 15, 1896. [6] Ibid., p. 111, July 11, 1896. [7] Pflüger's Archiv. Bd. lxv., p. 579.
[8] Arch. de Physiol., pp. 693, 724, July, 1896; p. 200, Jan., 1897; pp. 385, 398, Apr., 1897.

share in the synthesis of the hemoglobin and the development of the red corpuscles, although after its removal compensation is to a certain extent established, particularly by the increased hemopoietic activity of the bone-marrow. W. S. Hall and M. D. Eubank[1] state, among other interesting results, that regeneration of the blood after hemorrhage takes place more rapidly if the hemorrhage has been followed by **transfusion of an artificial serum.** [It is, indeed, well known that injections of this kind bring about, in addition to local effects within the vascular system, general metabolic changes. Thus] A. Charrin and A. Desgrez[2] assert that even solutions of the mineral constituents of serum cause when injected into the veins of rabbits a slight elevation in the quantity of urea excreted, while entire serum causes a marked increase; and they suppose that some of the common effects of the new serum-therapy may be due to the mineral substances, since these are practically the same in all artificial serums. [But the composition of the diet does not seem to have been sufficiently controlled; and it is hardly permissible in observations of this kind to be content with a mere estimation of urea.]

The effects of the introduction into the blood of large quantities of solutions of NaCl and Na_2CO_3 have been studied by Bosc and Vedel[3] in normal animals and in dogs affected by intravenous injections of bacillus coli.[4] They conclude that the 0.7% NaCl solution has the minimum harmful and the maximum physiologic effect, although much stronger solutions can be borne. [The writer of this abstract has found no harmful results in dogs after the injection of solutions of NaCl of the strength of 2% to 5% into the blood, and these strong solutions would seem to have the advantage of attracting water from the lymph-spaces, and thus for a considerable time of automatically increasing the volume of the circulating fluid.]

Otto Weiss[5] has made the remarkable observation that when the serum of a male rabbit was injected into the veins of a female rabbit albuminuria followed, while this was not the case when the serum was injected into a male animal. He believes that a true sexual difference is at the bottom of this phenomenon, and that it was not merely an accidental result. [The similar observation of Favoret, who saw albuminuria when the serum of a bitch was injected into a dog, certainly speaks in favor of this interpretation, but the number of experiments is too small to establish a definite conclusion.]

Permeability of the Corpuscles.—The relations between the corpuscles and the plasma have been illustrated by numerous researches since our last report. H. J. Hamburger[6] states that in the blood of the jugular vein the volume of the corpuscles, both colored and colorless, is greater than in the blood of the carotid artery, so that in the living body a rhythmic variation in the volume of the corpuscles takes place; they swell in the systemic and shrink in the pulmonary capillaries. He explains the phenomenon by the assumption that under the influence of CO_2 the substances which attract water increase to a greater degree in the corpuscles than in the serum, so that there is a disturbance of osmotic equilibrium. This can only be restored by the passage of water into the corpuscles. He attributes to these changes a certain significance in nutrition [which it is difficult to deny, if the variations in volume be admitted. And, indeed, there is no doubt that such variations can be produced outside the body by the alternate action of CO_2 and O, as v. Limbeck and Gürber had previously shown], and as G. N. Stewart[7] has incidentally

---

[1] Jour. Exper. Med., vol. i., No. 4, 1896, and N. Am. Pract., May, 1897.
[2] Arch. de Physiol., p. 780, Oct., 1896.   [3] Ibid., p. 937.   [4] Ibid., p. 44, Jan., 1897.
[5] Pflüger's Archiv, Bd lxv., p. 215.   [6] Zeit. f. Biol., Bd. xxxv., pp. 252 and 289, 1897.
[7] Jour. Boston Soc. of Med. Sci., June 3, 1897; Centralbl. f. Physiol., p. 332, Aug. 7, 1897.

to us that no theory can be complete whit does not take account of the facts, that injection of albumose may under ceain conditions, some of which are known and others as yet undiscovered, pr!uce not retardation, but hastening of coagulation, and that if a first injectioniuls to be followed by the ordinary anticoagulant effect, a second, repeated u ter conditions which would usually insure success, is equally ineffective. It night be plausibly suggested that if the immediate and most common effecof the presence of albumose in the blood be to stimulate the hepatic, or othei cells to the secretion of a substance that hinders coagulation, the organism in turn reacts against the presence of this substance, and makes an effort to rotect itself by the production of a second body with fibrinoplastic powers. n this case the final result of an injection of albumose would be determine, in any given case, by the relative intensity of two antagonistic processes.]

[The old statement of Claude Bernat and others that the blood of the hepatic vein coagulates more slowly than ie venous blood in general, which might seem to indicate that even under nmal circumstances, and in the absence of any artificial stimulus, the liver produces an anticoagulant substance, is put in doubt] by the experiments of N. 'aulesco,[1] who failed to detect any such difference in the blood of fasting do

· Arthus and Huber[2] show that the priary cleavage-products of the digestion of gelatin and casein have the same feet as the fibrin proteoses in preventing coagulation.

Pickering,[3] working with Norway hes, some specimens of which are albino in summer and pigmented in wter, has found that intravascular clotting is caused by the injection of n leoproteids or certain synthesized colloids during the pigmented, but not dung the albino condition. [This is an observation of great interest, because t brings the previously observed difference between albino and pigmentec rabbits in regard to intravascular coagulation into relation with a periodical recurring metabolic change. Not less curious, although strangely overlooke till this late day] are the facts reported by C. Delezenne,[4] that the blood obirds, when drawn without coming into contact with the tissues, coagulates wh marked slowness, and that coagulation is greatly hastened by the additionof extracts of the muscles or other organs.

Blood-pigment.—A. Gamgee[5] has investigated, by the aid of photography, and greatly extended Soret's discory of the absorption-band in the extreme violet, which, according to him, ismuch more characteristic of hemoglobin and several of its derivatives than ay of the bands in the less refrangible portions of the spectrum. [It is of nsiderable theoretic interest that] turaćin, the copper-containing pigment fir investigated by Church, shows a precisely similar band (Gamgee);[6] while some practical importance is the announcement by A. Jolles[7] of a methodadapted both to the scientific and the clinical estimation of the iron in sma quantities of blood. The method depends on a comparison of the color o a solution of ammonium sulphocyanid, to which a known amount of irl has been added, with that of a similar solution after addition of the ash c a known quantity of blood.

Hemopoiesis.—To the vexed questic of the part played by the spleen in the formation of the blood, J. Laudenich[8] makes an elaborate series of contributions. He supports the orthodox nclusion that the spleen takes a

[1] Arch. de Physiol., p. 21, Jan., 1897.   [2] Ibid., p. 857, Apr., 1897.
[3] Jour. of Physiol., vol. xx., p. 310.   Arch. de Physiol., p. 333, Apr., 1897.
[5] Lancet, Aug. 15, 1896.   [6] Ibid., p. 111, July 1 1896.   [7] Pflüger's Archiv. Bd. lxv., p. 579.
[8] Arch. de Physiol., pp. 693, 724, July, 1896; p200, Jan., 1897; pp. 385, 398, Apr., 1897.

share in the synthesis of the hæoglobin and the development of the red corpuscles, although after its remcal compensation is to a certain extent established, particularly by the incresed hemopoietic activity of the bone-marrow.
W. S. Hall and M. D. Euban,[1] state, among other interesting results, that
regeneration of the blood after hemorrhage takes place more rapidly if the
hemorrhage has been followed by **transfusion of an artificial serum.**
[It is, indeed, well known that injections of this kind bring about, in addition
to local effects within the vascul system, general metabolic changes. Thus]
A. Charrin and A. Desgrez[2] as rt that even solutions of the mineral constituents of serum cause when injcted into the veins of rabbits a slight elevation in the quantity of urea exreted, while entire serum causes a marked
increase; and they suppose that sue of the common effects of the new serum-
therapy may be due to the minerᵉ substances, since these are practically the
same in all artificial serums. [Bt the composition of the diet does not seem
to have been sufficiently controlleᶜ and it is hardly permissible in observations of this kind to be content wih a mere estimation of urea.]

The effects of the introduction nto the blood of large quantities of solutions of $NaCl$ and Na_2CO_3 have ben studied by Bosc and Vedel[3] in normal
animals and in dogs affected by intravenous injections of bacillus coli.[4] They
conclude that the 0.7 % $NaCl$ so tion has the minimum harmful and the
maximum physiologic effect. althorh much stronger solutions can be borne.
[The writer of this abstract has foıd no harmful results in dogs after the
injection of solutions of $NaCl$ of tl strength of 2 % to 5 % into the blood,
and these strong solutions would sm to have the advantage of attracting
water from the lvı phspaces. and ths for a considerable time of automatically
increasing the v f the circulaⁿg fluid.]

Otto Weiss ı rdłᵉ the remarkble observation that when the serum of
a male rabbı into the vıns of a female rabbit albuminuria followed. whi t casᵉ hen the serum was injected into a male
aniıal. Hᵉ tхtl difference is at the bottom of this phe-
nomeı m. aı lyın accidental result. [The similar observation ı ı mıuria when the serum of a bitch was injected ınto rᶜınly specaks in tᵣor of this interpretation, but the number of exⁱ ı snaı. tᵒ estʳlish a definite conclusion.]

Permeability of the Corpuscls.—The relations between the corpuscles and tl ı beᵉn illᵘstratᵗ by numerous researches since our last
report. H. J. H r statᵉ thᵉ in the blood of the jugular vein the
volum cı b thᵉ colᵣecand colorless, is greater than in the
blood cf tl ı rᵉıv. so that in he living body a rhythmic varia'
in the volu ı cf t comped cıkes ace; they swell in the systemic
shrink in thᵉ pıltı ıry capıllariᵉs. Ie explains the phenomenon by
assumption thıt uı lr the influᵉnce cf O, the substances whⁱch extract wate
incᵣeasᵉ to a grᵉ ıterᵈ gnᵉ in thᵉ corpules than in the s   there is
a dᵉsturbanᵉv cf entı tᵉᵉquilıʳıum. Tis can only be rᵉ   ssage
of water intᵒ thᵉᵉ rpısᵘlᵉs. Hᵉ attribᵤes to these chanᵍ   ᵗᵘⁱfi-
cnᵉ in nutritⁱ ıı [whⁱch iⁱ difficult tᵈeny, if the variᵃ   ᵛbe
admitted. Aı l. tl l. tlᵣˑ iˑ no dᵉbt that such varᵢ
dıᵈ outˑıdᵉ thᵉ lˑlˑ y thᵉ alternatᵉactⁱon of CO_2 and ˑ
and Gırlkᵣr h ł pᵉ ᵉ ˑˑ showⁿ]. anᶜas **G. N. Stewart**[7] ˑ

[1] r Fıper M   ˑˑ ł ˑand. **Am. Pract.,** May, 1897.
ˑˑ ˑˑ ˑ ˑ [3] Ił., p. **987.**   [4] Ibid., p. 44,
[5] Zk. f. **Biol.,** Bd. xxxv., pp. 252
ˑł r ˑ Ar   ˑˑ ˑˑ łtₑ 3. 1897 **Centralbl. f.** Physiol., p. 332, ˑ

demonstrated by a perfectly different method in the course of a research on the electric conductivity of blood. He finds that the conductivity of blood that has been reduced is somewhat less than that of the same blood when saturated with oxygen, and further that the conductivity of one and the same sample of defibrinated blood increases as the relative volume of the corpuscles in it decreases. The explanation of this is that, in comparison with the serum, the corpuscles are nonconductors. The electrical conductivity and, therefore, the molecular concentration (as regards the inorganic salts) of serum do not vary much in different animals of the same species, nor even in the different mammalian species investigated. On these facts Stewart has founded a method for rapidly estimating the relative volume of plasma and corpuscles in blood. His results have been confirmed by the independent investigations of W. Roth[1] and by those of St. Bugarsky and F. Tangl.[2] The fact that the red blood-corpuscles are nonconductors so long as they are intact, raises the question whether or not they are permeable to such ions as exist in serum. An answer to this question is attempted in the experiments of H. Koeppe,[3] S. G. Hedin,[4] and C. Eykman ;[5] and while they are all agreed that the ions Na, K, and SO_4 cannot pass through the corpuscles, there is still some dispute in regard to others.

Osmosis and Lymph-formation.—[There is apparently some slackening in the activity of research on this subject, and most of the papers that have appeared during the current year have been devoted to the discussion of facts already known or theories already formulated.] H. J. Hamburger[6] again takes up his parable in favor of the secretion-theory of Heidenhain. W. Cohnstein[7] endeavors to repel the assaults of Hamburger, Mendel, and others on the filtration-theory of Ludwig, while S. J. Meltzer and I. Adler,[8] on the cognate topic of absorption from the peritoneal cavity, assume a position midway between that of Heidenhain and that of Cohnstein (*Year-Book* for 1897, p. 1166). They insist on the importance of the part played by the tissue-spaces, which they look upon as a system of reservoirs anatomically independent of both blood-capillaries and lymph-capillaries, although capable of interchange with both. [We doubt, however, whether there is any good histologic basis for this view] Lazarus-Barlow[9] continues his work on the "initial rate of osmosis," which, however, Hamburger[10] criticises on the ground that in this "initial-rate of osmosis," as determined by Barlow, both the permeability of the membrane and the rate of diffusion are mixed up with the true power of attraction of water by the solution.

The Beat of the Heart.—[The proofs of the myogenic origin of the cardiac beat seem to be speedily accumulating.] Engelmann,[11] in a series of papers, accompanied by a colossal bibliography, works out in great detail the line of investigation so brilliantly begun, now more than a dozen years ago, by Gaskell, and concludes in favor of the muscular origin of the heart-beat both in the adult and in the embryo. W. T. Porter[12] makes the weighty observation that a portion of the apex of the ventricle (of the cat), presumably ganglion-free, connected with the rest of the heart only by its blood-vessels, continues to beat with a rhythm of its own for a considerable time. O. Lau-

[1] Centralbl. f. Physiol., p. 271, July 10, 1897.   [2] Ibid , pp. 297 and 301, July 24, 1897.
[3] Pflüger's Archiv, Bd. lxvii., p. 189.   [4] Ibid., Bd. lxviii., p. 229.
[5] Ibid., p. 58.   [6] Arch. f. (Anat. u) Physiol., p. 132. Apr 9. 1897.
[7] Verhandl. d. Berlin. Physiol. Ges. ; Arch. f. (Anat. u.) Physiol.. p. 379, July 2, 1896.
[8] Jour. Exper Med., p. 529, July. 1896.   [9] Jour. of Physiol., vol. xx., p. 145.
[10] Arch. f. (Anat. u.) Physiol., p 137, Apr. 9, 1897.
[11] Pflüger's Archiv, Bd. lxv., pp. 109 and 535.
[12] Jour. Exper. Med., vol. ii., No. 4, p. 391, 1897.

gendorff,[1] proceeding with his investigations on the action of the isolated mammalian heart, comes to the conclusion [an important one, if correct] that in fever the increase in the temperature of the blood is an influential factor in the acceleration of the heart. No removable heart-standstill, such as is readily induced in the frog's heart, can be caused in the heart of a warm-blooded animal. P. Botazzi[2] puts forward the ingenious theory [for which, however, we do not think he produces any real evidence] that the oscillations of tonus [previously described by others] in the auricles of the frog's heart are simply due to contractions and expansions of the sarcoplasmatic part of the muscular tissue, independent of the contractions of the fibrillæ [which almost everybody else believes to be the only contractile portions of the fiber].

Heart-sounds.—Sir Richard Quain[3] is responsible for the novel view that the first sound of the heart is due, not to vibrations of the auriculoventricular valves, nor to the muscle-sound of the contracting ventricles, but to the impact of the blood on the semilunar valves at the moment of the systole, and the resistance to its onward movement which it experiences there. [While great weight must be given to an authority so distinguished, and while some of the facts which he cites seem to favor such a theory, yet it appears to us that before it can be accepted it must be sufficiently elaborated to explain, among other things: 1. How it is that of two sounds produced (by hypothesis) in the same situation, one should be heard best over the position of the cardiac impulse and the other in the aortic area. 2. How it is that, since the auriculoventricular valves are during the ventricular systole exposed to the same conditions (high pressure on the ventricular, and low pressure on the auricular surface) as the semilunar valves are exposed to during the ventricular relaxation (high pressure on the arterial and low pressure on the ventricular surface), and since their structure is similar, and since both offer resistance to the effort of a stream of blood to regurgitate, a sound should arise only in the vicinity of one of the sets of valves. 3. How it is that the first sound is not *always* altered in aortic incompetence unaccompanied by aortic stenosis.] Possibly some light may be thrown upon such questions by the photographic method of recording the heart-sounds, which has been further elaborated by A. de Holowinski.[4]

Output of the Heart.—G. N. Stewart[5] has measured, by a new electric method, the output of the heart in more than 20 dogs, ranging in weight from less than 5 to about 35 kilos. He arrives at the conclusion that the older estimates of Vierordt, Volkmann, and others are too high, while the more modern estimates of Tigerstedt and Stolnikow are too low. He calculates that the average output of the left ventricle of a man weighing 70 kilos would, under the conditions of his experiments, not exceed 80 c.c. per beat. This agrees fairly well with the results of Zuntz and Schumburg,[6] who, comparing, by the aid of the *x*-rays, the size of the heart at rest and during severe muscular work, and using the data obtained by Zuntz on the horse, estimate that during work twice as much blood (120 c.c.) may be ejected from the left ventricle at each beat as during rest (60 c.c.).

The Cardiac Nerves.—[The common belief, founded on the experiments of Baxt, that there is no antagonism between the inhibitory and augmentor nerves of the heart must, so far as warm-blooded animals are concerned, be modified in the light of experiments of R. Hunt,[7] who states that

[1] Pflüger's Archiv, Bd. lxvi., p. 355.   [2] Jour. of Physiol., vol. xxi., p. 1.
[3] Lancet, p. 1672, June 19, 1897.   [4] Arch. de Physiol., p. 893, Oct., 1896.
[5] Science, Jan. 22, 1897; Brit. Assoc. Rep., 1897; Jour. of Physiol., vol. xxii, No. 3, 1897.
[6] Verhandl. d. Berlin. Physiol. Ges., Arch. f. (Anat. u.) Physiol., p. 550, Dec. 28, 1896.
[7] Jour. Exper. Med., p. 151, Mar., 1897.

in all cases the result of simultaneous stimulation of the two nerves is approximately the algebraic sum of the effects of stimulating them separately. [This result certainly does not hold in all its generality for an animal like the frog, for the author of this abstract[1] could only detect such an antagonism under special conditions, and then chiefly in the action of the nerves on the ventricle.] L. J. J. Muskens[2] believes he has proved the existence of **reflexes set up in the ventricle** of the frog's heart [as Knoll had previously done for the rabbit].

The **voluntary acceleration of the heart** is the theme of a paper by H. Van de Velde,[3] who asserts that the power is present, in rudiment at least, in a very large number of persons, and that it can be cultivated, although it is a dangerous acquisition.

Vasomotor Nerves.—Ch. A. François-Franck and L. Hallion[4] have made a beautiful series of experiments on the vasomotor innervation of the liver. They enclosed the organ in a plethysmograph, and recorded the blood-pressure at the same time in the portal vein and the hepatic artery. They find, among other results, that excitation of ordinary sensory nerves causes almost constantly, and excitation of the visceral sensory fibres in the vagus occasionally, a reflex constriction of the branches of the portal vein. A similar reflex regulation of the circulation in the pancreas has been demonstrated by the same observers;[5] while A. Biedl[6] announces the discovery in the splanchnics not only of vasodilator, but also of secretory fibers for the suprarenal capsules. [But we must say that the evidence he presents for the existence of this latter group is of the scantiest.]

METABOLISM, NUTRITION, AND DIETETICS.

Internal Secretion.—[No striking discovery in this subject has marked the past year, but our knowledge has been widened in various directions.]

Thyroid and Parathyroid.—[While it must be admitted, as Blumreich and Jacoby[7] assert, that there is a marked difference in histologic structure between the parathyroids and the thyroids, and while it has certainly not been proved that this difference diminishes when the thyroids proper are removed, yet we must characterize as too absolute the statement of these observers, that excision of the parathyroids in the rabbit has no influence on the result of thyroidectomy. For the experiments of Gley,[8] Moussu,[9] Vasalle and Generali,[10] and Rouxeau,[11] have shown [conclusively, in our opinion] that in the dog, cat, and rabbit the presence of the parathyroids is sufficient to prevent the appearance of the symptoms characteristic of complete thyroidectomy, while this is not the result if the parathyroids be removed and the thyroids proper retained. W. Edmunds[12] also finds that the presence of a single parathyroid in the dog is sufficient to prevent death, while in the absence of both parathyroids at least 40 % of the thyroid tissue must be left if life is to be maintained. [But he appears to speak only of the external parathyroids, and if he left 40 % of the thyroid, in all probability one or other of Kohn's "internal parathyroid bodies" would, sometimes at any rate, be included in this remnant.]

---

[1] Jour. of Physiol., vol. xiii., p. 117.   [2] Pflüger's Archiv, Bd. 66, p. 328.   [3] Ibid., p. 232.
[4] Arch. de Physiol., pp. 908 and 923, Oct., 1896; pp. 434 and 448, Apr., 1897.
[5] Ibid., p. 660, July, 1897.   [6] Pflüger's Archiv, Bd. 67, p. 443.
[7] Year-Book for 1897, p. 1169; Pflüger's Archiv, Bd. 64, p. 1, July 8, 1896.
[8] Ibid., Bd. 66, p. 308; Compt. rend., de la Soc. de Biol., p. 18, Jan. 9, 1897; Jan. 16, p. 46.
[9] Ibid., p. 44.   [10] Arch. Ital. de Biol., vols. xxv. and xxvi., 1896.
[11] Compt. rend. de la Soc. de Biol., p. 17, Jan. 9, 1897; Arch. de Physiol., p. 136, Jan., 1897.
[12] Proc. Physiol. Soc., June 27, 1896; Jour. of Physiol., vol. xx.

It is still uncertain what the active constituent of the thyroid secretion really is, although, for the moment, Baumann's thyriodin[1] has advanced to the place of honor among the artificial products. E. Wormser,[2] however, denies that it has any effect in preserving the life of dogs after thyroidectomy. He goes so far as to say that none of the substances as yet isolated from the thyroid is alone able to replace the gland itself, but that they must be all given together in order to do this. That thyriodin has a smaller effect on the general metabolism, as measured by the increased production of CO_2, than the fresh gland has, was shown by Magnus-Levy, and has been confirmed by F. Voit.[3] The excretion of nitrogen is markedly increased by both, but, according to B. Schöndorff,[4] only after a certain amount of the body-fat has first been used up. Hutchison[5] finds that the "colloid" can be split up by gastric digestion into a body consisting of a proteid in union with iodin, and another substance containing iodin but no proteid. The latter is less active than the former.

I. Ott[6] confirms the observation of Oliver and Schäfer that thyroid extract diminishes the rate of the heart and lowers the blood-pressure. It also produces a rise of temperature. A. Exner[7] has made the statement that after extirpation of one thyroid lobe (in the cat) division of the superior and inferior laryngeal nerves on the opposite side caused the tetany which is so characteristic a consequence of complete thyroidectomy. [This would be an important observation, if confirmed, as it would indicate the existence of a nervous control of the internal secretion of the thyroid, or at least the possibility of a loss of its function when its vasomotor nerves were paralyzed. But we confess that the experiments do not wear a very convincing aspect, even when taken in conjunction with] Katzenstein's discovery[8] that histologic changes are caused in the gland by section of these nerves.

Suprarenal Capsules.—N. de Dominicis[9] [with nearly the whole physiologic world against him] still defends the theory that the fatal result of extirpation of the suprarenals is due to what he calls a "neurotic cause," and not to any chemic action of poisons produced in the organism and normally neutralized or destroyed by the secretion of the glands. [It must be said, however, that the present trend of research is more and more in favor of the "chemic" theory. Thus] Szymonowicz[10] confirms in most essential particulars, in an independent research, the statements of Oliver and Schäfer,[11] and extends their work by showing that the blood coming from the veins of the capsules causes, when injected into the circulation, the same phenomena as the extracts of the organ, although [as was to be expected] in a less degree. It is true that Szymonowicz, like Cybulski, believes that the main action of the substance which causes a rise of blood-pressure is on the vasomotor center, and that Gottlieb[12] sees in the ganglion-cells of the heart its chief point of attack, while Oliver and Schäfer have demonstrated a vasoconstriction of peripheral origin, which has been confirmed by the observation of Bates[13] that long-continued pallor of the conjunctiva can be caused by dropping a small quantity of the extract into the eye. But in regard to the production of some active substance or substances by the capsules there is substantial agreement, and a certain degree of progress has even been made in their isolation and

[1] Year-Book for 1897, p. 1169. [2] Pflüger's Archiv, Bd. 67, p. 505.
[3] Zeit. f. Biol., xxxv., p. 116, 1897. [4] Pflüger's Archiv, Bd. 67, p. 395.
[5] Brit. Med. Jour., Jan. 23, 1897; Jour. of Physiol., vol. xx., p. 474.
[6] Med. Bull., Oct., 1896. [7] Pflüger's Archiv, Bd. 68, p. 100.
[8] Verhandl. d. Berlin. Physiol. Ges., Arch. f. (Anat. u.) Physiol., p. 371, July 30, 1897.
[9] Wien. med. Woch., No. 1, 1897. [10] Pflüger's Archiv, Bd. 64, p. 97.
[11] Year-Book for 1897, p. 1168. [12] Arch. f. Exper. Path. u. Pharmakol., p. 99, 1896.
[13] N. Y. Med. Jour., lxiii., p. 647.

recognition by chemic tests. J. J. Abel and A. C. Crawford, *e. g.*,[1] have shown, by separating the constituent which raises the blood-pressure in the form of a benzoyl compound, that it is a substance with basic properties, and must probably be classed with the pyrrol compounds or with the pyridin bases or alkaloids. B. Moore[2] also suggests that the active substance is a pyridin derivative. It seems certain that it is not a pyrocatechin compound, as Mühlmann[3] supposed, although it is possible that some pyrocatechin is present in the gland, but, in any case, according to P. Langlois,[4] not enough to produce the physiologic results observed.

The possible existence in the capsule of other substances capable of producing toxic effects is illustrated by the experiments of S. Vincent,[5] who finds that sufficiently large doses of the extract, injected subcutaneously, produce first slowness, then paresis, and finally paralysis of voluntary movement. [But it is hazardous to assume, without special proof, that such toxic effects are specific to the capsules. Bouchard and others, *e. g.*, have shown that extracts of the liver have toxic properties, and although it may be, as Vincent says, that this is not the case with the filtrate from the boiled extracts, yet the results of Mairet and Vires,[6] who found that hepatic extracts lose their power of inducing intravascular coagulation, but not their general toxic properties, by being heated to 60° C., emphasize the necessity for caution.] That the capsules, in addition to toxic, possess also, under certain circumstances, antitoxic properties, is suggested by the observation of Ed. Boinet,[7] that animals deprived of their capsules succumb to a smaller dose of a poison like strophanthin than normal animals. [But this might have been due merely to the general condition of the animals, and not to the removal of a specific antitoxic mechanism.]

Thymus.—Abeles and Billard[8] state that total ablation of the thymus in the frog [in which animal the organ persists in the adult condition] causes death, due, they believe, to a true autointoxication. The chief symptoms are muscular weakness, going on to paralysis, trophic disturbances including discoloration of the skin, and certain alterations in the blood. Subcutaneous implantation of the thymus does not sensibly prolong life.

Pituitary.—[It cannot be said that any real advance has been made in our knowledge of the function of this organ.] Mairet and Bosc[9] find that although ingestion or subcutaneous injection of pituitary extracts produces hardly any effect in healthy men and animals, intravenous injection (in animals) is followed by severe and even fatal symptoms. In epileptics ingestion of the gland causes delirious attacks 3 or 4 days after administration. [But we doubt whether they have succeeded in showing that these are at all different from the attacks commonly seen in persons suffering from epilepsy.]

General sketches of the present position of the doctrine of internal secretion will be found in papers by W. D. Halliburton,[10] J. W. Warren,[11] R. W. Chittenden,[12] W. H. Howell,[13] and J. G. Adami.[14] The last-named author deals particularly with the relations of internal secretion to pathologic anatomy.

---

[1] Johns Hopkins Hosp. Bull., No. 76, July, 1897.   [2] Jour. of Physiol., vol. xxi., 1897.
[3] Deutsch. med. Woch., No. 26, 1896.   [4] Arch. de Physiol., p. 152, Jan., 1897.
[5] Jour. of Physiol., vol. xxii., p. 111; Birmingham Med. Rev., Aug., 1896.
[6] Arch. de Physiol., p. 353, Apr., 1897.
[7] Ibid., p. 952, Oct., 1896.   [8] Ibid., p. 898.
[9] Ibid., p. 529, July, 1896.   [10] Practitioner, p. 34, Jan., 1897.
[11] Boston M. and S. Jour., July 30, 1896; Chicago Med. Rec., Aug., 1896.
[12] Boston M. and S. Jour., Aug. 20, 1896.   [13] Med. News, May 22, 1897.
[14] Montreal Med. Jour., May, 1897.

The Energy of Muscular Contraction.—[A crowd of writers have again attacked this ever-interesting problem, and while much yet remains obscure, we think that the tendency, noted by us in the *Year-Book* for 1897, to look upon the muscle as a machine which can and does make use of various kinds of food-substances, according as the supply of this or that material is plentiful or scanty, is becoming more and more pronounced.] Thus, J. Frentzel[1] shows [very clearly, we think] that both with a diet of pure fat and in hunger the energy corresponding to the work done by a dog could not possibly have come altogether from the combustion of proteids; some of it must have been due to the oxidation of fat. That fat can be burnt as such in the contracting muscle without undergoing a previous conversion into glycogen or glucose, as Chauveau and Seegen have contended, seems to follow from the experiments of Zuntz,[2] who finds that, had this conversion first to take place, about 30% more energy would be necessary to yield a given amount of work on a fatty than on a carbohydrate diet; and this is not the case. He concludes [and we think the conclusion not only just but inevitable] that all food-substances are alike capable of yielding the energy of muscular work without first being changed into sugar. This conclusion cannot be considered as in any way shaken by the observation of F. Laulanié,[3] that in animals on a diet free, or nearly free, from carbohydrates the respiratory quotient, after an increase during work which carries it nearly to unity, falls during the subsequent period of repose to less than its original value—an observation which he interprets [on insufficient grounds] as indicating the replacement of the glucose used up during work by glucose formed during the interval of rest by an incomplete oxidation of fat. [Nor does a second research by the same author,[4] on the changes that take place in the respiratory quotient during the digestion of a carbohydrate meal, lead to any more definite decision as to the immediate destiny of the carbohydrates absorbed from the alimentary canal, since its results can be harmonized either with the theory that some of the absorbed glucose is burnt as such without undergoing transformation, or with the counter-theory that it is first changed into fat, which is then partially oxidized to form glucose.] .The mere fact that sugar, as Schumburg[5] and others have shown, even in small quantities (30 gm. for a man), causes rapid restoration of exhausted muscles tells in reality neither for nor against the assumption that sugar plays the leading part in muscular metabolism.

Seegen[6] sees no contradiction [nor can we] between his view that the energy of muscular contraction comes mainly from carbohydrates, and the contention of Pflüger that the carbohydrate is united with proteid before it is oxidized in the muscle; for Seegen regards the ultimate, and Pflüger the proximate, source of the energy. That an increased amount of proteid is broken down during severe muscular exertion has long been known, and fresh evidence of it is afforded by the experiments of J. C. Dunlop, Noël Paton, R. Stockman, and I. Macadam,[7] who add the important observation that it is muscle-proteid which is broken down, because the increased excretion of nitrogen and sulphur is not accompanied by an increase in the uric acid, nitrogenous extractives, and phosphorus. Now these waste-products arise from nuclea proteids, in which muscle is poor. That the chemic change in contraction is essentially an oxidation is once more illustrated, and in a striking fashion,

[1] Pflüger's Archiv, Bd. 68, p. 191.
[2] Verhandl. d. Berlin. phvsiol. Ges., Arch. f. (Anat. u.) Physiol., p. 538, Dec. 28, 1896.
[3] Arch. de Physiol., p. 572, July, 1896.   [4] Ibid., p. 791, Oct., 1896.
[5] Verhandl. d. Berlin. physiol. Ges., Arch. f. (Anat. u.) Physiol., p. 537, Dec. 28, 1896.
[6] Arch. f. (Anat. u.) Physiol., p. 383, Dec. 28, 1896. Ibid., p. 465.
[7] Jour. of Physiol., vol. xxii., p. 68.

by the researches of A. Broca and Ch. Richet,[1] who find that when the muscles of a warm-blooded animal are caused to contract in the absence of oxygen (during asphyxia) they rapidly lose their contractility, and those of W. Kühne,[2] who shows that when all oxygen has been removed the protoplasmic movements of the staminal hairs of *Trodescantia* completely cease, and cannot be excited by electric stimulation when proper precautions are taken against the production of oxygen by electrolysis. But that even now much remains undetermined as to the precise seats of the oxidative processes in the body is emphasized by the results of Ch. Bohr and Henriques,[3] who [contrary to the prevailing opinion] appear to have demonstrated a considerable production of CO_2 and consumption of O within the pulmonary circulation, thus reviving [of course with quantitative modifications] the old theory of pulmonary combustion first put forward by Lavoisier.

As to the **quantitative relations between energy expended and work done** by a contracting muscle N. Zuntz[4] makes the important generalization that all mammals hitherto investigated use in normal work approximately the same quantity of chemic energy per unit of work. A little more than one-third of the energy expended can be transformed into mechanical work. A. Chauveau[5] and his pupil, J. Tissot,[6] have contributed an elaborate series of papers on the same subject, which, however, have been severely criticised by Zuntz[7] and by I. Munk,[8] and do not, at this stage of the controversy, call for further remark here.

Glycogenesis.—On the vexed question of the postmortem production of sugar in the liver Pavy[9] maintains his original view that it is due to the action of an unorganized ferment, while Noël Paton[10] believes that all the evidence shows that the conversion of the glycogen into glucose is a process bound up with katabolic changes in the "surviving" hepatic cells. [We think the truth is that both factors are concerned. It is certain that unaltered glycogen may sometimes be found in the liver many hours after the death of the animal even when the temperature has been artificially kept up. But we cannot follow Seegen[11] in his refusal to admit that the hepatic glycogen is the source of the hepatic glucose.]

Animal Heat.—J. Lefèvre[12] cites the results of experiments made on himself and on animals to determine the amount of heat lost under various conditions. The body was immersed in a bath of such dimensions that the quantity of water needed to cover it was a minimum. He finds that far from resisting cold by following a law the inverse of Newton's law of cooling, as Richet and others have asserted, the body loses more and more heat as the temperature of the bath is lowered. [If it should turn out that this statement is correct, the explanation will probably be found in such vasomotor changes in the skin as favor increased loss of heat, combined, at least in the case of the lower animals, with that reflex increase in the metabolism with which they confront a fall of external temperature. Lefèvre's final result, that the amount of heat lost depends only on the initial temperature of the bath, and is the same when that temperature is kept constant and when it is allowed to rise, is so

[1] Arch. de Physiol., p. 829, Oct., 1896.   [2] Zeit. f. Biol., xxxv., p. 43, 1897.
[3] Arch. de Physiol., p. 459, Apr., 1897; pp. 590 and 710, July, 1897.
[4] Verhandl. d. Berlin. physiol. Ges., Arch. f. (Anat. u.) Physiol., p. 358, July 2, 1896.
[5] Compt. rend. de la Soc. de Biol., tome cxxii., pp. 429 and 504; Arch. de Physiol., p. 229, Jan., 1897; p. 261, Apr., 1897.
[6] Ibid., p. 563, July, 1896; pp. 78, 90, Jan., 1897.   [7] Loc. cit.
[8] Arch. f. (Anat. u.) Physiol., p. 372, July 2, 1896.
[9] Proc. Physiol. Soc., June 27, 1896; Jour. of Physiol., vol. xx., p. ii.
[10] Ibid., vol. xxii., p. 121.   [11] Centralbl. f. Physiol., Bd. x., No. 17, Nov. 14, 1896.
[12] Arch. de Physiol., p. 537, July, 1896; p. 7, Jan., 1897; p. 317, Apr., 1897.

novel and unexpected that we hesitate to accept it without confirmation.] The existence of a chemic regulation of the heat-production in man has been investigated by Eykman[1] for inhabitants of the tropics (Dutch East Indies), as had previously been done by Loewy for inhabitants of the north temperate zone (Berlin), and with a like negative result. [While we are thus justified in concluding that at the top of the animal scale the chemic regulation of temperature so characteristic of the smaller animals is either altogether wanting or very feebly developed, it has been shown by H. M. Vernon[2] that even in such poikilothermal animals as the frog, newt, and earthworm the gaseous metabolism is to a certain extent independent of the external temperature and under the control of the nervous system.]

Among the numerous other researches in this department of physiology which the exigencies of space prevent us from referring to in detail, may be mentioned those of J. Rosenthal[3] on calorimetric technic; that of M. S. Pembrey[4] on the deep and surface-temperature in a case of traumatic section of the spinal cord; a paper by C. F. Hoover and T. Sollmann[5] on the temperature, pulse-rate, and nitrogenous metabolism during fasting in the hypnotic sleep; and one by J. Fawcett and W. Hale White[6] on the marked rise of temperature caused by β-hydronaphthylamin. [The statement in this last paper " that the rise of temperature cannot be due to diminution of the heat-loss, since the respiration is increased, and animals which, like rabbits do not perspire must lose most of the heat they part with by the lungs," has a medieval sound, and ought not to appear in a modern research.]

RESPIRATION.

Regulation of Respiratory Movements.—Boruttau[7] puts forward the theory that the variability in the effects of stimulation of the vagus on the respiratory movements [which has impressed everybody who has studied the subject] is due not to the existence in the nerve of two sets of fibers, but to a difference in the results of excitation of the same fibers according to the nature of the stimulus and the condition of the animal. All momentary stimuli, according to him, are inspiratory while all long-lasting stimuli are expiratory. M. Lewandowsky,[8] while agreeing with Boruttau, that only one set of respiratory fibers exists in the vagus, entertains a different view in regard to the manner in which they produce their effect. After section of both vagi the respiration is no longer permanently influenced by any reflex mechanism, but solely by the respiratory center. [This dominant role of the vagi was extended by Filehne and Kionka (*Year-Book* for 1897, p. 1178), even to that increase in the respiratory activity which is so constant an accompaniment of muscular exercise, the vagus-endings in the lungs, according to these observers, being stimulated by the excess of CO_2 in the blood.] C. Speck,[9] however, takes exception to these experiments, and concludes that the excitation is set up in the capillaries of the contracting muscles. [But Filehne and Kionka still saw increased respiratory activity on tetanizing a limb connected with the trunk only by its blood-vessels, and it seems to us to savor of special pleading to suggest, as Speck does, that the *nervi vasorum* might run for a

[1] Pflüger's Archiv, Bd. lxiv., p. 57.   [2] Jour. of Physiol., vol. xxi., p. 443.
[3] Arch. f. (Anat. u.) Physiol., p. 171, Apr. 9, 1897; p. 191, July 30, 1897.
[4] Proc. Physiol. Soc., Feb. 13, 1897; Jour. of Physiol., vol. xxi., p. xiii.
[5] Jour. Exper. Med., vol. ii., No. 4, p. 405.
[6] Jour. of Physiol., vol. xxi., p. 435.   [7] Pflüger's Archiv, Bd. lxv., p. 26.
[8] Arch. f. (Anat. u.) Physiol., p. 195, July 2, 1896; p. 483, Dec. 28, 1896.
[9] Arch. f. (Anat. u.) Physiol., p. 465, Dec. 28, 1896.

sufficiently great distance in the vascular walls to establish a nervous connection. At any rate, this has never been proved.]

[As to the direct action of the blood on the respiratory center, it is generally acknowledged that it may be stimulated both by deficiency of O and by excess of CO_2, but it has been a subject of long-continued discussion which of these factors is the more potent under normal conditions.] N. Zuntz and A. Loewy [1] now bring forward evidence that comparatively small alterations in the amount of CO_2 in the inspired air cause a relatively great increase in the respiration, while the deficiency of O must be much more decided to bring about any notable effect. It is, of course not at all out of harmony with this, that when very large quantities of CO_2 are inhaled (30% and upward in rabbits) a condition of narcosis comes on without any dyspnea (A. Benedicenti).[2]

The **influence of alterations in the atmospheric pressure** has been studied by Lewinstein,[3] who makes the remarkable observation that rabbits exposed continuously to a pressure of 300–400 mm. Hg die in 2 or at most 3 days, with widespread fatty degeneration (of heart, liver, kidneys, diaphragm, etc.). A. Loewy, J. Loewy, and L. Zuntz,[4] comparing their observations on men exposed to various pressures in the pneumatic cabinet with the effects of a mountain climate on the same individuals, have brought out the interesting [though not entirely novel] fact that the action of mountain air does not depend merely on its degree of rarefaction, but on other complex stimuli. They deny that any increase in the specific gravity of the blood takes place at high levels. [This is opposed to the experience of other observers, who have found an increase in the number of the red corpuscles.] Possibly the discrepancy is accounted for by the method (Hammerschlag's) which they used for determining the specific gravity, and which, despite the precautions adopted (L. Zuntz)[5] [the necessity for these we can vouch for from personal experience] would hardly reveal small differences of concentration. The effect of **rapid variations in atmospheric pressure**, such as workmen are exposed to in the air-lock of a caisson, has been investigated experimentally by R. Heller, W. Mager, and H. v. Schrötter,[6] with the result that all the serious permanent disturbances of the nervous and circulatory systems are believed to be due to the liberation of gas in the vessels when the pressure is suddenly reduced. The symptoms can in part be relieved by again raising the pressure. This is especially true of the circulatory troubles, and is of some therapeutic interest.

Types of Respiration.—An exhaustive study of the influence of sex, age, and race on the type of the respiratory movements has been made by G. W. Fitz.[7] [His work deals a final blow at the long-tottering theory that sexual differences in respiratory type exist. When women breathe differently from men this, according to Fitz, is due far more to peculiarities of dress than to peculiarities of organization.]

Oxygen-tension of Arterial Blood.—J. Haldane and J. L. Smith[8] have determined by means of a new method, first described by Haldane,[9] the oxygen-tension of human arterial blood as it leaves the lungs. Since it exceeds the partial pressure of the oxygen in the external air, and, *a fortiori*, that of the oxygen in the air of the alveoli, the gaseous exchange in the lungs cannot be explained by diffusion alone.

[1] Verhandl. d. Berlin. physiol. Ges., Arch. f. (Anat. u.) Physiol., p. 379, July 30, 1897.
[2] Ibid., p. 408, Dec. 28, 1896.   [3] Pflüger's Archiv, Bd. lxv., p. 278.
[4] Ibid., Bd. lxvi., p. 477.   [5] Ibid., p. 539.
[6] Ibid., Bd. lxvii., p. 1.   [7] Jour. Exper. Med., vol. i., p. 677, Nov., 1896.
[8] Jour. of Physiol., vol. xx., p. 497.   [9] Ibid., vol. xviii., p. 455.

Experimental Pneumothorax.—Rodet and Nicolas[1] show that a gas, such as CO_2, introduced into the pleural cavity is very soon replaced by a mixture of CO_2, N, and O, by exchange with the blood circulating in the pleural membrane.

DIGESTION AND ABSORPTION.

The influence of intraintestinal pressure on the **absorption of substances from the alimentary canal** has formed the subject of an investigation by H. J. Hamburger,[2] who asserts that a rise of pressure favors absorption, which completely ceases when the pressure falls to zero. This latter fact he considers a telling argument against the theory of " vital " absorption, which is further invalidated by his observation that an increase of intraabdominal pressure also hastens the disappearance of liquid from the peritoneal cavity, when it is not sufficiently great to obstruct the blood-flow by compressing the veins.[3] [We do not think, however, that Hamburger's conclusions necessarily follow from his premises, nor is it certain even that his premises are correct.] For Waymouth Reid[4] has demonstrated by careful experiments that the water, organic and inorganic solids of the serum of an animal are absorbed from a loop of its intestine when the hydrostatic pressure in the capillaries of the intestinal wall is considerably greater than that in the cavity of the intestine. Ligation of the lacteals does not affect the result. [It is difficult to harmonize this with any purely physical theory of absorption.] Reid,[5] however, sees no reason to suppose that the mesenteric nerves affect the absorption of such substances as peptone and water in any other way than by their influence on the caliber of the blood-vessels. The defensive function of the mucous membrane of the intestine against certain bacterial poisons (toxins of cholera, diphtheria, and pyogenic bacilli), which seems to be indicated by the researches of Charrin and Cassin,[6] is also, so far as it goes, in favor of the " vital " hypothesis of absorption. So, too, is the selection of the path of the lacteals by the fat in preference to the path of the blood-vessels, particularly if we accept the somewhat heretic doctrine put forward by B. Moore and D. P. Rockwood[7] that most, if not all, of the fat is absorbed in a soluble form (as soap or fatty acid) by the epithelial cells. That **fat-splitting** goes on energetically in the alimentary canal, even in the absence of the pancreas, has been shown by Abelmann, and this is confirmed by E. Hedon and J. Ville;[8] while S. Rosenberg[9] has found that after ligation and section of its ducts and blood-vessels, followed by almost complete degeneration of the pancreas, a large amount of fat was still absorbed. No sugar appeared in the urine; the animal lived for $10\frac{1}{2}$ months, and then died from a pneumonic affection. Even in the total absence of both bile and pancreatic juice Hedon and Ville saw absorption of the fat of milk to the extent of more than 20%. This explains the possibility of the absorption of fat from enemata, which has been carefully studied by P. Deucher.[10] To attain the best results the fat should be given in the form of an emulsion, heated to body-temperature, after previous evacuation of the bowel. The researches of

[1] Arch. de Physiol., p. 640. July, 1896.
[2] Arch. f. (Anat. u.) Physiol., p. 428, Dec. 28, 1896.
[3] Ibid., p. 332.   [4] Brit. Assoc. Rep., 1897.
[5] Jour. of Physiol., vol. xx., p. 298.   [6] Arch. de Physiol., p. 595, July, 1896.
[7] Jour. of Physiol., vol. xxi., p. 58.
[8] Arch. de Physiol., pp. 607 and 622, July, 1897.
[9] Arch. f. Anat. u. Physiol., p. 535, Dec. 28, 1896.
[10] Deutsch. Arch. f. klin. Med., Bd. lviii., H. 2 u. 3, 1897.

Hauriot[1] and of Cohnstein and Michaelis[2] render it probable that we must even extend the role of the fat-splitting ferments beyond the limits of the alimentary canal, for they bring forward evidence that fat-splitting goes on in the blood itself.

Cholagogue Action of Bile.—In a valuable investigation of the action of bile in a case of biliary fistula Pfaff and Balch[3] reinstate this medieval remedy as the only real cholagogue at present positively known. Doyon and Dufourt[4] confirm this conclusion. Salicylate of sodium may to a certain extent act as a cholagogue; calomel not at all.

With the view of elucidating the **mechanism of obstructive jaundice,** Wertheimer and Lepage[5] established a fistula of the thoracic duct in a dog, and then injected into the branch of bile-duct serving one lobe of the liver a quantity of sheep or ox-bile, which has a characteristic spectrum owing to the presence of cholohematin. They collected the bile secreted by another lobe, and found that it assumed the color and showed the spectrum of the foreign bile. They convinced themselves by postmortem injection that there was no direct communication between the two branches of bile-duct, and therefore concluded that the injected bile must have been absorbed into the blood in the one lobe and excreted by the other. [Should these experiments be confirmed, they would show that the importance of the lymphatics in the absorption of the bile in obstructive jaundice has been singularly exaggerated. It seems very possible, however, that in the injection the pressure was raised in the bile-ducts to a greater height than can *ever* be the case when they are simply ligated. And that actual injury was inflicted on the hepatic tissue is indicated by the fact that the lymph collected from the fistule was always deeply tinged with blood-pigment.]

Feces.—[It is well known that the feces represent not only the unabsorbed constituents of the food, but also, to an appreciable extent, the secretions of the alimentary canal.] An investigation by a quartette of observers, H. Hammerl,[6] F. Kermanner, J. Moeller and W. Prausnitz,[7] shows that the latter element is even more important than has been supposed. Indeed, it would appear more correct to speak of food-substances as causing the *formation* of a smaller or a greater amount of feces than of their being more or less completely absorbed. [Contrary to popular belief] there seems to be no essential difference in the completeness with which animal and vegetable food is taken up from the alimentary canal, nor does the number or kind of the intestinal bacteria appear to vary with the nature of the food.

Digestive Ferments.—R. Pfleiderer[8] finds, in confirmation of previous observers, that of all acids HCl is the best helpmate both of pepsin and of rennin. W. D. Halliburton and T. G. Brodie[9] state that a milk-curdling ferment, differing in certain respects from rennin, exists not only in extracts of pancreas, but in fresh pancreatic juice [a point on which there was some doubt]; and J. W. Warren,[10] bringing together the results of several of his pupils, shows that the zymogen of a milk-curdling ferment exists in the gastric mucous membrane of a very large number of vertebrates, although not in all that were examined.

Movements of the Stomach.—S. J. Meltzer[11] has continued his inter-

---

[1] Bull. de l'Acad. de Méd., Nov. 10, 1896.
[2] Sitz. d. Akad. d. Wiss. z. Berlin, p. 771, 1896, and Pflüger's Archiv, Bd. lxv., p. 473.
[3] Jour. Exper. Med., p. 49, Jan., 1897.   [4] Arch. de Physiol., p. 562, July, 1897.
[5] Ibid., p. 363, Apr., 1897.   [6] Zeit. f. Biol., Bd. xxxv., p. 287, 1897.
[7] Hammerl, Ibid., p. 355.   [8] Pflüger's Archiv, Bd. 66, p. 605.
[9] Jour. of Physiol., vol. xx., p. 97.   [10] Jour. Exper. Med., vol. ii., p. 475, 1897.
[11] N. Y. Med. Jour., Apr. 24, 1897.

esting researches on the movements of the stomach, and reports that stimulation of the peripheral end of either vagus in the dog causes contraction, which is always confined to the pyloric end and lesser curvature.

Innervation of Swallowing.—F. Lüscher[1] asserts that the recurrent laryngeal (in the rabbit), in addition to its motor fibres for the laryngeal muscles and the upper portion of the esophagus, contains afferent fibres, stimulation of which causes reflex swallowing movements. [These experiments support the older statements of Burkert and Krause, in opposition to those of Horsley and Semon, Hooper, etc.]

THE NERVOUS SYSTEM.

Nerve-cells.—Vitzou,[2] whose preliminary communication we noticed in the *Year-Book* for 1897, has now published his complete paper on the regeneration of nerve-cells. He concludes [and his work appears to be sound] that the brain in young monkeys possesses the power of reproducing the substance lost by operation. He removed completely the occipital lobes in a macaque monkey, and saw that the power of vision, lost for a time, was gradually regained. Histologic examination proved that new nerve-cells and nerve-fibers had made good the deficiency.

F. C. Eve[3] has reinvestigated the question whether functional activity produces any histologic change in lymphatic nerve-cells, and, unlike previous observers, comes to a negative conclusion. He thinks that the shrinking of the cell and nucleus which has been described is probably due to the reagents used in fixing the tissue. The only change of any kind he could detect was the occurrence of a slight, diffuse blue stain (with methylen-blue) in the cell-substance. [It is evident that such a conclusion, reached by a competent observer, renders a repetition of the well-known work of Hodge and others a desideratum. But evidence is gathering every year that the histologic structure of nerve-cells is actually affected by various circumstances] and Berkley[4] has even detected marked differences in the dendrites of the pyramidal cells of a man who, after a long course of addiction to alcohol and opium, died in an insane asylum, and those of a typical healthy brain.

A. Hill[5] has published an elaborate study of the conditions under which the chrome-silver (Golgi) method succeeds, with a criticism of its results, and announces the discovery in the granule-layer of the cerebellum of small "granule-cells" with *centripetal* axis-cylinder processes.

Spinal Paths.—E. Wertheimer and L. Lepage[6] state [although this is not new] that the integrity of the anterior pyramid is not essential for the conduction of impulses from the cerebral cortex to the muscles of the opposite side. According to them, the path by which the motor impulses pass from the cortex to the muscles of the same side ("homolateral" path) is direct, and not crossed. [This is a view which has been steadily growing in favor of late years, but the novel suggestion of M. Rothman,[7] that the pressure of degenerating on sound fibers at the decussation may cause the latter to degenerate, if it should prove to be correct, would again place the whole question in doubt, for the fibers that degenerate in the lateral pyramidal tract on the same side after removal of one Rolandic area might possibly belong to the motor cortex of the opposite side. The subject certainly requires renewed investigation.]

[1] Zeit. f. Biol., Bd. xxxv., p. 192, 1897.   [2] Arch. de Physiol., p. 29, Jan., 1897.
[3] Jour. of Physiol., vol. xx., p. 334.   [4] Boston M. and S. Jour., Mar. 18, 1897.
[5] Presidential Address before Neurol. Soc. of London, 1896; Brain, p. 125, 1897.
[6] Arch. de Physiol., p. 614, July, 1896.   [7] Arch. f. (Anat. u.) Physiol., p. 345, July 2, 1896.

Sherrington [1] makes a further contribution to our knowledge of the peripheral distribution of the fibers of the posterior roots and their cerebral homologues. One of his most interesting conclusions is that the sense of taste as well as of touch is destroyed in the monkey in the anterior two-thirds of the tongue after intracranial section of the fifth nerve. He definitely establishes the rule that the sensory nerves of a skeletal muscle are in all cases derived from the spinal ganglion corresponding to the segment of the cord containing its motor cells. The question whether any of the fibers of the posterior root are of intraspinal origin, he [2] also attacks, and comes to the conclusion, as Singer and Münzer had previously done, that in mammals the original negative result of Waller is correct. For the frog the same conclusion is reached by R. J. Horton-Smith.[3] [In the chick, however, it is generally admitted that a few of the posterior root-fibers do arise in intraspinal nerve-cells.]

Reflex Action.—F. Gotch [4] makes a noteworthy contribution to the long-standing controversy on the nature of the **knee-jerk.** He reaches the catholic conclusion that the tendon-tap causes two distinct effects, a direct stimulation of the vastus internus muscle on the same side and a reflex stimulation of this muscle, confined in the rabbit to the opposite side, but, possibly, in certain animals and under certain conditions, involving the same side also. P. Stewart [5] also furnishes evidence of the existence of a true crossed reflex knee-jerk, the average time elapsing between the tendon-tap and the appearance of the jerk on the opposite side being about 0.126 second.

Max Verworn [6] states that pressure or friction on the flanks of a frog whose cerebral hemispheres have been removed causes a tonic reflex contraction of muscles in all parts of the body, which outlasts the stimulus sometimes for as long as an hour. The reflex center is in the ventral portion of the mid-brain (optic lobes). [The author of this abstract has observed long-continued and general spasmodic contractions in frogs and also in Menobranchus after excision of the cerebral hemispheres, when the mucous membrane of the mouth was scratched with a pair of forceps. These phenomena are perhaps related to the reflex contractions noticed by Sherrington [7] in "brainless" monkeys and termed by him from their long duration "cataleptoid."]

Sherrington, in conjunction with H. E. Herring,[8] has continued his brilliant researches on the cortical inhibition of antagonistic muscles during the performance of coördinated movements, and brings forward numerous additional illustrations of such inhibition.

Cortical Localization.—Wesley Mills [9] concludes from his studies on the effects of stimulation of the cortex in a large number of animal groups that areas of the same name in different animals are not on the same functional plane [*i. e.*, have not attained the same level of organization]. In birds he finds no evidence of the existence of any "motor centers." Pitres [10] also raises his voice against the conventional view that the motor and sensory areas are separated from the rest of the cortex by hard-and-fast functional lines. In particular he sees no reason for supposing that any definite region is especially associated with the intellectual powers.

[1] Proc. Roy. Soc., vol. lx., p. 408, Jan. 21, 1897.   [2] Jour. of Physiol., vol. xxi., p. 209.
[3] Ibid., vol. xx., p. 101.   [4] Ibid., p. 322.
[5] Ibid., vol. xxii., p. 61.   [6] Pflüger's Archiv, Bd. lxv., p. 63.
[7] Lancet, Feb. 6, 1897 ; Proc. Roy. Soc., Dec. 29, 1896.
[8] Pflüger's Archiv, Bd. lxviii., p. 222.
[9] Trans. Roy. Soc. Can., vol. ii., sec. 4, pp. 3 and 25, 1896 ; N. Y. Med. Jour., Oct. 17, 1896
[10] Med. Congress, Nancy, Aug. 6, 1896 ; Pacific Med. Jour., Oct., 1896.

S. J. Sharkey[1] adds three interesting and well-studied cases to the precious, but as yet all too scanty, stock of evidence on the cortical localization in man. They corroborate the view, derived from experimental physiology, that the angular gyrus and occipital lobe are both concerned in vision, the former as a higher, the latter as an intermediate or lower center.

The Sympathetic System.—Langley and Anderson[2] complete their work on the innervation of the pelvic viscera by a paper dealing with the anatomy of the lumbar and sacral sympathetic nerves; while Langley[3] asserts, in opposition to the results of Schäfer and Moore [and the evidence he brings forward is undoubtedly strong], that the fibers which cause contraction of the spleen, like all or nearly all the fibers of the splanchnic nerves, make junction with the ganglion-cells in the solar plexus. And he takes the opportunity to reiterate his generalization that there is but one sympathetic cell on the course of each sympathetic fiber. A lucid account of our present knowledge of the constitution of the sympathetic system has been published by G. C. Huber.[4]

D. Courtade and J. F. Guyon[5] endeavor to rehabilitate the doctrine of v. Basch that the same nerve supplies the longitudinal muscular coat of such organs as the bladder and the intestines with inhibitory and the circular coat with motor fibers, and *vice versâ*. [It is an extraordinary circumstance that no reference is made by these writers to the well-known work of Langley, who has conclusively shown that there is no foundation for v. Basch's idea.]

SPECIAL SENSES.

Th. Beer,[6] in continuation of his remarkable investigations on the mechanism of accommodation in the lower animals, makes the further announcement that the cephalopod eye, like the eye of fishes, possesses a negative accommodation—*i. e.*, an accommodation for distance. From this he draws the general conclusion that all animals living in the water, when they possess the power of accommodation at all, have a negative and not a positive accommodation. The explanation he believes to be [and it is a very plausible one] that under water the greatest possible distance of distinct vision must be very much less than in air, and that, since water offers a relatively great resistance to locomotion, it is more important for the water-living animal to discern its prey or its enemy when it is near than when it is remote.

ELECTROPHYSIOLOGY.

A series of important contributions to the theory of **galvanotropism** has been made by J. Loeb,[7] among which is included[8] an examination of the question whether electromagnetic vibrations (Hertzian oscillations) have the power of stimulating such excitable tissues as the nerves of the frog. [So far as we can see at present, we think that more confidence is to be placed in the negative answer of Loeb than in the positive results of B. Danilewsky.[9]]

F. Gotch and G. J. Burch[10] have added largely to our knowledge of the electromotive properties of the *Malapterurus electricus ;* and F. S. Locke[11] has examined in detail the action of ether on contracture and on the so-called positive kathodic polarization.

[1] Lancet, p. 1399, May 22, 1897.　　　　[2] Jour. of Physiol., vol. xx., p. 372.
[3] Ibid., p. 223.　　　　[4] Jour. Compar. Neurol., vol. vii., No. 2, Sept., 1897.
[5] Arch. de Physiol., p. 622, July, 1896, p. 422, Apr., 1897.
[6] Pflüger's Archiv, Bd. 67, p. 541.　　　[7] Ibid., Bd. 65, pp. 41, 308, 518, etc.
[8] Ibid., Bd. 67, p. 483, June 18, 1897.　　[9] Arch. de Physiol., pp. 511 and 527, July, 1897.
[10] Phil. Trans., vol. 187 B., p. 347.　　[11] Jour. Exper. Med., vol. 1, p. 630, Nov., 1896.

LEGAL MEDICINE.

BY WYATT JOHNSTON, M. D.,

OF MONTREAL, CANADA.

Epitome.—The discovery by Florence of a characteristic chemical test for semen is a most important addition to medicolegal technic. The Röntgen photography has been quietly accepted by most courts as part of the regular medicolegal repertoire, perhaps with too little regard to the possible sources of error involved. Agitation in favor of a better system of appointing experts has been vigorously carried on in America during the year, but so far "much cry and little wool" appears to be the result. Even in France, where a much more satisfactory system exists, there has been a noteworthy amount of friction between the experts and the courts in recent years. Between the primitive state of affairs in which the dictum of the ordinary general practitioner is accepted as gospel, and the highly organized ones in which the decision of medical matters is left in the hands of medical men, the transition-stages are bound to be unsatisfactory, though the end is worth striving for. In the Luetgert *cause celèbre* the objectionable features of the present expert system were well shown. The Medicolegal Congress at Brussels and the Medicolegal Section of the Moscow International Congress brought out little that was novel. It is singular that neither in the American nor in the British Medical Association has legal medicine been allotted an independent section.

1. Literature.[1]—The admirable series of lectures by P. Brouardel [2] forms the most notable addition to the literature of the year on this subject. The very full reports of numerous cases, mostly personal, make these lectures of special value. The late E. v. Hofmann's parting gift to science was an excellent hand-atlas of legal medicine.[3] In America Witthaus's completing volume of the *System of Medical Jurisprudence and Toxicology*, edited by himself and Becker, gives the best statistical information available regarding toxicology. The deaths of E. v. Hofmann, G. Tarde, and A. Wernich have occurred during the year.

2. Criminology.—The increasing frequency of homicide in the United States is commented on by P. Bartholow,[4] who estimates the number of reported homicides as increasing from 1808 per annum in 1885 to 4292 in 1890, and to 10,500 in 1895. This latter rate of 15 per 100,000 population is said to be 25% higher than in Italy, double that in Spain, 5 times that of Austria, 9 times that of France, and 20 times that of England, Scotland, or

---

[1] The subject-matter has been divided as follows; 1, general medicolegal literature; 2, criminology; 3, medical jurisprudence; 4, medicolegal pathology, violent death and injuries; 5, medicolegal tests; 6, toxicology; 7, sexual; 8, mental. The abridgment needed to keep within the limits of space allowed was made at the expense of Nos. 2, 6, 7, and 8.

[2] La pendaison, la suffocation, la strangulation, la submersion, Paris, 1897; L'infanticide, Paris, 1897. Les explosifs et les explosions, Paris, 1897. La responsibilité médicale, Paris, Death and Sudden Death (translation), New York, 1897.

[3] Lehmann's Hand-atlanten, 1897.   [4] Jour. Am. Med. Assoc., Nov. 14, 1897.

Germany. [Some better system of collecting criminal statistics similar to those followed in Europe is needed in order to decide matters of such importance.]

Judicial castration as a punishment for rape is being regarded with increasing favor in districts where this crime is prevalent. In Kansas a bill to legalize it has been introduced. [It might advantageously be tried as a substitute for lynching in certain localities.]

3. Medical Jurisprudence.—[Judging by the titles of recent medico-legal text-books and of courses of lectures in the medical colleges, it is not yet generally understood that this term implies, strictly speaking, medical law and not legal medicine.]

Medical Secrecy.—The Playfair case, in which a distinguished physician took advantage of evidences of pregnancy gained during an operation upon a patient who happened also to be a family connection, to indulge in acts of persecution toward the lady, did not really open up any debatable points in reference to the relations of physician and patient. The opinions of the English Bench which were incidentally expressed during the trial shows that the absence of definite and fixed rules in the matter of secrecy is a decided source of danger to the physician. Although the award of $60,000 damages is large, there can be little doubt that the physician acted improperly. In France the secrecy enjoined by law is so great that even the public hospital records showing the dates of admission of patients cannot be used as evidence against criminals who have been treated in the institutions. W. Lefuel [1] deals very clearly with this phase of the subject.

Responsibility of Medical Men.—That this has become a very serious matter in France recent events have shown. In a recent case experts who had failed to recognize a typical case of coal-gas poisoning (and had given evidence whereby an innocent woman was sentenced to penal servitude for life and remained in prison till other similar deaths in the same dwelling led to an investigation) were ordered to pay jointly 40,000 fr. damages.[2] A more recent instance was that in which an expert directed to examine a woman charged with infanticide declared that she had recently been delivered. She was confined to prison, where 2 weeks later she gave birth to a child. The learned judge pronounced the expert's error to be inexcusable, "as he could have established the fact of pregnancy simply by examining the blood, which according to all standard authorities shows peculiar and characteristic alterations during pregnancy" (!). The decision of this modern Dogberry has led to a formal protest from the Société méd.-légale de France,[3] as it happens that no leading medicolegal work refers to the matter at all and the statements existing in medical literature are contradictory.

These occurrences have led A. Lacassagne to classify categorically the causes of experts' errors as follows:[4] 1. Of omission—forgetting a scientific rule, as in neglecting to open an important cavity, to note an important observation, or to make a necessary control. 2. Of commission—acting contrary to medicolegal practice, as in doing the docimasia-test wrongly; misinterpreting appearances, as in taking lividity for ecchymosis. Errors he considers excusable if they arise from want of scientific training or practice in medicolegal work, but inexcusable if they arise from presumption, exuberant imagination, or haste in drawing conclusions. The fact that in France any physician when ordered by a judge to make an *expertise* has no power to refuse, makes the matter a very serious one. A penalty of 3 months' imprisonment was meted out to Laporte[5] by a Paris court for having unskil-

[1] Ann. d'Hyg. pub., Jan., 1897.   [2] Druaux case, Rev. de Méd. légale, 1897.
[3] Ibid., July, 1897.   [4] Arch. d'Anthrop. crim., Jan., 1897.   [5] Sem. méd., Oct. 23, 1897.

fully caused the death of a woman through a bungling attempt to perform craniotomy with a large mattress-needle, after trying to use a cold chisel and mallet. As he rejected the offer of the family to obtain other medical aid, and as the case occurred in the heart of Paris under circumstances not specially urgent and not calling for improvised methods, he was certainly imprudent. The autopsy showed perforations of the bladder and peritonitis, but it was not clearly shown that these were caused by the instrument employed, and the exceptional severity of the sentence has been severely criticised. The case is mentioned as showing that a more uniform understanding on both sides should be had as to when a physician oversteps the limits of scientific practice. In America no cases having very important bearings in this direction have arisen during the year.

4. Medicolegal Pathology: Violent Death: Injuries.—Death. —A. Martin[1] considers that **cadaveric spasm** is totally distinct from post-mortem rigidity, and is due to the last vital act of the nervous system. The essential feature is an absolutely instantaneous death—too rapid even for a few minutes' agonal struggle. Precocious rigidity, on the other hand, depends for its causation on a special condition of the muscle-fiber. [It is not easy to see how the distinction could be so sharply made.]

F. Strassmann[2] has estimated quantitatively (by measuring the shortening which takes place in pins driven into the hearts of dogs 1 hour after death, and again examined 24 hours later) the extent of the alteration in the volume of the chambers due to **rigor mortis of the heart,** to which he was the first, in 1889, to direct attention.

A. Lacassagne[3] reports a case of a body found within a trunk, in which the symmetric distribution of ecchymoses about the shoulders, elbows, and knees led him to conclude that the **strangulation** which was the cause of death had actually taken place after the body had been placed in the trunk. P. Brouardel[4] reports the case of a boy who shut himself in a trunk to hide, and died from suffocation. When found the body was so much swollen that after removal it could not be replaced, giving rise to the wrong impression that it had been placed there originally by force.

R. Schultz[5] considers that in doubtful cases of strangulation microscopic examination of the skin for flattening of the papillæ and capillary hemorrhages may be necessary. The classic description of suggillation about the line of compression by a cord is never met with in practice. Any suffusion of the bridge of skin between two furrows is specially important, as this cannot be affected by hypostasis. Icard[6] discusses the Cauvin case, in which a young man received a life-sentence because certain experts had declared that fracture of the larynx could not be produced in the case of a woman of 82 by a young girl, using her hands alone. A new trial, ending in acquittal, was granted, when it was learned that a parallel lesion had without doubt been produced in another case by a young girl.

P. Dittrich[7] reports a case of **self-strangulation** done by an insane old man partly paralyzed in both legs and the right arm. An unsuccessful attempt to hang himself to the bedpost had immediately preceded the strangulation, which was by means of a cord.

Autoextirpation of the Larynx.—S. Szigeti[8] reports a suicide so

---

[1] Arch. d'Anthrop. crim., July, 1897.   [2] Vierteljahr. ger. Med., Supplement, 1896.
[3] Arch. d'Anthrop. crim., Jan., 1897.   [4] Ann. d'Hyg. pub., July, 1896.
[5] Vierteljahr. ger. Med., Jan. and July, 1897.
[6] Lyon méd., quoted in Rev. de Méd légale, Oct , 1896.
[7] Vierteljahr. ger. Med., Oct., 1896.   [8] Ibid.

remarkable that its possibility would hardly have been entertained had not the circumstances excluded homicide, in a woman of 42. The appearance of the injury is shown in Fig. 85. A table-knife was used, the first cut being made downward with the head thrown back, and the larynx being then probably grasped by the hand and excised by a series of sawing cuts. Death followed in 8 hours. The carotids, jugulars, and vagi were intact. One similar case is on record (by Jameson), in which the victim removed half one side of his larynx and brought it himself to the hospital where he sought relief.

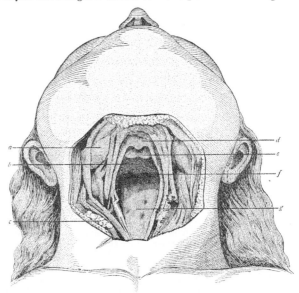

Fig. 85.—A case of suicide by excision of the larynx: *a*, submaxillary gland; *b*, soft palate; *c*, sternocleido-mastoid muscle; *d*, hyoid bone; *e*, epiglottis; *f*, pharynx; *g*, esophagus, posterior wall (Szigeti, Vierteljahr. f ger. Med., H. 2, 1896).

Electricity.—J. Kratter[1] has written a very complete monograph on this subject, with a very full bibliography.

Diagnosis of Vital from Postmortem Injuries.—R. Schultz[2] gives a lengthy review of the subject. The absence of ecchymosis and hemorrhage, where other extensive lesions exist and cause lowering of the general blood-pressure, is emphasized. Marked anemia of the organs is considered one of the most reliable signs of injuries having existed antemortem, as is also the occurrence of very profuse hemorrhages into the internal cavities, which cannot occur postmortem, and any appreciable suffusion about a large, gaping wound. Absence of signs of vital reaction by no means indicates that the lesions have been produced after death, and a knowledge of the conditions under which the body has remained since death may exclude the possibility of postmortem lesions, and so remove all doubt in the absence of positive signs of vital action. A. Lesser[3] has been able by interposing soft pads, when inflicting experimental injuries after death, to produce edema without ecchymosis.

[1] Deutke, Leipzig, 1896.   [2] Viertelj. ger. med. Supplement, 1896.   [3] Ibid., Jan., 1897.

Visceral changes in superficial burns have been studied experimentally by C. R. Bardeen,[1] who does not substantiate the statement that the essential cause of the lesions is capillary thrombosis, but finds them to be of the nature of focal necroses, similar to those occurring in infectious diseases, though cultures from the organs remain sterile. These focal necroses he was able to produce experimentally in animals.

Fat-embolism.—G. Puppe[2] finds that fat-emboli occur in subacute cases of phosphorus-poisoning, though absent in peracute cases, which die before the degenerative changes have time to develop fully.

Air-embolism.—J. Perkins[3] reports 2 cases of so-called uterine air-embolism, and also a doubtful case.[4] A review of the cases already recorded is given, and one is struck by two circumstances—that the patients died suddenly in the office of physicians or others who, rightly or wrongly, had acquired the name of being abortionists, and that where the instrument employed was known, it was a hollow one (syringe or catheter). He was able experimentally to admit sufficient air to kill a dog by simply opening the jugular and raising the head. [The pathologic proof of uterine air-embolism appears to be very defective in most of the cases. Although men of first-class scientific standing have reported cases, no one has yet taken the trouble to test the gas found and see what it really is. There is no evidence proving experimentally that uterine air-embolism is possible unless a hollow instrument is used.] Welch and Flexner[5] consider that many of the cases reported as air-embolism are really due to infection by the gas-bacillus (*b. aërogenes capsulatus*). This is the more likely to lead to confusion when the body is examined early, before decomposition has devoloped. [In the absence of the facilities or technical training necessary to make a complete bacteriologic examination there are two simple tests which any one can carry out—keeping the organs to see if gas-formation occurs, and keeping a drop or two of the blood dried for microscopic examination for bacilli. We have found it easy, by doing an autopsy carelessly, to enable small quantities of air to enter either the right or left heart from the cut vessels of the neck, if the blood be fluid and the shoulders slightly raised.]

Hiller, Meyer, and Schrotter[6] state that in **arterial air-embolism** (air in left circulation) death is not due to accumulation of air in the heart-cavities, but to obstruction of the coronary or cerebral arteries. The condition is rare, and chiefly occurs when gases expand in the blood from a lowering of the surrounding air-pressure (caisson-disease). Attention is also called to the possibility of its occurring through the coincidence of ordinary air-embolism and an abnormal communication between the two sides of the heart. The characteristic appearance of small air-bubbles is most distinctly seen in the coronary or mesenteric arteries.

Infanticide.—An unusual case is reported by F. Strassmann.[7] The mother endeavored to tear off the lower jaw and larynx of the child. The lower jaw was fractured in two places and a tear from each angle of the mouth extended down the neck, below the larynx. Death followed in two days, the autopsy showing that much blood had been aspirated and swallowed. H. Mittenzweig[8] reports a similar lesion as being caused by self-help during labor, though the child was strangled immediately after birth.

Accidental Death in Serum-therapy.—In the Langerhans child whose death occurred suddenly after a dose of diphtheria antitoxin, and

---

[1] Jour. Exper. Med., Sept., 1897.
[2] Viertelj. ger. med., Supplement, 1896.
[3] Boston M. and S. Jour., Feb. 18, 1897.
[4] New England Med. Monthly, June, 1897.
[5] Jour. Exper. Med., Jan., 1896.
[6] Zeit. f. klin. Med., Bd. 32, 1897.
[7] Viertelj. ger. Med., Oct , 1897.
[8] Ibid., 1897.

attracted much attention, F. Strassmann, after making an autopsy, found that death was due to inspiration of vomited matters into the air-passages. There was marked edema of the glottis and the suffocative attack commenced by a fit of coughing.

Destruction of Dead Body.—In the Luetgert trial at Chicago in Oct., 1897, it was alleged that a woman's body had been dissolved in a soap-vat into which 378 pounds of crude potash had been put and the solution heated with steam. Afterward cold water was run through the vat. The finding of fragments of bone, declared by one set of experts to be human, and to be parts of a femur, humerus, rib, phalanx, and temporal bone, as well as finding some corset-stays, false teeth, and some articles of jewelry recognized as belonging to the deceased, aroused suspicions. It was shown by the State that, under parallel conditions, solution of the body was possible in a few hours. [A really scientific and impartial study of this novel problem has not yet been made. From a scientific standpoint the verdict of the jury is immaterial, as the enduring triumphs of legal medicine are won in the laboratory and not in the court-room.]

Wounds and Injuries.—The zeal with which the medicolegal aspects of injuries are studied in Germany is shown by the publication of two special periodicals, a *Monatschrift* and an *Archiv für Unfallheilkunde*. In our own medical literature the work in this direction is scanty and singularly barren of scientific interest, largely no doubt because it is regarded from a business rather than a scientific standpoint. The duties and responsibilities of the official physicians of corporations are commercial and executive, rather than medical. While our railway surgery has advanced rapidly in the matter of organization, its contributions to science have been by comparison, disappointing.

Altman[1] concludes, in regard to **injuries of the lung** that, if the immediate effect is survived, the chances of recovery are relatively good. Punctured wounds are practically as serious as lacerated ones, the lesion of the pleura being the main consideration. Pneumonia and tuberculosis can often be traced to the result of trauma. Prolonged observation of a case is necessary before giving a prognosis, and this should always leave a wide margin for possibilities.

Important monographs on injuries of the **brain and nervous system** have been published by Crocq[2] and by C. Phelps,[3] the latter dealing especially with pistol-shot wounds.

Injuries of the diaphragm are considered medicolegally by L. Israel.[4] Lacerations usually occur on the left side, and affect middle-aged men. Diaphragmatic hernia is likely to happen, and is best diagnosed by Litten's sign.[5] The most serious results from this lesion are those which arise from constriction of the stomach and intestine.

A full discussion on **contusions of the abdomen** took place before the Eleventh French Congress of Surgery at Paris.[6]

A. Wegener[7] considers that in **injuries of the intestine** perforation must be regarded legally as a naturally fatal injury. In subcutaneous rupture of the intestine the abdominal walls are usually free from all marks of injury. Perforation, apart from other causes of shock, does not cause instant death. Omission to perform a laparotomy should not constitute malpractice.

Castex[8] deals with the legal bearing of **diseases and injuries of the**

[1] Viertelj. ger. Med., Supplement, 1897. [2] Paris, 1896.
[3] D. Appleton, New York, 1897. [4] Ibid. [5] Deutsch. med. Woch., No. 5, 1895.
[6] Sem. méd., Oct. 21, 1897. [7] Ibid. [8] Ann. d'Hyg. pub., June, 1897.

ear, nose, and throat; J. W. Park[1] with the eye and ear; F. Colley[2] with injuries of the tongue, especially with reference to the extent to which the functions of swallowing, taste, and speech remain after injury or removal. W. Ambrosius[3] considers very carefully the injuries of the male urinary tract, giving a very full bibliography and citing in particular a large number of cases of rupture of the bladder.

Trauma and carcinoma are studied by W. Berger,[4] who supports the usual view that repeated or continued slight injuries are most important in this respect. B. Schuchardt[5] gives a lengthy report of a case in which an affirmative report and superarbitrium were given in support of a traumatic origin for tuberculosis in a case in which a blow on the lumbar region was followed by neurasthenia and later by pulmonary tuberculosis.

Vaccination and Tuberculosis.—The following are the conclusions of a Prussian government report by Gerhardt and v. Leyden:[6] "Apart from the possibility that faulty technic leading to erysipelas, sepsis, or syphilis may produce a predisposition, through general weakening of the system, favorable to invasion of tubercle-bacilli; also the possibility that in children who have tuberculous glands, very exceptional cases with high fever might lead to generalization of the process, there is no ground for assuming that tuberculosis can occur through vaccination."

Interval before Death after Stab-wounds of the Heart.—M. Richter[7] reports that out of 27 cases periods of 5 minutes to 5 days elapsed in 10; in 10 others, owing to the bodies being found dead, the interval remained uncertain; 4 were able to walk into or from rooms to give alarm; 1 (suicide) closed the knife and put it in his pocket; in only 2 was death known to be instantaneous. Death from heart-wounds is thus less rapid than from those of large vascular trunks. The shape, size, situation, and direction of the wound are stated to have made little difference. [None of them, however, happened to involve the auricle, which we have found always to cause very rapid death.]

Accidental Gunshot-wounds.—J. N. Hall[8] gives a useful citation of the circumstances under which these occur, with especial reference to cases in which homicide was made to simulate accident. G. Corin[9] was able with small shot to produce experimentally fracture of the ulna at 12 meters distance.

5. Medicolegal Tests.—[The subjects comprised under this category become every year more varied. Bacteriology and photography have been the branches in which development has been most active during the year.]

X-rays in Legal Medicine.—The first recorded appearance of Röntgen photography in court was at Nottingham, England, in February, 1896, before Mr. Justice Hawkins, Miss Gladys Frolliot, an actress, promptly obtaining damages for an accident to her foot when the skiagraph was produced in court. Very few judges have objected to this form of evidence, though one court in New Jersey, finding that no precedent existed in that State, declined to establish one.[10] Doubtless, judging from the present tendency to give scientific demonstrations of all kinds before jurors, the fluoroscope will appear in evidence. That the skiagraph is not yet entitled to the same unhesitating credence granted to ordinary photographs is pointed out, amongst others, by E. A. Tracy,[11] who gives two photographs of the same hand (reproduced in

[1] Jour. Am. Med. Assoc., Dec. 12, 1896.　　　[2] Viertelj. ger. Med., Supplement, 1897.
[3] Ibid., July, 1897.　　[4] Ibid.　　[5] Ibid.　　[6] Ibid.　　[7] Ibid., Jan., 1896.
[8] Med. Rec., Sept. 19, 1896.　　　[9] Arch. Anthrop. crim., Mar., 1896.
[10] Med. News, Oct., 1897.　　　[11] Jour. Am. Med. Assoc., Nov. 5, 1897.

Figs. 86 and 87), showing well how pathologic changes may be accidentally (not to mention intentionally) simulated. The chief cause of error is due to the rays diverging from one point and not being refrangible.

Bordas and Ogier[1] utilized the process to detect the contents of "*inferdas machines*" sent by mail, also to show ossific points in the fetus. Bordas

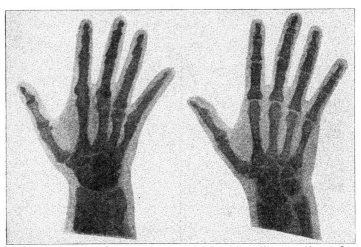

FIGS. 86 and 87.—Showing how pathologic changes may be accidentally simulated by a skiagraph (Jour. Am. Med. Assoc., Nov. 5, 1897).

claims that lungs of stillborn children appear opaque and expanded lungs transparent in skiagraphs.

Photography.—H. J. Gosse[2] emphasizes the importance of making the eyes of dead bodies look more lifelike before photographing. When this is not accomplished by a simple wet compress, moistening the conjunctiva (but not the cornea) with a weak alum solution or instilling a 25 % glycerin solution will often succeed. Where the globe is very flaccid, injection of glycerin into the posterior chamber with a hypodermic syringe is advised. Sir H. D. Littlejohn[3] insists on the importance of photographing the principal lesions found at each stage of medicolegal autopsies. [This is rendered specially necessary by the very thorough dissection-methods considered necessary in forensic cases, which make it almost impossible to preserve satisfactory specimens for future study without a feeling that one is neglecting some incision which may later on prove to have been essential.]

Blood-stains.—S. Szigeti[4] advises the use of hot concentrated carbolic acid as a solvent for old blood-stains in substances liable to be acted on by alkalies. It gives the acid hematin spectrum, and by diluting with alcohol it can be made to give that for reduced hematin. By adding concentrated H_2SO_4 hematoporphyrin can be obtained.

Iodin-test for Seminal Stains.—Florence's reaction,[5] obtained by bringing a drop of solution of iodin trichlorid (iodin, 2.5 ; potass. iodid, 1.65 ; water, 30) into contact with a moistened filament or a drop expressed

[1] Ann. d'Hyg. pub., May and Aug., 1896.   [2] Ibid., Dec., 1896.   [3] Lancet, Jan. 2, 1897.
[4] Viertelj. ger. Med., Supplement, 1896.   [5] See Arch. d' Anthrop. crim., 1895.

from a stain is recognized by prompt and abundant appearance of brown acicular and rhomboidal crystals, strongly resembling those of hemin in size, color, and appearance. The fixed alkalies and heat dissolve them, but they reappear on cooling, and are insoluble in weak ammonia. They are produced by contact of the solution with certain alkaloids, but not by any of the secretions or fluids of the body and not typically by the semen of animals. The test has been confirmed by a number of observers, who all agree as to its simplicity and usefulness as a preliminary test to see at once whether it is worth while examining for spermatozoa (for which Florence recommends employing a solution of crocein, producing double staining of the heads, best studied with a $\frac{1}{12}$ immersion-lens). We have found [1] that the prostatic and vesicular components of the semen tested separately do not give the reaction, and found it absent in 2 cases (advanced chronic vesiculitis and carcinoma of prostate), although spermatozoa were abundant. Lecao and Richter [2] have obtained the reaction from cholin. E. Posner [3] obtained it in a case of azoospermin, and thinks the prostatic element the essential one. E. di Mattei [4] had negative results with purely prostatic secretions. W. Florence [5] confirms Richter's statement that cholin gives the reaction, and has obtained it from putrefied alkaloidal bodies in egg yolks. W. F. Whitney [6] tested for the crystals, with negative results, in material containing Charcot-Leyden crystals (supposed to be identical with spermatic crystals). He recommends staining the film (obtained by pressing the moistened and disassociated filaments on a cover-glass and allowing it to dry) first with aqueous eosin and then with strong aqueous methyl-green, to obtain double staining of spermatozoa-heads. Mount in balsam.

American Observations on Entomology in Legal Medicine.—Results corresponding with those of Mégnin were obtained by G. Hough in Massachusetts, with bodies freely exposed to the air. He gives new points for the more ready classification of diptera.[7] M. G. Motter, in studying 150 buried bodies at Washington, D. C., found a much more varied and numerous fauna than that noted by Mégnin.[8] [We have personally [9] found that during the warm weather the results at Montreal are nearly, but not quite, in accord with Mégnin's statements. Montreal air- and soil-temperatures happen to correspond with those of Paris during the summer. Mégnin's publications chiefly refer to exposed and not to buried bodies.]

Glycogen-function of the Liver.—A. Lacassagne and E. Martin [10] have confirmed and extended some valuable forgotten observations of C. Bernard, showing that the livers of people meeting sudden or violent deaths contain 1% to 2% glucose—readily recognized by rubbing up the liver in water, boiling the emulsion, and testing the filtrate by Fehling's solution. An opalescent filtrate indicates unconverted glycogen. Two hundred bodies were examined. The test is negative in death from exhausting diseases and fevers, and hence, if positive, it implies that injuries to a sick person have been the immediate cause of death. Positive reactions are given in diabetes and deaths from apoplexy, hemoptysis, and hemorrhage. Stillborn children give positive reactions; but if syphilitic, negative ones. [We have tested the results and find them on the whole to be as stated.]

Bacteriology in Legal Medicine.—Bordas and Descoust [11] found that

1 Boston M. and S. Jour., Apr. 8, 1897.　　　 2 Wien. klin. Woch., No. 24, 1897.
3 Berlin. klin. Woch., No. 28, 1897.　　　　　 4 Cristalle del Florence, Naples, 1897.
5 Arch. d'Anthrop. crim., Nov., 1897.　　　　 6 Boston M. and S. Jour., Apr. 8, 1897.
7 Brit Med. Assoc., annual meeting, Sept. 2, 1897.　　　　8 Ibid.
9 Montreal Med. Jour., Aug., 1897.　　　　　 10 Arch. Anthrop. crim., July, 1897.
　　　　　　11 Rev. de Méd. légale., Mar., 1897.

gaseous decomposition did not occur in stillborn lungs exposed to spontaneous decomposition, and that when decomposing fluids were injected into the bronchi no gas was found unless air was injected at the same time. Malvoz[1] found absence of microorganisms in the tissues of healthy persons dying suddenly, and after the onset of putrefaction the deeper tissues remained free from bacteria for some time. In death from disease, the bacteria of terminal infections were present uniformly. [Our personal experience has been the same, the organs of healthy persons being often sterile some days after a violent death.] Wilman[2] considers the presence of the water-bacteria in the lung-alveoli and the stomach and intestines a valuable sign of drowning. Predominance of liquefying colonies is the distinguishing feature. [We presume the test would only be practicable during the early periods of immersion, when it is least needed. Further observations by bacteriologists are necessary to decide its practical value.]

G. Pouchet[3] reports an outbreak of sausage-poisoning in 1895 ; 11 cases, 1 death. No toxic substances could be isolated chemically, but virulent bacilli of the hog-cholera group were obtained in culture. [Pouchet's claim that this was the first successful application of bacteriology to legal medicine is too absurd to be seriously discussed. In any case his failure to obtain the bacilli from the dejecta leaves the chain of proof incomplete.]

Cicatrices as an Index of Right- and Left-handedness.—J. N.
Hall[4] found that cicatrices from whittling, etc., average from 4 to 12 on the opposite hand to that used habitually to hold the knife, as compared with 1 to 4 on the knife-hand. In women needle-pricks on the forefinger are equally significant. Of 100 persons examined, the results confirmed this in 91 ; in 8 the scars were too scanty to justify an opinion, and only 1 led to an error. Equal distribution of scars on both hands is suggestive of ambidexterity (left-handedness overcome). The test is more available than that of writing, as children naturally left-handed are taught to use the right hand for that purpose, though a weapon would still be held in the left.

Examination of Hairs.—P. Mimakow[5] found that dry heat below
150° C. produces no macro- or microscopic changes in hairs. At from 180° to 200° hairs are discolored red or black in 15 to 20 minutes. Hairs of normal appearance may show microscopically splitting and swelling at the tip and gas-bubbles in the shaft. This microscopic change was noticed after pistol-shots at a distance of 25 cm., where no change could be detected by the naked eye. Washing in water, then in alcohol, and mounting in balsam, are advised. F. Ringberg[6] found that changes may occur in the color of the hair many years after death from the effects of decomposition.

6. Toxicology.—E. Michel[7] found that **carbon monoxid** may persist
in blood-extravasations for from 2 to 5 days after it has disappeared from the circulating blood. Daniel[8] describes a simple modification of Haldane's quantitative colorimetry test for CO. A 1 % solution of normal blood in water is mixed with sufficient of a 1 % solution of blood previously saturated with CO from illuminating-gas to give the same tint as a 1 % solution of the blood to be tested. [A very full discussion of the whole subject of carbon monoxid took place at this congress, but the statements on many important points still remain irreconcilable.] I. Brouardel[9] has published a valuable monograph on arsenic-poisoning.

[1] Brussels méd.-leg. Congress, 1897. [2] Viertelj. ger. Med., Oct., 1896.
[3] Ann. d'Hyg. pub., Mar., 1897. [4] Boston M. and S. Jour., Dec. 17, 1896.
[5] Viertelj. ger. Med., Supplement, 1896. [6] Ibid., Oct., 1897. [7] Ibid., July, 1897.
[8] Brussels med.-lég. Congress, 1897. [9] Etude sur l'Arsenicesme, Paris, 1897.

7. The establishment of the special journal, *Annales de l' Unisexualité* (Leipzig), would serve a useful purpose if it relieves the scientific press from the necessity of publishing the endless supply of prurient detail having little novelty or scientific interest, which forms the bulk of the literature on sexual aberration.

There has been an increasing tendency to regard trauma as the cause of nervous and mental disturbances. More exact knowledge as to the anatomical and chemical conditions of the nervous and secretory organs has had a marked influence in the direction of transferring medicolegal problems in connection with this class of cases from the realms of hypothesis and metaphysics to those of tangible fact.

Absorption of Poisons.—J. S. Metzler[1] found that by ligating the stomachs of rabbits and dogs at cardia and pylorus strychnin could be retained for even 15 hours without producing any effect. Prussic acid under the same conditions was promptly toxic, ecchymoses of the mucosa leading to the inference that the difference was due to its direct absorption through lesions produced in the blood-vessels by contact.

The distribution of poisons in the body has been studied by A. Lesser[2] on a large scale (231 cases), his paper, however, not yet being completed. G. Miller[3] found that after a few days burial strychnin became diffused through all parts of the bodies of rabbits when injected after death into any of the body-cavities.

Effect of Bacteria on the Toxicity of Alkaloids.—S. Holenghi[4] found that the potency of weak atropin solutions in bouillon was progressively weakened by growth of B. coli and other putrefactive bacteria. Strychnin solutions at first showed an increase to double or treble the original toxicity (estimated by observing the degree of dilution in which a distinct physiologic effect was still obtainable), followed by a gradual diminution after the end of the first week.

[1] Jour. Exper. Med., July, 1896.
[2] Viertelj. ger. Med., Oct., 1897.
[3] Med.-Leg. Jour., Sept. and Dec., 1896.
[4] Viertelj. ger. Med., July, 1896.

PUBLIC HYGIENE AND PREVENTIVE MEDICINE.

By SAMUEL W. ABBOTT, M.D.,

OF BOSTON, MASS.

Introductory.—Progress in public hygiene in the United States has steadily advanced in the past thirty years or more. During that time nearly every State has established its Board of Health, and all the cities and many large towns now have local Boards of Health. Medical men have always constituted the most important factor in such boards, and will undoubtedly continue to fill such places in the future. The most important department of public hygiene is the management and control of infectious diseases, and one of the principal objects of preventive medicine is the limitation of the spread of those diseases which are preventable and are mostly of the infectious class. The subjects of isolation, quarantine, disinfection, notification of disease, hospital provisions, the supervision of water-supplies and systems of sewerage, plumbing-inspection, burial or disposal and transportation of the dead, and school-inspection, all are related more or less intimately with the general subject of disease-prevention. To these may be added such groupings or general topics as municipal hygiene, which embraces many of the foregoing subjects, the hygiene of occupations (industrial hygiene), food- and drug-inspection, the sale of poisons, and finally, as a basis of fixed and definite information as to the value of many of the foregoing measures, vital statistics.

THE MANAGEMENT AND CONTROL OF INFECTIOUS DISEASES.

Susceptibility to Infection in Relation to Age.—In his *Fourteenth Report for the City of Providence, R. I.* (1896), Chapin continues his researches on scarlet fever and diphtheria. These are directed to ascertaining the percentage of persons of different ages exposed to each of the above diseases who either contract them or fail to do so. The results are embodied in statistical tables, which possess a high etiologic value. It is obvious that the value of such tables depends on the care with which the data are obtained and the certainty that a uniform system of inquiry is pursued throughout. The headings of Chapin's returns are too copious to reproduce in their entirety; but the following will indicate the scope of the inquiries: number of families in which there was more than one susceptible child; number of families in which there was a second case; number of susceptible children in all the above families; number of these children who were attacked, etc., etc.

A separate table gives the ratio of cases to number of presumably susceptible persons exposed to infection. During the last ten years, for scarlet fever the ratio was as follows: for infants under one year, 26.3%; for the second year of life, 47.6; third year, 58.0; fourth year, 62.6; fifth year,

66.3; sixth year, 63.5; seventh year, 66.2; eighth year, 62.3; ninth year, 55.0; for adults over 20 years, 6.0. The percentage for scarlet fever at all ages was 38.4; that for diphtheria 30.6; the highest susceptibility for diphtheria (62.7 %) was at 4–5 years, and corresponded with the age at which the susceptibility was highest for scarlet fever.

The Value of Health-resorts for Consumptives.—The German Society of Public Health voted to recommend the collection of statistics of persons who have been treated at such homes or resorts, the inquiry to include a period of five years after leaving them.[1] The following conclusions were also presented for discussion at the same meeting: 1. Since neither the destruction of the specific cause of the disease nor the treatment of the sick by tuberculin has produced a demonstrable lessening of consumption, the health authorities turn to the hygienic and dietetic treatment, which can be conducted in sanitary homes or resorts. [This statement is altogether too dogmatic and exclusive. Lessening of the death-rate from phthisis **is** continually going on, and is due to a much greater number of factors than is admitted in the foregoing paragraph.] 2. Such resorts can only limit the spread of consumption, and that gradually, when they are erected in large numbers and are accessible to the poor. 3. The duty (of providing such resorts) rests upon those insurance companies which provide against disability from sickness and old age. These companies have the right to treat their insured before the period of breaking-down, in order to avoid that condition. In the effort to make use of this right, these societies should place the tuberculous patient as soon as possible in a health-resort, since it is only in the first stages of illness that the disease may be arrested and the working-powers of the sick man restored or preserved. Hence these organizations should aid in providing such resorts. 4. Sanitary homes for consumptives should be arranged and conducted on correct hygienic principles. They may be plainly furnished, but must contain everything that, according to experience, is necessary to increase the resistance of the human body against the development of tuberculosis. 5. These resorts should be provided with all the necessary apparatus for destroying the specific germs of tuberculosis, and making them innocuous to the neighborhood. 6. Without the constant services of a wise superintending physician the success of such treatment will be questionable. It is his duty to maintain the courage of the patient by the influence of his own personality, and to accustom him to that mode of life which is essential to his recovery, so that, after his dismissal, he will continue to practise the same mode of life at home.

The Imperial Board of Health of the German Empire, in a recent circular[2] upon the same subject, first calls attention to the prevalence of **tuberculosis in the German Empire** and **its incidence upon the wage-earning period of life**. (Out of a total of 268,500 deaths of persons between the ages of 15 and 60 years, 88,654, or almost one-third, were from tuberculosis.) It also calls attention to the proofs of the curability of the disease existing in the frequent occurrence of autopsies in which the evidence of cure is found. Furthermore, the circular cites the experience of the German Sanitaria, Görbersdorf and Falkenstein, and that of the large insurance companies which provide against disability from disease. The **value to the Empire of the added length of life** in persons who have been cured or whose health is improved is estimated at 7½ million marks, or a little less than 2 million dol-

---

[1] Deutsch. Vierteljahr. f. öff., Ges undheitspflege, 28, 1, 104, 1896.
[2] Ein Beitrag zur Beurtheilung des Nutzens von Heilstätten für Lungenkranke, Bearbeitet im Kaiserlichen Gesundheitsamte, Berlin, 1896.

lars annually. Hence the circular commends the establishment of homes for consumptives as a " blessing to mankind." [1]

Report of the Metropolitan Asylums Board (London) upon Antitoxin in Diphtheria.—The prominent point brought out in this report, as in nearly all recent reports upon the subject, is the necessity of beginning the antitoxin treatment as early in the course of the disease as possible. Comparing the results obtained under this treatment in 1896 with those of the non-antitoxin year 1894, the following figures are presented : Cases treated in 1894, 3042—fatality, 29.6 % ; in 1896, 4175—fatality, 20.8 %.

Fatality according to Day on which Treatment was Begun.

Day of first treatment.	Fatality (per cent.)		
	London.		Massachusetts.
	Antitoxin, 1896.	No antitoxin, 1894.	Antitoxin in 1895 and 1896.
First	4.7	22.5	1.5
Second	12.8	27.0	8.1
Third	17.7	29.4	9.5
Fourth	22.5	31.6	18.1
Fifth	24.6	30.8	16.0
All cases	20.8	29.6	11.8

The lowered rate of mortality represents 365 lives saved. The report concludes as follows : "We have only to add that we still hold to the opinion that in the antitoxic serum we possess a remedy of distinctly—we would now say much—greater value in the treatment of diphtheria than any other with which we are acquainted." The figures for Massachusetts are added to the foregoing table.

The following statement is made in the *Twenty-eighth Annual Report of the State Board of Health of Massachusetts* (1896) : "The most important lesson which is taught by these returns is the necessity of prompt administration of antitoxin in each and every case."

Conveyance of Typhoid-fever Infection by Means of the Air. —E. Gennano,[2] in a paper on the aërial convection of disease-germs, details the results of a series of experiments in which sterilized floor-dust, sand, peat, and loam were inoculated with a culture of the typhoid bacillus. Equal portions were dried, in some cases quickly, in others slowly, and in others but very little, and the length of time in which cultures might be obtained from them was compared. He concludes from these experiments that the typhoid-bacillus cannot live in the dried state, and hence dry dust cannot convey it. Moreover, it retains great vitality in moist places, and can exist in an *apparently* dried condition, such as is presented when it is surrounded by materials such as linen, articles of clothing, wood, and lumps of earth containing feces, which have moisture of their own, but as they become dry the bacilli perish. The danger is not that the bacilli pass into the air from them, but that particles of the materials containing bacilli are conveyed directly or indirectly to the mouth by the hand and by food and dishes. This character of the bacillus of retaining its vitality in a partially dried state must be considered as the chief source of infection. In his opinion, air-infection, especially from a dis-

[1] See also on the same subject, Recueil des Travaux de Comité Consultatif d'Hygiène publique de France, 25, p. 72, Melun, 1896. Also, Ueber Volksheilstätten für Lungenkranke, Georg Liebe, Breslau, 1896. [2] Zeit. f. Hyg., xxiv., 3, p. 423.

tance of several hundred meters, as maintained by Froid-boise,[1] must be absolutely impossible, and in this respect the typhoid-bacillus is like the cholera-germ. Air-infection by typhoid fever presupposes a mechanical attrition of material so fine that it becomes dry and consequently dies. [The chief method of transmission of typhoid fever infection is through the medium of water and milk, the latter being only a disguised form of the former. In a review of forty years' work of the Health Department of Glasgow, the author, J. B. Russell, says: "If we consider the history of enteric fever in detail, we observe that everything like an epidemic prevalence has been caused by the distribution of infected milk." [2]]

Unusual Sources of Typhoid Fever.—In addition to the recent attacks of illness due to the eating of oysters which had been gathered in waters polluted with sewage, reported in the special report of the Local Government Board,[3] another similar source is mentioned by Ramaroni,[4] of Bastia, Corsica. The author names five different kinds of shell-fish (mostly gasteropod mollusks, snails, limpets, etc.) which are usually eaten raw. These are collected near the mouths of sewers of the city and the public abattoir chiefly during the months of December to April, and in these months there has been during the past few years a decided increase in the prevalence of typhoid fever, contrary to the usual habit of prevalence in the autumn. The use of oysters as food increases largely in September, in accordance with a popular impression that they are not as healthful in the summer months. A writer in the *Boston Medical and Surgical Journal,* under the head of "Oysters and Typhoid Fever," calls attention to the fact that many cases of typhoid fever occurring in cities having good water-supplies are unexplained, and that their occurrence may be due to the increased consumption of oysters from bays and harbors largely polluted by sewage.[5] Geschwind[6] states that the kitchen gardeners of Bayonne are accustomed to sprinkle the foliage of certain leguminous plants with the contents of privy vaults diluted with water, and that the products are eaten raw as a salad. Several cases of typhoid fever among the officers of the garrison were traced to this source, and an expert found upon these plants the bacilli of typhoid fever, the coli communis, streptococci, staphylococci, the bacillus tuberculosis, and the joints of tenia.

The Notification of Measles.—With reference to the propriety of considering *measles* as a notifiable disease, English authorities appear to be divided in opinion.[7]

Transmission of Anthrax-infection by Hides and Leather.— G. Giuglio,[8] of Palermo, has demonstrated by experiment on guinea-pigs the possibility of transmission of anthrax-infection by hides and leather after they have been submitted to the ordinary processes of tanning.

Disinfection by Formaldehyd.—Recent valuable articles upon the efficiency of formaldehyd have been contributed by Walter,[9] Pfuhl,[10] Strüver,[11] and Kinyoun.[12]

[1] Bull. de l'Acad. royale de Méd. de Belgique, 1893.
[2] The Evolution of the Function of Public Health Administration. By J. B. Russell, B. A., M. D., LL. D., Glasgow, 1895.
[3] Oyster Culture and its Relation to Disease. Special Report of the Medical Officer to the Local Government Board, London, 1896; reports of H. W. Conn and C. J. Foote to the Connecticut Board of Health, 17th and 18th annual reports.
[4] Rev. d'Hyg.. p. 645, July, 1897.   [5] Boston M. and S. Jour., Sept. 23, 1897.
[6] Archiv. de méd. militaire, p. 313, May, 1897.
[7] See Kenwood's paper and discussion on the same in the Journal of the Sanitary Institute, p. 161, July, 1897.   [8] Ann. d'Igiene Sperimentale, p. 50, 1897.
[9] Zeit. f. Hyg., vol. xxi., p. 421, 1896.   [10] Ibid., vol. xxii., p. 330 and xxiv., p. 302.
[11] Ibid., vol. xxv., p. 386.   [12] Weekly Reports of Marine-Hospital Service, Jan. 29, 1897.

Walter's conclusions, from his investigations, are as follows: 1. Formalin in the strength of 1:10,000 arrests the growth of the germs of anthrax, cholera, typhoid fever, diphtheria, and staphylococcus pyogenes aureus. 2. In the gaseous form it arrests growth, even when greatly diluted. 3. In 1% solutions it kills pure cultures of pathogenic germs in an hour. In diluted alcoholic solutions the effect is more intense. 4. In 3% solutions, especially with the addition of alcohol, the hands may be freed from all germs. More extended investigations are necessary to show the degree to which the skin is affected. 5. By spraying artificially infected matter with formalin solution, and afterward enclosing it in air-tight vessels, such matter may be sterilized. 6. By means of formalin (or in other words formaldehyd) leather articles, uniforms, etc., may be thoroughly disinfected in large quantities, and without in any way injuring these articles; 24 hours' exposure are requisite for such disinfection. The possibility of disinfecting rooms may be considered as demonstrated by other experts. 7. Feces are almost instantly deodorized by a 1% solution, and are disinfected (germ-free) in ten minutes by a 10% solution. 8. Formalin acts well as a caustic. 9. It is an excellent preservative.

The Relation of Infectious Diseases to the Milk-supply.— W. T. Sedgwick[1] presents in a very clear manner the sanitary requirements of a good milk-supply.[2]

The Effect of Cemeteries upon Health.—Experiments conducted by Lösener for the Imperial Board of Health of Germany[3] showed that little harm need be feared in consequence of any escape of disease-germs from properly constructed graves to the surrounding soil or to neighboring water-supplies.

WATER AND WATER-SUPPLIES—SEWERAGE AND SEWAGE- AND REFUSE-DISPOSAL.

Treatment of Water Containing Lead.—The health officer of Pudsey, England, presents the results of experiments intended to remove the lead from the public water-supply of that town.[4] The method adopted was simply the addition of 3 gr. of chalk to each gallon of water. The water was drawn the first thing in the morning from a lead service-pipe 180 ft. in length. Lead-poisoning had been prevalent in that town. The following results were secured by the adoption of this treatment. The two years 1892 and 1896 are selected because in the former year no treatment was employed, while in 1896 it was employed throughout the year.

Months.	1892.	1896.
January	0.45	0.10
February	0.33	0.10
March	0.60	0.07
April	0.50	0.07
May	0.48	Trace
June	0.65	Trace
July	0.47	0.07
August	0.39	0.09
September	0.22	0.06
October	0.27	0.13
November	0.24	0.12
December	0.21	0.06

Monthly average grains of lead per gallon.

[1] Technology Quarterly, vol. x., No. 2, June, 1897.
[2] See also Ernest Hart's continuation of his summary of epidemics of illness traceable to milk-supplies in Brit. Med. Jour., p. 1167, May 8, 1897 ; also Fabre's experiments as to the source of the bacterial contamination of milk in Rev. d'Hyg., p. 721, Aug., 1897.
[3] Arbeiten aus dem Kaiserlichen Gesundheits., xii., 2, 448.
[4] Annual Report for 1896 of Medical Officer of Health, Pudsey, England.

The Softening of Hard Water.—The subject of softening hard water in those parts of the country which rest upon a stratum of limestone has not received in the United States the attention which it demands. The following statement,[1] however, shows that the question has decided economic value: "The hardness of the metropolitan water-supply is due almost entirely to the presence of the bicarbonate of lime in solution, which can readily be removed by treating the water with lime, as is successfully done by the Colne Valley Company. By this treatment with lime its hardness is reduced to about one-fourth of its original amount. This mode of softening water would appear to be the most economic, unless it can be shown that less than one-eighteeth of the total supply is used for washing, for it entails only about one-eighteeth of the expense incurred by the private consumers in the shape of additional soap."[2]

Sewer-gas and Sewer-ventilation.—Edward Walford[3] concludes, after a careful investigation of the subject of sewer-ventilation, "that there is very little reliable evidence to show that the ordinary specific infectious diseases are caused by inhaling sewer-gas, and that usually, where sewage is responsible for their causation, the mischief has arisen through swallowing either water or food which has become contaminated with sewage-matters."

FOOD- AND DRUG-INSPECTION.

The Practical Advantages of Food- and Drug-inspection.— The Food and Drug Statute of England was enacted in 1875, and the first full report of the Local Government Board upon its operations was for the year 1877, so that the people have had the protection which it affords for about 20 years. The following figures represent the improvement which has actually taken place, comparing the figures of the first report (1877) with those of the last published report (1895). They are as follows (condensed):

Percentage of Samples Adulterated, as found by the Government Analysts.[4]

	1877.	1895.
Milk	24.1	11.1
Flour	6.0	..
Coffee	17.5	10.0
Mustard	18.8	6.0
Butter	10.8	8.2
Bread	7.4	1.7
Wine	32.2	8.3
All articles	19.2	9.3

This very satisfactory result, a reduction of the actual ratio of adulteration by more than one-half, represents a very great gain to the general consumer in the quality of many of the ordinary articles of food which are subject to adulteration. The results obtained by a similar inspection in the continental cities, especially in Paris and the cities of the Swiss cantons, are very much of the same character. In Massachusetts a similar law has been in operation

[1] E. Frankland's Report on the Examination of the Water supplied by the Metropolitan Water Companies; Twenty-fifth Annual Report of Local Government Board, 1895–96, p. 279.

[2] For further valuable information upon this point, reference may be made to the two following treatises on water: Water and Water-supplies, by John C. Thresh, London, 1896; Chapter on water-softening. Water and its Purification, by S. Rideal, London, 1897.

[3] Sanitary Rec., p. 119, July 30, 1897.

[4] Reports of Local Government Board, England, for 1877 and 1895.

14 years, and the results of the examination of about 80,000 samples of food and drugs, with about 1200 prosecutions of offenders, have shown a marked reduction in adulteration and a consequent improvement in the food-supply. The following extract from the *Twenty-seventh Annual Report of the State Board of Health of Massachusetts*, p. 647, serves to illustrate the foregoing statement : " In 1884, soon after the enactment of the law and before an adequate appropriation had been provided for its enforcement, an examination of spices and cream of tartar, and other articles of food, as sold in open market in Massachusetts, gave the following results [examinations of similar articles made in 1896 showed a marked improvement in each instance] : Samples of spices collected in 1884, 431 ; number adulterated, 216, or 50.1 %. Samples of spices collected in July, 1896, 78 ; number adulterated, 2, or 2.6 %. Samples of cream of tartar collected in 1884, 232 ; number adulterated, 77, or 33.2 %. Samples of cream of tartar collected in July, 1896, 25, of which 1 was adulterated, or 4 %. Out of 123 samples of butter, cheese, tea, coffee, and confectionery collected in 1884, 15, or 12.2 %, were adulterated. Out of 82 samples of the same articles collected under similar conditions in July, 1896, all proved to be genuine.

INDUSTRIAL HYGIENE.

The Health of Zinc-workers.—The results of observations made upon the health of 1300 zinc-workmen by Seiffert[1] show that the blue line, the atrophy of parts about the mouth, the mucous membrane, adipose tissue, and muscular system, with changes in the tissues of the nervous and vascular systems and kidneys, point directly to lead-poisoning, and the actual use of 1% to 2% of lead as an alloy is sufficient to explain the trouble.

Prevention.—The author suggests the following remedies : 1. Among the young, only well-developed persons in perfect health and over 18 years of age should be employed. 2. The chief cause of the trouble is the dust of the workshops. Copious sprinkling of material, floors, and passage-ways should be done. 3. Gases and smoke should be carried away from the workmen. 4. Fresh water should be supplied in quantity sufficient for drinking-purposes. Drinking from open vessels exposed to the action of heat and dust should be forbidden. Water should be drawn from faucets and the mouth should be rinsed. Spittoons should be furnished for tuberculous workmen. Eating in the shops and the storage of food in them should be forbidden. Eating in rooms separate from the workshops should be encouraged. Other essential requirements are the provision of soap in abundance, the removal of sweat and poisonous dust from the body immediately after working-hours, changing of clothing after work, and the prevention of indulgence in drink. [Thus far very little has been accomplished in the way of investigations in industrial hygiene in America. There is here a wide and useful field for inquiry among the operatives in our manufacturing cities and mining districts.][2]

In treating of the frequency of **consumption among workmen** Sommerfeld[3] presents several tables. The following shows the mortality of such workmen from consumption as compared with the general mortality : the figures on the right show the deaths from consumption in each 1000 deaths

---

[1] Deutsch. Vierteljahrs. f. öff. Gesundheitspflege, 29, 3, 419, 1897.

[2] See also upon the same subject Hartmann's statement (Jahresber. d. preuss. Gewerberäthe, p. 187) that out of 2452 workmen in the zinc-works of Silesia (members of sick-benefit societies) there were 1382 cases of illness in 1893, or 56.3%, of which 11.9% were from diseases of the digestive organs, 1.6% from lead-poisoning, and 8.3% from rheumatism.

[3] Die Schwindsucht d. Arbeiter, Th. Sommerfeld, Berlin, 1895.

from all causes, and the other column the deaths from consumption in each 1000 living:[1]

Occupations not exposed to dust	2.39	381.0
Occupations exposed to dust	5.42	480.0
Dust-occupations:		
Metallic dust	5.83	470.6
Copper dust	5.31	520.5
Iron-dust	5.55	403.7
Lead-dust	7.79	501.0
Mineral dust	4.42	403.4
Organic dust	5.64	537.0
From leather and skins	4.45	565.9
From wool and cotton	5.35	554.1
From wood and paper	5.96	507.5
From tobacco	8.47	598.4
Mean	5.16	478.9
Mortality of the male population of Berlin over 15 years of age	4.93	332.3

The Ventilation of Railway Cars.—In a lecture before the Franklin Institute of Philadelphia C. B. Dudley,[2] Chemist of the Pennsylvania Railroad Company, admits "that it is not possible a the present time properly to ventilate a passenger-car on a railway." He states the problem as follows: "An ordinary passenger-coach contains about 400 cubic feet of space. It is proposed to take into this small space at least sixty persons: to keep them in this space continuously, without allowing them a chance to get out, for four hours or longer; to keep them warm enough for their comfort in winter; and to supply them with enough fresh air to ventilate the car properly and at the same time exclude, throughout the year, smoke and cinders, and in the summer season dust. No problem has ever been committed to the experimental and mechanical engineering departments of the railroad so difficult of solution as this problem of ventilation." By experiments with improved ventilators, plans of which were shown in the paper quoted, Dudley found that it was possible to take into the car 90,000 feet of fresh air in an hour; but this air could only be warmed about 40° above the temperature of the outer air. Hence, with an outdoor temperature of 0° such car would be uncomfortably cold. Experiments are still in progress to secure better results. As a result of the experiments already made, Dudley says, "It is possible to get much more air into a car than any system now takes in. If we could content ourselves with 20,000 to 40,000 feet of air per hour in severe weather, it is possible to have such a system put on the cars to-day. In milder weather this amount could be increased to the full capacity of the system."

VITAL STATISTIC.

Vital Statistics of the German Empire, 1894.—Rahts'[3] statement of the causes of death in the year 1894 in the German Empire, recently published, and contains in a condensed form very full statistics tl empire. It is illustrated with four excellent maps, bution of mortality from tuberculosis, acute lung dis-

he Parliamentary Committee upon Dangerous Trades (London, incident to the following occupations: bronzing, paper-staining omotives in factories. India-rubber manufacture, inflammable of aërated waters, electriconerating works, and woolsorting

", July, 1897.
_nstatistik, Medicinal-stistische Mittheilungen aus dem
) 129–181.

eases, and the diseases incient to childbirth, with the mortality of infants under one year. The result of the summary are stated as follows:

1. The deaths in 1894 ere less in number than those of 1892 or 1893, The difference between the mortality of 1893 and that of 1894 amounted to 2000 per million inhabitan. 2. The greatest decrease in the death-rate was among adults beyond the so of 60 years, and the principal decrease was in the deaths from acute lung diseases and influenza. The general death-rate was 22.4 per 1000. 3. There was a decrease in infant mortality (deaths under one year) which was coincidentwith a lessened birth-rate—the infant mortality amounted to 211 deaths (u ter 1 year) in 1000 births. About one-third of these deaths were due to intestinal catarrh. 4. The death-rate of childhood **(1–15 years)** has diminisht more noticeably than the general death-rate. **The mortal**ity from diphthem was less than that of the two previous years. Out of each 11 deaths at his time of life (1–15 years) 3 were from diphtheria. 5. More than one third of the deaths of adults (15–60) years) were deaths from tuberculosis . The lowest death-rate of adults (15–60 years) from tuberculosis occurredin three districts where the infant-mortality was high. Tuberculosis de troy the greatest relative number of adults in those districts where newborn infants survive in greatest numbers. 7. The increase of population in the course of one year was, therefore, more marked in districts having a high th n a ong thos having a low infantile death-rate.

The Decline in the Death-rate from Infectious or Preventable Diseases.—Krus ' show very conclusively the decline in the death-rate from typhoid fever, d rr a, small-pox, deaths in hospitals after surgical operations, etc., during 20 ears in Germany. The ratio in successive five-year periods for typhoid for per 10,000 living were as follows for 1875 to 1894: 6.17. 4 99, 2 7 and 1.86 Diarrhea, 1.63, 1.59, 0.45, and 0.3. Scarlet fever, erysipelas, consumptin, and deaths after surgical operations also showed a similar decline—that of consumption being from 52 to 36.

The saving of human life in consequence of the reduction in the mortality from infectious diseases in Prussia is estimated by him at 70,000 persons in one year

In Massachusetts the decline in the principal infectious diseases in the forty years 1856-95 was as f ow by five-year periods, including also the deaths from consumption and 4 fourth:

Death-rates from Cert Cases and Groups of Causes by Five-year Periods

from all causes, and the other column the deaths from consumption in each 1000 living:[1]

Occupations not exposed to dust	2.39	381.0
Occupations exposed to dust	5.42	480.0
Dust-occupations:		
Metallic dust	5.83	470.6
Copper dust	5.31	520.5
Iron-dust	5.55	403.7
Lead-dust	7.79	501.0
Mineral dust	4.42	403.4
Organic dust	5.64	537.0
From leather and skins	4.45	565.9
From wool and cotton	5.35	554.1
From wood and paper	5.96	507.5
From tobacco	8.47	598.4
Mean	5.16	478.9
Mortality of the male population of Berlin over 15 years of age	4.93	332.3

The Ventilation of Railway Cars.—In a lecture before the Franklin Institute of Philadelphia C. B. Dudley,[2] Chemist of the Pennsylvania Railroad Company, admits "that it is not possible at the present time properly to ventilate a passenger-car on a railway." He states the problem as follows: "An ordinary passenger-coach contains about 4000 cubic feet of space. It is proposed to take into this small space at least sixty persons: to keep them in this space continuously, without allowing them a chance to get out, for four hours or longer; to keep them warm enough for their comfort in winter; and to supply them with enough fresh air to ventilate the car properly and at the same time exclude, throughout the year, smoke and cinders, and in the summer season dust. No problem has ever been committed to the experimental and mechanical engineering departments of the railroad so difficult of solution as this problem of ventilation." By experiments with improved ventilators, plans of which were shown in the paper quoted, Dudley found that it was possible to take into the car 90,000 feet of fresh air in an hour; but this air could only be warmed about 40° above the temperature of the outer air. Hence, with an outdoor temperature of 0° such a car would be uncomfortably cold. Experiments are still in progress to secure better results. As a result of the experiments already made, Dudley says: "It is possible to get much more air into a car than any system now takes in. If we could content ourselves with 20,000 to 40,000 feet of air per hour in severe weather, it is possible to have such a system put on the cars to-day. In milder weather this amount could be increased to the full capacity of the system."

VITAL STATISTICS.

Vital Statistics of the German Empire in 1894.—Rahts'[3] statement of the causes of death in the year 1894 in the German Empire, recently published, is a model report, and contains in a condensed form very full statistics of the mortality of the empire. It is illustrated with four excellent maps, representing the distribution of mortality from tuberculosis, acute lung dis-

[1] See also the reports of the Parliamentary Committee upon Dangerous Trades (London, 1896 and 1897), upon the dangers incident to the following occupations: bronzing, paper-staining and -coloring, the use of locomotives in factories. India-rubber manufacture, inflammable paint, dry-cleaning, the bottling of aërated waters, electric generating works, and woolsorting and kindred industries.

[2] Jour. Franklin Institute, p. 3, July, 1897.

[3] Ergebnisse der Todesursachenstatistik, Medicinal-statistische Mittheilungen aus dem Kaiserlichen Gesundheitsamte, 3, pp. 129–181.

eases, and the diseases incident to childbirth, with the mortality of infants under one year. The results of the summary are stated as follows:

1. The deaths in 1894 were less in number than those of 1892 or 1893. The difference between the mortality of 1893 and that of 1894 amounted to 2000 per million inhabitants. 2. The greatest decrease in the death-rate was among adults beyond the age of 60 years, and the principal decrease was in the deaths from acute lung diseases and influenza. The general death-rate was 22.4 per 1000. 3. There was a decrease in infant mortality (deaths under one year) which was coincident with a lessened birth-rate—the infant mortality amounted to 211 deaths (under 1 year) in 1000 births. About one-third of these deaths were due to intestinal catarrh. 4. The death-rate of childhood (1-15 years) has diminished more noticeably than the general death-rate. The mortality from diphtheria was less than that of the two previous years. Out of each 11 deaths at this time of life (1-15 years) 3 were from diphtheria. 5. More than one-third of the deaths of adults (15-60 years) were deaths from tuberculosis. 6. The lowest death-rate of adults (15-60 years) from tuberculosis occurred in three districts where the infant-mortality was high. Tuberculosis destroys the greatest relative number of adults in those districts where newborn infants survive in greatest numbers. 7. The increase of population in the course of one year was, therefore, more marked in districts having a high than among those having a low infantile death-rate.

The Decline in the Death-rate from Infectious or Preventable Diseases.—Kruse[1] shows very conclusively the decline in the death-rate from typhoid fever, diarrhea, small-pox, deaths in hospitals after surgical operations, etc., during 20 years in Germany. The ratio in successive five-year periods for typhoid fever per 10,000 living were as follows for 1875 to 1894: 6.17, 4.99, 2.78, and 1.86. Diarrhea, 1.63, 1.59, 0.45, and 0.3. Scarlet fever, erysipelas, consumption, and deaths after surgical operations also showed a similar decline—that of consumption being from 52 to 36.

The saving of human life in consequence of the reduction in the mortality from infectious diseases in Prussia is estimated by him at 70,000 persons in one year.

In Massachusetts the decline in the principal infectious diseases in the forty years 1856-95 was as follows—by five-year periods, including also the deaths from consumption and childbirth:

Death-rates from Certain Causes and Groups of Causes by Five-year Periods (1856-95).[2]

Period.	Causes.	Death-rate in Massachusetts per 10,000 from these causes.
1856-60	Small-pox, measles, scarlet fever, diphtheria and croup, typhoid fever, cholera infantum, consumption, whooping-cough, dysentery, and childbirth.	81.7
1861-65		93.0
1866-70		74.8
1871-75		84.9
Mean		83.5
1876-80	Small-pox, measles, scarlet fever, diphtheria and croup, typhoid fever, cholera infantum, consumption, whooping-cough, dysentery, and childbirth.	73.1
1881-85		65.1
1886-90		56.8
1891-95		50.5
Mean		60.4

[1] Zeit. f. Hyg., xxv., 1.
[2] Twenty-eighth Report of State Board of Health of Mass., p. 816, 1896.

64

The Extent of the Losses due to Ill-health.—The great object and end of sanitary work are the diminution of disease and the consequent prolongation of human life. The actual magnitude of the losses due to impaired health is stated as follows, by the Imperial Board of Health of Germany.[1] The estimate is made from the statistical returns of the workingmen's clubs. In 1891, out of a total membership of 6½ millions, there were more than 2,000,000 cases of sickness, each of which lasted about 17 days, on an average. These clubs paid out for medical attendance nearly 22 million dollars. Since it is safe to assume that among the remainder of the German population 24 millions of whom are old enough to work, the cases of illness are quite as numerous and protracted as among the insured members of clubs, the expenses of sickness in Germany in one year is not reckoned too high at 120 million dollars. In this sum the loss due to the stoppage of wages is not included.

[1] Gesundheitsbüchlein, p. 1, 1896. Introductory remarks.

PHYSIOLOGIC CHEMISTRY.

By JOHN J. ABEL, M. D.,

OF BALTIMORE, MD.

During the Year.—Among the more valuable papers that have appeared are those of Mörner, on the proteids and proteid-precipitating substances of the normal urine; of Blumenthal and others, on animal substances which yield on decomposition one of the sugars; of Nencki and his pupils, and of Kaufmann and Schöndorff, on the distribution of ammonia and urea, and on the seat of formation of urea; of Siegfried, Witmaack, and Müller, on the occurrence of phosphosarcic acid, or nucleon, in human milk, etc.; of Schlossmann, on the separation of the proteids of milk; of Jaffé and Hirschl, on phenylhydrazin precipitates in the urine. Many papers describing methods, more or less useful to the physician, for the detection of albumin, albumoses, peptones, urea, etc. in the urine, have also been summarized or referred to. Some of the recent and most valuable investigations in physiologic chemistry are described in such voluminous and technical papers that it is impossible to incorporate their results in the space at our disposal.

Acetylene.—C. O. Southard [1] gives a short account of the properties of this hydrocarbon, C_2H_2, and of the methods for its manufacture, and thinks it ought to be of value as an illuminant for throat-work, etc., for physicians living in places where gas is not obtainable. Its explosive power is greater than that of gas, but it is no more dangerous when the proper precautions are taken. Brass should be avoided in pipes and burners intended for use with acetylene, as it unites with copper to form solid copper acetylene, which explodes violently on percussion or on heating to 200° C. The danger from poisoning is also pointed out, and it is asserted that the gas acts on blood similarly to carbonic oxid, only less energetically. This is, however, disproved by the recent excellent researches of Rosemann,[2] who finds, contrary to the older statements of Liebreich and Bistrow, that acetylene does not combine with hemoglobin, thus substantiating the experiments of Hermann and the more recent work of Ogier. Spectroscopic examination reveals no compound with hemoglobin. If such is formed, it is probably unstable and very different from carboxyhemoglobin. Conflicting statements as to the toxicity of acetylene having been made by previous investigators, Rosemann has made a considerable number of experiments, and finds that this gas is considerably less poisonous than pure carbonic oxid and also less poisonous than illuminating-gas. It should be borne in mind that Rosemann assumes that illuminating-gas contains only 8.88 % of carbonic oxid, whereas most of the gas now used in our cities contains as much as 30 %. Attention is also called to the toxicity of the products which may contaminate acetylene, such as sulphuretted and phosphoretted hydrogen. The recent experiments of the French authors, Gréhant, Berthelot, Moissan, and Brocinet,[3] also show that the poisonous action of acetylene has

---

[1] Pacific Med. Jour., Sept., 1896.
[2] On the toxicity of acetylene, Arch. f. exper. Path. u. Pharmakol., vol. xxxi., p. 179.
[3] Reviewed in Boston M. and S. Jour., July 30, 1896.

been greatly exaggerated, and when such was attributed to it, it was probably due to impure gas, CO or HCN.

Albumin-testing.—Tanret's Reagent.—A. R. Elliott[1] sets forth the delicacy and practicability of Tanret's method of detecting albumin, and points out to the practitioner how Tanret's reagent, which precipitates all modifications of albumin, as well as mucin, oleoresins, and alkaloids, may be made useful in a routine method for detecting and distinguishing different urinary proteids. Elliot, however, takes no note of the precipitation of bile-acids by Tanret's reagent, as was pointed out by Brasse[2] some years ago. Should such a precipitate be met with, it will be found to dissolve in ether; nor is mention made of the fact, to which attention is called in the treatise of Neubauer and Vogel, that uric acid may be precipitated by this reagent as above prepared.[3] This precipitate, which is perhaps rarely met with in actual urine-testing, is soluble on boiling and is easily distinguished from proteids. It may also be avoided by diluting before testing.

Jolles[4] announces a corrosive sublimate solution as a most delicate and practicable reagent for the detection of albumin in the urine. Glas,[5] Fürbringer,[6] and Spiegler,[7] have all preceded Jolles in setting forth the claims of corrosive sublimate as a proteid precipitant, but Spiegler's work in this field is alone referred to. Jolles's solution has the following composition : hydrarg. bichlor. corros., 10 ; natrium chloratum, 10 ; acidum succinic., 20 ; aqua distill., 500. This reagent has the great advantage of being colorless ; it may be applied to any urine, no matter what its composition may be, and when the result is negative one may rest assured that no traces of proteid, or at least none such as have a pathologic significance, are present. The test is made as follows : to 4 or 5 c.c. of filtered urine 1 c.c. of acetic acid (30%) and 4 c.c. of the reagent are added, and the whole is then shaken. To a second test-tube containing 4 or 5 c.c. of the same urine and 1 c.c. of acetic acid about 4 c.c. of distilled water are added and also shaken. This control-test is made to eliminate the disturbing action of mucin. A greater turbidity in the test-tube containing the reagent and urine indicates that albumin is present. The delicacy of the test is such that it still detects albumin when present in the proportion of 1 : 120,000. If iodids are present, a precipitate of mercuric iodid is formed, which is soluble in alcohol. The reagent has a specific gravity of 1040, and may be used in the "contact-method," a method which is especially serviceable when the urine is loaded with bacteria, as no attempt to clarify the urine need first be made if the test be applied in this way.

Asaprol.—Aseptol.—Refractometer Method.—E. Riegler[8] announces that asaprol in 10% solutions is a very delicate reagent for albumin. To 4 or 5 c.c. of urine 1 or 2 drops of hydrochloric acid and 10 drops of a 10% solution of asaprol are added. A precipitate indicates that albumins, albumoses, or peptones are present. Albumin is present if the contents of the test-tube remain cloudy on boiling. Aseptol, or orthophenolsulfonic acid, is, according to Riegler,[9] also well adapted to detect albumin when present in the proportion of 1 : 20,000. Like asaprol, this agent precipitates albumins and peptones, and the precipitates in this instance also clear up on heating. To 5 c.c. of urine 15 or 20 drops of the commercial solution of aseptol ($33\frac{1}{3}$%) are added ; the reagent is also serviceable in removing pro-

[1] N. Y. Med. Jour., Sept. 5, 1896.   [2] Maly's Jahresb., vol. xvii., p. 187.
[3] Neubauer and Vogel, Harn Analyse, p. 268.
[4] Zeit. f. Physiol. Chem., vol. xxi., p. 306.   [5] Maly's Jahresb., vol. vii., p. 17.
[6] Deutsch. med. Woch., vol. xxvii., p. 467, 1885.   [7] Wien. klin. Woch., No. 2, 1892.
[8] ibid., No. 54, 1894 ; Maly's Jahresb., vol. 25, p. 235.
[9] Wien. med. Blat., No. 35, 1895.

teids preparatory to making tests for sugar. Riegler prefers asaprol to aseptol because its solutions are less decomposable. In a later paper the author describes a quantitative method of estimating albumin, which is based on the examination of the precipitate obtained with asaprol. This precipitate is dissolved in $\frac{1}{10}$ normal alkali solution, and then tested with Pulfrich's refractometer. The index of refraction of the alkaline solution of the urinary albumin varies with the concentration of the solution, and hence when constants and standards are given it becomes a simple method to calculate the amount of proteid present.[1]

The Sulphosalicylic Acid Test.—R. Stein [2] sets forth the claims of the "sulpho-test" of Reoch and MacWilliams. Stein's method of employing this test is to add some crystals of sulphosalicylic acid to a small quantity of filtered urine in a test-tube. On shaking the tube a white homogeneous precipitate falls out instantly if considerable albumin is present, while with only very small quantities a cloudiness appears. Peptones and albumoses, which are also precipitated, are detected on boiling, when their precipitates will dissolve. The sulpho-test is thought by Stern to be of great value in cases with the small contracted kidney, when urine of low specific gravity is voided and when only very small quantities of albumin are present. Stein attributes to this test a very superior delicacy.

Ammonium Molybdate.—Yavorovsky [3] describes the following test. He "adds an excess of sodium carbonate to the urine, filters it, evaporates it to one-third of its volume, and then filters it again. To 4 c.c. of the filtrate is added one drop of a solution of 1 part of ammonium molybdate and 4 parts of citric acid in 40 parts of water. If albumin or peptone is present, cloudiness results either immediately or after a certain time. If this is due to peptone, it dissolves on warming and reappears on cooling." A. G. R. Foulerton [4] gives a study, for clinical purposes, of many of the methods in use for the detection of albumin and allied substances which occur in the urine in disease. The paper contains a table giving the reactions of albumin, albumoses, and peptones when nitric acid, Spiegler's solution, potassic ferrocyanid, metaphosphoric acid, picric acid, the biuret reaction, and the xanthoproteic reaction are used. It is also called to mind that the differentiation of proteoses and the separation of albumoses and peptones are by no means so simple a process as a tabular account of reactions might lead the physician to suppose. Foulerton also gives a list of many of the diseases in which proteosuria or peptonuria has been met with.

Albumosuria.—The recent investigations on albumosuria by Huppert,[5] Zeehuisen,[6] Haack,[7] and on the connection between circulating albumoses and febrile states, by Krehl and Matthes,[8] and Schultess,[9] and others all demonstrate the practical importance that attaches to a knowledge of methods for separating proteoses. Leick [10] has found that albumosuria occurs in fibrinous pneumonia at all stages of the disease.

Proteids and Proteid-like Substances in Normal Urine.—Many urinologists hold that the employment of exceedingly sensitive tests for albumin in the urine is to be criticised, not alone on the grounds that a mere trace of albumin is too readily accepted as the sign of a pathologic condition, but also because the sensitive tests so frequently require the exercise of a nice

[1] Wien. med. Blat., No. 48. [2] Med. Rec., Jan. 16, 1897.
[3] Med. News, Mar. 6, 1897, cited from Méd. moderne, No. 58, 1896.
[4] Practitioner, Dec., 1896. [5] Zeit. f. physiol. Chem., vol. 22, p. 500.
[6] Maly's Jahresb., vol. xxiii. [7] Arch. f. exper. Path. u. Pharmakol., vol. 38, p. 175.
[8] Deutsch. Arch. f. klin. Med., 1894. [9] Dissertation, Jena.
[10] Deutsch. med. Woch., No. 2, 1896.

chemic discrimination to decide whether the precipitate obtained is a normal constituent of the urine, albumin, a drug, or what not. The wide employment, however, of these sensitive tests gives new interest to the minute study of the urine. The distinguished physiologic chemist K. A. H. Mörner[1] has recently contributed an exhaustive study of the nature of the proteids and proteid-precipitating substances present in normal urine, and he concludes from his work that every so-called normal urine from adults of both sexes contains albumin, and also, as a rule, certain substances, chiefly chondroitin-sulphuric acid, which, when present in relatively large amount, may conceal the ordinary properties of the proteid, altering its coagulability and precipit-ability. Large quantities of urine, often as high as 250 liters, were required. The proteid-like material, always present in the form of a mucous cloud or nebecula, he collects as a sediment from urine preserved with chloroform, and finds that it consists of a *urine-mucoid* precipitated by acetic acid and a water-soluble mucin, which differs probably only in a minor way from the former. Both probably originate from the mucous membranes of the urinary passages. Boiling with mineral acids develops a strongly reducing-substance. The urine-mucoid is described as levo-rotatory (62° to 67°), has the percentage-composition C 49.4, N 12.74, S 2.3, and gives the proteid color-reactions. The results of certain experiments, such as boiling with hydrochloric acid, led Mörner to class this mucoid with the keratomucoids. The proteid matter which is held in solution in normal urine, hitherto described as "dissolved mucin," "mucin-like substance," or "nucleoalbumin," is found to consist chiefly of serum-albumin. The method employed to precipitate this serum-albumin was to shake dialyzed urine with chloroform, having previously added acetic acid. The proteid thus precipitated with acetic acid and chloro-form consisted of serum-albumin in combination with nucleinic acid, chon-droitin-sulphuric acid, and possibly other substances. In pathologic cases taurocholic acid may also acquire significance as entering into combina-tion with serum-albumin to form with it a precipitable compound like those just referred to. The serum-albumin present is referred to the blood for its origin.

On the Uric-acid Zone in Heller's Test for Albumin.—T. Husche[2]

has taken up the old question as to the composition of the white zone or cloud which more or less frequently interferes with the use of Heller's test. He finds that the uric-acid ring occurs only when highly concentrated urines are used, and that it agrees in appearance with Heller's description. It begins at a point a little above the line of contact of the acid and urine, has a sharply defined lower border, extending all throughout the supernatant layer of urine, and is completely dissolved by cautious heating. Sometimes the urates are thrown out in thick, flocculent streaks, gradually expanding as they extend upward; but more frequently, in place of these cloud-like streaks, a diffuse cloudiness is met with. According to Husche, most urines to which the test is applied show above the line of contact between acid and urine a fairly homogeneous cloudy layer, sharply outlined as to its lower surface, but extend-ing upward in the form of a cloud. Previous dilution of the urine makes no change in the appearance of this zone, and heating does not cause it to dis-appear entirely, while on cooling it is often more marked than before and lies at a higher level. The genuine uric-acid zone never appears after previous dilution. The spurious zone just referred to is supposed to be caused by nucleo-albumins. Further communications are promised on this point. When

---

[1] Maly's Jahresb., vol. 25, p. 263; Skandinav. Arch. f. Physiol., vol. 6, pp. 332–437.
[2] Wien. med. Woch., June 19, 1897.

the urine contains albumin and is concentrated and rich in urates one may observe, first, the albumin-zone, more or less dense at the line of union between acid and urine, above this again the turbidity due to uric acid, and in this turbid space a cloudy disk which Husche supposes to be caused by a nucleo-albumin.

Soluble Urates.—F. W. Tunicliffe[1] publishes a preliminary note on the solubility of piperidin urate and hexamethylenamin urate in distilled water, but states that the physical conditions obtaining in blood and other physiologic and pathologic fluids differ sufficiently from those in distilled water to render further research necessary before any statements can be made as to the usefulness of the above bases in the treatment of lithemia in the human subject. Piperidin urate is soluble in distilled water at 36° C. or 98° F. to the extent of 9.1 % ; hexamethylenamin urate at the same temperature is soluble to the extent of 3.3 %. At 17° C. the former salt is soluble to the extent of 5.3 % ; the latter to the extent of 0.7 %. For purposes of comparison the solubility of the following known urates is given: piperazin urate at 17° C. 2 % ; lithium urate, 20° C. 0.3 % ; at 39° C. 0.9 % ; potassium urate (acid salt), 20° C. 0.7 %-0.8 %. Further investigations are promised.

On the Danger of Filtering Urine with Talc.—Brandeth Symonds[2] finds by experiment that the use of purified talc for the purpose of clarifying urine and removing mucin and coloring-matters is to be avoided, since considerable albumin is also retained by the talc.

Ureometers.—Several ureometers have been described during the past few years, for each of which some special claim is made in the way of convenience, rapidity of manipulation, etc. G. A. Barbiera[3] describes a new mercury ureometer of simple design for use in the hypobromite method. G. Cavallero,[4] M. G. Mercier,[5] and Th. Lohnstein,[6] also describe forms devised by them. Linossier[7] describes a very simple apparatus which can be put together at trifling expense. The calculation of the amount of urea corresponding to the observed volume of nitrogen is made after data furnished by Yvon, "allowance having been made for incomplete decomposition of the urea and of other nitrogenous substances, for temperature and pressure, etc."

Estimation of Urea.—E. Riegler[8] describes a rapid and easy method of estimating urea based on the employment of Millon's reagent, which decomposes urea into equal volumes of carbon dioxid and nitrogen. The apparatus employed is simple. The results actually obtained vary from those required by theory by 0.01 % to 0.52 %. A. Kossel and H. Schmied[9] have compared the methods of estimating urea, which have been published by Gumlich, Mörner-Sjöqvist and Cazeneuve-Hugounenq, with a new method proposed by them. According to this method, 10 c.c. of urine to which a sufficient amount of barium carbonate has been added are put into a glass tube (sodium glass), which is then sealed and kept at 180 C. for one hour. The contents are then washed into a distilling-flask, barium hydrate is added, and the liberated ammonia is distilled into a $\frac{1}{10}$ normal hydrochloric acid solution, and thus estimated according to a well-known procedure. The new method was used in estimating the urea of normal and various pathologic urines, and was found to be satisfactory. The

[1] Brit. Med. Jour., Feb. 27, 1897.   [2] Med. Rec., Aug. 8, 1896.
[3] Maly's Jahresb., vol. xxiv., p. 71.   [4] Deutsch. med. Woch., p. 548, 1895.
[5] Chem. Centralb., ii., p. 410, 1895.
[6] Allg. medic. Central-zeitung, No. 31, 1894, Maly's Jahresb., vol. xxv., p. 231.
[7] Canad. Pract., Sept., 1896.   [8] Zeit. f. Analyt. Chemie, vol. xxxiii., p. 49.
[9] Du Bois Reymond's Arch., Physiol. Abth., p. 552, 1894.

results agreed with those obtained by the method of Gumlich ; those obtained by the method of Cazeneuve-Hugounenq were somewhat lower, and those by the Mörner-Sjöqvist method were slightly higher.   A point which may have to be borne in mind is that kreatin and kreatinin can be made to yield ammonia when treated by Kossel's method.

Bernhard Schöndorff's Method.[1]—This method, which requires considerable time, involves the precipitation and separation of compounds of the uric-acid series with the help of phosphotungstic acid, and determines the urea by decomposing it with phosphoric acid.   From the ammonia obtained the amount of urea present is readily calculated.   A second portion of the solution to be analyzed for urea is treated with an alkaline solution of barium chlorid and heated in sealed tubes to 150° C.   The carbonic acid thus obtained as a decomposition-product of the urea is determined in the gasometric way according to Pflüger's directions.   A control-analysis is also made to determine the amount of preformed carbonic acid present in the solution, and the amount thus found is deducted from that obtained (as above) by decomposition of the urea with barium chlorid.   It will thus be seen that Schöndorff estimates the urea present in animal fluids and tissues by decomposing it and estimating not only the obtained ammonia, but also the carbonic acid ; one serving as a control upon the other.   The details of the method, the points to be borne in mind when kreatin and amido-compounds are present, cannot be given here, but must be looked up in the original.   Further observations must determine the applicability of this method to the detection of very small quantities of urea.

Gréhant's Method.—M. Kaufmann [2] has examined the value of Gréhant's method for determining urea in blood and tissues.   Gréhant's method dates from 1870, and makes use of a solution of mercury, 1 gm. in 10 c.c. of pure nitric acid, for decomposing the urea, the CO_2 and N liberated enabling one to estimate the urea.   The method is well adapted to the estimation of urea in the blood, but in estimating urea in the tissues there is found to be a discrepancy in the amounts of CO_2 and N, other nitrogenous compounds being to some extent decomposed, yet even here the deviations from a standard estimation are not greater than when Schröder's method is used.

Urea in Animal Organs.—Making use of his method as just described, Schöndorff [3] has studied the distribution of urea in the blood, in the muscles, heart, kidneys, and other organs of dogs fed on large quantities of meat, and concludes that the muscle-tissue contains urea, the identity of the urea being made to rest on the melting-point and the nitrogen-determinations.   Urea was also found to be present in the red corpuscles, which contained as much as an equal amount of blood-serum.   With the exception of the muscles, heart, and kidneys, all the organs were found to contain urea in about the proportion in which it is present in blood.   M. Nencki and A. Kowarski,[4] on the other hand, making use of v. Schöndorff's method, were unable to isolate any urea from 2.5 kgm. of dog's muscle.   These investigators compare all past statements as to the normal occurrence of urea in muscle to accounts of the sea-serpent.   Their own method (stated in a few words) involves the use of phosphotungstic acid.   The filtrate from the precipitate thus induced is freed from phosphotungstic acid, an alcoholic solution of organic substances supposed to con-

---

[1] Pflüger's Archiv, vol. lxii., p. 1.
[2] Compt. rend. de la Soc. de Biol., vol. xlvii., pp. 145-147, and Maly's Jahresb., vol. xxv., p. 173.
[3] Pflüger's Archiv, vol. lxii., p. 332.
[4] Arch. f. exper. Path. u. Pharmakol., vol. xxxvi., p. 395.

tain the urea is obtained, and after evaporating this with an alcoholic solution of *ortho*-nitrobenzaldehyd, urea, if present, will be thrown out as a white crystalline compound, melting at 200° C. and having all the properties of

$$ortho\text{-nitrobenzylidendiureid, } C_6H_4(NO_2)CH\begin{cases} NH.CO.NH_2 \\ NH.CO.NH_2 \end{cases}$$

This method, as the writer can testify, is exceedingly delicate, and, using it, the authors in question were unable to detect urea in the acqueous extract from 850 gm. of dog's muscle, or in 450 gm. of Liebig's extract. On the other hand, using only 100 gm. of dog's blood, they could easily detect urea in the form of its compound with *ortho*-nitrobenzaldehyd. Inasmuch as urea can be separated by several methods from the muscles of the ray and shark, and only negative results are obtained when the same methods are applied to mammalian muscle, they conclude that the latter contains no urea.

Seat of Formation of Urea in the Body.—M. Nencki, I. Pawlow, and I. Zaleski,[1] continuing the splendid work of Nencki and his pupils, have made careful estimations of the ammonia-content of the blood and various tissues, and their results are such as to strengthen the view that the liver is the chief urea-forming organ of the body. Every 100 gm. of blood from the portal vein contain on the average 3.4 times as much as NH_3 as an equal amount of arterial blood, and 3.5 times as much as the blood of the hepatic veins. The amount of NH_3 in both the blood and the organs is dependent on the nature of the diet, being much increased, especially in the liver, spleen, mucous membranes of the stomach and intestines, and muscles, when the dogs are fed on an exclusive meat-diet. The ammonia-content of the gastric mucous membrane is twice as high as that of the gastric contents, and is the result of a series of changes effected in proteids when the mucous membranes are in a state of glandular activity. The decomposable ammonia-compounds thus formed (carbamates) are carried to the liver and there converted into urea. Directing the current of the portal vein into the inferior vena cava induces fatal ammonia-intoxication, on account of the accumulation of carbonic acid in the blood. Calculating from Cybulski's measurements of the velocity of the blood-flow in the portal vein and his own ammonia-estimations, Nencki concludes that the liver of the dog is able to hold back and convert into urea in the course of 10 hours as much as 4.72 gm. of ammonia, forming out of it 8.3 gm. of urea. It is admitted that the liver is not the only organ in which the formation of urea takes place; all the other organs of the body together, however, cannot compensate for the loss of the liver in regard to this function. The research in question is an exhaustive one, and note is taken of the objections that have been made by Pick, Lieblein, and Munzer to the view that the liver is the chief seat of urea-formation and to other points in the carbonic-acid theory of urea-function. M. Kaufmann[2] has also made, by means of Gréhant's and v. Schröder's methods, extensive experiments on the question as to where urea is mainly formed. He tied the aorta and vena cava in the thorax and kept the animals alive for from 30 to 105 minutes after the operation by means of artificial respiration. The blood after this operation sometimes contained considerably more urea than before, pointing to the formation of urea in other organs than the liver, this organ having been cut off from all connection with the blood by the above-explained operation. The urea-con-

[1] Arch. des Sci. biolog. de St. Petersburg, vol. iv., p. 197.
[2] Arch. de physiol., vol. xxvi., p. 531.

tent of the blood of a starving dog was also compared with that of the liver, brain, muscles, and spleen. The blood contained 32 mgm. urea in 100 gm., the brain 86 mgm., the spleen 62 mgm., the muscles 64 mgm., the liver 109 mgm. in every 100 gm. of substance. Kaufmann concludes that while the liver is the chief seat of the formation of urea, the other organs named also all take a part in this function. W. H. Thompson [1] concludes from a series of experiments on the nature of the work of the kidney as shown by the influence of atropin and morphin upon the secretion of the urine, that the kidney is a glandular organ, comparable to the true elaborating glands, and that it elaborates a part of the urea excreted by it out of other substances.

Urea in the Portal Blood.—E. Cavazzani and L. Salvatore [2] have determined the urea in aqueous extracts of fetal blood by means of the hypobromite method, previously removing the proteids. They found that the average amount of urea in the fetal blood in 32 determinations was 0.215%. The amount thus found does not tally with that found in the maternal blood, and the authors think it probable that the fetus itself produces urea.

Nitrogenous Compounds of the Urine.—At the second international congress for applied chemistry held in Paris from the 27th of July to the 5th of August, the section devoted to medical chemistry and pharmacy adopted the following statements with regard to the nitrogenous compounds of the urine: 1. In the present state of our knowledge, provided that the proper experimental precautions be observed, the hypobromite method of estimating urea is to be considered as sufficiently accurate for the purpose of clinical research. 2. The total nitrogen of the urine is to be estimated by Kjeldhal's method. The calculated difference between the total nitrogen found and the amount of nitrogen in urea represents nitrogen in the form of "incompletely oxidized substances." 3. When a rigorous estimation of the amount of uric acid present is required, the Salkowski-Ludwig method is adopted by most authors. For practical purposes the method of Deniges, possessing, as it does, sufficient exactitude and quickness of execution, deserves to be adopted.[3]

Clinical Significance of Casts.—G. Barrie [4] examined the urine of 50 inmates of a United States jail for albumin and casts, all the subjects being apparently in perfect health and varying from 15 to 65 years of age. In 40% of the cases casts of the hyaline and granular varieties were found, while in 1 case a few casts of the epithelial variety were found. The work of Gray, Shattuck, Brewer, Senator, Johnson, and others is commented on, and the general conclusion is arrived at that when apparently healthy persons exhibit both albumin and casts in their urine this state cannot safely be regarded as a truly physiologic condition, but in most such instances there is thought to be no doubt that the casts will disappear, the chances toward a serious result being about equal to those presented in a mild bronchitis. A few cases of renal insufficiency with all the symptoms of Bright's disease are also described, the outcome being sometimes fatal and again favorable, illustrating the fact that other things besides the mere urinary examination must be taken into account.

Preservation of Urinary Sediments.—Gumpricht [5] points out the value of a method of preserving urinary sediments for teachers of clinical medicine and for medical experts. He collects the sediment by centrifugation, using tubes with a constricted neck terminating in a small globular enlargement at the lower end, as these allow the supernatant fluid to be poured off without disturbing the sediment. When enough sediment has been gathered

[1] Jour. of Physiol., vol. xv., p. 433.   [2] Centralbl. f. Physiol, vol. ix., p. 25.
[3] Bull. de l'Acad. de Méd., Aug. 11, 1896.   [4] Med. Rec., Jan. 23, 1897.
                [5] Centralbl. f. innere Med., No. 30, 1896.

a quantity of a $\frac{2}{10}$ % solution of formalin is poured on it; the tube is shaken vigorously and then set aside. All constituents of the sediment retain their form and appearance. A series of sediments kept for a year were found to be unaltered, casts, epithelial cells, leucocytes, etc., retaining their original appearance. In order to avoid granular precipitations sediments from urines containing much albumin are washed once with physiologic salt-solution by the centrifugal method. Excess of urates may be removed by washing with warm water or concentrated solution of borax. In case red corpuscles or morphotic elements derived from erythrocytes are present in the sediment an aqueous solution of corrosive sublimate (1 : 20) is used for hardening. This solution is poured on the sediment prepared by centrifugation, the whole is shaken for five minutes, again precipitated, and washed six times by centrifugation with water or alcohol until all the sublimate has been removed, and then the formalin solution is added as already described.

Sugar in Urine.—Mark McDonald [1] points out the difficulties in deciding whether the urine contains a little sugar or whether it is simply that its normal reducing-substances are present in excessive quantity. The use of charcoal for removing the normal reducing-substances, as proposed by Sir William Roberts and by Seegen, is made the subject of a series of experiments. McDonald's results agree with those published by Seegen—namely, that filtration through animal charcoal leads to the loss of some sugar, the charcoal retaining it so firmly that even thorough washing will not remove all of it. The phenylhydrazin-test is also upheld by McDonald, who advises that small isolated crystals should be neglected in studying the precipitate produced by this reagent. The test may be rendered still more certain by treating a second portion of the urine with active yeast for from 12 to 24 hours, when on applying the test the result should be negative. J. Geyer [2] and others have attempted to show that the phenylhydrazin is poorly adapted to the determination of very small quantities of sugar. It must be admitted that the identity of the glycosazon-crystals can only be established with absolute certainty when melting-point determinations and analytical data are offered. J. A. Hirschl,[3] in a valuable paper, replies to previous attacks on this method, and shows how the observance of a number of precautions may give to this well-known test a high degree of certainty. The characteristic needle-shaped crystals of glycosazon can always be secured when the fermentation-test gives positive results. The crystalline compound which is often thrown out in normal urines during the first fifteen minutes of heating, and which may be mistaken for a glycosazon, probably consists only of the glycuronic acid compound of phenylhydrazin. In the course of further heating this disturbing precipitate turns into an amorphous brownish-yellow precipitate, which cannot be mistaken for the characteristic phenylglycosazon crystals.

Phenylhydrazin and Urea.—No one has yet determined in a satisfactory manner just what is the composition of the crystalline precipitate of needles, plates, burs, etc., which can be found in a large proportion of the urines of healthy people when this test is applied. M. Jaffé,[4] in a very recent paper, has attempted the analysis of this precipitate, but thus far without a satisfactory result. He has, however, isolated from a precipitate similarly obtained from the urine of the dog a crystalline compound of urea and phenylhydrazin, known as phenylsemicarbazid, $C_6H_5NHCONH_2$. This compound crystallizes in plates, is soluble in hot water and hot alcohol, reduces Fehling's solution on boiling, and melts at 172° C. Jaffé has found that this

---

[1] Lancet, Sept. 19, 1896.   [2] Wien. med. Presse, vol. 30.
[3] Zeit. f. physiol. Chemie, vol. 14, p. 377.   [4] Ibid., vol. 22, p. 532.

compound is readily thrown out of dog's urine when the animals are fed on meat, not when they are fed on bread or milk. He has not found it in the urine of human beings on a mixed diet.

On Substances in the Animal Body from which Sugar is Split Off.—Blumenthal [1] gives a succinct statement of the properties of glycoproteids, and shows how their study is destined to throw light on the origin of sugar in the body in pathologic conditions. The list of substances at present known to contain a carbohydrate group in their molecule includes the mucins, chondrosin, protagon, jecorin, phosphosarcic acid, adenylic acid, nucleohiston, and the nucleoproteids found by Hammersten to be present in the pancreas. From all of these substances it is possible to split off by chemical methods either a pentose or hexose, a galactose, etc., though in some instances the resulting carbohydrate has not been identified with certainty. In a broad way, therefore, all of these substances may be spoken of as compounds from which a sugar could be derived in the course of the metabolic processes taking place in the body. And of all the substances above named the nucleoproteid of the pancreas must be considered the most important from a clinical point of view, both because it occurs in relatively large quantity and because it yields much sugar (a pentose) on being decomposed. Blumenthal has discovered that certain nucleoproteids previously described by others as present in the liver, thymus, muscles, and pancreas, all yield a pentose when suitably treated, the osazone of which was isolated and found to melt at 153°–158° C. He has also isolated a new nucleoalbumin from the thyroid, from the spleen, and from brain-substance, which also yields a pentose. It is apparent, therefore, that such compounds are widely distributed in the animal organism. They are constituents of the cell-nucleus, and it is therefore possible that in the breaking down of cell-nuclei in the body sugar appears. The fact that the sugar which is split off in the laboratory from these compounds is a pentose acquires significance when the modern instances of pentosuria described by Salkowski, Külz and Vogel, and others, are borne in mind. How we can square the above laboratory achievement with the fact that the pathologic sugar-production seen in diabetes leads to a hexose, and only in a minor degree, or not at all, to a pentose, is at present not clear. Blumenthal thinks it is possible that the body splits up these nucleoalbumins in a different way, and that even if a pentose is first formed it might be changed either in a direct or in a more roundabout way into a hexose. He concludes, too, that it is not the proteid part of the nucleoalbumin, but the nucleinic acid contained in it from which the sugar is derived. He also does not think that Pavy has established the glucosidal nature of albumin, although he has rendered it probable, having obtained from egg-albumin a reducing-body whose osazone melts at 189°–190° C. That sugar can be formed in every cell of the body out of the nucleoalbumins contained in its nucleus is the author's final conclusion.

Mucin of White Fibrous Connective Tissue.—To the above may be added that R. H. Chittenden and W. J. Gies [2] have studied the cleavage-products of the mucin of white fibrous connective tissue, and have separated from these products a carbohydrate body which forms a well-defined and crystallized osazone which melts at 158°–160° C. They are at present unable to make definite statements as to the exact nature of this carbohydrate.

Chemistry of Colostrum Milk.—G. Woodward [3] reports analyses of 6 cases, and concludes that colostrum-corpuscles are not always found in so-called colostrum-milk; when they are present the percentage of proteids is

[1] Berlin. klin. Woch., Mar. 22, 1897.　　　　[2] Jour. Exper. Med., vol. i., p. 186.
[3] Ibid., Mar., 1897.

higher, and as they disappear the proteid percentage falls. The yellow color of colostrum-milk is especially marked in negro's milk; the specific gravity varies from 1024 to 1034, and this variation is chiefly due to the variation in the amount of fat present. The fat varies from 2% to 5.3%, the proteids from 1.64% to 2.22%, and the ash from 0.14% to 0.42%; total solids, from 10.18% to 13.65%; lactose from 5.6% to 7.4%. An average colostrum-milk contains 4% of fat, 1.9% of proteids, 6.5% of lactose, and 0.2% of ash, making the total solids 12.5% and water 87.5%.

Proteids of Milk.—A. Schlossmann[1] writes on the significance of the several proteids of milk and on the methods hitherto employed for separating them, and proposes a new method for effecting this separation. The new method precipitates the casein at 40° C. with a concentrated solution of potashalum, albumin and globulin not being precipitated by this reagent; globulin is precipitated with magnesium sulfate; the rest of the proteid is considered to be albumin. The precipitates after being properly treated are estimated by the Kjeldahl method. For practical purposes it is not necessary to separate albumin and globulin; the two are estimated together as " water-soluble proteid." Schlossmann protests vigorously against the view that the casein and albumin of milk have an equal nutritive value. The unequal value of nourishment at the mother's breast and by means of the flask is due to the fact, so Schlossmann thinks, that the child in drinking, say, 1105 gm. of mother's milk, avails itself of more than 5 gm. of very soluble and readily absorbable albumin, while in taking as a substitute for the above amount of mother's milk the usual equivalent, say, 600 gm. of cow's milk, it would get only 1.8 gm. of soluble albumin. That albumin is the chief proteid of colostrum, coupled with the fact that the newborn child has but little capacity for peptonizing casein, is also adduced as an argument in support of the view that the albumin of milk has a special value as compared with the casein.

The Nucleon of Milk.—M. Siegfried[2] has made the important observation that cow's milk contains a nucleon which is closely related to the nucleon or phosphosarcic acid of muscles. Further observations have been published by his pupil, Karl Witmaack,[3] showing that this substance is also present in human milk and in that of goats. Human milk contains more than twice as much of this physiologically important substance as cow's milk, and goat's milk about twice as much as cow's milk. The amount of nucleon in a liter of human milk varies from 1.1 gm. to 1.3 gm. M. Siegfried also comments in a recent paper on the very great physiologic importance which attaches to the new compound. Nucleon contains more phosphorus in organic combination than any other compound in milk. Cow's milk contains 0.6 gm. of this substance, while human milk contains 1.3 gm. Of the total phosphorus in cow's milk only 6% is present in nucleon, while in human milk 41.5% of the total phosphorus is present in the form of nucleon—indeed, almost all of the phosphorus contained in human milk is present as organically combined phosphorus in casein and nucleon. Although the total content of phosphorus is higher than in cow's milk, the preponderance of organically bound phosphorus in the latter is thought to be of great significance for boneformation in the infant. Martin Müller[4] has shown that the muscles of the newborn child contain at best only 0.057% of nucleon, as compared with the 0.11–0.22% found in the muscles of adults. This fact is also adduced to show the great significance of the new compound. Long-continued sterilization will decompose some of the nucleon contained in milk.

[1] Zeit. f. phyisol. Chemie, vol. xxii., p. 197.
[3] Ibid., vol. xxii., p. 567.
[2] Ibid., vol. xx., p. 373.
[4] Ibid., p. 561.

INDEX.

Étienne on hypertrophic osteoarthropathy, 91, 674.
Guiard on gonorrhea, 402.
Guilloz (T.) on photography of the eye, 836.
Guimaraes (P.) on hernia of the pancreas, 356.
Guinard (M. A.) on carcinoma of the uterus, 581.
Guinon and Meunier on Widal's reaction, 26.
Guiraud on typhoid fever, 36.
Guttéras (R.) on stricture, 415
Gulland (G. L.) on histologic technic, 703; on leukocytes, 102.
Gumma of the ciliary body, 814; of the iris, 814.
Gumprecht on leukocytic degenerations, 103; on urinary sediments, 1018.
Gunshot-wounds, 996; of the kidney, 439.
Guranowski on caries of the internal ear, 866; on cholesteatoma of the ear, 855.
Gurwitsch on balantidium coli, 221.
Gustin (P.) on superfetation, 452.
Guthrie (A.) on gonorrhea, 401.
Gutierrez (M.) on abortion, 474.
Gutmann (G.) on the ciliary nerves, 966; on holocain, 833.
Guyon on orchotomy, 420.
Gynecology, 521.
Gyromele, 190.

HAACK on albumosuria, 1013.
Haam on examination of the stomach, 174.
Habel on actinomycosis, 76.
Habermann (J.) on otorrhea, 851.
Habit-chorea, 739; -movements, 643.
Haegeler (C. S.) on airol, 228.
Haenel (W.) on tuberculosis of the ear, 865.
Haffkine (W. M.) on the plague, 45.
Haffkine's method, 38.
Hagelstam on bothriocephalus latus, 223
Haggard, Jr. (W. D.) on cystitis, 537; on vaginal section, 598; on vesicovaginal fistula, 536.
Hahn (M) on extravascular, blood, 650; on hyperleukocytosis, 693.
Haig (A.) on gout, 93.
Hair-cups, pitting about, 904.
Hairs, examination of, 999.
Halamon on albuminuria, 211.
Halbertsma on puerperal eclampsia, 495.
Haldane (J.) and Smith (J. L.) on arterial blood, 984.
Hall (J. N.) on cicatrices, 999; on gunshot-wounds, 996.
Hall (R. B.) on uterine anomalies, 552.
Hall (W. S.) and Eubank (M. D.) on hemopoiesis, 975.
Hallauer (O.) on cataract, 811.
Hallervorden on ammonia in the urine, 207.

Halliburton (W. D.) on internal secretion, 980; and Brodie (T. G.) on ferments, 986.
Hallucinations of hearing, 868.
Hallux valgus, 384, 774.
Halsted (W. S.) on metatarsalgia, 773.
Hamaide on formaldehyd, 939.
Hamburger (H. J.) on absorption from the alimentary canal, 985; on the blood, 975; on osmosis, 976.
Hamill (S. M.) on splenic hypertrophy, 639; on glandular fever, 630.
Hamilton (A. M.) on insanity, 754.
Hammerl (H.) on feces, 986.
Hammerschlag (A.) on carcinoma of the stomach, 183.
Hammerschlag (V.) on the membrana tympani, 840.
Hammerschlag's method, 100.
Hammer-toe springs, 774.
Hammock for typhoid fever, 36.
Hampeln on carcinoma of the lung, 166.
Hance (I. H.) on tuberculosis, 56.
Hand, diseases of, 776; disinfection of, 230; in idiocy, 763; sesamoid bones of, 960.
Handley (W. G.) on inguinal orchidectomy, 415.
Hankin (E. H.) on cholera, 38.
Hanley (J. J.) on calcareous degeneration of the heart, 656.
Hanna (W. J.) on traumatism of the heart, 144.
Hanot (V.) on pulmonary tuberculosis, 62; on rheumatism, 86; and Levy on tuberculosis of the aortic intima, 655.
Hanriot on digestion, 986.
Hansell (H. F.) on cyst of the brain, 797; on the eye in diabetes, 794; on the eye in kidney-disease, 793; on foreign body in the eye, 825; on glaucoma, 817; on gonorrheal conjunctivitis, 803; on homatropin, 784, 833.
Hansen on symphysiotomy, 507.
Hansmann on hematokolpos, 530; on myoma of the round ligament, 568.
Hanson (G. F.) on purity of drugs, 949.
Harding (G. F.) on congenital syphilis, 629.
Harding (L. A.) on mercurial ointment, 941.
Hard water, softening of, 1006.
Hare (H. A.) on diabetes mellitus, 67; on leukemia, 118; on pernicious anemia, 115; on toxemia, 84.
Hare (T. E.) on typhoid fever, 35.
Harlan and Woods on ocular statistics, 782.
Harley (G.) on gout, 95.
Harley (V.) on urobilin, 675.

Harnett (C. J.) on pneumonia, 164.
Harrington (F. B.) on intestinal obstruction, 297.
Harris (M. L.) on circular enterorrhaphy, 294; on fracture of the clavicle, 385.
Harris (T. J.) on syphilis of the internal ear, 866.
Harrison (G. T.) on inversion of the uterus, 500; on pelvic massage. 564.
Harrison (R.) on albuminuria, 434; on blood-erythema, 893; on extroversion of the bladder, 425; on gonorrhea, 403; on resection of the vas deferens, 420; on vesical calculus, 427.
Hart (B.) on fleshy mole, 473.
Hartcop (J. F.) on headache, 646.
Hartley-Krause operation, 409.
Hartmann (A.) on hyperostosis of the auditory meatus, 840; on wry-neck, 380; and Mignot on uterine fibroid, 569.
Hartridge on the eye, 799.
Hartzell (M. B.) on skin-diseases, 914.
Harvey (R. H.) on the constitutio lymphatica, 673; on the plague, 45.
Harvey (T. W.) on labor, 484.
Hasencamp (O.) on formaldehyd, 938.
Haslam (W. F.) on pyloric obstruction, 279.
Hatfield (A. C.) on maternal impressions, 458.
Haug on nephritis, 213; on the ear in nephritis, 846.
Haultain (F. W. N.) on fibroid tumor in pregnancy, 470.
Hausemann on carcinoma of the pleura, 668.
Hauser (A.) on typhoid fever, 11.
Haushalter (M. P.) on antitoxin in diphtheria, 615; on gonorrheal rheumatism, 631; on typhoid fever, 17, 19; and Étienne on tuberculosis, 60.
Havelburg on leprosy, 73; on yellow fever, 49.
Hawkes (C. S.) on scopolamin, 834.
Hawkins (H. P.) on appendicitis, 327; and Wallace (C. S.) on gastric ulcer, 283.
Hayden (M.) on trauma of the eye, 827.
Hayem on chlorosis. 110; on pyloric stenosis, 187.
Hayem's serum, 215.
Hay-fever, etiology, 874.
Haynes (W. H.) on ophthalmoplegia, 813.
Head, after-coming, perforation of, 506; diseases of, 768; fetal, retained in utero, 502; -presentations, mechanism of, 485; -swaying, 644.
Headaches of children, 646.
Heagler on typhoid fever, 13.
Healey (C. W. R.) on snakebite, 440.

1056

INDEX.

Moeller's superficial glossitis, 882.

Mohlau on *Anchylostomum duodenale*, 223.

Molderescu on heart-disease, 147.

Mole, fleshy, 473; tubal, 474.

Mollison on chloroform-anesthesia, 267.

Molluscum contagiosum of the lids. 800.

Monchet on operation during pregnancy, 470.

Moncorvo ou malaria, 645.

Mond on ovarian therapy, 547.

Moneret on ascites, 194.

Mongardi on otorrhea, 851.

Mongorvo on aualgene, 923.

Monin on hemorrhoids, 358.

Monocular blindness in hysteria, 752.

Monod on peritonitis. 595.

Monomphalic ischiopagus, 459.

Monro (T. K.) on paralysis of the iris, 813.

Monscourt (H.) on tuberculous otitis media, 849.

Monsonia in dysentery, 193.

Monstrosities, fetal, 459.

Montgomery on retinal detachment. 821.

Montgomery (E. E.) on neurasthenia in women. 523; on serum-therapy in puerperal sepsis. 512.

Monti (A.) on diphtheria, 616.

Moon-blindness, 809.

Moore (B.) on aneurysm, 371; on the suprarenal capsules, 980; on tuberculosis, 63; and Rockwood (D. P.) on digestion, 985.

Moore (J.) on gonorrhea, 402.

Moore (J. H.) on diphtheria, 621.

Moore (W.) on patent foramen ovale, 139.

Moorehead (T. H.) on puerperal sepsis. 513.

Mooren (A.) on myopia, 785.

Moorhouse (J. E.) on urticaria, 891.

Moraczewski on anemia, 108.

Morax on conjunctivitis, 802; on epithelioma of the orbit, 828.

Morcellement, 572.

Morgagni, hydatid of, 599.

Morgan (W. P.) on word-blindness, 798.

Morgenstern (M.) on the dentine, 963.

Moribund, delivery in. 499.

Morisani on contracted pelvis, 492; on puerperal eclampsia, 495.

Morison (A.) on the Schott method. 144.

Morison (A. E.) on the fissure of Rolando. 406.

Morison (J. R.) on ovariotomy in the aged, 588.

Morison (R) on appendicitis, 329; on pyloroplasty, 278.

Morner (K. A. H.) on the urine, 1014.

Morphea, symmetric, 906.

Morphin in angina pectoris. 717; in appendicitis, 317; in the plague, 45; in puerperal eclampsia, 493; in pulmonary hemorrhage. 70.

Morphinism, 756.

Morphology of the blood, 650; in tuberculosis, 60.

Morpurgo (E.) on ear-disease, 847.

Morris (H.) on vesical hematuria, 427; on *x*-rays, 444.

Morris (R. T.) on appendicitis, 324.

Morrow (P. A.) on lepra, 73; on symmetric morphea, 906.

Morrow (W. S.) on parotitis, 595.

Morse (J. L.) on melena, 638; on precocious maturity, 647; on rachitis, 632.

Morse (T. H.) on gastric ulcer, 281.

Mortality in labor, 483; puerperal, 510; of puerperal sepsis, 510; of tuberculosis, 59; of variola, 48.

Morton (C. A.) on appendicitis, 329; on goiter, 378; on irreducible hernia, 335.

Morvan's disease, 729.

Mosets (M.) on measles. 624.

Mosquito and malarial fever, 77; -theory of malarial fever, 78.

Moss (R. E.) on otorrhea, 849.

Mossé on glycosuria, 96; on typhoid fever, 626; and Daunic on typhoid fever, 25.

Mosso on salacetol, 952; and Ottolenghi on acetylene, 923; and Parletti on formalin, 230.

Motais on ptosis, 800.

Motor insufficiency of the stomach, 179.

Motter (M. G.) on entomology, 998.

Moullin (C. W. M.) on prostatic hypertrophy, 421; on wound of the heart, 370.

Moulton (H.) on corneal clouding, 808; on keratitis, 808.

Moute (E. J.) on deflected septum, 875; on otorrhea, 850, 851.

Moussu on the thyroid gland, 978.

Mouth, diseases of, 171; in influenza, 37.

Movable liver, 200.

Movements of the stomach, 986; "resisted," 145.

Mucin of white fibrous connective tissue, 1020.

Mucous colitis, 192.

Mucus, excretion of, from the bowel, 188.

Mühlmann on the suprarenal capsules, 980.

Müller (E.) on leukocythemia, 731; on nosophen, 231; on regeneration of the lens, 810; on secretion of saliva, 962; on sodium chlorid, 952.

Muller (H. F.) on the blood, 107.

Müller (M.) on the nucleon of milk, 102.

Müller-Kannberg on syphilis, 920.

Muetze (H.) on molluscum of the lids, 800.

Mules' operation. 830.

Mulford (H. J.) on acute rhinitis, 871.

Mullen (J. A.) on impaired auditory center, 846.

Mullins (G. L.) on carcinoma of the uterus, 576.

Multilocular ovarian cyst. 600.

Multiple echinococcus - cysts, 709; laryngeal papillomata, 644; myeloma, 99; neuritis, 727; peripheral perineuritis in rheumatism. 86; pregnancy, 500; spinal sclerosis, 738; tuberculous brain-tumor, 641.

Mumford (J. O.) on sprains, 394.

Mumps, 630; deafness from, 846; etiology, 688; of the lacrimal gland, 606.

Mundé (P. F.) on senile endometritis, 557; on virginal endometritis, 556.

Munk (J.) on muscular contraction, 982.

Munson (E. L.) on diabetes mellitus, 99.

Murawjew (W. W.) on encephalitis, 718.

Murdoch (R.) on the speculum, 836.

Muret on ovarian extract, 926.

Murmur, functional, 149; mitral systolic, 134; presystolic, 133; systolic, 134; tricuspid, 135; venous, in chlorosis, 111.

Murphy (J. B.) on end-to-end suture of vessels, 368; button, 279, 294, 295.

Murray (G. R.) on acromegaly, 745; on exophthalmic goiter, 669, 795.

Murray (R. M.) on axis-traction forceps, 504; on forceps in contracted pelvis, 492; on the uterus in pregnancy, 484.

Murrell (T. E.) on scopolamin hydrobromate, 784.

Murrell (W.) on acquired phthisis, 58.

Murri (A.) on cerebellar tumor, 725.

Muscle-affections of the eyes, 787.

Muscles, anatomy of, 968; diseases of, 380; displacements of, 381; injuries of, 381; innervation of, 968.

Muscle-transplantation, 383.

Muscular atrophy in coxalgia, 398; in hip-disease, 770; contraction, 981; dystrophy, progressive, 729.

Museum-specimens, preservation of, 700.

Muskens (L. J. J.) on the heart, 978.

Musser (J. H.) and Steele (J. D.) on aortic aneurysm, 156.

Mycoticopeptic ulcers, 664.

Mydriatics. 784.

Mydrol, 834.

Myelitis in measles, 624.

CATALOGUE

OF THE

MEDICAL PUBLICATIONS

OF

W. B. SAUNDERS,

No. 925 WALNUT STREET, PHILADELPHIA.

Arranged Alphabetically and Classified under Subjects.

THE books advertised in this Catalogue as being sold by subscription are usually to be obtained from traveling solicitors, but they will be sent direct from the office of publication (charges of shipment prepaid) upon receipt of the prices given. All the other books advertised are commonly for sale by booksellers in all parts of the United States; but any book will be sent by the publisher to any address, carriage prepaid, on receipt of the published price.

Money may be sent at the risk of the publisher in either of the following ways: A post-office money order, an express money order, a bank check, and in a registered letter. Money sent in any other way is at the risk of the sender.

See pages 30, 31, for a List of Contents classified according to subjects.

LATEST PUBLICATIONS.

SPECIAL ANNOUNCEMENT.

Mr. Saunders is pleased to announce that arrangements have been completed for the publication of an English edition of the world-famous

Lehmann medicinische Handatlanten.

For scientific accuracy, pictorial beauty, compactness, and cheapness these books surpass any similar volumes ever published. Each volume contains from

50 to 100 Colored Plates,

besides numerous other illustrations in the text. These colored plates have been executed by the most skilful German lithographers, in some cases twenty or more impressions being required to obtain the desired result. There is a full and appropriate description of each plate (printed, for convenience, opposite the plate), together with a condensed outline of the subject to which the book is devoted.

The same careful and competent editorial supervision will be secured in the English edition as in the originals. The translations will be directed and edited by the leading American specialists in the different subjects.

The great advantage of natural pictorial representation is indisputable. For lasting and practical knowledge, one accurate illustration is better than several pages of dry description.

These Atlases offer a ready and satisfactory substitute for clinical observation, available only to the residents of large medical centers; and with such persons the requisite variety is seen only after long years of routine hospital service.

By reason of their projected universal translation and reproduction, affording international distribution, the publishers have been enabled to secure for these Atlases the best artistic and professional talent, to produce them in the most elegant style, and yet to offer them at a price heretofore unapproached in cheapness. The success of the undertaking is demonstrated by the fact that volumes have already appeared in German, English, French, Italian, Russian, Spanish, Danish, Swedish, and Hungarian.

While appreciating the value of such colored plates, the profession has heretofore been practically debarred from purchasing similar works because of their extremely high price, made necessary by the limited sale and the enormous expense of production. The very low price of these Atlases will place them within the reach of even the novice in practice.

The following volumes are in active preparation and will be issued at an early date:

Atlas of Internal Medicine and Clinical Diagnosis. By Dr. Chr. Jakob, of Erlangen. Edited by Augustus A. Eshner, M.D., Professor of Clinical Medicine in the Philadelphia Polyclinic; Attending Physician to the Philadelphia Hospital. 68 colored plates, and 64 illustrations in the text.

Atlas of Legal Medicine. By Dr. E. R. von Hofmann, of Vienna. Edited by Frederick Peterson, M.D., Clinical Professor of Mental Diseases, Woman's Medical College, New York; Chief of Clinic, Nervous Dept., College of Physicians and Surgeons, New York. With 120 colored figures on 56 plates, and 193 beautiful half-tone illustrations.

Atlas of Operative Surgery. By Dr. O. Zuckerkandl, of Vienna. Edited by J. Chalmers DaCosta, M.D., Clinical Professor of Surgery, Jefferson Medical College, Philadelphia; Surgeon to the Philadelphia Hospital. With 24 colored plates, and 217 illustrations in the text.

Atlas of Laryngology. By Dr. L. Grünwald, of Munich. With 107 colored figures on 44 plates; 25 black-and-white illustrations.

Atlas of External Diseases of the Eye. By Dr. O. Haab, of Zurich. Edited by G. E. de Schweinitz, M.D., Professor of Ophthalmology, Jefferson Medical College, Philadelphia. With 100 colored illustrations.

Atlas of Venereal Diseases. By. Dr. Karl Kopp, of Munich. Edited by L. Bolton Bangs, M D., late Professor of Genito-Urinary and Venereal Diseases, New York Post-Graduate Medical School and Hospital. With 63 colored illustrations.

Atlas of Skin Diseases. By Dr. Karl Kopp, of Munich. With 90 colored and 17 black-and-white illustrations.

AN AMERICAN TEXT-BOOK OF APPLIED THERAPEUTICS.

Edited by JAMES C. WILSON, M.D., Professor of the Practice of Medicine and of Clinical Medicine in the Jefferson Medical College, Philadelphia. One handsome imperial octavo volume of 1326 pages. Illustrated. Cloth, $7.00 net; Sheep or Half Morocco, $8.00 net. *Sold by Subscription.*

"As a work either for study or reference it will be of great value to the practitioner, as it is virtually an exposition of such clinical therapeutics as experience has taught to be of the most value. Taking it all in all, no recent publication on therapeutics can be compared with this one in practical value to the working physician."—*Chicago Clinical Review.*

"The whole field of medicine has been well covered. The work is thoroughly practical, and while it is intended for practitioners and students, it is a better book for the general practitioner than for the student. The young practitioner especially will find it extremely suggestive and helpful."—*The Indian Lancet.*

AN AMERICAN TEXT-BOOK OF THE DISEASES OF CHILDREN.

Edited by LOUIS STARR, M.D., Physician to the Children's Hospital, Philadelphia, etc.; assisted by THOMPSON S. WESTCOTT, M.D., Attending Physician to the Dispensary for Diseases of Children, Hospital of the University of Pennsylvania. In one handsome imperial octavo volume of 1190 pages, profusely illustrated. Cloth, $7.00 net; Sheep or Half Morocco, $8.00 net. *Sold by Subscription.*

"This is far and away the best text-book on children's diseases ever published in the English language, and is certainly the one which is best adapted to American readers. We congratulate the editor upon the result of his work, and heartily commend it to the attention of every student and practitioner."—*American Journal of the Medical Sciences.*

"A condensation between the lids of a single volume of an amount of information upon childhood and its diseases which will be eagerly sought after by the profession."—*New York Medical Times.*

AN AMERICAN TEXT-BOOK OF DISEASES OF THE EYE, EAR, NOSE, AND THROAT.

Edited by G E. DE SCHWEINITZ, M.D., Professor of Ophthalmology in the Jefferson Medical College, Philadelphia; and B. ALEXANDER RANDALL, M.D., Professor of Diseases of the Ear in the University of Pennsylvania and in the Philadelphia Polyclinic. *In Preparation.*

AN AMERICAN TEXT-BOOK OF GENITO-URINARY AND SKIN DISEASES.

Edited by L. BOLTON BANGS, M.D., Late Professor of Genito-Urinary and Venereal Diseases, New York Post-Graduate Medical School and Hospital; and WILLIAM A. HARDAWAY, M.D., Professor of Diseases of the Skin, Missouri Medical College. *In Press. Ready soon.*

This latest addition to the series of "American Text-Books" it is confidently believed will meet the requirements of both students and practitioners, giving, as it does, a comprehensive and detailed presentation of the Diseases of the Genito-Urinary Organs, of the Venereal Diseases, and of the Affections of the Skin.

Having secured the collaboration of well-known authorities in the branches represented in the undertaking, the Editors have not restricted the Contributors in regard to the particular views set forth, but have offered every facility for the free expression of their individual opinions. The work will therefore be found to be original, yet homogeneous and fully representative of the several departments of medical science with which it is concerned.

Illustrated Catalogue of the "American Text-Books" sent free upon application.

AN AMERICAN TEXT-BOOK OF GYNECOLOGY, MEDICAL AND SURGICAL.

Edited by J. M. BALDY, M.D., Professor of Gynecology in the Philadelphia Polyclinic, etc.   Handsome imperial octavo volume of over 700 pages, with 360 illustrations in text, and 37 colored and half-tone plates.   Cloth, $6.00 net; Sheep or Half Morocco, $7.00 net.   *Sold by Subscription.*

"The nature of the text may be judged from its authorship; the distinguished American authorities who have compiled this publication have done their work well.   It is well indexed,—an important feature in a work essentially intended for reference.   .   .   .   The work is very fully illustrated, and the wood-cuts and plates are of high excellence.   .   .   . This addition to medical literature deserves favorable comment."—*British Medical Journal.*

"It is practical from beginning to end.   Its descriptions of conditions, its recommendations for treatment, and above all the necessary technique of different operations, are clearly and admirably presented.   .   .   .   It is well up to the most advanced views of the day, and embodies all the essential points of advanced American gynecology.   It is destined to make and hold a place in gynecological literature which will be peculiarly its own."— *Medical Record,* New York.

AN AMERICAN TEXT-BOOK OF LEGAL MEDICINE AND TOXICOLOGY.

Edited by FREDERICK PETERSON, M.D., Clinical Professor of Mental Diseases in the Woman's Medical College, New York; Chief of Clinic, Nervous Department, College of Physicians and Surgeons, New York; and WALTER S. HAINES, M.D., Professor of Chemistry, Pharmacy, and Toxicology in Rush Medical College, Chicago.   *In Preparation.*

AN AMERICAN TEXT-BOOK OF OBSTETRICS.

Edited by RICHARD C. NORRIS, M.D.; Art Editor, ROBERT L. DICKINSON, M.D.   One handsome imperial octavo volume of over 1000 pages, with nearly 900 beautiful colored and half-tone illustrations. Cloth, $7.00 net; Sheep or Half Morocco, $8.00 net.   *Sold by Subscription.*

"Permit me to say that your American Text-Book of Obstetrics is the most magnificent medical work that I have ever seen.   I congratulate you and thank you for this superb work, which alone is sufficient to place you first in the ranks of medical publishers."—ALEXANDER J C. SKENE, *Professor of Gynecology in the Long Island College Hospital, Brooklyn, N. Y.*

"This is the most sumptuously illustrated work on midwifery that has yet appeared.   In the number, the excellence, and the beauty of production of the illustrations it far surpasses every other book upon the subject.   This feature alone makes it a work which no medical library should omit to purchase."—*British Medical Journal.*

"The obstetrician and the general practitioner will find this book not only a pleasant and interesting volume, but the most valuable of its kind, both on account of the wide experience of the several authors and because of the attractiveness and accuracy of its illustrations.   .   .   .   As an authority, as a book of reference, as a 'working book' for the student or practitioner, we commend it because we believe there is no better."—*American Journal of the Medical Sciences.*

AN AMERICAN TEXT-BOOK OF PATHOLOGY.

Edited by JOHN GUITÉRAS, M.D., Professor of General Pathology and of Morbid Anatomy in the University of Pennsylvania; and DAVID RIESMAN, M.D., Demonstrator of Pathological Histology in the University of Pennsylvania.   *In Preparation.*

Illustrated Catalogue of the "American Text-Books" sent free upon application.

AN AMERICAN TEXT-BOOK OF PHYSIOLOGY.

Edited by WILLIAM H. HOWELL, PH.D., M.D., Professor of Physiology in the Johns Hopkins University, Baltimore, Md. One handsome imperial octavo volume of 1052 pages. Illustrated. Cloth, $6.00 net; Sheep or Half Morocco, $7.00 net. *Sold by Subscription.*

"The present volume constitutes practically a new departure in physiological text-books, on the lines which have already proved successful in medicine and surgery. Its value as a work of reference for the physician or pathologist is very great. We can commend it most heartily, not only to all students of physiology, but to every physician and pathologist, as a valuable and comprehensive work of reference, written by men who are of eminent authority in their own special subjects."—*London Lancet.*

"To the practitioner of medicine and to the advanced student this volume constitutes, we believe, the best exposition of the present status of the science of physiology in the English language."—*American Journal of the Medical Sciences.*

"The book is certainly the best thing in the way of physiological text-books that America has produced."—*Edinburgh Medical Journal.*

AN AMERICAN TEXT-BOOK OF SURGERY. Second Edition.

Edited by WILLIAM W. KEEN, M.D., LL.D., and J. WILLIAM WHITE, M.D., PH.D. Handsome imperial octavo volume of 1250 pages, with 500 wood-cuts in the text, and 39 colored and half-tone plates. Thoroughly revised and enlarged, with a section devoted to "The Use of the Röntgen Rays in Surgery." Cloth, $7.00 net; Sheep or Half Morocco, $8.00 net. *Sold by Subscription.*

"Personally, I should not mind it being called THE TEXT-BOOK (instead of A TEXT-BOOK), for I know of no single volume which contains so readable and complete an account of the science and art of Surgery as this does."—EDMUND OWEN, F.R.C.S., *Member of the Board of Examiners of the Royal College of Surgeons, England.*

"If this text-book is a fair reflex of the present position of American surgery, we must admit it is of a very high order of merit, and that English surgeons will have to look very carefully to their laurels if they are to preserve a position in the van of surgical practice."—*London Lancet.*

"This book marks an epoch in American book-making. All in all, the book is distinctly the most satisfactory work on modern surgery with which we are familiar. It is thorough, complete, and condensed."—*Boston Medical and Surgical Journal.*

AN AMERICAN TEXT-BOOK OF THE THEORY AND PRACTICE OF MEDICINE.

Edited by WILLIAM PEPPER, M.D., LL.D., Professor of the Theory and Practice of Medicine and of Clinical Medicine in the University of Pennsylvania. Two handsome imperial octavo volumes of about 1000 pages each. Illustrated. Prices per volume: Cloth, $5.00 net; Sheep or Half Morocco, $6.00 net. *Sold by Subscription.*

"I am quite sure it will commend itself both to practitioners and students of medicine, and become one of our most popular text-books."—ALFRED LOOMIS, M.D., LL.D., *Professor of Pathology and Practice of Medicine, University of the City of New York.*

"We reviewed the first volume of this work, and said: 'It is undoubtedly one of the best text-books on the practice of medicine which we possess.' A consideration of the second and last volume leads us to modify that verdict and to say that the completed work is in our opinion *the best* of its kind it has ever been our fortune to see."—*New York Medical Journal.*

"American physicians can look with pride upon the work of Dr. Pepper and his corps of associates. It brings our knowledge down to the present hour, and has been written from an eminently practical standpoint."—*Medical Record*, New York.

Illustrated Catalogue of the "American Text-Books" sent free upon application.

AN AMERICAN YEAR-BOOK OF MEDICINE AND SURGERY.

A Yearly Digest of Scientific Progress and Authoritative Opinion in all branches of Medicine and Surgery, drawn from journals, monographs, and text-books of the leading American and Foreign authors and investigators. Collected and arranged, with critical editorial comments, by eminent American specialists and teachers, under the general editorial charge of GEORGE M. GOULD, M.D. One handsome imperial octavo volume of about 1200 pages. Uniform in style, size, and general make-up with the "American Text-Book" Series. Cloth, $6.50 net; Half Morocco, $7.50 net. *Sold by Subscription.*

" It is difficult to know which to admire most—the research and industry of the distinguished band of experts whom Dr. Gould has enlisted in the service of the Year-Book, or the wealth and abundance of the contributions to every department of science that have been deemed worthy of analysis. . . . It is much more than a mere compilation of abstracts, for, as each section is entrusted to experienced and able contributors, the reader has the advantage of certain critical commentaries and expositions . . . proceeding from writers fully qualified to perform these tasks. . . . It is emphatically a book which should find a place in every medical library, and is in several respects more useful than the famous ' Jahrbücher ' of Germany."—*London Lancet.*

ANDERS' PRACTICE OF MEDICINE.

A Text-Book of the Practice of Medicine. By JAMES M. ANDERS, M.D., PH.D., LL.D., Professor of the Practice of Medicine and of Clinical Medicine, Medico-Chirurgical College, Philadelphia. In one handsome octavo volume of 1287 pages, fully illustrated. Cloth, $5.50 net; Sheep or Half Morocco, $6.50 net.

" We know of no recent author who has as effectively succeeded in bringing the new facts and ideas together, weaving them with the substantial realities of the old, in better form. The concise character of the text, the clearness with which its ideas are expressed, the ingenious arrangement of its data, the completeness of its detail, the order of sequence of its topics, and the whole general appearance of the volume tell of careful, conscientious work done by him. His tables for aiding in differential diagnosis, his association of clinical symptoms with the morbid lesions that accompany them, his tested therapeutic formulæ, his appropriate illustrations, his bacteriology, and his modern orthography have made of it a fully up-to-date, handy text-book for the general practitioner."—*American Medico-Surgical Bulletin.*

ASHTON'S OBSTETRICS. Third Edition, Revised.

Essentials of Obstetrics. By W. EASTERLY ASHTON, M.D., Professor of Gynecology in the Medico-Chirurgical College, Philadelphia. Crown octavo, 252 pages; 75 illustrations. Cloth, $1.00; interleaved for notes, $1.25.

[See *Saunders' Question-Compends*, page 21.]

" Embodies the whole subject in a nut-shell. We cordially recommend it to our readers."—*Chicago Medical Times.*

BALL'S BACTERIOLOGY. Third Edition, Revised.

Essentials of Bacteriology; a Concise and Systematic Introduction to the Study of Micro-organisms. By M. V. BALL, M.D., Bacteriologist to St. Agnes' Hospital, Philadelphia, etc. Crown octavo, 218 pages; 82 illustrations, some in colors, and 5 plates. Cloth, $1.00; interleaved for notes, $1.25.

[See *Saunders' Question-Compends*, page 21.]

" The student or practitioner can readily obtain a knowledge of the subject from a perusal of this book. The illustrations are clear and satisfactory."—*Medical Record*, New York.

BASTIN'S BOTANY.

Laboratory Exercises in Botany. By EDSON S. BASTIN, M.A., late Professor of Materia Medica and Botany, Philadelphia College of Pharmacy. Octavo volume of 536 pages, with 87 plates. Cloth, $2.50.

"It is unquestionably the best text-book on the subject that has yet appeared. The work is eminently a practical one. We regard the issuance of this book as an important event in the history of pharmaceutical teaching in this country, and predict for it an unqualified success."—*Alumni Report to the Philadelphia College of Pharmacy.*

"There is no work like it in the pharmaceutical or botanical literature of this country, and we predict for it a wide circulation."—*American Journal of Pharmacy.*

BECK'S SURGICAL ASEPSIS.

A Manual of Surgical Asepsis. By CARL BECK, M.D., Surgeon to St. Mark's Hospital and the New York German Poliklinik, etc. 306 pages; 65 text-illustrations, and 12 full-page plates. Cloth, $1.25 net.

"An excellent exposition of the 'very latest' in the treatment of wounds as practised by leading German and American surgeons."—*Birmingham* (Eng.) *Medical Review.*

"This little volume can be recommended to any who are desirous of learning the details of asepsis in surgery, for it will serve as a trustworthy guide."—*London Lancet.*

BOISLINIERE'S OBSTETRIC ACCIDENTS, EMERGENCIES, AND OPERATIONS.

Obstetric Accidents, Emergencies, and Operations. By L. CH. BOISLINIERE, M.D., late Emeritus Professor of Obstetrics, St. Louis Medical College. 381 pages, handsomely illustrated. Cloth, $2.00 net.

"It is clearly and concisely written, and is evidently the work of a teacher and practitioner of large experience."—*British Medical Journal.*

"A manual so useful to the student or the general practitioner has not been brought to our notice in a long time. The field embraced in the title is covered in a terse, interesting way."—*Yale Medical Journal.*

BROCKWAY'S MEDICAL PHYSICS. Second Edition, Revised.

Essentials of Medical Physics. By FRED J. BROCKWAY, M.D., Assistant Demonstrator of Anatomy in the College of Physicians and Surgeons, New York. Crown octavo, 330 pages; 155 fine illustrations. Cloth, $1.00 net; interleaved for notes, $1.25 net.

[See *Saunders' Question-Compends*, page 21.]

"The student who is well versed in these pages will certainly prove qualified to comprehend with ease and pleasure the great majority of questions involving physical principles likely to be met with in his medical studies."—*American Practitioner and News.*

"We know of no manual that affords the medical student a better or more concise exposition of physics, and the book may be commended as a most satisfactory presentation of those essentials that are requisite in a course in medicine."—*New York Medical Journal.*

"It contains all that one need know on the subject, is well written, and is copiously illustrated."—*Medical Record*, New York.

BURR ON NERVOUS DISEASES.

A Manual of Nervous Diseases. By CHARLES W. BURR, M.D., Clinical Professor of Nervous Diseases, Medico-Chirurgical College, Philadelphia; Pathologist to the Orthopedic Hospital and Infirmary for Nervous Diseases; Visiting Physician to St. Joseph's Hospital, etc. *In Preparation.*

BUTLER'S MATERIA MEDICA, THERAPEUTICS, AND PHAR-MACOLOGY.

A Text-Book of Materia Medica, Therapeutics, and Pharmacology. By GEORGE F. BUTLER, PH.G., M.D., Professor of Materia Medica and of Clinical Medicine in the College of Physicians and ∙ Surgeons, Chicago; Professor of Materia Medica and Therapeutics, Northwestern University, Woman's Medical School, etc. Octavo, 858 pages, illustrated. Cloth, $4.00 net; Sheep, $5.00 net.

A clear, concise, and practical text-book, adapted for permanent reference no less than for the requirements of the class-room. The arrangement (embodying the synthetic classification of drugs based upon therapeutic affinities) is believed to be at once the most philosophical and rational, as well as that best calculated to engage the interest of those to whom the academic study of the subject is wont to offer no little perplexity. Special attention has been given to the Pharmaceutical section, which is exceptionally lucid and complete.

CASSELBERRY ON THE NOSE AND THROAT.

Diseases of the Nose and Throat. By W. E. CASSELBERRY, Professor of Laryngology and Rhinology in the Northwestern University Medical School, Chicago. *In Preparation.*

CERNA ON THE NEWER REMEDIES. Second Edition, Revised.

Notes on the Newer Remedies, their Therapeutic Applications and Modes of Administration. By DAVID CERNA, M.D., PH.D., formerly Demonstrator of and Lecturer on Experimental Therapeutics in the University of Pennsylvania; Demonstrator of Physiology in the Medical Department of the University of Texas. Rewritten and greatly enlarged. Post-octavo, 253 pages. Cloth, $1.25.

"These ' Notes ' will be found very useful to practitioners who take an interest in the many newer remedies of the present day."—*Edinburgh Medical Journal.*

" The appearance of this new edition of Dr. Cerna's very valuable work shows that it is properly appreciated. The book ought to be in the possession of every practising physician."—*New York Medical Journal.*

CHAPIN ON INSANITY.

A Compendium of Insanity. By JOHN B. CHAPIN, M.D., LL.D., Physician-in-Chief, Pennsylvania Hospital for the Insane; late Physician-Superintendent of the Willard State Hospital, New York; Honorary Member of the Medico-Psychological Society of Great Britain, of the Society of Mental Medicine of Belgium, etc. *In Preparation.*

The author has given, in a condensed and concise form, a compendium of Diseases of the Mind, for the convenient use and aid of physicians and students. The work will also prove valuable to members of the legal profession and to those who, in their relations to the insane and to those supposed to be insane, often desire to acquire some practical knowledge of insanity presented in a form that may be understood by the non-professional reader.

CHAPMAN'S MEDICAL JURISPRUDENCE AND TOXICOLOGY. Second Edition, Revised.

Medical Jurisprudence and Toxicology. By HENRY C. CHAPMAN, M.D., Professor of Institutes of Medicine and Medical Jurisprudence in the Jefferson Medical College of Philadelphia. 254 pages, with 55 illustrations and 3 full-page plates in colors. Cloth, $1.50 net.

"The best book of its class for the undergraduate that we know of."—*New York Medical Times.*

CHURCH AND PETERSON'S NERVOUS AND MENTAL DISEASES.

Nervous and Mental Diseases. By ARCHIBALD CHURCH, M.D., Professor of Mental Diseases and Medical Jurisprudence in the Northwestern University Medical School, Chicago ; and FREDERICK PETERSON, M.D., Clinical Professor of Mental Diseases in the Woman's Medical College, New York ; Chief of Clinic, Nervous Department, College of Physicians and Surgeons, New York. *In Preparation.*

CLARKSON'S HISTOLOGY.

A Text-Book of Histology, Descriptive and Practical. By ARTHUR CLARKSON, M.B., C.M. Edin., formerly Demonstrator of Physiology in the Owen's College, Manchester ; late Demonstrator of Physiology in Yorkshire College, Leeds. Large octavo, 554 pages ; 22 engravings in the text, and 174 beautifully colored original illustrations. Cloth, strongly bound, $6.00 net.

" The work must be considered a valuable addition to the list of available text-books, and is to be highly recommended."—*New York Medical Journal.*

" This is one of the best works for students we have ever noticed. We predict that the book will attain a well-deserved popularity among our students."—*Chicago Medical Recorder.*

"The volume is a most valuable addition to the armamentarium of the teacher."—*Brooklyn Medical Journal.*

CLIMATOLOGY.

Transactions of the Eighth Annual Meeting of the American Climatological Association, held in Washington, September 22–25, 1891. Forming a handsome octavo volume of 276 pages, uniform with remainder of series. (A limited quantity only.) Cloth, $1.50.

COHEN AND ESHNER'S DIAGNOSIS.

Essentials of Diagnosis. By SOLOMON SOLIS-COHEN, M.D., Professor of Clinical Medicine and Applied Therapeutics in the Philadelphia Polyclinic; and AUGUSTUS A. ESHNER, M.D., Instructor in Clinical Medicine, Jefferson Medical College, Philadelphia. Post-octavo, 382 pages ; 55 illustrations. Cloth, $1.50 net.

[See *Saunders' Question-Compends,* page 21.]

" We can heartily commend the book to all those who contemplate purchasing a 'compend.' It is modern and complete, and will give more satisfaction than many other works which are perhaps too prolix as well as behind the times."—*Medical Review,* St. Louis.

CORWIN'S PHYSICAL DIAGNOSIS.

Essentials of Physical Diagnosis of the Thorax. By ARTHUR M. CORWIN, A.M., M.D., Demonstrator of Physical Diagnosis in Rush Medical College, Chicago ; Attending Physician to Central Free Dispensary, Department of Rhinology, Laryngology, and Diseases of the Chest, Chicago. 200 pages, illustrated. Cloth, flexible covers, $1.25 net.

" It is excellent. The student who shall use it as his guide to the careful study of physical exploration upon normal and abnormal subjects can scarcely fail to acquire a good working knowledge of the subject."—*Philadelphia Polyclinic.*

"A most excellent little work. It brightens the memory of the differential diagnostic signs, and it arranges orderly and in sequence the various objective phenomena to logical solution of a careful diagnosis."—*Journal of Nervous and Mental Diseases.*

CRAGIN'S GYNÆCOLOGY.   Fourth Edition, Revised.

Essentials of Gynæcology. By EDWIN B. CRAGIN, M.D., Attending Gynæcologist, Roosevelt Hospital, Out-Patients' Department, New York, etc.   Crown octavo, 200 pages; 62 fine illustrations.   Cloth, $1.00; interleaved for notes, $1.25.

[See *Saunders' Question-Compends*, page 21.]

"A handy volume, and a distinct improvement on students' compends in general. No author who was not himself a practical gynecologist could have consulted the student's needs so thoroughly as Dr. Cragin has done."—*Medical Record*, New York.

CROOKSHANK'S BACTERIOLOGY.

A Text-Book of Bacteriology. By EDGAR M. CROOKSHANK, M.B., Professor of Comparative Pathology and Bacteriology, King's College, London.   Octavo volume of 700 pages, with 273 engravings and 22 original colored plates.   Cloth, $6.50 net; Half Morocco, $7.50 net.

"To the student who wishes to obtain a good *résumé* of what has been done in bacteriology, or who wishes an accurate account of the various methods of research, the book may be recommended with confidence that he will find there what he requires."—*London Lancet.*

DaCOSTA'S SURGERY.

A Manual of Surgery, General and Operative. By JOHN CHALMERS DACOSTA, M.D., Clinical Professor of Surgery, Jefferson Medical College, Philadelphia; Surgeon to the Philadelphia Hospital, etc.   Handsome volume of 810 pages; 188 illustrations in the text, and 13 full-page plates in colors.   Cloth, $2.50 net.

"We know of no small work on surgery in the English language which so well fulfils the requirements of the modern student."—*Medico-Chirurgical Journal*, Bristol, England.

DE SCHWEINITZ ON DISEASES OF THE EYE.   Second Edition, Revised.

Diseases of the Eye. A Handbook of Ophthalmic Practice. By G. E. DE SCHWEINITZ, M.D., Professor of Ophthalmology in the Jefferson Medical College, Philadelphia, etc.   Handsome royal octavo volume of 679 pages, with 256 fine illustrations and 2 chromo-lithographic plates.   Cloth, $4.00 net; Sheep or Half Morocco, $5.00 net.

"A clearly written, comprehensive manual. One which we can commend to students as a reliable text-book, written with an evident knowledge of the wants of those entering upon the study of this special branch of medical science."—*British Medical Journal.*

"A work that will meet the requirements not only of the specialist, but of the general practitioner in a rare degree. I am satisfied that unusual success awaits it."—WILLIAM PEPPER, M.D., *Professor of the Theory and Practice of Medicine and Clinical Medicine, University of Pennsylvania.*

DORLAND'S OBSTETRICS.

A Manual of Obstetrics. By W. A. NEWMAN DORLAND, M.D., Assistant Demonstrator of Obstetrics, University of Pennsylvania; Instructor in Gynecology in the Philadelphia Polyclinic.   760 pages; 163 illustrations in the text, and 6 full-page plates.   Cloth, $2.50 net.

"By far the best book on this subject that has ever come to our notice."—*American Medical Review.*

"It has rarely been our duty to review a book which has given us more pleasure in its perusal and more satisfaction in its criticism. It is a veritable encyclopedia of knowledge, a gold mine of practical, concise thoughts."—*American Medico-Surgical Bulletin.*

FROTHINGHAM'S GUIDE FOR THE BACTERIOLOGIST.

Laboratory Guide for the Bacteriologist. By LANGDON FROTH-INGHAM, M.D.V., Assistant in Bacteriology and Veterinary Science, Sheffield Scientific School, Yale University. Illustrated. Cloth, 75 cts.

"It is a convenient and useful little work, and will more than repay the outlay necessary for its purchase in the saving of time which would otherwise be consumed in looking up the various points of technique so clearly and concisely laid down in its pages."—*American Medico-Surgical Bulletin.*

GARRIGUES' DISEASES OF WOMEN. Second Edition, Revised.

Diseases of Women. By HENRY J. GARRIGUES, A.M., M.D., Professor of Gynecology and Obstetrics in the New York School of Clinical Medicine; Gynecologist to St. Mark's Hospital and to the German Dispensary, New York City, etc. Handsome octavo volume of 728 pages, illustrated by 335 engravings and colored plates. Cloth, $4.00 net; Sheep or Half Morocco, $5.00 net.

"One of the best text-books for students and practitioners which has been published in the English language; it is condensed, clear, and comprehensive. The profound learning and great clinical experience of the distinguished author find expression in this book in a most attractive and instructive form. Young practitioners to whom experienced consultants may not be available will find in this book invaluable counsel and help."—THAD. A. REAMY, M.D., LL.D., *Professor of Clinical Gynecology, Medical College of Ohio.*

GLEASON'S DISEASES OF THE EAR. Second Edition, Revised.

Essentials of Diseases of the Ear. By E. B. GLEASON, S.B., M.D., Clinical Professor of Otology, Medico-Chirurgical College, Philadelphia; Surgeon-in-Charge of the Nose, Throat, and Ear Department of the Northern Dispensary, Philadelphia. 208 pages, with 114 illustrations. Cloth, $1.00; interleaved for notes, $1.25.

[See *Saunders' Question-Compends*, page 21.]

"It is just the book to put into the hands of a student, and cannot fail to give him a useful introduction to ear-affections; while the style of question and answer which is adopted throughout the book is, we believe, the best method of impressing facts permanently on the mind."—*Liverpool Medico-Chirurgical Journal.*

GOULD AND PYLE'S CURIOSITIES OF MEDICINE.

Anomalies and Curiosities of Medicine. By GEORGE M. GOULD, M.D., and WALTER L. PYLE, M.D. An encyclopedic collection of rare and extraordinary cases and of the most striking instances of abnormality in all branches of Medicine and Surgery, derived from an exhaustive research of medical literature from its origin to the present day, abstracted, classified, annotated, and indexed. Handsome imperial octavo volume of 968 pages, with 295 engravings in the text, and 12 full-page plates. Cloth, $6.00 net; Half Morocco, $7.00 net. *Sold by Subscription.*

"One of the most valuable contributions ever made to medical literature. It is, so far as we know, absolutely unique, and every page is as fascinating as a novel. Not alone for the medical profession has this volume value: it will serve as a book of reference for all who are interested in general scientific, sociologic, or medico-legal topics."—*Brooklyn Medical Journal.*

"This is certainly a most remarkable and interesting volume. It stands alone among medical literature, an anomaly on anomalies, in that there is nothing like it elsewhere in medical literature. It is a book full of revelations from its first to its last page, and cannot but interest and sometimes almost horrify its readers."—*American Medico-Surgical Bulletin.*

GRIFFIN'S MATERIA MEDICA AND THERAPEUTICS.

Manual of Materia Medica and Therapeutics. By HENRY A. GRIFFIN, A.B., M.D., Assistant Physician to the Roosevelt Hospital, Out-Patient Department, New York City. *In Preparation.*

GRIFFITH ON THE BABY.

The Care of the Baby. By J. P. CROZER GRIFFITH, M.D., Clinical Professor of Diseases of Children, University of Pennsylvania; Physician to the Children's Hospital, Philadelphia, etc. 12mo, 392 pages, with 67 illustrations in the text, and 5 plates. Cloth, $1.50.

"The best book for the use of the young mother with which we are acquainted. . . . There are very few general practitioners who could not read the book through with advantage."—*Archives of Pediatrics.*

"The whole book is characterized by rare good sense, and is evidently written by a master hand. It can be read with benefit not only by mothers but by medical students and by any practitioners who have not had large opportunities for observing children."—*American Journal of Obstetrics.*

GRIFFITH'S WEIGHT CHART.

Infant's Weight Chart. Designed by J. P. CROZER GRIFFITH, M.D., Clinical Professor of Diseases of Children in the University of Pennsylvania, etc. 25 charts in each pad. Per pad, 50 cents net.

A convenient blank for keeping a record of the child's weight during the first two years of life. Printed on each chart is a curve representing the average weight of a healthy infant, so that any deviation from the normal can readily be detected.

GROSS, SAMUEL D., AUTOBIOGRAPHY OF.

Autobiography of Samuel D. Gross, M.D., Emeritus Professor of Surgery in the Jefferson Medical College, Philadelphia, with Reminiscences of His Times and Contemporaries. Edited by his Sons, SAMUEL W. GROSS, M.D., LL.D., late Professor of Principles of Surgery and of Clinical Surgery in the Jefferson Medical College, and A. HALLER GROSS, A.M., of the Philadelphia Bar. Preceded by a Memoir of Dr. Gross, by the late AUSTIN FLINT, M.D., LL.D. In two handsome volumes, each containing over 400 pages, demy octavo, extra cloth, gilt tops, with fine Frontispiece engraved on steel. Price per volume, $2.50 net.

"Dr. Gross was perhaps the most eminent exponent of medical science that America has yet produced. His Autobiography, related as it is with a fulness and completeness seldom to be found in such works, is an interesting and valuable book. He comments on many things, especially, of course, on medical men and medical practice, in a very interesting way."—*The Spectator*, London, England.

HAMPTON'S NURSING.

Nursing: Its Principles and Practice. By ISABEL ADAMS HAMPTON, Graduate of the New York Training School for Nurses attached to Bellevue Hospital; Superintendent of Nurses, and Principal of the Training School for Nurses, Johns Hopkins Hospital, Baltimore, Md. 12mo, 484 pages, profusely illustrated. Cloth, $2.00 net.

"Seldom have we perused a book upon the subject that has given us so much pleasure as the one before us. We would strongly urge upon the members of our own profession the need of a book like this, for it will enable each of us to become a training school in himself."—*Ontario Medical Journal.*

HARE'S PHYSIOLOGY. Fourth Edition, Revised.

Essentials of Physiology. By H. A. HARE, M.D.; Professor of Therapeutics and Materia Medica in the Jefferson Medical College of Philadelphia; Physician to the Jefferson Medical College Hospital. Containing a series of handsome illustrations from the celebrated "Icones Nervorum Capitis" of Arnold. Crown octavo, 239 pages. Cloth, $1.00 net; interleaved for notes, $1.25 net.

[See *Saunders' Question-Compends*, page 21.]

" The best condensation of physiological knowledge we have yet seen."—*Medical Record*, New York.

HART'S DIET IN SICKNESS AND IN HEALTH.

Diet in Sickness and in Health. By MRS. ERNEST HART, formerly Student of the Faculty of Medicine of Paris and of the London School of Medicine for Women; with an INTRODUCTION by SIR HENRY THOMPSON, F.R.C.S., M.D., London. 220 pages; illustrated. Cloth, $1.50.

" We recommend it cordially to the attention of all practitioners; both to them and to their patients it may be of the greatest service."—*New York Medical Journal.*

HAYNES' ANATOMY.

A Manual of Anatomy. By IRVING S. HAYNES, M.D., Adjunct Professor of Anatomy and Demonstrator of Anatomy, Medical Department of the New York University, etc. 680 pages, illustrated with 42 diagrams in the text, and 134 full-page half-tone illustrations from original photographs of the author's dissections. Cloth, $2.50 net.

" This book is the work of a practical instructor—one who knows by experience the requirements of the average student, and is able to meet these requirements in a very satisfactory way. The book is one that can be commended."—*Medical Record*, New York.

HEISLER'S EMBRYOLOGY.

A Text-Book of Embryology. By JOHN C. HEISLER, M.D., Professor of Anatomy in the Medico-Chirurgical College, Philadelphia. *In Preparation.*

HIRST'S OBSTETRICS.

A Text-Book of Obstetrics. By BARTON COOKE HIRST, M.D., Professor of Obstetrics in the University of Pennsylvania. *In Preparation.*

HYDE AND MONTGOMERY ON SYPHILIS AND THE VENEREAL DISEASES.

Syphilis and the Venereal Diseases. By JAMES NEVINS HYDE, M.D., Professor of Skin and Venereal Diseases, and FRANK H. MONTGOMERY, M.D., Lecturer on Dermatology and Genito-Urinary Diseases in Rush Medical College, Chicago, Ill. 618 pages, profusely illustrated. Cloth, $2.50 net.

" We can commend this manual to the student as a help to him in his study of venereal diseases."—*Liverpool Medico-Chirurgical Journal.*

" The best student's manual which has appeared on the subject."—*St. Louis Medical and Surgical Journal.*

JACKSON AND GLEASON'S DISEASES OF THE EYE, NOSE, AND THROAT. Second Edition, Revised.

Essentials of Refraction and Diseases of the Eye. By EDWARD JACKSON, A.M., M.D., Professor of Diseases of the Eye in the Philadelphia Polyclinic and College for Graduates in Medicine; and— **Essentials of Diseases of the Nose and Throat.** By E. BALDWIN GLEASON, M.D., Surgeon-in-Charge of the Nose, Throat, and Ear Department of the Northern Dispensary of Philadelphia. Two volumes in one. Crown octavo, 290 pages; 124 illustrations. Cloth, $1.00; interleaved for notes, $1.25.

[See *Saunders' Question-Compends*, page 21.]

"Of great value to the beginner in these branches. The authors are both capable men, and know what a student most needs."—*Medical Record*, New York.

KEATING'S DICTIONARY. Second Edition, Revised.

A New Pronouncing Dictionary of Medicine, with Phonetic Pronunciation, Accentuation, Etymology, etc. By JOHN M. KEATING, M.D., LL.D., Fellow of the College of Physicians of Philadelphia; Vice-President of the American Pædiatric Society; Editor "Cyclopædia of the Diseases of Children," etc.; and HENRY HAMILTON, Author of "A New Translation of Virgil's Æneid into English Rhyme," etc.; with the collaboration of J. CHALMERS DACOSTA, M.D., and FREDERICK A. PACKARD, M.D. With an Appendix containing Tables of Bacilli, Micrococci, Leucomaïnes, Ptomaïnes; Drugs and Materials used in Antiseptic Surgery; Poisons and their Antidotes; Weights and Measures; Thermometric Scales; New Official and Unofficial Drugs, etc. One volume of over 800 pages. Prices, with Denison's Patent Ready-Reference Index: Cloth, $5.00 net; Sheep or Half Morocco, $6.00 net; Half Russia, $6.50 net. Without Patent Index: Cloth, $4.00 net; Sheep or Half Morocco, $5.00 net.

"I am much pleased with Keating's Dictionary, and shall take pleasure in recommending it to my classes."—HENRY M. LYMAN, M.D., *Professor of the Principles and Practice of Medicine, Rush Medical College, Chicago, Ill.*

"I am convinced that it will be a very valuable adjunct to my study-table, convenient in size and sufficiently full for ordinary use."—C. A. LINDSLEY, M.D., *Professor of the Theory and Practice of Medicine, Medical Dept. Yale University.*

KEATING'S LIFE INSURANCE.

How to Examine for Life Insurance. By JOHN M. KEATING, M.D., Fellow of the College of Physicians and Surgeons of Philadelphia; Vice-President of the American Pædiatric Society; Ex-President of the Association of Life Insurance Medical Directors. Royal octavo, 211 pages; with two large half-tone illustrations, and a plate prepared by Dr. McClellan from special dissections; also, numerous other illustrations. Cloth, $2.00 net.

"This is by far the most useful book which has yet appeared on insurance examination, a subject of growing interest and importance. Not the least valuable portion of the volume is Part II, which consists of instructions issued to their examining physicians by twenty-four representative companies of this country. If for these alone, the book should be at the right han of every physician interested in this special branch of medical science."—*The Medical News.*

KEEN ON THE SURGERY OF TYPHOID FEVER.

The Surgical Complications and Sequels of Typhoid Fever.
By WM. W. KEEN, M.D., LL.D., Professor of the Principles of Surgery and of Clinical Surgery, Jefferson Medical College, Philadelphia; Corresponding Member of the Société de Chirurgie, Paris; Honorary Member of the Société Belge de Chirurgie, etc. Octavo volume of about 400 pages. Cloth, $3.00 net. *Nearly Ready.*

This monograph is the only one in any language covering the entire subject of the Surgical Complications and Sequels of Typhoid Fever. It will prove to be of importance and interest not only to the general surgeon and physician, but also to many specialists—laryngologists, gynecologists, pathologists, and bacteriologists.

KEEN'S OPERATION BLANK. Second Edition, Revised Form.

An Operation Blank, with Lists of Instruments, etc. Required in Various Operations. Prepared by W. W. KEEN, M.D., LL.D., Professor of the Principles of Surgery in Jefferson Medical College, Philadelphia. Price per pad, containing blanks for fifty operations, 50 cents net.

KYLE ON THE NOSE AND THROAT.

Diseases of the Nose and Throat. By D. BRADEN KYLE, M.D., Chief Laryngologist to St. Agnes' Hospital, Philadelphia; Bacteriologist to the Orthopædic Hospital and Infirmary for Nervous Diseases; Instructor in Clinical Microscopy and Assistant Demonstrator of Pathology in the Jefferson Medical College, etc. *In Preparation.*

LAINÉ'S TEMPERATURE CHART.

Temperature Chart. Prepared by D. T. LAINÉ, M.D. Size 8 x 13½ inches. A conveniently arranged Chart for recording Temperature, with columns for daily amounts of Urinary and Fecal Excretions, Food, Remarks, etc. On the back of each chart is given in full the method of Brand in the treatment of Typhoid Fever. Price, per pad of 25 charts, 50 cents net.

"To the busy practitioner this chart will be found of great value in fever cases, and especially for cases of typhoid."—*Indian Lancet,* Calcutta.

LOCKWOOD'S PRACTICE OF MEDICINE.

A Manual of the Practice of Medicine. By GEORGE ROE LOCKWOOD, M.D., Professor of Practice in the Woman's Medical College of the New York Infirmary, etc. 935 pages, with 75 illustrations in the text, and 22 full-page plates. Cloth, $2.50 net.

"Gives in a most concise manner the points essential to treatment usually enumerated in the most elaborate works."—*Massachusetts Medical Journal.*

LONG'S SYLLABUS OF GYNECOLOGY.

A Syllabus of Gynecology, arranged in Conformity with "An American Text-Book of Gynecology." By J. W. LONG, M.D., Professor of Diseases of Women and Children, Medical College of Virginia, etc. Cloth, interleaved, $1.00 net.

"The book is certainly an admirable *résumé* of what every gynecological student and practitioner should know, and will prove of value not only to those who have the 'American Text-Book of Gynecology,' but to others as well."—*Brooklyn Medical Journal.*

Medical Publications of W. L Saunders.

MACDONALD'S SURGICAL DIAGNOSIS AND TREATMENT.

Surgical Diagnosis and Treatment. By J W. MACDONALD, M.D.
Edin., L.R.C.S., Edin., Professor of the Pratice of Surgery and of
Clinical Surgery in Hamline University; Visiting Surgeon to St.
Barnabas' Hospital, Minneapolis, etc. Handsome octavo volume of
800 pages, profusely illustrated. Cloth, $5.0 net; Half Morocco,
$6.00 net.

"The rapid advances made in the art of surgery have caused the literature of the science
to grow apace. Systems of surgery in many volumes, and te works of large dimensions,
are now deemed necessary to cover the field. The practical part of the surgeon's work is,
however, almost limited to two questions which he most answ every time his professional
advice or help is sought. The first question is, 'What is tt disease or injury?' The
second question is, 'What is the proper treatment?'
"While I would not for a moment underestimate the importance of a profound study
of the principles of surgery, of surgical pathology, or of bacteriology the present work will
be confined to a solution of the two questions just mentioned, ab the view of putting into
the hands of students and practitioners a single vol
of practical surgery."—*From the Author's Preface.*

MALLORY AND WRIGHT'S PATHOLOGICAL TECHNIQUE.

Pathological Technique. By FRANK B. MALORY, A.M., M.D.,
Assistant Professor of Pathology, Harvard University Medical School;
and JAMES H. WRIGHT, A.M., M.D., Instructor Pathology, Harvard
University Medical School. Octavo volume of 96 pages, handsomely
illustrated. Cloth, $2.50 net.

"I have been looking forward to the publication of this book, and I am glad to say that
I find it to be a most useful laboratory and post-mortem guide, full of practical information,
and well up to date."—WILLIAM H. WELCH, *Professor of Pathology, Johns Hopkins University, Baltimore, Md.*

MARTIN'S MINOR SURGERY, BANDAGING, AND VENEREAL DISEASES. Second Edition, Revised

**Essentials of Minor Surgery, Bandaging, and Venereal
Diseases.** By EDWARD MARTIN, A.M., M.D. Clinical Professor of
Genito-Urinary Diseases, University of Pennsylvania, etc. Crown
octavo, 166 pages, with 78 illustrations. Cloth, $1.00; interleaved for
notes, $1.25.

[See *Saunders' Question-Compends,* page 21.]

"A very practical and systematic study of the subjects, and shows the author's familiarity with the needs of students."—*Therapeutic Gazette.*

MARTIN'S SURGERY. Sixth Edition, Revised

Essentials of Surgery. Containing also Venereal Diseases, Surgical Landmarks, Minor and Operative Surgery, and a complete description, with illustrations, of the Handkerchief and Roller Bandages.
By EDWARD MARTIN, A.M., M.D., Clinical Professor of Genito-
rinary Diseases, University of Pennsylvania, etc. Crown octavo, 338
illustrated. With an Appendix containing ill directions for the
ials used in Antiseptic Surgery, etc. Cloth,
$1.25.

[See Saunders' Question-Compends, page 21.]

of modern surgery in a comparatively small space.
are admirable."—*Medical and Surgical Reporter.*

'A AND THERAPEUTICS. Fourth

dica, Therapeutics, and Prescription-
M D , late Demonstrator of Thera-
Philadelphia ; Fellow of the College
etc Crown octavo, 250 pages. Cloth,
$1.25

rition Compends, page 21.]

• old edition, has been largely improved by revi-

/ELL'S PRACTICE OF MEDICINE.

MACDONALD'S SURGICAL DIAGNOSIS AND TREATMENT.

Surgical Diagnosis and Treatment. By J. W. MACDONALD, M.D. Edin., L.R.C.S., Edin., Professor of the Practice of Surgery and of Clinical Surgery in Hamline University; Visiting Surgeon to St. Barnabas' Hospital, Minneapolis, etc. Handsome octavo volume of 800 pages, profusely illustrated. Cloth, $5.00 net; Half Morocco, $6.00 net.

"The rapid advances made in the art of surgery have caused the literature of the science to grow apace. Systems of surgery in many volumes, and text-books of large dimensions, are now deemed necessary to cover the field. The practical part of the surgeon's work is, however, almost limited to two questions which he must answer every time his professional advice or help is sought. The first question is, 'What is the disease or injury?' The second question is, 'What is the proper treatment?'

"While I would not for a moment underestimate the importance of a profound study of the principles of surgery, of surgical pathology, or of bacteriology, the present work will be confined to a solution of the two questions just mentioned, with the view of putting into the hands of students and practitioners a single volume containing the most practical part of practical surgery."—*From the Author's Preface.*

MALLORY AND WRIGHT'S PATHOLOGICAL TECHNIQUE.

Pathological Technique. By FRANK B. MALLORY, A.M., M.D., Assistant Professor of Pathology, Harvard University Medical School; and JAMES H. WRIGHT, A.M., M.D., Instructor in Pathology, Harvard University Medical School. Octavo volume of 396 pages, handsomely illustrated. Cloth, $2.50 net.

"I have been looking forward to the publication of this book, and I am glad to say that I find it to be a most useful laboratory and post-mortem guide, full of practical information, and well up to date."—WILLIAM H. WELCH, *Professor of Pathology, Johns Hopkins University, Baltimore, Md.*

MARTIN'S MINOR SURGERY, BANDAGING, AND VENEREAL DISEASES. Second Edition, Revised.

Essentials of Minor Surgery, Bandaging, and Venereal Diseases. By EDWARD MARTIN, A.M., M.D., Clinical Professor of Genito-Urinary Diseases, University of Pennsylvania, etc. Crown octavo, 166 pages, with 78 illustrations. Cloth, $1.00; interleaved for notes, $1.25.

[See *Saunders' Question-Compends*, page 21.]

"A very practical and systematic study of the subjects, and shows the author's familiarity with the needs of students."—*Therapeutic Gazette.*

MARTIN'S SURGERY. Sixth Edition, Revised.

Essentials of Surgery. Containing also Venereal Diseases, Surgical Landmarks, Minor and Operative Surgery, and a complete description, with illustrations, of the Handkerchief and Roller Bandages. By EDWARD MARTIN, A.M., M.D., Clinical Professor of Genito-Urinary Diseases, University of Pennsylvania, etc. Crown octavo, 338 pages, illustrated. With an Appendix containing full directions for the preparation of the materials used in Antiseptic Surgery, etc. Cloth, $1.00; interleaved for notes, $1.25.

[See *Saunders' Question-Compends*, page 21.]

"Contains all necessary essentials of modern surgery in a comparatively small space. Its style is interesting, and its illustrations are admirable."—*Medical and Surgical Reporter.*

MCFARLAND'S PATHOGENIC BACTERIA.

Text-Book upon the Pathogenic Bacteria. Specially written for Students of Medicine. By JOSEPH MCFARLAND, M.D., Professor of Pathology and Bacteriology in the Medico-Chirurgical College of Philadelphia, etc. Octavo volume of 359 pages, finely illustrated. Cloth, $2.50 net.

"Dr. McFarland has treated the subject in a systematic manner, and has succeeded in presenting in a concise and readable form the essentials of bacteriology up to date. Altogether, the book is a satisfactory one, and I shall take pleasure in recommending it to the students of Trinity College."—H. B. ANDERSON, M.D., *Professor of Pathology and Bacteriology, Trinity Medical College, Toronto.*

MEIGS ON FEEDING IN INFANCY.

Feeding in Early Infancy. By ARTHUR V. MEIGS, M.D. Bound in limp cloth, flush edges, 25 cents net.

"This pamphlet is worth many times over its price to the physician. The author's experiments and conclusions are original, and have been the means of doing much good."—*Medical Bulletin.*

MOORE'S ORTHOPEDIC SURGERY.

A Manual of Orthopedic Surgery. By JAMES E. MOORE, M.D., Professor of Orthopedics and Adjunct Professor of Clinical Surgery, University of Minnesota, College of Medicine and Surgery. Octavo volume of 356 pages, handsomely illustrated. Cloth, $2.50 net.

A practical book based upon the author's experience, in which special stress is laid upon early diagnosis, and treatment such as can be carried out by the general practitioner. The teachings of the author are in accordance with his belief that true conservatism is to be found in the middle course between the surgeon who operates too frequently and the orthopedist who seldom operates.

MORRIS'S MATERIA MEDICA AND THERAPEUTICS. Fourth Edition, Revised.

Essentials of Materia Medica, Therapeutics, and Prescription-Writing. By HENRY MORRIS, M.D., late Demonstrator of Therapeutics, Jefferson Medical College, Philadelphia; Fellow of the College of Physicians, Philadelphia, etc. Crown octavo, 250 pages. Cloth, $1.00; interleaved for notes, $1.25.

[See *Saunders' Question-Compends*, page 21.]

"This work, already excellent in the old edition, has been largely improved by revision."—*American Practitioner and News.*

MORRIS, WOLFF, AND POWELL'S PRACTICE OF MEDICINE. Third Edition, Revised.

Essentials of the Practice of Medicine. By HENRY MORRIS, M.D., late Demonstrator of Therapeutics, Jefferson Medical College, Philadelphia; with an Appendix on the Clinical and Microscopic Examination of Urine, by LAWRENCE WOLFF, M.D., Demonstrator of Chemistry, Jefferson Medical College, Philadelphia. Enlarged by some 300 essential formulæ collected and arranged by WILLIAM M. POWELL, M.D. Post-octavo, 488 pages. Cloth, $2.00.

[See *Saunders' Question-Compends*, page 21.]

"The teaching is sound, the presentation graphic; matter full as can be desired, and style attractive."—*American Practitioner and News.*

MORTEN'S NURSE'S DICTIONARY.

Nurse's Dictionary of Medical Terms and Nursing Treatment. Containing Definitions of the Principal Medical and Nursing Terms and Abbreviations; of the Instruments, Drugs, Diseases, Accidents, Treatments, Operations, Foods, Appliances, etc. encountered in the ward or in the sick-room. By HONNOR MORTEN, author of "How to Become a Nurse," etc. 16mo, 140 pages. Cloth, $1.00.

"A handy, compact little volume, containing a large amount of general information, all of which is arranged in dictionary or encyclopedic form, thus facilitating quick reference. It is certainly of value to those for whose use it is published."—*Chicago Clinical Review.*

NANCREDE'S ANATOMY. Fifth Edition.

Essentials of Anatomy, including the Anatomy of the Viscera. By CHARLES B. NANCREDE, M.D., Professor of Surgery and of Clinical Surgery in the University of Michigan, Ann Arbor. Crown octavo, 388 pages; 180 illustrations. With an Appendix containing over 60 illustrations of the osteology of the human body. Based upon *Gray's Anatomy.* Cloth, $1.00; interleaved for notes, $1.25.

[See *Saunders' Question-Compends,* page 21.]

"For self-quizzing and keeping fresh in mind the knowledge of anatomy gained at school, it would not be easy to speak of it in terms too favorable."—*American Practitioner.*

NANCREDE'S ANATOMY AND DISSECTION. Fourth Edition.

Essentials of Anatomy and Manual of Practical Dissection. By CHARLES B. NANCREDE, M.D., Professor of Surgery and of Clinical Surgery, University of Michigan, Ann Arbor. Post-octavo; 500 pages, with full-page lithographic plates in colors, and nearly 200 illustrations. Extra Cloth (or Oilcloth for the dissection-room), $2.00 net.

"It may in many respects be considered an epitome of Gray's popular work on general anatomy, at the same time having some distinguishing characteristics of its own to commend it. The plates are of more than ordinary excellence, and are of especial value to students in their work in the dissecting room."—*Journal of the American Medical Association.*

NORRIS'S SYLLABUS OF OBSTETRICS. Third Edition, Revised.

Syllabus of Obstetrical Lectures in the Medical Department of the University of Pennsylvania. By RICHARD C. NORRIS, A.M., M.D., Demonstrator of Obstetrics, University of Pennsylvania. Crown octavo, 222 pages. Cloth, interleaved for notes, $2.00 net.

"This work is so far superior to others on the same subject that we take pleasure in calling attention briefly to its excellent features. It covers the subject thoroughly, and will prove invaluable both to the student and the practitioner."—*Medical Record*, New York.

PENROSE'S DISEASES OF WOMEN.

A Text-Book of Diseases of Women. By CHARLES B. PENROSE, M.D., PH.D., Professor of Gynecology in the University of Pennsylvania; Surgeon to the Gynecean Hospital, Philadelphia. Octavo volume of 529 pages, handsomely illustrated. Cloth, $3.50 net.

"The book is to be commended without reserve, not only to the student but to the general practitioner who wishes to have the latest and best modes of treatment explained with absolute clearness."—*Therapeutic Gazette.*

"Taking it all in all, this is in our opinion one of the best works upon this subject that has appeared, and Mr. Saunders may feel justly proud of having the work issued from his press."—*Matthews' Quarterly Journal.*

POWELL'S DISEASES OF CHILDREN. Second Edition.

Essentials of Diseases of Children. By WILLIAM M. POWELL, M.D., Attending Physician to the Mercer House for Invalid Women at Atlantic City, N. J.; late Physician to the Clinic for the Diseases of Children in the Hospital of the University of Pennsylvania. Crown octavo, 222 pages. Cloth, $1.00; interleaved for notes, $1.25.

[See *Saunders' Question-Compends*, page 21.]

"Contains the gist of all the best works in the department to which it relates."— *American Practitioner and News.*

PRINGLE'S SKIN DISEASES AND SYPHILITIC AFFECTIONS.

Pictorial Atlas of Skin Diseases and Syphilitic Affections (American Edition). Translation from the French. Edited by J. J. PRINGLE, M.B., F.R.C.P., Assistant Physician to the Middlesex Hospital, London. Photo-lithochromes from the famous models in the Museum of the Saint-Louis Hospital, Paris, with explanatory wood-cuts and text. Complete in 12 Parts. Price per Part, $3.00.

"I strongly recommend this Atlas. The plates are exceedingly well executed, and will be of great value to all studying dermatology."— STEPHEN MACKENZIE, M.D. (London Hospital).

"The introduction of explanatory wood-cuts in the text is a novel and most important feature which greatly furthers the easier understanding of the excellent plates, than which nothing, we venture to say, has been seen better in point of correctness, beauty, and general merit."— *New York Medical Journal.*

PYE'S BANDAGING.

Elementary Bandaging and Surgical Dressing. With Directions concerning the Immediate Treatment of Cases of Emergency. For the use of Dressers and Nurses. By WALTER PYE, F.R.C.S., late Surgeon to St. Mary's Hospital, London. Small 12mo, with over 80 illustrations. Cloth, flexible covers, 75 cents net.

"The directions are clear and the illustrations are good."— *London Lancet.*

"The author writes well, the diagrams are clear, and the book itself is small and portable, although the paper and type are good."— *British Medical Journal.*

RAYMOND'S PHYSIOLOGY.

A Manual of Physiology. By JOSEPH H. RAYMOND, A.M., M.D., Professor of Physiology and Hygiene and Lecturer on Gynecology in the Long Island College Hospital; Director of Physiology in the Hoagland Laboratory, etc. 382 pages, with 102 illustrations in the text, and 4 full-page colored plates. Cloth, $1.25 net.

"Extremely well gotten up, and the illustrations have been selected with care. The text is fully abreast with modern physiology."— *British Medical Journal.*

RÖNTGEN RAYS.

Archives of the Röntgen Ray (Formerly Archives of Clinical Skiagraphy). Edited by SYDNEY ROWLAND, M.A., M.R.C.S., and W. S. HEDLEY, M.D., M.R.C.S. A series of collotype illustrations, with descriptive text, illustrating the applications of the new photography to Medicine and Surgery. Price per Part, $1.00. Now ready: Vol. I., Parts I. to IV.; Vol. II., Part I.

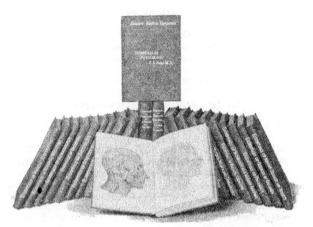

SAUNDERS' QUESTION COMPENDS

Arranged in Question and Answer Form.

THE MOST COMPLETE AND BEST ILLUSTRATED SERIES OF COMPENDS EVER ISSUED.

Now the Standard Authorities in Medical Literature . . . .

with Students and Practitioners in every City of the United States and Canada.

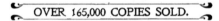

OVER 165,000 COPIES SOLD.

THE REASON WHY.

They are the advance guard of "Student's Helps"—that DO HELP. They are the leaders in their special line, well and authoritatively written by able men, who, as teachers in the large colleges, know exactly what is wanted by a student preparing for his examinations. The judgment exercised in the selection of authors is fully demonstrated by their professional standing. Chosen from the ranks of Demonstrators, Quiz-masters, and Assistants, most of them have become Professors and Lecturers in their respective colleges.

Each book is of convenient size (5 x 7 inches), containing on an average 250 pages, profusely illustrated, and elegantly printed in clear, readable type, on fine paper.

The entire series, numbering twenty-three volumes, has been kept thoroughly revised and enlarged when necessary, many of the books being in their fifth and sixth editions.

TO SUM UP.

Although there are numerous other Quizzes, Manuals, Aids, etc. in the market, none of them approach the "Blue Series of Question Compends;" and the claim is made for the following points of excellence :

    1. Professional distinction and reputation of authors.
    2. Conciseness, clearness, and soundness of treatment.
    3. Quality of illustrations, paper, printing, and binding.

Any of these Compends will be mailed on receipt of price (see next page for List).

Saunders' Question-Compend Series.

Price, Cloth, $1.00 per copy, except when otherwise noted.

"Where the work of preparing students' manuals is to end we cannot say, but the Saunders Series, in our opinion, bears off the palm at present."—*New York Medical Record.*

1. **ESSENTIALS OF PHYSIOLOGY.** By H. A. HARE, M.D. Fourth edition, revised and enlarged. ($1.00 net.)

2. **ESSENTIALS OF SURGERY.** By EDWARD MARTIN, M.D. Sixth edition, revised, with an Appendix on Antiseptic Surgery.

3. **ESSENTIALS OF ANATOMY.** By CHARLES B. NANCREDE, M.D. Fifth edition, with an Appendix.

4. **ESSENTIALS OF MEDICAL CHEMISTRY, ORGANIC AND INORGANIC.** By LAWRENCE WOLFF, M.D. Fourth edition, revised, with an Appendix.

5. **ESSENTIALS OF OBSTETRICS.** By W. EASTERLY ASHTON, M.D. Fourth edition, revised and enlarged.

6. **ESSENTIALS OF PATHOLOGY AND MORBID ANATOMY.** By C. E. ARMAND SEMPLE, M.D.

7. **ESSENTIALS OF MATERIA MEDICA, THERAPEUTICS, AND PRE-SCRIPTION-WRITING.** By HENRY MORRIS, M.D. Fourth edition, revised.

8, 9. **ESSENTIALS OF PRACTICE OF MEDICINE.** By HENRY MORRIS, M.D. An Appendix on URINE EXAMINATION. By LAWRENCE WOLFF, M.D. Third edition, enlarged by some 300 Essential Formulæ, selected from eminent authorities, by WM. M. POWELL, M.D. (Double number, $2.00.)

10. **ESSENTIALS OF GYNÆCOLOGY.** By EDWIN B. CRAGIN, M.D. Fourth edition, revised.

11. **ESSENTIALS OF DISEASES OF THE SKIN.** By HENRY W. STELWAGON, M.D. Third edition, revised and enlarged. ($1.00 net.)

12. **ESSENTIALS OF MINOR SURGERY, BANDAGING, AND VENEREAL DISEASES.** By EDWARD MARTIN, M.D. Second ed., revised and enlarged.

13. **ESSENTIALS OF LEGAL MEDICINE, TOXICOLOGY, AND HYGIENE.** By C. E. ARMAND SEMPLE, M.D.

14. **ESSENTIALS OF DISEASES OF THE EYE, NOSE, AND THROAT.** By EDWARD JACKSON, M.D., and E. B. GLEASON, M.D. Second ed., revised.

15. **ESSENTIALS OF DISEASES OF CHILDREN.** By WILLIAM M. POWELL, M.D. Second edition.

16. **ESSENTIALS OF EXAMINATION OF URINE.** By LAWRENCE WOLFF, M.D. Colored "VOGEL SCALE." (75 cents.)

17. **ESSENTIALS OF DIAGNOSIS.** By S. SOLIS COHEN, M.D., and A. A. ESHNER, M.D. ($1.50 net.)

18. **ESSENTIALS OF PRACTICE OF PHARMACY.** By LUCIUS E. SAYRE. Second edition, revised and enlarged.

20. **ESSENTIALS OF BACTERIOLOGY.** By M. V. BALL, M.D. Third edition, revised.

21. **ESSENTIALS OF NERVOUS DISEASES AND INSANITY.** By JOHN C. SHAW, M.D. Third edition, revised.

22. **ESSENTIALS OF MEDICAL PHYSICS.** By FRED J. BROCKWAY, M.D. Second edition, revised. ($1.00 net.)

23. **ESSENTIALS OF MEDICAL ELECTRICITY.** By DAVID D. STEWART, M.D., and EDWARD S LAWRANCE, M.D.

24. **ESSENTIALS OF DISEASES OF THE EAR.** By E. B. GLEASON, M.D. Second edition, revised and greatly enlarged.

Pamphlet containing specimen pages, etc. sent free upon application.

PRACTICAL, EXHAUSTIVE, AUTHORITATIVE.

SAUNDERS'

New Series of Manuals

FOR

STUDENTS AND PRACTITIONERS.

THAT there exists a need for thoroughly reliable hand-books on the leading branches of Medicine and Surgery is a fact amply demonstrated by the favor with which the SAUNDERS NEW SERIES OF MANUALS have been received by medical students and practitioners and by the Medical Press. These manuals are not merely condensations from present literature, but are ably written by well-known authors and practitioners, most of them being teachers in representative American colleges. Each volume is concisely and authoritatively written and exhaustive in detail, without being encumbered with the introduction of "cases," which so largely expand the ordinary text-book. These manuals will therefore form an admirable collection of advanced lectures, useful alike to the medical student and the practitioner: to the latter, too busy to search through page after page of elaborate treatises for what he wants to know, they will prove of inestimable value; to the former they will afford safe guides to the essential points of study.

The SAUNDERS NEW SERIES OF MANUALS are conceded to be superior to any similar books now on the market. No other manuals afford so much information in such a concise and available form. A liberal expenditure has enabled the publisher to render the mechanical portion of the work worthy of the high literary standard attained by these books.

Saunders' New Series of Manuals.

VOLUMES PUBLISHED.

PHYSIOLOGY. By JOSEPH HOWARD RAYMOND, A.M., M.D., Professor of Physiology and Hygiene and Lecturer on Gynecology in the Long Island College Hospital; Director of Physiology in the Hoagland Laboratory. etc. Illustrated. Cloth, $1.25 net.

SURGERY, General and Operative. By JOHN CHALMERS DACOSTA, M.D., Clinical Professor of Surgery, Jefferson Medical College, Philadelphia; Surgeon to the Philadelphia Hospital, etc. 188 illustrations and 13 plates. (Double number.) Cloth, $2.50 net.

DOSE-BOOK AND MANUAL OF PRESCRIPTION-WRITING. By E. Q. THORNTON, M.D., Demonstrator of Therapeutics, Jefferson Medical College, Philadelphia. Illustrated. Cloth, $1.25 net.

SURGICAL ASEPSIS. By CARL BECK, M.D., Surgeon to St. Mark's Hospital and to the New York German Poliklinik, etc. Illustrated. Cloth, $1.25 net.

MEDICAL JURISPRUDENCE. By HENRY C. CHAPMAN, M.D. Professor of Institutes of Medicine and Medical Jurisprudence in the Jefferson Medical College of Philadelphia. Illustrated. Cloth, $1.50 net.

SYPHILIS AND THE VENEREAL DISEASES. By JAMES NEVINS HYDE, M.D., Professor of Skin and Venereal Diseases, and FRANK H. MONTGOMERY, M.D., Lecturer on Dermatology and Genito-Urinary Diseases in Rush Medical College, Chicago. Profusely illustrated. (Double number.) Cloth, $2.50 net.

PRACTICE OF MEDICINE. By GEORGE ROE LOCKWOOD, M.D., Professor of Practice in the Woman's Medical College of the New York Infirmary; Instructor in Physical Diagnosis in the Medical Department of Columbia College, etc. Illustrated. (Double number.) Cloth, $2.50 net.

MANUAL OF ANATOMY. By IRVING S. HAYNES, M.D., Adjunct Professor of Anatomy and Demonstrator of Anatomy, Medical Department of the New York University, etc. Beautifully illustrated. (Double Number.) Cloth, $2.50 net.

MANUAL OF OBSTETRICS. By W. A. NEWMAN DORLAND, M.D., Assistant Demonstrator of Obstetrics, University of Pennsylvania; Chief of Gynecological Dispensary, Pennsylvania Hospital, etc. Profusely illustrated. (Double number.) Cloth, $2.50 net.

DISEASES OF WOMEN. By J. BLAND SUTTON, F.R.C.S., Assistant Surgeon to Middlesex Hospital and Surgeon to Chelsea Hospital, London; and ARTHUR E. GILES, M.D., B.Sc. Lond., F.R.C.S. Edin., Assistant Surgeon to Chelsea Hospital, London. Handsomely illustrated. (Double number.) Cloth, $2.50 net.

VOLUMES IN PREPARATION.

NOSE AND THROAT. By D. BRADEN KYLE, M.D., Chief Laryngologist to the St. Agnes Hospital, Philadelphia; Bacteriologist to the Orthopædic Hospital and Infirmary for Nervous Diseases; Instructor in Clinical Microscopy and Assistant Demonstrator of Pathology in the Jefferson Medical College, etc.

NERVOUS DISEASES. By CHARLES W. BURR, M.D., Clinical Professor of Nervous Diseases, Medico-Chirurgical College, Philadelphia; Pathologist to the Orthopædic Hospital and Infirmary for Nervous Diseases; Visiting Physician to the St. Joseph Hospital, etc.

*** There will be published in the same series, at short intervals, carefully-prepared works on various subjects by prominent specialists.

Pamphlet containing specimen pages, etc. sent free upon application.

SAUNDBY'S RENAL AND URINARY DISEASES.

Lectures on Renal and Urinary Diseases. By ROBERT SAUNDBY, M.D. Edin., Fellow of the Royal College of Physicians, London, and of the Royal Medico-Chirurgical Society; Physician to the General Hospital; Consulting Physician to the Eye Hospital and to the Hospital for Diseases of Women; Professor of Medicine in Mason College, Birmingham, etc. Octavo volume of 434 pages, with numerous illustrations and 4 colored plates. Cloth, $2.50 net.

" The volume makes a favorable impression at once. The style is clear and succinct. We cannot find any part of the subject in which the views expressed are not carefully thought out and fortified by evidence drawn from the most recent sources. The book may be cordially recommended."—*British Medical Journal.*

SAUNDERS' POCKET MEDICAL FORMULARY. Fourth Edition, Revised.

By WILLIAM M. POWELL, M.D., Attending Physician to the Mercer House for Invalid Women at Atlantic City, N. J. Containing 1750 formulæ selected from the best-known authorities. With an Appendix containing Posological Table, Formulæ and Doses for Hypodermic Medication, Poisons and their Antidotes, Diameters of the Female Pelvis and Fœtal Head, Obstetrical Table, Diet List for Various Diseases, Materials and Drugs used in Antiseptic Surgery, Treatment of Asphyxia from Drowning, Surgical Remembrancer, Tables of Incompatibles, Eruptive Fevers, Weights and Measures, etc. Handsomely bound in flexible morocco, with side index, wallet, and flap. $1.75 net.

" This little book, that can be conveniently carried in the pocket, contains an immense amount of material. It is very useful, and, as the name of the author of each prescription is given, is unusually reliable."—*Medical Record*, New York.

SAUNDERS' POCKET MEDICAL LEXICON. Fourth Edition, Revised.

A Dictionary of Terms and Words used in Medicine and Surgery. By JOHN M. KEATING, M.D., Fellow of the College of Physicians of Philadelphia; Editor of the " Cyclopædia of Diseases of Children," etc.; Author of the " New Pronouncing Dictionary of Medicine;" and HENRY HAMILTON, Author of "A New Translation of Virgil's Æneid into English Verse;" Co-Author of the "New Pronouncing Dictionary of Medicine." 32mo, 280 pages. Cloth, 75 cents; Leather Tucks, $1.00.

" Remarkably accurate in terminology, accentuation, and definition."—*Journal of the American Medical Association.*

SAYRE'S PHARMACY. Second Edition, Revised.

Essentials of the Practice of Pharmacy. By LUCIUS E. SAYRE, M.D., Professor of Pharmacy and Materia Medica in the University of Kansas. Crown octavo, 200 pages. Cloth, $1.00; interleaved for notes, $1.25.

[See *Saunders' Question-Compends*, page 21.]

" The topics are treated in a simple, practical manner. and the work forms a very useful student's manual."—*Boston Medical and Surgical Journal.*

SEMPLE'S LEGAL MEDICINE, TOXICOLOGY, AND HYGIENE.

Essentials of Legal Medicine, Toxicology, and Hygiene. By C. E. Armand Semple, B. A., M. B. Cantab., M. R. C. P. Lond., Physician to the Northeastern Hospital for Children, Hackney, etc. Crown octavo, 212 pages; 130 illustrations. Cloth, $1.00; interleaved for notes, $1.25.

[See *Saunders' Question-Compends*, page 21.]

"No general practitioner or student can afford to be without this valuable work. The subjects are dealt with by a masterly hand."—*London Hospital Gazette.*

SEMPLE'S PATHOLOGY AND MORBID ANATOMY.

Essentials of Pathology and Morbid Anatomy. By C. E. Armand Semple, B.A., M.B. Cantab., M.R.C.P. Lond., Physician to the Northeastern Hospital for Children, Hackney, etc. Crown octavo, 174 pages; illustrated. Cloth, $1.00; interleaved for notes, $1.25.

[See *Saunders' Question-Compends*, page 21.]

"Should take its place among the standard volumes on the bookshelf of both student and practitioner."—*London Hospital Gazette.*

SENN'S GENITO-URINARY TUBERCULOSIS.

Tuberculosis of the Genito-Urinary Organs, Male and Female. By Nicholas Senn, M.D., Ph.D., LL.D., Professor of the Practice of Surgery and of Clinical Surgery, Rush Medical College, Chicago. Handsome octavo volume of 320 pages, illustrated. Cloth, $3.00 net.

"An important book upon an important subject, and written by a man of mature judgment and wide experience. The author has given us an instructive book upon one of the most important subjects of the day."—*Clinical Reporter.*

"A work which adds another to the many obligations the profession owes the talented author."—*Chicago Medical Recorder.*

SENN'S SYLLABUS OF SURGERY.

A Syllabus of Lectures on the Practice of Surgery, arranged in conformity with "An American Text-Book of Surgery." By Nicholas Senn, M.D., Ph.D., Professor of the Practice of Surgery and of Clinical Surgery in Rush Medical College, Chicago. Cloth, $2.00.

"This syllabus will be found of service by the teacher as well as the student, the work being superbly done. There is no praise too high for it. No surgeon should be without it."—*New York Medical Times.*

SENN'S TUMORS.

Pathology and Surgical Treatment of Tumors. By N. Senn, M.D., Ph.D., LL.D., Professor of Surgery and of Clinical Surgery, Rush Medical College; Professor of Surgery, Chicago Polyclinic; Attending Surgeon to Presbyterian Hospital; Surgeon-in-Chief, St. Joseph's Hospital, Chicago. Octavo volume of 710 pages, with 515 engravings, including full-page colored plates. Cloth, $6.00 net; Half Morocco, $7.00 net.

"The most exhaustive of any recent book in English on this subject. It is well illustrated, and will doubtless remain as the principal monograph on the subject in our language for some years. The book is handsomely illustrated and printed, and the author has given a notable and lasting contribution to surgery."—*Journal of the American Medical Association.*

SHAW'S NERVOUS DISEASES AND INSANITY. Third Edition, Revised.

Essentials of Nervous Diseases and Insanity. By JOHN C. SHAW, M.D., Clinical Professor of Diseases of the Mind and Nervous System, Long Island College Hospital Medical School; Consulting Neurologist to St. Catherine's Hospital and to the Long Island College Hospital. Crown octavo, 186 pages; 48 original illustrations. Cloth, $1.00; interleaved for notes, $1.25.

[See *Saunders' Question-Compends*, page 21.]

" Clearly and intelligently written."—*Boston Medical and Surgical Journal.*

" There is a mass of valuable material crowded into this small compass."—*American Medico-Surgical Bulletin.*

STARR'S DIETS FOR INFANTS AND CHILDREN.

Diets for Infants and Children in Health and in Disease. By LOUIS STARR, M.D., Editor of "An American Text-Book of the Diseases of Children." 230 blanks (pocket-book size), perforated and neatly bound in flexible morocco. $1.25 net.

The first series of blanks are prepared for the first seven months of infant life ; each blank indicates the ingredients, but not the quantities, of the food, the latter directions being left for the physician. After the seventh month, modifications being less necessary, the diet lists are printed in full. Formulæ for the preparation of diluents and foods are appended.

STELWAGON'S DISEASES OF THE SKIN. Third Edition, Revised.

Essentials of Diseases of the Skin. By HENRY W. STELWAGON, M.D., Clinical Professor of Dermatology in the Jefferson Medical College, Philadelphia; Dermatologist to the Philadelphia Hospital; Physician to the Skin Department of the Howard Hospital, etc. Crown octavo, 270 pages; 86 illustrations. Cloth, $1.00 net; interleaved for notes, $1.25 net.

[See *Saunders' Question-Compends*, page 21.]

" The best student's manual on skin diseases we have yet seen."—*Times and Register.*

STENGEL'S PATHOLOGY.

A Manual of Pathology. By ALFRED STENGEL, M.D., Physician to the Philadelphia Hospital; Professor of Clinical Medicine in the Woman's Medical College; Physician to the Children's Hospital; late Pathologist to the German Hospital, Philadelphia, etc. *In Preparation.*

STEVENS' MATERIA MEDICA AND THERAPEUTICS. Second Edition, Revised.

A Manual of Materia Medica and Therapeutics. By A. A. STEVENS, A.M., M.D., Lecturer on Terminology and Instructor in Physical Diagnosis in the University of Pennsylvania; Demonstrator of Pathology in the Woman's Medical College of Philadelphia. Post-octavo, 445 pages. Cloth, $2.25.

" The author has faithfully presented modern therapeutics in a comprehensive work, and, while intended particularly for the use of students, it will be found a reliable guide and sufficiently comprehensive for the physician in practice."—*University Medical Magazine.*

STEVENS' PRACTICE OF MEDICINE. Fourth Edition, Revised.
A Manual of the Practice of Medicine. By A. A. STEVENS, A.M.,
M.D., Lecturer on Terminology and Instructor in Physical Diagnosis
in the University of Pennsylvania; Demonstrator of Pathology in
the Woman's Medical College of Philadelphia. Specially intended
for students preparing for graduation and hospital examinations. Post-
octavo, 511 pages; illustrated. Cloth, $2.50.

"The frequency with which new editions of this manual are demanded bespeaks its
popularity. It is an excellent condensation of the essentials of medical practice for the
student, and may be found also an excellent reminder for the busy physician."—*Buffalo
Medical Journal.*

STEWART'S PHYSIOLOGY.
A Manual of Physiology, with Practical Exercises. For
Students and Practitioners. By G. N. STEWART, M.A., M.D.,
D.Sc., lately Examiner in Physiology, University of Aberdeen, and
of the New Museums, Cambridge University; Professor of Physiology
in the Western Reserve University, Cleveland, Ohio. Octavo volume
of 800 pages; 278 illustrations in the text, and 5 colored plates.
Cloth, $3.50 net.

"It will make its way by sheer force of merit, and amply deserves to do so. It is one
of the very best English text-books on the subject."—*London Lancet.*

"Of the many text-books of physiology published, we do not know of one that so
nearly comes up to the ideal as does Prof. Stewart's volume."—*British Medical Journal.*

STEWART AND LAWRANCE'S MEDICAL ELECTRICITY.
Essentials of Medical Electricity. By D. D. STEWART, M.D.,
Demonstrator of Diseases of the Nervous System and Chief of the
Neurological Clinic in the Jefferson Medical College; and E. S.
LAWRANCE, M.D., Chief of the Electrical Clinic and Assistant Demon-
strator of Diseases of the Nervous System in the Jefferson Medical
College, etc. Crown octavo, 158 pages; 65 illustrations. Cloth,
$1.00; interleaved for notes, $1.25.

[See *Saunders' Question-Compends*, page 21.]

"Throughout the whole brief space at their command the authors show a discriminating
knowledge of their subject."—*Medical News.*

STONEY'S NURSING. Second Edition, Revised.
Practical Points in Nursing. For Nurses in Private Practice.
By EMILY A. M. STONEY, Graduate of the Training-School for Nurses,
Lawrence, Mass.; late Superintendent of the Training-School for
Nurses, Carney Hospital, South Boston, Mass. 456 pages, illustrated
with 73 engravings in the text, and 8 colored and half-tone plates.
Cloth, $1.75 net.

"There are few books intended for non-professional readers which can be so cordially
endorsed by a medical journal as can this one."—*Therapeutic Gazette.*

"This is a well-written, eminently practical volume, which covers the entire range of
private nursing as distinguished from hospital nursing, and instructs the nurse how best to
meet the various emergencies which may arise, and how to prepare everything ordinarily
needed in the illness of her patient."—*American Journal of Obstetrics and Diseases of
Women and Children.*

"It is a work that the physician can place in the hands of his private nurses with the
assurance of benefit."—*Ohio Medical Journal.*

SUTTON AND GILES' DISEASES OF WOMEN.

Diseases of Women. By J. BLAND SUTTON, F.R.C.S., Assistant Surgeon to Middlesex Hospital, and Surgeon to Chelsea Hospital, London; and ARTHUR E. GILES, M.D., B.Sc. Lond., F.R.C.S. Edin., Assistant Surgeon to Chelsea Hospital, London. 436 pages, handsomely illustrated. Cloth, $2.50 net.

" The book is very well prepared, and is certain to be well received by the medical public."—*British Medical Journal.*

" The text has been carefully prepared. Nothing essential has been omitted, and its teachings are those recommended by the leading authorities of the day."—*Journal of the American Medical Association.*

THOMAS'S DIET LISTS AND SICK-ROOM DIETARY.

Diet Lists and Sick=Room Dietary. By JEROME B. THOMAS, M.D., Visiting Physician to the Home for Friendless Women and Children and to the Newsboys' Home ; Assistant Visiting Physician to the Kings County Hospital. Cloth, $1.50. Send for sample sheet.

" The idea is good, and the lists are copious."—*London Lancet.*

" Its practical usefulness places it among the requirements of every practitioner."— *Chicago Medical Recorder.*

THORNTON'S DOSE-BOOK AND PRESCRIPTION-WRITING.

Dose=Book and Manual of Prescription=Writing. By E. Q. THORNTON, M.D., Demonstrator of ·Therapeutics, Jefferson Medical College, Philadelphia. 334 pages, illustrated. Cloth, $1.25 net.

" Full of practical suggestions; will take its place in the front rank of works of this sort."—*Medical Record*, New York.

VAN VALZAH AND NISBET'S DISEASES OF THE STOMACH.

Diseases of the Stomach. By WILLIAM W. VAN VALZAH, M.D., Professor of General Medicine and Diseases of the Digestive System and the Blood, New York Polyclinic; and J. DOUGLAS NISBET, M.D., Adjunct Professor of General Medicine and Diseases of the Digestive System and the Blood, New York Polyclinic. Octavo volume of about 600 pages. Cloth, $3.50 net. *Nearly Ready.*

VIERORDT'S MEDICAL DIAGNOSIS. Third Edition, Revised.

Medical Diagnosis. By Dr. OSWALD VIERORDT, Professor of Medicine at the University of Heidelberg. Translated, with additions, from the second enlarged German edition, with the author's permission, by FRANCIS H. STUART, A.M., M.D. Handsome royal octavo volume of 700 pages; 178 fine wood-cuts in text, many of them in colors. Cloth, $4.00 net; Sheep or Half Morocco, $5.00 net; Half Russia, $5.50 net.

" A treasury of practical information which will be found of daily use to every busy practitioner who will consult it."—C. A. LINDSLEY, M.D., *Professor of the Theory and Practice of Medicine, Yale University.*

" Rarely is a book published with which a reviewer can find so little fault as with the volume before us. Each particular item in the consideration of an organ or apparatus, which is necessary to determine a diagnosis of any disease of that organ, is mentioned; nothing seems forgotten. The chapters on diseases of the circulatory and digestive apparatus and nervous system are especially full and valuable. The reviewer would repeat that the book is one of the best—probably *the best*—which has fallen into his hands."—*University Medical Magazine.*

WARREN'S SURGICAL PATHOLOGY AND THERAPEUTICS.

Surgical Pathology and Therapeutics. By JOHN COLLINS WARREN, M.D., LL.D., Professor of Surgery, Medical Department Harvard University; Surgeon to the Massachusetts General Hospital, etc. Handsome octavo volume of 832 pages; 136 relief and lithographic illustrations, 33 of which are printed in colors, and all of which were drawn by William J. Kaula from original specimens. Cloth, $6.00 net; Half Morocco, $7.00 net.

"There is the work of Dr. Warren, which I think is the most creditable book on Surgical Pathology, and the most beautiful medical illustration of the bookmaker's art, that has ever been issued from the American press."—DR. ROSWELL PARK, *in the Harvard Graduate Magazine.*

"The handsomest specimen of bookmaking that has ever been issued from the American medical press."—*American Journal of the Medical Sciences.*

"A most striking and very excellent feature of this book is its illustrations. Without exception, from the point of accuracy and.artistic merit, they are the best ever seen in a work of this kind. Many of those representing microscopic pictures are so perfect in their coloring and detail as almost to give the beholder the impression that he is looking down the barrel of a microscope at a well-mounted section."—*Annals of Surgery.*

WEST'S NURSING.

An American Text=Book of Nursing. By AMERICAN TEACHERS. Edited by ROBERTA M. WEST, late Superintendent of Nurses in the Hospital of the University of Pennsylvania. *In Preparation.*

WOLFF ON EXAMINATION OF URINE.

Essentials of Examination of Urine. By LAWRENCE WOLFF, M.D., Demonstrator of Chemistry, Jefferson Medical College, Philadelphia, etc. Colored (Vogel) urine scale and numerous illustrations. Crown octavo. Cloth, 75 cents.

[See *Saunders' Question-Compends,* page 21.]

"A very good work of its kind—very well suited to its purpose."—*Times and Register.*

WOLFF'S MEDICAL CHEMISTRY. Fourth Edition, Revised.

Essentials of Medical Chemistry, Organic and Inorganic. Containing also Questions on Medical Physics, Chemical Physiology, Analytical Processes, Urinalysis, and Toxicology. By LAWRENCE WOLFF, M.D., Demonstrator of Chemistry, Jefferson Medical College, Philadelphia, etc. Crown octavo, 218 pages. Cloth, $1.00; interleaved for notes, $1.25.

[See *Saunders' Question-Compends,* page 21.]

"The scope of this work is certainly equal to that of the best course of lectures on Medical Chemistry."—*Pharmaceutical Era.*

CLASSIFIED LIST

OF THE

MEDICAL PUBLICATIONS

OF

W. B. SAUNDERS,

925 Walnut Street, Philadelphia.

ANATOMY, EMBRYOLOGY, HISTOLOGY.

Clarkson—A Text-Book of Histology, 9
Haynes—A Manual of Anatomy, . . . 13
Heisler—A Text-Book of Embryology, 13
Nancrede—Essentials of Anatomy, . . 18
Nancrede—Essentials of Anatomy and Manual of Practical Dissection, . . . 18
Semple—Essentials of Pathology and Morbid Anatomy, ... 25

BACTERIOLOGY.

Ball—Essentials of Bacteriology, . . . 6
Crookshank—A Text-Book of Bacteriology, ... 10
Frothingham—Laboratory Guide, . . 11
Mallory and Wright — Pathological Technique, ... 16
McFarland—Pathogenic Bacteria, . . 17

CHARTS, DIET-LISTS, ETC.

Griffith—Infant's Weight Chart, . . 12
Hart—Diet in Sickness and in Health, . 13
Keen—Operation Blank, ... 15
Lainé—Temperature Chart, ... 15
Meigs—Feeding in Early Infancy, . . 17
Starr—Diets for Infants and Children, . 26
Thomas—Diet-Lists and Sick-Room Dietary, ... 28

CHEMISTRY AND PHYSICS.

Brockway—Essentials of Medical Physics, ... 7
Wolff—Essentials of Medical Chemistry, 29

CHILDREN.

An American Text-Book of Diseases of Children. 3
Griffith—Care of the Baby, ... 12
Griffith—Infant's Weight Chart, . . . 12
Meigs—Feeding in Early Infancy, . . 17
Powell—Essentials of Dis. of Children, 19
Starr—Diets for Infants and Children, . 26

DIAGNOSIS.

Cohen and Eshner—Essentials of Diagnosis, ... 9
Corwin—Physical Diagnosis, ... 9
Macdonald—Surgical Diagnosis and Treatment, ... 16
Vierordt—Medical Diagnosis, ... 28

DICTIONARIES.

Keating—Pronouncing Dictionary, . . 14
Morten—Nurse's Dictionary, ... 18
Saunders' Pocket Medical Lexicon, . 24

EYE, EAR, NOSE, AND THROAT.

An American Text-Book of Diseases of the Eye, Ear, Nose, and Throat, . 3
Casselberry—Dis. of Nose and Throat, 8
De Schweinitz—Diseases of the Eye, 10
Gleason—Essentials of Dis. of the Ear, 11
Jackson and Gleason—Essentials of Diseases of the Eye, Nose, and Throat, 14
Kyle—Diseases of the Nose and Throat, 15

GENITO-URINARY.

An American Text-Book of Genito-Urinary and Skin Diseases, ... 3
Hyde and Montgomery—Syphilis and the Venereal Diseases, ... 13
Martin—Essentials of Minor Surgery, Bandaging, and Venereal Diseases, . 16
Saundby—Renal and Urinary Diseases, 24
Senn—Genito-Urinary Tuberculosis, . 25

GYNECOLOGY.

American Text-Book of Gynecology, 4
Cragin—Essentials of Gynecology, . . 10
Garrigues—Diseases of Women, . . . 11
Long—Syllabus of Gynecology, . . . 15
Penrose—Diseases of Women, ... 18
Sutton and Giles—Diseases of Women, 28

MATERIA MEDICA, PHARMACOLOGY, AND THERAPEUTICS.

An American Text-Book of Applied Therapeutics, ... 3
Butler—Text-Book of Materia Medica, Therapeutics and Pharmacology, . . 8
Cerna—Notes on the Newer Remedies, 8
Griffin—Materia Med. and Therapeutics, 12
Morris—Essentials of Materia Medica and Therapeutics, ... 17
Saunders' Pocket Medical Formulary, 24
Sayre—Essentials of Pharmacy, . . . 24
Stevens—Essentials of Materia Medica and Therapeutics, ... 26
Thornton—Dose-Book and Manual of Prescription-Writing, ... 28
Warren—Surgical Pathology and Therapeutics, ... 29

MEDICAL JURISPRUDENCE AND TOXICOLOGY.

An American Text-Book of Legal Medicine and Toxicology, ... 4
Chapman—Medical Jurisprudence and Toxicology, ... 8
Semple—Essentials of Legal Medicine, Toxicology, and Hygiene, ... 25

In Preparation for Early Publication.

AN AMERICAN TEXT-BOOK OF DISEASES OF THE EYE, EAR, NOSE, AND THROAT.

Edited by G. E. DE SCHWEINITZ, M.D., Professor of Ophthalmology in the Jefferson Medical College, Philadelphia; and B. ALEXANDER RANDALL, M.D., Professor of Diseases of the Ear in the University of Pennsylvania and in the Philadelphia Polyclinic.

AN AMERICAN TEXT-BOOK OF PATHOLOGY.

Edited by JOHN GUITÉRAS, M.D., Professor of General Pathology and of Morbid Anatomy in the University of Pennsylvania; and DAVID RIESMAN, M.D., Demonstrator of Pathological Histology in the University of Pennsylvania.

PETERSON AND HAINES' LEGAL MEDICINE AND TOXICOLOGY.

An American Text-Book of Legal Medicine and Toxicology. Edited by FREDERICK PETERSON, M.D., Clinical Professor of Mental Diseases in the Woman's Medical College, New York; Chief of Clinic, Nervous Department, College of Physicians and Surgeons, New York; and WALTER S. HAINES, M.D., Professor of Chemistry, Pharmacy, and Toxicology in Rush Medical College, Chicago.

STENGEL'S PATHOLOGY.

A Manual of Pathology. By ALFRED STENGEL, M.D., Physician to the Philadelphia Hospital; Professor of Clinical Medicine in the Woman's Medical College; Physician to the Children's Hospital; late Pathologist to the German Hospital, Philadelphia, etc.

CHURCH AND PETERSON'S NERVOUS AND MENTAL DISEASES.

Nervous and Mental Diseases. By ARCHIBALD CHURCH, M.D., Professor of Mental Diseases and Medical Jurisprudence in the Northwestern University Medical School, Chicago; and FREDERICK PETERSON, M.D., Clinical Professor of Mental Diseases in the Woman's Medical College, New York; Chief of Clinic, Nervous Department, College of Physicians and Surgeons, New York.

HEISLER'S EMBRYOLOGY.

A Text-Book of Embryology. By JOHN C. HEISLER, M.D., Professor of Anatomy in the Medico-Chirurgical College, Philadelphia.

KYLE ON THE NOSE AND THROAT.

Diseases of the Nose and Throat. By D. BRADEN KYLE, M.D., Chief Laryngologist to St. Agnes' Hospital; Bacteriologist to the Orthopedic Hospital and Infirmary for Nervous Diseases; Instructor in Clinical Microscopy and Assistant Demonstrator of Pathology, Jefferson Medical College, Philadelphia.

HIRST'S OBSTETRICS.

A Text-Book of Obstetrics. By BARTON COOKE HIRST, M.D., Professor of Obstetrics in the University of Pennsylvania.

WEST'S NURSING.

An American Text-Book of Nursing. By AMERICAN TEACHERS. Edited by ROBERTA M. WEST, Late Superintendent of Nurses in the Hospital of the University of Pennsylvania.

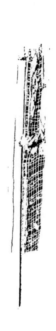

SOLD BY SUBSCRIPTION.

JUST PUBLISHED.

THE

CARE OF THE BABY.

A MANUAL

FOR

MOTHERS AND NURSES.

BY

J. P. CROZER GRIFFITH, M. D.,

Clinical Professor of Diseases of Children in the Hospital
of the University of Pennsylvania; Professor of
Clinical Medicine in the Philadelphia Polyclinic;
Physician to the Children's, to St. Agnes',
and to the Methodist Hospital, etc.

400 PAGES. PROFUSELY ILLUSTRATED.

PRICE, $1.50.

This work contains practical directions for the care
and management of children in health and disease.
It is written from the standpoint of the physician,
but is adapted to the use of the mother and the
nurse, and includes such advice as is required in
treating minor ailments, and what to do until the
doctor comes in serious disease.

Sent post-paid on receipt of price.

W. B. SAUNDERS, Publisher,
925 Walnut Street, Philadelphia, Pa.

"It is no book . . . characterized by rare good sense, and is evidently written by . . . master a d . . ."—*An Jo of Obstetrics.*

. . . the English